HARRISON'S
Cardiovascular Medicine

Derived from Harrison's Principles of Internal Medicine, 17th Edition

Editors

ANTHONY S. FAUCI, MD

Chief, Laboratory of Immunoregulation;
Director, National Institute of Allergy and Infectious Diseases,
National Institutes of Health, Bethesda

DENNIS L. KASPER, MD

William Ellery Channing Professor of Medicine, Professor of
Microbiology and Molecular Genetics, Harvard Medical School;
Director, Channing Laboratory, Department of Medicine,
Brigham and Women's Hospital, Boston

DAN L. LONGO, MD

Scientific Director, National Institute on
Aging, National Institutes of Health,
Bethesda and Baltimore

EUGENE BRAUNWALD, MD

Distinguished Hersey Professor of Medicine,
Harvard Medical School; Chairman, TIMI Study Group,
Brigham and Women's Hospital, Boston

STEPHEN L. HAUSER, MD

Robert A. Fishman Distinguished Professor and Chairman,
Department of Neurology, University of California, San Francisco

J. LARRY JAMESON, MD, PhD

Professor of Medicine;
Vice President for Medical Affairs and Lewis
Landsberg Dean,
Northwestern University Feinberg School of
Medicine, Chicago

JOSEPH LOSCALZO, MD, PhD

Hersey Professor of Theory and Practice of Medicine,
Harvard Medical School; Chairman, Department of Medicine;
Physician-in-Chief, Brigham and Women's Hospital, Boston

HARRISON'S
Cardiovascular Medicine

Editor

Joseph Loscalzo, MD, PhD
Hersey Professor of Theory and Practice of Medicine,
Harvard Medical School; Chairman, Department of Medicine;
Physician-in-Chief, Brigham and Women's Hospital, Boston

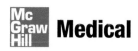

New York   Chicago   San Francisco   Lisbon   London   Madrid
Mexico City   Milan   New Delhi   San Juan   Seoul   Singapore   Sydney   Toronto

The McGraw·Hill Companies

Harrison's Cardiovascular Medicine

1 2 3 4 5 6 7 8 9 0   CTP/CTP   14 13 12 11 10

ISBN 978-0-07-170291-1
MHID 0-07-170291-1

This book was set in Bembo by Glyph International. The editors were James Shanahan and Kim J. Davis. The production supervisor was Catherine H. Saggese. Project management was provided by Smita Rajan of Glyph International. The cover design was by Thomas DePierro. Cover, section, and chapter opener illustrations © MedicalRF.com. All rights reserved.

China Translation & Printing Services Ltd. was the printer and binder.

Library of Congress Cataloging-in Publication Data

Harrison's cardiovascular medicine / editor, Joseph Loscalzo.
    p. ; cm.
    "Comprises the key cardiovascular chapters contained in Harrison's Principles of Internal Medicine, 17e"—Pref.
    Includes bibliographical references and index.
    ISBN 978-0-07-170291-1 (pbk. : alk. paper)
    1. Cardiology.   2. Cardiovascular system–Diseases.   I. Loscalzo, Joseph.
II. Harrison's principles of internal medicine.   IV. Title: Cardiovascular medicine.
    [DNLM: 1. Cardiovascular Diseases. WG 100 H323   2010].
RC667.H356   2010
616.1'2—dc22
                                                                2009042895

CONTENTS

Numbers in brackets refer to the chapter(s) written or co-written by the contributor.

ELLIOTT M. ANTMAN, MD
Professor of Medicine, Harvard Medical School; Director, Samuel L. Levine Cardiac Unit, and Senior Investigator, TIMI Study Group, Brigham and Women's Hospital, Boston [33, 35]

ERIC H. AWTRY, MD
Assistant Professor of Medicine, Boston University School of Medicine, Boston [23, 24]

DONALD S. BAIM, MD†
Professor of Medicine, Harvard Medical School; Executive Vice President, Chief Medical and Scientific Officer, Boston Scientific Corporation, Natick [13, 36, 44]

GERALD BLOOMFIELD, MD, MPH
Department of Internal Medicine, The Johns Hopkins University School of Medicine, Baltimore [Review and Self-Assessment]

EUGENE BRAUNWALD, MD, MA (Hon), ScD (Hon)
Distinguished Hersey Professor of Medicine, Harvard Medical School; Chairman, TIMI Study Group, Brigham and Women's Hospital, Boston [1, 3, 6, 7, 9, 10, 20, 21, 22, 33, 34, 35]

CYNTHIA D. BROWN, MD
Department of Internal Medicine, The Johns Hopkins University School of Medicine, Baltimore [Review and Self-Assessment]

CHRISTOPHER P. CANNON, MD
Associate Professor of Medicine, Harvard Medical School; Associate Physician, Cardiovascular Division, Senior Investigator, TIMI Study Group, Brigham and Women's Hospital, Boston [34]

JONATHAN R. CARAPETIS, MBBS, PhD
Director, Menzies School of Health Research; Professor, Charles Darwin University, Australia [26]

AGUSTIN CASTELLANOS, MD
Professor of Medicine; Director, Clinical Electrophysiology, University of Miami Miller School of Medicine, Miami [29]

JOHN S. CHILD, MD
Director, Ahmanson-UCLA Adult Congenital Heart Disease Center; Streisand Professor of Medicine and Cardiology, David Geffen School of Medicine at UCLA, Los Angeles [19]

WILSON S. COLUCCI, MD
Thomas J. Ryan Professor of Medicine, Boston University School of Medicine; Chief, Cardiovascular Medicine, Boston University Medical Center, Boston [23, 24]

MARK A. CREAGER, MD
Professor of Medicine, Harvard Medical School; Simon C. Fireman Scholar in Cardiovascular Medicine; Director, Vascular Center, Brigham and Women's Hospital, Boston [38, 39]

ROBERT H. ECKEL, MD
Professor of Medicine, Division of Endocrinology, Metabolism and Diabetes, Division of Cardiology; Professor of Physiology and Biophysics; Charles A. Boettcher II Chair in Atherosclerosis; Program Director, Adult General Clinical Research Center, University of Colorado at Denver and Health Sciences Center; Director Lipid Clinic, University Hospital, Aurora [32]

DANIEL J. FINK,† MD, MPH
Associate Professor of Clinical Pathology, College of Physicians and Surgeons, Columbia University, New York [Appendix]

J. MICHAEL GAZIANO, MD, MPH
Chief, Division of Aging, Brigham and Women's Hospital; Director, Massachusetts Veterans Epidemiology, Research and Information Center (MAVERIC) and Geriatric Research, Education and Clinical Center (GRECC), Boston VA Healthcare System; Associate Professor of Medicine, Harvard Medical School, Boston [2]

THOMAS A. GAZIANO, MD, MSc
Instructor in Medicine, Harvard Medical School; Associate Physician of Cardiovascular Medicine, Brigham and Women's Hospital, Boston [2]

RAYMOND J. GIBBONS, MD
Arthur M. and Gladys D. Gray Professor of Medicine, Mayo Clinic College of Medicine; Consultant, Cardiovascular Diseases, Mayo Clinic, Rochester [12, 42]

JAMES F. GLOCKNER, MD
Assistant Professor of Radiology, Mayo Clinic College of Medicine, Rochester [12, 42]

ARY L. GOLDBERGER, MD
Professor of Medicine, Harvard Medical School; Associate Director, Division of Interdisciplinary Medicine and Biotechnology, Beth Israel Deaconess Medical Center, Boston [11, 41, 43]

HELEN H. HOBBS, MD
Investigator, Howard Hughes Medical Institute; Professor of Internal Medicine and Molecular Genetics, University of Texas Southwestern Medical Center, Dallas [31]

JUDITH S. HOCHMAN, MD
Harold Synder Family Professor of Cardiology; Clinical Chief, the Leon H. Charney Division of Cardiology; New York University School of Medicine; Director, Cardiovascular Clinical Research, New York [28]

SHARON A. HUNT, MD
Professor, Cardiovascular Medicine, Stanford University, Palo Alto [18]

DAVID H. INGBAR, MD
Professor of Medicine, Physiology & Pediatrics; Director, Pulmonary, Allergy, Critical Care & Sleep Division; Executive Director, Center for Lung Science & Health, University of Minnesota School of Medicine; Co-Director, Medical ICU & Respiratory Care, University of Minnesota Medical Center, Fairview [28]

ADOLF W. KARCHMER, MD
Professor of Medicine, Harvard Medical School, Boston [25]

LOUIS V. KIRCHHOFF, MD, MPH
Professor, Departments of Internal Mediciene and Epidemiology, University of Iowa; Staff Physician, Department of Veterans Affairs Medical Center, Iowa City [27]

†Deceased

THEODORE A. KOTCHEN, MD
Associate Dean for Clinical Research; Director, General Clinical
Research Center, Medical College of Wisconsin, Wisconsin [37]

ALEXANDER KRATZ, MD, PhD, MPH
Assistant Professor of Clinical Pathology, Columbia University College
of Physicians and Surgeons; Associate Director, Core Laboratory,
Columbia University Medical Center, New York-Presbyterian
Hospital; Director, Allen Pavilion Laboratory, New York [Appendix]

THOMAS H. LEE, MD
Professor of Medicine, Harvard Medical School; Chief Executive
Officer, Partners Community Health Care, Inc; Network President,
Partners Health Care, Boston [4]

PETER LIBBY, MD
Mallinckrodt Professor of Medicine, Harvard Medical School;
Chief, Cardiovascular Medicine, Brigham and Women's Hospital,
Boston [1, 30]

JOSEPH LOSCALZO, MD, PhD, MA (Hon)
Hersey Professor of the Theory and Practice of Medicine, Harvard
Medical School; Chairman, Department of Medicine, Physician-in-
Chief, Brigham and Women's Hospital, Boston [1, 7, 8, 33, 38, 39]

DOUGLAS L. MANN, MD
Professor of Medicine, Molecular Physiology and Biophysics; Chief,
Section of Cardiology, Baylor College of Medicine, St. Luke's
Episcopal Hospital and Texas Heart Institute, Houston [17]

FRANCIS MARCHLINSKI, MD
Professor of Medicine; Director of Cardiac Electrophysiology,
University of Pennsylvania Health System, University of
Pennsylvania School of Medicine, Philadelphia [16]

ROBERT J. MYERBERG, MD
Professor of Medicine and Physiology; AHA Chair in Cardiovascular
Research, University of Miami Miller School of Medicine, Miami [29]

RICK A. NISHIMURA, MD
Judd and Mary Morris Leighton Professor of Cardiovascular
Diseases; Professor of Medicine, Mayo Clinic College of Medicine,
Rochester [12, 42]

PATRICK T. O'GARA, MD
Associate Professor of Medicine, Harvard Medical School; Director,
Clinical Cardiology, Brigham and Women's Hospital, Boston [10, 20]

ROBERT A. O'ROURKE, MD
Distinguished Professor of Medicine Emeritus, University of Texas
Health Science Center, San Antonio [9]

MICHAEL A. PESCE, PhD
Clinical Professor of Pathology, Columbia University College of
Physicians and Surgeons; Director of Specialty Laboratory, New York
Presbyterian Hospital, Columbia University Medical Center,
New York [Appendix]

DANIEL J. RADER, MD
Cooper-McClure Professor of Medicine, University of Pennsylvania
School of Medicine, Philadelphia [31]

STUART RICH, MD
Professor of Medicine, Section of Cardiology, University of Chicago,
Chicago [40]

JOSHUA SCHIFFER, MD
Department of Internal Medicine, The Johns Hopkins University
School of Medicine, Baltimore [Review and Self-Assessment]

RICHARD M. SCHWARTZSTEIN, MD
Professor of Medicine, Harvard Medical School; Associate Chair,
Pulmonary and Critical Care Medicine; Vice-President for
Education, Beth Israel Deaconess Medical Center, Boston [5]

ANDREW P. SELWYN, MA, MD
Professor of Medicine, Harvard Medical School, Boston [33]

ADAM SPIVAK, MD
Department of Internal Medicine, The Johns Hopkins University
School of Medicine, Baltimore [Review and Self-Assessment]

A. JAMIL TAJIK, MD
Thomas J. Watson, Jr., Professor; Professor of Medicine and
Pediatrics; Chairman (Emeritus), Zayed Cardiovascular Center, Mayo
Clinic, Rochester, Minnesota; Consultant, Cardiovascular Division,
Mayo Clinic, Scottsdale [12, 42]

GORDON F. TOMASELLI, MD
David J. Carver Professor of Medicine, Vice Chairman, Department
of Medicine for Research, The Johns Hopkins University, Baltimore
[14, 15]

CHARLES WIENER, MD
Professor of Medicine and Physiology; Vice Chair, Department of
Medicine; Director, Osler Medical Training Program, The Johns
Hopkins University School of Medicine, Baltimore [Review and
Self-Assessment]

JOSHUA WYNNE, MD, MBA, MPH
Executive Associate Dean, Professor of Medicine, University of
North Dakota School of Medicine and Health Sciences,
Grand Forks [21]

PREFACE

Cardiovascular disease is the leading cause of death in the United States, and is rapidly becoming a major cause of death in the developing world. Advances in the therapy and prevention of cardiovascular diseases have clearly improved the lives of patients with these common, potentially devastating disorders; yet, the disease prevalence and the risk factor burden for disease (especially obesity in the United States and smoking worldwide) continue to increase globally. Cardiovascular medicine is, therefore, of crucial importance to the field of internal medicine.

Cardiovascular medicine is a large and growing subspecialty, and comprises a number of specific subfields, including coronary heart disease, congenital heart disease, valvular heart disease, cardiovascular imaging, electrophysiology, and interventional cardiology. Many of these areas involve novel technologies that facilitate diagnosis and therapy. The highly specialized nature of these disciplines within cardiology and the increasing specialization of cardiologists argue for the importance of a broad view of cardiovascular medicine by the internist in helping to guide the patient through illness and the decisions that arise in the course of its treatment.

The scientific underpinnings of cardiovascular medicine have also been evolving rapidly. The molecular pathogenesis and genetic basis for many diseases are now known and, with this knowledge, diagnostics and therapeutics are becoming increasingly individualized. Cardiovascular diseases are largely complex phenotypes, and this structural and physiological complexity recapitulates the complex molecular and genetic systems that underlie it. As knowledge about these complex systems expands, the opportunity for identifying unique therapeutic targets increases, holding great promise for definitive interventions in the future. Regenerative medicine is another area of cardiovascular medicine that is rapidly achieving translation. Recognition that the adult human heart can repair itself, albeit sparingly with typical injury, and that cardiac precursor (stem) cells reside within the myocardium to do this can be expanded, and can be used to repair if not regenerate a normal heart is an exciting advance in the field. These concepts represent a completely novel paradigm that will revolutionize the future of the subspecialty.

In view of the importance of cardiovascular medicine to the field of internal medicine, and the rapidity with which the scientific basis for the discipline is advancing, *Harrison's Cardiovascular Medicine* was developed. The purpose of this sectional is to provide the readers with a succinct overview of the field of cardiovascular medicine. To achieve this goal, *Harrison's Cardiovascular Medicine* comprises the key cardiovascular chapters contained in *Harrison's Principles of Internal Medicine, 17e*, contributed by leading experts in the field. This sectional is designed not only for physicians-in-training on cardiology rotations, but also for practicing clinicians, other health care professionals, and medical students who seek to enrich and update their knowledge of this rapidly changing field. The editors trust that this book will increase both the readers' knowledge of the field, and their appreciation for its importance.

Joseph Loscalzo, MD, PhD

Review and self-assessment questions and answers were taken from Wiener C, Fauci AS, Braunwald E, Kasper DL, Hauser SL, Longo DL, Jameson JL, Loscalzo J (editors) Bloomfield G, Brown CD, Schiffer J, Spivak A (contributing editors). *Harrison's Principles of Internal Medicine Self-Assessment and Board Review*, 17th ed. New York, McGraw-Hill, 2008, ISBN 978-0-07-149619-3.

 The global icons call greater attention to key epidemiologic and clinical differences in the practice of medicine throughout the world.

 The genetic icons identify a clinical issue with an explicit genetic relationship.

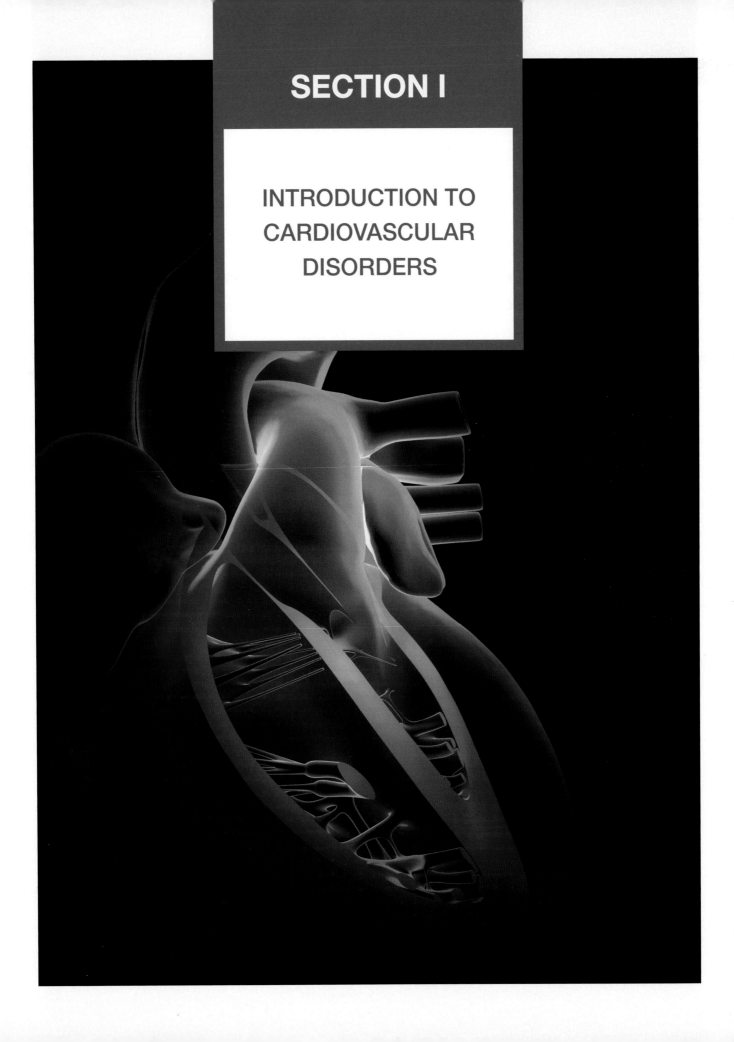

SECTION I

INTRODUCTION TO CARDIOVASCULAR DISORDERS

CHAPTER 1

BASIC BIOLOGY OF THE CARDIOVASCULAR SYSTEM

Joseph Loscalzo ■ Peter Libby ■ Eugene Braunwald

THE BLOOD VESSEL

VASCULAR ULTRASTRUCTURE

Blood vessels participate in homeostasis on a moment-to-moment basis and contribute to the pathophysiology of diseases of virtually every organ system. Hence, an understanding of the fundamentals of vascular biology furnishes a foundation for understanding normal function of all organ systems and many diseases. The smallest blood vessels, capillaries, consist of a monolayer of endothelial cells in close juxtaposition with occasional smooth-muscle–like cells known as *pericytes* (**Fig. 1-1***A*). Unlike larger vessels, pericytes do not invest the entire microvessel to form a continuous sheath. Veins and arteries typically have a trilaminar structure (**Fig. 1-1***B*–*E*). The *intima* consists of a monolayer of endothelial cells continuous with those of the capillary trees. The middle layer, or *tunica media*, consists of layers of smooth-muscle cells; in veins, this layer can contain just a few layers of smooth-muscle cells (Fig. 1-1*B*). The outer layer, the *adventitia*, consists of looser extracellular matrix with occasional fibroblasts, mast cells, and nerve terminals. Larger arteries have their own vasculature, the *vasa vasorum*, which nourish the outer aspects of the tunica media. The adventitia of many veins surpasses the intima in thickness.

The tone of muscular arterioles regulates blood pressure and flow through various arterial beds. These smaller arteries have relatively thick tunica media in relation to the adventitia (Fig. 1-1*C*). Medium-size muscular arteries likewise contain a prominent tunica media (Fig. 1-1*D*). Atherosclerosis commonly affects this type of muscular artery. The larger elastic arteries have a much more structured tunica media consisting of concentric bands of smooth-muscle cells interspersed with strata of elastin-rich extracellular matrix sandwiched between continuous layers of smooth-muscle cells (Fig. 1-1*E*). Larger arteries have a clearly demarcated internal elastic lamina that forms the barrier between the intima and media. An external elastic lamina demarcates the media of arteries from the surrounding adventitia.

ORIGIN OF VASCULAR CELLS

The intima in human arteries often contains occasional resident smooth-muscle cells beneath the monolayer of vascular endothelial cells. The embryonic origin of smooth-muscle cells in various types of artery differs. Some upper-body arterial smooth-muscle cells derive from the neural crest, whereas lower-body arteries generally recruit smooth-muscle cells during development from neighboring mesodermal structures, such as the

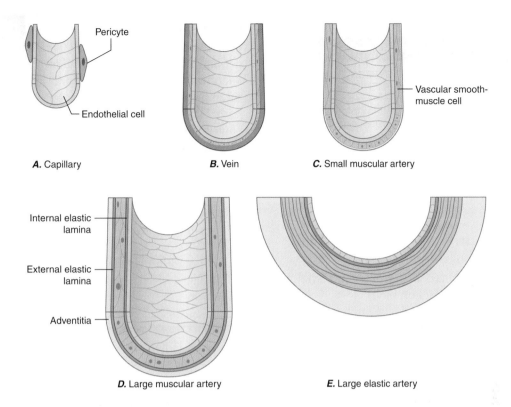

FIGURE 1-1
Schematics of the structures of various types of blood vessels. A. Capillaries consist of an endothelial tube in contact with a discontinuous population of pericytes. **B.** Veins typically have thin medias and thicker adventitias. **C.** A small muscular artery consists of a prominent tunica media.

D. Larger muscular arteries have a prominent media with smooth-muscle cells embedded in a complex extracellular matrix. **E.** Larger elastic arteries have circular layers of elastic tissue alternating with concentric rings of smooth-muscle cells.

somites. Recent evidence suggests that the bone marrow may give rise to both vascular endothelial cells and smooth-muscle cells, particularly under conditions of repair of injury or vascular lesion formation. Indeed, the ability of bone marrow to repair an injured endothelial monolayer may contribute to maintenance of vascular health and may promote arterial disease when this reparative mechanism fails due to injurious stimuli or age. The precise sources of endothelial and mesenchymal progenitor cells or their stem cell precursors remain the subject of active investigation.

VASCULAR CELL BIOLOGY

Endothelial Cell

The key cell of the vascular intima, the endothelial cell, has manifold functions in health and disease. Most obviously, the endothelium forms the interface between tissues and the blood compartment. It must, therefore, regulate the entry of molecules and cells into tissues in a selective manner. The ability of endothelial cells to serve as a permselective barrier fails in many vascular disorders, including atherosclerosis and hypertension. This dysregulation of permselectivity also occurs in pulmonary edema and other situations of "capillary leak."

The endothelium also participates in the local regulation of blood flow and vascular caliber. Endogenous substances produced by endothelial cells, such as prostacyclin, endothelium-derived hyperpolarizing factor, and nitric oxide (NO), provide tonic vasodilatory stimuli under physiologic conditions in vivo (**Table 1-1**). Impaired production or excess catabolism of NO impairs this endothelium-dependent vasodilator function and may contribute to excessive vasoconstriction under various pathologic situations. By contrast, endothelial cells also produce potent vasoconstrictor substances such as endothelin in a regulated fashion. Excessive production of reactive oxygen species, such as superoxide anion (O_2^-), by endothelial or smooth-muscle cells under pathologic conditions (e.g., excessive exposure to angiotensin II) can promote local oxidative stress and inactivate NO.

The endothelial monolayer contributes critically to inflammatory processes involved in normal host defenses and pathologic states. The normal endothelium resists prolonged contact with blood leukocytes; however, when activated by bacterial products, such as endotoxin or proinflammatory cytokines released during infection or injury, endothelial cells express an array of leukocyte adhesion molecules that bind various classes of leukocytes. The endothelial cells appear to recruit selectively

TABLE 1-1

ENDOTHELIAL FUNCTIONS IN HEALTH AND DISEASE

HOMEOSTATIC PHENOTYPE	DYSFUNCTIONAL PHENOTYPE
Vasodilatation	Impaired dilatation, vasoconstriction
Antithrombotic, profibrinolytic	Prothrombotic, antifibrinolytic
Anti-inflammatory	Proinflammatory
Antiproliferative	Proproliferative
Antioxidant	Prooxidant

different classes of leukocytes under different pathologic conditions. The gamut of adhesion molecules and chemokines generated during acute bacterial processes tends to recruit granulocytes. In chronic inflammatory diseases, such as tuberculosis or atherosclerosis, endothelial cells express adhesion molecules that favor the recruitment of mononuclear leukocytes that characteristically accumulate in these conditions.

The endothelial monolayer also dynamically regulates thrombosis and hemostasis. NO, in addition to its vasodilatory properties, can limit platelet activation and aggregation. Like NO, prostacyclin produced by endothelial cells under normal conditions not only provides a vasodilatory stimulus but also antagonizes platelet activation and aggregation. Thrombomodulin expressed on the surface of endothelial cells binds thrombin at low concentrations and inhibits coagulation through activation of the protein C pathway, leading to enhanced catabolism of clotting factors Va and VIIIa, thereby combating thrombus formation. The surface of endothelial cells contains heparan sulfate glycosaminoglycans that furnish an endogenous antithrombin coating to the vasculature. Endothelial cells also participate actively in fibrinolysis and its regulation. They express receptors for plasminogen activators and produce tissue-type plasminogen activator. Through local generation of plasmin, the normal endothelial monolayer can promote the lysis of nascent thrombi.

When activated by inflammatory cytokines—bacterial endotoxin, or angiotensin II, for example—endothelial cells can produce substantial quantities of the major inhibitor of fibrinolysis, plasminogen activator inhibitor 1 (PAI-1). Thus, under pathologic circumstances, the endothelial cell may promote local thrombus accumulation rather than combat it. Inflammatory stimuli also induce the expression of the potent procoagulant tissue factor, a contributor to disseminated intravascular coagulation in sepsis.

Endothelial cells also participate in the pathophysiology of a number of immune-mediated diseases. Lysis of endothelial cells mediated by complement provides an example of immunologically mediated tissue injury.

Presentation of foreign histocompatibility complex antigens by endothelial cells in solid organ allografts can trigger immunologic rejection. In addition, immune-mediated endothelial injury may contribute in some patients with thrombotic thrombocytopenic purpura and in patients with hemolytic uremic syndrome. Thus, in addition to contributing to innate immune responses, endothelial cells participate actively in both humoral and cellular limbs of the immune response.

Endothelial cells can also regulate growth of the subjacent smooth-muscle cells. Heparan sulfate glycosaminoglycans elaborated by endothelial cells can hold smooth-muscle proliferation in check. In contrast, when exposed to various injurious stimuli, endothelial cells can elaborate growth factors and chemoattractants, such as platelet-derived growth factor, that can promote the migration and proliferation of vascular smooth-muscle cells. Dysregulated elaboration of these growth-stimulatory molecules may promote smooth-muscle accumulation in arterial hyperplastic diseases, including atherosclerosis and in-stent stenosis.

Clinical Assessment of Endothelial Function

Endothelial function can be assessed noninvasively and invasively, and typically involves evaluating one measure of endothelial behavior in vivo, viz., endothelium-dependent vasodilation. Using either pharmacologic or mechanical agonists, the endothelium is stimulated to release acutely molecular effectors that alter underlying smooth-muscle cell tone. Invasively, endothelial function can be assessed with the use of agonists that stimulate release of endothelial NO, such as the cholinergic agonists acetylcholine and methacholine. The typical approach involves measuring quantitatively the change in coronary diameter in response to an intracoronary infusion of these short-lived, rapidly acting agents. Noninvasively, endothelial function can be assessed in the forearm circulation by performing occlusion of brachial artery blood flow with a blood pressure cuff, after which the cuff is deflated and the change in brachial artery blood flow and diameter are measured ultrasonographically (**Fig. 1-2**). This approach depends upon shear stress-dependent changes in endothelial release of NO following restoration of blood flow, as well as the effect of adenosine released (transiently) from ischemic tissue in the forearm.

Typically, the change in vessel diameter detected by these invasive and noninvasive approaches is ~10%. In individuals with frank atherosclerosis or risk factors for atherosclerosis (especially hypertension, hypercholesterolemia, diabetes mellitus, and smoking), such studies can detect endothelial dysfunction as defined by a smaller change in diameter and, in the extreme case, a so-called paradoxical vasoconstrictor response owing to the direct effect of cholinergic agonists on vascular smooth-muscle cell tone.

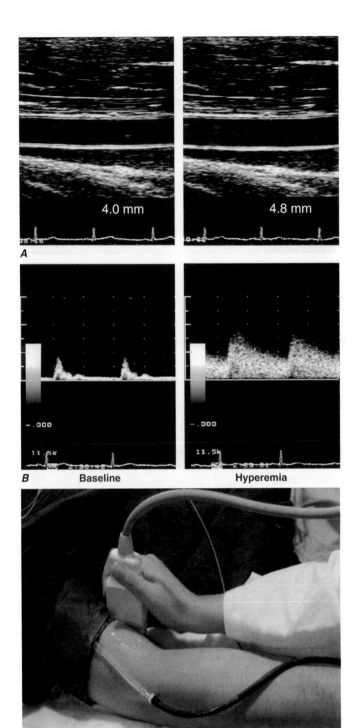

C

FIGURE 1-2

Assessment of endothelial function in vivo using blood pressure cuff-occlusion and release. Upon deflation of the cuff, changes in diameter (**A**) and blood flow (**B**) of the brachial artery are monitored with an ultrasound probe (**C**). *(Reproduced with permission of J. Vita, MD.)*

smooth-muscle cells at the level of the muscular arteries controls blood pressure and, hence, regional blood flow and the afterload experienced by the left ventricle (see later). The vasomotor tone of veins, governed by smooth-muscle cell tone, regulates the capacitance of the venous tree and influences the preload experienced by both ventricles. Smooth-muscle cells in the adult vessel seldom replicate. This homeostatic quiescence of smooth-muscle cells changes under conditions of arterial injury or inflammatory activation. Proliferation and migration of arterial smooth-muscle cells can contribute to the development of arterial stenoses in atherosclerosis, of arteriolar remodeling that can sustain and propagate hypertension, and of the hyperplastic response of arteries injured by angioplasty or stent deployment. In the pulmonary circulation, smooth-muscle migration and proliferation contribute decisively to the pulmonary vascular disease that gradually occurs in response to sustained high-flow states, such as left-to-right shunts. Such pulmonary vascular disease provides a major obstacle to the management of many patients with adult congenital heart disease.

Smooth-muscle cells also secrete the bulk of vascular extracellular matrix. Excessive production of collagen and glycosaminoglycans contributes to the remodeling and altered biology and biomechanics of arteries affected by hypertension or atherosclerosis. In larger elastic arteries, the elastin synthesized by smooth-muscle cells serves to maintain not only normal arterial structure but also hemodynamic function. The ability of the larger arteries, such as the aorta, to store the kinetic energy of systole promotes tissue perfusion during diastole. Arterial stiffness associated with aging or disease, as manifested by a widening pulse pressure, increases left ventricular afterload and portends a poor prognosis.

Like endothelial cells, vascular smooth-muscle cells do not merely respond to vasomotor or inflammatory stimuli elaborated by other cell types but can themselves serve as a source of such stimuli. For example, when stimulated by bacterial endotoxin, smooth-muscle cells can elaborate large quantities of proinflammatory cytokines, such as interleukin 6, as well as lesser quantities of many other proinflammatory mediators. Like endothelial cells, upon inflammatory activation, arterial smooth-muscle cells can produce prothrombotic mediators, such as tissue factor, the antifibrinolytic protein PAI-1, and other molecules that modulate thrombosis and fibrinolysis. Smooth-muscle cells may also elaborate autocrine growth factors that can amplify hyperplastic responses to arterial injury.

VASCULAR SMOOTH-MUSCLE CELL

The vascular smooth-muscle cell, the major cell type of the media layer of blood vessels, also actively contributes to vascular pathobiology. Contraction and relaxation of

Vascular Smooth-Muscle Cell Function

A principal function of vascular smooth-muscle cells is to maintain vessel tone. Vascular smooth-muscle cells contract when stimulated by a rise in intracellular calcium

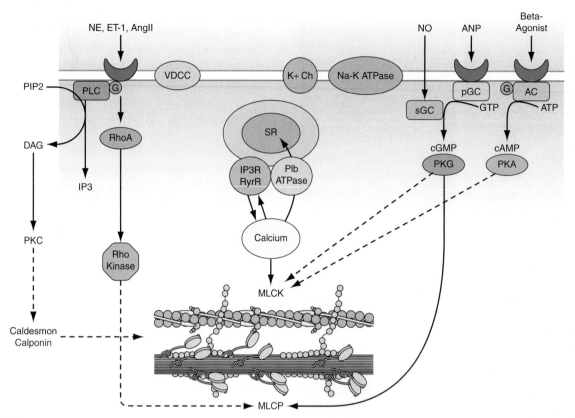

FIGURE 1-3

Regulation of vascular smooth-muscle cell calcium concentration and actomyosin ATPase-dependent contraction. NE, norepinephrine; ET-1, endothelin-1; AngII, angiotensin II; PIP_2, phosphatidylinositol 4,5-biphosphate; PLC, phospholipase C; DAG, diacylglycerol; G, G-protein; VDCC, voltage-dependent calcium channel; IP_3, inositol 1,4,5-trisphosphate; PKC, protein kinase C; SR, sarcoplasmic reticulum; NO, nitric oxide; ANP, antrial natriuretic peptide; pGC, particular guanylyl cyclase; AC, adenylyl cyclase; sGC, soluble guanylyl cyclase; PKG, protein kinase G; PKA, protein kinase A; MLCK, myosin light chain kinase; MLCP, myosin light chain phosphatase. *(Modified from B Berk, in Vascular Medicine, 3d ed, p 23. Philadelphia, Saunders, Elsevier, 2006; with permission.)*

concentration by calcium influx through the plasma membrane and by calcium release from intracellular stores (**Fig. 1-3**). In vascular smooth-muscle cells, voltage-dependent L-type calcium channels open with membrane depolarization, which is regulated by energy-dependent ion pumps such as the Na^+,K^+-ATPase and ion channels such as the Ca^{2+}-sensitive K^+ channel. Local changes in intracellular calcium concentration, termed *calcium sparks*, result from the influx of calcium through the voltage-dependent calcium channel and are caused by the coordinated activation of a cluster of ryanodine-sensitive calcium release channels in the sarcoplasmic reticulum (see later). Calcium sparks lead to a further direct increase in intracellular calcium concentration and indirectly increases intracellular calcium concentration by activating chloride channels. In addition, calcium sparks reduce contractility by activating large-conductance calcium-sensitive K^+ channels, hyperpolarizing the cell membrane and thereby limiting further voltage-dependent increases in intracellular calcium.

Biochemical agonists also increase intracellular calcium concentration, doing so by receptor-dependent activation of phospholipase C with hydrolysis of phosphatidylinositol 4,5-bisphosphate with generation of diacylglycerol (DAG) and inositol 1,4,5-trisphosphate (IP_3). These membrane lipid derivatives, in turn, activate protein kinase C and increase intracellular calcium concentration. In addition, IP_3 binds to its specific receptor found in the sarcoplasmic reticulum membrane to increase calcium efflux from this calcium storage pool into the cytoplasm.

Vascular smooth-muscle cell contraction is principally controlled by the phosphorylation of myosin light chain, which, in the steady state, depends on the balance between the actions of myosin light chain kinase and myosin light chain phosphatase. Myosin light chain kinase is activated by calcium through the formation of a calcium-calmodulin complex; with phosphorylation of myosin light chain by this kinase, the myosin ATPase activity is increased and contraction sustained. Myosin light chain phosphatase dephosphorylates myosin light chain, reducing myosin ATPase activity and contractile force. Phosphorylation of the myosin binding subunit (thr695) of myosin light chain phosphatase by Rho kinase inhibits phosphatase activity and induces calcium sensitization of the contractile apparatus. Rho kinase is itself activated by the small GTPase RhoA, which is stimulated by guanosine exchange factors and inhibited by GTPase-activating proteins.

Both cyclic AMP and cyclic GMP relax vascular smooth-muscle cells, doing so by complex mechanisms. β-Agonists acting through their G-protein-coupled receptors activate adenylyl cyclase to convert ATP to cyclic AMP; NO and atrial natriuretic peptide acting directly and via a G-protein-coupled receptor, respectively, activate guanylyl cyclase to convert GTP to cyclic GMP. These agents, in turn, activate protein kinase A and protein kinase G, respectively, which inactivates myosin light chain kinase and decreases vascular smooth-muscle cell tone. In addition, protein kinase G can directly interact with the myosin-binding substrate subunit of myosin light chain phosphatase, increasing phosphatase activity and decreasing vascular tone. Lastly, several mechanisms drive NO-dependent, protein kinase G–mediated reductions in vascular smooth-muscle cell calcium concentration, including phosphorylation-dependent inactivation of RhoA; decreased IP_3 formation; phosphorylation of the IP_3 receptor–associated cyclic GMP kinase substrate, with subsequent inhibition of IP_3 receptor function; phosphorylation of phospholamban, which increases calcium ATPase activity and sequestration of calcium in the sarcoplasmic reticulum; and protein kinase G–dependent stimulation of plasma membrane calcium ATPase activity, perhaps by activation of the Na^+,K^+-ATPase or hyperpolarization of the cell membrane by activation of calcium-dependent K^+ channels.

Control of Vascular Smooth-Muscle Cell Tone

Vascular smooth-muscle cell tone is governed by the autonomic nervous system and by the endothelium in tightly regulated control networks. Autonomic neurons enter the blood vessel media from the adventitia and modulate vascular smooth-muscle cell tone in response to baroreceptors and chemoreceptors within the aortic arch and carotid bodies, and in response to thermoreceptors in the skin. These regulatory components comprise rapidly acting reflex arcs modulated by central inputs that respond to sensory inputs (olfactory, visual, auditory, and tactile) as well as emotional stimuli. Autonomic regulation of vascular tone is mediated by three classes of nerves: *sympathetic*, whose principal neurotransmitters are epinephrine and norepinephrine; *parasympathetic*, whose principal neurotransmitter is acetylcholine; and *nonadrenergic/noncholinergic*, which include two subgroups—nitrergic, whose principal neurotransmitter

is NO; and peptidergic, whose principal neurotransmitters are substance P, vasoactive intestinal peptide, calcitonin gene-related peptide, and ATP.

Each of these neurotransmitters acts through specific receptors on the vascular smooth-muscle cell to modulate intracellular calcium and, consequently, contractile tone. Norepinephrine activates α receptors and epinephrine activates α and β receptors (adrenergic receptors); in most blood vessels, norepinephrine activates postjunctional α_1 receptors in large arteries, and α_2 receptors in small arteries and arterioles, leading to vasoconstriction. Most blood vessels express β_2 adrenergic receptors on their vascular smooth-muscle cells and respond to β agonists by cyclic AMP–dependent relaxation. Acetylcholine released from parasympathetic neurons binds to muscarinic receptors (of which there are five subtypes, M_1–M_5) on vascular smooth-muscle cells to yield vasorelaxation. In addition, NO stimulates presynaptic neurons to release acetylcholine, which can stimulate release of NO from the endothelium. Nitrergic neurons release NO produced by neuronal NO synthase, which causes vascular smooth-muscle cell relaxation via the cyclic GMP–dependent and –independent mechanisms described above. The peptidergic neurotransmitters all potently vasodilate, acting either directly or through endothelium-dependent NO release to decrease vascular smooth-muscle cell tone.

The endothelium modulates vascular smooth-muscle tone by the direct release of several effectors, including NO, prostacyclin, and endothelium-derived hyperpolarizing factor, all of which cause vasorelaxation; and endothelin, which causes vasoconstriction. The release of these endothelial effectors of vascular smooth-muscle cell tone is stimulated by mechanical (shear stress, cyclic strain, etc.) and biochemical mediators (purinergic agonists, muscarinic agonists, peptidergic agonists), with the biochemical mediators acting through endothelial receptors specific to each class.

In addition to these local, paracrine modulators of vascular smooth-muscle cell tone, circulating mediators can also affect tone, including norepinephrine and epinephrine, vasopressin, angiotensin II, bradykinin, and the natriuretic peptides (ANP, BNP, CNP, and DNP), as discussed above.

VASCULAR REGENERATION

Growing new blood vessels can occur in response to conditions such as chronic hypoxia or tissue ischemia. Growth factors, including vascular endothelial growth factor, activate a signaling cascade that stimulates endothelial proliferation and tube formation, defined as *angiogenesis*. The development of collateral vascular networks in the ischemic myocardium reflects this process and can result from selective activation of endothelial progenitor cells, which may reside in the blood vessel wall or home to the ischemic tissue subtended by an occluded or severely stenotic vessel from the bone marrow. True arteriogenesis, or the development of a new blood vessel comprising all three cell layers, does not normally occur in the cardiovascular system of mammals. Recent insights into the molecular determinants and progenitor cells that can recapitulate blood vessel development de novo is the subject of ongoing and rapidly advancing study.

VASCULAR PHARMACOGENOMICS

The past decade has witnessed considerable progress in efforts to define genetic differences underlying individual differences in vascular pharmacologic responses. Many investigators have focused on receptors and enzymes associated with neurohumoral modulation of vascular function, as well as hepatic enzymes that metabolize drugs affecting vascular tone. The genetic polymorphisms thus far associated with differences in vascular response often (but not invariably) relate to functional differences in the activity or expression of the receptor or enzyme of interest. Some of these polymorphisms appear to be differentially expressed in specific ethnic groups or by sex. A summary of recently identified polymorphisms defining these vascular pharmacogenomic differences is provided in Table 1-2.

CELLULAR BASIS OF CARDIAC CONTRACTION

THE CARDIAC ULTRASTRUCTURE

About three-fourths of the ventricle is composed of individual striated muscle cells (myocytes), normally 60–140 μm in length and 17–25 μm in diameter (Fig. 1-4A). Each cell contains multiple, rodlike cross-banded strands (myofibrils) that run the length of the cell and are, in turn, composed of serially repeating structures, the sarcomeres. The cytoplasm between the myofibrils contains other cell constituents, including the single centrally located nucleus, numerous mitochondria, and the intracellular membrane system, the sarcoplasmic reticulum.

The *sarcomere*, the structural and functional unit of contraction, lies between two adjacent dark lines, the Z lines. The distance between Z lines varies with the degree of contraction or stretch of the muscle and ranges between 1.6 and 2.2 μm. Within the confines of the sarcomere are alternating light and dark bands, giving the myocardial fibers their striated appearance under the light microscope. At the center of the sarcomere is a dark band of constant length (1.5 μm), the A band, which is flanked by two lighter bands, the I bands, which are of variable length. The sarcomere of heart

TABLE 1-2

GENETIC POLYMORPHISMS IN VASCULAR FUNCTION AND DISEASE RISK		
GENE	**POLYMORPHIC ALLELE**	**CLINICAL IMPLICATIONS**
α-adrenergic receptors		
α-1A	Arg492Cys	None
α-2B	Glu9/G1712	Increased CHD events
α-2C	A2cDcl3232-325	Ethnic differences in risk of hypertension or heart failure
Angiotensin-converting enzyme (ACE)	Insertion/deletion polymorphism in intron 16	D allele or DD genotype–increased response to ACE inhibitors; inconsistent data for increased risk of atherosclerotic heart disease, and hypertension
Ang II type I receptor	1166A → C Ala-Cys	Increased response to Ang II and increased risk of pregnancy-associated hypertension
β-Adrenergic receptors		
β-1		
	Ser49Gly	Increased HR and DCM risk
	Arg389Gly	Increased heart failure in blacks
β-2		
	Arg16Gly	Familial hypertension, increased obesity risk
	Glu27Gln	Hypertension in white type II diabetics
	Thr164Ile	Decreased agonist affinity and worse HF outcome
B2-Bradykinin receptor	Cys58Thr, Cys412Gly, Thr21Met	Increased risk of hypertension in some ethnic groups
Endothelial nitric oxide synthase (eNOS)	Nucleotide repeats in introns 4 and 13, Glu298Asp	Increased MI and venous thrombosis
	Thr785Cys	Early coronary artery disease

Note: CHD, coronary heart disease; HR, heart rate; DCM, dilated cardiomyopathy; HF, heart failure; MI, myocardial infarction.
Source: Adapted From B Schaefer et al: Heart Dis 5:129, 2003.

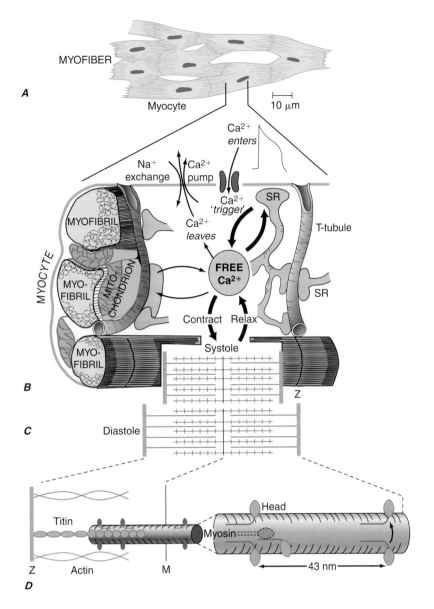

FIGURE 1-4

A shows the branching myocytes making up the cardiac myofibers. **B** illustrates the critical role played by the changing [Ca^{2+}] in the myocardial cytosol. Ca^{2+} ions are schematically shown as entering through the calcium channel that opens in response to the wave of depolarization that travels along the sarcolemma. These Ca^{2+} ions "trigger" the release of more calcium from the sarcoplasmic reticulum (SR) and thereby initiate a contraction-relaxation cycle. Eventually the small quantity of Ca^{2+} that has entered the cell leaves predominantly through an Na$^+$/Ca^{2+} exchanger, with a lesser role for the sarcolemmal Ca^{2+} pump. The varying actin-myosin overlap is shown for (**B**) systole, when [Ca^{2+}] is maximal, and (**C**) diastole, when [Ca^{2+}] is minimal. **D.** The myosin heads, attached to the thick filaments, interact with the thin actin filaments. *(From LH Opie, Heart Physiology, reprinted with permission. Copyright LH Opie, 2004.)*

muscle, like that of skeletal muscle, consists of two sets of interdigitating myofilaments. Thicker filaments, composed principally of the protein myosin, traverse the A band. They are about 10 nm (100 Å) in diameter, with tapered ends. Thinner filaments, composed primarily of actin, course from the Z line through the I band into the A band. They are approximately 5 nm (50 Å) in diameter and 1.0 μm in length. Thus, thick and thin filaments overlap only within the (dark) A band, while the (light) I band contains only thin filaments. On electron-microscopic examination, bridges may be seen to extend between the thick and thin filaments within the A band; these comprise myosin heads (see later) bound to actin filaments.

THE CONTRACTILE PROCESS

The sliding filament model for muscle contraction rests on the fundamental observation that both the thick and thin filaments are constant in overall length during both contraction and relaxation. With activation, the actin filaments are propelled further into the A band. In the process, the A band remains constant in length, whereas the I band shortens and the Z lines move toward one another.

The *myosin* molecule is a complex, asymmetric fibrous protein with a molecular mass of about 500,000 Da; it has a rodlike portion that is about 150 nm (1500 Å) in length with a globular portion (head) at its end. These globular portions of myosin form the bridges between the myosin and actin molecules and are the site of ATPase activity. In forming the thick myofilament, which is composed of ~300 longitudinally stacked myosin molecules, the rodlike segments of the myosin molecules are laid down in an orderly, polarized manner, leaving the globular portions projecting outward so that they can interact with actin to generate force and shortening (**Fig. 1-4B**).

Actin has a molecular mass of about 47,000 Da. The thin filament consists of a double helix of two chains of actin molecules wound about each other on a larger molecule, tropomyosin. A group of regulatory proteins—troponins C, I, and T—are spaced at regular intervals on this filament (**Fig. 1-5**). In contrast to myosin, actin lacks intrinsic enzymatic activity but does combine reversibly with myosin in the presence of ATP and Ca^{2+}. The calcium ion activates the myosin ATPase, which in turn breaks down ATP, the energy source for contraction (Fig. 1-5). The activity of myosin ATPase determines the rate of forming and breaking of the actomyosin cross-bridges and, ultimately, the velocity of muscle contraction. In relaxed muscle, tropomyosin inhibits this interaction. *Titin* (**Fig. 1-4D**) is a large, flexible, myofibrillar protein that connects myosin to the Z line. Its stretching contributes to the elasticity of the heart.

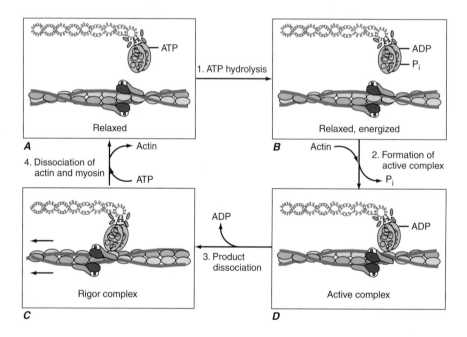

FIGURE 1-5

Four steps in cardiac muscle contraction and relaxation. In relaxed muscle (**A**), ATP bound to the myosin cross-bridge dissociates the thick and thin filaments. **Step 1:** Hydrolysis of myosin-bound ATP by the ATPase site on the myosin head transfers the chemical energy of the nucleotide to the activated cross-bridge (**B**). When cytosolic Ca^{2+} concentration is low, as in relaxed muscle, the reaction cannot proceed because tropomyosin and the troponin complex on the thin filament do not allow the active sites on actin to interact with the cross-bridges. Therefore, even though the cross-bridges are energized, they cannot interact with actin. **Step 2:** When Ca^{2+} binding to troponin C has exposed active sites on the thin filament, actin interacts with the myosin cross-bridges to form an active complex (**D**) in which the energy derived from ATP is retained in the actin-bound cross-bridge, whose orientation has not yet shifted.

Step 3: The muscle contracts when ADP dissociates from the cross-bridge. This step leads to the formation of the low-energy rigor complex (**C**) in which the chemical energy derived from ATP hydrolysis has been expended to perform mechanical work (the "rowing" motion of the cross-bridge). **Step 4:** The muscle returns to its resting state, and the cycle ends when a new molecule of ATP binds to the rigor complex and dissociates the cross-bridge from the thin filament. This cycle continues until calcium is dissociated from troponin C in the thin filament, which causes the contractile proteins to return to the resting state with the cross-bridge in the energized state. ATP, adenosine triphosphate; ATPase, adenosine triphosphatase; ADP, adenosine disphosphate. *[From AM Katz: Heart failure: Cardiac function and dysfunction, in Atlas of Heart Diseases, 3d ed, WS Colucci (ed). Philadelphia, Current Medicine, 2002. Reprinted with permission.]*

During activation of the cardiac myocyte, Ca^{2+} becomes attached to troponin C, which results in a conformational change in the regulatory protein tropomyosin; the latter, in turn, exposes the actin cross-bridge interaction sites (Fig. 1-5). Repetitive interaction between myosin heads and actin filaments is termed *cross-bridge cycling*, which results in sliding of the actin along the myosin filaments, ultimately causing muscle shortening and/or the development of tension. The splitting of ATP then dissociates the myosin cross-bridge from actin. In the presence of ATP (Fig. 1-5), linkages between actin and myosin filaments are made and broken cyclically as long as sufficient Ca^{2+} is present; these linkages cease when $[Ca^{2+}]$ falls below a critical level, and the troponin-tropomyosin complex once more prevents interactions between the myosin cross-bridges and actin filaments (**Fig. 1-6**).

Intracytoplasmic Ca^{2+} is a principal mediator of the inotropic state of the heart. The fundamental action of most agents that stimulate myocardial contractility (positive inotropic stimuli), including the digitalis glycosides and β-adrenergic agonists, is to raise the $[Ca^{2+}]$ in the vicinity of the myofilaments, which, in turn, triggers cross-bridge cycling. Increased impulse traffic in the cardiac adrenergic nerves stimulates myocardial contractility as a consequence of the release of norepinephrine from cardiac adrenergic nerve endings. Norepinephrine activates myocardial β receptors and, through the G_s-stimulated guanine nucleotide binding protein, activates the enzyme adenylyl cyclase, which leads to the formation of the intracellular second messenger cyclic AMP from ATP (Fig. 1-6). Cyclic AMP, in turn, activates protein kinase A (PKA), which phosphorylates the Ca^{2+} channel in the myocardial sarcolemma, thereby enhancing the influx of Ca^{2+} into the myocyte. Other functions of PKA are discussed below.

The *sarcoplasmic reticulum* (SR) (**Fig. 1-7**) is a complex network of anastomosing intracellular channels that invests the myofibrils. Its longitudinally disposed membrane-lined tubules closely invest the surfaces of individual sarcomeres but have no direct continuity with the outside of the cell. However, closely related to the SR, both structurally and functionally, are the transverse tubules, or T system, formed by tubelike invaginations of the sarcolemma that extend into the myocardial fiber along the Z lines, i.e., the ends of the sarcomeres.

CARDIAC ACTIVATION

In the inactive state, the cardiac cell is electrically polarized, i.e., the interior has a negative charge relative to the outside of the cell, with a transmembrane potential of −80 to −100 mV (Chap. 14). The sarcolemma, which in the resting state is largely impermeable to Na^+, has a Na^+- and K^+-stimulating pump energized by ATP that extrudes Na^+ from the cell; this pump plays a critical role in establishing the resting potential. Thus, intracellular $[K^+]$ is

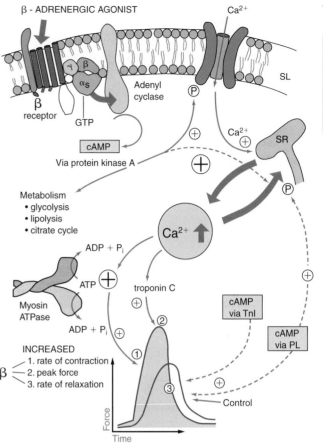

FIGURE 1-6

Signal systems involved in positive intropic and lusitropic (enhanced relaxation) effects of β-adrenergic stimulation. When the β-adrenergic agonist interacts with the β receptor, a series of G-protein–mediated changes leads to activation of adenylyl cyclase and formation of cyclic adenosine monophosphate (cAMP). The latter acts via protein kinase A to stimulate metabolism (*left*) and to phosphorylate the Ca^{2+} channel protein (*right*). The result is an enhanced opening probability of the Ca^{2+} channel, thereby increasing the inward movement of Ca^{2+} ions through the sarcolemma (SL) of the T tubule. These Ca^{2+} ions release more calcium from the sarcoplasmic reticulum (SR) to increase cytosolic Ca^{2+} and to activate troponin C. Ca^{2+} ions also increase the rate of breakdown of adenosine triphosphate (ATP) to adenosine diphosphate (ADP) and inorganic phosphate (Pi). Enhanced myosin ATPase activity explains the increased rate of contraction, with increased activation of troponin C explaining increased peak force development. An increased rate of relaxation is explained because cAMP also activates the protein phospholamban, situated on the membrane of the SR, that controls the rate of uptake of calcium into the SR. The latter effect explains enhanced relaxation (lusitropic effect). P, phosphorylation; PL, phospholamban; TnI, troponin I. (*Modified from LH Opie, Heart Physiology, reprinted with permission. Copyright LH Opie, 2004.*)

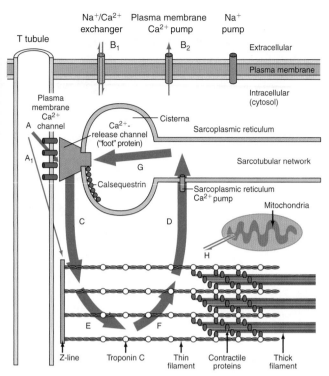

FIGURE 1-7

The Ca²⁺ fluxes and key structures involved in cardiac excitation-contraction coupling. The arrows denote the direction of Ca²⁺ fluxes. The thickness of each arrow indicates the magnitude of the calcium flux. Two Ca²⁺ cycles regulate excitation-contraction coupling and relaxation. The larger cycle is entirely intracellular and involves Ca²⁺ fluxes into and out of the sarcoplasmic reticulum, as well as Ca²⁺ binding to and release from troponin C. The smaller extracellular Ca²⁺ cycle occurs when this cation moves into and out of the cell. The action potential opens plasma membrane Ca²⁺ channels to allow passive entry of Ca²⁺ into the cell from the extracellular fluid (***arrow A***). Only a small portion of the Ca²⁺ that enters the cell directly activates the contractile proteins (***arrow A1***). The extracellular cycle is completed when Ca²⁺ is actively transported back out to the extracellular fluid by way of two plasma membrane fluxes mediated by the sodium-calcium exchanger (***arrow B1***) and the plasma membrane calcium pump (***arrow B2***). In the intracellular Ca²⁺ cycle, passive Ca²⁺ release occurs through channels in the cisternae (***arrow C***) and initiates contraction; active Ca²⁺ uptake by the Ca²⁺ pump of the sarcotubular network (***arrow D***) relaxes the heart. Diffusion of Ca²⁺ within the sarcoplasmic reticulum (***arrow G***) returns this activator cation to the cisternae, where it is stored in a complex with calsequestrin and other calcium-binding proteins. Ca²⁺ released from the sarcoplasmic reticulum initiates systole when it binds to troponin C (***arrow E***). Lowering of cytosolic [Ca²⁺] by the sarcoplasmic reticulum (SR) cause this ion to dissociate from troponin (***arrow F***) and relaxes the heart. Ca²⁺ may also move between mitochondria and cytoplasm (H). (*Adapted from Katz, with permission.*)

relatively high and [Na⁺] is far lower, while, conversely, extracellular [Na⁺] is high and [K⁺] is low. At the same time, in the resting state, extracellular [Ca²⁺] greatly exceeds free intracellular [Ca²⁺].

The four phases of the action potential are illustrated in Fig. 14-1*B*. During the plateau of the action potential (phase 2), there is a slow inward current through L-type Ca²⁺ channels in the sarcolemma (Fig. 1-7). The depolarizing current not only extends across the surface of the cell but penetrates deeply into the cell by way of the ramifying T tubular system. The absolute quantity of Ca²⁺ that crosses the sarcolemma and T system is relatively small and itself appears to be insufficient to bring about full activation of the contractile apparatus. However, this Ca²⁺ current triggers the release of much larger quantities of Ca²⁺ from the SR, a process termed *Ca²⁺-induced Ca²⁺ release*. The latter is a major determinant of intracytoplasmic [Ca²⁺] and therefore of myocardial contractility.

Ca²⁺ is released from the SR through a Ca²⁺ release channel, a cardiac isoform of the ryanodine receptor (RyR2), which controls intracytoplasmic [Ca²⁺] and, as in vascular smooth-muscle cells, leads to the local changes in intracellular [Ca²⁺] called calcium sparks. A number of regulatory proteins, including *calstabin 2*, inhibit RyR2 and, thereby, the release of Ca²⁺ from the SR. PKA dissociates calstabin from the RyR2, enhancing Ca²⁺ release and, thereby, myocardial contractility. Excessive plasma catecholamine levels and cardiac sympathetic neuronal release of norepinephrine cause hyperphosphorylation of PKA, leading to calstabin 2–depleted RyR2. The latter depletes SR Ca²⁺ stores and, thereby, impairs cardiac contraction, leading to heart failure, and also triggers ventricular arrhythmias.

The Ca²⁺ released from the SR then diffuses toward the myofibrils, where, as already described, it combines with troponin C (Fig. 1-6). By repressing this inhibitor of contraction, Ca²⁺ activates the myofilaments to shorten. During repolarization, the activity of the Ca²⁺ pump in the SR, the SR Ca²⁺ ATPase (SERCA₂A), reaccumulates Ca²⁺ against a concentration gradient, and the Ca²⁺ is stored in the SR by its attachment to a protein, *calsequestrin*. This reaccumulation of Ca²⁺ is an energy (ATP) requiring process that lowers the cytoplasmic [Ca²⁺] to a level that inhibits the actomyosin interaction responsible for contraction and in this manner leads to myocardial relaxation. Also, there is an exchange of Ca²⁺ for Na⁺ at the sarcolemma (Fig. 1-7), reducing the cytoplasmic [Ca²⁺]. Cyclic AMP–dependent PKA phosphorylates the SR protein *phospholamban*; the latter, in turn, permits activation of the Ca²⁺ pump, thereby increasing the uptake of Ca²⁺ by the SR, accelerating the rate of relaxation and providing larger quantities of Ca²⁺ in the SR for release by subsequent depolarization, thereby stimulating contraction.

Thus, the combination of the cell membrane, transverse tubules, and SR, with their ability to transmit the action potential and to release and then reaccumulate Ca^{2+}, play a fundamental role in the rhythmic contraction and relaxation of heart muscle. Genetic or pharmacologic alterations of any component, whatever its etiology, can disturb these functions.

CONTROL OF CARDIAC PERFORMANCE AND OUTPUT

The extent of shortening of heart muscle and, therefore, the stroke volume of the ventricle in the intact heart depend on three major influences: (1) the length of the muscle at the onset of contraction, i.e., the preload; (2) the tension that the muscle is called upon to develop during contraction, i.e., the afterload; and (3) the contractility of the muscle, i.e., the extent and velocity of shortening at any given preload and afterload. The major determinants of preload, afterload, and contractility are shown in Table 1-3.

TABLE 1-3

DETERMINANTS OF STROKE VOLUME

I. Ventricular Preload
  A. Blood volume
  B. Distribution of blood volume
    1. Body position
    2. Intrathoracic pressure
    3. Intrapericardial pressure
    4. Venous tone
    5. Pumping action of skeletal muscles
  C. Atrial contraction
II. Ventricular Afterload
  A. Systemic vascular resistance
  B. Elasticity of arterial tree
  C. Arterial blood volume
  D. Ventricular wall tension
    1. Ventricular radius
    2. Ventricular wall thickness
III. Myocardial Contractility[a]
  A. Intramyocardial $[Ca^{2+}]$ ↑↓
  B. Cardiac adrenergic nerve activity ↑↓[b]
  C. Circulating catecholamines ↑↓[b]
  D. Cardiac rate ↑↓[b]
  E. Exogenous inotropic agents ↑
  F. Myocardial ischemia ↓
  G. Myocardial cell death (necrosis, apoptosis, autophagy) ↓
  H. Alterations of sarcomeric and cytoskeletal proteins ↓
    1. Genetic
    2. Hemodynamic overload
  I. Myocardial fibrosis ↓
  J. Chronic overexpression of neurohormones ↓
  K. Ventricular remodeling ↓
  L. Chronic and/or excessive myocardial hypertrophy ↓

[a]Arrows indicate directional effects of determinants of contractility.
[b]Contractility rises initially but later becomes depressed.

The Role of Muscle Length (Preload)

The preload determines the length of the sarcomeres at the onset of contraction. The length of the sarcomeres associated with the most forceful contraction is ~2.2 μm. At this length, the two sets of myofilaments are configured so as to provide the greatest area for their interaction. The length of the sarcomere also regulates the extent of activation of the contractile system, i.e., its sensitivity to Ca^{2+}. According to this concept, termed *length-dependent activation*, the myofilament sensitivity to Ca^{2+} is also maximal at the optimal sarcomere length. The relation between the initial length of the muscle fibers and the developed force has prime importance for the function of heart muscle. This relationship forms the basis of Starling's law of the heart, which states that, within limits, the force of ventricular contraction depends on the end-diastolic length of the cardiac muscle; in the intact heart the latter relates closely to the ventricular end-diastolic volume.

Cardiac Performance

The ventricular end-diastolic or "filling" pressure is sometimes used as a surrogate for the end-diastolic volume. In isolated heart and heart-lung preparations, the stroke volume varies directly with the end-diastolic fiber length (preload) and inversely with the arterial resistance (afterload), and as the heart fails—i.e., as its contractility declines—it delivers a progressively smaller stroke volume from a normal or even elevated end-diastolic volume. The relation between the ventricular end-diastolic pressure and the stroke work of the ventricle (the ventricular function curve) provides a useful definition of the level of contractility of the heart in the intact organism. An increase in contractility is accompanied by a shift of the ventricular function curve upward and to the left (greater stroke work at any level of ventricular end-diastolic pressure, or lower end-diastolic volume at any level of stroke work), while a shift downward and to the right characterizes depression of contractility (Fig. 1-8).

Ventricular Afterload

In the intact heart, as in isolated cardiac muscle, the extent (and velocity) of shortening of ventricular muscle fibers at any level of preload and of myocardial contractility relate inversely to the afterload, i.e., the load that opposes shortening. In the intact heart, the afterload may be defined as the tension developed in the ventricular wall during ejection. Afterload is determined by the aortic pressure as well as by the volume and thickness of the ventricular cavity. Laplace's law indicates that the tension of the myocardial fiber is a function of the product of the intracavitary ventricular pressure and ventricular radius divided by the wall thickness.

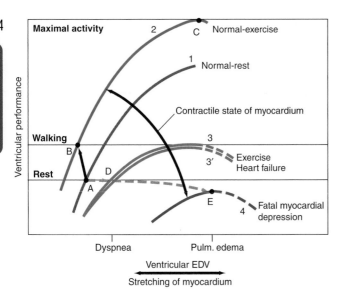

FIGURE 1-8

The interrelations among influences on ventricular end-diastolic volume (EDV) through stretching of the myocardium and the contractile state of the myocardium. Levels of ventricular EDV associated with filling pressures that result in dyspnea and pulmonary edema are shown on the abscissa. Levels of ventricular performance required when the subject is at rest, while walking, and during maximal activity are designated on the ordinate. The broken lines are the descending limbs of the ventricular-performance curves, which are rarely seen during life but show the level of ventricular performance if end-diastolic volume could be elevated to very high levels. For further explanation, see text. *[Modified from WS Colucci and E Braunwald: Pathophysiology of Heart Failure, in Braunwald's Heart Disease, 7th ed, DP Zipes et al (eds). Philadelphia, Elsevier, 2005.]*

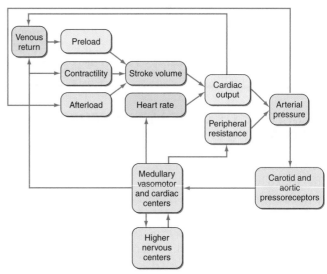

FIGURE 1-9

Interactions in the intact circulation of preload, contractility, and afterload in producing stroke volume. Stroke volume combined with heart rate determines cardiac output, which, when combined with peripheral vascular resistance, determines arterial pressure for tissue perfusion. The characteristics of the arterial system also contribute to afterload, an increase of which reduces stroke volume. The interaction of these components with carotid and aortic arch baroreceptors provides a feedback mechanism to higher medullary and vasomotor cardiac centers and to higher levels in the central nervous system to affect a modulating influence on heart rate, peripheral vascular resistance, venous return, and contractility. *[From MR Starling: Physiology of myocardial contraction, in Atlas of Heart Failure: Cardiac Function and Dysfunction, 3d ed, WS Colucci and E Braunwald (eds). Philadelphia, Current Medicine, 2002.]*

Therefore, at any given level of aortic pressure, the afterload on a dilated left ventricle is higher than that on a normal-sized ventricle. Conversely, at the same aortic pressure and ventricular diastolic volume, the afterload on a hypertrophied ventricle is lower than of a normal chamber. The aortic pressure, in turn, depends on the peripheral vascular resistance, the physical characteristics of the arterial tree, and the volume of blood it contains at the onset of ejection.

Ventricular afterload critically regulates cardiovascular performance (**Fig. 1-9**). As already noted, elevations of both preload and contractility increase myocardial fiber shortening, while increases in afterload reduce it. The extent of myocardial fiber shortening and left ventricular size determines stroke volume. An increase in arterial pressure induced by vasoconstriction, for example, augments afterload, which opposes myocardial fiber shortening, reducing stroke volume.

When myocardial contractility becomes impaired and the ventricle dilates, afterload rises (Laplace's law) and limits cardiac output. Increased afterload may also result from neural and humoral stimuli that occur in response to a fall in cardiac output. This increased afterload may reduce cardiac output further, thereby increasing ventricular volume and initiating a vicious circle, especially in patients with ischemic heart disease and limited myocardial O_2 supply. Treatment with vasodilators has the opposite effect; by reducing afterload, cardiac output rises (Chap. 17).

Under normal circumstances, the various influences acting on cardiac performance enumerated above interact in a complex fashion to maintain cardiac output at a level appropriate to the requirements of the metabolizing tissues (Fig. 1-9); interference with a single mechanism may not influence the cardiac output. For example, a moderate reduction of blood volume or the loss of the atrial contribution to ventricular contraction can ordinarily be sustained without a reduction in the cardiac output at rest. Under these circumstances, other factors, such as increases in the frequency of adrenergic nerve impulses to the heart, in heart rate, and in venous tone, will serve as compensatory mechanisms and sustain cardiac output in a normal individual.

Exercise

The integrated response to exercise illustrates the interactions among the three determinants of stroke volume, i.e., preload, afterload, and contractility (Fig. 1-8). Hyperventilation, the pumping action of the exercising muscles, and venoconstriction during exercise all augment venous return and, hence, ventricular filling and preload (Table 1-3). Simultaneously, the increase in the adrenergic nerve impulse traffic to the myocardium, the increased concentration of circulating catecholamines, and the tachycardia that occur during exercise combine to augment the contractility of the myocardium (Fig. 1-8, curves 1 and 2) and together elevate stroke volume and stroke work, without a change or even a reduction of end-diastolic pressure and volume (Fig. 1-8, points A and B). Vasodilatation occurs in the exercising muscles, thus tending to limit the increase in arterial pressure that would otherwise occur as cardiac output rises to levels as high as five times greater than basal levels during maximal exercise. This vasodilatation ultimately allows the achievement of a greatly elevated cardiac output during exercise, at an arterial pressure only moderately higher than in the resting state.

ASSESSMENT OF CARDIAC FUNCTION

Several techniques can define impaired cardiac function in clinical practice. The cardiac output and stroke volume may be depressed in the presence of heart failure, but, not uncommonly, these variables are within normal limits in this condition. A somewhat more sensitive index of cardiac function is the ejection fraction, i.e., the ratio of stroke volume to end-diastolic volume (normal value = $67 \pm 8\%$), which is frequently depressed in systolic heart failure, even when the stroke volume itself is normal. Alternatively, abnormally elevated ventricular end-diastolic volume (normal value = 75 ± 20 mL/m^2) or end-systolic volume (normal value = 25 ± 7 mL/m^2) signify impairment of left ventricular systolic function.

Noninvasive techniques, particularly echocardiography as well as radionuclide scintigraphy and cardiac MRI (Chap. 12), have great value in the clinical assessment of myocardial function. They provide measurements of end-diastolic and end-systolic volumes, ejection fraction, and systolic shortening rate, and they allow assessment of ventricular filling (see later) as well as regional contraction and relaxation. The latter measurements are particularly important in ischemic heart disease, as myocardial infarction causes regional myocardial damage.

A limitation of measurements of cardiac output, ejection fraction, and ventricular volumes in assessing cardiac function is that ventricular loading conditions strongly influence these variables. Thus, a depressed ejection fraction and lowered cardiac output may be observed in patients with normal ventricular function but with reduced preload, as occurs in hypovolemia, or with increased afterload, as occurs in acutely elevated arterial pressure.

The end-systolic left ventricular pressure-volume relationship is a particularly useful index of ventricular performance since it does not depend on preload and afterload (Fig. 1-10). At any level of myocardial contractility, left ventricular end-systolic volume varies inversely with end-systolic pressure; as contractility declines, end-systolic volume (at any level of end-systolic pressure) rises.

DIASTOLIC FUNCTION

Ventricular filling is influenced by the extent and speed of myocardial relaxation, which in turn is determined by the rate of uptake of Ca^{2+} by the SR; the latter may be enhanced by adrenergic activation and reduced by ischemia, which reduces the ATP available for pumping Ca^{2+} into the SR (see earlier). The stiffness of the ventricular wall may also impede filling. Ventricular stiffness increases

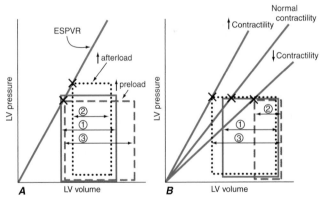

FIGURE 1-10

The responses of the left ventricle to increased afterload, increased preload, and increased and reduced contractility are shown in the pressure-volume plane. **A.** Effects of increases in preload and afterload on the pressure-volume loop. Since there has been no change in contractility, ESPVR (the end-systolic pressure volume relation) is unchanged. With an increase in afterload, stroke volume falls (1 → 2); with an increase in preload, stroke volume rises (1 → 3). **B.** With increased myocardial contractility and constant LV end-diastolic volume, the ESPVR moves to the left of the normal line (lower end-systolic volume at any end-systolic pressure) and stroke volume rises (1 → 3). With reduced myocardial contractility, the ESPVR moves to the right; end-systolic volume is increased and stroke volume falls (1 → 2).

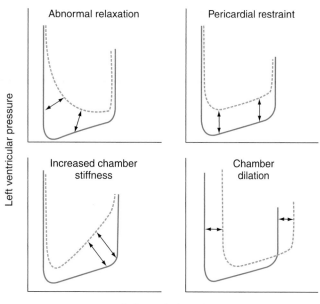

FIGURE 1-11

Mechanisms that cause diastolic dysfunction reflected in the pressure-volume relation. The bottom half of the pressure-volume loop is depicted. Solid lines represent normal subjects; broken lines represent patients with diastolic dysfunction. *(From JD Carroll et al: The differential effects of positive inotropic and vasodilator therapy on diastolic properties in patients with congestive cardiomyopathy. Circulation 74:815, 1986; with permission.)*

with hypertrophy and conditions that infiltrate the ventricle, such as amyloid, or by an extrinsic constraint (e.g., pericardial compression) (Fig. 1-11).

Ventricular filling can be assessed by continuously measuring the velocity of flow across the mitral valve using Doppler ultrasound. Normally, the velocity of inflow is more rapid in early diastole than during atrial systole; with mild to moderately impaired relaxation, the rate of early diastolic filling declines, while the rate of presystolic filling rises. With further impairment of filling, the pattern is "pseudo-normalized," and early ventricular filling becomes more rapid as left atrial pressure upstream to the stiff left ventricle rises.

CARDIAC METABOLISM

The heart requires a continuous supply of energy (in the form of ATP) not only to perform its mechanical pumping functions but also to regulate intracellular and transsarcolemmal ionic movements and concentration gradients. Among its pumping functions, the development of tension, the frequency of contraction, and the level of myocardial contractility are the principal determinants of the heart's substantial energy needs, making its O_2 requirements approximately 15% of that of the entire organism.

Most ATP production depends on the oxidation of substrate [glucose and free fatty acids (FFAs)]. Myocardial FFAs are derived from circulating FFAs, which result principally from lipolysis of adipose tissue, while the myocyte's glucose is obtained from plasma as well as from the cell's breakdown of its glycogen stores (glycogenolysis). There is a reciprocal relation between the utilization of these two principal sources of acetyl CoA in cardiac muscle. Glucose is broken down in the cytoplasm into a three-carbon product, pyruvate, which passes into the mitochondria, where it is metabolized to the two-carbon fragment, acetyl coenzyme A, and undergoes oxidation. FFAs are converted to acyl-CoA in the cytoplasm and acetyl coenzyme A (Co-A) in the mitochondria. Acetyl Co-A enters the citric acid (Krebs) cycle to produce ATP by oxidative phosphorylation within the mitochondria; ATP then enters the cytoplasm from the mitochondrial compartment. Intracellular ADP, resulting from the breakdown of ATP, enhances mitochondrial ATP production.

In the fasted, resting state, circulating FFA concentrations and their myocardial uptake are high, and they are the principal source of acetyl CoA (~70%). In the fed state, with elevations of blood glucose and insulin, glucose oxidation increases and FFA oxidation subsides. Increased cardiac work, the administration of inotropic agents, hypoxia, and mild ischemia all enhance myocardial glucose uptake, glucose production resulting from glycogenolysis, and glucose metabolism to pyruvate (glycolysis). By contrast, β-adrenergic stimulation, as occurs during stress, raises the circulating levels and metabolism of FFAs in favor of glucose. Severe ischemia inhibits the cytoplasmic enzyme pyruvate dehydrogenase, and despite both glycogen and glucose breakdown, glucose is metabolized only to lactic acid (anaerobic glycolysis), which does not enter the citric acid cycle. Anaerobic glycolysis produces much less ATP than aerobic glucose metabolism, in which glucose is metabolized to pyruvate and subsequently oxidized to CO_2. High concentrations of circulating FFAs, which can occur when adrenergic stimulation is superimposed on severe ischemia, reduce oxidative phosphorylation and also cause ATP wastage; the myocardial content of ATP declines, and myocardial contraction becomes impaired. In addition, products of FFA breakdown can exert toxic effects on cardiac cell membranes and may be arrhythmogenic.

Myocardial energy is stored as creatine phosphate (CP), which is in equilibrium with ATP, the immediate source of energy. In states of reduced energy availability, the CP stores decline first. Cardiac hypertrophy, fibrosis, tachycardia, increased wall tension resulting from ventricular dilatation, and increased intracytoplasmic [Ca^{2+}] all contribute to increased myocardial energy needs. When coupled with reduced coronary flow reserve, as occurs with obstruction of coronary arteries or abnormalities of the coronary microcirculation, an imbalance in myocardial ATP production relative to demand may occur, and the resulting ischemia can worsen or cause heart failure.

REGENERATING CARDIAC TISSUE

Until very recently, the mammalian myocardium was viewed as an end-differentiated organ without regeneration potential. Resident and bone marrow–derived stem cells have now been identified, are currently being evaluated as sources of regenerative potential for the heart, and offer the exciting possibility of reconstructing an infarcted or failing ventricle.

FURTHER READINGS

COLUCCI WS, BRAUNWALD E (eds): *Atlas of Heart Failure: Cardiac Function and Dysfunction*, 4th ed. Philadelphia, Current Medicine, 2004

DEANFIELD JE et al: Endothelial function and dysfunction: Testing and clinical relevance. Circulation 115:1285, 2007

KATZ AM: *Physiology of the Heart*, 4th ed. Philadelphia, Lippincott Williams and Wilkins, 2005

KIRBY ML: *Cardiac Development*, New York, Oxford University Press, 2007

LIBBY P et al: The vascular endothelium and atherosclerosis, in *The Handbook of Experimental Pharmacology*, S Moncada and EA Higgs (eds). Berlin-Heidelberg, Springer-Verlag, 2006

MAHONEY WM, SCHWARTZ SM: Defining smooth muscle cells and smooth muscle cell injury. J Clin Invest 15:221, 2005

OPIE LH: *Heart Physiology: From Cell to Circulation*, 4th ed. Philadelphia, Lippincott, Williams and Wilkins, 2004

———: Mechanisms of cardiac contraction and relaxation, in *Braunwald's Heart Disease*, 8th ed, P Libby et al (eds). Philadelphia, Elsevier, 2008

WEHRENS XH et al: Intracellular calcium release and cardiac disease. Annu Rev Physiol 67:69, 2005

CHAPTER 2

EPIDEMIOLOGY OF CARDIOVASCULAR DISEASE

Thomas A. Gaziano ■ J. Michael Gaziano

Cardiovascular disease (CVD) is now the most common cause of death worldwide. Before 1900, infectious diseases and malnutrition were the most common causes of death throughout the world, and CVD was responsible for <10% of all deaths. Today CVD accounts for ~30% of deaths worldwide, including nearly 40% in high-income countries and about 28% in low- and middle-income countries.

THE EPIDEMIOLOGIC TRANSITION

The global rise in CVD is the result of an unprecedented transformation in the causes of morbidity and mortality during the twentieth century. Known as the *epidemiologic transition*, the shift is driven by industrialization, urbanization, and associated lifestyle changes, and it is taking place in every part of the world among all races, ethnic groups, and cultures. The transition is divided into four basic stages: pestilence and famine, receding pandemics, degenerative and human-made diseases, and delayed degenerative diseases. A fifth stage, characterized by an epidemic of inactivity and obesity, may be emerging in some countries (Table 2-1).

Malnutrition, infectious diseases, and high infant and child mortality that are offset by high fertility mark the *age of pestilence and famine*. Tuberculosis, dysentery, cholera, and influenza are often fatal, resulting in a mean life expectancy of about 30 years. Cardiovascular disease, which accounts for <10% of deaths, takes the form of rheumatic heart disease and cardiomyopathies caused by infection and malnutrition. Approximately 10% of the world's population remains in the age of pestilence and famine.

Per capita income and life expectancy increase during the *age of receding pandemics* as the emergence of public health systems, cleaner water supplies, and improved nutrition combine to drive down deaths from infectious disease and malnutrition. Infant and childhood mortality also decline, but deaths resulting from CVD increase to between 10 and 35% of all deaths. Rheumatic valvular disease, hypertension, coronary heart disease, and stroke are the predominant forms of CVD. Almost 40% of the world's population is currently in this stage.

The *age of degenerative and human-made diseases* is distinguished by mortality from noncommunicable diseases—primarily CVD—surpassing mortality from malnutrition and infectious diseases. Caloric intake, particularly from animal fat, increases. Coronary heart disease and stroke are prevalent, and between 35 and 65% of all deaths can be traced to CVD. Typically, the rate of death from coronary heart disease (CHD) exceeds that of stroke by a ratio of 2:1–3:1. During this period, average life expectancy surpasses 50 years. Roughly 35% of the world's population falls into this category.

In the *age of delayed degenerative diseases*, CVD and cancer remain the major causes of morbidity and mortality, with CVD accounting for 40–50% of all deaths.

TABLE 2-1

FIVE STAGES OF EPIDEMIOLOGIC TRANSITION

STAGE	DESCRIPTION	DEATHS RELATED TO CVD	PREDOMINANT CVD TYPE
Pestilence and famine	Predominance of malnutrition and infectious diseases as causes of death; high rates of infant and child mortality; low mean life expectancy	< 10%	Rheumatic heart disease, cardiomyopathies caused by infection and malnutrition
Receding pandemics	Improvements in nutrition and public health, leading to decrease in rates of deaths related to malnutrition and infection; precipitous decline in infant and child mortality rates	10–35%	Rheumatic valvular disease, hypertension, CHD, and stroke (predominantly hemorrhagic)
Degenerative and human-made diseases	Increased fat and caloric intake and decrease in physical activity, leading to emergence of hypertension and atherosclerosis; with increase in life expectancy, mortality from chronic, noncommunicable diseases exceeds mortality from malnutrition and infectious disease	35–65%	CHD and stroke (ischemic and hemorrhagic)
Delayed degenerative diseases	CVD and cancer the major causes of morbidity and mortality; fewer deaths among those with disease and primary events delayed due to better treatment and prevention efforts; decline of age-adjusted CVD mortality; CVD affecting older and older individuals	40–50%	CHD, stroke, and congestive heart failure
Inactivity and obesity	Overweight and obesity increase at alarming rate; diabetes and hypertension increase; leveling off of decline in smoking-rate; physical activity recommendations met by a minority of the population	Possible reversal of age-adjusted declines in mortality	CHD, stroke, and congestive heart failure, peripheral vascular disease

Note: CHD, coronary heart disease; CVD, cardiovascular disease.
Source: Adapted from AR Omran: Milbank Mem Fund Q 49:509, 1971; and SJ Olshansky, AB Ault: Milbank Q 64:355, 1986.

However, age-adjusted CVD mortality declines, aided by preventive strategies, such as smoking cessation programs and effective blood pressure control; by acute hospital management; and by technological advances, such as the availability of bypass surgery. CHD, stroke, and congestive heart failure are the primary forms of CVD. About 15% of the world's population is now in the age of delayed degenerative diseases or is exiting this age and moving into the fifth stage of the epidemiologic transition.

In the industrialized world, physical activity continues to decline although total caloric intake increases. The resulting epidemic of overweight and obesity may signal the start of the *age of inactivity and obesity*. Rates of type 2 diabetes mellitus, hypertension, and lipid abnormalities are on the rise, trends that are particularly evident in children. If these risk factor trends continue, age-adjusted CVD mortality rates could increase in the coming years.

THE EPIDEMIOLOGIC TRANSITION IN THE UNITED STATES

The United States, like other high-income countries, has proceeded through four stages of the epidemiologic transition. Recent trends, however, suggest that the rates of decline of some chronic and degenerative diseases have slowed. Given the large amount of available data, the United States serves as a useful reference point for comparisons.

The Age of Pestilence and Famine (Before 1900)

The American colonies were born into pestilence and famine, with half of the original Pilgrims who arrived in 1620 dying of infection and malnutrition by the following spring. At the end of the 1800s, the U.S. economy was still largely agrarian, with >60% of the population living in rural settings. By 1900, average life expectancy had increased to about 50 years. However, tuberculosis, pneumonia, and other infectious diseases still accounted for more deaths than any other cause. CVD accounted for <10% of all deaths.

The Age of Receding Pandemics (1900–1930)

By 1900, a public health infrastructure was in place: 40 states had health departments, many larger towns had major public works efforts to improve the water supply and sewage systems, municipal use of chlorine to disinfect water was widespread, pasteurization and other improvements in food handling were introduced, and the educational quality of health care personnel improved. These changes led to dramatic declines in infectious disease mortality rates. However, the continued shift from a rural, agriculture-based economy to an urban, industrial economy had a number of consequences for risk behaviors and factors for CVD. In particular, consumption of fresh fruits and vegetables declined and consumption of meat and grains increased, resulting in diets that were higher in animal fat and processed carbohydrates. In addition, the availability of factory-rolled cigarettes made them more accessible and affordable for the mass population. Age-adjusted CVD mortality rates rose from 300 per 100,000 persons in 1900 to approximately 390 per 100,000 persons during this period, driven by rapidly rising CHD rates.

The Age of Degenerative and Human-Made Diseases (1930–1965)

During this period, deaths from infectious diseases fell to fewer than 50 per 100,000 persons per year, and life expectancy increased to almost 70 years. At the same time, the country became increasingly urbanized and industrialized, precipitating a number of important lifestyle changes. By 1955, 55% of adult men were smoking, and fat consumption represented ~40% of total calories. Lower activity levels, high-fat diets, and increased smoking pushed CVD death rates to their peak levels.

The Age of Delayed Degenerative Diseases (1965–)

Substantial declines in age-adjusted CVD mortality rates began in the mid-1960s. In the 1970s and 1980s, age-adjusted CHD mortality rates fell ~2% per year, and stroke rates fell 3% per year. A main characteristic of this phase is the steadily rising age at which a first CVD event occurs. Two significant advances have been attributed to the decline in CVD mortality rates: new therapeutic approaches and the implementation of prevention measures. Treatments once considered advanced, such as angioplasty, bypass surgery, and implantation of defibrillators, are now considered the standard of care. Treatment for hypertension and elevated cholesterol along with the widespread use of aspirin has also made major contributions to reducing deaths from CVD. In addition, Americans were exposed to public health campaigns promoting lifestyle modifications effective at reducing the prevalence of smoking, hypertension, and dyslipidemia.

Is the United States Entering a Fifth Age?

Starting in the 1990s, the age-standardized death rate had decreased to an average of about 2% per year for CHD and 1% for stroke. In 2003, the age-standardized death rate for total CVD was 306 per 100,000. The slowing of the decline may be due, in part, to a slowing of the rate of decline in risk factors, such as smoking, and alarming increases in other risk factors, such as obesity and physical inactivity.

CURRENT WORLDWIDE VARIATIONS

An epidemiologic transition similar to that which occurred in the United States is occurring throughout the world, but unique regional features have modified aspects of the transition in various parts of the world. In terms of economic development, the world can be divided into two broad categories: (1) high-income countries; and (2) low- and middle-income countries, which can be further subdivided into six distinct economic/geographic regions. Currently, 85% of the world's population lives in low- and middle-income countries, and it is these countries that are driving the rates of change in the global burden of CVD (Fig. 2-1). Three million CVD deaths occurred in high-income countries in 2001, in comparison with 13 million in the rest of the world.

High-Income Countries

Approximately 940 million persons live in the high-income countries, where CHD is the dominant form of CVD, with rates that tend to be twofold to fivefold higher than stroke rates. The rates of CVD in Canada, New Zealand, Australia, and Western Europe tend to be similar to those in the United States; however, among the countries of Western Europe, the absolute rates vary threefold with a clear north/south gradient. The highest CVD death rates are in the northern countries, such as Finland, Ireland, and Scotland, with the lowest CVD

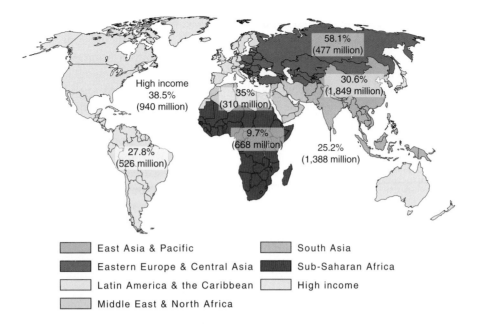

FIGURE 2-1

CVD death as a percentage of total deaths, and total population, in seven economic regions of the world defined by the World Bank. *(Based on data from CD Mathers et al: Deaths and* *Disease Burden by Cause: Global Burden of Disease Estimates for 2001 by World Bank Country Groups. Disease Control Priorities Working Paper 18. April 2004, revised January 2005.)*

rates in the Mediterranean countries of France, Spain, and Italy. Japan is unique among the high-income countries: stroke rates increased dramatically over the last century, but CHD rates did not rise as sharply. This difference may stem in part from genetic factors, but it is more likely that the fish- and plant-based, low-fat diet and resulting low cholesterol levels have played a larger role. Importantly, Japanese dietary habits are undergoing substantial changes, reflected in an increase in cholesterol levels.

Low- and Middle-Income Countries

The World Bank groups the low- and middle-income countries (gross national income per capita lower than U.S. $9200) into six geographic regions: East Asia and the Pacific, (Eastern) Europe and Central Asia, Latin America and the Caribbean, Middle East and North Africa, South Asia, and Sub-Saharan Africa. Although communicable diseases continue to be a major cause of death, CVD has emerged as a significant health concern in the low- and middle-income countries (**Fig. 2-2**).

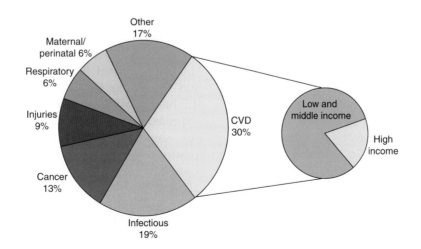

FIGURE 2-2

CVD compared with other causes of death. CVD, cardiovascular disease. *(Based on data from CD Mathers et al: Deaths and Disease Burden by Cause: Global Burden of* *Disease Estimates for 2001 by World Bank Country Groups. Disease Control Priorities Working Paper 18. April 2004, revised January 2005.)*

In most of these countries, there is an urban/rural gradient for CHD, stroke, and hypertension, with higher rates in urban centers.

Although CVD rates are rapidly rising, there are vast differences among the regions and countries, as well as within the countries. Many factors contribute to the heterogeneity. First, the regions are at various stages of the epidemiologic transition. Second, vast differences in lifestyle and behavioral risk factors exist. Third, racial and ethnic differences may lead to altered susceptibilities to various forms of CVD. In addition, it should be noted that for most countries in these regions, accurate country-wide data on cause-specific mortality are not precise, as death certificate completion is not routine, and most countries do not have a centralized registry for deaths.

The *East Asia and Pacific* region appears to be straddling the second and third phases of the epidemiologic transition, with China, Indonesia, and Sri Lanka's large combined population driving most of the trends. Overall, CVD is a major cause of death in China, but like Japan, stroke (particularly hemorrhagic) causes more deaths than CHD. China also appears to have a geographic gradient like that of Western Europe, with higher CVD rates in northern China than in southern China. Other countries, such as Vietnam and Cambodia, are just emerging from the pestilence and famine stage.

The *Eastern Europe and Central Asia* region is firmly in the peak of the third phase, with the highest death rates (58%) due to CVD in the world, nearly double the rate of high-income countries. There is, however, also regional variability. In Russia, increased CVD rates have contributed to falling life expectancy, particularly for men, whose life expectancy has dropped from 71.6 years in 1986 to 59 years today. In Poland, by contrast, the age-adjusted mortality rate decreased by ~30% for men during the 1990s, and slightly more among women.

In general, the *Latin America and Caribbean* region appears to be in the third phase of the epidemiologic transition, although as in other low- and middle-income regions, there is vast regional heterogeneity, with some areas in the second phase of the transition and some in the fourth. Today, ~28% of all deaths in this region are attributable to CVD, with CHD rates higher than stroke rates. Approximately 25% of the citizens live in poverty, and many are still dealing with infectious diseases and malnutrition as major problems.

The *Middle East and North Africa* region appears to be entering the third phase of the epidemiologic transition, with rates just below high-income nations. In this region, increasing economic wealth has been accompanied characteristically by urbanization but uncharacteristically by increasing fertility rates as infant and childhood mortality rates have declined. The traditional high-fiber diet, low in fat and cholesterol, has changed rapidly. Over the past few decades, daily fat consumption has increased in most of these countries, ranging from a 13.6% increase in Sudan to a 143.3% increase in Saudi Arabia.

Most persons in *South Asia* live in rural India, a country that is experiencing an alarming increase in heart disease. CVD accounted for 32% of all deaths in 2000, and the World Health Organization (WHO) estimates that 60% of the world's cardiac patients will be Indian by 2010. The transition appears to be in the Western style, with CHD as the dominant form of CVD. In 1960, CHD represented 4% of all CVD deaths in India, whereas in 1990 the proportion was >50%. This is somewhat unexpected because stroke tends to be a more dominant factor early in the epidemiologic transition. This finding may reflect inaccuracies in cause-specific mortality estimates or possibly an underlying genetic component. It has been suggested that Indians have exaggerated insulin insensitivity in response to the Western lifestyle pattern that may differentially increase rates of CHD over stroke. Certain remote areas, however, are still emerging from the age of pestilence and famine, with CVD accounting for <10% of total deaths. Rheumatic heart disease continues to be a major cause of morbidity and mortality.

Sub-Saharan Africa remains largely in the first phase of the epidemiologic transition, with CVD rates half of those in high-income nations. Life expectancy has decreased by an average of 5 years since the early 1990s largely because of HIV/AIDS and other chronic diseases, according to the World Bank; life expectancies are the lowest in the world. Although HIV/AIDS is the leading overall cause of death in this region, CVD is the third leading killer and is first among those older than 30 years. Hypertension is now a major public health concern and has resulted in stroke being the dominant form of CVD. Rheumatic heart disease remains an important cause of CVD mortality and morbidity.

GLOBAL TRENDS IN CARDIOVASCULAR DISEASE

In 1990, CVD accounted for 28% of the world's 50.4 million deaths and 9.7% of the 1.4 billion lost disability-adjusted life years (DALYs). By 2001, CVD was responsible for 29% of all deaths and 14% of the 1.5 billion lost DALYs. By 2030, when the population is expected to reach 8.2 billion, 32.5% of all deaths will be the result of CVD (Table 2-2). Of these, 14.9% of deaths in men and 13.1% of deaths in women will be caused by CHD. Stroke will be responsible for 10.4% of all male deaths and 11.8% of all female deaths.

In *high-income countries*, population growth will be fueled by emigration from low- and middle-income countries, but the population of high-income countries will shrink as a proportion of the world's population. In high-income countries, the modest decline in CVD death rates begun in the latter third of the twentieth century

TABLE 2-2

ESTIMATED MORBIDITY RELATED TO HEART DISEASE: 2010–2030

DEATHS	BY 2010	BY 2030
CVD deaths: annual number of all deaths	18.1 million	24.2 million
CVD deaths: percentage of all deaths	30.8%	32.5%
CHD deaths: percentage of all male deaths	13.1%	14.9%
CHD deaths: percentage of all female deaths	13.6%	13.1%
Stroke deaths: percentage of all male deaths	9.2%	10.4%
Stroke deaths: percentage of all female deaths	11.5%	11.8%

Note: CVD, cardiovascular disease; CHD, coronary heart disease.
Source: Adapted from Mackay and Mensah.

will continue, but the rate of decline appears to be slowing. However, these countries are expected to see an increase in the prevalence of CVD as well as the absolute number of deaths as the population ages.

Significant portions of the population living in *low- and middle-income countries* have entered the third phase of the epidemiologic transition, and some are entering the fourth stage. Changing demographics play a significant role in future predictions for CVD throughout the world. For example, between 1990 and 2001, the population of Eastern Europe and Central Asia grew by 1 million persons per year, whereas South Asia added 25 million persons each year.

Higher CVD rates will also have an economic impact. Even assuming no increase in CVD risk factors, most countries, but especially India and South Africa, will see a large number of individuals between 35 and 64 years die of CVD over the next 30 years, as well as an increasing level of morbidity among middle-aged individuals related to heart disease and stroke. It is estimated that in China, there will be 9 million deaths from CVD in 2030—up from 2.4 million in 2002—with half occurring in individuals between 35 and 64 years.

REGIONAL TRENDS IN RISK FACTORS

As indicated earlier, the global variation in CVD rates is related to temporal and regional variations in known risk behaviors and factors. Ecologic analyses of major CVD risk factors and mortality demonstrate high correlations between expected and observed mortality rates for the three main risk factors—smoking, serum cholesterol, and hypertension—and suggest that many of the regional variations are based on differences in conventional risk factors.

BEHAVIORAL RISK FACTORS

Tobacco

Every year, more than 5.5 trillion cigarettes are produced—enough to provide every person on the planet with 1,000 cigarettes. Worldwide, 1.2 billion persons smoked in 2000, a number that is projected to increase to 1.6 billion by 2030. Tobacco currently causes an estimated 5 million deaths annually (9% of all deaths). If current smoking patterns continue, by 2030 the global burden of disease attributable to tobacco will reach 10 million deaths annually. A unique feature of low- and middle-income countries is easy access to smoking during the early stages of the epidemiologic transition because of the availability of relatively inexpensive tobacco products.

Diet

Total caloric intake per capita increases as countries develop. With regard to CVD, a key element of dietary change is an increase in intake of saturated animal fats and hydrogenated vegetable fats, which contain atherogenic *trans* fatty acids, along with a decrease in intake of plant-based foods and an increase in simple carbohydrates. Fat contributes less than 20% of calories in rural China and India, less than 30% in Japan, and well above 30% in the United States. Caloric contributions from fat appear to be falling in the high-income countries. In the United States, between 1971 and 2000, the percentage of calories derived from saturated fat decreased from 13 to 11%.

Physical Inactivity

The increased mechanization that accompanies the economic transition leads to a shift from physically demanding, agriculture-based work to largely sedentary industry- and office-based work. In the United States, ~25% of the population does not participate in any leisure-time physical activity, and only 22% report engaging in sustained physical activity for at least 30 minutes on 5 or more days per week (the current recommendation). In contrast, in countries like China, physical activity is still integral to everyday life. Approximately 90% of the urban population walks or rides a bicycle daily to work, shopping, or school.

METABOLIC RISK FACTORS

Lipid Levels

Worldwide, high cholesterol levels are estimated to cause 56% of ischemic heart disease and 18% of strokes, amounting to 4.4 millions deaths annually. As countries move through the epidemiologic transition, mean population plasma cholesterol levels tend to rise. Social and individual changes that accompany urbanization clearly play a role because plasma cholesterol levels tend to be higher among urban residents than among rural residents. This shift is largely driven by greater consumption of dietary fats—primarily from animal products and processed vegetable oils—and decreased physical activity. In high-income countries, mean population cholesterol levels are generally falling, but in low- and middle-income countries, there is wide variation in these levels.

Hypertension

Elevated blood pressure is an early indicator of the epidemiologic transition. Worldwide, ~62% of strokes and 49% of cases of ischemic heart disease are attributable to suboptimal (>115 mmHg systolic) blood pressure, which is believed to account for more than 7 million deaths annually. Rising mean blood pressure is apparent as populations industrialize and move from rural to urban settings. Among urban-dwelling men and women in India, for example, the prevalence of hypertension is 25.5% and 29.0%, respectively, whereas it is 14.0% and 10.8%, respectively, in rural communities. One major concern in low- and middle-income countries is the high rate of undetected, and therefore untreated, hypertension. This may explain, at least in part, the higher stroke rates in these countries in relation to CHD rates during the early stages of the transition. The high rates of hypertension, especially undiagnosed hypertension, throughout Asia probably contribute to the high prevalence of hemorrhagic stroke in the region.

Obesity

Although clearly associated with increased risk of CHD, much of the risk posed by obesity may be mediated by other CVD risk factors, including hypertension, diabetes mellitus, and lipid profile imbalances. In the mid-1980s, the WHO's MONICA (multinational *moni*toring of trends and determinants in *ca*rdiovascular disease) project sampled 48 populations for cardiovascular risk factors. In all but one male population (China) and in most of the female populations, between 50 and 75% of adults aged 35–64 years were overweight or obese. In addition, the prevalence of extreme obesity (BMI ≥ 40 kg/m^2) more than tripled over a decade, increasing from 1.3 to 4.9%. In many of the low- and middle-income countries, obesity appears to coexist with undernutrition and malnutrition. Although the prevalence of obesity in low- and middle-income countries is certainly less than among high-income countries, it is on the rise in the former, as well. For example, a survey undertaken in 1998 found that as great as 58% of African women living in South Africa may be overweight or obese.

Diabetes Mellitus

As a consequence of, or in addition to, increasing body mass index and decreasing levels of physical activity, worldwide rates of diabetes—predominantly type 2 diabetes—are on the rise. In 2003, 194 million adults, or 5% of the world's population, had diabetes, with nearly three-quarters living in high-income countries. By 2025, the number is predicted to increase 72% to 333 million. By 2025, the number of individuals with type 2 diabetes is projected to double in three of the six low- and middle-income regions: Middle East and North Africa, South Asia, and Sub-Saharan Africa. There appear to be clear genetic susceptibilities to diabetes mellitus in various racial and ethnic groups. For example, migration studies suggest that South Asians and Indians tend to be at higher risk than those of European descent.

SUMMARY

Although CVD rates are declining in high-income countries, they are increasing in every other region of the world. The consequences of this preventable epidemic will be substantial on many levels—individual mortality and morbidity, family suffering, and staggering economic costs.

Three complementary strategies can be used to lessen the impact. First, the overall burden of CVD risk factors can be lowered through population-wide public health measures, such as national campaigns against cigarette smoking, unhealthy diets, and physical inactivity. Second, it is important to identify higher-risk subgroups of the population who stand to benefit the most from specific, low-cost prevention interventions, including screening for and treatment of hypertension and elevated cholesterol. Simple, low-cost interventions, such as the "polypill," a regimen of aspirin, a statin, and an antihypertensive agent, also need to be explored. Third, resources should be allocated to acute as well as secondary prevention interventions. For countries with limited resources, a critical first step in developing a comprehensive plan is better assessment of cause-specific mortality and morbidity, as well as the prevalence of the major preventable risk factors.

In the meantime, the high-income countries must continue to bear the burden of research and development aimed at prevention and treatment, being mindful of the economic limitations of many countries. The concept of the epidemiologic transition provides insight into how to alter the course of the CVD epidemic. The efficient transfer of low-cost preventive and therapeutic strategies could alter the natural course of this epidemic and thereby reduce the excess global burden of preventable CVD.

FURTHER READINGS

GAZIANO JM: Global burden of cardiovascular disease, in *Braunwald's Heart Disease: A Textbook of Cardiovascular Medicine*, 8th ed. Philadelphia, Elsevier Saunders, 2008

JAMISON DT et al (eds): *Disease Control Priorities in Developing Countries*, 2d ed. Washington, DC, Oxford University Press, 2006

LEEDER S et al: *A Race against Time: The Challenge of Cardiovascular Disease in Developing Economies*. New York, Columbia University Press, 2004

LOPEZ AD et al (eds): *Global Burden of Disease and Risk Factors*. Washington, DC, Oxford University Press, 2006

MACKAY J, MENSAH G: *Atlas of Heart Disease and Stroke*. Geneva, World Health Organization, 2004

Epidemiology of Cardiovascular Disease

CHAPTER 3

APPROACH TO THE PATIENT WITH POSSIBLE CARDIOVASCULAR DISEASE

Eugene Braunwald

THE MAGNITUDE OF THE PROBLEM

Cardiovascular diseases comprise the most prevalent serious disorders in industrialized nations and are a rapidly growing problem in developing nations (Chap. 2). Although age-adjusted death rates for coronary heart disease have declined by two-thirds in the past four decades in the United States, cardiovascular diseases remain the most common causes of death, responsible for 40% of all deaths, almost 1 million deaths each year. Approximately one-fourth of these deaths are sudden. The growing prevalence of obesity, type 2 diabetes mellitus, and metabolic syndrome (Chap. 32), which are important risk factors for atherosclerosis, now threatens to reverse the progress that has been made in the age-adjusted reduction of mortality of coronary heart disease.

For many years cardiovascular disease was considered to be more frequent in men than in women. In fact, the percentage of all deaths secondary to cardiovascular disease is greater among women (43%) than among men (37%). In addition, whereas the absolute number of deaths secondary to cardiovascular disease has declined over the past decades in men, the number has risen in women. Inflammation and the above-mentioned risk factors, i.e., obesity, type 2 diabetes mellitus, and the metabolic syndrome, appear to play a more prominent role in the development of coronary atherosclerosis in women than in men. Coronary artery disease (CAD) is more frequently associated with dysfunction of the coronary microcirculation in women than in men. Exercise electrocardiography has a lower diagnostic accuracy in the prediction of epicardial obstruction in women.

CARDIAC SYMPTOMS

The symptoms caused by heart disease result most commonly from myocardial ischemia, from disturbance of the contraction and/or relaxation of the myocardium, from obstruction to blood flow, or from an abnormal cardiac rhythm or rate.

Ischemia, which is caused by an imbalance between the heart's oxygen supply and demand, is manifest most frequently as chest discomfort (Chap. 4), whereas reduction of the pumping ability of the heart commonly leads to fatigue and elevated intravascular pressure upstream to the failing ventricle. The latter results in abnormal fluid accumulation, with peripheral edema (Chap. 7) or pulmonary congestion and dyspnea (Chap. 5). Obstruction to blood flow, as occurs in valvular stenosis, can cause symptoms that resemble those resulting from myocardial failure (Chap. 17). Cardiac arrhythmias often develop suddenly, and the resulting symptoms and signs—palpitations (Chap. 8), dyspnea, hypotension, and syncope—generally occur abruptly and may disappear as rapidly as they develop.

Although dyspnea, chest discomfort, edema, and syncope are cardinal manifestations of cardiac disease, they occur in other conditions as well. Thus, dyspnea is observed in disorders as diverse as pulmonary disease, marked obesity, and anxiety (Chap. 5). Similarly, chest discomfort may result from a variety of noncardiac and cardiac causes other than myocardial ischemia (Chap. 4). Edema, an important finding in untreated or inadequately treated heart failure, may also occur with primary renal disease and in hepatic cirrhosis (Chap. 7). Syncope occurs not only with serious cardiac arrhythmias but also in a number of neurologic conditions. Whether or not heart disease is responsible for these symptoms can frequently be determined by carrying out a careful clinical examination (Chap. 9), supplemented by noninvasive testing using electrocardiography at rest and during exercise (Chap. 11), echocardiography, roentgenography, and other forms of myocardial imaging (Chap. 12).

Myocardial or coronary function that may be adequate at rest may be insufficient during exertion. Thus, dyspnea and/or chest discomfort that appear during activity are characteristic of patients with heart disease, while the opposite pattern, i.e., the appearance of these symptoms at rest and their remission during exertion, is rarely observed in such patients. It is important, therefore, to question the patient carefully about the relation of symptoms to exertion.

Many patients with cardiovascular disease may be asymptomatic, both at rest and during exertion, but may present an abnormal physical finding, such as a heart murmur, elevated arterial pressure, or an abnormality of the ECG or of the cardiac silhouette on the chest roentgenogram or other imaging test. It is important to assess the global risk of CAD in asymptomatic individuals, using a combination of clinical assessment and measurement of cholesterol and its fractions, as well as other biomarkers such as C-reactive protein (CRP) in some patients (Chap. 30). Because the first clinical manifestation of CAD may be catastrophic—sudden cardiac death, acute myocardial infarction, or stroke in previous asymptomatic persons—it is mandatory to identify those at high risk of such events and institute further testing and preventive measures.

DIAGNOSIS

As outlined by the New York Heart Association, the elements of a complete cardiac diagnosis include the systematic consideration of the following:

1. *The underlying etiology.* Is the disease congenital, hypertensive, ischemic, or inflammatory in origin?
2. *The anatomic abnormalities.* Which chambers are involved? Are they hypertrophied, dilated, or both? Which valves are affected? Are they regurgitant and/or stenotic? Is there pericardial involvement? Has there been a myocardial infarction?
3. *The physiologic disturbances.* Is an arrhythmia present? Is there evidence of congestive heart failure or of myocardial ischemia?
4. *Functional disability.* How strenuous is the physical activity required to elicit symptoms? The classification provided by the New York Heart Association is useful in describing functional disability (Table 3-1).

One example may serve to illustrate the importance of establishing a complete diagnosis. In a patient who presents with exertional chest discomfort, the identification of myocardial ischemia as the etiology is of great clinical importance. However, the simple recognition of ischemia is insufficient to formulate a therapeutic strategy or prognosis until the underlying anatomic abnormalities responsible for the myocardial ischemia, e.g., coronary atherosclerosis or aortic stenosis, are identified and a judgment is made as to whether other physiologic disturbances that cause an imbalance between myocardial oxygen supply and demand, such as severe anemia, thyrotoxicosis, or supraventricular tachycardia, play a contributory role. Finally, the severity of the disability should govern the extent and tempo of the workup and strongly influence the therapeutic strategy that is selected.

The establishment of a correct and complete cardiac diagnosis usually commences with the history and physical examination (Chap. 9). Indeed, the clinical examination remains the basis for the diagnosis of a wide variety of disorders. The clinical examination may then be supplemented by five types of laboratory tests: (1) ECG

TABLE 3-1

NEW YORK HEART ASSOCIATION FUNCTIONAL CLASSIFICATION	
Class I	Class III
No limitation of physical activity	Marked limitation of physical activity
No symptoms with ordinary exertion	Less than ordinary activity causes symptoms
Class II	Asymptomatic at rest
Slight limitation of physical activity	Class IV
Ordinary activity causes symptoms	Inability to carry out any physical activity without discomfort
	Symptoms at rest

Source: Modified from The Criteria Committee of the New York Heart Association.

(Chap. 11); (2) noninvasive imaging examinations (chest roentgenogram, echocardiogram, radionuclide, computer tomographic and magnetic resonance imaging; Chap. 12); (3) blood tests to assess risk [e.g., lipid determinations, CRP (Chap. 30)], or cardiac function [e.g., brain natriuretic peptide (BNP); Chap. 17]; (4) occasionally specialized invasive examinations, i.e., cardiac catheterization and coronary arteriography (Chap. 13); and (5) genetic tests to identify monogenic cardiac diseases [e.g., hypertrophic cardiomyopathy (Chap. 21), Marfan syndrome, and abnormalities of cardiac ion channels that lead to prolongation of the QT interval and an increase in risk of sudden death (Chap. 16)]. These tests are becoming more widely available.

FAMILY HISTORY

In eliciting the history of a patient with known or suspected cardiovascular disease, particular attention should be directed to the family history. Familial clustering is common in many forms of heart disease. Mendelian transmission of single-gene defects may occur, as in hypertrophic cardiomyopathy (Chap. 21), Marfan syndrome, and sudden death associated with a prolonged QT syndrome (Chap. 16). Premature coronary disease and essential hypertension, type 2 diabetes mellitus, and hyperlipidemia (the most important risk factors for coronary artery disease) are usually polygenic disorders. Although familial transmission may be less obvious than in the single-gene disorders, it is also helpful in assessing risk and prognosis in polygenic disorders. Familial clustering of cardiovascular diseases may occur not only on a genetic basis but may also be related to familial dietary or behavior patterns, such as excessive ingestion of salt or calories or cigarette smoking.

ASSESSMENT OF FUNCTIONAL IMPAIRMENT

When an attempt is made to determine the severity of functional impairment in a patient with heart disease, it is helpful to ascertain the level of activity and the rate at which it is performed before symptoms develop. Thus, it is not sufficient to state that the patient complains of dyspnea. The breathlessness that occurs after running up two long flights of stairs denotes far less functional impairment than similar symptoms occurring after taking a few steps on level ground. Also, the degree of customary physical activity at work and during recreation should be considered. The development of two-flight dyspnea in a well-conditioned marathon runner may be far more significant than the development of one-flight dyspnea in a previously sedentary person. The history should include a detailed consideration of the patient's therapeutic regimen. For example, the persistence or development of edema, breathlessness, and other

manifestations of heart failure in a patient whose diet is rigidly restricted in sodium content and who is receiving optimal doses of diuretics and other therapies for heart failure (Chap. 17) is far graver than are similar manifestations in the absence of these measures. Similarly, the presence of angina pectoris despite treatment with optimal doses of multiple antianginal drugs (Chap. 33) is more serious than it is in a patient on no therapy. In an effort to determine the progression of symptoms, and thereby the severity of the underlying illness, it may be useful to ascertain what, if any, specific tasks the patient could have carried out 6 months or 1 year earlier that he or she cannot carry out at present.

ELECTROCARDIOGRAM

(See also Chap. 11) Although an ECG should usually be recorded in patients with known or suspected heart disease, with the exception of the identification of arrhythmias, of ventricular hypertrophy, and of acute myocardial infarction, it rarely permits establishment of a specific diagnosis. The range of normal electrocardiographic findings is wide, and the tracing can be affected significantly by many noncardiac factors, such as age, body habitus, and serum electrolyte concentrations. In the absence of other abnormal findings, electrocardiographic changes must not be overinterpreted.

ASSESSMENT OF THE PATIENT WITH A HEART MURMUR

(Fig. 3-1) The cause of a heart murmur can often be readily elucidated from a systematic evaluation of its major attributes: timing, duration, intensity, quality, frequency, configuration, location, and radiation when considered in the light of the history, general physical examination, and other features of the cardiac examination, as described in Chap. 9.

The majority of heart murmurs are mid-systolic and soft (grades I to II/VI). When such a murmur occurs in an asymptomatic child or young adult *without* other evidence of heart disease on clinical examination, it is usually benign and echocardiography is not generally required. On the other hand, two-dimensional and Doppler echocardiography (Chap. 12) are indicated in patients with loud systolic murmurs (grades ≥III/VI), especially those that are holosystolic or late systolic, and in most patients with diastolic or continuous murmurs.

NATURAL HISTORY

Cardiovascular disorders often present acutely, as in a previously asymptomatic person who develops an acute myocardial infarction (Chap. 35) or the previously asymptomatic patient with hypertrophic cardiomyopathy (Chap. 21) or with a prolonged QT interval (Chap. 16)

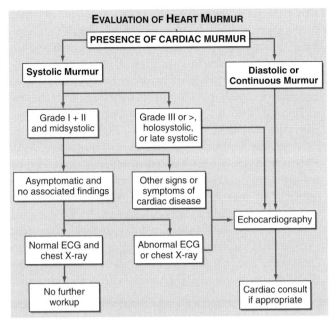

EVALUATION OF HEART MURMUR

FIGURE 3-1

An alternative "echocardiography first" approach to the evaluation of a heart murmur that also uses the results of the electrocardiogram (ECG) and chest x-ray in asymptomatic patients with soft midsystolic murmurs and no other physical findings. The algorithm is useful for patients older than 40 years in whom the prevalence of coronary artery disease and aortic stenosis increases as the cause of systolic murmur. [From RA O'Rourke, in Primary Cardiology, 2d ed, E Braunwald, L Goldman (eds). Philadelphia, Saunders, 2003.]

whose first clinical manifestation is syncope or even sudden death. However, the alert physician may recognize the patient at risk of these complications long before they occur and can often take measures to prevent their occurrence. For example, the patient with acute myocardial infarction will often have had risk factors for atherosclerosis for many years. Had these been recognized, their elimination or reduction might have delayed or even prevented the infarction. Similarly, the patient with hypertrophic cardiomyopathy may have had a heart murmur for years, and a family history of this disorder. These findings could have led to an echocardiographic examination and the recognition of the condition and appropriate therapy long before the occurrence of a serious acute manifestation.

Patients with valvular heart disease or idiopathic dilated cardiomyopathy, on the other hand, may have a prolonged course of gradually increasing dyspnea and other manifestations of chronic heart failure that is punctuated by episodes of acute deterioration only late in the course of the disease. It is of great importance to understand the natural history of various cardiac disorders so as to apply diagnostic and therapeutic measures that are appropriate to each stage of the condition as well as to provide the patient and family with an estimate of the prognosis.

PITFALLS IN CARDIOVASCULAR MEDICINE

Increasing subspecialization in internal medicine and the perfection of advanced diagnostic techniques in cardiology can lead to several undesirable consequences. Examples include:

1. Failure by the *noncardiologist* to recognize important cardiac manifestations of systemic illnesses, e.g., the presence of mitral stenosis, patent foramen ovale, and/or transient atrial arrhythmia in a patient with stroke or the presence of pulmonary hypertension and cor pulmonale in a patient with scleroderma or Raynaud's syndrome. A cardiovascular examination should be carried out to identify and estimate the severity of cardiovascular involvement that accompanies many noncardiac disorders.

2. Failure by the *cardiologist* to recognize underlying systemic disorders in patients with heart disease. For example, hyperthyroidism should be tested for in an elderly patient with atrial fibrillation and unexplained heart failure. Similarly, Lyme disease should be considered in a patient with unexplained fluctuating atrioventricular block. A cardiovascular abnormality may provide the clue critical to the recognition of some systemic disorders. For instance, an unexplained pericardial effusion may provide an early clue to the diagnosis of tuberculosis or neoplasm.

3. Overreliance on and overutilization of laboratory tests, particularly invasive techniques for the examination of the cardiovascular system. Cardiac catheterization and coronary arteriography (Chap. 13) provide precise diagnostic information that is critical to clinical evaluation which may be crucial in developing a therapeutic plan in patients with known or suspected CAD. Although a great deal of attention has been directed to these examinations, it is important to recognize that they serve to *supplement*, not *supplant*, a careful examination carried out by clinical and noninvasive techniques. A coronary arteriogram should not be carried out in lieu of a careful history in patients with chest pain suspected of having ischemic heart disease. Although coronary arteriography may establish whether the coronary arteries are obstructed, and if so the severity of the obstruction, the results of the procedure by themselves often do not provide a definite answer to the question of whether a patient's complaint of chest discomfort is attributable to coronary arteriosclerosis and whether or not revascularization is indicated.

Despite the value of invasive tests in certain circumstances, they entail some small risk to the patient, involve discomfort and substantial cost, and place a strain on medical facilities. Therefore, they should be carried out only if, after the results of clinical examination and assessment by noninvasive tests have been considered, the results (of the invasive examination) can be expected to modify the patient's management.

DISEASE PREVENTION AND MANAGEMENT

The prevention of heart disease, especially of CAD, is one of the most important tasks of primary care health givers as well as cardiologists. Prevention begins with risk assessment, followed by attention to lifestyle, such as achieving optimal weight and discontinuing smoking, and aggressive treatment of all abnormal risk factors, such as hypertension, hyperlipidemia, and diabetes mellitus.

After a complete diagnosis has been established in patients with known heart disease, a number of management options are usually available. Several examples may be used to demonstrate some of the principles of cardiovascular therapeutics:

1. In the absence of evidence of heart disease, a clear, definitive statement to that effect should be made and the patient should *not* be asked to return at intervals for repeated examinations. If there is no evidence for disease, such continued attention may lead to the patient developing inappropriate anxiety and fixation on the heart.

2. If there is no evidence of cardiovascular disease but the patient has one or more risk factors for the development of ischemic heart disease (Chap. 33), a plan for risk reduction should be developed and the patient should be retested at intervals to assess compliance and that the risk factors are being reduced.

3. Asymptomatic or mildly symptomatic patients with valvular heart disease that is anatomically severe should be evaluated periodically, every 6 to 12 months, by clinical and noninvasive examinations. Early signs of deterioration of ventricular function may signify the need for surgical treatment before the development of disabling symptoms, irreversible myocardial damage, and excessive risk of surgical treatment (Chap. 20).

4. In patients with CAD (Chap. 33), available practice guidelines should be considered in the decision on the form of treatment (medical, percutaneous coronary intervention, or surgical revascularization). Mechanical revascularization, i.e., the latter two modalities, may be employed too frequently in the United States and perhaps too infrequently in Eastern Europe and developing nations. The mere presence of angina pectoris and/or the demonstration of critical coronary arterial narrowing at angiography should not reflexly evoke a decision to treat the patient by revascularization. Instead, these procedures should be limited to patients with CAD whose angina has not responded adequately to medical treatment or in whom revascularization has been shown to improve the natural history (e.g., acute coronary syndrome, or multivessel CAD with left ventricular dysfunction).

FURTHER READINGS

ABRAMS J: *Synopsis of Cardiac Physical Diagnosis*, 2d ed. Oxford, Butterworth Heinemann, 2001

AMERICAN HEART ASSOCIATION: *Heart Disease and Stroke Statistics, 2006 Update.* Dallas, TX, American Heart Association, *www.americanheart.org*

AMERICAN HEART ASSOCIATION: *Heart Disease and Stroke Statistics, 2009 Update.* Dallas, TX, American Heart Association, *www.americanheart.org*

MORROW DA et al: Chronic coronary artery disease, in *Braunwald's Heart Disease,* 8th ed, P Libby et al (eds). Philadelphia, Saunders, 2008

NATIONAL HEART, LUNG AND BLOOD INSTITUTE: *FY 2005 Fact Book.* Bethesda, MD, National Heart, Lung and Blood Institute, 2006

THE CRITERIA COMMITTEE OF THE NEW YORK HEART ASSOCIATION: *Nomenclature and Criteria for Diagnosis*, 9th ed. Boston, Little, Brown, 1994

THE NHLBI-SPONSORED WOMEN'S ISCHEMIA SYNDROME EVALUATION (WISE): Challenging existing paradigms in ischemic heart disease. J Am Coll Cardiol 47(Suppl S):1, 2006

VANDEN BELT J: The history, in Classic *Teachings in Clinical Cardiology: A Tribute to W. Proctor Harvey*, M Chizner (ed). Cedar Grove, NJ, Laennec, 1996, pp 41–54

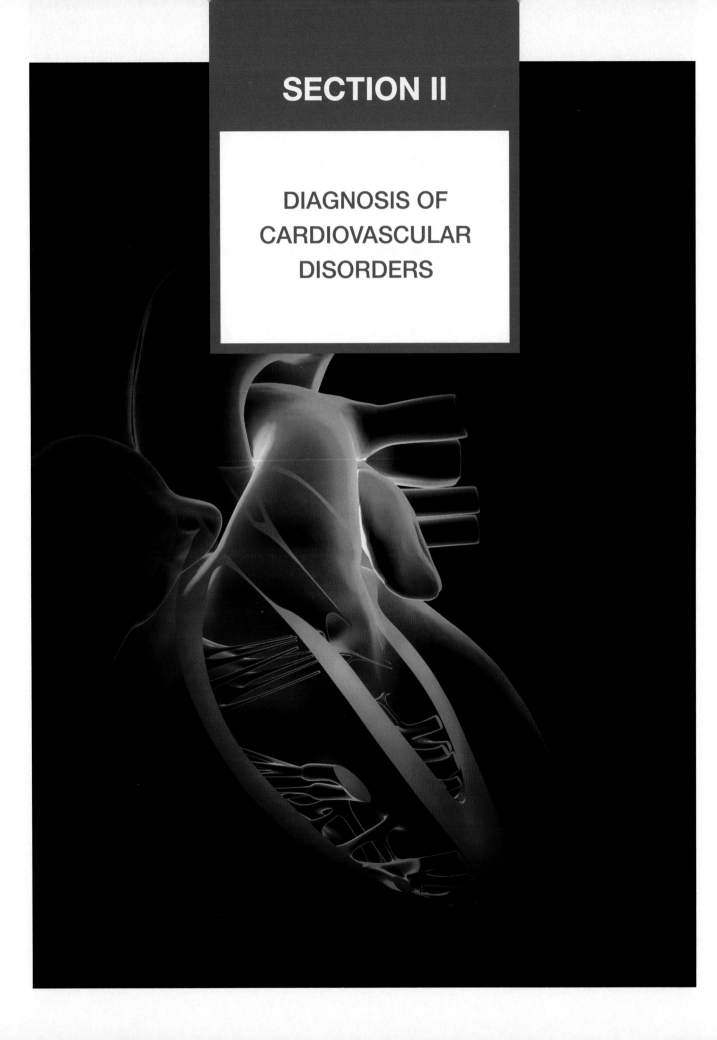

SECTION II

DIAGNOSIS OF CARDIOVASCULAR DISORDERS

CHAPTER 4

CHEST DISCOMFORT

Thomas H. Lee

Chest discomfort is one of the most common challenges for clinicians in the office or emergency department. The differential diagnosis includes conditions affecting organs throughout the thorax and abdomen, with prognostic implications that range from benign to life-threatening (Table 4-1). Failure to recognize potentially serious conditions such as acute ischemic heart disease, aortic dissection, tension pneumothorax, or pulmonary embolism can lead to serious complications, including death. Conversely, overly conservative management of low-risk patients leads to unnecessary hospital admissions, tests, procedures, and anxiety.

CAUSES OF CHEST DISCOMFORT

Myocardial Ischemia and Injury

Myocardial ischemia occurs when the oxygen supply to the heart is not sufficient to meet metabolic needs. This mismatch can result from a decrease in oxygen supply, a rise in demand, or both. The most common underlying cause of myocardial ischemia is obstruction of coronary arteries by atherosclerosis; in the presence of such obstruction, transient ischemic episodes are usually precipitated by an increase in oxygen demand as a result of physical exertion. However, ischemia can also result from psychological stress, fever, or large meals or from compromised oxygen delivery due to anemia, hypoxia, or hypotension. Ventricular hypertrophy due to valvular heart disease, hypertrophic cardiomyopathy, or hypertension can predispose the myocardium to ischemia because of impaired penetration of blood flow from epicardial coronary arteries to the endocardium.

▪ Angina Pectoris

(See also Chap. 33) The chest discomfort of myocardial ischemia is a visceral discomfort that is usually described as a heaviness, pressure, or squeezing (Table 4-2). Other common adjectives for anginal pain are burning and aching. Some patients deny any "pain" but may admit to dyspnea or a vague sense of anxiety. The word "sharp" is sometimes used by patients to describe intensity rather than quality.

The location of angina pectoris is usually retrosternal; most patients do not localize the pain to any small area. The discomfort may radiate to the neck, jaw, teeth, arms, or shoulders, reflecting the common origin in the posterior horn of the spinal cord of sensory neurons supplying the heart and these areas. Some patients present with aching in sites of radiated pain as their only symptoms of ischemia. Occasional patients report epigastric distress with ischemic episodes. Less common is radiation to below the umbilicus or to the back.

Stable angina pectoris usually develops gradually with exertion, emotional excitement, or after heavy meals. Rest or treatment with sublingual nitroglycerin typically leads to relief within several minutes. In contrast, pain that is fleeting (lasting only a few seconds) is rarely ischemic in origin. Similarly, pain that lasts for several hours is unlikely to represent angina, particularly if the patient's electrocardiogram (ECG) does not show evidence of ischemia.

Anginal episodes can be precipitated by any physiologic or psychological stress that induces tachycardia. Most myocardial perfusion occurs during diastole, when there is minimal pressure opposing coronary artery flow

TABLE 4-1

DIFFERENTIAL DIAGNOSES OF PATIENTS ADMITTED TO HOSPITAL WITH ACUTE CHEST DISCOMFORT RULED NOT MYOCARDIAL INFARCTION

DIAGNOSIS	PERCENT
Gastroesophageal disease[a]	42
Gastroesophageal reflux	
Esophageal motility disorders	
Peptic ulcer	
Gallstones	
Ischemic heart disease	31
Chest wall syndromes	28
Pericarditis	4
Pleuritis/pneumonia	2
Pulmonary embolism	2
Lung cancer	1.5
Aortic aneurysm	1
Aortic stenosis	1
Herpes zoster	1

[a]In order of frequency.
Source: P Fruergaard et al: Eur Heart J 17:1028, 1996.

from within the left ventricle. Since tachycardia decreases the percentage of the time in which the heart is in diastole, it decreases myocardial perfusion.

Unstable Angina and Myocardial Infarction

(See also Chaps. 34 and 35) Patients with these acute ischemic syndromes usually complain of symptoms similar in quality to angina pectoris, but more prolonged and severe. The onset of these syndromes may occur with the patient at rest, or awakened from sleep, and sublingual nitroglycerin may lead to transient or no relief. Accompanying symptoms may include diaphoresis, dyspnea, nausea, and light-headedness.

The physical examination may be completely normal in patients with chest discomfort due to ischemic heart disease. Careful auscultation during ischemic episodes may reveal a third or fourth heart sound, reflecting myocardial systolic or diastolic dysfunction. A transient murmur of mitral regurgitation suggests ischemic papillary muscle dysfunction. Severe episodes of ischemia can lead to pulmonary congestion and even pulmonary edema.

Other Cardiac Causes

Myocardial ischemia caused by hypertrophic cardiomyopathy or aortic stenosis leads to angina pectoris similar to that caused by coronary atherosclerosis. In such cases, a loud systolic murmur or other findings usually suggest that abnormalities other than coronary atherosclerosis may be contributing to the patient's symptoms. Some patients with chest pain and normal coronary angiograms have functional abnormalities of the coronary circulation, ranging from coronary spasm visible on coronary angiography to abnormal vasodilator responses and

heightened vasoconstrictor responses. The term "cardiac syndrome X" is used to describe patients with angina-like chest pain and ischemic-appearing ST-segment depression during stress despite normal coronary arteriograms. Some data indicate that many such patients have limited changes in coronary flow in response to pacing stress or coronary vasodilators. Despite the possibility that chest pain may be due to myocardial ischemia in such patients, their prognosis is excellent.

Pericarditis

(See also Chap. 22) The pain in pericarditis is believed to be due to inflammation of the adjacent parietal pleura, since most of the pericardium is believed to be insensitive to pain. Thus, infectious pericarditis, which usually involves adjoining pleural surfaces, tends to be associated with pain, while conditions that cause only local inflammation (e.g., myocardial infarction or uremia) and cardiac tamponade tend to result in mild or no chest pain.

The adjacent parietal pleura receives its sensory supply from several sources, so the pain of pericarditis can be experienced in areas ranging from the shoulder and neck to the abdomen and back. Most typically, the pain is retrosternal and is aggravated by coughing, deep breaths, or changes in position—all of which lead to movements of pleural surfaces. The pain is often worse in the supine position and relieved by sitting upright and leaning forward. Less common is a steady aching discomfort that mimics acute myocardial infarction.

Diseases of the Aorta

(See also Chap. 38) *Aortic dissection* is a potentially catastrophic condition that is due to spread of a subintimal hematoma within the wall of the aorta. The hematoma may begin with a tear in the intima of the aorta or with rupture of the vasa vasorum within the aortic media. This syndrome can occur with trauma to the aorta, including motor vehicle accidents or medical procedures in which catheters or intraaortic balloon pumps damage the intima of the aorta. Nontraumatic aortic dissections are rare in the absence of hypertension and/or conditions associated with deterioration of the elastic or muscular components of the media within the aorta's wall. Cystic medial degeneration is a feature of several inherited connective tissue diseases, including Marfan and Ehlers-Danlos syndromes. About half of all aortic dissections in women younger than 40 years occur during pregnancy.

Almost all patients with acute dissections present with severe chest pain, although some patients with chronic dissections are identified without associated symptoms. Unlike the pain of ischemic heart disease, symptoms of aortic dissection tend to reach peak severity immediately, often causing the patient to collapse from its intensity. The classic teaching is that the adjectives used to

TABLE 4-2

TYPICAL CLINICAL FEATURES OF MAJOR CAUSES OF ACUTE CHEST DISCOMFORT

CONDITION	DURATION	QUALITY	LOCATION	ASSOCIATED FEATURES
Angina	More than 2 and less than 10 min	Pressure, tightness, squeezing, heaviness, burning	Retrosternal, often with radiation to or isolated discomfort in neck, jaw, shoulders, or arms—frequently on left	Precipitated by exertion, exposure to cold, psychologic stress S4 gallop or mitral regurgitation murmur during pain
Unstable angina	10–20 min	Similar to angina but often more severe	Similar to angina	Similar to angina, but occurs with low levels of exertion or even at rest
Acute myocardial infarction	Variable; often more than 30 min	Similar to angina but often more severe	Similar to angina	Unrelieved by nitroglycerin May be associated with evidence of heart failure or arrhythmia
Aortic stenosis	Recurrent episodes as described for angina	As described for angina	As described for angina	Late-peaking systolic murmur radiating to carotid arteries
Pericarditis	Hours to days; may be episodic	Sharp	Retrosternal or toward cardiac apex; may radiate to left shoulder	May be relieved by sitting up and leaning forward Pericardial friction rub
Aortic dissection	Abrupt onset of unrelenting pain	Tearing or ripping sensation; knifelike	Anterior chest, often radiating to back, between shoulder blades	Associated with hypertension and/or underlying connective tissue disorder, e.g., Marfan syndrome Murmur of aortic insufficiency, pericardial rub, pericardial tamponade, or loss of peripheral pulses
Pulmonary embolism	Abrupt onset; several minutes to a few hours	Pleuritic	Often lateral, on the side of the embolism	Dyspnea, tachypnea, tachycardia, and hypotension
Pulmonary hypertension	Variable	Pressure	Substernal	Dyspnea, signs of increased venous pressure including edema and jugular venous distention
Pneumonia or pleuritis	Variable	Pleuritic	Unilateral, often localized	Dyspnea, cough, fever, rales, occasional rub
Spontaneous pneumothorax	Sudden onset; several hours	Pleuritic	Lateral to side of pneumothorax	Dyspnea, decreased breath sounds on side of pneumothorax
Esophageal reflux	10–60 min	Burning	Substernal, epigastric	Worsened by postprandial recumbency Relieved by antacids
Esophageal spasm	2–30 min	Pressure, tightness, burning	Retrosternal	Can closely mimic angina
Peptic ulcer	Prolonged	Burning	Epigastric, substernal	Relieved with food or antacids
Gallbladder disease	Prolonged	Burning, pressure	Epigastric, right upper quadrant, substernal	May follow meal
Musculoskeletal disease	Variable	Aching	Variable	Aggravated by movement May be reproduced by localized pressure on examination
Herpes zoster	Variable	Sharp or burning	Dermatomal distribution	Vesicular rash in area of discomfort
Emotional and psychiatric conditions	Variable; may be fleeting	Variable	Variable; may be retrosternal	Situational factors may precipitate symptoms Anxiety or depression often detectable with careful history

describe the pain reflect the process occurring within the wall of the aorta—"ripping" and "tearing"—but more recent data suggest that the most common presenting complaint is sudden onset of severe, sharp pain. The location often correlates with the site and extent of the dissection. Thus, dissections that begin in the ascending aorta and extend to the descending aorta tend to cause pain in the front of the chest that extends into the back, between the shoulder blades.

Physical findings may also reflect extension of the aortic dissection that compromises flow into arteries branching off the aorta. Thus, loss of a pulse in one or both arms, cerebrovascular accident, or paraplegia can all be catastrophic consequences of aortic dissection. Hematomas that extend proximally and undermine the coronary arteries or aortic valve apparatus may lead to acute myocardial infarction or acute aortic insufficiency. Rupture of the hematoma into the pericardial space leads to pericardial tamponade.

Another abnormality of the aorta that can cause chest pain is a *thoracic aortic aneurysm*. Aortic aneurysms are frequently asymptomatic but can cause chest pain and other symptoms by compressing adjacent structures. This pain tends to be steady, deep, and sometimes severe.

Pulmonary Embolism

Chest pain caused by pulmonary embolism is believed to be due to distention of the pulmonary artery or infarction of a segment of the lung adjacent to the pleura. Massive pulmonary emboli may lead to substernal pain that is suggestive of acute myocardial infarction. More commonly, smaller emboli lead to focal pulmonary infarctions that cause pain that is lateral and pleuritic. Associated symptoms include dyspnea and, occasionally, hemoptysis. Tachycardia is usually present. Although not always present, certain characteristic ECG changes can support the diagnosis.

Pneumothorax

Sudden onset of pleuritic chest pain and respiratory distress should lead to consideration of spontaneous pneumothorax, as well as pulmonary embolism. Such events may occur without a precipitating event in persons without lung disease, or as a consequence of underlying lung disorders.

Pneumonia or Pleuritis

Lung diseases that damage and cause inflammation of the pleura of the lung usually cause a sharp, knifelike pain that is aggravated by inspiration or coughing.

Gastrointestinal Conditions

Esophageal pain from acid reflux from the stomach, spasm, obstruction, or injury can be difficult to discern from myocardial syndromes. Acid reflux typically causes a deep burning discomfort that may be exacerbated by alcohol, aspirin, or some foods; the discomfort is often relieved by antacid or other acid-reducing therapies. Acid reflux tends to be exacerbated by lying down and may be worse in early morning when the stomach is empty of food that might otherwise absorb gastric acid.

Esophageal spasm may occur in the presence or absence of acid reflux and leads to a squeezing pain indistinguishable from angina. Prompt relief of esophageal spasm is often provided by antianginal therapies such as sublingual nifedipine, further promoting confusion between these syndromes. Chest pain can also result from injury to the esophagus, such as a Mallory-Weiss tear caused by severe vomiting.

Chest pain can result from diseases of the gastrointestinal tract below the diaphragm, including *peptic ulcer disease*, *biliary disease*, and *pancreatitis*. These conditions usually cause abdominal pain as well as chest discomfort; symptoms are not likely to be associated with exertion. The pain of ulcer disease typically occurs 60 to 90 min after meals, when postprandial acid production is no longer neutralized by food in the stomach. Cholecystitis usually causes a pain that is described as aching, occurring an hour or more after meals.

Neuromusculoskeletal Conditions

Cervical disk disease can cause chest pain by compression of nerve roots. Pain in a dermatomal distribution can also be caused by *intercostal muscle cramps* or by *herpes zoster*. Chest pain symptoms due to herpes zoster may occur before skin lesions are apparent.

Costochondral and *chondrosternal syndromes* are the most common causes of anterior chest musculoskeletal pain. Only occasionally are physical signs of costochondritis such as swelling, redness, and warmth (Tietze's syndrome) present. The pain of such syndromes is usually fleeting and sharp, but some patients experience a dull ache that lasts for hours. Direct pressure on the chondrosternal and costochondral junctions may reproduce the pain from these and other musculoskeletal syndromes. Arthritis of the shoulder and spine and bursitis may also cause chest pain. Some patients who have these conditions and myocardial ischemia blur and confuse symptoms of these syndromes.

Emotional and Psychiatric Conditions

As great as 10% of patients who present to emergency departments with acute chest discomfort have panic disorder or other emotional conditions. The symptoms in these populations are highly variable, but frequently the discomfort is described as visceral tightness or aching that lasts more than 30 min. Some patients offer other atypical descriptions, such as pain that is fleeting, sharp, and/or localized to a small region. The ECG in patients with emotional conditions may be difficult to interpret if hyperventilation causes ST-T-wave abnormalities. A careful history may elicit clues of depression, prior panic attacks, somatization, agoraphobia, or other phobias.

Approach to the Patient:
CHEST DISCOMFORT

The evaluation of the patient with chest discomfort must accommodate two goals—determining the diagnosis and assessing the safety of the immediate management plan. The latter issue is often dominant when the patient has acute chest discomfort, such as patients seen in the emergency department. In such settings, the clinician must focus first on identifying patients who require aggressive interventions to diagnose or manage potentially life-threatening conditions, including acute ischemic heart disease, acute aortic dissection, pulmonary embolism, and tension pneumothorax. If such conditions are unlikely, the clinician must address questions such as the safety of discharge to home, admission to a non-coronary care unit facility, or immediate exercise testing. Table 4-3 displays a sequence of questions that can be used in the evaluation of the patient with chest discomfort, with the diagnostic entities that are most important for consideration at each stage of the evaluation.

ACUTE CHEST DISCOMFORT In patients with acute chest discomfort, the clinician must first assess the patient's respiratory and hemodynamic status. If either is compromised, initial management should focus on stabilizing the patient before the diagnostic evaluation is pursued. If, however, the patient does not require emergent interventions, a focused history, physical examination, and laboratory evaluation should then be performed to assess the patient's risk of life-threatening conditions.

Clinicians who are seeing patients in the office setting should not assume that they do not have acute ischemic heart disease, even if the prevalence may be lower. Malpractice litigation related to myocardial infarctions that were missed during office evaluations is becoming increasingly common, and ECGs were not performed in many such cases. The prevalence of high-risk patients seen in office settings may be increasing due to congestion in emergency departments.

In either setting, the *history* should include questions about the quality and location of the chest discomfort (Table 4-2). The patient should also be asked about the nature of onset of the pain and its duration. Myocardial ischemia is usually associated with a gradual intensification of symptoms over a period of minutes. Pain that is fleeting or that lasts hours without being associated with electrocardiographic changes is not likely to be ischemic in origin. Although the presence of risk factors for coronary artery disease may heighten concern for this diagnosis,

---

TABLE 4-3

CONSIDERATIONS IN THE ASSESSMENT OF THE PATIENT WITH CHEST DISCOMFORT

1. Could the chest discomfort be due to an acute, potentially life-threatening condition that warrants immediate hospitalization and aggressive evaluation?

Acute ischemic heart disease	Pulmonary embolism
Aortic dissection	Spontaneous pneumothorax

2. If not, could the discomfort be due to a chronic condition likely to lead to serious complications?

   Stable angina
   Aortic stenosis
   Pulmonary hypertension

3. If not, could the discomfort be due to an acute condition that warrants specific treatment?

   Pericarditis
   Pneumonia/pleuritis
   Herpes zoster

4. If not, could the discomfort be due to another treatable chronic condition?

Esophageal reflux	Cervical disk disease
Esophageal spasm	Arthritis of the shoulder or spine
Peptic ulcer disease	Costochondritis
Gallbladder disease	Other musculoskeletal disorders
Other gastrointestinal conditions	Anxiety state

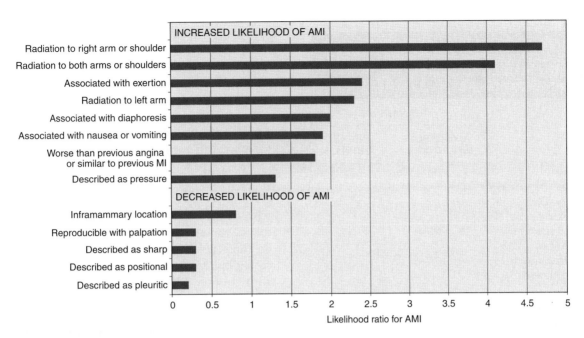

FIGURE 4-1

Impact of chest pain characteristics on odds of acute myocardial infarction (AMI). *(Figure prepared from data in Swap and Nagurney.)*

the absence of such risk factors does not lower the risk for myocardial ischemia enough to be used to justify a decision to discharge a patient.

Wide radiation of chest pain increases probability that pain is due to myocardial infarction. Radiation of chest pain to the left arm is common with acute ischemic heart disease, but radiation to the right arm is also highly consistent with this diagnosis. **Figure 4-1** shows estimates derived from several studies of the impact of various clinical features from the history on the probability that a patient has an acute myocardial infarction.

Right shoulder pain is also common with acute cholecystitis, but this syndrome is usually accompanied by pain that is located in the abdomen rather than chest. Chest pain that radiates between the scapulae raises the question of aortic dissection.

The *physical examination* should include evaluation of blood pressure in both arms and of pulses in both legs. Poor perfusion of a limb may be due to an aortic dissection that has compromised flow to an artery branching from the aorta. Chest auscultation may reveal diminished breath sounds; a pleural rub; or evidence of pneumothorax, pulmonary embolism, pneumonia, or pleurisy. Tension pneumothorax may lead to a shift in the trachea from the midline, away from the side of the pneumothorax. The cardiac examination should seek pericardial rubs, systolic and diastolic murmurs, and third or fourth heart sounds. Pressure on the chest wall may reproduce symptoms

in patients with musculoskeletal causes of chest pain; it is important that the clinician ask the patient if the chest pain syndrome is being completely reproduced before drawing too much reassurance that more serious underlying conditions are not present.

An *ECG* is an essential test for adults with chest discomfort that is not due to an obvious traumatic cause. In such patients, the presence of electrocardiographic changes consistent with ischemia or infarction (Chap. 11) is associated with high risks of acute myocardial infarction or unstable angina (**Table 4-4**); such patients should be admitted to a unit with electrocardiographic monitoring and the capacity to respond to a cardiac arrest. The absence of such changes does not exclude acute ischemic heart disease, but the risk of life-threatening complications is low for patients with normal electrocardiograms or only nonspecific ST-T-wave changes. If these patients are not considered appropriate for immediate discharge, they are often candidates for early or immediate exercise testing.

Markers of myocardial injury are often obtained in the emergency department evaluation of acute chest discomfort. The most commonly used markers are creatine kinase (CK), CK-MB, and the cardiac troponins (I and T). Rapid bedside assays of the cardiac troponins have been developed and shown to be sufficiently accurate to predict prognosis and guide management. Some data support the use of other markers, such as serum myoglobin, C-reactive protein (CRP), placental

TABLE 4-4

PREVALENCE OF MYOCARDIAL INFARCTION AND UNSTABLE ANGINA AMONG SUBSETS OF PATIENTS WITH ACUTE CHEST DISCOMFORT IN THE EMERGENCY DEPARTMENT

	PREVALENCE	
FINDING	**MYOCARDIAL INFARCTION, %**	**UNSTABLE ANGINA, %**
ST elevation (≥1 mm) or Q waves on ECG not known to be old	79	12
Ischemia or strain on ECG not known to be old (ST depression ≥1 mm or ischemic T waves)	20	41
None of the preceding ECG changes but a prior history of angina or myocardial infarction (history of heart attack or nitroglycerin use)	4	51
None of the preceding ECG changes and no prior history of angina or myocardial infarction (history of heart attack or nitroglycerin use)	2	14

Note: ECG, electrocardiogram.
Source: Unpublished data from Brigham and Women's Hospital Chest Pain Study, 1997–1999.

growth factor, myeloperoxidase, and B-type natriuretic peptide (BNP); their roles are the subject of ongoing research. Single values of any of these markers do not have high sensitivity for acute myocardial infarction or for prediction of complications. Hence, decisions to discharge patients home should not be made on the basis of single negative values of these tests.

Provocative tests for coronary artery disease are not appropriate for patients with ongoing chest pain. In such patients, rest myocardial perfusion scans can be considered; a normal scan reduces the likelihood of coronary artery disease and can help avoid admission of low-risk patients to the hospital. Promising early results suggest that 64-slice computed tomography (CT) and cardiac magnetic resonance imaging (MRI) may be of sufficient accuracy for diagnosis of coronary disease that these technologies may become widely used for patients with acute chest pain in whom the diagnosis is not clear.

Clinicians frequently employ therapeutic trials with sublingual nitroglycerin or antacids or, in the stable patient seen in the office setting, a proton pump inhibitor. A common error is to assume that a response to any of these interventions clarifies the diagnosis. While such information is often helpful, the patient's response may be due to the placebo effect. Hence, myocardial ischemia should never be considered excluded solely because of a response to antacid therapy. Similarly, failure of nitroglycerin to relieve pain does not exclude the diagnosis of coronary disease.

If the patient's history or examination is consistent with aortic dissection, imaging studies to evaluate the aorta must be pursued promptly because of the high risk of catastrophic complications with this condition. Appropriate tests include a chest CT scan with contrast, MRI, or transesophageal echocardiography (TEE).

Acute pulmonary embolism should be considered in patients with respiratory symptoms, pleuritic chest pain, hemoptysis, or a history of venous thromboembolism or coagulation abnormalities. Initial tests usually include CT angiography or a lung scan, which are sometimes combined with lower extremity venous ultrasound or D-dimer testing.

If patients with acute chest discomfort show no evidence of life-threatening conditions, the clinician should then focus on serious chronic conditions with the potential to cause major complications, the most common of which is stable angina. Early use of exercise electrocardiography, stress echocardiography, or stress perfusion imaging for such patients, whether in the office or the emergency department, is now an accepted management strategy for low-risk patients. Exercise testing is not appropriate, however, for patients who (1) report pain that is believed to be ischemic occurring at rest or (2) have electrocardiographic changes not known to be old that are consistent with ischemia.

Patients with sustained chest discomfort who do not have evidence for life-threatening conditions should be evaluated for evidence of conditions likely to benefit from acute treatment (Table 4-3). Pericarditis may be suggested by the history, physical examination, and ECG (Table 4-2). Clinicians should carefully assess blood pressure patterns and consider echocardiography in such patients to detect evidence of impending pericardial tamponade. Chest x-rays can be used to evaluate the possibility of pulmonary disease.

GUIDELINES AND CRITICAL PATHWAYS FOR ACUTE CHEST DISCOMFORT

Guidelines for the initial evaluation for patients with acute chest pain have been developed by the American College of Cardiology, American Heart Association, and other organizations. These guidelines recommend performance of an ECG for all patients with chest pain who do not have an obvious noncardiac cause of their pain, and performance of a chest x-ray for patients with signs or symptoms consistent with congestive heart failure, valvular heart disease, pericardial disease, or aortic dissection or aneurysm.

The American College of Cardiology/American Heart Association guidelines on exercise testing support its use in low-risk patients presenting to the emergency department, as well as in selected intermediate-risk patients. However, these guidelines emphasize that exercise tests should be performed only after patients have been screened for high-risk features or other indicators for hospital admission.

Many medical centers have adopted critical pathways and other forms of guidelines to increase efficiency and to expedite the treatment of patients with high-risk acute ischemic heart disease syndromes. These guidelines emphasize the following strategies:

- Rapid identification and treatment of patients for whom emergent reperfusion therapy, either via percutaneous coronary interventions or thrombolytic agents, is likely to lead to improved outcomes.
- Triage to non-coronary care unit monitored facilities such as intermediate-care units or chest pain units of patients with a low risk for complications, such as patients without new ischemic changes on their ECGs and without ongoing chest pain. Such patients can usually be safely observed in non-coronary care unit settings, undergo early exercise testing, or be discharged home. Risk stratification can be assisted through use of prospectively validated multivariate algorithms that have been published for acute ischemic heart disease and its complications.
- Shortening lengths of stay in the coronary care unit and hospital. Recommendations regarding the minimum length of stay in a monitored bed for a patient who has no further symptoms have decreased in recent years to 12 h or less if exercise testing or other risk stratification technologies are available.

NONACUTE CHEST DISCOMFORT

The management of patients who do not require admission to the hospital or who no longer require inpatient observation includes identification of the cause of the symptoms and the likelihood of major complications. Noninvasive tests for coronary disease serve to diagnose the condition and to identify patients with high-risk forms of coronary disease who may benefit from revascularization. Gastrointestinal causes of chest pain can be evaluated via endoscopy or radiology studies, or with trials of medical therapy. Emotional and psychiatric conditions warrant appropriate evaluation and treatment; randomized trial data indicate that cognitive therapy and group interventions lead to decreases in symptoms for such patients.

FURTHER READINGS

BRENNAN ML et al: Prognostic value of myeloperoxidase in patients with chest pain. N Engl J Med 349:1595, 2003

GIBBONS RJ et al: ACC/AHA 2002 guideline update for exercise testing. A report of the American College of Cardiology/American Heart Association Task Force on Practice Guidelines (Committee on Exercise Testing). Available at *www.acc.org/qualityandscience/clinical/guidelines/exercise/dirindex.htm*. Accessed on January 22, 2006

GIBSON PB et al: Low event rate for stress-only perfusion imaging in patients evaluated for chest pain. J Am Coll Cardiol 39:999, 2002

HEESCHEM C et al: Prognostic value of placental growth factor in patients with chest pain. JAMA 291:435, 2004

KWONG RY et al: Detecting acute coronary syndrome in the emergency department with cardiac magnetic resonance imaging. Circulation 197:531, 2003

LEBER AW et al: Quantification of obstructive and nonobstructive coronary lesions of 64-slice computed tomography. J Am Coll Cardiol 46:147, 2005

MILLER JM et al: Diagnostic performance of coronary angiography by 64-row CT. N Engl J Med 359:2324, 2008

SAENGER AK, JAFFE AS: Requiem for a heavyweight: the demise of ceratin kinase-MB. Circulation 118:2200, 2008

SEQUIST T, LEE TH: Prediction of missed myocardial infarction among symptomatic outpatients without coronary heart disease. Am Heart J 149:74, 2005

SEQUIST TD et al: Missed opportunities in the primary care management of early acute ischemic heart disease. Arch Intern Med 166: 2237, 2006

SUZUKI T et al: Diagnosis of acute aortic dissection by D-dimer. Circulation 119:2702, 2009

SWAP CJ, NAGURNEY JT: Value and limitations of chest pain history in the evaluation of patients with suspected acute coronary syndromes. JAMA 294:2623, 2005

TONG KL et al: Myocardial contrast echocardiography versus Thrombolysis in Myocardial Infarction score in patients presenting to the emergency department with chest pain and a nondiagnostic electrocardiogram. J Am Coll Cardiol 46:928, 2005

TSAI TT et al: Acute aortic syndromes. Circulation 205:3802, 2005

CHAPTER 5

DYSPNEA AND PULMONARY EDEMA

Richard M. Schwartzstein

DYSPNEA

The American Thoracic Society defines *dyspnea* as a "subjective experience of breathing discomfort that consists of qualitatively distinct sensations that vary in intensity. The experience derives from interactions among multiple physiological, psychological, social, and environmental factors, and may induce secondary physiological and behavioral responses." Dyspnea, a symptom, must be distinguished from the signs of increased work of breathing.

MECHANISMS OF DYSPNEA

Respiratory sensations are the consequence of interactions between the *efferent*, or outgoing, motor output from the brain to the ventilatory muscles (feed-forward) and the *afferent*, or incoming, sensory input from receptors throughout the body (feedback), as well as the integrative processing of this information that we infer must be occurring in the brain (Fig. 5-1). A given disease state may lead to dyspnea by one or more mechanisms, some of which may be operative under some circumstances but not others.

Motor Efferents

Disorders of the ventilatory pump are associated with increased work of breathing or a sense of an increased effort to breathe. When the muscles are weak or fatigued, greater effort is required, even though the mechanics of the system are normal. The increased neural output from the motor cortex is thought to be sensed due to a corollary discharge that is sent to the sensory cortex at the same time that signals are sent to the ventilatory muscles.

Sensory Afferents

Chemoreceptors in the carotid bodies and medulla are activated by hypoxemia, acute hypercapnia, and acidemia. Stimulation of these receptors, as well as others that lead to an increase in ventilation, produce a sensation of air hunger. Mechanoreceptors in the lungs, when stimulated by bronchospasm, lead to a sensation of chest tightness. J receptors, sensitive to interstitial edema, and pulmonary vascular receptors, activated by acute changes in pulmonary artery pressure, appear to contribute to air hunger. Hyperinflation is associated with the sensation of an inability to get a deep breath or of an unsatisfying breath. It is not clear if this sensation arises from receptors in the lungs or chest wall, or if it is a variant of the sensation of air hunger. Metaboreceptors, located in skeletal muscle, are believed to be activated by changes in the local biochemical milieu of the tissue active during exercise and, when stimulated, contribute to the breathing discomfort.

Integration: Efferent-Reafferent Mismatch

A discrepancy or mismatch between the feed-forward message to the ventilatory muscles and the feedback

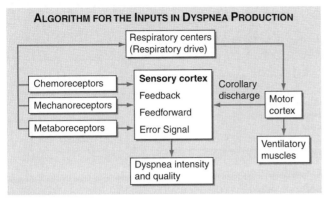

ALGORITHM FOR THE INPUTS IN DYSPNEA PRODUCTION

FIGURE 5-1

Hypothetical model for integration of sensory inputs in the production of dyspnea. Afferent information from the receptors throughout the respiratory system projects directly to the sensory cortex to contribute to primary qualitative sensory experiences and provide feedback on the action of the ventilatory pump. Afferents also project to the areas of the brain responsible for control of ventilation. The motor cortex, responding to input from the control centers, sends neural messages to the ventilatory muscles and a corollary discharge to the sensory cortex (feed-forward with respect to the instructions sent to the muscles). If the feed-forward and feedback messages do not match, an error signal is generated and the intensity of dyspnea increases. *(Adapted from Gillette and Schwartzstein.)*

TABLE 5-1

ASSOCIATION OF QUALITATIVE DESCRIPTORS AND PATHOPHYSIOLOGIC MECHANISMS OF SHORTNESS OF BREATH

DESCRIPTOR	PATHOPHYSIOLOGY
Chest tightness or constriction	Bronchoconstriction, interstitial edema (asthma, myocardial ischemia)
Increased work or effort of breathing	Airway obstruction, neuromuscular disease (COPD, moderate to severe asthma, myopathy, kyphoscoliosis)
Air hunger, need to breathe, urge to breathe	Increased drive to breathe (CHF, pulmonary embolism, moderate to severe airflow obstruction)
Cannot get a deep breath, unsatisfying breath	Hyperinflation (asthma, COPD) and restricted tidal volume (pulmonary fibrosis, chest wall restriction)
Heavy breathing, rapid breathing, breathing more	Deconditioning

Note: CHF, congestive heart failure; COPD, chronic obstructive pulmonary disease.
Source: From Schwartzstein and Feller-Kopman.

from receptors that monitor the response of the ventilatory pump increases the intensity of dyspnea. This is particularly important when there is a mechanical derangement of the ventilatory pump, such as in asthma or chronic obstructive pulmonary disease (COPD).

Anxiety

Acute anxiety may increase the severity of dyspnea either by altering the interpretation of sensory data or by leading to patterns of breathing that heighten physiologic abnormalities in the respiratory system. In patients with expiratory flow limitation, for example, the increased respiratory rate that accompanies acute anxiety leads to hyperinflation, increased work of breathing, a sense of an increased effort to breathe, and a sense of an unsatisfying breath.

ASSESSING DYSPNEA

Quality of Sensation

As with pain, dyspnea assessment begins with a determination of the quality of the discomfort (Table 5-1). Dyspnea questionnaires, or lists of phrases commonly used by patients, assist those who have difficulty describing their breathing sensations.

Sensory Intensity

A modified Borg scale or visual analogue scale can be utilized to measure dyspnea at rest, immediately following exercise, or on recall of a reproducible physical task, e.g., climbing the stairs at home. An alternative approach is to inquire about the activities a patient can do, i.e., to gain a sense of the patient's disability. The Baseline Dyspnea Index and the Chronic Respiratory Disease Questionnaire are tools commonly used for this purpose.

Affective Dimension

For a sensation to be reported as a symptom, it must be perceived as unpleasant and interpreted as abnormal. We are still in the early stages of learning the best ways to assess the affective dimension of dyspnea. Some therapies for dyspnea, such as pulmonary rehabilitation, may reduce breathing discomfort, in part, by altering this dimension.

DIFFERENTIAL DIAGNOSIS

Dyspnea is the consequence of deviations from normal function in the cardiopulmonary systems. Alterations in the

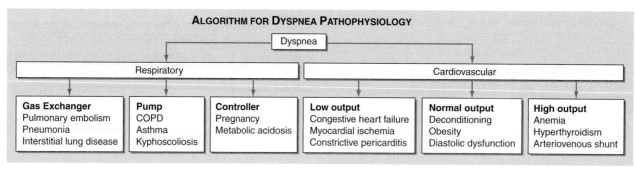

ALGORITHM FOR DYSPNEA PATHOPHYSIOLOGY

FIGURE 5-2

Pathophysiology of dyspnea. When confronted with a patient with shortness of breath of unclear cause, it is useful to begin the analysis with a consideration of the broad pathophysiologic categories that explain the vast majority of cases. COPD, chronic obstructive pulmonary disease. *(Adapted from Schwartzstein and Feller-Kopman.)*

respiratory system can be considered in the context of the controller (stimulation of breathing); the ventilatory pump (the bones and muscles that form the chest wall, the airways, and the pleura); and the gas exchanger (the alveoli, pulmonary vasculature, and surrounding lung parenchyma). Similarly, alterations in the cardiovascular system can be grouped into three categories: conditions associated with high, normal, and low cardiac output (Fig. 5–2).

Respiratory System Dyspnea

Controller

Acute hypoxemia and hypercapnia are associated with increased activity in the controller. Stimulation of pulmonary receptors, as occurs in acute bronchospasm, interstitial edema, and pulmonary embolism, also leads to hyperventilation and air hunger, as well as a sense of chest tightness in the case of asthma. High altitude, high progesterone states such as pregnancy, and drugs such as aspirin stimulate the controller and can cause dyspnea even when the respiratory system is normal.

Ventilatory Pump

Disorders of the airways (e.g., asthma, emphysema, chronic bronchitis, bronchiectasis) lead to increased airway resistance and work of breathing. Hyperinflation further increases the work of breathing and can produce a sense of an inability to get a deep breath. Conditions that stiffen the chest wall, such as kyphoscoliosis, or those that weaken ventilatory muscles, such as myasthenia gravis or the Guillain-Barré syndrome, are also associated with an increased effort to breathe. Large pleural effusions may contribute to dyspnea, both by increasing the work of breathing and by stimulating pulmonary receptors if there is associated atelectasis.

Gas Exchanger

Pneumonia, pulmonary edema, and aspiration all interfere with gas exchange. Pulmonary vascular and interstitial lung disease and pulmonary vascular congestion may produce dyspnea by direct stimulation of pulmonary receptors. In these cases, relief of hypoxemia typically has only a small impact on the intensity of dyspnea.

Cardiovascular System Dyspnea

High Cardiac Output

Mild to moderate anemia is associated with breathing discomfort during exercise. Left-to-right intracardiac shunts may lead to high cardiac output and dyspnea, although in their later stages the conditions may be complicated by the development of pulmonary hypertension, which contributes to dyspnea. The breathlessness associated with obesity is probably due to multiple mechanisms, including high cardiac output and impaired ventilatory pump function.

Normal Cardiac Output

Cardiovascular deconditioning is characterized by early development of anaerobic metabolism and stimulation of chemoreceptors and metaboreceptors. Diastolic dysfunction—due to hypertension, aortic stenosis, or hypertrophic cardiomyopathy—is an increasingly frequent recognized cause of exercise-induced breathlessness. Pericardial disease, e.g., constrictive pericarditis, is a relatively rare cause of chronic dyspnea.

Low Cardiac Output

Diseases of the myocardium resulting from coronary artery disease and nonischemic cardiomyopathies result in a greater left ventricular end-diastolic volume and an elevation of the left ventricular end-diastolic as well as pulmonary capillary pressures. Pulmonary receptors are stimulated by the elevated vascular pressures and resultant interstitial edema, causing dyspnea.

Approach to the Patient:
DYSPNEA

(**Fig. 5-3**) In obtaining a *history*, the patient should be asked to describe in his/her own words what the discomfort feels like, as well as the effect of position, infections, and environmental stimuli on the dyspnea. Orthopnea is a common indicator of congestive heart failure, mechanical impairment of the diaphragm associated with obesity, or asthma triggered by esophageal reflux. Nocturnal dyspnea suggests congestive heart failure or asthma. Acute, intermittent episodes of dyspnea are more likely to reflect episodes of myocardial ischemia, bronchospasm, or pulmonary embolism, while chronic persistent dyspnea is typical of COPD, and interstitial lung disease. Risk factors for occupational lung disease and for coronary artery disease should be solicited. Left atrial myxoma or hepatopulmonary syndrome should be considered when the patient complains of *platypnea*, defined as dyspnea in the upright position with relief in the supine position.

The *physical examination* should begin during the interview of the patient. Inability of the patient to speak in full sentences before stopping to get a deep breath suggests a condition that leads to stimulation of the controller or an impairment of the ventilatory pump with reduced vital capacity. Evidence for increased work of breathing (supraclavicular retractions, use of accessory muscles of ventilation, and the tripod position, characterized by sitting with one's hands braced on the knees) is indicative of disorders of the ventilatory pump, most commonly increased airway resistance or stiff lungs and chest wall. When measuring the vital signs, an accurate assessment of the respiratory rate should be obtained and examination for a pulsus paradoxus carried out (Chap. 22); if it is >10 mmHg, consider the presence of COPD. During the general examination, signs of anemia

CHAPTER 5   Dyspnea and Pulmonary Edema

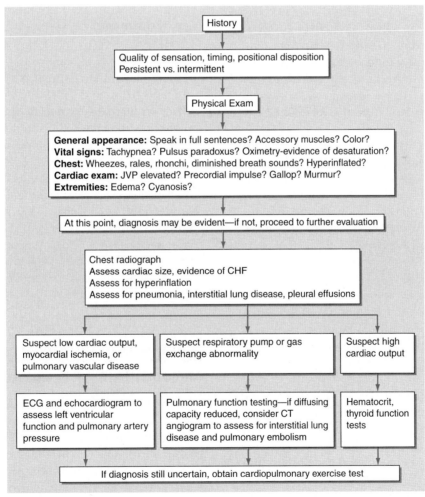

FIGURE 5-3

An algorithm for the evaluation of the patient with dyspnea. JVP, jugular venous pulse; CHF, congestive heart failure; ECG, electrocardiogram; CT, computed tomography. (*Adapted from Schwartzstein and Feller-Kopman.*)

(pale conjunctivae), cyanosis, and cirrhosis (spider angiomata, gynecomastia) should be sought. Examination of the chest should focus on symmetry of movement; percussion (dullness indicative of pleural effusion, hyper-resonance a sign of emphysema); and auscultation (wheezes, rales, rhonchi, prolonged expiratory phase, diminished breath sounds, which are clues to disorders of the airways, and interstitial edema or fibrosis). The cardiac examination should focus on signs of elevated right heart pressures (jugular venous distention, edema, accentuated pulmonic component to the second heart sound); left ventricular dysfunction (S3 and S4 gallops); and valvular disease (murmurs). When examining the abdomen with the patient in the supine position, it should be noted whether there is paradoxical movement of the abdomen (inward motion during inspiration), a sign of diaphragmatic weakness. Clubbing of the digits may be an indication of interstitial pulmonary fibrosis, and the presence of joint swelling or deformation as well as changes consistent with Raynaud's disease may be indicative of a collagen-vascular process that can be associated with pulmonary disease.

Patients with exertional dyspnea should be asked to walk under observation in order to reproduce the symptoms. The patient should be examined for new findings that were not present at rest and for oxygen saturation. A "picture" of the patient while symptomatic may be worth thousands of dollars in laboratory tests.

Following the history and physical examination, a *chest radiograph* should be obtained. The lung volumes should be assessed (hyperinflation indicates obstructive lung disease, low lung volumes suggest interstitial edema or fibrosis, diaphragmatic dysfunction, or impaired chest wall motion). The pulmonary parenchyma should be examined for evidence of interstitial disease and emphysema. Prominent pulmonary vasculature in the upper zones indicates pulmonary venous hypertension, while enlarged central pulmonary arteries suggest pulmonary artery hypertension. An enlarged cardiac silhouette suggests a dilated cardiomyopathy or valvular disease. Bilateral pleural effusions are typical of congestive heart failure and some forms of collagen vascular disease. Unilateral effusions raise the specter of carcinoma and pulmonary embolism but may also occur in heart failure. *Computed tomography* (CT) *of the chest* is generally reserved for further evaluation of the lung parenchyma (interstitial lung disease) and possible pulmonary embolism.

Laboratory studies should include an electrocardiogram to look for evidence of ventricular hypertrophy and prior myocardial infarction. Echocardiography is indicated in patients in whom systolic dysfunction, pulmonary hypertension, or valvular heart disease is suspected.

DISTINGUISHING CARDIOVASCULAR FROM RESPIRATORY SYSTEM DYSPNEA If a patient has evidence of both pulmonary and cardiac disease, a cardiopulmonary exercise test should be carried out to determine which system is responsible for the exercise limitation. If, at peak exercise, the patient achieves predicted maximal ventilation, demonstrates an increase in dead space or hypoxemia (oxygen saturation below 90%), or develops bronchospasm, the respiratory system is probably the cause of the problem. Alternatively, if the heart rate is >85% of the predicted maximum, if anaerobic threshold occurs early, if the blood pressure becomes excessively high or drops during exercise, if the O_2 pulse (O_2 consumption/heart rate, an indicator of stroke volume) falls, or if there are ischemic changes on the electrocardiogram, an abnormality of the cardiovascular system is likely the explanation for the breathing discomfort.

℞ **Treatment:**
DYSPNEA

The first goal is to correct the underlying problem responsible for the symptom. If this is not possible, one attempts to lessen the intensity of the symptom and its effect on the patient's quality of life. Supplemental O_2 should be administered if the resting O_2 saturation is ≤90% or if the patient's saturation drops to these levels with activity. For patients with COPD, pulmonary rehabilitation programs have demonstrated positive effects on dyspnea, exercise capacity, and rates of hospitalization. Studies of anxiolytics and antidepressants have not demonstrated consistent benefit. Experimental interventions—e.g., cold air on the face, chest wall vibration, and inhaled furosemide—to modulate the afferent information from receptors throughout the respiratory system are being studied.

PULMONARY EDEMA

MECHANISMS OF FLUID ACCUMULATION

The extent to which fluid accumulates in the interstitium of the lung depends on the balance of hydrostatic and oncotic forces within the pulmonary capillaries and in the surrounding tissue. Hydrostatic pressure favors movement of fluid from the capillary into the interstitium. The oncotic pressure, which is determined by the protein concentration in the blood, favors movement of fluid into the vessel. Albumin, the primary protein in the plasma, may be low in conditions such as cirrhosis and nephrotic syndrome. Although hypoalbuminemia favors movement of fluid into the tissue for any given hydrostatic pressure in the capillary, it is usually not sufficient by itself to cause interstitial edema. In a healthy individual, the tight junctions of the capillary endothelium are impermeable to proteins, and the lymphatics in the tissue carry away the small amounts of protein that may leak out; together these factors result in an oncotic force that maintains fluid in the capillary. Disruption of the endothelial barrier, however, allows protein to escape the capillary bed and enhances the movement of fluid into the tissue of the lung.

Cardiogenic Pulmonary Edema

(See also Chap. 28) Cardiac abnormalities that lead to an increase in pulmonary venous pressure shift the balance of forces between the capillary and the interstitium. Hydrostatic pressure is increased and fluid exits the capillary at an increased rate, resulting in interstitial and, in more severe cases, alveolar edema. The development of pleural effusions may further compromise respiratory system function and contribute to breathing discomfort.

Early signs of pulmonary edema include exertional dyspnea and orthopnea. Chest radiographs show peribronchial thickening, prominent vascular markings in the upper lung zones, and Kerley B lines. As the pulmonary edema worsens, alveoli fill with fluid; the chest radiograph shows patchy alveolar filling, typically in a perihilar distribution, which then progresses to diffuse alveolar infiltrates. Increasing airway edema is associated with rhonchi and wheezes.

Noncardiogenic Pulmonary Edema

By definition, hydrostatic pressures are normal in noncardiogenic pulmonary edema. Lung water increases due to damage of the pulmonary capillary lining with leakage of proteins and other macromolecules into the tissue; fluid follows the protein as oncotic forces are shifted from the vessel to the surrounding lung tissue. This process is associated with dysfunction of the surfactant lining the alveoli, increased surface forces, and a propensity for the alveoli to collapse at low lung volumes. Physiologically, noncardiogenic pulmonary edema is characterized by intrapulmonary shunt with hypoxemia and decreased pulmonary compliance. Pathologically, hyaline membranes are evident in the alveoli, and inflammation leading to pulmonary fibrosis may be seen. Clinically, the picture ranges from mild dyspnea to respiratory failure. Auscultation of the lungs may be relatively normal despite chest radiographs that show diffuse alveolar infiltrates. CT scans demonstrate that the distribution of alveolar edema is more heterogeneous than was once thought.

It is useful to categorize the causes of noncardiogenic pulmonary edema in terms of whether the injury to the lung is likely to result from direct, indirect, or pulmonary

TABLE 5-2

COMMON CAUSES OF NONCARDIOGENIC PULMONARY EDEMA

Direct Injury to Lung
Chest trauma, pulmonary contusion
Aspiration
Smoke inhalation
Pneumonia
Oxygen toxicity
Pulmonary embolism, reperfusion
Hematogenous Injury to Lung
Sepsis
Pancreatitis
Nonthoracic trauma
Leukoagglutination reactions
Multiple transfusions
Intravenous drug use, e.g., heroin
Cardiopulmonary bypass
Possible Lung Injury Plus Elevated Hydrostatic Pressures
High altitude pulmonary edema
Neurogenic pulmonary edema
Reexpansion pulmonary edema

vascular causes (Table 5-2). Direct injuries are mediated via the airways (e.g., aspiration) or as the consequence of blunt chest trauma. Indirect injury is the consequence of mediators that reach the lung via the blood stream. The third category includes conditions that may be the consequence of acute changes in pulmonary vascular pressures, possibly the result of sudden autonomic discharge in the case of neurogenic and high-altitude pulmonary edema, or sudden swings of pleural pressure, as well as transient damage to the pulmonary capillaries in the case of reexpansion pulmonary edema.

Distinguishing Cardiogenic from Noncardiogenic Pulmonary Edema

The *history* is essential for assessing the likelihood of underlying cardiac disease as well as for identification of one of the conditions associated with noncardiogenic pulmonary edema. The *physical examination* in cardiogenic pulmonary edema is notable for evidence of increased intracardiac pressures (S_3 gallop, elevated jugular venous pulse, peripheral edema), and rales and/or wheezes on auscultation of the chest. In contrast, the physical examination in noncardiogenic pulmonary edema is dominated by the findings of the precipitating condition; pulmonary findings may be relatively normal in the early stages. The *chest radiograph* in cardiogenic pulmonary edema typically shows an enlarged cardiac silhouette, vascular redistribution, interstitial thickening, and perihilar alveolar infiltrates; pleural effusions are common. In noncardiogenic pulmonary edema, heart size is normal, alveolar infiltrates are distributed more uniformly throughout the lungs, and pleural effusions are uncommon. Finally, the *hypoxemia* of cardiogenic pulmonary edema is due largely to ventilation-perfusion mismatch and responds to the administration of supplemental oxygen. In contrast, hypoxemia in noncardiogenic pulmonary edema is due primarily to intrapulmonary shunting and typically persists despite high concentrations of inhaled O_2.

FURTHER READINGS

AARON SD et al: Overdiagnosis of asthma in obese and nonobese adults. CMAJ 179:1121, 2008

ABIDOV A et al: Prognostic significance of dyspnea in patients referred for cardiac stress testing. N Engl J Med 353:1889, 2005

BANZETT RB et al: The affective dimension of laboratory dyspnea: Air hunger is more unpleasant than work/effort. Am J Respir Crit Care Med 177:1384, 2008

Dyspnea mechanisms, assessment, and management: A consensus statement. Am Rev Resp Crit Care Med 159:321, 1999

GILLETTE MA, SCHWARTZSTEIN RM: Mechanisms of dyspnea, in *Supportive Care in Respiratory Disease*, SH Ahmedzai and MF Muer (eds). Oxford, Oxford University Press, 2005

MAHLER DA et al: Descriptors of breathlessness in cardiorespiratory diseases. Am J Respir Crit Care Med 154:1357, 1996

———, O'DONNELL DE (eds): *Dyspnea: Mechanisms, Measurement, and Management*. New York, Marcel Dekker, 2005

SCHWARTZSTEIN RM. The language of dyspnea, in *Dyspnea: Mechanisms, Measurement, and Management*, DA Mahler and DE O'Donnell (eds). New York, Marcel Dekker, 2005

———, FELLER-KOPMAN D: Shortness of breath, in *Primary Care Cardiology*, 2d ed, E Braunwald and L Goldman (eds). Philadelphia: WB Saunders, 2003

CHAPTER 6

HYPOXIA AND CYANOSIS

Eugene Braunwald

HYPOXIA

The fundamental task of the cardiorespiratory system is to deliver O_2 (and substrates) to the cells and to remove CO_2 (and other metabolic products) from them. Proper maintenance of this function depends on intact cardiovascular and respiratory systems, an adequate number of red blood cells and hemoglobin, and a supply of inspired gas containing adequate O_2.

EFFECTS

Decreased O_2 availability to cells results in an inhibition of the respiratory chain and increased anaerobic glycolysis. This switch from aerobic to anaerobic metabolism, Pasteur's effect, maintains some, albeit markedly reduced, adenosine triphosphate (ATP) production. In severe hypoxia, when ATP production is inadequate to meet the energy requirements of ionic and osmotic equilibrium, cell membrane depolarization leads to uncontrolled Ca^{2+} influx and activation of Ca^{2+}-dependent phospholipases and proteases. These events, in turn, cause cell swelling and ultimately cell necrosis.

The adaptations to hypoxia are mediated, in part, by the upregulation of genes encoding a variety of proteins, including glycolytic enzymes such as phosphoglycerate kinase and phosphofructokinase, as well as the glucose transporters GLUT-1 and GLUT-2; and by growth factors, such as vascular endothelial growth factor (VEGF) and erythropoietin, which enhance erythrocyte production.

During hypoxia systemic arterioles dilate, at least in part, by opening of K_{ATP} channels in vascular smooth-muscle cells due to the hypoxia-induced reduction in ATP concentration. By contrast, in pulmonary vascular smooth-muscle cells, inhibition of K^+ channels causes depolarization which, in turn, activates voltage-gated Ca^{2+} channels raising the cytosolic $[Ca^{2+}]$ and causing smooth-muscle cell contraction. Hypoxia-induced pulmonary arterial constriction shunts blood away from poorly ventilated toward better-ventilated portions of the lung; however, it also increases pulmonary vascular resistance and right ventricular afterload.

Effects on the Central Nervous System

Changes in the central nervous system, particularly the higher centers, are especially important consequences of hypoxia. Acute hypoxia causes impaired judgment, motor incoordination, and a clinical picture resembling acute alcoholism. High-altitude illness is characterized by headache secondary to cerebral vasodilatation, and by gastrointestinal symptoms, dizziness, insomnia, and fatigue, or somnolence. Pulmonary arterial and sometimes venous constriction cause capillary leakage and high-altitude pulmonary edema (HAPE) (Chap. 5), which intensifies hypoxia and can initiate a vicious circle. Rarely, high-altitude cerebral edema (HACE) develops. This is manifest by severe headache and papilledema and can cause coma. As hypoxia becomes more severe, the centers of the brainstem are affected, and death usually results from respiratory failure.

CAUSES OF HYPOXIA

Respiratory Hypoxia

When hypoxia occurs consequent to respiratory failure, Pa_{O2} declines, and when respiratory failure is persistent, the hemoglobin-oxygen (Hb-O_2) dissociation curve is displaced to the right, with greater quantities of O_2 released at any level of tissue P_{O2}. Arterial hypoxemia, i.e., a reduction of O_2 saturation of arterial blood (Sa_{O2}), and consequent cyanosis are likely to be more marked when such depression of Pa_{O2} results from pulmonary disease than when the depression occurs as the result of a decline in the fraction of oxygen in inspired air (F_{IO2}). In the latter situation, Pa_{CO2} falls secondary to anoxia-induced hyperventilation and the Hb-O_2 dissociation curve is displaced to the left, limiting the decline in Sa_{O2} at any level of Pa_{O2}.

The most common cause of respiratory hypoxia is *ventilation-perfusion mismatch* resulting from perfusion of poorly ventilated alveoli. Respiratory hypoxemia may also be caused by *hypoventilation*, and it is then associated with an elevation of Pa_{CO2}. The two forms of respiratory hypoxia are usually correctable by inspiring 100% O_2 for several minutes. A third cause is shunting of blood across the lung from the pulmonary arterial to the venous bed (*intrapulmonary right-to-left shunting*) by perfusion of nonventilated portions of the lung, as in pulmonary atelectasis or through pulmonary arteriovenous connections. The low Pa_{O2} in this situation is correctable only in part by an F_{IO2} of 100%.

Hypoxia Secondary to High Altitude

As one ascends rapidly to 3000 m (~10,000 ft), the reduction of the O_2 content of inspired air (F_{IO2}) leads to a decrease in alveolar P_{O2} to about 60 mmHg, and a condition termed *high-altitude illness* develops (see earlier). At higher altitudes, arterial saturation declines rapidly and symptoms become more serious; and at 5000 m, unacclimatized individuals usually cease to be able to function normally.

Hypoxia Secondary to Right-to-Left Extrapulmonary Shunting

From a physiologic viewpoint, this cause of hypoxia resembles intrapulmonary right-to-left shunting but is caused by congenital cardiac malformations such as tetralogy of Fallot, transposition of the great arteries, and Eisenmenger's syndrome (Chap. 19). As in pulmonary right-to-left shunting, the Pa_{O2} cannot be restored to normal with inspiration of 100% O_2.

Anemic Hypoxia

A reduction in hemoglobin concentration of the blood is attended by a corresponding decline in the O_2-carrying capacity of the blood. Although the Pa_{O2} is normal in anemic hypoxia, the absolute quantity of O_2 transported per unit volume of blood is diminished. As the anemic blood passes through the capillaries and the usual quantity of O_2 is removed from it, the P_{O2} and saturation in the venous blood decline to a greater degree than normal.

Carbon Monoxide (CO) Intoxication

Hemoglobin that is combined with CO [carboxyhemoglobin (COHb)] is unavailable for O_2 transport. In addition, the presence of COHb shifts the Hb-O_2 dissociation curve to the left so that O_2 is unloaded only at lower tensions, contributing further to tissue hypoxia.

Circulatory Hypoxia

As in anemic hypoxia, the Pa_{O2} is usually normal, but venous and tissue P_{O2} values are reduced as a consequence of reduced tissue perfusion and greater tissue O_2 extraction. This pathophysiology leads to an increased arterial–mixed venous O_2 difference, or $(a - \bar{v})$ gradient. Generalized circulatory hypoxia occurs in heart failure (Chap. 17) and in most forms of shock.

Specific Organ Hypoxia

Localized circulatory hypoxia may occur consequent to decreased perfusion secondary to organic arterial obstruction, as in localized atherosclerosis in any vascular bed, or as a consequence of vasoconstriction, as observed in Raynaud's phenomenon (Chap. 39). Localized hypoxia may also result from venous obstruction and the resultant expansion of interstitial fluid causing arterial compression and, thereby, reduction of arterial inflow. Edema, which increases the distance through which O_2 must diffuse before it reaches cells, can also cause localized hypoxia. In an attempt to maintain adequate perfusion to more vital organs in patients with reduced cardiac output secondary to heart failure or hypovolemic shock, vasoconstriction may reduce perfusion in the limbs and skin, causing hypoxia of these regions.

Increased O_2 Requirements

If the O_2 consumption of tissues is elevated without a corresponding increase in perfusion, tissue hypoxia ensues and the P_{O_2} in venous blood declines. Ordinarily, the clinical picture of patients with hypoxia due to an elevated metabolic rate, as in fever or thyrotoxicosis, is quite different from that in other types of hypoxia; the skin is warm and flushed owing to increased cutaneous blood flow that dissipates the excessive heat produced, and cyanosis is usually absent.

Exercise is a classic example of increased tissue O_2 requirements. These increased demands are normally met by several mechanisms operating simultaneously: (1) increasing the cardiac output and ventilation and, thus, O_2 delivery to the tissues; (2) preferentially directing the blood to the exercising muscles by changing vascular resistances in the circulatory beds of exercising tissues, directly and/or reflexly; (3) increasing O_2 extraction from the delivered blood and widening the arteriovenous O_2 difference; and (4) reducing the pH of the tissues and capillary blood, shifting the Hb-O_2 curve to the right and unloading more O_2 from hemoglobin. If the capacity of these mechanisms is exceeded, then hypoxia, especially of the exercising muscles, will result.

Improper Oxygen Utilization

Cyanide and several other similarly acting poisons cause cellular hypoxia. The tissues are unable to utilize O_2, and as a consequence, the venous blood tends to have a high O_2 tension. This condition has been termed *histotoxic hypoxia*.

ADAPTATION TO HYPOXIA

An important component of the respiratory response to hypoxia originates in special chemosensitive cells in the carotid and aortic bodies and in the respiratory center in the brainstem. The stimulation of these cells by hypoxia increases ventilation, with a loss of CO_2, and can lead to respiratory alkalosis. When combined with the metabolic acidosis resulting from the production of lactic acid, the serum bicarbonate level declines.

With the reduction of Pa_{O_2}, cerebrovascular resistance decreases and cerebral blood flow increases in an attempt to maintain O_2 delivery to the brain. However, when the reduction of Pa_{O_2} is accompanied by hyperventilation and a reduction of Pa_{CO_2}, cerebrovascular resistance rises, cerebral blood flow falls, and hypoxia is intensified.

The diffuse, systemic vasodilation that occurs in generalized hypoxia raises the cardiac output. In patients with underlying heart disease, the requirements of peripheral tissues for an increase of cardiac output with hypoxia may precipitate congestive heart failure. In patients with ischemic heart disease, a reduced Pa_{O_2} may intensify myocardial ischemia and further impair left ventricular function.

One of the important mechanisms of compensation for chronic hypoxia is an increase in the hemoglobin concentration and in the number of red blood cells in the circulating blood, i.e., the development of polycythemia secondary to erythropoietin production. In persons with chronic hypoxemia secondary to prolonged residence at a high altitude (4200 m, >13,000 ft), a condition termed *chronic mountain sickness* develops. It is characterized by a blunted respiratory drive, reduced ventilation, erythrocytosis, cyanosis, weakness, right ventricular enlargement secondary to pulmonary hypertension, and even stupor.

CYANOSIS

Cyanosis refers to a bluish color of the skin and mucous membranes resulting from an increased quantity of reduced hemoglobin, or of hemoglobin derivatives, in the small blood vessels of those areas. It is usually most marked in the lips, nail beds, ears, and malar eminences. Cyanosis, especially if developed recently, is more commonly detected by a family member than the patient. The florid skin characteristic of polycythemia vera must be distinguished from the true cyanosis discussed here. A cherry-colored flush, rather than cyanosis, is caused by carboxyhemoglobin (COHb).

The degree of cyanosis is modified by the color of the cutaneous pigment and the thickness of the skin, as well as by the state of the cutaneous capillaries. The accurate clinical detection of the presence and degree of cyanosis is difficult, as proved by oximetric studies. In some instances, central cyanosis can be detected reliably when the Sa_{O_2} has decreased to 85%; in others, particularly in dark-skinned persons, it may not be detected until it has decreased to 75%. In the latter case, examination of the mucous membranes in the oral cavity and the conjunctivae rather than examination of the skin is more helpful in the detection of cyanosis.

The increase in the quantity of reduced hemoglobin in the mucocutaneous vessels that produces cyanosis may be brought about either by an increase in the quantity of venous blood as a result of dilation of the venules and venous ends of the capillaries or by a reduction in the Sa_{O_2} in the capillary blood. In general, cyanosis becomes apparent when the concentration of reduced hemoglobin in capillary blood exceeds 40 g/L (4 g/dL).

It is the *absolute*, rather than the *relative*, quantity of reduced hemoglobin that is important in producing cyanosis. Thus, in a patient with severe anemia, the *relative* quantity of reduced hemoglobin in the venous blood may be very large when considered in relation to the total quantity of hemoglobin in the blood. However, since the concentration of the latter is markedly reduced, the *absolute* quantity of reduced hemoglobin may still be small, and, therefore, patients with severe anemia and even *marked* arterial desaturation may not display cyanosis. Conversely, the higher the total hemoglobin content, the greater is the tendency toward cyanosis; thus, patients with marked polycythemia tend to be cyanotic at higher levels of Sa_{O2} than patients with normal hematocrit values. Likewise, local passive congestion, which causes an increase in the total quantity of reduced hemoglobin in the vessels in a given area, may cause cyanosis. Cyanosis is also observed when nonfunctional hemoglobin, such as methemoglobin or sulfhemoglobin, is present in blood.

Cyanosis may be subdivided into central and peripheral types. In the *central* type, the Sa_{O2} is reduced or an abnormal hemoglobin derivative is present, and the mucous membranes and skin are both affected. *Peripheral* cyanosis is due to a slowing of blood flow and abnormally great extraction of O_2 from normally saturated arterial blood. It results from vasoconstriction and diminished peripheral blood flow, such as occurs in cold exposure, shock, congestive failure, and peripheral vascular disease. Often in these conditions, the mucous membranes of the oral cavity or those beneath the tongue may be spared. Clinical differentiation between central and peripheral cyanosis may not always be simple, and in conditions such as cardiogenic shock with pulmonary edema there may be a mixture of both types.

DIFFERENTIAL DIAGNOSIS

Central Cyanosis

(Table 6-1) Decreased Sa_{O2} results from a marked reduction in the Pa_{O2}. This reduction may be brought about by a decline in the FI_{O2} without sufficient compensatory alveolar hyperventilation to maintain alveolar P_{O2}. Cyanosis usually becomes manifest in an ascent to an altitude of 4000 m (13,000 ft).

Seriously *impaired pulmonary function*, through perfusion of unventilated or poorly ventilated areas of the lung or alveolar hypoventilation, is a common cause of central cyanosis. The condition may occur acutely, as in extensive pneumonia or pulmonary edema, or chronically with chronic pulmonary diseases (e.g., emphysema). In the latter situation, secondary polycythemia is generally present and clubbing of the fingers (see later) may occur. Another cause of reduced Sa_{O2} is *shunting of systemic venous blood into the arterial circuit*. Certain forms of congenital heart disease are associated with cyanosis on this basis (see above and Chap. 19).

Pulmonary arteriovenous fistulae may be congenital or acquired, solitary or multiple, microscopic or massive. The severity of cyanosis produced by these fistulae depends on their size and number. They occur with some frequency in hereditary hemorrhagic telangiectasia. Sa_{O2} reduction and cyanosis may also occur in some patients with

TABLE 6-1

CAUSES OF CYANOSIS
Central Cyanosis
Decreased arterial oxygen saturation
Decreased atmospheric pressure—high altitude
Impaired pulmonary function
Alveolar hypoventilation
Uneven relationships between pulmonary ventilation and perfusion (perfusion of hypoventilated alveoli)
Impaired oxygen diffusion
Anatomic shunts
Certain types of congenital heart disease
Pulmonary arteriovenous fistulas
Multiple small intrapulmonary shunts
Hemoglobin with low affinity for oxygen
Hemoglobin abnormalities
Methemoglobinemia—hereditary, acquired
Sulfhemoglobinema—acquired
Carboxyhemoglobinemia (not true cyanosis)
Peripheral Cyanosis
Reduced cardiac output
Cold exposure
Redistribution of blood flow from extremities
Arterial obstruction
Venous obstruction

cirrhosis, presumably as a consequence of pulmonary arteriovenous fistulae or portal vein–pulmonary vein anastomoses.

In patients with cardiac or pulmonary right-to-left shunts, the presence and severity of cyanosis depend on the size of the shunt relative to the systemic flow as well as on the Hb-O_2 saturation of the venous blood. With increased extraction of O_2 from the blood by the exercising muscles, the venous blood returning to the right side of the heart is more unsaturated than at rest, and shunting of this blood intensifies the cyanosis. Secondary polycythemia occurs frequently in patients with arterial O_2 unsaturation and contributes to the cyanosis.

Cyanosis can be caused by small quantities of circulating methemoglobin and by even smaller quantities of sulfhemoglobin. Although they are uncommon causes of cyanosis, these abnormal oxyhemoglobin derivatives should be sought by spectroscopy when cyanosis is not readily explained by malfunction of the circulatory or respiratory systems. Generally, digital clubbing does not occur with them.

Peripheral Cyanosis

Probably the most common cause of peripheral cyanosis is the normal vasoconstriction resulting from exposure to cold air or water. When cardiac output is reduced, cutaneous vasoconstriction occurs as a compensatory mechanism so that blood is diverted from the skin to more vital areas such as the central nervous system and heart, and cyanosis of the extremities may result even though the arterial blood is normally saturated.

Arterial obstruction to an extremity, as with an embolus, or arteriolar constriction, as in cold-induced vasospasm (Raynaud's phenomenon, Chap. 39), generally results in pallor and coldness, and there may be associated cyanosis. Venous obstruction, as in thrombophlebitis, dilates the subpapillary venous plexuses and thereby intensifies cyanosis.

Approach to the Patient:
CYANOSIS

Certain features are important in arriving at the cause of cyanosis:

1. It is important to ascertain the time of onset of cyanosis. Cyanosis present since birth or infancy is usually due to congenital heart disease.
2. Central and peripheral cyanosis must be differentiated. Evidences of disorders of the respiratory or cardiovascular systems are helpful. Massage or gentle warming of a cyanotic extremity will increase peripheral blood flow and abolish peripheral, but not central, cyanosis.
3. The presence or absence of clubbing of the digits (see later) should be ascertained. The combination of cyanosis and clubbing is frequent in patients with congenital heart disease and right-to-left shunting, and is seen occasionally in patients with pulmonary disease such as lung abscess or pulmonary arteriovenous fistulae. In contrast, peripheral cyanosis or acutely developing central cyanosis is *not* associated with clubbed digits.
4. Pa_{O_2} and Sa_{O_2} should be determined, and in patients with cyanosis in whom the mechanism is obscure, spectroscopic examination of the blood performed to look for abnormal types of hemoglobin (critical in the differential diagnosis of cyanosis).

CLUBBING

The selective bulbous enlargement of the distal segments of the fingers and toes due to proliferation of connective tissue, particularly on the dorsal surface, is termed *clubbing*;

there is also increased sponginess of the soft tissue at the base of the nail. Clubbing may be hereditary, idiopathic, or acquired and associated with a variety of disorders, including cyanotic congenital heart disease (see earlier), infective endocarditis, and a variety of pulmonary conditions (among them primary and metastatic lung cancer, bronchiectasis, lung abscess, cystic fibrosis, and mesothelioma), as well as with some gastrointestinal diseases (including inflammatory bowel disease and hepatic cirrhosis). In some instances it is occupational, e.g., in jackhammer operators.

Clubbing in patients with primary and metastatic lung cancer, mesothelioma, bronchiectasis, and hepatic cirrhosis may be associated with *hypertrophic osteoarthropathy*. In this condition, the subperiosteal formation of new bone in the distal diaphyses of the long bones of the extremities causes pain and symmetric arthritis-like changes in the shoulders, knees, ankles, wrists, and elbows. The diagnosis of hypertrophic osteoarthropathy may be confirmed by bone radiographs. Although the mechanism of clubbing is unclear, it appears to be secondary to a humoral substance that causes dilation of the vessels of the fingertip.

FURTHER READINGS

BANSAL S et al: Sodium retention in heart failure and cirrhosis. Potential role of natriuretic doses of mineralocorticoid antagonist Circ Hear Fail 2:370, 2009

FAWCETT RS et al: Nail abnormalities: Clues to systemic disease. Am Fam Physician 69:1417, 2004

GIORDANO FJ: Oxygen, oxidative stress, hypoxia, and heart failure. J Clin Invest 115:500, 2005

GRIFFEY RT et al: Cyanosis. J Emerg Med 18:369, 2000

HACKETT PH, ROACH RC: Current concepts: High altitude illness. N Engl J Med 345:107, 2001

LEVY MM: Pathophysiology of oxygen delivery in respiratory failure. Chest 128(Suppl 2):547S, 2005

MCCULLOUGH JC: Renal disorders and heart disease, in *Braunwald's Heart Disease*, 8th ed, P. Libby et al (eds). Philadelphia, Saunders Elsevier, 2008

MICHIELS C: Physiological and pathological responses to hypoxia. Am J Pathol 164:1875, 2004

SCHRIER RW: Decreased effective blood volume in edematous disorders: What does this mean? J Am Soc Nephrol 18:2028, 2007

SEMENZA GL: Involvement of oxygen-sensing pathways in physiological and pathological erythropoiesis. Blood, e-published, 2009

SKORECKI KL et al: Extracellular fluid and edema formation, in Brenner and Rector's The Kidney, 8th ed, Philadelphia, Elsevier, 2008

SPICKNALL KE, ZIRWAS MJ: English JC 3rd. Clubbing: an update on diagnosis, differential diagnosis, pathophysiology, and clinical relevance. J Am Acad Dermatol 52:1020, 2005

TSAI BM et al: Hypoxic pulmonary vasoconstriction in cardiothoracic surgery: Basic mechanisms to potential therapies. Ann Thorac Surg 78:360, 2004

CHAPTER 7

EDEMA

Eugene Braunwald ■ Joseph Loscalzo

Edema is defined as a clinically apparent increase in the interstitial fluid volume, which may expand by several liters before the abnormality is evident. Therefore, a weight gain of several kilograms usually precedes overt manifestations of edema, and a similar weight loss from diuresis can be induced in a slightly edematous patient before "dry weight" is achieved. *Anasarca* refers to gross, generalized edema. *Ascites* and *hydrothorax* refer to accumulation of excess fluid in the peritoneal and pleural cavities, respectively, and are considered to be special forms of edema.

Depending on its cause and mechanism, edema may be localized or have a generalized distribution; it is recognized in its generalized form by puffiness of the face, which is most readily apparent in the periorbital areas, and by the persistence of an indentation of the skin following pressure; this is known as "pitting" edema. In its more subtle form, edema may be detected by noting that after the stethoscope is removed from the chest wall, the rim of the bell leaves an indentation on the skin of the chest for a few minutes. When the ring on a finger fits more snugly than in the past or when a patient complains of difficulty in putting on shoes, particularly in the evening, edema may be present.

PATHOGENESIS

About one-third of total-body water is confined to the extracellular space. Approximately 75% of the extracellular space is interstitial fluid and the remainder is the plasma.

Starling Forces

The forces that regulate the disposition of fluid between the two components of the extracellular compartment are frequently referred to as the *Starling forces*. The hydrostatic pressure within the vascular system and the colloid oncotic pressure in the interstitial fluid tend to promote movement of fluid from the vascular to the extravascular space. On the other hand, the colloid oncotic pressure contributed by plasma proteins and the hydrostatic pressure within the interstitial fluid, referred to as the *tissue tension*, promote the movement of fluid into the vascular compartment.

As a consequence of these forces, there is a movement of water and diffusible solutes from the vascular space at the arteriolar end of the capillaries. Fluid is returned from the interstitial space into the vascular system at the venous end of the capillaries and by way of the lymphatics. Unless these channels are obstructed, lymph flow rises with increases in net movement of fluid from the vascular compartment to the interstitium. The flows are usually balanced so that a steady state exists in the sizes of the intravascular and interstitial compartments, and, yet, a large exchange between them occurs. However, should either the hydrostatic or oncotic pressure gradient be altered significantly, a further net movement of fluid between the two components of the extracellular space will take place. The development of edema, then, depends on one or more alterations in the Starling forces so that there is increased flow of fluid from the vascular system into the interstitium or into a body cavity.

Edema due to an increase in capillary pressure may result from an elevation of venous pressure due to obstruction to venous and/or lymphatic drainage. An increase in capillary pressure may be generalized, as occurs in congestive heart failure (see below). The Starling forces may also be imbalanced when the colloid oncotic pressure of the plasma is reduced, owing to any factor that may induce hypoalbuminemia, such as severe malnutrition, liver disease, loss of protein into the urine or into the gastrointestinal tract, or a severe catabolic state. Edema may be localized to one extremity when venous pressure is elevated due to unilateral thrombophlebitis (see later in the chapter).

Capillary Damage

Edema may also result from damage to the capillary endothelium, which increases its permeability and permits the transfer of protein into the interstitial compartment. Injury to the capillary wall can result from drugs, viral or bacterial agents, and thermal or mechanical trauma. Increased capillary permeability may also be a consequence of a hypersensitivity reaction and is characteristic of immune injury. Damage to the capillary endothelium is presumably responsible for inflammatory edema, which is usually nonpitting, localized, and accompanied by other signs of inflammation—redness, heat, and tenderness.

Reduction of Effective Arterial Volume

In many forms of edema, the effective arterial blood volume, a parameter that represents the filling of the arterial tree, is reduced. Underfilling of the arterial tree may be caused by a reduction of cardiac output and/or systemic vascular resistance. As a consequence of underfilling, a series of physiologic responses designed to restore the effective arterial volume to normal are set into motion. A key element of these responses is the retention of salt and, therefore, of water, ultimately leading to edema.

Renal Factors and the Renin-Angiotensin-Aldosterone (RAA) System

In the final analysis, renal retention of Na^+ is central to the development of generalized edema. The diminished renal blood flow characteristic of states in which the effective arterial blood volume is reduced is translated by the renal juxtaglomerular cells (specialized myoepithelial cells surrounding the afferent arteriole) into a signal for increased renin release. Renin is an enzyme with a molecular mass of about 40,000 Da that acts on its substrate, angiotensinogen, an α_2-globulin synthesized by the liver, to release angiotensin I (AI), a decapeptide, which is broken down to angiotensin II (AII), an octapeptide.

AII has generalized vasoconstrictor properties; it is especially active on the efferent arterioles. This efferent arteriolar constriction reduces the hydrostatic pressure in the peritubular capillaries, while the increased filtration fraction raises the colloid osmotic pressure in these vessels, thereby enhancing salt and water reabsorption in the proximal tubule as well as in the ascending limb of the loop of Henle.

The RAA system has long been recognized as a hormonal system; however, it also operates locally. Intrarenally produced AII contributes to glomerular efferent arteriolar constriction, and this "tubuloglomerular feedback" causes salt and water retention. These renal effects of AII are mediated by activation of AII type 1 receptors, which can be blocked by specific antagonists [angiotensin receptor blockers (ARBs)].

The mechanisms responsible for the increased release of renin when renal blood flow is reduced include: (1) a baroreceptor response in which reduced renal perfusion results in incomplete filling of the renal arterioles and diminished stretch of the juxtaglomerular cells, a signal that increases the elaboration and/or release of renin; (2) reduced glomerular filtration, which lowers the NaCl load reaching the distal renal tubules and the macula densa, cells in the distal convoluted tubules that act as chemoreceptors and that signal the neighboring juxtaglomerular cells to secrete renin; and (3) activation of the β-adrenergic receptors in the juxtaglomerular cells by the sympathetic nervous system and by circulating catecholamines, which also stimulates renin release. The three mechanisms generally act in concert to enhance Na^+ retention and, thereby, contribute to the formation of edema.

AII that enters the systemic circulation stimulates the production of aldosterone by the zona glomerulosa of the adrenal cortex. Aldosterone, in turn, enhances Na^+ reabsorption (and K^+ excretion) by the collecting tubule. In patients with heart failure, not only is aldosterone secretion elevated but the biologic half-life of aldosterone is prolonged, which increases further the plasma level of the hormone. A depression of hepatic blood flow, especially during exercise, is responsible for reduced hepatic catabolism of aldosterone. The activation of the RAA system is most striking in the early phase of acute, severe heart failure and is less intense in patients with chronic, stable, compensated heart failure.

Increased quantities of aldosterone are secreted in heart failure and in other edematous states, and blockade of the action of aldosterone by spironolactone (an aldosterone antagonist) or amiloride (a blocker of epithelial Na^+ channels) often induces a moderate diuresis in edematous states. Yet, persistently augmented levels of aldosterone (or other mineralocorticoids) alone do not always promote accumulation of edema, as witnessed by the lack of striking fluid retention in most instances of primary aldosteronism. Furthermore, although normal individuals retain some NaCl and water with the administration of potent mineralocorticoids, such as deoxycorticosterone acetate or fludrocortisone, this accumulation is self-limiting, despite continued exposure to the steroid, a phenomenon known as *mineralocorticoid escape*. The failure of normal individuals who receive large doses of mineralocorticoids to accumulate large quantities of extracellular fluid and to develop edema is probably a consequence of an increase in glomerular filtration rate (pressure natriuresis) and the action of natriuretic substance(s) (see later). The continued secretion of aldosterone may be more important in the accumulation of fluid in edematous states because patients with edema secondary to heart failure, nephrotic syndrome, and hepatic cirrhosis are generally unable to repair the deficit in effective arterial blood volume. As a consequence, they do not develop pressure natriuresis.

Arginine Vasopressin (AVP)

The secretion of AVP occurs in response to increased intracellular osmolar concentration, and by stimulating V_2 receptors, AVP increases the reabsorption of free water in the renal distal tubule and collecting duct, thereby increasing total-body water. Circulating AVP is elevated in many patients with heart failure secondary to a nonosmotic stimulus associated with decreased effective arterial volume. Such patients fail to show the normal reduction of AVP with a reduction of osmolality, contributing to edema formation and hyponatremia.

Endothelin

This potent peptide vasoconstrictor is released by endothelial cells; its concentration is elevated in heart failure and contributes to renal vasoconstriction, Na^+ retention, and edema in heart failure.

Natriuretic Peptides

Atrial distention and/or a Na^+ load cause release into the circulation of atrial natriuretic peptide (ANP), a polypeptide; a high-molecular-weight precursor of ANP is stored in secretory granules within atrial myocytes. Release of ANP causes (1) excretion of sodium and water by augmenting glomerular filtration rate, inhibiting sodium reabsorption in the proximal tubule, and inhibiting release of renin and aldosterone; and (2) arteriolar and venous dilation by antagonizing the vasoconstrictor actions of AII, AVP, and sympathetic stimulation. Thus, ANP has the capacity to oppose Na^+ retention and arterial pressure elevation in hypervolemic states.

The closely related brain natriuretic peptide (BNP) is stored primarily in ventricular myocardium and is released when ventricular diastolic pressure rises. Its actions are similar to those of ANP. Circulating levels of ANP and BNP are elevated in congestive heart failure and in cirrhosis with ascites, but obviously not sufficiently to prevent edema formation. In addition, in edematous states there is abnormal resistance to the actions of natriuretic peptides.

CLINICAL CAUSES OF EDEMA

Obstruction of Venous (and Lymphatic) Drainage of a Limb

In this condition the hydrostatic pressure in the capillary bed upstream (proximal) to the obstruction increases so that an abnormal quantity of fluid is transferred from the vascular to the interstitial space. Since the alternative route (i.e., the lymphatic channels) may also be obstructed or maximally filled, an increased volume of interstitial fluid in the limb develops, i.e., there is trapping of fluid in the extremity. Tissue tension rises in the affected limb until it counterbalances the primary alterations in the Starling forces, at which time no further fluid accumulates. The net effect is a local increase in the volume of interstitial fluid, causing local edema. The displacement of fluid into a limb may occur at the expense of the blood volume in the remainder of the body, thereby reducing effective arterial blood volume and leading to the retention of NaCl and H_2O until the deficit in plasma volume has been corrected. This sequence occurs in ascites and hydrothorax, in which fluid is trapped or accumulates in the cavitary space, depleting the intravascular volume and leading to secondary salt and fluid retention.

Congestive Heart Failure

(See also Chap. 17) In this disorder the impaired systolic emptying of the ventricle(s) and/or the impairment of ventricular relaxation promotes an accumulation of blood in the venous circulation at the expense of the effective arterial volume, and the aforementioned sequence of events (**Fig. 7–1**) is initiated. In mild heart failure, a small increment of total blood volume may repair the deficit of arterial volume and establish a new steady state. Through the operation of Starling's law of the heart, an increase in ventricular diastolic volume promotes a more forceful contraction and may thereby restore the cardiac output. However, if the cardiac disorder is more severe, fluid retention continues, and the increment in blood volume accumulates in the venous circulation. With reduction in cardiac output, a decrease in baroreflex-mediated inhibition of the vasomotor center activates renal vasoconstrictor nerves and the RAA system, causing Na^+ and H_2O retention.

Incomplete ventricular emptying (systolic heart failure) and/or inadequate ventricular relaxation (diastolic heart failure) both lead to an elevation of ventricular diastolic pressure. If the impairment of cardiac function primarily involves the right ventricle, pressures in the

55

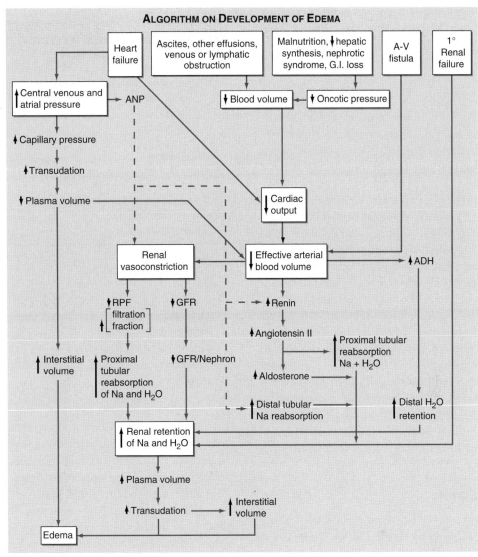

FIGURE 7-1

Sequence of events leading to the formation and retention of salt and water and the development of edema. ANP, atrial natriuretic peptide; RPF, renal plasma flow; GFR, glomerular filtration rate; ADH, antidiuretic hormone. Inhibitory influences are shown by broken lines.

systemic veins and capillaries rise, augmenting the transudation of fluid into the interstitial space and enhancing the likelihood of peripheral edema. The elevated systemic venous pressure is transmitted to the thoracic duct with consequent reduction of lymph drainage, further increasing the accumulation of edema.

If the impairment of cardiac function (incomplete ventricular emptying and/or inadequate relaxation) involves the left ventricle primarily, then, pulmonary venous and capillary pressures rise. Pulmonary artery pressure rises and this, in turn, interferes with the emptying of the right ventricle, leading to an elevation of right ventricular diastolic and of central and systemic venous pressures, thereby enhancing the likelihood of the formation of peripheral edema. The elevation of pulmonary capillary pressure may cause pulmonary edema, which impairs gas exchange. The resultant hypoxemia may impair cardiac function further, sometimes causing a vicious circle.

Nephrotic Syndrome and Other Hypoalbuminemic States

The primary alteration in this disorder is a diminished colloid oncotic pressure due to losses of large quantities of protein into the urine. With severe hypoalbuminemia and the consequent reduced colloid osmotic pressure, the NaCl and H₂O that are retained cannot be restrained within the vascular compartment, and total and effective arterial blood volumes decline. This process initiates the edema-forming sequence of events described above, including activation of the RAA system. Impaired renal function contributes further to the formation of edema. A similar sequence of events occurs in other conditions that lead to *severe* hypoalbuminemia, including (1) severe nutritional deficiency states; (2) severe, chronic liver disease (see later); and (3) protein-losing enteropathy.

Cirrhosis

This condition is characterized by hepatic venous outflow blockade, which, in turn, expands the splanchnic blood volume and increases hepatic lymph formation. Intrahepatic hypertension acts as a potent stimulus for renal Na^+ retention and a reduction of effective arterial blood volume. These alterations are frequently complicated by hypoalbuminemia secondary to reduced hepatic synthesis, as well as systemic vasodilation, which reduce the effective arterial blood volume further, leading to activation of the RAA system, of renal sympathetic nerves, and of other NaCl- and H_2O-retaining mechanisms. The concentration of circulating aldosterone is often elevated by the liver's failure to metabolize this hormone. Initially, the excess interstitial fluid is localized preferentially proximal (upstream) to the congested portal venous system and obstructed hepatic lymphatics, i.e., in the peritoneal cavity (ascites). In later stages, particularly when there is severe hypoalbuminemia, peripheral edema may develop. The excess production of prostaglandins (PGE_2 and PGI_2) in cirrhosis attenuates renal Na^+ retention. When the synthesis of these substances is inhibited by nonsteroidal anti-inflammatory drugs (NSAIDs), renal function deteriorates and Na^+ retention increases.

Drug-Induced Edema

A large number of widely used drugs can cause edema (Table 7-1). Mechanisms include renal vasoconstriction (NSAIDs and cyclosporine), arteriolar dilatation (vasodilators), augmented renal Na^+ reabsorption (steroid hormones), and capillary damage (interleukin 2).

Idiopathic Edema

This syndrome, which occurs almost exclusively in women, is characterized by periodic episodes of edema (unrelated to the menstrual cycle), frequently accompanied by abdominal distention. Diurnal alterations in weight occur with orthostatic retention of NaCl and H_2O, so that the patient may weigh several pounds more after having been in the upright posture for several hours. Such large diurnal weight changes suggest an increase in capillary permeability that appears to fluctuate in severity and to be aggravated by hot weather. There is some evidence that a reduction in plasma volume occurs in this condition with secondary activation of the RAA system and impaired suppression of AVP release.

Idiopathic edema should be distinguished from cyclical or premenstrual edema, in which the NaCl and H_2O retention may be secondary to excessive estrogen stimulation. There are also some cases in which the edema appears to be diuretic-induced. It has been postulated

TABLE 7-1

DRUGS ASSOCIATED WITH EDEMA FORMATION
Nonsteroidal anti-inflammatory drugs
Antihypertensive agents
Direct arterial/arteriolar vasodilators
Hydralazine
Clonidine
Methyldopa
Guanethidine
Minoxidil
Calcium channel antagonists
α-Adrenergic antagonists
Thiazolidinediones
Steroid hormones
Glucocorticoids
Anabolic steroids
Estrogens
Progestins
Cyclosporine
Growth hormone
Immunotherapies
Interleukin 2
OKT3 monoclonal antibody

Source: From Chertow.

that in these patients chronic diuretic administration leads to mild blood volume depletion, which causes chronic hyperreninemia and juxtaglomerular hyperplasia. Salt-retaining mechanisms appear to overcompensate for the direct effects of the diuretics. *Acute* withdrawal of diuretics can then leave the Na^+-retaining forces unopposed, leading to fluid retention and edema. Decreased dopaminergic activity and reduced urinary kallikrein and kinin excretion have been reported in this condition and may also be of pathogenetic importance.

℞ Treatment: IDIOPATHIC EDEMA

The treatment of idiopathic cyclic edema includes a reduction in NaCl intake, rest in the supine position for several hours each day, and the wearing of elastic stockings (which should be put on before arising in the morning). A variety of pharmacologic agents including angiotensin-converting enzyme inhibitors, progesterone, the dopamine receptor agonist bromocriptine, and the sympathomimetic amine dextroamphetamine, have all been reported to be useful when administered to patients who do not respond to simpler measures. Diuretics may be helpful initially but may lose their effectiveness with continuous administration; accordingly, they should be employed sparingly, if at all. Discontinuation of diuretics paradoxically leads to diuresis in diuretic-induced edema, described above.

DIFFERENTIAL DIAGNOSIS

LOCALIZED EDEMA

(See also Chap. 39) Edema originating from inflammation or hypersensitivity is usually readily identified. Localized edema due to venous or lymphatic obstruction may be caused by thrombophlebitis, chronic lymphangitis, resection of regional lymph nodes, filariasis, etc. Lymphedema is particularly intractable because restriction of lymphatic flow results in increased protein concentration in the interstitial fluid, a circumstance that aggravates retention of fluid.

GENERALIZED EDEMA

The differences among the three major causes of generalized edema are shown in (Table 7-2).

The great majority of patients with generalized edema suffer from advanced cardiac, renal, hepatic, or nutritional disorders. Consequently, the differential diagnosis of generalized edema should be directed toward identifying or excluding these several conditions.

Edema of Heart Failure

(See also Chap. 17) The presence of heart disease, as manifested by cardiac enlargement and a gallop rhythm, together with evidence of cardiac failure, such as dyspnea, basilar rales, venous distention, and hepatomegaly, usually indicate that edema results from heart failure. Noninvasive tests, such as echocardiography, may be helpful in establishing the diagnosis of heart disease. The edema of heart failure typically occurs in the dependent portions of the body.

Edema of the Nephrotic Syndrome

Marked proteinuria (>3.5 g/d), hypoalbuminemia (<35 g/L), and, in some instances, hypercholesterolemia are present.

TABLE 7-2

PRINCIPAL CAUSES OF GENERALIZED EDEMA: HISTORY, PHYSICAL EXAMINATION, AND LABORATORY FINDINGS

ORGAN SYSTEM	HISTORY	PHYSICAL EXAMINATION	LABORATORY FINDINGS
Cardiac	Dyspnea with exertion prominent—often associated with orthopnea—or paroxysmal nocturnal dyspnea	Elevated jugular venous pressure, ventricular (S_3) gallop; occasionally with displaced or dyskinetic apical pulse; peripheral cyanosis, cool extremities, small pulse pressure when severe	Elevated urea nitrogen-to-creatinine ratio common; elevated uric acid; serum sodium often diminished; liver enzymes occasionally elevated with hepatic congestion
Hepatic	Dyspnea infrequent, except if associated with significant degree of ascites; most often a history of ethanol abuse	Frequently associated with ascites; jugular venous pressure normal or low; blood pressure lower than in renal or cardiac disease; one or more additional signs of chronic liver disease (jaundice, palmar erythema, Dupuytren's contracture, spider angiomata, male gynecomastia; asterixis and other signs of encephalopathy) may be present	If severe, reductions in serum albumin, cholesterol, other hepatic proteins (transferrin, fibrinogen); liver enzymes elevated, depending on the cause and acuity of liver injury; tendency toward hypokalemia, respiratory alkalosis; macrocytosis from folate deficiency
Renal	Usually chronic: may be associated with uremic signs and symptoms, including decreased appetite, altered (metallic or fishy) taste, altered sleep pattern, difficulty concentrating, restless legs or myoclonus; dyspnea can be present, but generally less prominent than in heart failure	Blood pressure may be elevated; hypertensive or diabetic retinopathy in selected cases; nitrogenous fetor; periorbital edema may predominate; pericardial friction rub in advanced cases with uremia	Albuminuria, hypoalbuminemia; sometimes, elevation of serum creatinine and urea nitrogen; hyperkalemia, metabolic acidosis, hyperphosphatemia, hypocalcemia, anemia (usually normocytic)

Source: From Chertow.

This syndrome may occur during the course of a variety of kidney diseases, which include glomerulonephritis, diabetic glomerulosclerosis, and hypersensitivity reactions. A history of previous renal disease may or may not be elicited.

Edema of Acute Glomerulonephritis and Other Forms of Renal Failure

The edema occurring during the acute phases of glomerulonephritis is characteristically associated with hematuria, proteinuria, and hypertension. Although some evidence supports the view that the fluid retention is due to increased capillary permeability, in most instances the edema results from primary retention of $NaCl$ and H_2O by the kidneys owing to renal insufficiency. This state differs from congestive heart failure in that it is characterized by a normal (or sometimes even increased) cardiac output and a normal arterial–mixed venous oxygen difference. Patients with edema due to renal failure commonly have evidence of arterial hypertension as well as pulmonary congestion on chest roentgenograms even without cardiac enlargement, but they may not develop orthopnea. Patients with *chronic* renal failure may also develop edema due to primary renal retention of $NaCl$ and H_2O.

Edema of Cirrhosis

Ascites and biochemical and clinical evidence of hepatic disease (collateral venous channels, jaundice, and spider angiomas) characterize edema of hepatic origin. The ascites is frequently refractory to treatment because it collects as a result of a combination of obstruction of hepatic lymphatic drainage, portal hypertension, and hypoalbuminemia. A sizable accumulation of ascitic fluid may increase intraabdominal pressure and impede venous return from the lower extremities; hence, it tends to promote accumulation of edema in this region as well.

Edema of Nutritional Origin

A diet grossly deficient in protein over a prolonged period may produce hypoproteinemia and edema. The latter may be intensified by the development of beriberi heart disease, also of nutritional origin, in which multiple peripheral arteriovenous fistulae result in reduced effective systemic perfusion and effective arterial blood volume, thereby enhancing edema formation. Edema may actually become intensified when famished subjects are first provided with an adequate diet. The ingestion of more food may increase the quantity of $NaCl$ ingested, which is then retained along with H_2O. So-called refeeding edema may also be linked to increased release of insulin, which directly increases tubular Na^+ reabsorption. In addition to hypoalbuminemia, hypokalemia and caloric deficits may be involved in the edema of starvation.

Other Causes of Edema

Other causes include hypothyroidism, in which the edema (myxedema) is located typically in the pretibial region and which may also be associated with periorbital puffiness; exogenous hyperadrenocortism; pregnancy; and administration of estrogens and vasodilators, particularly dihydropyridines such as nifedipine.

DISTRIBUTION OF EDEMA

The distribution of edema is an important guide to its cause. Thus, edema limited to one leg or to one or both arms is usually the result of venous and/or lymphatic obstruction. Edema resulting from hypoproteinemia characteristically is generalized, but it is especially evident in the very soft tissues of the eyelids and face and tends to be most pronounced in the morning because of the recumbent posture assumed during the night. Less common causes of facial edema include trichinosis, allergic reactions, and myxedema. Edema associated with heart failure, by contrast, tends to be more extensive in the legs and to be accentuated in the evening, a feature also determined largely by posture. When patients with heart failure have been confined to bed, edema may be most prominent in the presacral region. Paralysis reduces lymphatic and venous drainage on the affected side and may be responsible for unilateral edema.

ADDITIONAL FACTORS IN DIAGNOSIS

The color, thickness, and sensitivity of the skin are significant. Local tenderness and warmth suggest inflammation. Local cyanosis may signify venous obstruction. In individuals who have had repeated episodes of prolonged edema, the skin over the involved areas may be thickened, indurated, and often red.

Estimation of the venous pressure is of importance in evaluating edema. Ordinarily, a significant generalized increase in venous pressure can be recognized by the level at which cervical veins collapse (Chap. 9). In patients with obstruction of the superior vena cava, edema is confined to the face, neck, and upper extremities, in which the venous pressure is elevated compared with that in the lower extremities. Severe heart failure may cause ascites that may be distinguished from the ascites caused by hepatic cirrhosis by the jugular venous pressure, which is usually elevated in heart failure and normal in cirrhosis.

Determination of the concentration of serum albumin aids importantly in identifying those patients, in whom edema is due, at least in part, to diminished intravascular colloid oncotic pressure. The presence of proteinuria also affords useful clues. The absence of proteinuria excludes nephrotic syndrome but cannot exclude nonproteinuric causes of renal failure. Slight to moderate proteinuria is the rule in patients with heart failure.

Approach to the Patient:
EDEMA

An important first question is whether the edema is localized or generalized. If it is localized, those local phenomena that may be responsible should be considered. If the edema is generalized, it should be determined, first, if there is serious hypoalbuminemia, e.g., serum albumin <25 g/L. If so, the history, physical examination, urinalysis, and other laboratory data will help evaluate the question of cirrhosis, severe malnutrition, or the nephrotic syndrome as the underlying disorder. If hypoalbuminemia is not present, it should be determined if there is evidence of congestive heart failure of a severity to promote generalized edema. Finally, it should be determined whether the patient has an adequate urine output, or if there is significant oliguria or anuria.

FURTHER READINGS

ABASSI ZA et al: Control of extracellular fluid volume and the pathophysiology of edema formation, in *The Kidney*, 7th ed, BM Brenner (ed). Philadelphia, Saunders, 2004, pp 777–856

BANSAL S et al: Sodium retention in heart failure and cirrhosis. Potential role of natriuretic doses of mineralocorticoid antagonist? Circ Heart Fail 2:370, 2009

CHERTOW GM: Approach to the patient with edema, in *Cardiology for the Primary Care Physician*, 2d ed, E Braunwald, L Goldman (eds). Philadelphia, Saunders, 2003, pp 117–128

DISKIN CJ et al: Edema, oncotic pressure, and free entropy: Novel considerations for treatment of edema through attention to thermodynamics. Nephron 78:131, 1998

MCCULLOUGH JC: Renal disorders and heart disease, in *Braunwald's Heart Disease*, 7th ed, D Zipes et al (eds). Philadelphia, Saunders, 2005

——: Renal disorders and heart disease, in *Braunwald's Heart Disease*, 8th ed, P. Libby et al (eds). Philadelphia, Saunders Elsevier, 2008

O'BRIEN JG et al: Treatment of edema. Am Fam Physician 71:2111, 2005

SCHRIER RW: Decreased effective blood volume in edematous disorders: What does this mean? J Am Soc Nephrol 18:2028, 2007

SKORECKI KL et al: Extracellular fluid and edema formation, in Brenner and Rector's The Kidney, 8th ed, Philadelphia, Elsevier, 2008

STREETEN DH: Idiopathic edema. Pathogenesis, clinical features, and treatment. Endocrinol Metab Clin North Am 24:531, 1995

CHAPTER 8

PALPITATIONS

Joseph Loscalzo

Palpitations are extremely common among patients who present to their caregiver and can best be defined as an intermittent "thumping," "pounding," or "fluttering" sensation in the chest. The sensation can be either intermittent or sustained, and either regular or irregular. Most patients interpret palpitations as an unusual awareness of the heartbeat and become especially concerned when they sense that they have had "skipped" or "missing" heartbeats. Palpitations are often noted when the patient is resting quietly, during which time other stimuli are minimal. Palpitations that are positional may reflect a structural process within (e.g., atrial myxoma) or adjacent to (e.g., mediastinal mass) the heart.

Palpitations are brought about by cardiac (43%), psychiatric (31%), miscellaneous (10%), and unknown (16%) causes, according to one large series. Cardiac causes include premature atrial and ventricular contractions, supraventricular and ventricular arrhythmias, mitral valve prolapse, aortic regurgitation, and atrial myxoma. Intermittent palpitations are commonly caused by premature atrial or ventricular contractions: the postextrasystolic beat is sensed by the patient owing to the increase in ventricular end-diastolic dimension following the pause in the cardiac cycle and the increased strength of contraction (*postextrasystolic potentiation*) of that beat. Regular, sustained palpitations can be caused by regular supraventricular and ventricular tachycardias (Chap. 16). Irregular, sustained palpitations can be caused by atrial fibrillation.

It is important to note that most arrhythmias are not associated with palpitations. In those that are, it is often useful either to ask the patient to "tap out" the rhythm of the palpitations or to take his or her pulse while palpitations are occurring. In general, hyperdynamic cardiovascular states caused by catecholaminergic stimulation from exercise, stress, or pheochromocytoma can lead to palpitations. In addition, the enlarged ventricle of aortic regurgitation and accompanying hyperdynamic precordium frequently lead to the sensation of palpitations. Other factors that enhance the strength of myocardial contraction, including tobacco, caffeine, aminophylline, atropine, thyroxine, cocaine, and amphetamines, can cause palpitations.

Psychiatric causes of palpitations include panic attack or disorder, anxiety states, and somatization, alone or in combination. Patients with psychiatric causes for palpitations more commonly report a longer duration of the sensation (>15 min) and other accompanying symptoms than do patients with other causes. Among the miscellaneous causes of palpitations are included thyrotoxicosis, drugs (see earlier) and ethanol, spontaneous skeletal muscle contractions of the chest wall, pheochromocytoma, and systemic mastocytosis.

Approach to the Patient:
PALPITATIONS

The principal goal in assessing patients with palpitations is to determine if the symptom is caused by a life-threatening arrhythmia. Patients with preexisting coronary artery disease (CAD) or risk factors for CAD are at greatest risk for ventricular arrhythmias as a cause for palpitations. In addition, the association of palpitations with other symptoms suggesting hemodynamic compromise, including syncope or lightheadedness, supports this diagnosis. Palpitations caused by sustained tachyarrhythmias in patients with CAD can be accompanied by angina pectoris or dyspnea.

In patients with ventricular dysfunction (systolic or diastolic), aortic stenosis, hypertrophic cardiomyopathy, or mitral stenosis, with or without CAD, palpitations can be accompanied by dyspnea from increased left atrial and pulmonary capillary wedge pressure.

Key features of the physical examination that will help confirm or refute the presence of an arrhythmia as a cause for the palpitations and its adverse hemodynamic consequences include measurement of the vital signs, assessment of the jugular venous pressure and pulse, and auscultation of the chest and precordium. A resting electrocardiogram can be used to document the arrhythmia. If exertion is known to induce the arrhythmia and accompanying palpitations, exercise electrocardiography can be used to make the diagnosis. If the arrhythmia is sufficiently infrequent, other methods must be used, including continuous electrocardiographic (Holter) monitoring; telephonic monitoring, through which the patient can transmit an electrocardiographic tracing during a sensed episode; and loop recordings (external or implantable), which can capture the electrocardiographic event for later review.

Most patients with palpitations do not have serious arrhythmias or underlying structural heart disease. Occasional benign atrial or ventricular premature contractions can often be managed with beta blocker therapy if sufficiently troubling to the patient. Palpitations incited by alcohol, tobacco, or illicit drugs need to be managed by abstention, while those caused by pharmacologic agents should be addressed by considering alternative therapies. Psychiatric causes of palpitations may benefit from cognitive or pharmacotherapies. The physician should note that palpitations are at the very least bothersome and, on occasion, frightening to the patient. Once serious causes for the symptom have been excluded, the patient should be reassured the palpitations will not adversely affect his or her prognosis.

ACKNOWLEDGMENT

Dr. Thomas Lee authored this chapter in previous editions. Some of the material from the 16th edition of Harrison's Principles of Internal Medicine has been carried forward.

FURTHER READINGS

ABBOTT AV: Diagnostic approach to palpitations. Am Fam Physician 71:743, 2005

GIADA F et al: Recurrent unexplained palpitations (RUP) study. J Am Coll Cardiol 49:1951, 2007

LAWLESS CE, BRINER W: Palpitations in athletes. Sports Med 38:687, 2008

OLSON JA et al: Utility of mobile cardiac outpatient telemetry for the diagnosis of palpitations, presyncope, syncope, and the assessment of therapy efficacy. J Cardiovasc Electrophysiol 18:473, 2007

PICKETT CC, ZIMETBAUM PJ: Palpitations: A proper evaluation and approach to effective medical therapy. Curr Cardiol Rep 7:362, 2005

SULFI S et al: Limited clinical utility of Holter monitoring in patients with palpitations or altered consciousness: analysis of 8973 recordings in 7394 patients. Ann Noninvasive Electrocardiol 13:39, 2008

WEBER BE, KAPOOR WN: Evaluation and outcomes of patients with palpitations. Am J Med 100:138, 1996

CHAPTER 9

PHYSICAL EXAMINATION OF THE CARDIOVASCULAR SYSTEM

Robert A. O'Rourke ■ Eugene Braunwald

A precise and detailed physical examination is an often underutilized low-cost method for assessing the cardiovascular system. It frequently provides important information for the appropriate selection of additional noninvasive or invasive tests. First, the general physical appearance should be evaluated. The patient may appear tired because of a chronic low cardiac output; the respiratory rate may be rapid in cases of pulmonary venous congestion. Central cyanosis, often associated with clubbing of the fingers and toes, indicates right-to-left cardiac or extracardiac shunting or inadequate oxygenation of blood by the lungs. Cyanosis in the distal extremities, cool skin, and increased sweating result from vasoconstriction in patients with severe heart failure (Chap. 6). Noncardiovascular details can be equally important. For example, infective endocarditis is the likely diagnosis in patients with petechiae, Osler's nodes, and Janeway lesions (Chap. 25).

The blood pressure should be taken in both arms and with the patient supine and upright; the heart rate should be timed for 30 s. Orthostatic hypotension and tachycardia may indicate a reduced blood volume, while resting tachycardia may be due to heart failure or hypovolemia.

EXAMINATION OF THE RETINA

Visualization of the smaller vessels of the body is possible in the retina. The optic disc should be observed first, with a search for evidence of edema and blurred margins and for cupping with sharp contours. Neovascularization or the pallor of optic atrophy should be excluded. Next, the examiner should scan along the superior temporal arcade, inspecting the arteries for embolic plaques at each bifurcation and noting the arteriovenous crossings for evidence of obscuration of the vein and for marked nicking and narrowing of the vessels, as occurs in hypertension (Chap. 37).

Early diabetic microaneurysms, a manifestation of diabetic microvascular disease, are found just temporal to the fovea, along the horizontal raphe, and cotton-wool infarcts are found circularly around the disc. Thus, the retina can be searched efficiently for evidence of cardiovascular disease.

Variations in the caliber of a single vessel are more important than arteriovenous ratios. These occur in the form of focal narrowing, or *beading*, and are seen in hypercholesterolemia or spasm. In severe hypertension, hypertensive retinopathy with scattered flame-shaped hemorrhages, very constricted arterioles, and cotton-wool spots are evident.

Retinal emboli have particular cardiovascular importance. Of these, platelet emboli are both the most common and the most evanescent. Hollenhorst cholesterol plaques may be detected at the same bifurcations for months to years after the embolic shower. Platelet emboli, Hollenhorst plaques, and calcium emboli are usually seen along the course of a retinal artery, and their presence indicates that a patient is shedding from the heart, aorta, great vessels, or carotid arteries.

EXAMINATION OF THE ABDOMEN

The diameter of the *abdominal* aorta should be estimated. A pulsatile, expansible mass is indicative of an abdominal aortic aneurysm (Chap. 38). An abdominal aortic aneurysm may be missed if the examiner does not assess the area above the umbilicus.

Specific abnormalities of the abdomen may be secondary to heart disease. A large, tender liver is common in patients with heart failure or constrictive pericarditis. Systolic hepatic pulsations are frequent in patients with tricuspid regurgitation. A palpable spleen is a late sign in patients with severe heart failure and is also often evident in patients with infective endocarditis. Ascites may occur with heart failure alone, but it is less common with the use of diuretic therapy. Constrictive pericarditis should be considered when the ascites is out of proportion to peripheral edema. When there is an arteriovenous fistula, a continuous murmur may be heard over the abdomen. A systolic bruit heard over the kidney areas may signify renal artery stenosis in patients with systemic hypertension.

EXAMINATION OF THE EXTREMITIES

Examination of the upper and lower extremities may provide important diagnostic information. Palpation of the peripheral arterial pulses in the upper and lower extremities is necessary to define the adequacy of systemic blood flow and to detect the presence of occlusive arterial lesions. Atherosclerosis of the peripheral arteries may produce intermittent claudication of the buttock, calf, thigh, or foot, with severe disease resulting in tissue damage of the toes. Peripheral atherosclerosis is an important risk factor for coincident ischemic heart disease.

The ankle-brachial index (ABI) is useful in cardiovascular risk assessment. The ABI is the ratio of the systolic blood pressure at the ankle divided by the higher of the two arm systolic blood pressures. It reflects the degree of lower-extremity arterial occlusive disease, which is manifest by reduced blood pressure distal to stenotic lesions. Either posterior tibial or dorsalis pedis artery pressures can be used. It is important to note that each equally reflects the status of the aortoiliac and femoropopliteal segments but different tibial arteries; therefore, the resulting ABIs may differ. An arm systolic pressure of 120 mmHg and an ankle systolic pressure of 60 mmHg yields an ABI of 0.5 (60/120). The ABI is inversely related to disease severity. A resting ABI <0.9 is considered abnormal. Lower values correspond to progressively more severe occlusive peripheral arterial disease (PAD) and disabling claudication. An ABI <0.3 is consistent with critical ischemia, rest pain, and tissue loss.

Thrombophlebitis often causes pain (in the calf or thigh) or edema, and when present, pulmonary emboli should be considered as well. Edema of the lower extremities is a sign of heart failure but may also be secondary to local factors, such varicose veins or thrombophlebitis, or to the removal of veins at coronary artery bypass surgery. Under such circumstances, the edema is often unilateral.

ARTERIAL PRESSURE PULSE

The normal central aortic pulse wave is characterized by a fairly rapid rise to a somewhat rounded peak (**Fig. 9-1**). The anacrotic shoulder, present on the ascending limb, occurs at the time of peak rate of aortic flow just before maximum pressure is reached. The less-steep descending limb is interrupted by a sharp downward deflection, coincident with aortic valve closure, called the *incisura*. As the pulse wave is transmitted distally, the initial upstroke becomes steeper, the anacrotic shoulder becomes less apparent, and the smoother dicrotic notch replaces the

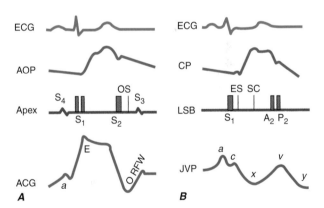

FIGURE 9-1

A. Schematic representation of electrocardiogram, aortic pressure pulse (AOP), phonocardiogram recorded at the apex, and apex cardiogram (ACG). On the phonocardiogram, S_1, S_2, S_3, and S_4 represent the first through fourth heart sounds; OS represents the opening snap of the mitral valve, which occurs coincident with the O point of the apex cardiogram. S_3 occurs coincident with the termination of the rapid-filling wave (RFW) of the ACG, while S_4 occurs coincident with the *a* wave of the ACG. **B.** Simultaneous recording of electrocardiogram, indirect carotid pulse (CP), phonocardiogram along the left sternal border (LSB), and indirect jugular venous pulse (JVP). ES, ejection sound; SC, systolic click.

64 incisure. Accordingly, palpation of a peripheral arterial pulse (e.g., the radial pulse) frequently gives less information than examination of a more central pulse (e.g., the carotid pulse) regarding alterations in left ventricular ejection or aortic valve function. However, certain findings, such as the bisferiens pulse of aortic regurgitation or pulsus alternans, are more evident in peripheral arteries (**Fig. 9-2**).

The carotid pulse is best examined with the sternocleidomastoid muscle relaxed and with the patient's head rotated slightly toward the examiner. In palpating

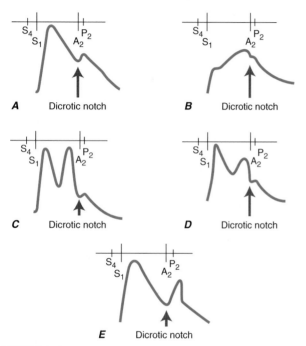

FIGURE 9-2

Schematic diagrams of the configurational changes in carotid pulse and their differential diagnoses. Heart sounds are also illustrated. **A.** Normal. A$_2$, aortic component of the second heart sound; S$_1$, first heart sound; S$_4$, atrial sound. **B.** Anacrotic pulse with a slow initial upstroke. The peak is close to S$_2$. These features suggest fixed left ventricular outflow obstruction, such as occurs with valvular aortic stenosis. **C.** Pulsus bisferiens with both percussion and tidal waves occurring during systole. This type of carotid pulse contour is most frequently observed in patients with hemodynamically significant aortic regurgitation or combined aortic stenosis and regurgitation with dominant regurgitation. It is rarely appreciated at the bedside by palpation. **D.** In hypertrophic obstructive cardiomyopathy, the pulse wave upstroke rises rapidly and the trough is followed by a smaller slowly rising positive pulse. **E.** A dicrotic pulse results from an accentuated dicrotic wave and tends to occur in patients with sepsis, severe heart failure, hypovolemic shock, cardiac tamponade, and aortic valve replacement. *[From K Chatterjee: Bedside evaluation of the heart: The physical examination, in Cardiology: An Illustrated Text/Reference, K Chatterjee, W Parmley (eds). Philadelphia, JB Lippincott, 1991.]*

the brachial arterial pulse, the examiner can support the patient's relaxed elbow with the right arm while compressing the brachial pulse with the thumb. The usual technique is to compress the artery with the thumb or forefinger until the maximum pulse is sensed. Varying degrees of pressure should then be applied while concentrating on the separate phases of the pulse wave. This method, known as *trisection*, is useful for assessing the sharpness of the upstroke, systolic peak, and diastolic slope of the arterial pulse. In most normal persons, a dicrotic wave is not palpable.

A small weak pulse, *pulsus parvus*, is common in conditions with a diminished left ventricular stroke volume, a narrow pulse pressure, and increased peripheral vascular resistance. A *hypokinetic* pulse may be due to hypovolemia, to left ventricular failure, to restrictive pericardial disease, or to mitral valve stenosis. In aortic valve stenosis, the delayed systolic peak, *pulsus tardus*, results from obstruction to left ventricular ejection (Fig. 9-2B). In contrast, a large, bounding (hyperkinetic) pulse is usually associated with an increased left ventricular stroke volume, a wide pulse pressure, and a decrease in peripheral vascular resistance. This pattern occurs characteristically in patients with an elevated stroke volume, as in complete heart block; with hyperkinetic circulation due to anxiety, anemia, exercise, or fever; or with a rapid runoff of blood from the arterial system (due to a patent ductus arteriosus or peripheral arteriovenous fistula). Patients with mitral regurgitation or a ventricular septal defect (VSD) may also have a bounding pulse, since vigorous left ventricular ejection produces a rapid upstroke in the arterial pulse, even though the duration of systole and the forward stroke volume may be reduced. In aortic regurgitation, the rapidly rising, bounding arterial pulse results from an increased left ventricular stroke volume and an increased rate of ventricular ejection.

The *bisferiens pulse*, which has two systolic peaks (Fig. 9-2C), is characteristic of aortic regurgitation (with or without accompanying stenosis) and of hypertrophic cardiomyopathy (Chap. 21). In the latter condition, the pulse wave upstroke rises rapidly and forcefully, producing the first systolic peak ("percussion wave") (Fig. 9-2D). A brief decline in pressure follows because of the sudden midsystolic decrease in the rate of left ventricular ejection, when severe obstruction often develops. This pressure trough is followed by a smaller and more slowly rising positive pulse wave ("tidal wave") produced by continued ventricular ejection and by reflected waves from the periphery. The dicrotic pulse has two palpable waves, one in the systole and one in diastole (Fig. 9-2E). It usually denotes a very low stroke volume, particularly in patients with dilated cardiomyopathy.

Pulsus alternans is a pattern in which there is regular alteration of the pressure pulse amplitude, despite a regular rhythm. It is due to alternating left ventricular contractile force, usually indicates severe impairment of left ventricular function, and commonly occurs in patients who also have a loud third heart sound. Pulsus alternans may also occur during or following paroxysmal tachycardia or for several beats following a premature beat in patients without heart disease. In *pulsus bigeminus*, there is also a regular alteration of pressure pulse amplitude, but it is caused by a premature ventricular contraction that follows each regular beat. In *pulsus paradoxus*, the decrease in systolic arterial pressure that normally accompanies the reduction in arterial pulse amplitude during inspiration is accentuated. In patients with pericardial tamponade (Chap. 22), airway obstruction, or superior vena cava obstruction, the decrease in systolic arterial pressure frequently exceeds the normal decrease of 10 mmHg and the peripheral pulse may disappear completely during inspiration.

Simultaneous palpation of the radial and femoral arterial pulses, which normally are virtually coincident, is important to rule out aortic coarctation, in which the latter pulse is weakened and delayed (Chap. 19).

JUGULAR VENOUS PULSE (JVP)

The two main objectives of the examination of the neck veins are inspection of their waveform and estimation of the central venous pressure (CVP). In most patients, the right internal jugular vein is best for both purposes. Usually, the pulsation of the internal jugular vein is greatest when the trunk is inclined by <30°. In patients with elevated venous pressure, it may be necessary to elevate the trunk further, sometimes to as great as 90°. When the neck muscles are relaxed, shining a beam of light tangentially across the skin overlying the vein exposes the pulsations of the internal jugular vein. Simultaneous palpation of the left carotid artery aids the examiner in deciding which pulsations are venous and in relating the venous pulsations to their timing in the cardiac cycle.

The normal JVP reflects phasic pressure changes in the right atrium and consists of two or sometime three positive waves and two negative troughs (Figs. 9-1*B* and 9-3). The positive presystolic *a* wave is produced by venous distention due to right atrial contraction and is the dominant wave in the JVP, particularly during inspiration. Large *a* waves indicate that the right atrium is contracting against an increased resistance, such as occurs with tricuspid stenosis (Fig. 9-3) or more commonly with increased resistance to right ventricular filling (pulmonary hypertension or pulmonic stenosis). Large *a* waves also occur during arrhythmias whenever the right atrium contracts while the tricuspid valve is closed by right ventricular systole. Such "cannon" *a* waves may occur regularly (as during junctional rhythm) or irregularly (as in atrioventricular (AV) dissociation with ventricular tachycardia or complete heart block). The *a* wave is absent in patients with atrial fibrillation, and there is an increased delay

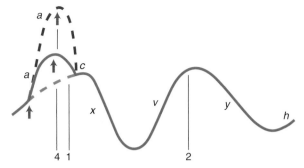

FIGURE 9-3

Jugular venous pulse. The normal contour is shown by the solid red line. The *a* wave (a) is absent in atrial fibrillation (dashed green line). The *a* wave becomes large when the right atrium contracts against a greater than normal volume of blood, a noncompliant or hypertrophied right ventricle, or a closing or closed tricuspid valve (dashed blue line). Arrows indicate the beginning and the peak of the *a* wave. The numbers represent the heart sounds. The fourth heart sound coincides with the peak of the large or giant *a* wave. *[From TC Evans et al: Physical examination, in Cardiology: Fundamentals and Practice, 2d ed, ER Giuliani (ed). St. Louis, Mosby-Year Book, 1991, by permission of the Mayo Foundation.]*

between the *a* wave and the carotid arterial pulse in patients with first-degree AV block.

The *c* wave, often observed in the JVP (Fig. 9-1), is a positive wave produced by the bulging of the tricuspid valve into the right atrium during right ventricular isovolumetric systole and by the impact of the carotid artery adjacent to the jugular vein. The *x* descent is due both to atrial relaxation and to the downward displacement of the tricuspid valve during ventricular systole. The *x* descent wave during systole is often accentuated in patients with constrictive pericarditis (Fig. 9-3), but the nadir of this wave is reduced with right ventricular dilation and is often reversed in tricuspid regurgitation. The positive, late systolic *v* wave results from the increasing volume of blood in the right atrium during ventricular systole when the tricuspid valve is closed. Tricuspid regurgitation causes the *v* wave to be more prominent; when tricuspid regurgitation becomes severe, the combination of a prominent *v* wave and obliteration of the *x* descent results in a single large positive systolic wave. After the *v* wave peaks, the right atrial pressure falls because of the decreased bulging of the tricuspid valve into the right atrium as right ventricular pressure declines and tricuspid valve opens (Fig. 9-3).

This negative descending limb—the *y* descent of the JVP—is produced mainly by the opening of the tricuspid valve and the subsequent rapid inflow of blood into the right ventricle. A rapid, deep *y* descent in early diastole occurs with severe tricuspid regurgitation. A venous pulse characterized by a sharp *y* descent, a deep *y* trough, and a rapid ascent to the baseline is seen in patients with constrictive pericarditis or with severe right-sided heart failure and a high venous pressure. A slow γ descent in the JVP suggests an obstruction to right ventricular filling, as occurs with tricuspid stenosis or right atrial myxoma.

The right internal jugular is the best vein to use for accurate estimation of the CVP. The sternal angle is used as the reference point because the center of the right atrium lies ~5 cm below the sternal angle in the average patient, regardless of body position. The patient is examined at the optimal degree of trunk elevation for visualization of venous pulsations. The vertical distance between the top of the oscillating venous column and the level of the sternal angle is determined; generally it is <3 cm (3 cm + 5 cm = 8 cm blood). The most common cause of a high venous pressure is an elevated right ventricular diastolic pressure.

In patients suspected of having right ventricular failure who have a normal CVP at rest, the *abdomino-jugular reflux test* may be helpful. The palm of the examiner's hand is placed over the abdomen, and firm pressure is applied for 10 s or more. In normal persons, this maneuver does not alter the jugular venous pressure significantly, but when right heart function is impaired, the upper level of venous pulsation usually increases. A positive abdominojugular test is best defined as an increase in JVP during 10 s of firm midabdominal compression followed by a rapid drop in pressure of 4 cm blood on release of the compression. The most common cause of a positive test is right-sided heart failure secondary to elevated left heart filling pressures. Also, abdominal compression may elicit the JVP pattern typical of tricuspid regurgitation when the resting pulse wave is normal. *Kussmaul's sign*—an increase rather than the normal decrease in the CVP during inspiration—is caused most often by severe right-sided heart failure; it is a frequent finding in patients with constrictive pericarditis or right ventricular infarction.

PRECORDIAL PALPATION

The location, amplitude, duration, and direction of the cardiac impulse usually can be best appreciated with the fingertips. The normal left ventricular apex impulse is located at or medial to the left midclavicular line in the fourth or fifth intercostal space. Left ventricular hypertrophy results in exaggeration of the amplitude, duration, and often size of the normal left ventricular thrust. The impulse may be displaced laterally and downward into the sixth or seventh intercostal space, particularly in patients with a left ventricular volume load such as occurs in cases of aortic regurgitation or dilated cardiomyopathy. Right ventricular hypertrophy often results in a sustained systolic lift at the lower left parasternal area, which starts in early systole and is synchronous with the left ventricular apical impulse.

Abnormal precordial pulsations occur during systole in patients with left ventricular dyssynergy due to ischemic heart disease or to diffuse myocardial disease from some other cause. They are most commonly felt in the left midprecordium one or two interspaces above the left ventricular apex.

A left parasternal lift is frequently present in patients with severe mitral regurgitation and is due to anterior displacement of the right ventricle by an enlarged, expanding left atrium. Pulmonary artery pulsation is often visible and palpable in the second left intercostal space. This pulsation usually denotes pulmonary hypertension or increased pulmonary blood flow.

Thrills are palpable, low frequency vibrations associated with heart murmurs. The systolic murmur of mitral regurgitation may be palpated at the cardiac apex. When the palm of the hand is placed over the precordium, the thrill of aortic stenosis crosses the palm toward the right side of the neck, while the thrill of pulmonic stenosis radiates more often to the left side of the neck. The thrill due to a VSD is usually located in the third or fourth intercostal spaces near the left sternal border.

Percussion should be performed to identify normal or abnormal position of the heart, stomach, and liver.

CARDIAC AUSCULTATION

To obtain the most information from cardiac auscultation, the observer should keep in mind several principles: (1) Auscultation should be performed in a quiet room to avoid the distracting noises of normal activity. (2) For optimal auscultation, attention must be focused on the phase of the cardiac cycle during which the auscultatory event is expected to occur. (3) The timing of a heart sound or murmur can be determined accurately from its relation to other observable events in the cardiac cycle—the carotid arterial pulse, the apical impulse, or the JVP.

HEART SOUNDS

The major components of heart sounds are vibrations associated with the abrupt acceleration or deceleration of blood in the cardiovascular system. Studies using simultaneous echocardiographic-phonocardiographic recordings indicate that the first and second heart sounds are produced primarily by the closure of the AV and semilunar valves and the events that accompany these closures. The intensity of the *first heart sound* (S_1) is influenced by (1) the position of the mitral leaflets at the onset of ventricular systole; (2) the rate of rise of the left ventricular pressure pulse; (3) the presence or absence of structural disease of the mitral valve; and (4) the amount of tissue, air, or fluid between the heart and the stethoscope. S_1 is louder if diastole is shortened because of tachycardia, if AV flow is increased because of high cardiac output or prolonged because of mitral stenosis, or if atrial contraction precedes ventricular contraction by an unusually short interval, reflected in a short PR interval. The loud S_1 in mitral stenosis usually signifies that the valve is pliable and that it remains open at the onset of isovolumetric contraction because of the elevated left atrial pressure. A soft S_1 may be due to poor conduction of sound through the chest wall, a slow rise of the left ventricular pressure pulse, a long PR interval, or imperfect closure due to reduced valve substance, as in mitral regurgitation. S_1 is also soft when the anterior mitral leaflet is immobile because of rigidity and calcification, even in the presence of predominant mitral stenosis.

Splitting of the two high-pitched components of S_1 by 10–30 ms is a normal phenomenon (Fig. 9-1A). The first component of S_1 is usually attributed to mitral valve closure, and the second to tricuspid valve closure. Widening of the S_1 is due most often to complete right bundle branch block and the resulting delay in onset of the right ventricular pressure pulse.

Splitting of the Second Heart Sound

This sound (S_2) normally splits into audibly distinct aortic (A_2) and pulmonic (P_2) components during inspiration, when the augmented inflow into the right ventricle increases its stroke volume and ejection period and thus delays closure of the pulmonic valve. P_2 is coincident with the incisura of the pulmonary artery pressure curve, which is separated from the right ventricular pressure tracing by an interval termed the *hangout time*. The absolute value of this interval reflects the resistance to pulmonary vascular bed. This interval is prolonged, and physiologic splitting of S_2 is accentuated, in conditions associated with right ventricular volume overload and a distensible pulmonary vascular bed. However, in patients with an increase in pulmonary vascular resistance, the hangout time is markedly reduced, and narrow splitting of S_2 is present. Splitting that persists with expiration (heard best at the pulmonic area or left sternal border) is usually abnormal when the patient is in the upright position. Such splitting may be due to many causes: delayed activation of the right ventricle (right bundle branch block); left ventricular ectopic beats; a left ventricular pacemaker; prolongation of right ventricular contraction with an increased right ventricular pressure load (pulmonary embolism or pulmonic stenosis); or delayed pulmonic valve closure because of right ventricular volume overload associated with right ventricular failure or diminished impedance of the pulmonary vascular bed and a prolonged hangout time [atrial septal defect (ASD)].

In pulmonary hypertension, P_2 is loud, and splitting of S_2 may be diminished, normal, or accentuated, depending on the cause of the pulmonary hypertension, the pulmonary vascular resistance, and the presence or absence of right ventricular decompensation. Early aortic valve closure, occurring with mitral regurgitation or a VSD, may also produce splitting that persists during expiration. In patients with an ASD, the proportion of right atrial filling contributed by the left atrium and the venae cavae varies reciprocally during the respiratory cycle, so that right atrial inflow remains relatively constant. Therefore, the volume and duration of right ventricular ejection are not significantly increased by inspiration, and there is little inspiratory exaggeration of the splitting of S_2. The phenomenon, termed *fixed splitting* of the second heart sound, is of considerable diagnostic value.

A delay in aortic valve closure causing P_2 to precede A_2 results in so-called reversed (paradoxic) splitting of S_2. Splitting is then maximal in expiration and decreases during inspiration with the normal delay of pulmonic valve closure. The most common causes of reversed splitting of S_2 are left bundle branch block and delayed excitation of the left ventricle from a right ventricular ectopic beat. Mechanical prolongation of left ventricular systole, resulting in reversed splitting of S_2, may also be caused by severe aortic outflow obstruction, a large aorta-to-pulmonary artery shunt, systolic hypertension, and ischemic heart disease or cardiomyopathy with left ventricular failure. P_2 is normally softer than A_2 in the second left intercostal space; a P_2 that is greater than A_2 in this area suggests pulmonary hypertension (except in patients with ASD).

Systolic Sounds

The *ejection sound* (ES) is a sharp, high-pitched event occurring in early systole and closely following the first heart sound (Fig. 9-1B). Ejection sounds occur in the presence of semilunar valve stenosis and in conditions associated with dilation of the aorta or pulmonary artery. *Nonejection clicks*, or *midsystolic clicks*, occurring with or without a late systolic murmur, often denote prolapse of one or both leaflets of the mitral valve (Chap. 20). They probably result from chordae tendineae that are functionally unequal in length and are best heard along the lower left sternal border and at the left ventricular apex. Systolic clicks usually occur later than the systolic ejection sound.

Diastolic Sounds

The *opening snap* (OS) (Fig. 9-1A) is a brief, high-pitched, early diastolic sound, which is usually due to stenosis of an AV valve, most often the mitral valve. It is generally heard best at the lower left sternal border and radiates well to the base of the heart. The A_2-OS interval is inversely related to the height of the mean left atrial pressure and ranges from 0.04–0.12 s. The OS of tricuspid stenosis occurs later in diastole than the mitral

OS and is often overlooked. A tumor plop in patients with left atrial myxoma may have the timing of an opening snap, but it is usually lower-pitched.

The *third heart sound* (S$_3$) (Fig. 9-1*A*) is a low-pitched sound produced in the ventricle 0.14–0.16 s after A$_2$, at the termination of rapid filling. This sound is frequent in normal children and in patients with high cardiac output. However, in patients older than 40 years, an S$_3$ usually indicates impairment of ventricular function, AV valve regurgitation, or other conditions that increase the rate or volume of ventricular filling. The left-sided S$_3$ is best heard with the bell piece of the stethoscope at the left ventricular apex during expiration and with the patient in the left lateral position. The right-sided S$_3$ is best heard at the left sternal border or just beneath the xiphoid and is usually louder with inspiration. Third heart sounds often disappear with treatment of heart failure. An S$_3$ that is earlier (0.10–0.12 s after A$_2$) and higher-pitched than normal (a pericardial knock) often occurs in patients with constrictive pericarditis (Chap. 22); its presence depends on the restrictive effect of the adherent pericardium, which abruptly halts diastolic filling.

The *fourth heart sound* (S$_4$) (Fig. 9-1*A*) is a low-pitched, presystolic sound produced in the ventricle during ventricular filling; it is associated with an effective atrial contraction and is best heard with the bell piece of the stethoscope. The sound is absent in patients with atrial fibrillation. The S$_4$ occurs when diminished ventricular compliance increases the resistance to ventricular filling; it is frequently present in patients with systemic hypertension, aortic stenosis, hypertrophic cardiomyopathy, ischemic heart disease, and acute mitral regurgitation. Most patients with an acute myocardial infarction and sinus rhythm have an audible S$_4$. The S$_4$ is loudest at the left ventricular apex when the patient is in the left lateral position and is accentuated by mild isotonic or isometric exercise in the supine position. The right-sided S$_4$ is present in patients with right ventricular hypertrophy secondary to either pulmonic stenosis or pulmonary hypertension and frequently accompanies a prominent presystolic *a* wave in the JVP. An S$_4$ frequently accompanies delayed AV conduction, even in the absence of clinically detectable heart disease. The incidence of an audible S$_4$ increases with increasing age. Whether an audible S$_4$ in adults without other evidence of cardiac disease is abnormal remains controversial.

HEART MURMURS

(See also Chap. 10) The evaluation of the patient with a heart murmur may vary greatly depending on its intensity, timing, location and radiation, and response to various physiologic maneuvers. The intensity (loudness) of murmurs may be graded from I to VI. A grade I murmur is so faint that it can be heard only with special effort; a grade IV murmur is commonly accompanied by a thrill; and a grade VI murmur is audible with the stethoscope

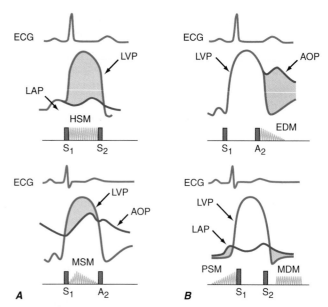

FIGURE 9-4

A. Schematic representation of ECG, aortic pressure (AOP), left ventricular pressure (LVP), and left atrial pressure (LAP). The shaded areas indicate a transvalvular pressure difference during systole. HSM, holosystolic murmur; MSM, midsystolic murmur. *B.* Graphic representation of ECG, aortic pressure (AOP), left ventricular pressure (LVP), and left atrial pressure (LAP) with shaded areas indicating transvalvular diastolic pressure difference. EDM, early diastolic murmur; PSM, presystolic murmur; MDM, mid-diastolic murmur.

removed from contact with the chest. The configuration of a murmur may be crescendo, decrescendo, crescendo-decrescendo (diamond-shaped), or plateau (**Fig. 9-4**). The precise time of onset and time of cessation of a murmur depend on the instant in the cardiac cycle at which an adequate pressure difference between two chambers arises and disappears.

The location on the chest wall where the murmur is best heard and the areas to which it radiates can aid in identifying the cardiac structure from which the murmur originates. For example, the murmur of aortic valve stenosis is usually loudest in the second right intercostal space and radiates to the carotid arteries. By contrast, the murmur of mitral regurgitation is most often loudest at the cardiac apex, but it may radiate to the left sternal border and base of the heart when the posterior mitral leaflet is predominantly involved or to the axilla and back when the anterior leaflet is more severely affected.

Effects of Physiologic Interventions

By noting changes in the characteristics of the murmur during maneuvers that alter cardiac hemodynamics, its correct origin and significance can usually be identified (**Table 9-1**).

TABLE 9-1

EFFECTS OF PHYSIOLOGIC AND PHARMACOLOGIC INTERVENTIONS ON THE INTENSITY OF HEART MURMURS AND SOUNDS

Respiration   Systolic murmurs due to TR or pulmonic blood flow through a normal or stenotic valve and diastolic murmurs of TS or PR generally increase with inspiration, as do right-sided S_3 and S_4. Left-sided murmurs and sounds usually are louder during expiration, as is the PES.

Valsalva maneuver   Most murmurs decrease in length and intensity. Two exceptions are the systolic murmur of HCM, which usually becomes much louder, and that of MVP, which becomes longer and often louder. Following release of the Valsalva maneuver, right-sided murmurs tend to return to control intensity earlier than left-sided murmurs.

After VPB or AF   Murmurs originating at normal or stenotic semilunar valves increase in the cardiac cycle following a VPB or in the cycle after a long cycle length in AF. By contrast, systolic murmurs due to AV valve regurgitation either do not change, diminish (papillary muscle dysfunction), or become shorter (MVP).

Positional changes   With *standing*, most murmurs diminish, two exceptions being the murmur of HCM, which becomes louder, and that of MVP, which lengthens and often is intensified. With *squatting*, most murmurs become louder, but those of HCM and MVP usually soften and may disappear. Passive leg raising usually produces the same results.

Exercise   Murmurs due to blood flow across normal or obstructed valves (e.g., PS, MS) become louder with both isotonic and submaximal isometric (handgrip) exercise. Murmurs of MR, VSD, and AR also increase with handgrip exercise. However, the murmur of HCM often decreases with near maximum handgrip exercise. Left-sided S4 and S3 are often accentuated by exercise, particularly when due to ischemic heart disease.

Note: TR, tricuspid regurgitation; TS, tricuspid stenosis; PR, pulmonic regurgitation; HCM, hypertrophic cardiomyopathy; MVP, mitral valve prolapse; PS, pulmonic stenosis; MS, mitral stenosis; MR, mitral regurgitation; PES, pulmonic ejection sound; VSD, ventricular septal defect; AR, aortic regurgitation; VPB, ventricular premature beat; AF, atrial fibrillation.

Systolic Murmurs

Holosystolic (Pansystolic) Murmurs

These are generated when there is flow between two chambers that have widely different pressures throughout systole, such as the left ventricle and either the left atrium or the right ventricle. The pressure gradient occurs early in contraction and lasts until relaxation is almost complete. Therefore, holosystolic murmurs begin before aortic ejection, and at the area of maximal intensity they begin with S_1 and end after S_2. Holosystolic murmurs accompany mitral or tricuspid regurgitation and VSD.

The murmur of tricuspid regurgitation associated with pulmonary hypertension is holosystolic and frequently increases during inspiration. Not all patients with mitral or tricuspid regurgitation or VSD have holosystolic murmurs. Often, a mild valvular regurgitant jet, detected by color-flow Doppler techniques (Chap. 12), is not associated with an audible murmur.

Midsystolic Murmurs

These are also called *systolic ejection murmurs*, which are often crescendo-decrescendo in shape and occur when blood is ejected across the aortic or pulmonic outflow tracts (Fig. 9-4). The murmur starts shortly after S_1, when the ventricular pressure becomes high enough to open the semilunar valve. As the velocity of ejection increases, the murmur gets louder; as ejection declines, it diminishes. The murmur ends before the ventricular pressure falls enough to permit closure of the aortic or pulmonic leaflets. When the semilunar valves are normal, an increased flow rate (as occurs in states of elevated cardiac output), ejection into a dilated vessel beyond the valve, or increased transmission of sound through a thin chest wall may be responsible for this murmur. Most benign, functional murmurs are midsystolic and originate from the pulmonary outflow tract. Valvular or subvalvular obstruction of either ventricle may also cause such a midsystolic murmur, the intensity being related to the flow rate.

The murmur of aortic stenosis is the prototype of the left-sided midsystolic murmur. The location and radiation of this murmur are influenced by the direction of the high-velocity jet within the aortic root. In *valvular aortic stenosis*, the murmur is usually maximal in the second right intercostal space, with radiation into the neck. The murmur may disappear over the sternum and reappear at the apex, leaving a false impression that mitral regurgitation is present (Gallavardin Phenomenon). In hypertrophic cardiomyopathy, the midsystolic murmur originates in the left ventricular cavity and is usually maximal at the lower left sternal edge and apex, with relatively little radiation to the carotids. When the aortic valve is immobile (calcified), the aortic closure sound (A_2) may be soft and inaudible so that the length and configuration of the murmur are difficult to determine.

The patient's age and the area of maximal intensity aid in determining the significance of midsystolic murmurs. Thus, in a young adult with a thin chest and a high velocity of blood flow, a faint or moderate midsystolic murmur heard only in the pulmonic area is usually without clinical significance, while a somewhat louder murmur in the aortic area may indicate congenital aortic stenosis. In elderly patients, pulmonic flow murmurs are rare, while aortic systolic murmurs are common and may be due to aortic dilation, a significant degree of valvular aortic stenosis, or nonstenotic thickening of the aortic valve leaflets. Midsystolic aortic and pulmonic murmurs are intensified during the cardiac cycle following a premature ventricular beat, while those due to mitral regurgitation are unchanged or softer. Echocardiography may be necessary to separate a prominent and exaggerated functional murmur from one due to congenital or acquired semilunar valve stenosis.

Early Systolic Murmurs

These murmurs begin with the first heart sound and end in midsystole. In *large VSDs with pulmonary hypertension*, the shunting at the end of systole may be small or absent, resulting in an early systolic murmur. A similar murmur may occur with very small *muscular VSDs*. An early systolic murmur is a feature of *tricuspid regurgitation occurring in the absence of pulmonary hypertension*, a lesion that is common in narcotics abusers with infective endocarditis. Patients with acute mitral regurgitation into a noncompliant left atrium and a large *v* wave often have a loud early systolic murmur that diminishes as the pressure gradient between the left ventricle and left atrium decreases the late systole (Chap. 20).

Late Systolic Murmurs

These murmurs are faint or moderately loud, high-pitched apical murmurs that start well after ejection and do not mask either heart sound. They are probably related to papillary muscle dysfunction caused by infarction or ischemia of these muscles or to their distortion by left ventricular dilation. They may appear only during angina but are common in patients with myocardial infarction or diffuse myocardial disease. Late systolic murmurs following midsystolic clicks are due to late systolic mitral regurgitation caused by prolapse of the mitral valve into the left atrium (Chap. 20).

Diastolic Murmurs

Early Diastolic Murmurs

These murmurs begin with or shortly after S_2, as soon as the corresponding ventricular pressure falls enough below that in the aorta or pulmonary artery. The high-pitched murmurs of aortic regurgitation or of pulmonic regurgitation due to pulmonary hypertension are generally decrescendo, since there is a progressive decline in the volume or rate of regurgitation during diastole. Faint, high-pitched murmurs of aortic regurgitation are difficult to hear unless they are specifically sought by applying firm pressure with the diaphragm over the left midsternal border while the patient sits leaning forward and holds a breath in full expiration. The diastolic murmur of aortic regurgitation is enhanced by an acute elevation of the arterial pressure, such as occurs with handgrip.

Mid-diastolic Murmurs

These murmurs usually arise from the mitral or tricuspid valves, occur during early ventricular filling, and are due to disproportion between valve orifice sizes and flow rate. Such murmurs may be quite loud (grade III/VI), despite only slight AV valve stenosis, when there is normal or increased blood flow. Conversely, the murmurs may be soft or even absent despite severe obstruction if the cardiac output is markedly reduced. When stenosis is marked, the diastolic murmur is prolonged, and the duration of the murmur is more reliable than its intensity as an index of the severity of valve obstruction.

The low-pitched, mid-diastolic murmur of mitral stenosis characteristically follows the OS. It should be specifically sought by placing the bell of the stethoscope at the site of the left ventricular impulse, which is best localized with the patient on the left side. Frequently, the murmur of mitral stenosis is present only at the left ventricular apex, and it may be increased in intensity by mild supine exercise. In tricuspid stenosis, the mid-diastolic murmur is localized to a relatively limited area along the left sternal edge and may be louder during inspiration.

Mid-diastolic murmurs may be generated across the mitral valve in cases of mitral regurgitation, patent ductus arteriosus, or VSD, and across the tricuspid valve in cases of tricuspid regurgitation or ASD. These murmurs are related to the very rapid flow across an AV valve, usually follow an S_3, and tend to occur with large left-to-right shunts or severe AV valve regurgitation.

In acute, severe aortic regurgitation, the left ventricular diastolic pressure may exceed the left atrial pressure, resulting in a mid-diastolic murmur due to "diastolic mitral regurgitation." In severe, chronic aortic regurgitation, a murmur is frequently present that may be either mid-diastolic or presystolic (Austin-Flint murmur). This murmur appears to originate at the anterior mitral valve leaflet when blood enters the left ventricle simultaneously from both the aortic root and the left atrium.

Presystolic Murmurs

These murmurs begin during the period of ventricular filling that follows atrial contraction and therefore occur in sinus rhythm. They are usually due to AV valve stenosis and have the same quality as the mid-diastolic-filling rumble, but they are usually crescendo, reaching peak intensity at the time of a loud S_1. The presystolic murmur corresponds to the AV valve gradient, which may be minimal until the moment of right or left atrial contraction. It is the presystolic murmur that is most characteristic of tricuspid stenosis and sinus rhythm. A right or left *atrial myxoma* may occasionally cause either mid-diastolic or presystolic murmurs that resemble the murmurs of mitral or tricuspid stenosis.

Continuous Murmurs

These murmurs begin in systole, peak near S_2, and continue into all or part of diastole. They result from continuous flow due to a communication between high- and low-pressure areas that persists through the end of systole and the beginning of diastole. A *patent ductus arteriosus* causes a continuous murmur as long as the pressure in the pulmonary artery is much below that in the aorta. When pulmonary hypertension is present, the diastolic portion may disappear, leaving the murmur confined to systole. Surgically produced connections and the subclavian-pulmonary artery anastomosis result in murmurs similar to that of a patent ductus.

Continuous murmurs may result from congenital or acquired *systemic arteriovenous fistula, coronary arteriovenous fistula,* anomalous origin of the left coronary artery from the pulmonary artery, and *communications between the sinus of Valsalva and the right side of the heart.* Murmurs associated with *pulmonary arteriovenous fistulas* may be continuous but are usually only systolic. Continuous murmurs may also be due to disturbances of flow pattern in constricted systemic (e.g., renal) or pulmonary arteries when marked pressure differences between the two sides of the narrow segment persist; a continuous murmur in the back may be present in *coarctation of the aorta; pulmonary embolism* may cause continuous murmurs in partially occluded vessels.

The "mammary souffle," an innocent murmur heard over the breasts during late pregnancy and in the early postpartum period, may be systolic or continuous. The innocent cervical venous hum is a continuous murmur usually audible over the medial aspect of the right supraclavicular fossa with the patient upright. The hum is usually louder during diastole and can be abolished instantaneously by digital compression of the ipsilateral internal jugular vein. Transmission of a loud venous hum to the area below the clavicles may result in a mistaken diagnosis of patent ductus arteriosus.

Pericardial Friction Rub

(See also Chap. 22) These adventitious sounds may have presystolic, systolic, and early diastolic scratchy components and may be confused with a murmur or extracardiac sound when heard only in systole. A pericardial friction rub is best appreciated with the patient upright and leaning forward and may be accentuated during expiration.

FURTHER READINGS

BRAUNWALD E, PERLOFF JK: Physical examination of the heart and circulation, in *Braunwald's Heart Disease*, 7th ed, D Zipes et al (eds). Philadelphia, Saunders, 2005

GOSWAMI MJ et al: The history, physical examination and cardiac auscultation, in *Hurst's The Heart Manual of Cardiology*, 11th ed, RA O'Rourke et al (eds). New York, McGraw Hill, 2006

JAVHAR S: The demise of the physical exam. N Engl J Med 354:548, 2006

MARKEL H: The stethoscope and the art of listening. N Engl J Med 354:551, 2006

O'ROURKE RA: Approach to a patient with a heart murmur, in *Primary Cardiology*, 2d ed, E Braunwald, L Goldman (eds). Philadelphia, Saunders, 2003

PERLOFF JK (ed): *Physical Examination of the Heart and Circulation*, 3d ed. Philadelphia, Saunders, 2000

VLACHOPOULOUS C, O'ROURKE MF: Genesis of the normal and abnormal arterial pulse. Curr Probl Cardiol 25:297, 2000

CHAPTER 10

APPROACH TO THE PATIENT WITH A HEART MURMUR

Patrick T. O'Gara ■ Eugene Braunwald

The differential diagnosis of a heart murmur begins with a careful assessment of its major attributes and response to bedside maneuvers. The history, clinical context, and associated findings provide additional clues by which the significance of a heart murmur is established. Following completion of these initial steps, noninvasive testing can be pursued to clarify any remaining ambiguity and to provide additional anatomic and physiologic information that will impact patient management. Accurate bedside identification of a heart murmur can also inform decisions regarding referral to a cardiovascular specialist, the indications for antibiotic or rheumatic fever prophylaxis, and the need to restrict various forms of physical activity.

Heart murmurs are caused by audible vibrations that are due to increased turbulence from accelerated blood flow through normal or abnormal orifices; flow through a narrowed or irregular orifice into a dilated vessel or chamber; or backward flow through an incompetent valve, ventricular septal defect, or patent ductus arteriosus. They are traditionally defined in terms of their timing within the cardiac cycle (Fig. 10-1). *Systolic murmurs* begin with or after the first heart sound (S_1) and terminate at or before the component (A_2 or P_2) of the second

heart sound (S_2) that corresponds to their side of origin (left or right, respectively). *Diastolic murmurs* begin with or after the associated component of S_2 and end at or before the subsequent S_1. *Continuous murmurs* are not confined to either phase of the cardiac cycle, but rather begin in early systole and proceed through S_2 into all or part of diastole. The accurate timing of heart murmurs is the first step in their identification. The distinction between S_1 and S_2, and therefore systole and diastole, is usually a straightforward process, but can be difficult in the setting of a tachyarrhythmia, in which case the heart sounds can be distinguished by simultaneous palpation of the carotid arterial pulse. The upstroke should closely follow S_1.

DURATION

The duration of a heart murmur depends on the length of time in the cardiac cycle over which a pressure difference exists between two cardiac chambers, the left ventricle and the aorta, the right ventricle and the pulmonary artery, or the great vessels. The magnitude and variability of this pressure difference dictate the velocity of flow; the degree of turbulence; and the resulting frequency, configuration,

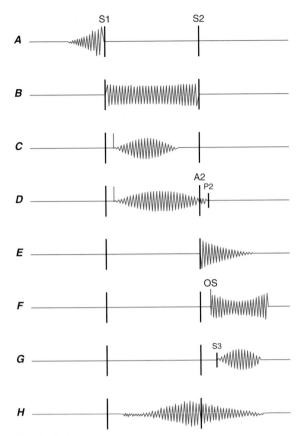

FIGURE 10-1

Diagram depicting principal heart murmurs. A. Presystolic murmur of mitral or tricuspid stenosis. **B.** Holosystolic (pansystolic) murmur of mitral or tricuspid regurgitation or of ventricular septal defect. **C.** Aortic ejection murmur beginning with an ejection click and fading before the second heart sound. **D.** Systolic murmur in pulmonic stenosis spilling through the aortic second sound, pulmonic valve closure being delayed. **E.** Aortic or pulmonary diastolic murmur. **F.** Long diastolic murmur of mitral stenosis following the opening snap. **G.** Short mid-diastolic inflow murmur following a third heart sound. **H.** Continuous murmur of patent ductus arteriosus. *(Adapted from P Wood, Diseases of the Heart and Circulation, London, Eyre & Spottiswood, Ltd.,1968.)*

and intensity of the murmur. The diastolic murmur of chronic aortic regurgitation (AR) is a blowing, high-frequency event, whereas the murmur of mitral stenosis (MS), indicative of the left atrial–left ventricular diastolic pressure gradient, is a low-frequency event, heard as a rumbling sound with the bell of the stethoscope. The frequency components of a heart murmur may vary at different sites of auscultation. The coarse systolic murmur of aortic stenosis (AS) may sound higher-pitched and more acoustically pure at the apex, a phenomenon eponymously referred to as the *Gallavardin effect*. Some murmurs may have a distinct or unusual quality, such as the "honking" sound appreciated in some patients with mitral regurgitation (MR) due to mitral valve prolapse (MVP).

The configuration of a heart murmur may be crescendo, decrescendo, crescendo-decrescendo, or plateau. The decrescendo configuration of the murmur of chronic AR (Fig. 10-1*E*) can be understood in terms of the progressive decline in the diastolic pressure gradient between the aorta and the left ventricle. The crescendo-decrescendo configuration of the murmur of AS reflects the changes in the systolic pressure gradient between the left ventricle and the aorta as ejection occurs, whereas the plateau configuration of the murmur of chronic rheumatic MR (Fig. 10-1*B*) is consistent with the large and nearly constant pressure difference between the left ventricle and the left atrium.

INTENSITY

The intensity of a heart murmur is graded on a scale of 1–6 (or I–VI). A grade 1 murmur is very soft and is heard with great effort. A grade 2 murmur is easily heard, but not particularly loud. A grade 3 murmur is loud, but is not accompanied by a palpable thrill over the site of maximal intensity. A grade 4 murmur is very loud and accompanied by a thrill. A grade 5 murmur is loud enough to be heard with only the edge of the stethoscope touching the chest, whereas a grade 6 murmur is loud enough to be heard with the stethoscope slightly off the chest. Murmurs of grade 3 or greater intensity usually signify important structural heart disease and indicate high blood flow velocity at the site of murmur production. Small ventricular septal defects (VSDs), for example, are accompanied by loud, usually grade 4 or greater, systolic murmurs as blood is ejected at high velocity from the left to the right ventricle. Low velocity events, such as left-to-right shunting across an atrial septal defect (ASD), are usually silent. The intensity of a heart murmur may also be diminished by any process that increases the distance between the intracardiac source and the stethoscope on the chest wall, such as obesity, obstructive lung disease, and a large pericardial effusion. The intensity of a murmur may also be misleadingly soft when cardiac output is significantly reduced.

LOCATION AND RADIATION

Recognition of the location and radiation of the murmur helps facilitate its accurate identification (**Fig. 10-2**). Adventitious sounds, such as a systolic click or diastolic snap, or abnormalities of S_1 or S_2, may provide additional clues. Careful attention to the characteristics of the murmur and other heart sounds during the respiratory cycle and the performance of simple bedside maneuvers when indicated complete the auscultatory examination. These features, and recommendations for further testing, are discussed below in the context of specific systolic, diastolic, and continuous heart murmurs (**Table 10-1**).

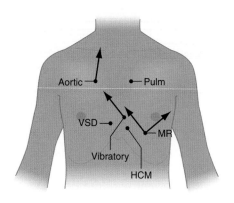

FIGURE 10-2

Maximal intensity and radiation of six isolated systolic murmurs. HOCM, hypertrophic obstructive cardiomyopathy; MR, mitral regurgitation; Pulm, pulmonary stenosis; Aortic, aortic stenosis; VSD, ventricular septal defect. *(From JB Barlow, Perspectives on the Mitral Valve. Philadelphia, FA Davis, 1987, p 140.)*

SYSTOLIC HEART MURMURS

Early Systolic Murmurs

Early systolic murmurs begin with S_1 and extend for a variable period of time, ending well before S_2. Their causes are relatively few in number. *Acute severe MR* into a normal-sized, relatively noncompliant left atrium results in an early, decrescendo systolic murmur best heard at or just medial to the apical impulse. These characteristics reflect the progressive attenuation of the pressure gradient between the left ventricle and the left atrium during systole due to the rapid rise in left atrial pressure caused by the sudden volume load into an unprepared chamber, and contrast sharply with the auscultatory features of chronic MR. Clinical settings in which acute, severe MR occur include: (1) papillary muscle rupture complicating acute myocardial infarction (MI) (Chap. 35), (2) rupture of chordae tendineae in the setting of myxomatous mitral valve disease (MVP, Chap. 20), (3) infective endocarditis (Chap. 25), and (4) blunt chest wall trauma.

Acute, severe MR from papillary muscle rupture usually accompanies an inferior, posterior, or lateral MI and occurs 2–7 days after presentation. It is often signaled by chest pain, hypotension, and pulmonary edema, but a murmur may be absent in up to 50% of cases. The posteromedial papillary muscle is involved 6–10 times more frequently than the anterolateral papillary muscle. The murmur is to be distinguished from that associated with post-MI ventricular septal rupture, which is accompanied by a systolic thrill at the left sternal border in nearly all patients and is holosystolic in duration. A new heart murmur following MI is an indication for transthoracic echocardiography (TTE) (Chap. 12), which

allows bedside delineation of its etiology and pathophysiologic significance. The distinction between acute MR and ventricular septal rupture can also be achieved with right heart catheterization, sequential determination of oxygen saturations, and analysis of the pressure waveforms (tall *v* wave in the pulmonary artery wedge pressure in MR). Post-MI mechanical complications of this nature mandate aggressive medical stabilization and prompt referral for surgical repair.

Spontaneous chordal rupture can complicate the course of myxomatous mitral valve disease (MVP) and result in new-onset or "acute on chronic" severe MR. MVP may occur as an isolated phenomenon or the lesion may be part of a more generalized connective tissue disorder as seen, for example, in patients with Marfan syndrome. Acute severe MR as a consequence of infective endocarditis results from destruction of leaflet tissue, chordal rupture, or both. Blunt chest wall trauma is usually self-evident, but may be disarmingly trivial. It can result in papillary muscle contusion and rupture, chordal detachment, or leaflet avulsion. TTE is indicated in all cases of suspected acute severe MR to define its mechanism and severity, delineate left ventricular size and systolic function, and provide an assessment of suitability for primary valve repair.

A congenital, small muscular VSD (Chap. 19) may be associated with an early systolic murmur. The defect closes progressively during septal contraction and thus the murmur is confined to early systole. It is localized to the left sternal border (Fig. 10-2) and is usually of grade 4 or 5 intensity. Signs of pulmonary hypertension or left ventricular volume overload are absent. Anatomically large and uncorrected VSDs, which usually involve the membranous portion of the septum, may lead to pulmonary hypertension. The murmur associated with the left-to-right shunt, which may earlier have been holosystolic, becomes limited to the first portion of systole as the elevated pulmonary vascular resistance leads to an abrupt rise in right ventricular pressure and an attenuation of the interventricular pressure gradient during the remainder of the cardiac cycle. In such instances, signs of pulmonary hypertension (right ventricular lift, loud and single or closely split S_2) may predominate. The murmur is best heard along the left sternal border but is softer. Suspicion of a VSD is an indication for TTE.

Tricuspid regurgitation (TR) with normal pulmonary artery pressures, as may occur with infective endocarditis, may produce an early systolic murmur. The murmur is soft (grade 1 or 2), best heard at the lower left sternal border, and may increase in intensity with inspiration (Carvallo's sign). Regurgitant "*c-v*" waves may be visible in the jugular venous pulse (JVP). TR in this setting is not associated with signs of right heart failure.

TABLE 10-1

PRINCIPAL CAUSES OF HEART MURMURS

Systolic Murmurs

Early systolic
  Mitral
  Acute MR
  VSD
  Muscular
  Nonrestrictive with pulmonary hypertension
  Tricuspid
  TR with normal pulmonary artery pressure
Midsystolic
  Aortic
  Obstructive
  Supravalvular—supravalvular aortic stenosis, coarctation of the aorta
  Valvular—AS and aortic sclerosis
  Subvalvular—discrete, tunnel or HOCM
  Increased flow, hyperkinetic states, AR, complete heart block
  Dilatation of ascending aorta, atheroma, aortitis
  Pulmonary
  Obstructive
  Supravalvular—pulmonary artery stenosis
  Valvular—pulmonic valve stenosis
  Subvalvular—infundibular stenosis (dynamic)
  Increased flow, hyperkinetic states, left-to-right shunt (e.g., ASD)
  Dilatation of pulmonary artery
Late systolic
  Mitral
  MVP, acute myocardial ischemia
  Tricuspid
  TVP
  Holosystolic
  Atrioventricular valve regurgitation (MR, TR)
  Left-to-right shunt at ventricular level (VSD)

Diastolic Murmurs

Early diastolic
  Aortic regurgitation
  Valvular: congenital (bicuspid valve), rheumatic deformity, endocarditis, prolapse, trauma,
    post-valvulotomy
  Dilatation of valve ring: aorta dissection, annulo-aortic ectasia, cystic medial degeneration,
    hypertension, ankylosing spondylitis
  Widening of commissures: syphilis
  Pulmonic regurgitation
  Valvular: post-valvulotomy, endocarditis, rheumatic fever, carcinoid
  Dilatation of valve ring: pulmonary hypertension; Marfan syndrome
  Congenital: isolated or associated with tetralogy of Fallot, VSD, pulmonic stenosis
Mid-diastolic
  Mitral
  Mitral stenosis
  Carey-Coombs murmur (mid-diastolic apical murmur in acute rheumatic fever)
  Increased flow across nonstenotic mitral valve (e.g., MR, VSD, PDA, high-output states, and
    complete heart block)
  Tricuspid
  Tricuspid stenosis
  Increased flow across nonstenotic tricuspid valve (e.g., TR, ASD, and anomalous pulmonary
    venous return)
  Left and right atrial tumors (myxoma)
  Severe AR (Austin Flint murmur)

(Continued)

CHAPTER 10 Approach to the Patient with a Heart Murmur

TABLE 10-1 *(CONTINUED)*

PRINCIPAL CAUSES OF HEART MURMURS

Continuous Murmurs

Patent ductus arteriosus	Proximal coronary artery stenosis
Coronary AV fistula	Mammary souffle of pregnancy
Ruptured sinus of Valsalva aneurysm	Pulmonary artery branch stenosis
Aortic septal defect	Bronchial collateral circulation
Cervical venous hum	Small (restrictive) ASD with MS
Anomalous left coronary artery	Intercostal AV fistula

Note: AR, aortic regurgitation; AS, aortic stenosis; ASD, atrial septal defect; AV, arteriovenous; HOCM, hypertrophic obstructive cardiomyopathy; MR, mitral regurgitation; MS, mitral stenosis; MVP, mitral valve prolapse; PDA, patent ductus arteriosus; TR, tricuspid regurgitation; TVP, tricuspid valve prolapse; VSD, ventricular septal defect.

Source: E Braunwald, JK Perloff, in D Zipes et al (eds): *Braunwald's Heart Disease*, 7th ed. Philadelphia, Elsevier, 2005; PJ Norton, RA O'Rourke, in E Braunwald, L Goldman (eds): *Primary Cardiology*, 2d ed. Philadelphia, Elsevier, 2003.

Midsystolic Murmurs

Midsystolic murmurs begin at a short interval following S_1, end before S_2 (Fig. 10-1C), and are usually crescendo-decrescendo in configuration. Aortic stenosis is the most common cause of a midsystolic murmur in an adult. The murmur of AS is usually loudest to the right of the sternum in the second intercostal space (aortic area, Fig. 10-2) and radiates into the carotids. Transmission of the midsystolic murmur to the apex, where it becomes higher pitched, is common (Gallavardin effect, see earlier in this chapter).

Differentiation of this apical systolic murmur from MR can be difficult. The murmur of AS will increase in intensity, or become louder, in the beat following a premature beat, whereas the murmur of MR will remain of constant intensity from beat to beat. The intensity of the AS murmur also varies directly with the cardiac output. With a normal cardiac output, a systolic thrill and grade 4 or higher murmur suggest severe AS. The murmur is softer in the setting of heart failure and low cardiac output. Other auscultatory findings of severe AS include a soft or absent A_2, paradoxical splitting of S_2, an apical S_4, and a late-peaking systolic murmur. In children, adolescents, and young adults with congenital valvular AS, an early ejection sound (click) is usually audible, more often along the left sternal border than at the base. Its presence signifies a flexible, noncalcified bicuspid valve (or one of its variants) and localizes the left ventricular outflow obstruction to the valvular (rather than sub- or supravalvular) level.

Assessment of the volume and rate of rise of the carotid pulse can provide additional information. A small and delayed upstroke (*parvus et tardus*) is consistent with severe AS. The carotid pulse examination is less discriminatory, however, in older patients with stiffened arteries.

The electrocardiogram (ECG) shows signs of left ventricular hypertrophy (LVH) as the severity of the stenosis increases. TTE is indicated to assess the anatomic features of the aortic valve, the severity of the stenosis, left ventricular size, wall thickness and function, and the size and contour of the aortic root and proximal ascending aorta.

The obstructive form of hypertrophic cardiomyopathy (HOCM) is associated with a midsystolic murmur that is usually loudest along the left sternal border or between the left lower sternal border and the apex (Chap. 21, Fig. 10-2). The murmur is produced by both dynamic left ventricular outflow tract obstruction and MR, and thus its configuration is a hybrid between ejection and regurgitant phenomena. The intensity of the murmur may vary from beat to beat, and following provocative maneuvers, but usually does not exceed grade 3. The murmur will classically increase in intensity with maneuvers that result in increasing degrees of outflow tract obstruction, such as a reduction in preload or afterload (Valsalva, standing, vasodilators) or to an augmentation of contractility (inotropic stimulation). Maneuvers that increase preload (squatting, passive leg raising, volume administration) or afterload (squatting, vasopressors) or that reduce contractility (β-adrenoreceptor blockers) decrease the intensity of the murmur. In rare patients, there may be reversed splitting of S_2. A sustained left ventricular apical impulse and an S_4 may be appreciated. In contrast to AS, the carotid upstroke is rapid and of normal volume. Rarely, it is bisferiens or bifid in contour (see Fig. 9-2D) due to midsystolic closure of the aortic valve. LVH is present on the ECG and the diagnosis is confirmed by TTE. Although the systolic murmur associated with MVP behaves similarly to that due to HOCM in response to the Valsalva maneuver and to standing/squatting (Fig. 10-3), the two lesions can be distinguished on the basis of their associated findings, such as the presence of LVH in HOCM or a non-ejection click in MVP.

The midsystolic, crescendo-decrescendo murmur of congenital pulmonic stenosis (PS, Chap. 19), is best appreciated in the second and third left intercostal spaces (pulmonic area) (Figs. 10-2 and 10-4). The duration of the murmur lengthens and the intensity of P_2 diminishes with increasing degrees of valvular stenosis (Fig. 10-1D). An early ejection sound, the intensity of which decreases with inspiration, is heard in younger patients. A parasternal lift and ECG evidence of right ventricular hypertrophy indicate severe pressure overload. If obtained, the chest x-ray may show poststenotic dilatation of the main pulmonary artery. TTE is recommended for complete characterization.

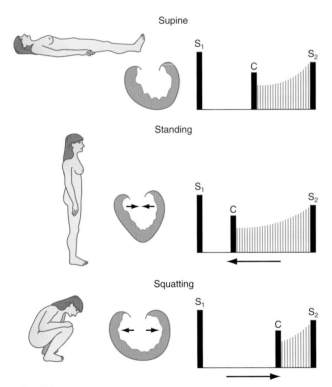

FIGURE 10-3

A midsystolic nonejection sound (C) occurs in mitral valve prolapse and is followed by a late systolic murmur that crescendos to the second heart sound (S_2). Standing decreases venous return; the heart becomes smaller; C moves closer to the first heart sound (S_1) and the mitral regurgitant murmur has an earlier onset. With prompt squatting, venous return increases; the heart becomes larger; C moves toward S_2, and the duration of the murmur shortens. *(From JA Shaver, JJ Leonard, DF Leon, Examination of the Heart, Part IV, Auscultation of the Heart. Dallas, American Heart Association, 1990, p 13. Copyright, American Heart Association.)*

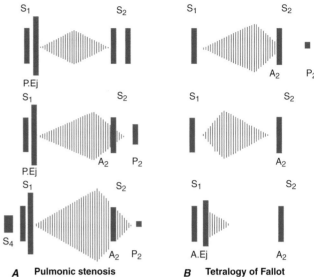

A Pulmonic stenosis   **B** Tetralogy of Fallot

FIGURE 10-4

A. In valvular pulmonic stenosis with intact ventricular septum, right ventricular systolic ejection becomes progressively longer, with increasing obstruction to flow. As a result, the murmur becomes longer and louder, enveloping the aortic component of the second heart sound (A_2). The pulmonic component (P_2) occurs later, and splitting becomes wider but more difficult to hear because A_2 is lost in the murmur and P_2 becomes progressively fainter and lower pitched. As the pulmonic gradient increases, isometric contraction shortens until the pulmonary valvular ejection sound fuses with the first heart sound (S_1). In severe pulmonic stenosis with concentric hypertrophy and decreasing right ventricular compliance, a fourth heart sound appears. **B.** In tetralogy of Fallot with increasing obstruction at pulmonic infundibular area, an increasing amount of right ventricular blood is shunted across the silent ventricular septal defect and flow across the obstructed outflow tract decreases. Therefore, with increasing obstruction the murmur becomes shorter, earlier, and fainter. P_2 is absent in severe tetralogy of Fallot. A large aortic root receives almost all cardiac output from both ventricular chambers, and the aorta dilates and is accompanied by a root ejection sound that does not vary with respiration. P.Ej, pulmonary ejection (valvular); A.Ej, aortic ejection (root). *(From JA Shaver, JJ Leonard, DF Leon, Examination of the Heart, Part IV, Auscultation of the Heart. Dallas, American Heart Association, 1990, p 45. Copyright, American Heart Association.)*

Significant left-to-right intracardiac shunting due to an ASD (Chap. 19) leads to an increase in pulmonary blood flow and a grade 2–3 midsystolic murmur at the mid- to upper left sternal border with fixed splitting of S_2. Ostium secundum ASDs are most common. Features suggestive of a primum ASD include the coexistence of MR due to a cleft anterior mitral valve leaflet and left axis deviation of the QRS complex on ECG. With sinus venosus ASDs, the left-to-right shunt is usually not large enough to result in a systolic murmur, though the ECG may show abnormalities of sinus node function. A grade 2 or 3 midsystolic murmur may also be heard best at the upper left sternal border in patients with idiopathic dilatation of the pulmonary artery. A pulmonary ejection sound is present. TTE is indicated to evaluate a grade 2 or 3 midsystolic murmur when there are other signs of cardiac disease.

An isolated grade 1 or 2 midsystolic murmur, heard in the absence of symptoms or signs of heart disease, is most often a benign finding for which no further evaluation, including TTE, is necessary. The most common example of a murmur of this type in an older adult patient is the crescendo-decrescendo murmur of aortic valve sclerosis, heard at the second right interspace (Fig. 10-2). Aortic sclerosis is defined as focal thickening and calcification of the aortic valve to a degree that does not interfere with leaflet opening. The carotid upstrokes are normal and electrocardiographic LVH is not present. A grade 1 or 2 midsystolic murmur can often be heard at the left sternal border with pregnancy, hyperthyroidism, or anemia, physiologic states that are associated with accelerated blood flow. *Still's murmur* refers to a benign grade 2, vibratory midsystolic murmur at the lower left sternal border in normal children and adolescents (Fig. 10-2).

Late Systolic Murmurs

A late systolic murmur that is best heard at the left ventricular apex is often due to MVP (Chap. 20). Often, this murmur is introduced by one or more nonejection clicks. The radiation of the murmur can help identify the specific mitral leaflet involved in the process of prolapse or flail. The term *flail* refers to the movement made by an unsupported portion of the leaflet after loss of its chordal attachment(s). With posterior leaflet prolapse or flail, the resultant jet of MR is directed anteriorly and medially, as a result of which the murmur radiates to the base of the heart and masquerades as AS. Anterior leaflet prolapse or flail results in a posteriorly directed MR jet that radiates to the axilla or left infrascapular region. Leaflet flail is associated with a murmur of grade 3 or 4 intensity that can be heard throughout the precordium in thin-chested patients. The presence of an S_3 or a short, rumbling mid-diastolic murmur, signifies severe MR.

Bedside maneuvers that decrease left ventricular preload, such as standing, will cause the click and murmur of MVP to move closer to the first heart sound, as leaflet prolapse occurs earlier in systole. Standing also causes the murmur to become louder and longer. With squatting, left ventricular preload and afterload are increased abruptly, and the click and murmur move away from the first heart sound, as leaflet prolapse is delayed. The murmur becomes softer and shorter in duration (Fig. 10-3). As noted above, the responses to standing and squatting are similar to those observed in patients with HOCM.

A late, apical systolic murmur indicative of MR may be heard transiently in the setting of acute myocardial ischemia. It is due to apical tethering and malcoaptation of the leaflets in response to structural and functional changes of the ventricle and mitral annulus. The intensity of the murmur varies as a function of left ventricular afterload and will increase in the setting of hypertension. TTE is recommended for assessment of late systolic murmurs.

Holosystolic Murmurs

(Figs. 10-1B and 10-5) Holosystolic murmurs begin with S_1 and continue through systole to S_2. They are usually indicative of chronic mitral or tricuspid valve regurgitation or a VSD, and warrant TTE for further characterization. The holosystolic murmur of chronic MR is best heard at the left ventricular apex and radiates to the axilla (Fig. 10-2). It is usually high pitched and plateau in configuration because of the wide difference between left ventricular and left atrial pressure throughout systole. In contrast to acute MR, left atrial compliance is normal or even increased in chronic MR. As a result, there is only a small increase in left atrial pressure for any increase in regurgitant volume.

There are several conditions associated with chronic MR and an apical holosystolic murmur, including rheumatic scarring of the leaflets, mitral annular calcification, and severe left ventricular chamber enlargement. The circumference of the mitral annulus increases as the left ventricle enlarges and leads to failure of leaflet coaptation with central MR in patients with dilated cardiomyopathy (Chap. 21). The severity of the MR is worsened by any contribution from apical displacement of the papillary muscles and leaflet tethering. Because the mitral annulus is contiguous with the left atrial endocardium, gradual enlargement of the left atrium from chronic MR will result in further stretching of the annulus and more MR and thus, "MR begets MR." Chronic severe MR results in enlargement and leftward displacement of the left ventricular apex beat and, in some patients, a diastolic filling complex as described previously.

The holosystolic murmur of chronic TR is generally softer than that of MR, is loudest at the left lower sternal border, and usually increases in intensity with inspiration (Carvallo's sign). Associated signs include "c-v" waves in the JVP, an enlarged and pulsatile liver, ascites, and peripheral edema. The abnormal jugular venous wave forms are the predominant finding and are very often seen in the absence of an audible murmur, despite Doppler echocardiographic verification of TR. Causes of primary TR include myxomatous disease (prolapse), endocarditis, rheumatic disease, carcinoid, Ebstein's anomaly, and chordal detachment following the performance of

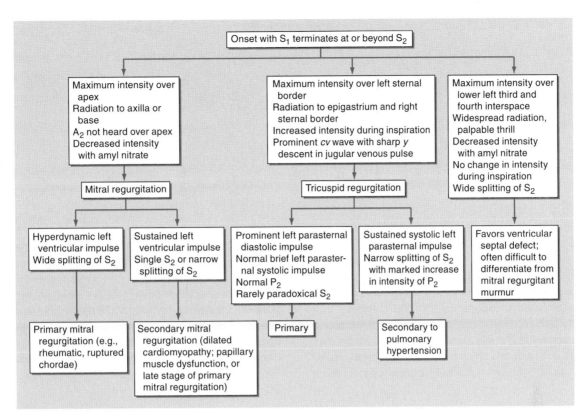

FIGURE 10-5
Differential diagnostic of a holosystolic murmur.

right ventricular endomyocardial biopsy. TR is more commonly a passive process that results secondarily from chronic elevations of pulmonary artery and right ventricular pressures, leading to right ventricular enlargement, annular dilatation, papillary muscle displacement, and failure of leaflet coaptation.

The holosystolic murmur of a VSD is loudest at the mid- to lower left sternal border (Fig. 10-2) and radiates widely. A thrill is present at the site of maximal intensity in the majority of patients. There is no change in the intensity of the murmur with inspiration. The intensity of the murmur varies as a function of the anatomic size of the defect. Small, restrictive VSDs, as exemplified by the *maladie de Roger*, create a very loud murmur due to the significant and sustained systolic pressure gradient between the left and right ventricles. With large defects, the ventricular pressures tend to equalize, shunt flow is balanced, and a murmur is not appreciated. The distinction between post-MI ventricular septal rupture and MR has been reviewed previously.

DIASTOLIC HEART MURMURS

Early Diastolic Murmurs

(Fig. 10-1*E*) Chronic AR results in a high-pitched, blowing, decrescendo, early to mid-diastolic murmur

that begins following the aortic component of S_2 (A_2) and is best heard at the second right interspace (**Fig. 10-6**). The murmur may be soft and difficult to hear, unless auscultation is performed with the patient leaning forward at end-expiration. This maneuver brings the aortic root closer to the anterior chest wall. Radiation of the murmur may provide a clue as to the cause of the AR. With primary valve disease, such as that due to congenital bicuspid disease, prolapse, or endocarditis, the diastolic murmur tends to radiate along the left sternal border. When AR is caused by aortic root disease, the diastolic murmur may radiate along the right sternal border. Diseases of the aortic root cause dilatation or distortion of the aortic annulus and failure of leaflet coaptation. Causes include Marfan syndrome with aneurysm formation, annulo-aortic ectasia, ankylosing spondylitis, and aortic dissection.

Chronic, severe AR may also produce a lower pitched mid- to late, grade 1 or 2 diastolic murmur at the apex (Austin Flint murmur), which is thought to reflect turbulence at the mitral inflow area from the admixture of regurgitant (aortic) and forward (mitral) blood flow (Fig. 10-1*G*). This lower pitched apical diastolic murmur can be distinguished from that due to MS by the absence of an opening snap and the response of the murmur to a vasodilator challenge. Lowering afterload with an agent such as amyl nitrite will decrease the

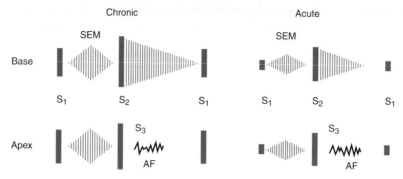

FIGURE 10-6

Contrast between the auscultatory findings in chronic and acute aortic regurgitation. In chronic aortic regurgitation, a prominent systolic ejection murmur resulting from the large forward stroke volume is heard at the base and the apex and ends well before the second heart sound (S_2). The aortic diastolic regurgitant murmur begins with S_2 and continues in a decrescendo fashion, terminating before the first heart sound (S_1). At the apex, the mid-diastolic component of Austin Flint murmur (AF) is introduced by a prominent third heart sound (S_3). A presystolic component of the AF is also heard. In acute aortic regurgitation there is a significant decrease in the intensity of the systolic ejection murmur compared with that of chronic aortic regurgitation because of the decreased forward stroke volume. S_1 is markedly decreased in intensity because of premature closure of the mitral valve, and at the apex the presystolic component of the AF murmur is absent. The early diastolic murmur at the base ends well before S_1 because of equilibration of the left ventricle and aortic end-diastolic pressure. Significant tachycardia is usually present. *(From JA Shaver: Heart Dis Stroke 2:100, 1994.)*

duration and magnitude of the aortic–left ventricular diastolic pressure gradient, and thus the Austin Flint murmur of severe AR will become shorter and softer. The intensity of the diastolic murmur of mitral stenosis (**Fig. 10-7**) may either remain constant or increase with afterload reduction because of the reflex increase in cardiac output and mitral valve flow.

Although AS and AR may coexist, a grade 2 or 3 crescendo-decrescendo midsystolic murmur is frequently heard at the base of the heart in patients with isolated severe AR, and is due to an increased volume and rate of systolic flow. Accurate bedside identification of coexistent AS can be difficult, unless the carotid pulse examination is abnormal or the midsystolic murmur is of grade 4 or greater intensity. In the absence of heart failure, chronic severe AR is accompanied by several peripheral signs of significant diastolic run-off, including a wide pulse pressure, a water-hammer carotid upstroke (Corrigan's pulse), and Quincke's pulsations of the nail beds. The diastolic murmur of *acute severe AR* (Fig. 10-6) is notably shorter in duration and lower pitched than the murmur of chronic AR. It can be very difficult to appreciate in the presence of a rapid heart rate. These attributes reflect the abrupt rate of rise of diastolic pressure within the unprepared and noncompliant left ventricle, and the correspondingly rapid decline in the aortic–left ventricular diastolic pressure gradient. Left ventricular diastolic pressure may increase sufficiently to result in premature closure of the mitral valve and a soft first heart sound. Peripheral signs of significant diastolic run-off are absent.

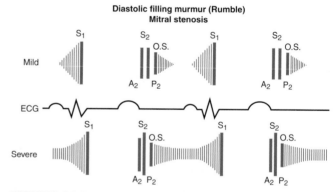

FIGURE 10-7

Diastolic filling murmur (rumble) in mitral stenosis. In mild mitral stenosis, the diastolic gradient across the valve is limited to the two phases of rapid ventricular filling in early diastole and presystole. The rumble may occur during either or both periods. As the stenotic process becomes severe, a large pressure gradient exists across the valve during the entire diastolic filling period, and the rumble persists throughout diastole. As the left atrial pressure becomes greater, the interval between A_2 and the opening snap shortens. In severe mitral stenosis, secondary pulmonary hypertension develops and results in a loud P_2 and the splitting interval usually narrows. ECG, electrocardiogram. *(From JA Shaver, JJ Leonard, DF Leon, Examination of the Heart, Part IV, Auscultation of the Heart. Dallas, American Heart Association, 1990, p 55. Copyright, American Heart Association.)*

Pulmonic regurgitation (PR) results in a decrescendo, early to mid-diastolic murmur (*Graham Steell murmur*) that begins after the pulmonic component of S_2 (P_2), is best heard at the second left interspace, and radiates along the left sternal border. The intensity of the murmur may increase with inspiration. PR is most commonly due to dilatation of the valve annulus from chronic elevation of the pulmonary artery pressure. Signs of pulmonary hypertension, including a right ventricular lift and a loud, single or narrowly split S_2, are present. These features also help distinguish PR from AR as the cause of a decrescendo diastolic murmur heard along the left sternal border. PR in the absence of pulmonary hypertension can occur with endocarditis or a congenitally deformed valve. It is usually present following repair of tetralogy of Fallot in childhood. When pulmonary hypertension is not present, the diastolic murmur is softer and lower pitched than the classic Graham Steell murmur, and the examiner can be misled as to the severity of the PR.

TTE is indicated for the further evaluation of the patient with an early to mid-diastolic murmur. Longitudinal assessment of the severity of the valve lesion and ventricular size and systolic function help guide the decision for surgical management. TTE can also provide anatomic information regarding the root and proximal ascending aorta, though computed tomographic or magnetic resonance angiography may be indicated for more precise characterization (Chap. 12).

Mid-Diastolic Murmurs

(Figs. 10-1*G* and 10-1*H*) Mid-diastolic murmurs result from obstruction and/or augmented flow at the level of the mitral or tricuspid valve. Rheumatic fever is the most common cause of MS (Fig. 10-7). In younger patients with pliable valves, S_1 is loud and the murmur begins after an opening snap, which is a high-pitched sound that occurs shortly after S_2. The distance between the pulmonic component of the second heart sound (P_2) and the opening snap is inversely related to the magnitude of the left atrial to left ventricular pressure gradient. The murmur of MS is low pitched and thus is best heard with the bell of the stethoscope. It is loudest at the left ventricular apex and often only appreciated when the patient is turned in the left lateral decubitus position. It is usually of grade 1 or 2 intensity, but may be absent when the cardiac output is severely reduced despite significant obstruction. The intensity of the murmur increases during maneuvers that increase cardiac output and mitral valve flow, such as exercise. The duration of the murmur reflects the length of time over which left atrial pressure exceeds left ventricular pressure. An increase in the intensity of the murmur just before S_1, a phenomenon known as *presystolic accentuation* (Figs. 10-1*A* and 10-7), occurs in patients in sinus rhythm

and is due to a late increase in transmitral flow with atrial contraction. Presystolic accentuation does not occur in patients with atrial fibrillation.

The mid-diastolic murmur associated with tricuspid stenosis is best heard at the lower left sternal border and increases in intensity with inspiration. A prolonged γ descent may be visible in the jugular venous wave form. This murmur is very difficult to hear and often obscured by left-sided acoustical events.

There are several other causes of mid-diastolic murmurs. Large left atrial myxomas may prolapse across the mitral valve and cause variable degrees of obstruction to left ventricular inflow (Chap. 23). The murmur associated with an atrial myxoma may change in duration and intensity with changes in body position. An opening snap is not present and there is no presystolic accentuation. Augmented mitral diastolic flow can occur with isolated severe MR or with a large left-to-right shunt at the ventricular or great vessel level and produce a soft, rapid filling sound (S_3) followed by a short, low-pitched mid-diastolic apical murmur. The Austin Flint murmur of severe, chronic AR has already been described.

A short mid-diastolic murmur is rarely heard during an episode of acute rheumatic fever (Carey-Coombs murmur) and is due to enhanced flow through an edematous mitral valve. An opening snap is not present in the acute phase and the murmur dissipates with resolution of the acute attack. Complete heart block with dyssynchronous atrial and ventricular activation may be associated with intermittent mid- tolate diastolic murmurs if atrial contraction occurs when the mitral valve is partially closed. Mid-diastolic murmurs indicative of increased tricuspid valve flow can occur with severe, isolated TR and with large ASDs and significant left-to-right shunting. Other signs of an ASD are present (Chap. 19), including fixed-splitting of S_2 and a midsystolic murmur at the mid- to upper left sternal border. TTE is indicated for evaluation of the patient with a mid- to late diastolic murmur. Findings specific to the diseases discussed above will help guide management.

Continuous Murmurs

(Figs. 10-1*H* and 10-8) Continuous murmurs begin in systole, peak near the second heart sound, and continue into all or part of diastole. Their presence throughout the cardiac cycle implies a pressure gradient between two chambers or vessels during both systole and diastole. The continuous murmur associated with a patent ductus arteriosus is best heard at the upper left sternal border. Large, uncorrected shunts may lead to pulmonary hypertension, attenuation or obliteration of the diastolic component of the murmur, reversal of shunt flow, and differential cyanosis of the lower extremities. A ruptured sinus of Valsalva aneurysm creates a continuous murmur of abrupt onset at the upper right sternal border.

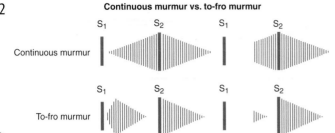

Continuous murmur vs. to-fro murmur

FIGURE 10-8

Comparison of the continuous murmur and the to-fro murmur. During abnormal communication between high-pressure and low-pressure systems, a large pressure gradient exists throughout the cardiac cycle, producing a continuous murmur. A classic example is patent ductus arteriosus. At times, this type of murmur can be confused with a to-fro murmur, which is a combination of systolic ejection murmur and a murmur of semilunar valve incompetence. A classic example of a to-fro murmur is aortic stenosis and regurgitation. A continuous murmur crescendos to around the second heart sound (S_2), whereas a to-fro murmur has two components. The midsystolic ejection component decrescendos and disappears as it approaches S_2. *(From JA Shaver, JJ Leonard, DF Leon, Examination of the Heart, Part IV, Auscultation of the Heart. Dallas, American Heart Association, 1990, p 55. Copyright, American Heart Association.)*

Rupture typically occurs into a right heart chamber, and the murmur is indicative of a continuous pressure difference between the aorta and either the right ventricle or right atrium. A continuous murmur may also be audible along the left sternal border with a coronary arteriovenous fistula and at the site of an arteriovenous fistula used for hemodialysis access. Enhanced flow through enlarged intercostal collateral arteries in patients with aortic coarctation may produce a continuous murmur along the course of one or more ribs. A cervical bruit with both systolic and diastolic components (a to-fro murmur, Fig. 10-8) usually indicates a high-grade carotid artery stenosis.

Not all continuous murmurs are pathologic. A continuous venous hum can be heard in healthy children and young adults, especially during pregnancy. It is best appreciated in the right supraclavicular fossa and can be obliterated by pressure over the right internal jugular vein or by having the patient turn his/her head toward the examiner. The continuous mammary souffle of pregnancy is created by enhanced arterial flow through engorged breasts and usually appears during the late third trimester or early puerperium. The murmur is louder in systole. Firm pressure with the diaphragm of the stethoscope can eliminate the diastolic portion of the murmur.

TABLE 10-2

DYNAMIC AUSCULTATION: BEDSIDE MANEUVERS THAT CAN BE USED TO CHANGE THE INTENSITY OF CARDIAC MURMURS (SEE TEXT)

1. Respiration
2. Isometric exercise (handgrip)
3. Transient arterial occlusion
4. Pharmacologic manipulation of preload and/or afterload
5. Valsalva maneuver
6. Rapid standing/squatting
7. Post-premature beat

Dynamic Auscultation

(**Tables 10–2** and 9–1) Careful attention to the behavior of heart murmurs during simple maneuvers that alter cardiac hemodynamics can provide important clues as to their cause and significance.

RESPIRATION

Auscultation should be performed during quiet respiration or with a modest increase in inspiratory effort, as more forceful movement of the chest tends to obscure the heart sounds. Left-sided murmurs may be best heard at end-expiration, when lung volumes are minimized and the heart and great vessels are brought closer to the chest wall. This phenomenon is characteristic of the murmur of AR. Murmurs of right-sided origin, such as tricuspid or pulmonic regurgitation, increase in intensity during inspiration. The intensity of left-sided murmurs either remains constant or decreases with inspiration.

Bedside assessment should also account for the behavior of S_2 with respiration and the dynamic relationship between the aortic and pulmonic components (**Fig. 10-9**). Reversed splitting can be a feature of severe AS, HOCM, left bundle branch block, right ventricular apical pacing, or acute myocardial ischemia. Fixed splitting of S_2 in the presence of a grade 2 or 3 midsystolic murmur at the mid- or upper left sternal border indicates an ASD. Physiologic but wide splitting during the respiratory cycle implies either premature aortic valve closure, as can occur with severe MR, or delayed pulmonic valve closure due to PS or right bundle branch block.

ALTERATIONS OF SYSTEMIC VASCULAR RESISTANCE

Murmurs can change characteristics following maneuvers that alter systemic vascular resistance and left ventricular afterload. The systolic murmurs of MR and VSD become louder during sustained handgrip, simultaneous inflation of blood pressure cuffs on both upper extremities to pressures 20–40 mmHg above systolic pressure for 20 s,

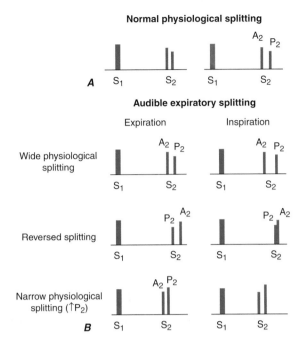

Normal physiological splitting

Audible expiratory splitting

FIGURE 10-9

A. Normal physiologic splitting. During expiration, the aortic (A_2) and pulmonic (P_2) components of the second heart sound are separated by <30 ms and are appreciated as a single sound. During inspiration, the splitting interval widens, and A_2 and P_2 are clearly separated into two distinct sounds. *B.* Audible expiratory splitting. Wide physiologic splitting is caused by a delay in P_2. Reversed splitting is caused by a delay in A_2, resulting in paradoxical movement; i.e., with inspiration P_2 moves towards A_2, and the splitting interval narrows. Narrow physiologic splitting occurs in pulmonary hypertension, and both A_2 and P_2 are heard during expiration at a narrow splitting interval because of the increased intensity and high-frequency composition of P_2. *(From JA Shaver, JJ Leonard, DF Leon, Examination of the Heart, Part IV, Auscultation of the Heart. Dallas, American Heart Association, 1990, p 17. Copyright, American Heart Association.)*

or infusion of a vasopressor agent. The murmurs associated with AS or HOCM will either become softer or remain unchanged with these maneuvers. The diastolic murmur of AR becomes louder in response to interventions that raise systemic vascular resistance.

Opposite changes in systolic and diastolic murmurs may occur with the use of pharmacologic agents that lower systemic vascular resistance. Inhaled amyl nitrite is now rarely used for this purpose but can help to distinguish the murmur of AS or HOCM from that of either MR or VSD. The former two murmurs increase in intensity, whereas the latter two become softer after exposure to amyl nitrite. As noted previously, the Austin Flint murmur of severe AR becomes softer, but the mid-diastolic rumble of MS becomes louder, in response to the abrupt lowering of systemic vascular resistance with amyl nitrite.

The Valsalva maneuver results in an increase in intrathoracic pressure, followed by a decrease in venous return, ventricular filling, and cardiac output. The majority of murmurs decrease in intensity during the strain phase of the maneuver. Two notable exceptions are the murmurs associated with MVP and obstructive HOCM, both of which become louder during the Valsalva maneuver. The murmur of MVP may also become longer as leaflet prolapse occurs earlier in systole at smaller ventricular volumes. These murmurs behave in a similar and parallel fashion with standing. Both the click and the murmur of MVP move closer in timing to S_1 on rapid standing (Fig. 10-3). The increase in the intensity of the murmur of HOCM is predicated on the augmentation of the dynamic left ventricular outflow tract gradient that occurs with reduced ventricular filling. Squatting results in abrupt increases in both venous return and left ventricular afterload, changes that predictably cause a decrease in the intensity and duration of the murmurs associated with MVP and HOCM. The click and murmur of MVP move away from S_1 with squatting.

POST-PREMATURE VENTRICULAR CONTRACTION

A change in the intensity of a systolic murmur in the first beat after a premature beat, or in the beat after a long cycle length in patients with atrial fibrillation, can help distinguish AS from MR, particularly in an older patient in whom the murmur of AS is well transmitted to the apex. Systolic murmurs due to left ventricular outflow obstruction, including that due to AS, increase in intensity in the beat following a premature beat because of the combined effects of enhanced left ventricular filling and post-extrasystolic potentiation of contractile function. Forward flow accelerates, causing an increase in the gradient and a louder murmur. The intensity of the murmur of MR does not change in the post-premature beat as there is relatively little further increase in mitral valve flow or change in the left ventricular to left atrial gradient.

The Clinical Context

Additional clues as to the etiology and importance of a heart murmur can be gleaned from the history and other physical examination findings. Symptoms suggestive of cardiovascular, neurologic, or pulmonary disease should help focus the differential diagnosis, as should findings relevant to the jugular venous pressure and wave forms, the arterial pulses, other heart sounds, the lungs, abdomen, skin, and extremities. In many instances, laboratory studies, an ECG, and/or a chest x-ray may have been obtained earlier and may contain valuable

CHAPTER 10 Approach to the Patient with a Heart Murmur

information. A patient with suspected infective endocarditis, for example, may have a murmur in the setting of fever, chills, anorexia, fatigue, dyspnea, splenomegaly, petechiae, and positive blood cultures. A new systolic murmur in a patient with a marked fall in blood pressure after a recent MI suggests myocardial rupture. On the other hand, an isolated grade 1 or 2 midsystolic murmur at the left sternal border in a healthy, active, and asymptomatic young adult is most likely a benign finding for which no further evaluation is indicated. The context in which the murmur is appreciated often dictates the need for further testing.

Echocardiography

(See **Fig. 10-10**, Chaps. 9 and 12) Echocardiography with color flow and spectral Doppler is a valuable tool for the assessment of cardiac murmurs. Information regarding valve structure and function, chamber size, wall thickness, ventricular function, estimated pulmonary artery pressures, intracardiac shunt flow, pulmonary and hepatic vein flow, and aortic flow can be readily ascertained. It is important to note that Doppler signals of trace or mild valvular regurgitation of no clinical consequence can be detected with structurally normal tricuspid, pulmonic, and mitral valves. Such signals are not likely to generate enough turbulence to create a murmur.

Echocardiography is indicated for the evaluation of patients with early, late, or holosystolic murmurs, and for patients with grade 3 or louder midsystolic murmurs.

Patients with grade 1 or 2 midsystolic murmurs, but other symptoms or signs of cardiovascular disease, including those from ECG or chest x-ray, should also undergo echocardiography. Echocardiography is indicated for the evaluation of any patient with a diastolic murmur and for patients with continuous murmurs not due to a venous hum or mammary souffle. Echocardiography should also be considered when there is a clinical need to verify normal cardiac structure and function in a patient whose symptoms and signs are likely noncardiac in origin. The performance of serial echocardiography to follow the course of asymptomatic individuals with valvular heart disease is a central feature of their longitudinal assessment and provides valuable information that may impact on decisions regarding the timing of surgery. Routine echocardiography is *not* recommended for asymptomatic patients with a grade 1 or 2 midsystolic murmur without other signs of heart disease. For this category of patients, referral to a cardiovascular specialist should be considered if doubt exists regarding the significance of the murmur after the initial examination.

The selective use of echocardiography outlined above has not been subjected to rigorous cost-effective analysis. At least one study has suggested that initial referral of pediatric patients with heart murmurs to a specialist results in modest cost savings. For some clinicians, handheld or miniaturized cardiac ultrasound devices have replaced the stethoscope. Although several reports attest to the improved sensitivity of such devices for the detection of valvular heart disease, accuracy is highly

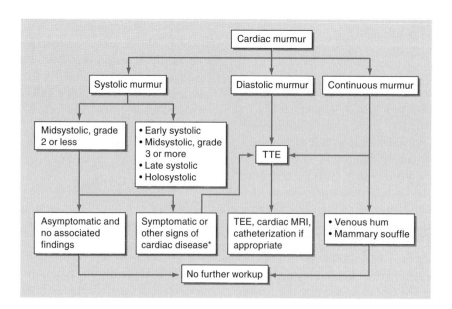

FIGURE 10-10

Strategy for evaluating heart murmurs. *If an electrocardiogram or chest x-ray has been obtained and is abnormal, echocardiography is indicated. TTE, transthoracic echocardiography; TEE, transesophageal echocardiography; MRI, magnetic resonance imaging. *(Adapted from Bonow et al.)*

operator dependent and incremental cost considerations have not been adequately addressed. The use of electronic or digital stethoscopes with spectral display capabilities has also been proposed as a method to improve the characterization of heart murmurs and the teaching of cardiac auscultation.

Other Cardiac Testing

(Chap. 12, Fig. 10-10) In relatively few patients, clinical assessment and TTE do not adequately characterize the origin and significance of a heart murmur. Transesophageal echocardiography (TEE) can be considered for further evaluation, especially when the TTE windows are limited by body size, chest configuration, or intrathoracic pathology. TEE offers enhanced sensitivity for the detection of a wide range of structural cardiac disorders. Electrocardiographically gated cardiac magnetic resonance imaging (MRI), although limited in its ability to display valvular morphology, can provide quantitative information regarding valvular function, stenosis severity, regurgitant fraction, shunt flow, chamber and great vessel size, ventricular function, and myocardial perfusion. Cardiac MRI has greater capability than cardiac computed tomography (CCT) in this regard and has largely supplanted the need for cardiac catheterization and invasive hemodynamic assessment when there is a discrepancy between the clinical and echocardiographic findings. Coronary angiography is performed routinely in most adult patients prior to valve surgery, especially when there is a suspicion of coronary artery disease predicated on symptoms, risk factors, and/or age.

Integrated Approach

The accurate identification of a heart murmur begins with a systematic approach to cardiac auscultation. Characterization of its major attributes, as reviewed above, allows the examiner to construct a preliminary differential diagnosis, which is then refined by integration of information available from the history, associated cardiac findings, the general physical examination, and the clinical context. The need for and urgency of further testing follow sequentially. Correlation of the findings on auscultation with the noninvasive data provides an educational feedback loop and an opportunity for improving physical examination skills. Cost constraints mandate that noninvasive imaging be justified on the basis of its incremental contribution to diagnosis, treatment, and outcome. Additional study is required to assess the cost-effective application of newer imaging technology.

FURTHER READINGS

BARRETT MJ et al: Mastering cardiac murmurs: The power of repetition. Chest 126(2):470, 2004

BONOW RO et al: ACC/AHA 2006 Guidelines for the management of patients with valvular heart disease: A report of the American College of Cardiology/American Heart Association Task Force on Practice Guidelines (Committee on Management of Patients with Valvular Heart Disease). American College of Cardiology Web Site. Available at *http://www.acc.org/clinical/guidelines/valvular/index.pdf*

CHOUNDHRY NK, ETCHELLS EE: Does this patient have aortic regurgitation? JAMA 281:2231, 1999

ETCHELLS E et al: Does this patient have an abnormal systolic heart murmur? JAMA 277(7):564, 1997

FANG J, O'GARA P: The history and physical examination, in *Braunwald's Heart Disease. A Textbook of Cardiovascular Medicine*, 8th ed, P Libby et al (eds). Philadelphia, Saunders Elsevier, 2008

MURGO JP: Systolic ejection murmurs in the era of modern cardiology. What do we really know? J Am Coll Cardiol 32(6): 1596, 1998

TAVEL ME: Cardiac auscultation: A glorious past—and it does have a future! Circulation 113:1255, 2006

VUKANOVIC-CRILEY JM et al: Competency in cardiac examination skills in medical students, trainees, physicians and faculty: A multicenter study. Arch Intern Med 166(6):610, 2006

CHAPTER 11

ELECTROCARDIOGRAPHY

Ary L. Goldberger

The electrocardiogram (ECG) is a graphic recording of electric potentials generated by the heart. The signals are detected by means of metal electrodes attached to the extremities and chest wall and are then amplified and recorded by the electrocardiograph. ECG *leads* actually display the instantaneous *differences* in potential between these electrodes.

The clinical utility of the ECG derives from its immediate availability as a noninvasive, inexpensive, and highly versatile test. In addition to its use in detecting arrhythmias, conduction disturbances, and myocardial ischemia, electrocardiography may reveal other findings related to life-threatening metabolic disturbances (e.g., hyperkalemia) or increased susceptibility to sudden cardiac death (e.g., QT prolongation syndromes). The widespread use of coronary fibrinolysis and acute percutaneous coronary interventions in the early therapy of acute myocardial infarction (Chap. 35) has refocused attention on the sensitivity and specificity of ECG signs of myocardial ischemia.

ELECTROPHYSIOLOGY

(See also Chaps. 15 and 16) Depolarization of the heart is the initiating event for cardiac contraction. The electric currents that spread through the heart are produced by three components: cardiac pacemaker cells, specialized conduction tissue, and the heart muscle itself. The ECG, however, records only the depolarization (stimulation) and repolarization (recovery) potentials generated by the atrial and ventricular myocardium.

The depolarization stimulus for the normal heartbeat originates in the *sinoatrial* (SA) *node* (**Fig. 11-1**), or *sinus node*, a collection of *pacemaker cells*. These cells fire spontaneously; that is, they exhibit *automaticity*. The first phase of cardiac electrical activation is the spread of the depolarization wave through the right and left atria, followed by atrial contraction. Next, the impulse stimulates pacemaker and specialized conduction tissues in the atrioventricular (AV) nodal and His-bundle areas; together, these two regions constitute the AV junction. The bundle of His bifurcates into two main branches, the right and left bundles, which rapidly transmit depolarization wavefronts to the right and left ventricular myocardium by way of Purkinje fibers. The main left bundle bifurcates into two primary subdivisions, a left anterior fascicle and a left posterior fascicle. The depolarization wavefronts then spread through the ventricular wall, from endocardium to epicardium, triggering ventricular contraction.

Since the cardiac depolarization and repolarization waves have direction and magnitude, they can be represented by vectors. *Vectorcardiograms* that measure and display these instantaneous potentials are no longer used much in clinical practice. However, the general principles of vector analysis remain fundamental to understanding the genesis

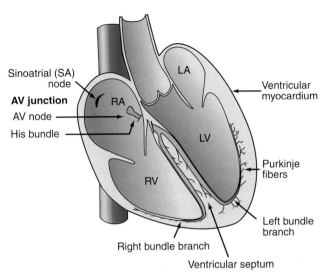

FIGURE 11-1
Schematic of the cardiac conduction system.

ECG WAVEFORMS AND INTERVALS

The ECG waveforms are labeled alphabetically, beginning with the P wave, which represents atrial depolarization (**Fig. 11-2**). The QRS complex represents

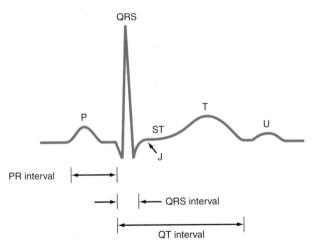

FIGURE 11-2
Basic ECG waveforms and intervals. Not shown is the R-R interval, the time between consecutive QRS complexes.

ventricular depolarization, and the ST-T-U complex (ST segment, T wave, and U wave) represents ventricular repolarization. The J point is the junction between the end of the QRS complex and the beginning of the ST segment. Atrial repolarization is usually too low in amplitude to be detected, but it may become apparent in such conditions as acute pericarditis or atrial infarction.

The QRS-T waveforms of the surface ECG correspond in a general way with the different phases of simultaneously obtained ventricular *action potentials*, the intracellular recordings from single myocardial fibers (Chap. 15). The rapid upstroke (phase 0) of the action potential corresponds to the onset of QRS. The plateau (phase 2) corresponds to the isoelectric ST segment, and active repolarization (phase 3) to the inscription of the T wave. Factors that decrease the slope of phase 0 by impairing the influx of Na^+ (e.g., hyperkalemia, or drugs such as flecainide) tend to increase QRS duration. Conditions that prolong phase 2 (use of amiodarone, hypocalcemia) increase the QT interval. In contrast, shortening of ventricular repolarization (phase 2), as by digitalis administration or hypercalcemia, abbreviates the ST segment.

The electrocardiogram is ordinarily recorded on special graph paper which is divided into 1 mm^2 gridlike boxes. Since the ECG paper speed is generally 25 mm/s, the smallest (1 mm) horizontal divisions correspond to 0.04 (40 ms), with heavier lines at intervals of 0.20 s (200 ms). Vertically, the ECG graph measures the amplitude of a given wave or deflection (1 mV = 10 mm with standard calibration; the voltage criteria for hypertrophy mentioned below are given in millimeters). There are four major ECG intervals: R-R, PR, QRS, and QT (Fig. 11-2). The heart rate (beats per minute) can be readily computed from the interbeat (R-R) interval by dividing the number of large (0.20 s) time units between consecutive R waves into 300 or the number of small (0.04 s) units into 1500. The PR interval measures the time (normally 120–200 ms) between atrial and ventricular depolarization, which includes the physiologic delay imposed by stimulation of cells in the AV junction area. The QRS interval (normally 100–110 ms or less) reflects the duration of ventricular depolarization. The QT interval includes both ventricular depolarization and repolarization times and varies inversely with the heart rate. A rate-related ("corrected") QT interval, QT_c, can be calculated as $QT/\sqrt{RR}$ and normally is ≤0.44 s. (Some references give QT_c upper normal limits as 0.43 s in men and 0.45 s in women.)

The QRS complex is subdivided into specific deflections or waves. If the initial QRS deflection in a given lead is negative, it is termed a Q *wave*; the first positive deflection is termed an R *wave*. A negative deflection after an R wave is an S *wave*. Subsequent positive or negative waves are labeled R′ and S′, respectively.

of normal and pathologic ECG waveforms. Vector analysis illustrates a central concept of electrocardiography—that the ECG records the complex spatial and temporal summation of electrical potentials from multiple myocardial fibers conducted to the surface of the body. This principle accounts for inherent limitations in both ECG *sensitivity* (activity from certain cardiac regions may be canceled out or may be too weak to be recorded) and *specificity* (the same vectorial sum can result from either a selective gain or a loss of forces in opposite directions).

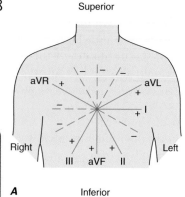

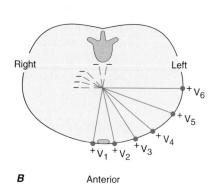

FIGURE 11-3

The six frontal plane (A) and six horizontal plane (B) leads provide a three-dimensional representation of cardiac electrical activity.

Lowercase letters (qrs) are used for waves of relatively small amplitude. An entirely negative QRS complex is termed a *QS wave*.

ECG LEADS

The 12 conventional ECG leads record the difference in potential between electrodes placed on the surface of the body. These leads are divided into two groups: six limb (extremity) leads and six chest (precordial) leads. The limb leads record potentials transmitted onto the *frontal plane* (**Fig. 11-3A**), and the chest leads record potentials transmitted onto the *horizontal plane* (**Fig. 11-3B**). The six limb leads are further subdivided into three standard "*bipolar*" leads (I, II, and III) and three augmented "*unipolar*" leads (aVR, aVL, and aVF). Each standard lead measures the difference in potential between electrodes at two extremities: lead I = left arm – right arm voltages, lead II = left leg – right arm, and lead III = left leg – left arm. The unipolar leads measure the voltage (V) at one locus relative to an electrode (called the *central terminal* or *indifferent electrode*) that has approximately zero potential. Thus, aVR = right arm, aVL = left arm, and aVF = left leg (foot). The lowercase *a* indicates that these unipolar potentials are electrically augmented by 50%. The right leg electrode functions as a ground. The spatial orientation and polarity of the six frontal plane leads is represented on the hexaxial diagram (**Fig. 11-4**).

The six chest leads (**Fig. 11-5**) are unipolar recordings obtained by electrodes in the following positions: lead V_1, fourth intercostal space, just to the right of the sternum; lead V_2, fourth intercostal space, just to the left of the sternum; lead V_3, midway between V_2 and V_4; lead V_4, midclavicular line, fifth intercostal space; lead V_5, anterior axillary line, same level as V_4; and lead V_6, midaxillary line, same level as V_4 and V_5.

Together, the frontal and horizontal plane electrodes provide a three-dimensional representation of cardiac electrical activity. Each lead can be likened to a different camera angle "looking" at the same events—atrial and ventricular depolarization and repolarization—from different spatial orientations. The conventional 12-lead ECG can be supplemented with additional leads under special circumstances. For example, right precordial leads V_3R, V_4R, etc., are useful in detecting evidence of acute right ventricular ischemia. Bedside monitors and ambulatory ECG (Holter) recordings usually employ only one or two modified leads. **Intracardiac electrocardiography and electrophysiologic testing are discussed in Chaps. 15 and 16.**

The ECG leads are configured so that a positive (upright) deflection is recorded in a lead if a wave of depolarization spreads toward the positive pole of that lead, and

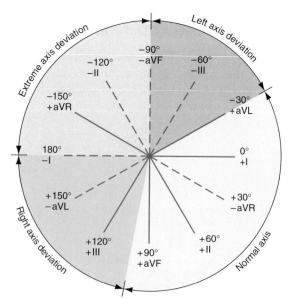

FIGURE 11-4

The frontal plane (limb or extremity) leads are represented on a hexaxial diagram. Each ECG lead has a specific spatial orientation and polarity. The positive pole of each lead axis (*solid line*) and negative pole (*hatched line*) are designated by their angular position relative to the positive pole of lead I (0°). The mean electrical axis of the QRS complex is measured with respect to this display.

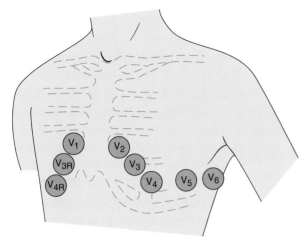

FIGURE 11-5

The horizontal plane (chest or precordial) leads are obtained with electrodes in the locations shown.

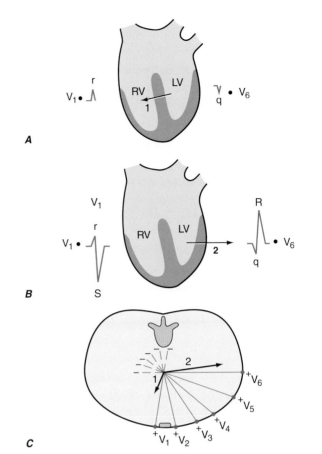

FIGURE 11-6

Ventricular depolarization can be divided into two major phases, each represented by a vector. *A*. The first phase (*arrow 1*) denotes depolarization of the ventricular septum, beginning on the left side and spreading to the right. This process is represented by a small "septal" r wave in lead V_1 and a small septal q wave in lead V_6. ***B*.** Simultaneous depolarization of the left and right ventricles (LV and RV) constitutes the second phase. Vector 2 is oriented to the left and posteriorly, reflecting the electrical predominance of the LV. ***C*.** Vectors (*arrows*) representing these two phases are shown in reference to the horizontal plane leads. (*After Goldberger, 2006.*)

a negative deflection if the wave spreads toward the negative pole. If the mean orientation of the depolarization vector is at right angles to a given lead axis, a biphasic (equally positive and negative) deflection will be recorded.

GENESIS OF THE NORMAL ECG

P WAVE

The normal atrial depolarization vector is oriented downward and toward the subject's left, reflecting the spread of depolarization from the sinus node to the right and then the left atrial myocardium. Since this vector points toward the positive pole of lead II and toward the negative pole of lead aVR, the normal P wave will be positive in lead II and negative in lead aVR. By contrast, activation of the atria from an ectopic pacemaker in the lower part of either atrium or in the AV junction region may produce retrograde P waves (negative in lead II, positive in lead aVR). The normal P wave in lead V_1 may be biphasic with a positive component reflecting right atrial depolarization, followed by a small (<1 mm^2) negative component reflecting left atrial depolarization.

QRS COMPLEX

Normal ventricular depolarization proceeds as a rapid, continuous spread of activation wavefronts. This complex process can be divided into two major, sequential phases, and each phase can be represented by a mean vector (**Fig. 11-6**). The first phase is depolarization of the interventricular septum from the left to the right and anteriorly (vector 1). The second results from the simultaneous depolarization of the right and left ventricles; it is normally dominated by the more massive left ventricle, so that vector 2 points leftward and posteriorly.

Therefore, a right precordial lead (V_1) will record this biphasic depolarization process with a small positive deflection (septal r wave) followed by a larger negative deflection (S wave). A left precordial lead, e.g. V_6, will record the same sequence with a small negative deflection (septal q wave) followed by a relatively tall positive deflection (R wave). Intermediate leads show a relative increase in R-wave amplitude (normal R-wave progression) and a decrease in S-wave amplitude progressing across the chest from the right to left. The precordial lead where the R and S waves are of approximately equal amplitude is referred to as the *transition zone* (usually V_3 or V_4) (**Fig. 11-7**).

The QRS pattern in the extremity leads may vary considerably from one normal subject to another

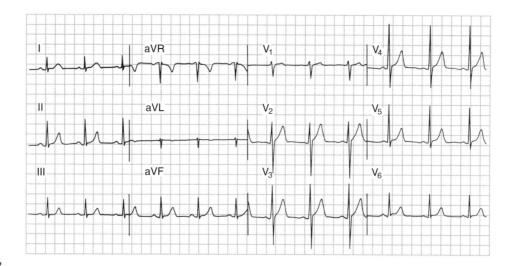

FIGURE 11-7

Normal electrocardiogram from a healthy subject. Sinus rhythm is present with a heart rate of 75 beats per minute. PR interval is 0.16 s; QRS interval (duration) is 0.08 s; QT interval is 0.36 s; QT_c is 0.40 s; the mean QRS axis is about +70°. The precordial leads show normal R-wave progression with the transition zone (R wave = S wave) in lead V_3.

depending on the *electrical axis* of the QRS, which describes the mean orientation of the QRS vector with reference to the six frontal plane leads. Normally, the QRS axis ranges from −30° to +100° (Fig. 11-4). An axis more negative than −30° is referred to as *left axis deviation*, while an axis more positive than +100° is referred to as *right axis deviation*. Left axis deviation may occur as a normal variant but is more commonly associated with left ventricular hypertrophy, a block in the anterior fascicle of the left bundle system (left anterior fascicular block or hemiblock), or inferior myocardial infarction. Right axis deviation may also occur as a normal variant (particularly in children and young adults); as a spurious finding due to reversal of the left and right arm electrodes; or in conditions such as right ventricular overload (acute or chronic), infarction of the lateral wall of the left ventricle, dextrocardia, left pneumothorax, or left posterior fascicular block.

T WAVE AND U WAVE

Normally, the mean T-wave vector is oriented roughly concordant with the mean QRS vector (within about 45° in the frontal plane). Since depolarization and repolarization are electrically opposite processes, this normal QRS–T-wave vector concordance indicates that repolarization must normally proceed in the reverse direction from depolarization (i.e., from ventricular epicardium to endocardium). The normal U wave is a small, rounded deflection (≤1 mm) that follows the T wave and usually has the same polarity as the T wave. An abnormal increase in U-wave amplitude is most commonly due to drugs (e.g., dofetilide, amiodarone, sotalol, quinidine, procainamide, disopyramide) or to hypokalemia. Very prominent U waves are a marker of increased susceptibility to

the *torsades de pointe* type of ventricular tachycardia (Chap. 16). Inversion of the U wave in the precordial leads is abnormal and may be a subtle sign of ischemia.

MAJOR ECG ABNORMALITIES

CARDIAC ENLARGEMENT AND HYPERTROPHY

Right atrial overload (acute or chronic) may lead to an increase in P-wave amplitude (≥2.5 mm) (**Fig. 11-8**). Left atrial overload typically produces a biphasic P wave in V_1 with a broad negative component or a broad (≥120 ms), often notched P wave in one or more limb leads (Fig. 11-8). This pattern may also occur with left atrial conduction delays in the absence of actual atrial enlargement, leading to the more general designation of *left atrial abnormality*.

Right ventricular hypertrophy due to a pressure load (as from pulmonic valve stenosis or pulmonary artery hypertension) is characterized by a relatively tall R wave in lead V_1 (R ≥ S wave), usually with right axis deviation (**Fig. 11-9**); alternatively, there may be a qR pattern in V_1 or V_3R. ST depression and T-wave inversion in the right to midprecordial leads are also often present. This pattern, formerly called right ventricular "strain," is attributed to repolarization abnormalities in acutely or chronically overloaded muscle. Prominent S waves may occur in the left lateral precordial leads. Right ventricular hypertrophy due to ostium secundum–type atrial septal defects, with the accompanying right ventricular volume overload, is commonly associated with an incomplete or complete right bundle branch block pattern with a rightward QRS axis.

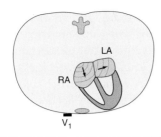

FIGURE 11-8

Right atrial (RA) overload may cause tall, peaked P waves in the limb or precordial leads. Left atrial (LA) abnormality may cause broad, often notched P waves in the limb leads and a biphasic P wave in lead V_1 with a prominent negative component representing delayed depolarization of the LA. *(After MK Park, WG Guntheroth: How to Read Pediatric ECGs, 4th ed. St. Louis, Mosby/Elsevier, 2006.)*

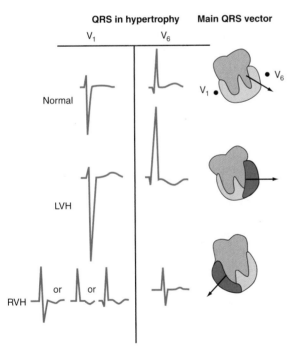

FIGURE 11-9

Left ventricular hypertrophy (LVH) increases the amplitude of electrical forces directed to the left and posteriorly. In addition, repolarization abnormalities may cause ST-segment depression and T-wave inversion in leads with a prominent R wave. Right ventricular hypertrophy (RVH) may shift the QRS vector to the right; this effect usually is associated with an R, RS, or qR complex in lead V_1. T-wave inversions may be present in right precordial leads.

Acute cor pulmonale due to pulmonary embolism, for example, may be associated with a normal ECG or a variety of abnormalities. Sinus tachycardia is the most common arrhythmia, although other tachyarrhythmias, such as atrial fibrillation or flutter, may occur. The QRS axis may shift to the right, sometimes in concert with the so-called $S_1Q_3T_3$ pattern (prominence of the S wave in lead I, Q wave in lead III, with T-wave inversion in lead III). Acute right ventricular dilation may also be associated with slow R-wave progression and T-wave inversions in V_1–V_4 simulating acute anterior infarction. A right ventricular conduction disturbance may appear.

Chronic cor pulmonale due to obstructive lung disease (Chap. 17) usually does not produce the classic ECG patterns of right ventricular hypertrophy noted above. Instead of tall right precordial R waves, chronic lung disease more typically is associated with small R waves in right-to-midprecordial leads (slow R-wave progression) due in part to downward displacement of the diaphragm and the heart. Low-voltage complexes are commonly present, owing to hyperaeration of the lungs.

A number of different voltage criteria for *left ventricular hypertrophy* (Fig. 11-9) have been proposed on the basis of the presence of tall left precordial R waves and deep right precordial S waves [e.g., SV_1 + (RV_5 or RV_6) >35 mm]. Repolarization abnormalities (ST depression with T-wave inversions, formerly called the left ventricular "strain" pattern) may also appear in leads with prominent R waves. However, prominent precordial voltages may occur as a normal variant, especially in athletic or young individuals. Left ventricular hypertrophy may increase limb lead voltage with or without increased precordial voltage (e.g., $RaVL + SV_3 > 20$ mm in women and >28 mm in men). The presence of left atrial abnormality increases the likelihood of underlying left ventricular hypertrophy in cases with borderline voltage criteria. Left ventricular hypertrophy often progresses to incomplete or complete left bundle branch block. The sensitivity of conventional voltage criteria for left ventricular hypertrophy is decreased in obese persons and in smokers. ECG evidence for left ventricular hypertrophy is a major noninvasive marker of increased risk of cardiovascular morbidity and mortality, including sudden cardiac death. However, because of false-positive and false-negative diagnoses, the ECG is of limited utility in diagnosing atrial or ventricular enlargement. More definitive information is provided by echocardiography (Chap. 12).

BUNDLE BRANCH BLOCKS

Intrinsic impairment of conduction in either the right or left bundle system (intraventricular conduction disturbances) leads to prolongation of the QRS interval. With complete bundle branch blocks, the QRS interval

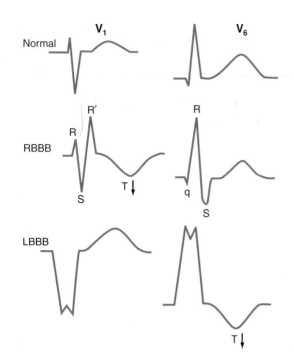

FIGURE 11-10

Comparison of typical QRS-T patterns in right bundle branch block (RBBB) and left bundle branch block (LBBB) with the normal pattern in leads V₁ and V₆. Note the secondary T-wave inversions (*arrows*) in leads with an rSR′ complex with RBBB and in leads with a wide R wave with LBBB.

is ≥120 ms in duration; with incomplete blocks the QRS interval is between 100 and 120 ms. The QRS vector is usually oriented in the direction of the myocardial region where depolarization is delayed (**Fig. 11-10**). Thus, with right bundle branch block, the terminal QRS vector is oriented to the right and anteriorly (rSR′ in V₁ and qRS in V₆, typically). Left bundle branch block alters both early and later phases of ventricular depolarization. The major QRS vector is directed to the left and posteriorly. In addition, the normal early left-to-right pattern of septal activation is disrupted such that septal depolarization proceeds from right to left as well. As a result, left bundle branch block generates wide, predominantly negative (QS) complexes in lead V₁ and entirely positive (R) complexes in lead V₆. A pattern identical to that of left bundle branch block, preceded by a sharp spike, is seen in most cases of electronic right ventricular pacing because of the relative delay in left ventricular activation.

Bundle branch block may occur in a variety of conditions. In subjects without structural heart disease, right bundle branch block is seen more commonly than left bundle branch block. Right bundle branch block also occurs with heart disease, both congenital (e.g., atrial septal defect) and acquired (e.g., valvular, ischemic). Left bundle branch block is often a marker of one of four underlying conditions associated with increased risk of

cardiovascular morbidity and mortality: coronary heart disease (frequently with impaired left ventricular function), hypertensive heart disease, aortic valve disease, and cardiomyopathy. Bundle branch blocks may be chronic or intermittent. A bundle branch block may be rate-related; for example, it often occurs when the heart rate exceeds some critical value.

Bundle branch blocks and depolarization abnormalities secondary to artificial pacemakers not only affect ventricular depolarization (QRS) but are also characteristically associated with *secondary repolarization* (ST-T) abnormalities. With bundle branch blocks, the T wave is typically opposite in polarity to the last deflection of the QRS (Fig. 11-10). This discordance of the QRS–T-wave vectors is caused by the altered sequence of repolarization that occurs secondary to altered depolarization. In contrast, *primary repolarization* abnormalities are independent of QRS changes and are related instead to actual alterations in the electrical properties of the myocardial fibers themselves (e.g., in the resting membrane potential or action potential duration), not just to changes in the sequence of repolarization. Ischemia, electrolyte imbalance, and drugs such as digitalis all cause such primary ST–T-wave changes. Primary and secondary T-wave changes may coexist. For example, T-wave inversions in the right precordial leads with left bundle branch block or in the left precordial leads with right bundle branch block may be important markers of underlying ischemia or other abnormalities. A distinctive abnormality simulating right bundle branch block with ST-segment elevations in the right chest leads is seen with the Brugada pattern (Chap. 16).

Partial blocks (fascicular or "hemiblocks") in the left bundle system (left anterior or posterior fascicular blocks) generally do not prolong the QRS duration substantially but instead are associated with shifts in the frontal plane QRS axis (leftward or rightward, respectively). More complex combinations of fascicular and bundle branch blocks may occur involving the left and right bundle system. Examples of *bifascicular block* include right bundle branch block and left posterior fascicular block, right bundle branch block with left anterior fascicular block, and complete left bundle branch block. Chronic bifascicular block in an asymptomatic individual is associated with a relatively low risk of progression to high-degree AV heart block. In contrast, new bifascicular block with acute anterior myocardial infarction carries a much greater risk of complete heart block. Alternation of right and left bundle branch block is a sign of *trifascicular disease*. However, the presence of a prolonged PR interval and bifascicular block does not necessarily indicate trifascicular involvement, since this combination may arise with AV node disease and bifascicular block. Intraventricular conduction delays can also be caused by extrinsic (toxic) factors that slow ventricular conduction, particularly hyperkalemia or drugs (e.g., class 1 antiarrhythmic agents, tricyclic antidepressants, phenothiazines).

Prolongation of QRS duration does not necessarily indicate a conduction delay but may be due to *preexcitation* of the ventricles via a bypass tract, as in Wolff–Parkinson–White (WPW) patterns (Chap. 16) and related variants. The diagnostic triad of WPW consists of a wide QRS complex associated with a relatively short PR interval and slurring of the initial part of the QRS (delta wave), the latter effect due to aberrant activation of ventricular myocardium. The presence of a bypass tract predisposes to reentrant supraventricular tachyarrhythmias.

MYOCARDIAL ISCHEMIA AND INFARCTION

(See also Chap. 35) The ECG is a cornerstone in the diagnosis of acute and chronic ischemic heart disease. The findings depend on several key factors: the nature of the process [reversible (i.e., ischemia) versus irreversible (i.e., infarction)], the duration (acute versus chronic), extent (transmural versus subendocardial), and localization (anterior versus inferoposterior), as well as the presence of other underlying abnormalities (ventricular hypertrophy, conduction defects).

Ischemia exerts complex time-dependent effects on the electrical properties of myocardial cells. Severe, acute ischemia lowers the resting membrane potential and shortens the duration of the action potential. Such changes cause a voltage gradient between normal and ischemic zones. As a consequence, current flows between these regions. These currents of injury are represented on the surface ECG by deviation of the ST segment (**Fig. 11-11**). When the acute ischemia is *transmural*, the ST vector is usually shifted in the direction of the outer (epicardial) layers, producing ST elevations and sometimes, in the earliest stages of ischemia, tall, positive so-called hyperacute T waves over the ischemic zone. With ischemia confined primarily to the *subendocardium*, the ST vector typically shifts toward the subendocardium and ventricular cavity, so that overlying (e.g., anterior precordial) leads show ST-segment depression (with ST elevation in lead aVR). Multiple factors affect the amplitude of acute ischemic ST deviations. Profound ST elevation or depression in multiple leads usually indicates very severe ischemia. From a clinical viewpoint, the division of acute myocardial infarction into ST segment elevation and non-ST elevation types is useful since the efficacy of acute reperfusion therapy is limited to the former group.

The ECG leads are more helpful in localizing regions of ST elevation than non-ST elevation ischemia. For example, acute transmural anterior (including apical and lateral) wall ischemia is reflected by ST elevations or increased T-wave positivity in one or more of the precordial leads (V_1–V_6) and leads I and aVL. Inferior wall ischemia produces changes in leads II, III, and aVF. Posterior wall ischemia may be indirectly recognized by *reciprocal* ST depressions in leads V_1–V_3. Prominent reciprocal ST depressions in these leads also occur with certain inferior wall infarcts, particularly those with posterior or lateral wall extension. Right ventricular ischemia usually produces ST elevations in right-sided chest leads (Fig. 11-5). When ischemic ST elevations occur as the earliest sign of acute infarction, they are typically followed within a period ranging from hours to days by evolving T-wave inversions and often by Q waves occurring in the same lead distribution. (T-wave inversions due to evolving or chronic ischemia correlate with prolongation of repolarization and are often associated with QT lengthening.) Reversible transmural ischemia, for example, due to coronary vasospasm (Prinzmetal's variant angina, and possibly the tako-tsubo cardiomyopathy syndrome), may cause transient ST-segment elevations without development of Q waves. Depending on the severity and duration of such ischemia, the ST elevations may either resolve completely in minutes or be followed by T-wave inversions that persist for hours or even days. Patients with ischemic chest pain who present with deep T-wave inversions in multiple precordial leads (e.g., V_1–V_4) with or without cardiac enzyme elevations typically have severe obstruction in the left anterior descending coronary artery system (**Fig. 11-12**). In contrast, patients whose baseline ECG already shows abnormal T-wave inversions may develop T-wave normalization (pseudonormalization) during episodes of acute transmural ischemia.

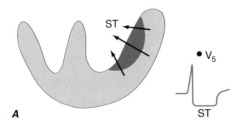 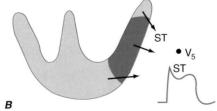

FIGURE 11-11
Acute ischemia causes a current of injury. With predominant subendocardial ischemia (**A**), the resultant ST vector will be directed toward the inner layer of the affected ventricle and the ventricular cavity. Overlying leads therefore will record ST depression. With ischemia involving the outer ventricular layer (**B**) (transmural or epicardial injury), the ST vector will be directed outward. Overlying leads will record ST elevation.

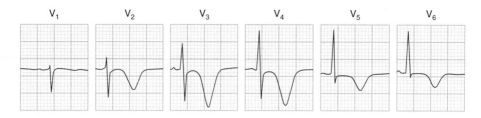

FIGURE 11-12

Severe anterior wall ischemia (with or without infarction) may cause prominent T-wave inversions in the precordial leads. This pattern is usually associated with a high-grade stenosis of the left anterior descending coronary artery.

With infarction, depolarization (QRS) changes often accompany repolarization (ST-T) abnormalities. Necrosis of sufficient myocardial tissue may lead to decreased R-wave amplitude or abnormal Q waves in the anterior or inferior leads (**Fig. 11-13**). Previously, abnormal Q waves were considered to be markers of transmural myocardial infarction, while subendocardial infarcts were thought not to produce Q waves. However, careful ECG-pathology correlative studies have indicated that transmural infarcts may occur without Q waves and that subendocardial (nontransmural) infarcts may sometimes be associated with Q waves. Therefore, infarcts are more appropriately classified as "Q-wave" or "non-Q-wave." The major acute ECG changes in syndromes of ischemic heart disease are summarized schematically in **Fig. 11-14**. Loss of depolarization forces due to posterior or lateral infarction may cause reciprocal increases in R-wave amplitude in leads V_1 and V_2 without diagnostic Q waves in any of the conventional leads. Atrial infarction may be associated with PR-segment deviations due to an atrial current of injury, changes in P-wave morphology, or atrial arrhythmias.

In the weeks and months following infarction, these ECG changes may persist or begin to resolve. Complete normalization of the ECG following Q-wave infarction is uncommon but may occur, particularly with smaller infarcts. In contrast, ST-segment elevations that persist for several weeks or more after a Q-wave infarct usually correlate with a severe underlying wall motion disorder (akinetic or dyskinetic zone), although not necessarily a frank ventricular aneurysm.

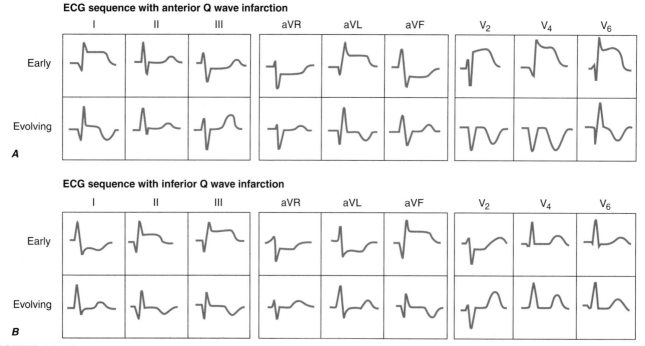

FIGURE 11-13

Sequence of depolarization and repolarization changes with (**A**) acute anterior and (**B**) acute inferior wall Q-wave infarctions. With anterior infarcts, ST elevation in leads I, aVL, and the precordial leads may be accompanied by reciprocal ST depressions in leads II, III, and aVF. Conversely, acute inferior (or posterior) infarcts may be associated with reciprocal ST depressions in leads V_1 to V_3. *(After Goldberger, 2006.)*

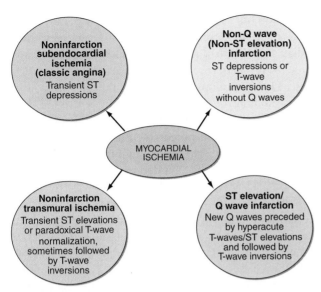

FIGURE 11-14

Variability of ECG patterns with acute myocardial ischemia. The ECG also may be normal or nonspecifically abnormal. Furthermore, these categorizations are not mutually exclusive. For example, a non-ST elevation infarct may evolve into a Q-wave infarct; ST elevations may be followed by a non-Q-wave infarct; or ST depressions and T-wave inversions may be followed by a Q-wave infarct. *(After Goldberger, 2006.)*

TABLE 11-1

DIFFERENTIAL DIAGNOSIS OF ST SEGMENT ELEVATIONS

Ischemia/myocardial infarction
   Noninfarction, transmural ischemia (Prinzmetal's angina, and possibly tako-tsubo syndrome)
   Acute myocardial infarction
   Postmyocardial infarction (ventricular aneurysm pattern)
Acute pericarditis
Normal variant ("early repolarization" pattern)
Left ventricular hypertrophy/left bundle branch block[a]
Other (rarer)
   Brugada pattern (right bundle branch block-like pattern with ST elevations in right precordial leads)[a]
   Class 1C antiarrhythmic drugs[a]
   DC cardioversion
   Hypercalcemia[a]
   Hyperkalemia[a]
   Hypothermia (J wave/Osborn waves)
   Myocardial injury
      Myocarditis
      Tumor invading left ventricle
      Trauma to ventricles

[a]Usually localized to V_1-V_2 or V_3.
Source: Modified from Goldberger, 2006.

ECG changes due to ischemia may occur spontaneously or may be provoked by various exercise protocols (stress electrocardiography) (Chap. 33). In patients with severe ischemic heart disease, exercise testing is most likely to elicit signs of subendocardial ischemia (horizontal or downsloping ST depression in multiple leads). ST-segment elevation during exercise is most often observed after a Q-wave infarct. This repolarization change does not necessarily indicate active ischemia but correlates strongly with the presence of an underlying ventricular wall motion abnormality. However, in patients *without* prior infarction, transient ST-segment elevation with exercise is a reliable sign of transmural ischemia.

The ECG has important limitations in both sensitivity and specificity in the diagnosis of ischemic heart disease. Although a single normal ECG does not exclude ischemia or even acute infarction, a normal ECG *throughout* the course of an acute infarct is distinctly uncommon. Prolonged chest pain without diagnostic ECG changes, therefore, should always prompt a careful search for other noncoronary causes of chest pain (Chap. 4). Furthermore, the diagnostic changes of acute or evolving ischemia are often masked by the presence of left bundle branch block, electronic ventricular pacemaker patterns, and WPW pre-excitation. On the other hand, clinicians may overdiagnose ischemia or infarction based on the presence of ST-segment elevations or depressions, T-wave inversions, tall positive T waves, or Q waves *not* related to ischemic heart disease (pseudoinfarct patterns). For example, ST-segment elevations simulating ischemia may occur with acute pericarditis or myocarditis, as a normal variant ("early repolarization" pattern), or in a variety of other conditions (Table 11-1). Similarly, tall, positive T waves do not invariably represent hyperacute ischemic changes but may also be caused by normal variants, hyperkalemia, cerebrovascular injury, and left ventricular volume overload due to mitral or aortic regurgitation, among other causes.

ST-segment elevations and tall, positive T waves are common findings in leads V_1 and V_2 in left bundle branch block or left ventricular hypertrophy in the absence of ischemia. The differential diagnosis of Q waves (Table 11-2) includes physiologic or positional variants, ventricular hypertrophy, acute or chronic noncoronary myocardial injury, hypertrophic cardiomyopathy, and ventricular conduction disorders. Digoxin, ventricular hypertrophy, hypokalemia, and a variety of other factors may cause ST-segment depression mimicking subendocardial ischemia. Prominent T-wave inversion may occur with ventricular hypertrophy, cardiomyopathies, myocarditis, and cerebrovascular injury (particularly intracranial bleeds), among many other conditions.

METABOLIC FACTORS AND DRUG EFFECTS

A variety of metabolic and pharmacologic agents alter the ECG and, in particular, cause changes in repolarization (ST-T-U) and sometimes QRS prolongation. Certain life-threatening electrolyte disturbances

TABLE 11-2

DIFFERENTIAL DIAGNOSIS OF Q WAVES (WITH SELECTED EXAMPLES)

Physiologic or positional factors
    Normal variant "septal" q waves
    Normal variant Q waves in V_1 to V_2, aVL, III, and aVF
    Left pneumothorax or dextrocardia: loss of lateral
        R-wave progression
Myocardial injury or infiltration
    Acute processes: myocardial ischemia or infarction,
        myocarditis, hyperkalemia
    Chronic processes: myocardial infarction, idiopathic
        cardiomyopathy, myocarditis, amyloid, tumor, sarcoid,
        scleroderma, Chagas' disease, echinococcus cyst
Ventricular hypertrophy/enlargement
    Left ventricular (slow R-wave progression[a])
    Right ventricular (reversed R-wave progression[b] or
        slow R-wave progression[a], particularly with chronic
        obstructive lung disease)
    Hypertrophic cardiomyopathy (may simulate anterior,
        inferior, posterior, or lateral infarcts)
Conduction abnormalities
    Left bundle branch block (slow R-wave progression[a])
    Wolff-Parkinson-White patterns

[a]Small or absent R waves in the right to midprecordial leads.
[b]Progressive decrease in R-wave amplitude from V_1 to the mid- or lateral precordial leads.
Source: After Goldberger, 2006.

may be diagnosed initially and monitored from the ECG. *Hyperkalemia* produces a sequence of changes (**Fig. 11-15**), usually beginning with narrowing and peaking (tenting) of the T waves. Further elevation of extracellular K^+ leads to AV conduction disturbances, diminution in P-wave amplitude, and widening of the QRS interval. Severe hyperkalemia eventually causes cardiac arrest with a slow sinusoidal type of mechanism ("sine-wave" pattern) followed by asystole. *Hypokalemia* (**Fig. 11-16**) prolongs ventricular repolarization, often with prominent U waves. Prolongation of the QT interval is also seen with drugs that increase the duration of the ventricular action potential—class 1A antiarrhythmic agents and related drugs (e.g., quinidine, disopyramide, procainamide, tricyclic antidepressants, phenothiazines) and class III agents [amiodarone (Fig. 11-16), sotalol, ibutilide]. Marked QT prolongation, sometimes with deep, wide T-wave inversions, may occur with intracranial bleeds, particularly subarachnoid hemorrhage ("CVA T-wave" pattern) (Fig. 11-16). Systemic *hypothermia* also prolongs repolarization, usually with a distinctive convex elevation of the J point (Osborn wave). *Hypocalcemia* typically prolongs the QT interval (ST portion), while *hypercalcemia* shortens it (**Fig. 11-17**). Digitalis glycosides also shorten the QT interval, often with a characteristic "scooping" of the ST–T-wave complex (*digitalis effect*).

Many other factors are associated with ECG changes, particularly alterations in ventricular repolarization. T-wave flattening, minimal T-wave inversions, or slight ST-segment depression ("nonspecific ST–T-wave changes") may occur with a variety of electrolyte and acid-base disturbances, a variety of infectious processes, central nervous system disorders, endocrine abnormalities, many drugs, ischemia, hypoxia, and virtually any type of cardiopulmonary abnormality. While subtle ST–T-wave changes may be markers of ischemia, transient nonspecific repolarization changes may also occur following a meal or with postural (orthostatic) change, hyperventilation, or exercise in healthy individuals.

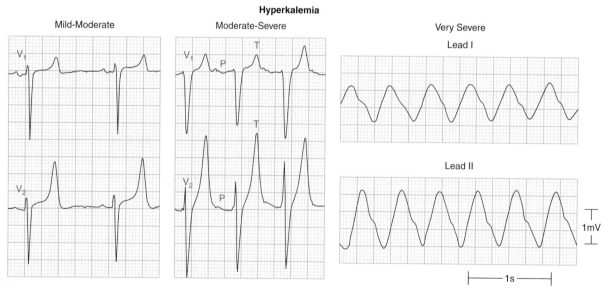

Hyperkalemia

Mild-Moderate   Moderate-Severe   Very Severe

Lead I

Lead II

1mV

1s

FIGURE 11-15

The earliest ECG change with hyperkalemia is usually peaking ("tenting") of the T waves. With further increases in the serum potassium concentration, the QRS complexes widen, the P waves decrease in amplitude and may disappear, and finally a sine-wave pattern leads to asystole unless emergency therapy is given. (*After Goldberger, 2006.*)

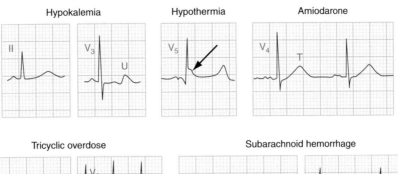

Hypokalemia   Hypothermia   Amiodarone

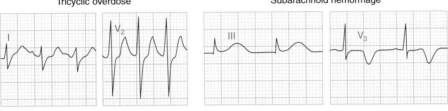

Tricyclic overdose   Subarachnoid hemorrhage

FIGURE 11-16

A variety of metabolic derangements, drug effects, and other factors may prolong ventricular repolarization with QT prolongation or prominent U waves. Prominent repolarization prolongation, particularly if due to hypokalemia, inherited "channelopathies," or certain pharmacologic agents, indicates increased susceptibility to torsades de pointes–type ventricular tachycardia (Chap. 16). Marked systemic hypothermia is associated with a distinctive convex "hump" at the J point (Osborn wave, *arrow*) due to altered ventricular action potential characteristics. Note QRS and QT prolongation along with sinus tachycardia in the case of tricyclic antidepressant overdose.

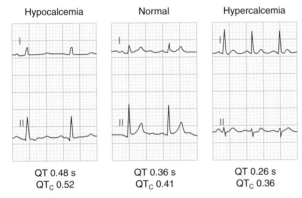

Hypocalcemia   Normal   Hypercalcemia

QT 0.48 s   QT 0.36 s   QT 0.26 s
QT$_C$ 0.52   QT$_C$ 0.41   QT$_C$ 0.36

FIGURE 11-17

Prolongation of the Q-T interval (ST-segment portion) is typical of hypocalcemia. Hypercalcemia may cause abbreviation of the ST segment and shortening of the QT interval.

ELECTRICAL ALTERNANS

Electrical alternans—a beat-to-beat alternation in one or more components of the ECG signal—is a common type of nonlinear cardiovascular response to a variety of hemodynamic and electrophysiologic perturbations. Total electrical alternans (P-QRS-T) with sinus tachycardia is a relatively specific sign of pericardial effusion, usually with cardiac tamponade. The mechanism relates to a periodic swinging motion of the heart in the effusion at a frequency exactly one-half the heart rate. Repolarization (ST-T or U wave) alternans is a sign of electrical instability and may precede ventricular tachyarrhythmias.

CLINICAL INTERPRETATION OF THE ECG

Accurate analysis of ECGs requires thoroughness and care. The patient's age, gender, and clinical status should always be taken into account. For example, T-wave inversions in leads V_1–V_3 are more likely to represent a normal variant in a healthy young adult woman ("persistent juvenile T-wave pattern") than in an elderly man with chest discomfort. Similarly, the likelihood that ST-segment depression during exercise testing represents ischemia depends partly on the prior probability of coronary artery disease.

Many mistakes in ECG interpretation are errors of omission. Therefore, a systematic approach is essential. The following 14 points should be analyzed carefully in every ECG: (1) standardization (calibration) and technical features (including lead placement and artifacts); (2) rhythm; (3) heart rate; (4) PR interval/AV conduction; (5) QRS interval; (6) QT/QT$_c$ interval; (7) mean QRS electrical axis; (8) P waves; (9) QRS voltages; (10) precordial R-wave progression; (11) abnormal Q waves; (12) ST segments; (13) T waves; (14) U waves.

Only after analyzing all these points should the interpretation be formulated. Where appropriate, important clinical correlates or inferences should be mentioned. For example, the combination of left atrial abnormality (enlargement) and signs of right ventricular hypertrophy suggests mitral stenosis. Low voltage with sinus tachycardia raises the possibility of pericardial tamponade or chronic obstructive lung disease. Sinus tachycardia with QRS and QT-(U) prolongation, especially in the context of mental status changes, suggests tricyclic antidepressant overdose (Fig. 11-16). The triad of peaked T waves (hyperkalemia), a long QT due to ST segment lengthening (hypocalcemia) and left ventricular hypertrophy (systemic hypertension) suggests chronic renal failure. Comparison with previous ECGs is essential. **The diagnosis and management of specific cardiac arrhythmias and conduction disturbances are discussed in Chaps. 15 and 16.**

COMPUTERIZED ELECTROCARDIOGRAPHY

Computerized ECG systems are widely used. Digital systems provide for convenient storage and immediate retrieval of thousands of ECG records. Despite advances, computer interpretation of ECGs has important limitations. Incomplete or inaccurate readings are most likely with arrhythmias and complex abnormalities. Therefore, computerized interpretation (including measurements of basic ECG intervals) should not be accepted without careful clinician review.

FURTHER READINGS

ASHLEY EA et al: An evidence-based review of the resting electrocardiogram as a screening technique for heart disease. Prog Cardiovasc Dis 44:55, 2001

GOLDBERGER AL: *Clinical Electrocardiography: A Simplified Approach*, 7th ed. St. Louis, Mosby/Elsevier, 2006

GUGLIN MF, THATAI D: Common errors in computer electrocardiogram interpretation. Int J Cardiol 106:232, 2006

KRIGFIELD P, et al: Recommendations for the standardization and interpretation of the electrocardiogram. Part I: The electrocardiogram and its standardization. J Am Coll Cardiol 49:1109, 2007

MIRVIS DM, GOLDBERGER AL: Electrocardiography, in *Braunwald's Heart Disease: A Textbook of Cardiovascular Medicine*, 8th ed, P Libby et al (eds). Philadelphia, Saunders, 2008

SURAWICZ B, KNILANS TK: *Chou's Electrocardiography in Clinical Practice*, 5th ed. Philadelphia, Saunders, 2001

WAGNER G, et al: Recommendations for the standardization and interpretation of the electrocardiogram. Part VI: Acute myocardial ischemia. J Am Coll Cardiol 53:1003, 2009

CHAPTER 12

NONINVASIVE CARDIAC IMAGING: ECHOCARDIOGRAPHY, NUCLEAR CARDIOLOGY, AND MRI/CT IMAGING

Rick A. Nishimura ■ Raymond J. Gibbons ■ James F. Glockner ■ A. Jamil Tajik

Cardiovascular imaging has significantly enhanced the practice of cardiology over the past few decades. Two-dimensional echocardiography (2DE) is able to visualize the heart directly in real time using ultrasound, providing instantaneous assessment of the myocardium, cardiac chambers, valves, pericardium, and great vessels. Doppler echocardiography measures the velocity of moving red blood cells and has become a noninvasive alternative to cardiac catheterization for assessment of hemodynamics. Transesophageal echocardiography (TEE) provides a unique window for high-resolution imaging of posterior structures of the heart, particularly the left atrium, mitral valve, and aorta. Nuclear cardiology uses isotopes to assess myocardial perfusion and ventricular function and has contributed greatly to the evaluation of patients with ischemic heart disease. Cardiac magnetic resonance imaging (MRI) and computed tomography (CT) can delineate cardiac structure and function with high resolution. They are particularly useful in the examination of cardiac masses, the pericardium, and the great vessels. MRI stress testing is now possible examining both ventricular function and perfusion. Detection of coronary calcification by CT as well as by direct visualization of coronary

arteries by CT angiography (CTA) are of growing utility in patients with suspected coronary artery disease (CAD). This chapter provides an overview of the basic concepts of these cardiac imaging modalities, as well as the clinical indications for each procedure. The illustrations in this chapter are supplemented by static images in Chap. 42.

ECHOCARDIOGRAPHY

TWO-DIMENSIONAL ECHOCARDIOGRAPHY

Basic Principles

Two-dimensional echocardiography (2DE) uses the principle of ultrasound reflection off cardiac structures to produce images of the heart (Table 12-1). For a transthoracic echocardiogram (TTE), the imaging is performed with a handheld transducer placed directly on the chest wall. In selected patients, a TEE may be performed, in which an ultrasound transducer is mounted on the tip of an endoscope placed in the esophagus and directed toward the cardiac structures.

Current echocardiographic machines are portable and can be wheeled directly to the patient's bedside. Thus,

TABLE 12-1

CLINICAL USES OF ECHOCARDIOGRAPHY	
Two-Dimensional Echocardiography	**Doppler Echocardiography**
Cardiac chambers	Valve stenosis
Chamber size	Gradient
Left ventricular	Valve area
Hypertrophy	Valve regurgitation
Regional wall motion	Semiquantitation
abnormalities	Intracardiac pressures
Valve	Volumetric flow
Morphology and motion	Diastolic filling
Pericardium	Intracardiac shunts
Effusion	**Transesophageal**
Tamponade	**Echocardiography**
Masses	Inadequate transthoracic
Great vessels	images
Stress Echocardiography	Aortic disease
Two-dimensional	Infective endocarditis
Myocardial ischemia	Source of embolism
Viable myocardium	Valve prosthesis
Doppler	Intraoperative
Valve disease	

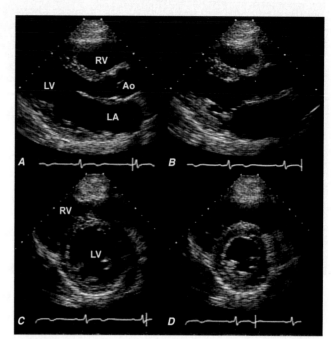

FIGURE 12-1

Two-dimensional echocardiographic still-frame images from a normal patient with a normal heart. Parasternal long axis view during systole and diastole (***A***) and systole (***B***). During systole, there is thickening of the myocardium and reduction in the size of the left ventricle (LV). The valve leaflets are thin and open widely. Parasternal short axis view during diastole (***C***) and systole (***D***) demonstrating a decrease in the left ventricular cavity size during systole as well as an increase in wall thickening. LA, left atrium; RV, right ventricle; Ao, aorta.

a major advantage of echocardiography over other imaging modalities is the ability to obtain instantaneous images of the cardiac structures for immediate interpretation. Handheld echocardiographic units weighing 6 lb (<2.7 kg) have now become available, further enhancing the ease and portability of echocardiography. They are becoming an essential initial diagnostic modality for the critically ill patient in the emergency room and critical care setting.

A limitation of TTE is the inability to obtain high-quality images in all patients, especially those with a thick chest wall or severe lung disease, as ultrasound waves are poorly transmitted through lung parenchyma. New technology such as harmonic imaging and IV contrast agents (which traverse the pulmonary circulation) can now be used to enhance endocardial borders in patients with poor acoustic windows.

Chamber Size and Function

2DE is an ideal imaging modality for assessing left ventricular (LV) size and function (Fig. 12-1). A qualitative assessment of the cavity sizes of the ventricles and systolic function can be made directly from the 2-D image by experienced observers. 2DE is useful in the diagnosis of LV hypertrophy and is the imaging modality of choice for the diagnosis of hypertrophic cardiomyopathy. Other chamber sizes are assessed by visual analysis, including the left atrium and right-sided chambers.

Valve Abnormalities

(See Chap. 20) 2DE is the "gold standard" for imaging valve morphology and motion. Leaflet thickness and

mobility, valve calcification, and the appearance of sub-valvular and supravalvular structures can be assessed. Valve stenosis is reliably diagnosed by the thickening and decreased mobility of the valve. 2DE is also the gold standard for the diagnosis of mitral stenosis, which produces typical tethering and diastolic doming, and the severity of the stenosis can be ascertained from a direct planimeter measurement of the mitral valve orifice. The presence and often the etiology of stenosis of the semilunar valves can be made by 2DE (Fig. 12-2), but evaluation of the severity of the stenosis requires Doppler echocardiography (see later). The diagnosis of valvular regurgitation must be made by Doppler echocardiography, but 2DE is valuable for determining the etiology of the regurgitation, as well as its effects on ventricular dimensions, shape, and function.

Pericardial Disease

(See Chap. 22) 2DE is the imaging modality of choice for the detection of pericardial effusion, which is easily visualized as a black echolucent ovoid structure surrounding the heart (Fig. 22-4). In the hemodynamically unstable patient with pericardial tamponade, typical echo

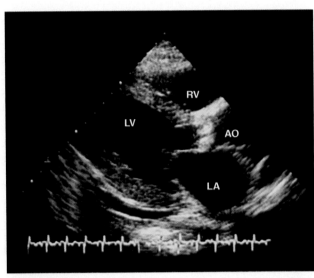

FIGURE 12-2

Still frame two-dimensional echocardiographic image from the parasternal long axis view of a patient with aortic stenosis. The aortic valve is calcified with restricted opening during systole. Ao, aorta; RV, right ventricle; LA, left atrium; LV, left ventricle.

findings include a dilated inferior vena cava, right atrial collapse, and then right ventricular collapse, usually at the base of the ventricle. Echocardiographically guided pericardiocentesis has now become a standard of care. A 2DE can directly visualize the location of the pericardial fluid to guide the entry point of the needle.

Intracardiac Masses

(See Chap. 23) Intracardiac masses can be visualized on 2DE, provided that image quality is adequate. Solid masses appear as echo-dense structures, which can be located inside the cardiac chambers or infiltrating into the myocardium or pericardium. LV thrombus appears as an echo-dense structure, usually in the apical region associated with regional wall motion abnormalities. The appearance and mobility of the thrombus are predictive of embolic events. Vegetations appear as mobile linear echo densities attached to valve leaflets. Atrial myxoma can be diagnosed by the appearance of a well-circumscribed mobile mass with attachments to the atrial septum (Fig. 23-1). The high-resolution images provided by TEE may be required for further delineation of myocardial masses, especially those <1 cm in diameter.

Aortic Disease

(See Chap. 38) 2DE can provide extremely useful information on diseases of the aorta. The proximal ascending aorta, the arch, and the distal descending aorta can usually be visualized via the transthoracic approach. The definitive diagnosis of a suspected aortic dissection usually requires a TEE, which can rapidly provide high-resolution images of the proximal ascending and descending thoracic aorta (Fig. 12-3).

DOPPLER ECHOCARDIOGRAPHY

Basic Principles

Doppler echocardiography uses ultrasound reflecting off moving red blood cells to measure the velocity of blood flow across valves, within cardiac chambers, and through the great vessels. Normal and abnormal blood flow patterns can be assessed noninvasively. *Color-flow Doppler* imaging displays the blood velocities in real time superimposed upon a 2-D echocardiographic image. The different colors indicate the direction of blood flow (red toward and blue away from the transducer), with

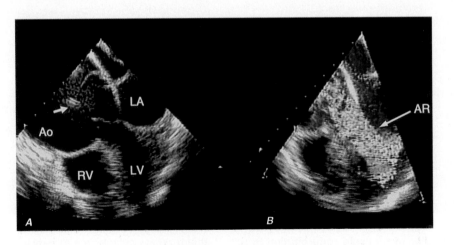

FIGURE 12-3

Transesophageal echocardiographic view of a patient with a dilated aorta, aortic dissection, and severe aortic regurgitation. **A.** The long axis apex-down view of the black and white two-dimensional image in diastole. The arrow points to the intimal flap that is seen in the dilated ascending aorta. **B.** Color-flow imaging that demonstrates a large mosaic jet of aortic regurgitation. Ao, aorta; LA, left atrium; LV, left ventricle; RV, right ventricle; AR, aortic regurgitation.

green superimposed when there is turbulent flow. *Pulsed-wave Doppler* measures the blood flow velocity in a specific location on the 2-D echocardiographic image. *Continuous-wave Doppler* echocardiography can measure high velocities of blood flow directed along the line of the Doppler beam, such as occur in the presence of valve stenosis, valve regurgitation, or intracardiac shunts. The high velocities can be used to determine intracardiac pressure gradients by a modified Bernoulli equation:

$$\text{Pressure change} = 4 \times (\text{velocity})^2$$

The derived pressure gradient can be used to determine intracardiac pressures and stenosis severity.

Tissue Doppler echocardiography measures the velocity of myocardial motion. The velocity of myocardium is several magnitudes lower than the velocity of moving red blood cells. Myocardial velocities can be used to determine myocardial strain rate, which is a quantitative measure of regional myocardial contraction and relaxation.

Valve Gradients

In the presence of valvular stenosis, there is an increase in the velocity of blood flow across the stenotic valve. A continuous-wave Doppler beam is used to determine an instantaneous gradient across the valve.

Valvular Regurgitation

Valvular regurgitation is diagnosed by Doppler echocardiography when there is abnormal retrograde flow across the valve. Color-flow imaging is the Doppler method used most frequently to detect valve regurgitation by visualization of a high-velocity turbulent jet in the chamber proximal to the regurgitant valve (Fig. 12-3). The size and extent of the color-flow jet into the receiving cardiac chamber provide a semiquantitative estimate of the severity of regurgitation.

Intracardiac Pressures

These can be calculated from the peak continuous-wave Doppler signal of a regurgitant lesion. The Bernoulli equation is applied to the peak velocity to obtain the pressure gradient between two cardiac chambers. This is commonly applied to a tricuspid regurgitant jet, from which the systolic pressure gradient between the right atrium and right ventricle can be calculated. Adding an assumed right atrial pressure to this gradient will give a derived right ventricular systolic pressure. In the absence of right ventricular outflow tract obstruction, the latter provides the pulmonary artery systolic pressure (**Fig. 12-4**).

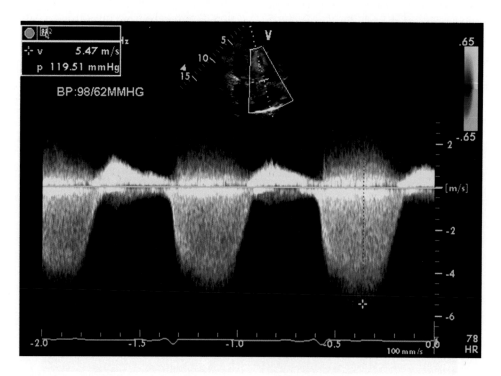

FIGURE 12-4

Continuous-wave Doppler of tricuspid regurgitation in a patient with pulmonary hypertension. There is an increase in the velocity of flow from the right ventricle into the right atrium to 5.4 m/s. Using the modified Bernoulli equation, the peak pressure gradient between the right ventricle and right atrium during systole is 120 mmHg. Assuming a right atrial pressure of 10 mmHg, the right ventricular systolic pressure is 130 mmHg. In the absence of right ventricular outflow tract obstruction, this indicates there is severe pulmonary hypertension with a pulmonary artery systolic pressure of 130 mmHg.

Cardiac Output

Volume flow rates (or stroke volume and cardiac output) can be reliably measured noninvasively by Doppler echocardiography. Flow is calculated as the product of the cross-sectional area of the vessel or chamber through which blood moves and the velocity of blood flow as assessed by continuous-wave Doppler determination. The time-velocity integral can be used to calculate pulsatile flow, and that integral multiplied by the cross-sectional area of, for example, the aortic root yields the stroke volume which, when multiplied by the heart rate, provides an estimate of the cardiac output.

Diastolic Filling

Doppler echocardiography allows noninvasive evaluation of ventricular diastolic filling. The transmitral velocity curves reflect the relative pressure gradients between the left atrium and ventricle throughout diastole. They are influenced by the rate of ventricular relaxation, the driving force across the valve, and the compliance of the ventricle. There is a progression of diastolic dysfunction, which can be assessed by Doppler flow velocity curves. In the early phase of diastolic dysfunction there is primarily an impairment of LV relaxation, with reduced early transmitral flow and a compensatory increase in flow during atrial contraction (**Fig. 12-5**). As disease progresses, and ventricular compliance declines, left atrial pressure rises, resulting in a higher early transmitral velocity and shortening of the deceleration of flow in early diastole so that the filling pattern becomes normal, termed *pseudonormalization*. In patients with the most severe diastolic dysfunction and further elevation of left atrial pressure, early diastolic flow velocity rises further, termed the *restrictive filling pattern*. The addition of analysis of Doppler tissue velocities of annular motion provides further information concerning the diastolic properties.

Congenital Heart Disease

(See Chap. 19) 2DE and Doppler echocardiography have been useful in the evaluation of patients with congenital heart disease. Congenital stenotic or regurgitant valve lesions can be assessed. The detection of intracardiac shunts is possible by 2DE and Doppler echocardiography (Fig. 19-1). Patency of surgical shunts and conduits can be determined.

STRESS ECHOCARDIOGRAPHY

2DE and Doppler echocardiography are usually performed with the patient in the resting state. Further information can be obtained by reimaging during either exercise or pharmacologic stress. The primary indications for stress echocardiography are to confirm the suspicion of ischemic heart disease and estimate its severity (see later).

A decrease in systolic contraction of an ischemic area of myocardium, termed a *regional wall motion abnormality*, occurs before symptoms or electrocardiographic changes. New regional wall motion abnormalities, a decline in ejection fraction, and an increase in end-systolic volume with stress are all indicators of myocardial ischemia. Exercise stress testing is usually done with exercise protocols using either upright treadmill or bicycle exercise. The echocardiographic imaging is done at baseline and then immediately after exercise. In patients who are not able to exercise, pharmacologic testing can be performed by infusion of dobutamine to increase myocardial oxygen demand. Dobutamine echocardiography has

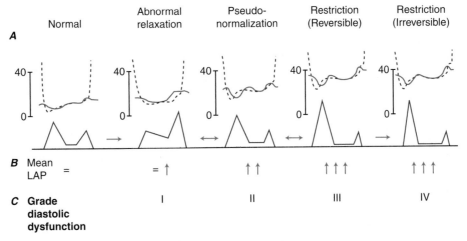

FIGURE 12-5
Diagrammatic illustration indicating the progression of diastolic dysfunction. A. Left atrial and ventricular pressures; **B.** Transmitral flow velocity as measured by Doppler echocardiography; **C.** Grade of diastolic dysfunction. LAP, left atrial pressure.

also been used to assess myocardial viability in patients with poor systolic function and concomitant CAD.

Doppler echocardiography can be used at rest and during exercise in patients with valvular heart disease to determine the hemodynamic response to stress. In patients with low-output, low-gradient aortic stenosis, the response of the gradient to dobutamine stimulation is of diagnostic and therapeutic value.

TRANSESOPHAGEAL ECHOCARDIOGRAPHY

When limited information is obtained from a TTE due to poor imaging windows, TEE can be useful. Diseases of the aorta, such as aortic dissection, can be readily diagnosed by TEE (Fig. 12-3). Defining the source of embolism is a common indication for TEE, as abnormalities such as atrial thrombi, patent foramen ovale, and aortic plaques can be detected. Other masses, particularly those in the atria, can be visualized. The presence of vegetations for the diagnosis of infective endocarditis and its complications can be assessed by TEE. The technique has been used before cardioversion in patients with atrial fibrillation to detect a thrombus in the left atrium or left atrial appendage. If no thrombus is present, cardioversion can be safely performed, as long as there is full-dose anticoagulation before, during, and after the procedure.

EMERGENCY ECHOCARDIOGRAPHY

A major advantage of echocardiography is the ability to obtain instantaneous images of the cardiac structures for immediate interpretation at the patient's bedside. Thus, echocardiography has become an ideal imaging modality for cardiac emergencies.

Unstable Hemodynamics

For the patient with unstable hemodynamics, echocardiography can determine LV size and function, right ventricular size and function, and the presence of acute valvular regurgitation and pericardial tamponade. Echocardiography is especially useful in the hemodynamically unstable patient following myocardial infarction (Chaps. 35 and 28), in whom acute mechanical complications (e.g., papillary muscle rupture, ventricular septal defect, myocardial perforation with tamponade, and right ventricular infarction) that need to be differentiated from severe LV systolic dysfunction can be diagnosed.

Chest Pain Syndromes

(See Chap. 4) Echocardiography can be useful in selected patients with chest pain syndromes. For those patients who have an equivocal electrocardiogram, the presence

of regional wall motion abnormalities on an echocardiogram can lead to the diagnosis of myocardial ischemia as an etiology for the pain. Other etiologies of chest pain, such as acute dissection or pericarditis with effusion, can also be diagnosed by echocardiography.

NUCLEAR CARDIOLOGY

BASIC PRINCIPLES OF NUCLEAR CARDIOLOGY

All nuclear cardiology studies depend on the injection into the patient of an isotope that emits photons, generally gamma rays generated during radioactive decay when the nucleus of an isotope changes from one energy level to a lower one. Radionuclide imaging uses a special camera that images these photons.

ASSESSMENT OF VENTRICULAR FUNCTION

Equilibrium radionuclide angiography, also known as *multiple-gated blood pool imaging*, involves the imaging of ^{99m}Tc-labeled albumin or red cells that are uniformly distributed throughout the blood volume. Resting images of the blood pool of isotopes within the cardiac chambers are obtained by electrocardiographic gating through multiple cycles, so that sufficient counts can be detected to obtain an image. This requires that the heart rate be reasonably constant. It provides an accurate, reproducible method for assessment of LV function. It is most commonly used when echocardiography is technically difficult or when poor LV function requires accurate quantitation.

Gated single-photon emission computed tomography (SPECT) is the nuclear cardiology technique that is most commonly utilized to assess ejection fraction and regional wall motion. This is usually performed post-stress by gating the acquisition of SPECT myocardial perfusion images using ^{99m}Tc- labeled compounds (see later). An automated technique determines the endocardial borders of the LV cavity, and a geometric model is used to calculate the ejection fraction.

ASSESSMENT OF MYOCARDIAL PERFUSION BY SPECT

(See Chap. 33) Myocardial perfusion imaging by nuclear techniques is now widely applied for the evaluation of ischemic heart disease. Injection of radioisotopes at rest and during stress is performed to produce images of myocardial regional uptake proportional to regional blood flow. With maximal exercise, myocardial blood flow is increased up to fivefold above the resting condition. In the presence of a fixed coronary stenosis, there is an inability to increase myocardial perfusion in the territory supplied by the stenosis, creating a flow differential and inhomogeneous distribution of the isotope. In patients who are unable to exercise, pharmacologic agents are used to increase blood flow and create similar inhomogeneities. The preferred pharmacologic agents are adenosine or dipyridamole, which increase blood flow to a similar degree as exercise. In patients with bronchospastic lung disease, which is a contraindication to the use of adenosine or dipyridamole, dobutamine may be used as an alternative, although it does not increase myocardial blood flow to the same extent.

^{201}Tl (thallium) was the first isotope used for this purpose. It has been largely replaced by ^{99m}Tc, which has a higher photon energy and shorter half-life, permitting the injection of larger doses resulting in scans of higher quality (Fig. 12-6). Two technetium-labeled myocardium perfusion agents are in common use: tetrofosmin and sestamibi. Like thallium, tetrofosmin and sestamibi distribute to the myocardium in relation to blood flow, and their uptake requires an intact cell membrane and a viable myocardial cell. Both agents are bound within the cell in a nearly irreversible fashion. As a result, these agents must generally be injected twice—once at rest and once during stress.

POSITRON EMISSION TOMOGRAPHY

The underlying physics of positron emission tomography (PET) scanning differs from that involved in the standard radionuclide techniques described above. Positron emission

is a type of beta-decay of an unstable isotope. In this unstable isotope, a proton undergoes spontaneous decay into a neutron, a neutrino, and a β$^+$ particle (positron). The spontaneous release of positrons from these unstable nuclei leads to their interaction with electrons, which cause the release of gamma-radiation (photons) upon collision with tissue. It is this gamma emission that is detected by the gamma camera in the PET scanner. The very high energy of the photons results in far less scatter than with conventional nuclear cardiology techniques. PET cameras are considerably more expensive than conventional nuclear cardiology cameras. Rubidium-82 is the most commonly used positron emitter, as it is available from a generator and does not require a nearby cyclotron. Pharmacologic stress with dipyridamole, adenosine, or dobutamine is preferred for PET scanning.

Positron emitters can be employed to study myocardial blood flow and myocardial metabolism. Nitrogen-13 ammonia, oxygen-15 water, and rubidium-82 have all been employed to assess myocardial blood flow. They permit measurement of absolute regional blood flows, in contrast to the relative blood flows that are assessed with ^{201}Tl- or ^{99m}Tc-labeled compounds. This advantage has been utilized for research purposes but has generally not been exploited clinically. Myocardial metabolism is most often assessed using fluorine-18 deoxyglucose. The agent permits the detection and quantification of exogenous glucose utilization in areas of hypoperfused myocardium.

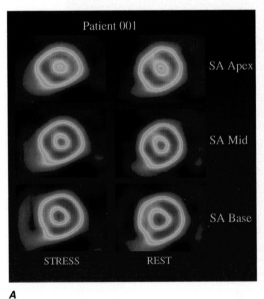

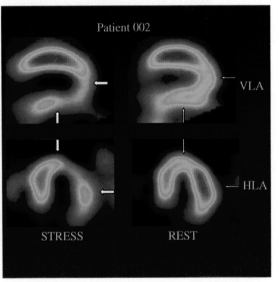

FIGURE 12-6

Exercise studies of atypical and typical angina. A. Exercise ^{99m}Tc sestamibi study of a 71-year-old white female with atypical angina. **Left:** Stress images; **Right:** rest images. The images are normal. There is uniform sestamibi uptake throughout the myocardium at rest and during stress. **B.** Exercise sestamibi study of a 75-year-old male with a history of typical angina. **Left:** Stress images; **Right:** rest images. The stress images show a large defect involving the apex, lateral, and inferior walls (thick arrows), which improves at rest (thin arrows). Subsequent coronary angiography demonstrates severe three-vessel coronary artery disease.

The clinical application of PET scanning that has been best studied is the assessment of myocardial viability. The pattern of enhanced fluorodeoxyglucose uptake in regions of decreased perfusion (termed *glucose/blood flow "mismatch"*) indicates the presence of ischemic myocardium that has preferentially shifted its metabolic substrate toward glucose rather than fatty acid or lactate. This pattern identifies regions of ischemic or hibernating myocardium that are likely to improve in function after revascularization (Fig. 12-7).

Comparative studies have consistently shown the ability of PET to identify ischemic or hibernating myocardium in 10–20% of regions that would be classified as fibrotic (infarcted) by ^{201}Tl- or ^{99m}Tc-labeled compounds. For that reason, this technique is generally regarded as the gold standard for the assessment of myocardial viability. When large fixed defects (infarcts) are detected by ^{201}Tl- or ^{99m}Tc labeled compounds in patients who are candidates for coronary revascularization, PET imaging can help in the decision whether the risk of revascularization is justified by the potential benefit.

The technical limitations of ^{201}Tl- and ^{99m}Tc-labeled compounds in obese patients, and the increasing prevalence of patient obesity, are contributing to the increasing use of PET scanning for the assessment of myocardial perfusion.

MRI AND CT IMAGING

MAGNETIC RESONANCE IMAGING

Basic Principles

MRI is a technique based on the magnetic properties of hydrogen nuclei. In the presence of a large magnetic field, nuclear spin transitions from the ground state to excited states can be induced, and as the nuclei relax and return to their ground state, they release energy in the form of electromagnetic radiation that is detected and processed into an image. Contrast agents, such as gadolinium, are frequently employed to produce magnetic resonance angiograms (MRAs). These agents provide enhanced soft tissue contrast as well as the opportunity to obtain rapid angiographic images during the first pass of contrast through the vascular system. Cardiac MRI is particularly challenging because of the rapid motion of the heart and coronary arteries. Static and cine images can be obtained using electrocardiographic triggering, often within a short breath-hold of 10–15 s. Cine images can be acquired in any plane with excellent blood-myocardial contrast, and these images can be used to quantify ejection fraction, end-systolic and end-diastolic volumes, and cardiac mass with high accuracy, reliability, and reproducibility, without the need for ionizing radiation.

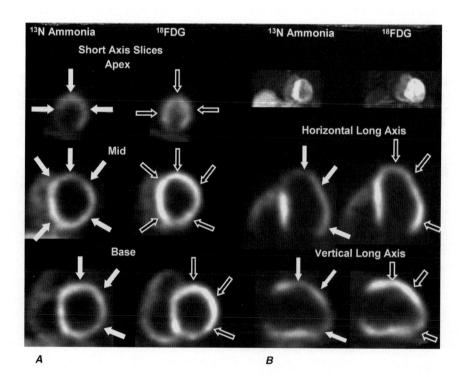

FIGURE 12-7

Positron emission tomography (PET). Short-axis PET resting ammonia image (**A**) and FDG image (**B**) of a 63-year-old diabetic female with dyspnea on exertion, a fixed SPECT defect, severe LV dysfunction, and severe coronary artery disease. The ammonia images show a very large apical, septal, anterior and lateral perfusion defect, which improves on the FDG images. This is consistent with hibernating myocardium. The patient underwent CABG with subsequent dramatic improvement in LV function. FDG, fluorodeoxyglucose; SPECT, single-photon emission CT; CABG, coronary artery bypass grafting; LV, left ventricular.

Clinical Utility

The multiplanar capabilities of MRI, coupled with excellent contrast and spatial resolution, are often valuable in defining anatomic relationships in patients with complex congenital heart disease and cardiomyopathies (Fig. 21-2). Cardiac masses can be characterized and their relationship to normal anatomic structures defined. Likewise, MRI is often the examination of choice to determine whether a mediastinal or pulmonary mass has invaded the pericardium or heart. The entire pericardium can be visualized in multiple planes, and MRI has proved useful in characterizing pericardial effusions or pericardial thickening in patients with indeterminate results on echocardiography. Specialized pulse sequences have been designed to measure the velocity of blood in each pixel of the image, so that flow across valves and within blood vessels may be determined with accuracy. These techniques may allow characterization of the severity of valvular disease as well as quantification of shunt volumes.

MRA is a standard technique for imaging the aorta and large vessels of the chest and abdomen, with results essentially identical to conventional catheter-based angiography (Fig. 12-8). MRA of the coronary arteries is a much more difficult challenge, because of the small size of these vessels and because of their rapid and complex motion during the cardiac cycle. Although promising results have been achieved, coronary MRA is not yet an accurate and reliable clinical technique.

MRI is a promising technology for the evaluation of patients with suspected or known coronary disease. Ventricular function and wall motion can be assessed at rest and during infusion of inotropic agents. Assessment of myocardial perfusion can be performed by injecting a bolus of gadolinium contrast and then continuously scanning the heart as the gadolinium passes through the cardiac chambers and into the myocardium. Relative perfusion deficits are reflected as regions of low signal intensity within the myocardium. Pharmacologic stress (typically achieved with vasodilators) can be applied during perfusion imaging to detect physiologically significant coronary artery lesions. Myocardial perfusion imaging with cardiac MRI is more sensitive then SPECT imaging for detecting subendocardial ischemia due to its enhanced spatial resolution. Myocardial viability may be determined by imaging the heart 10–20 min after gadolinium injection, as infarcted tissue retains contrast by virtue of its larger extracellular volume.

Limitations of MRI

Relative contraindications include the presence of pacemakers, internal defibrillators, or cerebral aneurysm clips. A small percentage of patients are claustrophobic and unable to tolerate the examination within the relatively confined quarters of the magnet bore. However, open-bore magnets are now available to deal with this problem. Examination of clinically unstable patients is problematic, because close monitoring is difficult. Image quality in patients with significant arrhythmias is often limited.

COMPUTED TOMOGRAPHIC IMAGING

Basic Principles

CT is fast, simple, noninvasive, and provides images with excellent spatial resolution and good soft tissue contrast. Cardiac CT has long been technically challenging because image acquisition times for conventional CT were too long to freeze cardiac motion. The development of electron-beam CT and multislice spiral (helical) CT have led to improved temporal resolution and routine imaging of the beating heart.

Clinical Applications

Cardiac CT has several clinical applications. Pericardial calcification is an important sign of constrictive pericarditis and is easily detected by CT (Fig. 12-9). CT is useful in characterizing cardiac masses, particularly those containing fat or calcium. The ability to detect small amounts of fat with high spatial resolution makes CT an attractive technique for imaging patients with suspected arrhythmogenic right ventricular dysplasia (Chap. 21). Cine images can be used to evaluate wall motion and to

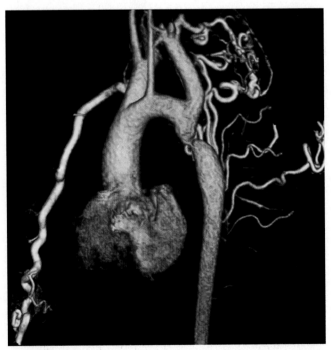

FIGURE 12-8
Still frame of an MR angiogram showing a severe coarctation of the descending aorta, with abundant collateral arteries.

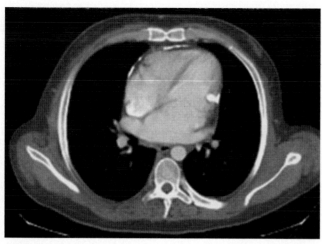

FIGURE 12-9

CT scan demonstrating calcium in a thickened pericardium in a patient with constrictive pericarditis. The calcium is shown as white densities.

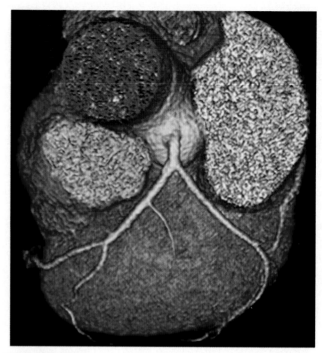

FIGURE 12-10

Three-dimensional reconstruction of a CT angiogram demonstrating a normal main left coronary artery arising from the aorta, and its two branches, the left anterior descending artery (*left*) and the left circumflex artery (*right*).

determine ejection fraction, end-diastolic and end-systolic volumes, and cardiac mass.

CT angiography (CTA) has demonstrated accuracy similar to MRA in imaging the aorta and great vessels, and CTA is rapidly becoming the examination of choice in the evaluation of patients with suspected pulmonary embolus. CTA is an excellent imaging modality for the diagnosis of aortic dissection or penetrating ulcers. Visualization of the entire aorta is possible by CTA, so that the initial diagnosis as well as follow-up of patients with aortic aneurysmal disease can be done.

Coronary Calcification

Calcium in the coronary arteries occurs in atherosclerosis and is absent in the normal coronary artery. CT is very sensitive for the detection of coronary artery calcification and is being promoted as a noninvasive modality for the screening and diagnosis of CAD. The quantity of coronary calcification (coronary calcium score) is related to the severity of CAD. However, although CT has a very high sensitivity for the detection of CAD, it has a low specificity. The overall predictive accuracy for angiographic obstructive coronary disease in a typical population of patients with CAD is similar to other imaging modalities, such as SPECT. Due to its low specificity, CT should not be used for the diagnosis of obstructive coronary disease.

Contrast-Enhanced CTA

With the high temporal and spatial resolution of multi-slice spiral CT, accurate assessment of luminal narrowing in the major branches of the coronary arteries is possible in selected patients. Studies at experienced centers have shown a high sensitivity (>85%), and specificity (>90%)

of CTA as compared to cardiac catheterization. The highest accuracy has been noted in the left main and the proximal portions of the left anterior descending and left circumflex arteries (**Fig. 12-10**), probably due to the rapid motion of the right and circumflex arteries. Fast, irregular heart rates and body motion limit the accuracy of CTA.

The concept of "noninvasive coronary angiography" has generated great interest in the widespread utility of CTA. However, at present, the major well-accepted indication for coronary CTA is in the evaluation of suspected coronary anomalies. CTA may also be of use in patients with chest pain syndromes who have an intermediate pretest probability of CAD who are unable to exercise or have an uninterpretable or equivocal stress test.

Limitations of CT

Limitations of CT include its dependence on ionizing radiation (in contrast to MRI) and the need for iodinated contrast, which is problematic in patients with renal insufficiency or contrast allergy. While radiation doses for some applications (such as coronary calcification scoring) are relatively low, doses tend to increase as the spatial resolution improves, and the doses for coronary CTA generally exceed those delivered during standard diagnostic cardiac catheterization.

SELECTION OF IMAGING TESTS

BASIC PREMISE

The choice of the optimal imaging modality for a particular patient should be based upon the major problem being addressed, other concomitant clinical questions, as well as the local expertise and equipment available in an institution. The clinical urgency and costs need to be considered, because of the high costs of some of these modalities (Table 12–2).

Left Ventricular Size and Function

2DE is the primary imaging modality obtained for assessment of LV cavity size, systolic function, and wall thickness. It is widely available, portable, and provides an instantaneous view of the heart. Echocardiography can also provide concomitant information on valve function, pulmonary artery pressures, and diastolic filling, which are valuable in the patient presenting with possible heart failure. The disadvantage is poor endocardial resolution in some patients and the lack of reproducible quantitative measurements.

Equilibrium radionuclide angiography can provide an accurate quantitative measurement of LV function but is not widely available and cannot be used in patients with irregular rhythms. Gated SPECT can measure ejection fraction as a part of stress imaging. MRI and CT scanning provide the highest quality resolution of endocardial border and thus are the most accurate of all modalities. However, they are of higher cost, lack portability, and do not provide concomitant hemodynamic information as echocardiography does.

Valvular Heart Disease

2DE and Doppler echocardiography provide anatomic and hemodynamic information regarding valve disease, thus echocardiography is the first test of choice. MRI can also visualize valve motion and determine abnormal flow velocities across valves, but there is less validation of quantitative hemodynamic measurements in comparison to echocardiography.

Pericardial Disease

Echocardiography is the first imaging modality of choice in patients with suspected pericardial effusion and tamponade, due to its rapid image display and portability. For patients with suspected constrictive pericarditis, either MRI or CT scanning is the imaging modality that best delineates pericardial thickness. Hemodynamic analysis of the enhancement of ventricular interaction that occurs in pericardial constriction can be assessed by Doppler echocardiography.

TABLE 12-2

SELECTION OF IMAGING TESTS				
	ECHO	**NUCLEAR**	**CT**[a]	**MRI**[b]
LV Size/function	Initial modality of choice Low cost, portable Provides ancillary structural and hemodynamic information	Available from gated SPECT stress imaging	Best resolution Highest cost	Best resolution Highest cost
Valve disease	Initial modality of choice Valve motion Doppler hemodynamics			Visualize valve motion Delineate abnormal flow
Pericardial disease	Pericardial effusion Doppler hemodynamics		Pericardial thickening	Pericardial thickening
Aortic disease	TEE rapid diagnosis[c] Acute dissection		Image entire aorta Acute aneurysm Aortic dissection	Image entire aorta Aortic aneurysm Chronic dissection
Cardiac masses	TTE—large intracardiac masses TEE—smaller intracardiac massesc	Extracardiac masses	Extracardiac masses Myocardial masses	Myocardiac masses

[a]Contrast required.
[b]Relative contraindication: pacemakers, metallic objects, claustrophobic.
[c]When not seen on TTE.
Note: Echo, echocardiography; SPECT, single-photon emission CT; TEE, transesophageal echocardiography; TTE, transthoracic echocardiogram.

CT scanning and MRI are the imaging modalities of choice for the evaluation of the stable patient with suspected aortic aneurysm or aortic dissection. In the acutely ill patient with suspected aortic dissection, either TEE or CT scanning is a reliable imaging modality.

Cardiac Masses

2-D TTE is the first test to rule out an intracardiac mass; masses >1.0 cm in diameter are usually well visualized. Intracardiac masses of smaller size may be visualized by TEE. CT scanning and MRI are optimal for evaluating masses extrinsic to the heart or involving the myocardium.

CHOOSING THE APPROPRIATE STRESS TEST

The choice of an initial stress testing modality should be based on the evaluation of the patient's resting electrocardiogram, the ability to perform exercise, and the available local expertise and technology (**Fig. 12-11**).

For the standard assessment of CAD, the exercise electrocardiographic test should be the initial stress test in patients with an interpretable electrocardiogram who are able to exercise. If there are resting electrocardiographic abnormalities (ST depression >1 mm, LV hypertrophy, bundle branch block, paced rhythm, preexcitation), if the patient is taking digoxin, or if the patient has had a prior coronary revascularization, an imaging modality (either nuclear imaging or echocardiography) should be used for initial evaluation. Pharmacologic stress testing with imaging should be used in patients who are unable to exercise.

When an imaging modality is indicated, the decision to use an echocardiographic or a nuclear test depends not only on the clinical features but also on the available local expertise and technology. Both echocardiography and nuclear imaging require expertise in the performance and interpretation of the tests, and the patient is often best evaluated with the imaging modality for which the most expertise and experience are available. There are, however, certain situations in which one imaging modality has an advantage over the other.

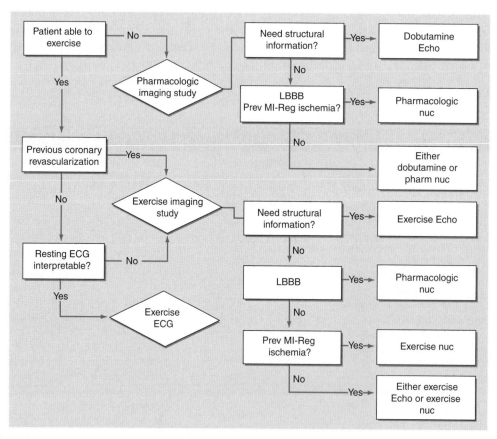

FIGURE 12-11

Flow diagram showing selection of initial stress test in a patient with chest pain. Patients who are able to exercise, without previous revascularization, and with an interpretable resting ECG can be tested with an exercise ECG. The appropriate imaging study for other patients depends on multiple factors (see text). LBBB, left bundle branch block; Prev MI-Reg ischemia, previous MI with a need to detect regional ischemia; Nuc, SPECT nuclear imaging study; Pharm, pharmacologic.

Echocardiography provides additional structural information. Therefore, if there is a question of concomitant valve disease, pericardial disease, or aortic disease, echocardiography is able to provide information regarding these issues. The major limitation of echocardiography is the inability to obtain diagnostic images in all patients, especially those with chronic obstructive pulmonary disease or severe obesity. If there is inadequate definition of endocardial motion on the resting echocardiogram, stress echocardiography should not be performed unless contrast enhancement can be used. If the patient has had a previous infarction and one needs to determine whether a specific region of the myocardium is ischemic, nuclear imaging is the preferred modality. Nuclear imaging using ^{99m}Tc-labeled compounds is preferred in obese patients and those with severe lung disease. Nuclear imaging is more sensitive and less specific than echocardiography for the detection of myocardial ischemia.

The imaging tests can add prognostic information, especially when the results of an exercise electrocardiogram fall into an intermediate risk category. For nuclear imaging, a normal stress (exercise or pharmacologic) myocardial perfusion scan is highly predictive of the absence of significant artery disease and a low risk of subsequent cardiac death. Similarly, for stress (exercise or dobutamine) echocardiography, an increase in ejection fraction and a decrease in end-systolic volume at a high workload predict the absence of significant CAD and a low risk of subsequent cardiac death. On the other hand, for nuclear imaging, large or multiple stress-induced defects, or a large fixed defect with LV dilatation or increased ^{201}Tl lung uptake are high-risk findings. For stress echocardiography, patients with a decrease in ejection fraction, multiple new regional wall motion abnormalities, and an increase in end-systolic volume at a low workload are at high risk. Investigations are underway to determine the clinical value of stress MRI.

FURTHER READINGS

ACHENBACH S, DANIEL WG: Computed tomography of the heart, in P Libby et al (eds): *Braunwald's Heart Disease*, 8th ed, Philadelphia, Elsevier, 2008

CHEITLIN MD et al: ACC/AHA/ASE 2003 Guideline Update for the Clinical Application of Echocardiography: A Report of the American College of Cardiology/American Heart Association Task Force on Practice Guidelines (ACC/AHA/ASE Committee to Update the 1997 Guidelines for the Clinical Application of Echocardiography). Circulation 108:1146, 2003

CONSTANTINE G et al: Role of MRI in clinical cardiology. Lancet 363:2162, 2004

GIBBONS RJ et al: ACC/AHA 2002 Guideline Update for Exercise Testing: A Report of the American College of Cardiology/American Heart Association Task Force on Practice Guidelines (Committee on Exercise Testing). J Am Coll Cardiol 40:1531, 2002

HENDEL RC et al: ACCF Appropriateness criteria for cardiac computed tomography and cardiac magnetic resonance imaging: A report of the American College of Cardiology Foundation. J Am Coll Cardiol 48:1475, 2006

KLOCKE FJ et al: ACC/AHA/ASNC Guidelines for the Clinical Use of Cardiac Radionuclide Imaging-Executive Summary: A Report of the American College of Cardiology/American Heart Association Task Force on Practice Guidelines (ACC/AHA/ASNC Committee to Revise the 1995 Guidelines for the Clinical Use of Cardiac Radionuclide Imaging). J Am Coll Cardiol 42:1318, 2003

MARWICK TH: Measurement of strain and strain rate by echocardiography: Ready for prime time? J Am Coll Cardiol 47:1313, 2006

PENNELL D: Cardiovascular magnetic resonance, in P Libby et al (eds): *Braunwald's Heart Disease*, 8th ed, Philadelphia, Elsevier, 2008

CHAPTER 13

DIAGNOSTIC CARDIAC CATHETERIZATION AND ANGIOGRAPHY

Donald S. Baim[†]

Despite progressive improvements in noninvasive techniques, cardiac catheterization remains a key clinical tool for assessing the anatomy and physiology of the heart and its associated vasculature. It involves the insertion of catheters (2-mm diameter hollow plastic tubes) into a peripheral artery or vein under local anesthesia, and their passage into the heart for the purposes of intracardiac pressure measurement or the injection of a liquid radiographic contrast agent. The findings of diagnostic cardiac catheterization characterize the extent and severity of cardiac disease and thereby can help to determine the most appropriate plan for medical, surgical, or catheter-based treatment. Although the majority of patients with coronary artery disease (CAD) or valvular disease can be managed medically using only clinical and noninvasive data (e.g., exercise testing, echocardiography, and MRI), >2 million patients each year undergo cardiac catheterization and angiographic procedures for diagnostic or interventional purposes, or both. This chapter focuses on the uses of cardiac catheterization as a diagnostic tool. For further discussion of catheter-based interventions, see Chap. 36.

BASIC PRINCIPLES

Given the expense and small but real risks of cardiac catheterization, the procedure is not indicated routinely whenever cardiac disease is diagnosed or suspected. Instead, cardiac catheterization is reserved for situations where there is a need to confirm the presence of a clinically suspected condition, define its anatomic and physiologic severity, and determine the presence or absence of important associated conditions. This situation arises most commonly when a patient experiences limiting or escalating symptoms of cardiac dysfunction (Chap. 17) that may include acute coronary syndromes, such as unstable angina or acute myocardial infarction (Chap. 34), or when objective measures (such as exercise testing or echocardiography) suggest that the patient has findings (such as an early positive exercise test or worsening ventricular function) that signal a high risk of progressing to rapid functional deterioration, myocardial infarction, or other adverse events. Under these circumstances, diagnostic catheterization may not only identify the culprit coronary lesions, but in ~40% of procedures may progress seamlessly into a catheter-based therapeutic procedure

[†]Recently deceased.

[percutaneous coronary intervention (PCI); Chap. 36] that can provide definitive correction. Alternatively, diagnostic catheterization may demonstrate only less critical lesions that can be managed medically or severe lesions poorly suited to PCI that may be referred for treatment by cardiac surgery (e.g., coronary bypass surgery, valve replacement, or valve repair).

While cardiac catheterization was once considered mandatory in *all* patients being considered for cardiac surgery, currently many patients with congenital or valvular heart disease undergo surgical correction based solely on clinical and noninvasive test data [e.g., echocardiography and MRI (Chap. 12)], with diagnostic coronary angiography performed in older patients or those with risk factors for or non-invasive testing suggesting coronary disease, prior to surgery.

When there is a clinical "need to know," there are very few absolute contraindications to diagnostic cardiac catheterization in a patient who understands and accepts the associated risks. The risk of death from elective cardiac catheterization approaches 1 in 10,000 (0.01%), but the procedure does carry a small (~1 in 1000) risk of stroke or myocardial infarction, transient tachy- or bradyarrhythmias, or bruising or bleeding at the catheter insertion site. These complications respond to drug therapy, countershock, or vascular surgical repair, without long-term sequelae. About 1% of patients used to experience *allergic reactions* to iodinated contrast agents, ranging from urticaria to frank anaphylaxis in sensitive patients, but these have become rare events with current nonionic low-osmolar contrast agents.

Other patients (particularly those with baseline renal dysfunction or proteinuria) may develop transient deterioration in renal function, the chance of which may be further reduced by adequate prehydration (50% normal saline, or D_5W with 154 meq/L of sodium bicarbonate added, given at 3 mL/kg for 1 h prior to and 1 mL/kg for 6 h following the procedure, absent congestive heart failure), preprocedure administration of N-acetylcysteine (Mucomist, 600 mg orally before and twice a day after the procedure), or the use of an iso-osmolar contrast agent (iodixanol). Newer low- or iso-osmolar contrast agents also reduce the chance of myocardial depression and other side effects (hypotension, nausea, bradycardia, or a sensation of marked warmth following injection) that were once common when earlier high-osmolar contrast agents were used.

Cardiac catheterization is generally performed with the patient fasting for the previous 6 h and awake but lightly sedated. The desired level of sedation may be achieved with preprocedure sedatives such as oral diazepam (Valium, 5–10 mg), or with IV conscious sedation using midazolam (Versed, 1 mg) or fentanyl (25–50 µg) following guidelines for conscious sedation. Most elective procedures are performed on an *outpatient* basis, with the patient discharged with instructions regarding maintenance of a liberal oral fluid intake, avoidance of strenuous activity, and self-monitoring for access site complications, following 2–4 h of postprocedure bed rest. If required by associated medical conditions or complications, or if a PCI has been performed, overnight hospitalization may be recommended.

To minimize the risks of bleeding at the local catheter insertion site, patients who have been anticoagulated chronically with warfarin should have this agent discontinued at least 48 h prior to the procedure, so that the INR falls below 2. Oral aspirin (325 mg/d) is routinely administered to patients undergoing diagnostic catheterization for suspected coronary disease, since aspirin pretreatment is desired if a coronary intervention is to be performed. Since cardiac catheterization is a sterile procedure, prophylactic antibiotics are not necessary.

Most (>95%) cardiac catheterizations are performed by the percutaneous femoral technique that begins with needle puncture of the common femoral artery or (for right heart catheterization) the femoral vein. A flexible guidewire is inserted through this needle and supports insertion of a vascular access sheath, through which the desired catheters can be advanced. This percutaneous technique can be adapted to other arterial sites such as (1) the brachial and radial artery in patients with peripheral vascular disease involving the abdominal aorta and iliac or femoral arteries or in whom immediate postprocedure ambulation is desired, or (2) the internal jugular vein for right heart catheterization in patients who may require prolonged hemodynamic monitoring.

Cardiac catheterization may include a variety of different measurements of pressure and flow (hemodynamics) as well as a variety of different contrast injections recorded as x-ray movies (angiography), determined by the nature of the clinical problem being evaluated, and the extent of information available from prior noninvasive evaluation of left ventricular and valvular function. Full left and right heart hemodynamic studies are generally reserved for patients in whom the noninvasive data are unclear, or in whom intra- and postprocedural hemodynamic monitoring of unstable circulatory status may be desired.

Right Heart Catheterization

This procedure involves measurement of the pressures in the right side of the heart. It was once a routine component of cardiac catheterization but is now used in <25% of procedures, especially when significant left and/or right ventricular dysfunction, valve disease, myopericardial disease, or intracardiac shunting is suspected. The right heart catheterization procedure is similar to the placement of a Swan-Ganz catheter at the bedside (except that it is performed under fluoroscopic guidance). A balloon flotation catheter is inserted percutaneously into a suitable vein (femoral, brachial, subclavian, or internal jugular) and advanced sequentially into the right atrium, right ventricle, pulmonary artery, and pulmonary artery wedge position. Pressure is recorded at each of these locations, and after recording the pulmonary wedge pressure (which approximates left atrial pressure), the balloon is deflated so that blood samples can be obtained for oxygen saturation measurement to screen for intracardiac shunts and to estimate the cardiac output by the Fick principle (Table 13-1). Alternatively, the cardiac output may be estimated by the thermodilution method, using a thermistor on the catheter to analyze the temperature deviations in the pulmonary artery that occur following a 10-mL bolus injection of room-temperature IV solution into the right atrium.

Left Heart Catheterization

This procedure may be performed by percutaneous access of the femoral, brachial, or radial arteries. The left heart catheter is advanced under fluoroscopic guidance into the central aorta and then retrograded across the aortic valve into the left ventricle. If a right heart catheter is in place, simultaneous measurement and recording of left heart, right heart, and peripheral arterial pressures, together with a determination of cardiac output by either thermodilution or the Fick method, can capture a comprehensive hemodynamic profile. When valvular stenosis is present, the measurements of the pressures in the upstream and downstream chambers (e.g., in the left ventricle and ascending aorta for aortic stenosis, or the pulmonary capillary wedge pressure and left ventricle in mitral stenosis) can be combined with the measurement of flow from the cardiac output measurement to allow calculation of the stenotic valve orifice area.

An example of normal pressure tracings is shown in **Fig. 13-1**. In contrast, the characteristic hemodynamic tracings of mitral stenosis, with a diastolic pressure gradient between the left atrium (or pulmonary capillary wedge pressure) and the left ventricle, is seen in **Fig. 13-2**, and the findings of significant mitral regurgitation with a prominent *v* wave in the pulmonary capillary wedge pressure that increases substantially during modest exercise in **Fig. 13-3**. Severe *aortic stenosis* results in a systolic gradient between the left ventricular cavity and the ascending aorta, as shown in **Fig. 13-4**, whereas severe *aortic regurgitation* produces a widening of the aortic pulse pressure, with equilibration of aortic and left ventricular pressures in diastole as seen in **Fig. 13-5**. Valvular heart disease affecting the tricuspid or pulmonic valves results in similar deformities of the right-sided pressures, i.e., in patients with severe *tricuspid regurgitation*, the right atrial pressure resembles the right ventricular pressure closely in appearance, whereas in *tricuspid stenosis*, there is a pressure gradient between the right atrium and ventricle during diastole.

TABLE 13-1

NORMAL VALUES FOR HEMODYNAMIC PARAMETERS	
Pressures (mmHg)	
Systemic arterial	
Peak systolic/end-diastolic	100–140/60–90
Mean	70–105
Left ventricle	
Peak systolic/end-diastolic	100–140/3–12
Left atrium (or pulmonary capillary wedge)	
Mean	2–10
a wave	3–15
v wave	3–15
Pulmonary artery	
Peak systolic/end-diastolic	15–30/4–12
Mean	9–18
Right ventricle	
Peak systolic/end-diastolic	15–30/2–8
Right atrium	
Mean	2–8
a wave	2–10
v wave	2–10
Resistances [(dyn·s)/cm^5]	
Systemic vascular resistance	700–1600
Pulmonary vascular resistance	20–130
Cardiac index [(L/min)/m^2]	2.6–4.2
Oxygen consumption index [(L/min)/m^2]	110–150
Arteriovenous oxygen difference (mL/L)	30–50

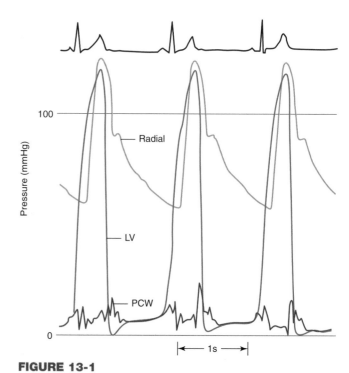

FIGURE 13-1

Left ventricular (LV), radial artery, and pulmonary capillary wedge (PCW) pressures in a patient with normal cardiovascular function. Note the absence of a pressure gradient between the LV and radial artery in systole and between the LV and PCW in diastole.

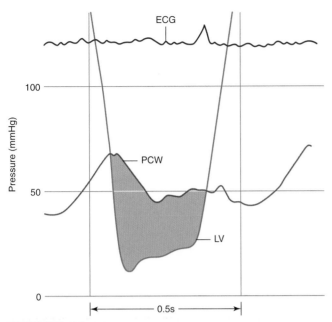

FIGURE 13-2

Pulmonary capillary wedge (PCW) and left ventricular (LV) pressure tracings in a 40-year-old woman with mitral stenosis. The patient also had systemic hypertension and significant elevation of her LV diastolic pressure. ECG, electrocardiogram. *[From BA Carabello, W Grossman, in Grossman's Cardiac Catheterization, Angiography, and Intervention, 7th ed, DS Baim (ed). Baltimore, Lippincott Williams & Wilkins, 2006.]*

LEFT VENTRICULAR AND AORTIC ANGIOGRAPHY

If left ventricular size and function have not been previously assessed by noninvasive means, left ventriculography may be performed by power injection through a suitable

catheter (usually a pigtail shape) of 30–45 mL of radiographic contrast material into the left ventricular chamber at a rate of 10–12 mL/s. The resulting radiographic images define the left ventricular cavity silhouette throughout the cardiac cycle, and tracing of that silhouette at end-diastole and end-systole permits calculation of the absolute left ventricular chamber volumes and the ejection fraction (the fraction of end-diastolic volume ejected during systole; normally 50–80%), as well as qualitative assessment of regional wall motion abnormalities. Regional abnormalities of wall motion include diminished inward motion of a myocardial segment (*hypokinesis*), absence of inward movement of a myocardial segment (*akinesis*), and paradoxical systolic expansion of a regional myocardial segment (*dyskinesis*) (**Fig. 13-6**).

Mitral regurgitation is also easily visualized during left ventriculography as the leakage of radiographic contrast material back into the left atrium during left ventricular systole (**Fig. 13-7**). Its severity can be estimated qualitatively using a grading system of 1+ (mild; radiographic contrast material clears with each beat and never opacifies the entire left atrium) to 4+ (severe; opacification of the entire left atrium occurs within one beat, and contrast material can be seen refluxing into the pulmonary veins).

Aortography involves rapid injection of radiographic contrast material into the ascending aorta, to detect abnormalities of the ascending aorta and aortic valve. It allows qualitative assessment abnormalities such as aortic regurgitation, which is graded using a 1+ to 4+ scale, similar to that used for mitral regurgitation (see above). Aortography can permit identification of aortic aneurysm and/or aortic dissection in which external compression of the aortic true lumen is caused by displacement of an

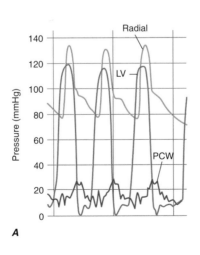

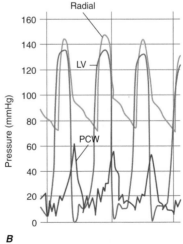

FIGURE 13-3

Hemodynamic findings at rest and during exercise in a patient with mitral regurgitation. Left ventricular (LV), pulmonary capillary wedge (PCW), and radial artery pressure tracings are shown before (**A**) and during (**B**) the sixth minute of supine bicycle exercise. PCW mean pressure and

v wave increase substantially with exercise. *[From W Grossman, in Grossman's Cardiac Catheterization, Angiography, and Intervention, 7th ed, DS Baim (ed). Baltimore, Lippincott Williams & Wilkins, 2006.]*

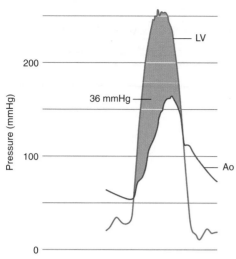

FIGURE 13-4

Severe aortic stenosis. Hemodynamic findings show the left ventricular (LV), and aortic (Ao) pressure with a slow systolic rise and large (96 mmHg) systolic gradient (shaded area) corresponding to critical aortic stenosis (aortic valve area 0.5 cm²). *[From BA Carabello, W Grossman, in Grossman's Cardiac Catheterization, Angiography, and Intervention, 7th ed, DS Baim (ed). Baltimore, Lippincott Williams & Wilkins, 2006.]*

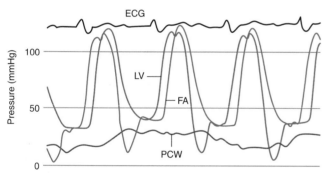

FIGURE 13-5

Severe aortic regurgitation. There is equilibration between the left ventricular (LV) and aortic or femoral artery (FA) pressures in diastole. Also, LV diastolic pressure exceeds pulmonary capillary wedge (PCW) pressure early in diastole, indicating premature closure of the mitral valve (a characteristic feature of severe aortic regurgitation). ECG, electrocardiogram. *[From W Grossman, in Grossman's Cardiac Catheterization, Angiography, and Intervention, 7th ed, DS Baim, W Grossman (eds). Baltimore, Lippincott Williams & Wilkins, 2006.]*

intimal flap separating the true and false aortic lumina (Chap. 38). Aortography may also be used to identify the origin of patent saphenous vein grafts which cannot be cannulated selectively and have not been identified by the cardiac surgeon by placement of a radiopaque marker at the graft origin.

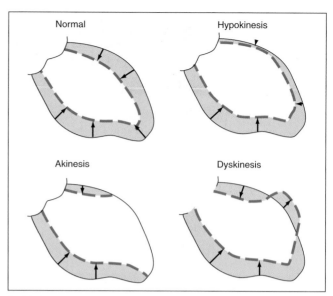

FIGURE 13-6

Diagrammatic representation of end-diastolic (*solid line*) and end-systolic (*dashed line*) silhouettes of left ventricular cineangiograms. These represent various forms of localized wall motion disorder in patients with coronary heart disease. Normal wall motion is symmetric; a patient with *hypokinesis* exhibits reduced contraction, seen here over the anterior and apical surfaces; a patient with *akinesis* exhibits absent wall motion, seen here over the anteroapical surface; a patient with *dyskinesis* exhibits paradoxic bulging of a small portion of the anterior wall with systole.

CORONARY ANGIOGRAPHY

While the aspects of cardiac catheterization described above may be performed in specific clinical situations, the essence of modern catheterization is high-quality coronary angiography. The tips of specially shaped catheters are placed into the left and then the right coronary artery, and any surgical bypass grafts, under fluoroscopic guidance. Hand injection of a radiographic contrast agent allows opacification of their lumina, with those images recorded at 15 frames per second on a radiographic image (*cine angiography*). Each coronary artery is usually viewed in several projections to permit assessment of the location and severity of any stenosis relative to the adjacent "normal" vessel segments (**Fig. 13-8**). In addition to the detection of coronary artery stenoses, coronary angiography evaluates the rapidity of coronary flow, the blush of capillary filling in the myocardium, collateral pathways that perfuse myocardial territories supplied by an occluded vessel, the presence of congenital abnormalities of the coronary circulation (e.g., coronary fistulae), and patency of any previously constructed coronary artery bypass grafts.

The degree of stenosis is typically evaluated by visual estimation of percent diameter stenosis of each lesion relative to the "uninvolved" adjacent reference segment, with 50% diameter stenosis representing the minimal

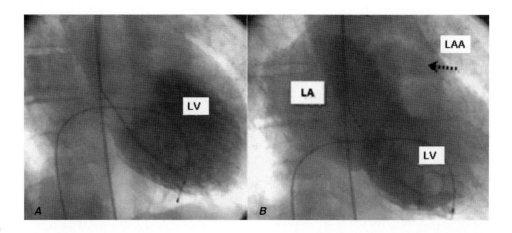

FIGURE 13-7

Left ventricular angiogram showing end-diastole (A) and end-systole (B). Left ventricular ejection fraction remains normal, but the calculated ventricular volumes are increased, due to severe chronic mitral regurgitation [note dense opacification of the left atrium (LA) and left atrial appendage (*arrow*) on the systolic frame]. *(From D Baim, in Grossman's Cardiac Catheterization, Angiography, and Intervention, 7th ed, DS Baim (ed). Baltimore, Lippincott Williams & Wilkins, 2006.)*

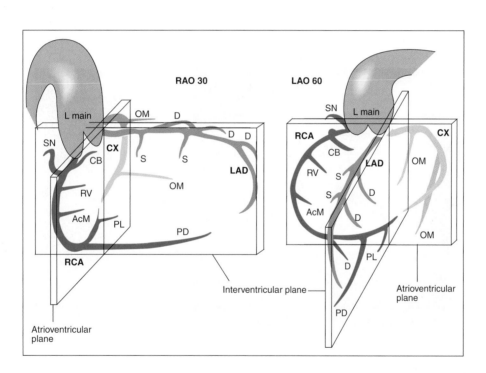

FIGURE 13-8

Representation of coronary anatomy relative to the interventricular and atrioventricular valve planes. Coronary branches are indicated as L main (left main), LAD (left anterior descending), D (diagonal), S (septal), CX (circumflex), OM (obtuse marginal), RCA (right coronary artery), CB (conus branch), SN (sinus node), AcM (acute marginal), PD (posterior descending), PL (posterolateral left ventricular). RAO, right anterior oblique; LAO, left anterior oblique. *[From DS Baim in Grossman's Cardiac Catheterization, Angiography, and Intervention, 7th ed, DS Baim (ed). Baltimore, Lippincott Williams & Wilkins, 2006.]*

lesion severity that is capable of interfering with maximal increases in perfusion of the related myocardial territory during stress (**Fig. 13-9**). Borderline lesions (i.e., those between 40 and 70% diameter stenosis) that are not clearly related to the clinical ischemic syndrome may be further assessed by the following:

(1) measurement of the pressure gradient between the segments proximal and distal to the stenosis; (2) measurement of the increase in distal coronary blood flow during maximal coronary vasodilatation using adenosine; and (3) use of intravascular ultrasound (IVUS), which has the advantage of imaging the underlying plaque as well as

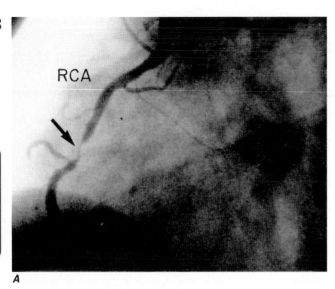

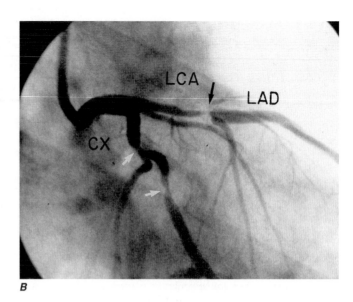

FIGURE 13-9

A. Coronary angiogram showing a right coronary artery (RCA) with a severe (95%) stenosis at its midpoint (*arrow*). **B.** Coronary angiogram of a left coronary artery (LCA) with a tight stenosis in the proximal left anterior descending (LAD) artery (*black arrow*) immediately prior to the origin of a large septal branch. The circumflex artery (CX) has two moderately severe stenoses (*white arrows*).

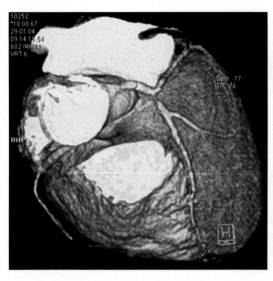

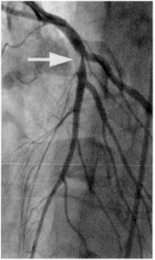

FIGURE 13-10

Comparison of 64-slice multidetector CT imaging to contrast coronary angiography in a patient with severe stenosis of the proximal left anterior descending (*arrow*). This technique may supplant screening coronary angiography in patients who do not have clinical indications for percutaneous coronary intervention. *(Images provided by Thomas J. Brady, M.D.)*

precisely measuring the luminal cross-sectional area at the point of a borderline lesion. Despite recent progress in multidetector computed tomography (MDCT) that suggests this evolving technique (Chap. 12) may ultimately replace screening pre-surgical coronary angiography (Fig. 13-10), coronary arteriography remains the most definitive diagnostic tool for evaluation of the *coronary anatomy* with sufficient precision to inform decisions regarding coronary surgery vs. catheter-based interventions in patients with CAD.

POSTPROCEDURE CARE

The average diagnostic cardiac catheterization procedure takes ~30 min and ~60 mL of contrast (increased to ~90 mL by contrast left ventriculography). No anticoagulant agents are usually administered for a purely diagnostic procedure, and the vascular sheaths are removed at the end of the procedure. Hemostasis may be achieved by applying local pressure over the puncture site for 10–15 min, followed by a 2- to 4-h period of bed rest before ambulation and discharge. Alternatively, a variety of vascular closure devices (sutures or external clips or collagen plugs) are now available to seal the arterial puncture site, allowing a shorter period of bed rest and earlier ambulation. Most patients with suitable anatomy, however, will go on seamlessly to undergo PCI following the diagnostic catheterization procedure before the sheaths are removed, followed by an overnight hospital stay (Chap. 36).

FURTHER READINGS

BAIM DS (ed): *Grossman's Cardiac Catheterization, Angiography, and Intervention*, 7th ed. Baltimore, Lippincott Williams & Wilkins, 2006

BERRY C: Comparison of intravascular ultrasound and quantitative coronary angiography for the assessment of coronary artery disease progression. Circulation 115:1851, 2007

BUDOFF MJ: Clinical utility of computed tomography and magnetic resonance techniques for noninvasive coronary angiography. J Am Coll Cardiol 42:1867, 2003

DAVIDSON CJ et al: Cardiac catheterization, in *Braunwald's Heart Disease*, 7th ed, D Zipes et al (eds). Philadelphia, Saunders, 2005

KERN MJ (ed): Hemodynamic Rounds, *Interpretation of Cardiac Pathophysiology from Pressure Waveform Analysis*, 3d ed. Hoboken, Wiley-Blackwell, 2009

NICHOLLS SJ et al: Exploring the natural history of atherosclerosis with intravascular ultrasound. Expert Rev Cardiovasc Ther 5:295, 2007

RYAN TJ: The coronary angiogram and its seminal contributions to cardiovascular medicine over five decades. Circulation 106:752, 2002

TOBIS J: Assessment of intermediate severity coronary lesions in the catheterization laboratory. J Am Coll Cardiol 49:839, 2007

Diagnostic Cardiac Catheterization and Angiography

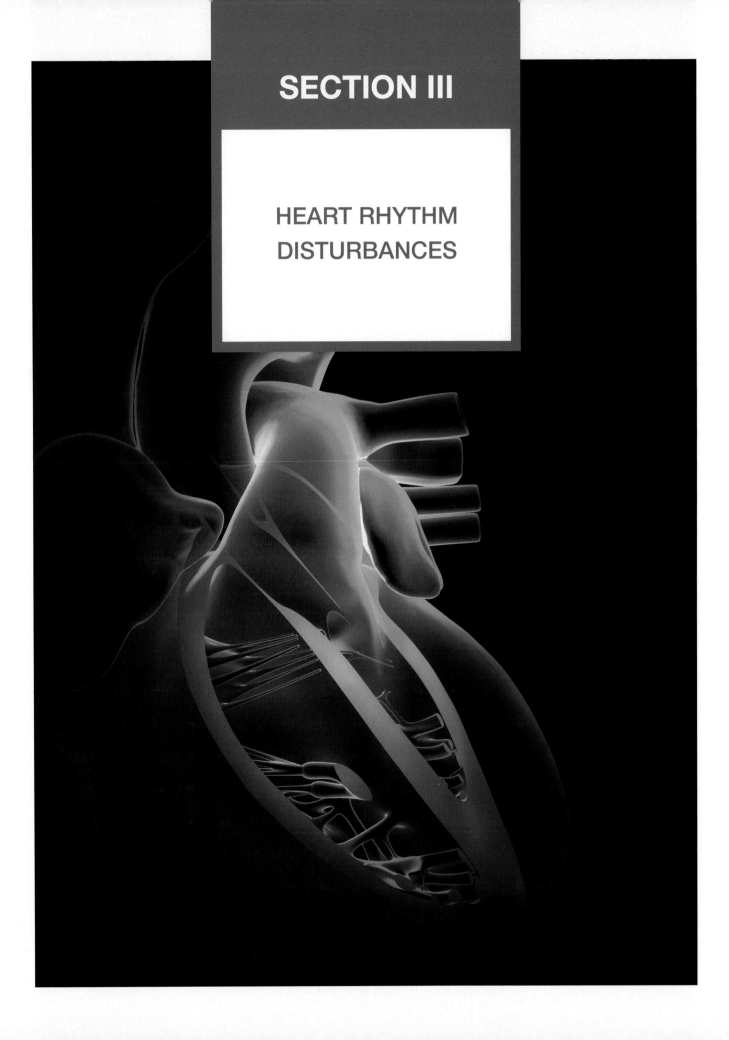

SECTION III

HEART RHYTHM
DISTURBANCES

CHAPTER 14

PRINCIPLES OF ELECTROPHYSIOLOGY

Gordon F. Tomaselli

HISTORY AND INTRODUCTION

The field of cardiac electrophysiology was ushered in with the development of the electrocardiogram (ECG) by Einthoven at the turn of the twentieth century. The recording of cellular membrane currents revealed that the body surface ECG is the timed sum of the cellular action potentials in the atria and ventricles. In the late 1960s, the development of intracavitary recording, and in particular the ability to record His-bundle electrograms with programmed stimulation of the heart, marked the beginning of contemporary clinical electrophysiology. Adoption of radiofrequency technology to ablate cardiac tissue in the early 1990s heralded the birth of interventional cardiac electrophysiology.

The clinical problem of sudden death caused by ventricular arrhythmias, most commonly in the setting of coronary obstruction, was recognized as early as the late nineteenth century. The problem was vexing and led to the development of pharmacologic and nonpharmacologic therapies, including transthoracic defibrillators, cardiac massage, and, most recently, implantable defibrillators. Over time the limitations of antiarrhythmic drug therapy have been repeatedly highlighted in clinical trials, such that ablation and devices are first-line therapy for a number of cardiac arrhythmias.

In the past decade the genetic basis of a number of heritable arrhythmias has been elucidated, revealing important insights into the mechanisms not only of these rare arrhythmias, but also of similar rhythm disturbances observed in more common forms of heart disease.

DESCRIPTIVE PHYSIOLOGY

The normal cardiac impulse is generated by pacemaker cells in the sinoatrial node located at the junction of the right atrium and superior vena cava (Fig. 11-1). This impulse is slowly transmitted through nodal tissue to the anatomically complex atria, where it is more rapidly conducted to the atrioventricular node (AVN) inscribing the P wave of the ECG (Fig. 11-2). There is a perceptible delay in conduction through the anatomically and functionally heterogeneous AVN. The time needed for activation of the atria and the AVN delay is represented as the PR interval of the ECG. The AVN is the only electrical connection between the atria and ventricles in the normal heart. The electrical impulse emerges from the AVN and is transmitted to the His–Purkinje system, specifically the common bundle of His, then the left and right bundle branches, and hence to the Purkinje network, facilitating activation of ventricular muscle. Under normal circumstances, the ventricles are rapidly activated in a well-defined fashion that is determined by the course of the Purkinje network and inscribes the QRS complex (Fig. 11-2). Recovery of electrical excitability occurs more slowly and is governed by the time of activation and duration of regional action potentials. The relative brevity of epicardial action potentials in the ventricle results in repolarization occurring first on the epicardial surface then proceeding to the endocardium, which inscribes a T wave normally of the same polarity as the QRS complex. The duration of activation and recovery is determined by the action potential duration represented on the body surface ECG by the QT interval (Fig. 11-2).

The gross anatomic features of the heart—the extracellular matrix and intramural vasculature—create both macro- and microanatomic barriers that are central to both the normal electrophysiology of the heart and clinically important arrhythmias. Cardiac myocytes exhibit a characteristically long action potential (200–400 ms) compared to neurons or skeletal muscle cells (1–5 ms). The action potential profile is sculpted by the orchestrated activity of multiple distinctive time- and voltage-dependent ionic currents (Fig. 14-1A). The currents, in turn, are carried by complex transmembrane proteins that passively conduct ions down their electrochemical gradients through selective pores (ion channels), actively transport ions against their electrochemical gradient (pumps, transporters), or electrogenically exchange ionic species (exchangers).

Action potentials in the heart are regionally distinct. The regional variability in cardiac action potentials is the result of differences in the number and types of ion channel proteins expressed by different cell types in the heart. Further, unique sets of ionic currents are active in pacemaking and muscle cells, and the relative contributions of these currents may vary in the same cell type in different regions of the heart (Fig. 14-1A).

Ion channels are complex, multisubunit transmembrane glycoproteins that open and close in response to a

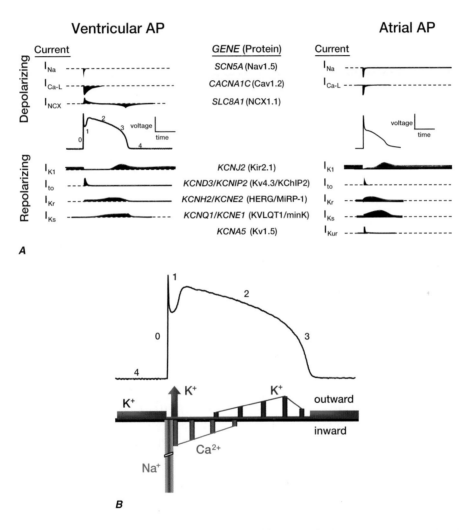

FIGURE 14-1

A. Cellular atrial and ventricular action potentials. Schematic atrial and ventricular action potentials with the phases are shown in the top portion of the figure. Phases 0–4 are the rapid upstroke, early repolarization, plateau, late repolarization, and diastole respectively. The ionic currents and the genes that generate the currents with schematics of the current trajectories are shown above and below the action potentials. The active currents and their densities vary in atrial and ventricular myocytes. **B.** A ventricular action potential with a schematic of the ionic currents flowing during the phases of the action potential. Potassium current (I_{K1}) is the principal current during phase 4 and determines the resting membrane potential of the myocyte. Sodium current generates the upstroke of the action potential (phase 0), activation of I_{to} with inactivation of the Na current inscribes early repolarization (phase 1). The plateau phase (2) is generated by a balance of repolarizing potassium currents and depolarizing calcium current. Inactivation of the calcium current with persistent activation of potassium currents (predominantly I_{Kr} and I_{Ks}) cause phase 3 repolarization.

number of biologic stimuli, including a change in membrane voltage, ligand binding (directly to the channel or to a G protein–coupled receptor), and mechanical deformation (**Fig. 14-2**). Other ion motive transmembrane proteins, such as exchangers and transporters, contribute

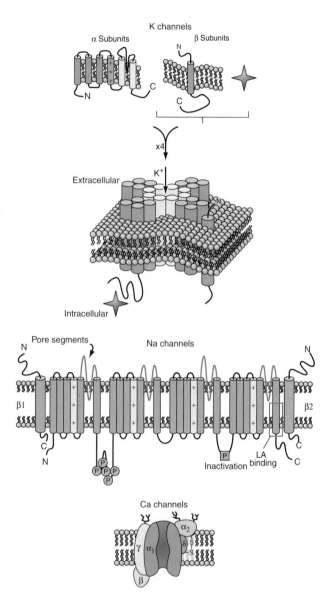

FIGURE 14-2

Topology and subunit composition of the voltage dependent ion channels. (*Top panel*) Potassium channels are formed by the tetramerization of α or pore-forming subunits and one or more β subunits, only single β subunits are shown for clarity. (***Bottom panel***) Sodium and calcium channels are composed of α subunits with four homologous domains and one or more ancillary subunits. In all channel types the loop of protein between the fifth and sixth membrane spanning repeat in each subunit or domain forms the ion-selective pore. In the case of the sodium channel, the channel is a target for phosphorylation, the linker between the third and fourth homologous domain is critical to inactivation, and the sixth membrane-spanning repeat in the fourth domain is important in local anesthetic antiarrhythmic drug binding.

importantly to cellular excitability in the heart. Ion pumps establish and maintain the ionic gradients across the cell membrane that serve as the driving force for current flow through ion channels. Transporters or exchangers that do not move ions in an electrically neutral manner (e.g., the sodium-calcium exchanger transports three Na^+ for one Ca^{2+}) are termed *electrogenic*, and contribute directly to the action potential profile.

The most abundant superfamily of ion channels expressed in the heart is voltage-gated. Several structural themes are common to all voltage-dependent ion channels. First, the architecture is modular, consisting either of four homologous subunits (e.g., K^+ channels) or of four internally homologous domains (e.g., Na^+ and Ca^{2+} channels). Second, the proteins fold around a central pore lined by amino acids that exhibit exquisite conservation within a given channel family of like selectivity (e.g., jellyfish, eel, fruit fly, and human Na channels have very similar P segments). Third, the general strategy for activation gating (opening and closing in response to changes in membrane voltage) is highly conserved: the fourth transmembrane segment (S4), studded with positively charged residues, lies within the membrane field and moves in response to depolarization, opening the channel. Fourth, most ion channel complexes include not only the pore-forming proteins (α subunits) but also auxiliary subunits (e.g., β subunits) that modify channel function (Fig. 14-2).

Na^+ and Ca^{2+} channels are the primary carriers of depolarizing current in both the atrium and ventricles; inactivation of these currents and activation of repolarizing K^+ currents hyperpolarize the heart cell, reestablishing the negative resting membrane potential (**Fig. 14-1B**). The *plateau phase* is a time when little current is flowing, and relatively minor changes in depolarizing or repolarizing currents can have profound effects on the action potential shape and duration. Mutations in subunits of these channel proteins produce arrhythmogenic alterations in the action potentials that cause long and short QT syndrome, idiopathic ventricular fibrillation, familial atrial fibrillation, and some forms of conduction system disease.

MECHANISMS OF CARDIAC ARRHYTHMIAS

Cardiac arrhythmias result from abnormalities of impulse generation, conduction, or both. It is, however, difficult to establish with certainty an underlying mechanism for many clinical arrhythmias. The response of a tachycardia to pacing (initiation, termination, entrainment) is used in the clinical electrophysiology laboratory to make the diagnosis of reentry. There are even fewer specific tools available to diagnose non-reentrant arrhythmias. It is clear that molecular changes in the heart predispose to the development of abnormalities of cardiac rhythm. However, an exclusively molecular approach to understanding

TABLE 14-1

ARRHYTHMIA MECHANISMS

ELECTROPHYSIOLOGIC PROPERTY	MOLECULAR COMPONENTS	MECHANISM	PROTOTYPIC ARRHYTHMIAS
Cellular			
Impulse Initiation			
Automaticity	I_f, I_{Ca-L}, I_{Ca-T}, I_K, I_{K1}	Suppression/acceleration of phase 4	Sinus bradycardia, sinus tachycardia
Triggered automaticity	Calcium overload, I_{TI}	DADs	Digitalis toxicity, reperfusion VT
	I_{Ca-L}, I_K, I_{Na}	EADs	Torsades des pointes, congenital and acquired
Excitation	I_{Na}	Suppression of phase 0	Ischemic VF
	I_{K-ATP}	AP shortening, inexcitability	
	I_{Ca-L}	Suppression	AV block
Repolarization	I_{Na}, I_{Ca-L}, I_K, I_{K1}, Ca^{2+} homeostasis	AP prolongation, EADS, DADs	Polymorphic VT (HF, LVH)
	I_{Ca-L}, K channels, Ca^{2+} homeostasis	AP shortening	Atrial fibrillation
Multicellular			
Cellular coupling	Connexins (Cx43), I_{Na}, I_{K-ATP}	Decreased coupling	Ischemic VT/VF
Tissue Structure	Extracellular matrix, collagen	Excitable gap and functional reentry	Monomorphic VT, atrial fibrillation

Note: DAD, delayed afterdepolarization; VT, ventricular tachyarrhythmia; IVR, idioventricular rhythm; EAD, early afterdepolarization; VF, ventricular fibrillation; AV, atrioventricular; HF, heart failure; AP, action potential.

arrhythmia mechanisms is limited by failure to include cellular and network properties of the heart. A summary of the cellular and molecular changes that underlie prototypic arrhythmias and their putative mechanisms is given in Table 14-1.

Alterations in Impulse Initiation: Automaticity

Spontaneous (phase 4) diastolic depolarization underlies the property of automaticity (pacemaking) characteristic of cells in the sinoatrial (SA) and atrioventricular (AV) nodes, His-Purkinje system, coronary sinus, and pulmonary veins. Phase 4 depolarization results from the concerted action of a number of ionic currents including the inward rectifier (I_{K1}) and delayed rectifier (rapid I_{Kr} and slow I_{Ks} components) K^+ currents, Ca^{2+} currents, electrogenic Na^+,K^+-ATPase, the Na^+-Ca^{2+} exchanger, and the so-called funny, or pacemaker, current (I_f); however, the relative importance of these currents remains controversial.

The rate of phase 4 depolarization and, therefore, the firing rate of pacemaker cells are dynamically regulated. Prominent among the factors that modulate phase 4 is autonomic nervous system tone. The negative chronotropic effect of activation of the parasympathetic nervous system is the result of release of acetylcholine that binds to muscarinic receptors, releasing G protein βγ subunits that activate a potassium current (I_{KACh}) in nodal and

atrial cells. The resulting increase in K^+ conductance opposes membrane depolarization, slowing the rate of rise of phase 4 of the action potential. Conversely, augmentation of sympathetic nervous system tone increases myocardial catecholamine concentrations, which activate both α and β receptors. The effect of β$_1$-adrenergic stimulation predominates in pacemaking cells, augmenting both L-type Ca current (I_{Ca-L}) and I_f, thus increasing the slope of phase 4. Enhanced sympathetic nervous system activity can dramatically increase the rate of firing of SA nodal cells, producing sinus tachycardia with rates >200 beats/min. By contrast, the increased rate of firing of Purkinje cells is more limited, rarely producing ventricular tachyarrhythmias >120 beats/min.

Normal automaticity may be affected by a number of other factors associated with heart disease. Hypokalemia and ischemia may reduce the activity of the Na^+,K^+-ATPase, thereby reducing the background repolarizing current and enhancing phase 4 diastolic depolarization. The end result would be an increase in the spontaneous firing rate of pacemaking cells. Modest increases in extracellular potassium may render the maximum diastolic potential more positive, thereby also increasing the firing rate of pacemaking cells. A more significant increase in $[K^+]_o$, however, renders the heart inexcitable by depolarizing the membrane potential.

Normal or enhanced automaticity of subsidiary latent pacemakers produces escape rhythms in the setting of failure of more dominant pacemakers. Suppression of a pacemaker cell by a faster rhythm leads to an increased intracellular Na^+ load ($[Na^+]_i$), and extrusion of Na^+ from the cell by the Na^+,K^+-ATPase produces an increased background repolarizing current that slows phase 4 diastolic depolarization. At slower rates, the $[Na^+]_i$ is decreased, as is the activity of the Na^+,K^+-ATPase, resulting in progressively more rapid diastolic depolarization and warm-up of the tachycardia rate. Overdrive suppression and warm-up are characteristic of, but may not be observed in, all automatic tachycardias. Abnormal conduction into tissue with enhanced automaticity (*entrance block*) may blunt or eliminate the phenomena of overdrive suppression and warm-up of automatic tissue.

Abnormal automaticity may underlie atrial tachycardia, accelerated idioventricular rhythms, and ventricular tachycardia, particularly that associated with ischemia and reperfusion. It has also been suggested that injury currents at the borders of ischemic myocardium may depolarize adjacent non-ischemic tissue, predisposing to automatic ventricular tachycardia.

Afterdepolarizations and Triggered Automaticity

Triggered automaticity or activity refers to impulse initiation that is dependent on afterdepolarizations (Fig. 14-3). Afterdepolarizations are membrane voltage oscillations that occur during [early afterdepolarizations (EADs)] or following [delayed afterdepolarizations (DADs)] an action potential.

The cellular feature common to the induction of DADs is the presence of increased Ca^{2+} load in the cytosol and

sarcoplasmic reticulum. Inhibition of the Na^+,K^+-ATPase by digitalis glycosides facilitates, but is not necessary for creating, the Ca^{2+} overload that predisposes to DADs. Catecholamines and ischemia sufficiently enhance Ca^{2+} loading to produce DADs. Accumulation of lysophospholipids in ischemic myocardium with consequent Na^+ and Ca^{2+} overload has been suggested as a mechanism for DADs and triggered automaticity. Cells from damaged areas or surviving a myocardial infarction may display spontaneous release of calcium from the sarcoplasmic reticulum, and this may generate "waves" of intracellular calcium elevation and arrhythmias.

EADs occur during the action potential and interrupt the orderly repolarization of the myocyte. It has been traditionally held that, unlike DADs, EADs do not depend on a rise in intracellular Ca^{2+}, and that, instead, action potential prolongation and reactivation of depolarizing currents are fundamental to their production. More recent experimental evidence suggests a previously unappreciated interrelationship between intracellular calcium loading and EADs. Cytosolic calcium may increase when action potentials are prolonged. This, in turn, appears to enhance L-type Ca current, further prolonging action potential duration as well as providing the inward current driving EADs. Intracellular calcium loading by action potential prolongation may also enhance the likelihood of DADs. The interrelationship among intracellular $[Ca^{2+}]$, EADs, and DADs may be one explanation for the susceptibility of hearts that are calcium loaded (e.g., in ischemia or congestive heart failure) to develop arrhythmias, particularly on exposure to action potential–prolonging drugs.

EAD-triggered arrhythmias exhibit rate dependence. In general, the amplitude of an EAD is augmented at slow rates when action potentials are longer. Rapid pacing will shorten the action potential duration and reduce EAD amplitude, likely due to augmentation of delayed rectifier K^+ currents and, perhaps, hastening of Ca^{2+}-induced inactivation of L-type Ca currents. Similarly, catecholamines increase heart rate and decrease action potential duration and EAD amplitude, despite the well-described effect of β-adrenergic stimulation on increasing L-type Ca current. A fundamental condition that underlies the development of EADs is action potential and QT prolongation. Hypokalemia, hypomagnesemia, bradycardia, and, most commonly, drugs can predispose to the generation of EADs, invariably in the context of prolonging the action potential. Antiarrhythmics with class IA and III action (see later) produce action potential and QT prolongation intended to be therapeutic, but frequently causing arrhythmias. Noncardiac drugs, such as phenothiazines, nonsedating antihistamines, and some antibiotics can also prolong the action potential duration and predispose to EAD-mediated triggered arrhythmias. Decreased $[K^+]_o$ may paradoxically decrease membrane potassium currents (particularly I_{Kr}) in the ventricular

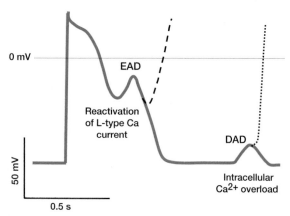

FIGURE 14-3

Schematic action potentials with early (EAD) and delayed afterdepolarizations (DAD). Afterdepolarizations are spontaneous depolarizations in cardiac myocytes. EADs occur before the end of the action potential (phases 2 and 3), interrupting repolarization. DADs occur during phase 4 of the action potential after completion of repolarization. The cellular mechanisms of EADs and DADs differ (see text).

myocyte, explaining why hypokalemia causes action potential prolongation and EADs. In fact, potassium infusions in patients with the congenital long QT syndrome (LQTS) and in those with drug-induced acquired QT prolongation shorten the QT interval.

EAD-mediated triggered activity likely underlies initiation of the characteristic polymorphic ventricular tachycardia, torsade de pointes, seen in patients with congenital and acquired forms of the LQTS. Structural heart disease, such as cardiac hypertrophy and failure, may also delay ventricular repolarization (so-called electrical remodeling) and predispose to arrhythmias related to abnormalities of repolarization. The abnormalities of repolarization in hypertrophy and failure are often magnified by concomitant drug therapy or electrolyte disturbances.

Abnormal Impulse Conduction: Reentry

The most common arrhythmia mechanism is reentry. Reentry is a property of networks of myocytes. Fundamentally, reentry is defined as circulation of an activation wave around an inexcitable obstacle. Thus, the requirements for reentry are two electrophysiologically dissimilar pathways for impulse propagation around an inexcitable region such that unidirectional block occurs in one of the pathways and a region of excitable tissue exists at the head of the propagating wavefront (Fig. 14-4). Structural and electrophysiologic properties of the heart may contribute to the development of the inexcitable obstacle and of

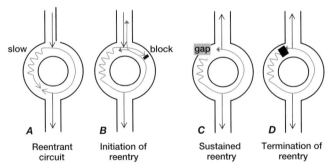

FIGURE 14-4

Schematic diagram of reentry. A. The circuit comprises two limbs, one with slow conduction. **B.** A premature impulse blocks in the fast pathway and conducts over the slow pathway, allowing the fast pathway to recover so that the activation wave can reenter the fast pathway from the retrograde direction. **C.** During sustained reentry utilizing such a circuit, a gap (excitable gap) exists between the activating head of the wave and the recovering tail. **D.** One mechanism of termination of reentry is when the conduction and recovery characteristics of the circuit change, and the activating head of the wave collides with the tail, extinguishing the tachycardia.

unidirectional block. The complex geometry of muscle bundles in the heart and spatial heterogeneity of cellular coupling or other active membrane properties (i.e., ionic currents) appear to be critical.

A key feature in classifying reentrant arrhythmias, particularly for therapy, is the presence and size of an excitable gap. An excitable gap exists when the tachycardia circuit is longer than the tachycardia wavelength (λ = conduction velocity $\times$ refractory period, representing the size of the circuit that can sustain reentry), allowing appropriately timed stimuli to reset propagation in the circuit. Reentrant arrhythmias may exist in the heart in the absence of an excitable gap and with a tachycardia wavelength nearly the same size as the path length. In this case, the wavefront propagates through partially refractory tissue with no anatomic obstacle and no fully excitable gap; this is referred to as *leading circle reentry*, a form of functional reentry (reentry that depends on functional properties of the tissue). Unlike excitable gap reentry, there is no fixed anatomic circuit in leading circle reentry, and it may therefore not be possible to disrupt the tachycardia with pacing or destruction of a part of the circuit. Furthermore, the circuit in leading circle reentry tends to be less stable than that in excitable gap reentrant arrhythmias, with large variations in cycle length and predilection to termination.

Anatomically determined, excitable gap reentry can explain several clinically important tachycardias, such as AV reentry, atrial flutter, bundle branch reentry ventricular tachycardia, and ventricular tachycardia in scarred myocardium. Atrial flutter represents an example of a reentrant tachycardia with a large excitable gap not always due to an anatomic constraint but to functional block (reflecting the special properties of the crista terminalis discussed above). There is strong evidence to suggest that arrhythmias, such as atrial and ventricular fibrillation, are associated with more complex activation of the heart and are due to functional reentry.

Structural heart disease is associated with changes in conduction and refractoriness that increase the risk of reentrant arrhythmias. Chronically ischemic myocardium exhibits a down-regulation of the gap junction channel protein (connexin 43) that carries intercellular ionic current. The border zones of infarcted and failing ventricular myocardium exhibit not only functional alterations of ionic currents but also remodeling of tissue and altered distribution of gap junctions. The changes in gap junction channel expression and distribution, in combination with macroscopic tissue alterations, support a role for slowed conduction in reentrant arrhythmias that complicate chronic coronary artery disease. Aged human atrial myocardium exhibits altered conduction, manifest as highly fractionated atrial electrograms, producing an ideal substrate for the reentry that may underlie the very common development of atrial fibrillation in the elderly.

Approach to the Patient:
CARDIAC ARRHYTHMIA

The evaluation of patients with suspected cardiac arrhythmias is highly individualized; however, two key features, the history and ECG, are pivotal in directing the diagnostic workup and therapy. Patients with cardiac arrhythmias exhibit a wide spectrum of clinical presentations from asymptomatic ECG abnormalities to survival from cardiac arrest. In general, the more severe the presenting symptoms, the more aggressive are the evaluation and treatment. Loss of consciousness that is believed to be of cardiac origin typically mandates an exhaustive search for the etiology and often requires invasive, device-based therapy. The presence of structural heart disease and prior myocardial infarction dictates a change in the approach to the management of syncope or ventricular arrhythmias. The presence of a family history of serious ventricular arrhythmias or premature sudden death will influence the evaluation of presumed heritable arrhythmias.

The physical examination is focused on determining if there is cardiopulmonary disease that is associated with specific cardiac arrhythmias. The absence of significant cardiopulmonary disease often, but not always, suggests benignity of the rhythm disturbance. In contrast, palpitations, syncope, or near syncope in the setting of significant heart or lung disease has more ominous implications. In addition, the physical examination may reveal the presence of a persistent arrhythmia such as atrial fibrillation.

The judicious use of noninvasive diagnostic tests is an important element in the evaluation of patients with arrhythmias, and there is none more important that the ECG, particularly if recorded at the time of symptoms. Uncommon but diagnostically important signatures of electrophysiologic disturbances may be unearthed on the resting ECG, such as delta waves in Wolff-Parkinson-White (WPW) syndrome, prolongation or shortening of the QT interval, right precordial ST-segment abnormalities in Brugada syndrome, and epsilon waves in arrhythmogenic right ventricular dysplasia. Variants of body surface ECG recording can provide important information about arrhythmia substrates and triggers. Holter monitoring and event recording, either continuous or intermittent, record the body surface ECG over longer periods of time, enhancing the possibility of observing the cardiac rhythm during symptoms. Implantable long-term monitors and commercial ambulatory ECG monitoring services exist that permit prolonged telemetric monitoring for both diagnosis and to assess the efficacy of therapy.

Long-term recordings permit the assessment of the time-varying behavior of the heart rhythm. Heart rate variability (HRV) and QT interval variability (QTV) provide noninvasive methods to assess autonomic nervous system influence on the heart. HRV arises because of subtle changes in sinus rate due to changes in sympathovagal input to the sinus node. Normal time domain, frequency domain, and geometric methods metrics have been established for HRV; a decrease in HRV and an increase in low-frequency power have been associated with increased sympathetic nervous system tone and increased mortality in patients after myocardial infarction. Signal-averaged electrocardiography (SAECG) uses signal-averaging techniques to amplify small potentials in the body surface ECG that are associated with slow conduction in the myocardium. The presence of these small potentials, referred to as *late potentials* because of their timing with respect to the QRS complex, and prolongation of the filtered (or averaged) QRS duration are indicative of slowed conduction in the ventricle and have been associated with an increased risk of ventricular arrhythmias after myocardial infarction. Exercise electrocardiography is important in determining the presence of myocardial demand ischemia; more recently, analysis of the morphology of the QT interval with exercise has been used to assess the risk of serious ventricular arrhythmias. Microscopic alterations in the T wave [T wave alternans (TWA)] at low heart rates identify patients at risk for ventricular arrhythmias. A number of other tests of the variability in the T-wave morphology or duration of the QT interval have been used to assess instability in repolarization of the ventricle and an increased risk of arrhythmias.

Head-up tilt (HUT) testing is a useful in the evaluation of some patients with syncope. The physiologic response to HUT is incompletely understood; however, redistribution of blood volume and increased ventricular contractility occur consistently. Exaggerated activation of a central reflex in response to HUT produces a stereotypic response of an initial increase in heart rate, then a drop in blood pressure followed by a reduction in heart rate characteristic of neurally mediated hypotension. Other responses to HUT may be observed in patients with orthostatic hypotension and autonomic insufficiency. HUT is most often used in patients with recurrent syncope, although it may be useful in patients with single syncopal episodes with associated injury, particularly in the absence of structural heart disease. In patients with structural heart disease, HUT may be indicated in those with syncope, in whom other causes (e.g., asystole, ventricular tachyarrhythmias) have been excluded. HUT has been suggested as a useful tool in the diagnosis and therapy of recurrent idiopathic vertigo, chronic fatigue syndrome, recurrent transient ischemic attacks, and repeated falls of unknown etiology in the elderly. Importantly, HUT is relatively contraindicated in the presence of severe coronary artery disease with proximal coronary stenoses, known severe cerebrovascular disease, severe mitral stenosis, and obstruction to left ventricular outflow (e.g., aortic stenosis). The method of HUT is variable, but the angle of tilt and the duration of upright posture are central to the diagnostic utility of the test. The use of pharmacologic provocation of orthostatic stress with isoproterenol, nitrates, adenosine, and edrophonium have been used to shorten the test and enhance specificity.

Electrophysiologic testing is central to the understanding and treatment of many cardiac arrhythmias. Indeed, most frequently electrophysiologic testing is interventional, providing both diagnosis and therapy. The components of the electrophysiologic test are baseline measurements of conduction under resting and stressed (rate or pharmacologic) conditions and maneuvers, both pacing and pharmacologic, to induce arrhythmias. A number of sophisticated electrical mapping and catheter-guidance techniques have been developed to facilitate catheter-based therapeutics in the electrophysiology laboratory.

℞ Treatment: CARDIAC ARRHYTHMIAS

ANTIARRHYTHMIC DRUG THERAPY The interaction of antiarrhythmic drugs with cardiac tissues and the resulting electrophysiologic changes are complex. An incomplete understanding of the effects of these drugs has produced serious missteps that have had adverse effects on patient outcomes and the development of newer pharmacologic agents. Currently, antiarrhythmic drugs have been relegated to an ancillary role in the treatment of most cardiac arrhythmias.

There are several explanations for the complexity of antiarrhythmic drug action: the structural similarity of target ion channels; regional differences in the levels of expression of channels and transporters, which change with disease; time and voltage dependence of drug action; and the effect of these drugs on targets other than ion channels. Recognizing the limitations of any scheme to classify antiarrhythmic agents, a shorthand that is useful in describing the major mechanisms of action is of some utility. Such a classification scheme was proposed in 1970 by Vaughan-Williams and later modified by Singh and Harrison. The classes of antiarrhythmic action are: class I, local anesthetic effect due to blockade of Na^+ current; class II, interference with the action of catecholamines at the β-adrenergic receptor; class III, delay of repolarization due to inhibition of K^+ current or activation of depolarizing current; class IV, interference with calcium conductance (Table 14-2). The limitations of the Vaughan-Williams classification

TABLE 14-2

ANTIARRHYTHMIC DRUG ACTIONS

DRUG	CLASS ACTIONS				MISCELLANEOUS ACTION
	I	II	III	IV	
Quinidine	++		++		α-Adrenergic blockade
Procainamide	++		++		Ganglionic blockade
Flecainide	+++		+		
Propafenone	++	+			
Sotalol		++	+++		
Dofetilide			+++		
Amiodarone	++	++	+++	+	α-Adrenergic blockade
Ibutilide			+++		Na^+ channel activator

scheme include multiple actions of most drugs, overwhelming consideration of antagonism as a mechanism of action, and the fact that several agents have none of the four classes of action in the scheme.

CATHETER ABLATION The use of catheter ablation is based on the principle that there is a critical anatomic region of impulse generation or propagation required for the initiation and maintenance of cardiac arrhythmias. Destruction of such a critical region results in the elimination of the arrhythmia. The use of radiofrequency (RF) energy in clinical medicine is nearly a century old. The first catheter ablation using a DC energy source was performed in the early 1980s by Scheinman and colleagues. By the early 1990s, RF had been adapted for use in catheter-based ablation in the heart (Fig. 14-5).

The RF frequency band (300–30,000 kHz) is used to generate energy for several biomedical applications, including coagulation and cauterizing tissues. Energy of this frequency will not stimulate skeletal muscle or the heart and heats tissue by a resistive mechanism, with the intensity of heating being proportional to the delivered power. The density of power in the tissue falls off rapidly (with the 4th power of the radius or distance), as does the temperature, allowing for the production of small-volume lesions. The applied power, energy, or current are not good predictors of lesion size; temperature at the electrode-tissue interface is the best predictor, with temperatures >55°C consistently producing tissue necrosis. The temperature rise at the tissue-electrode interface is rapid, but heating is slower in the tissue, and steady-state lesion size may be not achieved for ≥40 s of radiofrequency energy application. Notably, tissue temperature may remain high for many seconds despite cessation of energy delivery, producing undesired ablation of cardiac structures. Alternative, less frequently used energy sources for catheter ablation of cardiac arrhythmias

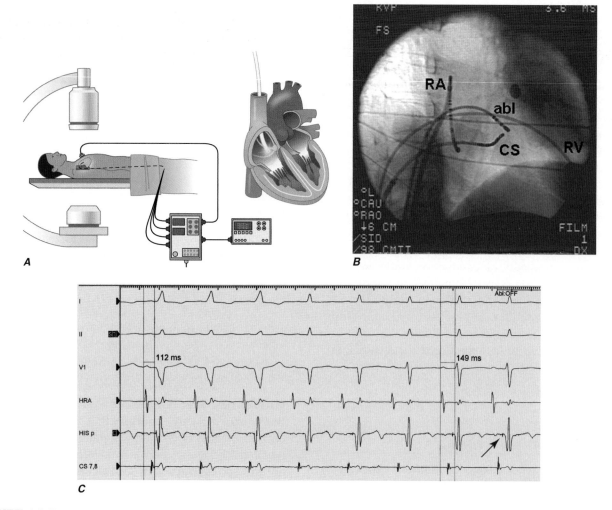

FIGURE 14-5

Catheter ablation of cardiac arrhythmias. *A.* A schematic of the lead system and generator in a patient undergoing radiofrequency catheter ablation (RFA); the circuit involves the lead in the heart and a dispersive patch placed on the body surface (usually the back). The inset shows a diagram of the heart with a catheter located at the AV valve ring for ablation of an accessory pathway. ***B.*** A right anterior oblique fluoroscopic image of the catheter position for ablation of a left-sided accessory pathway. A catheter is placed in the atrial side of the mitral valve ring (abl) via a transseptal puncture; other catheters are placed in the coronary sinus (CS) to record intracardiac electrograms around the mitral annulus; a circumferential catheter in the right atrium (RA) and a catheter in the right ventricular apex (RV). ***C.*** Body surface ECG recordings (I, II, V1) and endocardial electrograms (HRA: high right atrium; HISp: proximal His-bundle electrogram; CS 7,8 recordings from poles 7 and 8 of a decapolar catheter placed in the coronary sinus) during RFA of a left-sided accessory pathway in a patient with WPW syndrome. The QRS narrows at the fourth complex, the arrow shows the His-bundle electrogram, which becomes apparent with elimination of ventricular preexcitation over the accessory pathway.

include microwaves (915 MHz or 2450 MHz), lasers, ultrasound, or freezing (cryoablation). In addition to RF energy, cryoablation is being used clinically and is a safe and effective alternative to RF, especially with ablation in the region of the AV node. At temperatures just below 32°C, membrane ion transport is disrupted, producing depolarization of cells, decreased action potential amplitude and duration, and slowed conduction velocity (resulting in local conduction block)—all of which are reversible, if the tissue is rewarmed in a timely fashion. Tissue cooling can be used for mapping and ablation. Cryomapping can be used to confirm the location of a desired ablation target, such as an accessory pathway in WPW syndrome, or can be used to determine the safety of ablation around the AV node by monitoring AV conduction during cooling. Another advantage of cryoablation is that once the catheter tip cools below freezing, it adheres to the tissue, increasing catheter stability independent of the rhythm or pacing.

FURTHER READINGS

AKAR FG, TOMASELLI GF: Genetic basis of cardiac arrhythmias, in *Hurst's The Heart*, 11th ed, V Fuster et al (eds). New York, McGraw-Hill, 2004

———: Genetic basis of cardiac arrhythmias, in *Hurst's The Heart*, 12th ed, V Fuster et al (eds). New York, McGraw-Hill, 2007

HILLE B: *Ion Channels of Excitable Membranes*, 3d ed. Sunderland, MA, Sinauer Associates, Inc, 2001, Chaps 1, 3, 4, 21, 22

JOSEPHSON ME: *Clinical Cardiac Electrophysiology: Techniques and Interpretations*, 3d ed. Philadelphia, Lippincott Williams & Wilkins, 2002

———: *Clinical Cardiac Electrophysiology: Techniques and Interpretations*, 4th ed. Philadelphia, Lippincott Williams & Wilkins, 2008

SAKSENA S, CAMM AJ (eds): *Electrophysiological Disorders of the Heart*. Philadelphia, Elsevier Churchill Livingstone, 2005

ZIPES DP, JALIFE J (eds): *Cardiac Electrophysiology: From Cell to Bedside*, 4th ed. Philadelphia, Elsevier, 2004

——— (eds): *Cardiac Electrophysiology: From Cell to Bedside*, 5th ed. Philadelphia, Elsevier, 2009

CHAPTER 15

THE BRADYARRHYTHMIAS

Gordon F. Tomaselli

Electrical activation of the heart normally originates in the sinoatrial (SA) node, the predominant pacemaker. Other subsidiary pacemakers in the atrioventricular (AV) node, specialized conducting system, and muscle may initiate electrical activation if the SA node is dysfunctional or suppressed. Typically subsidiary pacemakers discharge at a slower rate and, in the absence of an appropriate increase in stroke volume, may result in tissue hypoperfusion.

Spontaneous activation and contraction of the heart are the consequence of the specialized pacemaking tissue found within these anatomic locales. As described in Chap. 14, action potentials in the heart are regionally heterogeneous. The action potentials in cells isolated from nodal tissue are distinct from those recorded from atrial and ventricular myocytes (Fig. 15-1). The complement of ionic currents present in nodal cells results in a less negative resting membrane potential compared with atrial or ventricular myocytes. Electrical diastole in nodal cells is characterized by slow diastolic depolarization (phase 4), which generates an action potential as the membrane voltage reaches threshold. The action potential upstrokes (phase 0) are slow compared with atrial or ventricular myocytes, being mediated by calcium rather than sodium current. Cells with properties of SA and AV nodal tissue are electrically connected to the remainder of the myocardium by cells with an electrophysiologic phenotype between that of nodal cells and atrial or ventricular myocytes. Cells in the SA node exhibit the most rapid phase 4 depolarization and thus are the dominant pacemakers in the normal heart.

Bradycardia results from either a failure of impulse initiation or impulse conduction. Failure of impulse initiation may be caused by depressed automaticity resulting from a slowing or failure of phase 4 diastolic depolarization (Fig. 15-2), which may result from disease or exposure to drugs. Prominently, the autonomic nervous system modulates the rate of phase 4 diastolic depolarization and, thus, the firing rate of both primary (SA node) and subsidiary pacemakers. Failure of conduction of an impulse from nodal tissue to atrial or ventricular myocardium may produce bradycardia as a result of exit block. Conditions that alter activation and connectivity of cells (e.g., fibrosis) in the heart may result in failure of impulse conduction.

SA node dysfunction and AV conduction block are the most common causes of pathologic bradycardia. SA node dysfunction may be difficult to distinguish from physiologic sinus bradycardia, particularly in the young. SA node dysfunction increases in frequency between the fifth and sixth decades of life and should be considered in patients with fatigue, exercise intolerance, or syncope and sinus bradycardia. Transient AV block is common in the young and likely the result of the high vagal tone found in up to 10% of young adults. Acquired and persistent failure of AV conduction is decidedly rare in healthy adult populations, with an estimated incidence of ~200/million population per year.

Permanent pacemaking is the only reliable therapy for symptomatic bradycardia in the absence of extrinsic and reversible etiologies such as increased vagal tone, hypoxia, hypothermia, and drugs (Table 15-1). Approximately 50% of the 150,000 permanent pacemakers implanted in the United States and 20–30% of the 150,000 of those implanted in Europe were implanted for SA node disease.

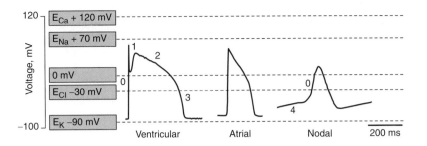

FIGURE 15-1

Action potential profiles recorded in cells isolated from SA or AV nodal tissue compared to that of cells from atrial or ventricular myocardium. Nodal cell action potentials exhibit more depolarized resting membrane potentials, slower phase 0 upstrokes, and phase 4 diastolic depolarization.

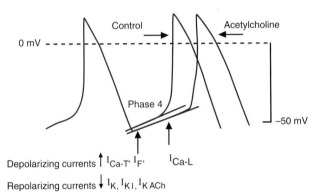

FIGURE 15-2

Schematics of nodal action potentials and the currents that contribute to phase 4 depolarization. Relative increases in depolarizing L- (I_{Ca-L}) and T- (I_{Ca-T}) type calcium and pacemaker currents (I_f) along with a reduction in repolarizing inward rectifier (I_{K1}) and delayed rectifier (I_K) potassium currents result in depolarization. Activation of ACh-gated (I_{KACh}) potassium current and beta blockade slows the rate of phase 4 and decreases the pacing rate. *(Modified from J Jalife et al: Basic Cardiac Electrophysiology for the Clinician, Blackwell Publishing, 1999.)*

SA NODE DISEASE

Structure and Physiology of the SA Node

The SA node is composed of a cluster of small fusiform cells located in the sulcus terminalis on the epicardial surface of the heart at the right atrial–superior vena caval junction, where they envelop the SA nodal artery. The SA node is structurally heterogeneous, but the central prototypic nodal cells have fewer distinct myofibrils than the surrounding atrial myocardium, no intercalated disks visible on light microscopy, a poorly developed sarcoplasmic reticulum, and no T-tubules. Cells in the peripheral regions of the SA node are transitional in both structure and function. The SA nodal artery arises from the right coronary artery in 55–60% and left circumflex artery in 40–45% of persons. The SA node is richly innervated by sympathetic and parasympathetic nerves and ganglia.

Irregular and slow propagation of impulses from the SA node can be explained by the electrophysiology of nodal cells and the structure of the SA node itself. The action potentials of SA nodal cells are characterized by a relatively depolarized membrane potential (Fig. 15-1) of −40 to −60 mV, slow phase 0 upstroke, and relatively rapid phase 4 diastolic depolarization compared to the action potentials recorded in cardiac muscle cells. The relative absence of inward rectifier potassium current (I_{K1}) accounts for the depolarized membrane potential; the slow upstroke of phase 0 is the result of the absence of available fast sodium current (I_{Na}) and is mediated by L-type calcium current (I_{Ca-L}); and phase 4 depolarization is the result of the aggregate activity of a number of ionic currents. Prominently, both L- and T-type (I_{Ca-T}) calcium currents, the pacemaker current (so-called funny current, or I_f) formed by the tetramerization of hyperpolarization-activated cyclic nucleotide-gated channels, and the electrogenic sodium-calcium exchanger provide depolarizing current that is antagonized by delayed rectifier (I_{Kr}) and acetylcholine-gated (I_{KACh}) potassium currents. I_{Ca-L}, I_{Ca-T}, and I_f are modulated by β–adrenergic stimulation and I_{KACh} by vagal stimulation, explaining the exquisite sensitivity of diastolic depolarization to autonomic nervous system activity. The slow conduction within the SA node is explained by the absence of I_{Na} and poor electrical coupling of cells in the node, resulting from sizeable amounts of interstitial tissue and a low abundance of gap junctions. The poor coupling allows for graded electrophysiological properties within the node, with the peripheral transitional cells being silenced by electrotonic coupling to atrial myocardium.

Etiology of SA Nodal Disease

SA nodal dysfunction has been classified as intrinsic or extrinsic. The distinction is important because extrinsic dysfunction is often reversible and should generally be corrected before considering pacemaker therapy (Table 15-1). The most common causes of extrinsic SA node dysfunction are drugs and autonomic nervous system

TABLE 15-1

ETIOLOGIES OF SA NODE DYSFUNCTION

EXTRINSIC	INTRINSIC
Autonomic	Sick sinus syndrome (SSS)
Carotid sinus hypersensitivity	Coronary artery disease (chronic and acute MI)
Vasovagal (cardioinhibitory) stimulation	Inflammatory
Drugs	Pericarditis
Beta blockers	Myocarditis (including viral)
Calcium channel blockers	Rheumatic heart disease
Digoxin	Collagen vascular diseases
Antiarrhythmics (class I and III)	Lyme disease
Adenosine	Senile amyloidosis
Clonidine (other sympatholytics)	Congenital heart disease
Lithium carbonate	TGA/Mustard and Fontan repairs
Cimetidine	Iatrogenic
Amitriptyline	Radiation therapy
Phenothiazines	Post surgical
Narcotics (methadone)	Chest trauma
Pentamidine	Familial
Hypothyroidism	AD SSS, OMIM #163800 (15q24-25)
Sleep apnea	AR SSS, OMIM #608567 (3p21)
Hypoxia	SA node disease with myopia, OMIM 182190
Endotracheal suctioning (vagal maneuvers)	Kearns-Sayre syndrome, OMIM #530000
Hypothermia	Myotonic dystrophy
Increased intracranial pressure	Type 1, OMIM #160900 (19q13.2-13.3)
	Type 2, OMIM #602668 (3q13.3-q24)
	Friedreich's ataxia, OMIM #229300 (9q13, 9p23-p11)

Note: MI, myocardial infarction; TGA, transposition of the great arteries; AD, autosomal dominant; AR, autosomal recessive; OMIM, Online Mendelian Inheritance in Man (database).

influences that suppress automaticity and/or compromise conduction. Other extrinsic causes include hypothyroidism, sleep apnea, and conditions likely to occur in critically ill patients such as hypothermia, hypoxia, increased intracranial pressure (Cushing's response), and endotracheal suctioning via activation of the vagus nerve.

Intrinsic sinus node dysfunction is degenerative and often characterized pathologically by fibrous replacement of the SA node or its connections to the atrium. Acute and chronic coronary artery disease (CAD) may be associated with SA node dysfunction, although in the setting of acute myocardial infarction (MI; typically inferior), the abnormalities are transient. Inflammatory processes may alter SA node function, ultimately producing replacement fibrosis. Pericarditis, myocarditis, and rheumatic heart disease have been associated with SA nodal disease with sinus bradycardia, sinus arrest, and exit block. Carditis associated with systemic lupus erythematosus (SLE), rheumatoid arthritis (RA), and mixed connective tissue disorders (MCTDs) may also affect SA node structure and function. Senile amyloidosis is an infiltrative disorder in patients typically in their ninth decade of life; deposition of amyloid protein in the atrial myocardium can impair SA node function. Some SA node disease is iatrogenic and the result of surgical correction of congenital heart disease, particularly palliative repair of corrected transposition of the great arteries by the Mustard procedure.

Rare heritable forms of sinus node disease have been described, and several have been genetically characterized. Autosomal dominant sinus node dysfunction in conjunction with supraventricular tachycardia (i.e., tachycardia-bradycardia variant of sick-sinus syndrome, SSS) has been linked to mutations in the pacemaker current (I_f) subunit gene *HCN4* on chromosome 15. An autosomal recessive form of SSS with the prominent feature of atrial inexcitability and absence of P waves on the electrocardiogram (ECG) is caused by mutations in the cardiac sodium channel gene, *SCN5A*, on chromosome 3. SSS associated with myopia has been described but not genetically characterized. There are several neuromuscular diseases including Kearns-Sayre syndrome (ophthalmoplegia, pigmentary degeneration of the retina, and cardiomyopathy) and myotonic dystrophy that have a predilection for the conducting system and SA node.

SSS in both the young and the elderly is associated with an increase in fibrous tissue in the SA node. The onset of SSS may be hastened by coexisting disease, such as CAD, diabetes mellitus, hypertension, and valvular diseases and cardiomyopathies.

Clinical Features of SA Node Disease

SA node dysfunction may be completely asymptomatic and manifest as an ECG anomaly such as sinus bradycardia; sinus arrest and exit block; or alternating supraventricular tachycardia, usually atrial fibrillation, and bradycardia. Symptoms associated with SA node dysfunction, and in particular tachycardia-bradycardia syndrome, may be related to both bradycardia and tachycardia. For example, tachycardia may be associated with palpitations, angina pectoris, and heart failure; and bradycardia may be associated with hypotension syncope, presyncope, fatigue, and weakness. In the setting of SSS, overdrive suppression of the SA node may result in prolonged pauses and syncope upon termination of the tachycardia. In many patients, symptoms associated with SA node dysfunction are the result of concomitant cardiovascular disease. A significant minority of patients with SSS will develop signs and symptoms of heart failure that may be related to slow or fast heart rates.

One-third to one-half of patients with SA node dysfunction will develop supraventricular tachycardia, usually atrial fibrillation or atrial flutter. The incidence of chronic atrial fibrillation in patients with SA node dysfunction increases with advanced age, hypertension, diabetes mellitus, left ventricular dilation, valvular heart disease, and ventricular pacing. Remarkably, some symptomatic patients may experience an improvement in symptoms with the development of atrial fibrillation, presumably from an increase in their average heart rate. Patients with the tachycardia-bradycardia variant of SSS, similar to patients with atrial fibrillation, are at risk for thromboembolism, and *those at greatest risk*, including patients ≥65 years, or patients with a prior history of stroke, valvular heart disease, left ventricular dysfunction, or atrial enlargement, should be treated with anticoagulants. Up to one-quarter of patients with SA node disease will have concurrent AV conduction disease; although only a minority will require specific therapy for high-grade AV block.

The natural history of SA node dysfunction is one of varying intensity of symptoms even in patients who present with syncope. Symptoms related to SA node dysfunction may be significant, but overall mortality is usually not compromised in the absence of other significant comorbid conditions. These features of the natural history need to be taken into account when considering therapy in these patients.

Electrocardiography of SA Node Disease

The electrocardiographic manifestations of SA node dysfunction include sinus bradycardia, sinus pauses, sinus arrest, sinus exit block, tachycardia (in SSS), and chronotropic incompetence. It is often difficult to distinguish pathologic from physiologic sinus bradycardia. By definition sinus bradycardia is a rhythm driven by the SA node with a rate of <60 beats/min; sinus bradycardia is very common and typically benign. Resting heart rates of <60 beats/min are very common in young healthy individuals and physically conditioned subjects. A sinus rate of <40 beats/min in the awake state in the absence of physical conditioning is generally considered abnormal. Sinus pauses and sinus arrest result from the failure of the SA node to discharge, producing a pause without P waves visible on the ECG (**Fig. 15-3**). Sinus pauses of up to 3 s are common in the awake athlete, and pauses of this duration or longer may be observed in asymptomatic elderly subjects. Intermittent failure of conduction from the SA node produces sinus exit block. The severity of sinus exit block may vary in a manner similar to that of AV block (see later). Prolongation of conduction from the sinus node will not be apparent on the ECG; second-degree SA block will produce intermittent conduction from the SA node and a regularly irregular atrial rhythm.

Second degree SA block appears on the ECG as an intermittent absence of P waves. Type I second degree SA block results from progressive prolongation of SA node conduction and appears on the ECG as a progressive shortening of the P-P interval, followed by a pause

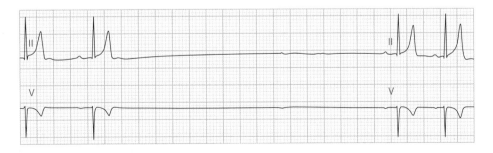

FIGURE 15-3

Sinus slowing and pauses on the ECG. The ECG is recorded during sleep in a young patient without heart disease. The heart rate before the pause is slow, and the PR interval is prolonged consistent with an increase in vagal tone.

The P waves have a morphology consistent with sinus rhythm. The recording is from a two-lead telemetry system where the tracing labeled II mimics frontal lead II and V represents lead MCL 1 which mimics lead V1 of the standard 12-lead ECG.

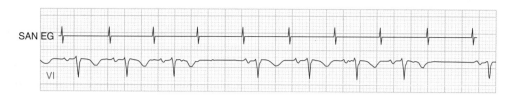

FIGURE 15-4

Mobitz type I SA nodal exit block. A theoretical SA node electrogram (SAN EG) is shown. Note that there is grouped beating producing a regularly irregular heart rhythm. The SA node EG rate is constant with progressive delay in exit from the node, and activation of the atria, inscribing the P wave. This produces subtly decreasing P-P intervals prior to the pause, and the pause is less that twice the cycle length of the last sinus interval.

(Fig. 15-4). In type II second degree SA block there is no change in the P-P interval before the pause. Complete or third degree SA block results in no P waves on the ECG. Tachycardia-bradycardia syndrome is manifest as alternating sinus bradycardia and atrial tachyarrhythmias. Although atrial tachycardia, atrial flutter, and atrial fibrillation may be observed, the latter is the most common tachycardia. Chronotropic incompetence is the inability to increase the heart rate in response to exercise or other stress appropriately and is defined in greater detail below.

Diagnostic Testing

SA node dysfunction is most commonly a clinical or electrocardiographic diagnosis. Sinus bradycardia or pauses on the resting ECG are rarely sufficient to diagnose SA node disease, and longer-term recording and symptom correlation are generally required. Symptoms in the absence of sinus bradyarrhythmias may be sufficient to exclude a diagnosis of SA node dysfunction.

Electrocardiographic recording plays a central role in the diagnosis and management of SA node dysfunction. Despite the limitations of the resting ECG, longer-term recording employing Holter or event monitors may permit correlation of symptoms with the cardiac rhythm. Many contemporary event monitors may be automatically triggered to record the ECG when certain programmed heart rate criteria are met. Implantable ECG monitors permit long-term recording (12–18 months) in particularly challenging patients.

Failure to increase the heart rate with exercise is referred to as *chronotropic incompetence*. This is alternatively defined as a failure to reach 85% of predicted maximal heart rate at peak exercise, or failure to achieve a heart rate >100 beats/min with exercise or a maximal heart rate with exercise less than two standard deviations below that of an age-matched control population. Exercise testing may be useful in discriminating chronotropic incompetence from resting bradycardia and may aid in the identification of the mechanism of exercise intolerance.

Autonomic nervous system testing is useful in diagnosing carotid sinus hypersensitivity; pauses >3 s are consistent with the diagnosis but may be present in asymptomatic elderly subjects. Determining the intrinsic heart rate (IHR) may distinguish SA node dysfunction from slow heart rates resulting from high vagal tone. The normal IHR after administration of 0.2 mg/kg propranolol and 0.04 mg/kg atropine is 117.2 − (0.53 × age) in beats/min; a low IHR is indicative of SA disease.

Electrophysiologic testing may play a role in the assessment of patients with presumed SA node dysfunction and in the evaluation of syncope, particularly in the setting of structural heart disease. In this circumstance, electrophysiologic testing is used to rule out more malignant etiologies of syncope such as ventricular tachyarrhythmias and AV conduction block. There are several ways to assess SA node function invasively. They include the sinus node recovery time (SNRT), defined as the longest pause after cessation of overdrive pacing of the right atrium near the SA node (normal: <1500 ms or, corrected for sinus cycle length, <550 ms); and the sinoatrial conduction time (SACT), defined as one-half the difference between the intrinsic sinus cycle length and a noncompensatory pause after a premature atrial stimulus (normal <125 ms). The combination of an abnormal SNRT, an abnormal SACT, and a low IHR is a sensitive and specific indicator of intrinsic SA node disease.

℞ Treatment:
SINOATRIAL NODE DYSFUNCTION

Since SA node dysfunction is not associated with increased mortality, the aim of therapy is alleviation of symptoms. Exclusion of extrinsic causes of SA node dysfunction and correlation of the cardiac rhythm with symptoms is an essential part of patient management. Pacemaker implantation is the primary therapeutic intervention in patients with symptomatic SA node dysfunction. Pharmacologic considerations are important in the evaluation and management of patients with SA nodal disease. A number of drugs modulate SA node function and are extrinsic causes of dysfunction (Table 15-1). Beta blockers and calcium channel blockers increase SNRT in patients with SA node dysfunction, and antiarrhythmic drugs with class I and III action may promote SA node exit block. In general such agents should be discontinued prior to making decisions regarding the need for permanent pacing in patients with SA node disease. Chronic pharmacologic therapy for sinus bradyarrhythmias is limited. Some pharmacologic agents may improve SA node function; digitalis, for example, has been shown to shorten SNRT in patients with SA node dysfunction. Isoproterenol or atropine administered IV may increase the sinus rate acutely. Theophylline has been used both acutely and chronically to increase heart rate but has liabilities when used in patients with tachycardia-bradycardia syndrome, increasing the frequency of supraventricular tachyarrhythmias; and in patients with structural heart disease, increasing the risk of potentially serious ventricular arrhythmias. At the current time, there is only a single randomized study of therapy for SA node dysfunction. In patients with resting heart rates <50 and >30 beats/min on a Holter monitor, patients who received dual-chamber pacemakers experienced significantly fewer syncopal episodes and had symptomatic improvement compared to patients randomized to theophylline or no treatment.

In certain circumstances, sinus bradycardia requires no specific treatment or only temporary rate support. Sinus bradycardia is common in patients with acute inferior or posterior MI and can be exacerbated by vagal activation induced by pain or the use of drugs such as morphine. Ischemia of the SA nodal artery probably occurs in acute coronary syndromes more typically with involvement with the right coronary artery, and even with infarction, the effect on SA node function is most often transient.

Sinus bradycardia is a prominent feature of carotid sinus hypersensitivity and neurally mediated hypotension associated with vasovagal syncope that responds to pacemaker therapy. Carotid hypersensitivity with recurrent syncope or presyncope associated with a predominant cardioinhibitory component responds to pacemaker implantation. Several randomized trials have demonstrated that patients with drug-refractory vasovagal syncope have fewer recurrences and longer time to recurrence of symptoms with permanent pacing.

The details of pacing modes and indications for pacing in SA node dysfunction are discussed later in the chapter.

ATRIOVENTRICULAR CONDUCTION DISEASE

Structure and Physiology of the AV Node

The AV conduction axis is structurally complex, involving the atria and ventricles as well as the AV node. Unlike the SA node, the AV node is a subendocardial structure originating in the transitional zone, which is composed of aggregates of cells in the posterior–inferior right atrium. Superior, medial, and posterior transitional atrionodal bundles converge on the compact AV node. The compact AV node (~1 × 3 × 5 mm) is located at the apex of the triangle of Koch, which is defined by the coronary sinus ostium posteriorly, the septal tricuspid valve annulus anteriorly, and the tendon of Todaro superiorly. The compact AV node continues as the penetrating AV bundle where it immediately traverses the central fibrous body and is in close proximity to the aortic, mitral, and tricuspid valve annuli; thus, it is subject to injury in the setting of valvular heart disease or its surgical treatment. The penetrating AV bundle continues through the annulus fibrosis and emerges along the ventricular septum adjacent to the membranous septum as the bundle of His. The right bundle branch (RBB) emerges from the distal AV bundle in a band that traverses the right ventricle (moderator band). In contrast, the left bundle branch (LBB) is a broad subendocardial sheet of tissue on the septal left ventricle. The Purkinje fiber network emerges from the RBB and LBB and extensively ramifies on the endocardial surfaces of the right and left ventricles, respectively.

The blood supply to the penetrating AV bundle is from the AV nodal artery and first septal perforator of the left anterior descending coronary artery. The bundle branches also have a dual blood supply from the septal perforators of the left anterior descending coronary artery and branches of the posterior descending coronary artery. The AV node is highly innervated with postganglionic sympathetic and parasympathetic nerves. The bundle of His and distal conducting system are minimally influenced by autonomic tone.

The cells that comprise the AV node complex are heterogeneous with a range of action potential profiles. In the transitional zones, the cells have an electrical phenotype between atrial myocytes and cells of the compact node (Fig. 15-1). Atrionodal transitional connections may exhibit *decremental conduction*, defined as slowing of conduction with increasingly rapid rates of stimulation. Fast and slow AV nodal pathways have been described, but controversy remains as to whether these two types of pathway are anatomically distinct or represent functional heterogeneities in different regions of the AV nodal complex. Myocytes that comprise the compact node are depolarized (resting membrane potential ~ −60 mV); exhibit action potentials with low amplitudes, slow upstrokes of phase 0 (<10 V/s), and phase 4 diastolic depolarization; high-input resistance; and relative insensitivity to external [K$^+$]. The action potential phenotype is explained by the complement of ionic currents expressed. AV nodal cells lack I_{K1} and I_{Na}; I_{Ca-L} is responsible for phase 0; and phase 4 depolarization reflects the composite activity of the depolarizing currents I_f, I_{Ca-L}, I_{Ca-T}, and I_{NCX} and the repolarizing currents I_{Kr} and I_{KACh}. Electrical coupling between cells in the AV node is tenuous due to the relatively sparse expression of gap junction channels (predominantly connexin-40) and increased extracellular volume.

The His bundle and bundle branches are insulated from ventricular myocardium. The most rapid conduction in the heart is observed in these tissues. The action potentials exhibit very rapid upstrokes (phase 0), prolonged plateaus (phase 2), and modest automaticity (phase 4 depolarization). Gap junctions, composed largely of connexin-40, are abundant but bundles are poorly connected transversely to ventricular myocardium.

Etiology of AV Conduction Disease

Conduction block from the atrium to the ventricle can occur for a variety of reasons in a number of clinical situations, and AV conduction block may be classified in a number of ways. The etiologies may be functional or structural, in part analogous to extrinsic and intrinsic causes of SA nodal dysfunction. The block may be classified by its severity from first to third degree or complete AV block, or by the location of block within the AV conduction system. Table 15-2 summarizes the etiologies of AV conduction block, those that are functional (autonomic, metabolic/endocrine, and drug-related) tend to be reversible. Most other etiologies produce structural changes, typically fibrosis, in segments of the AV conduction axis that are generally permanent. Heightened vagal tone during sleep or in well-conditioned individuals can be associated with all grades of AV block. Carotid sinus hypersensitivity, vasovagal syncope, and cough and micturition syncope may be associated with SA node slowing and AV conduction block. Transient metabolic and endocrinologic disturbances as well as a number of pharmacologic agents may also produce reversible AV conduction block.

Several infectious diseases have a predilection for the conducting system. Lyme disease may involve the heart in up to 50% of cases; 10% of patients with Lyme carditis develop AV conduction block, which is generally reversible but may require temporary pacing support. Chagas disease, common in Latin America and syphilis may produce more persistent AV conduction disturbances. Some autoimmune and infiltrative diseases may produce AV conduction block including SLE, RA, MCTD, scleroderma, amyloidosis (primary and secondary), sarcoidosis, and hemochromatosis; rare malignancies may also impair AV conduction.

Idiopathic progressive fibrosis of the conduction system is one of the more common and degenerative causes of AV conduction block. Aging is associated with degenerative changes in the summit of the ventricular septum, central fibrous body, and aortic and mitral annuli and has been described as "sclerosis of the left cardiac skeleton." The process typically begins in the

TABLE 15-2

ETIOLOGIES OF ATRIOVENTRICULAR BLOCK	
Autonomic	
Carotid sinus hypersensitivity	Vasovagal
Metabolic/endocrine	
Hyperkalemia	Hypothyroidism
Hypermagnesemia	Adrenal insufficiency
Drug-related	
Beta blockers	Adenosine
Calcium channel blockers	Antiarrhythmics (class I & III)
Digitalis	Lithium
Infectious	
Endocarditis	Tuberculosis
Lyme disease	Diphtheria
Chagas disease	Toxoplasmosis
Syphilis	
Heritable/congenital	
Congenital heart disease	Facioscapulohumeral MD, OMIM #158900 (4q35)
Maternal SLE	
Kearns-Sayre syndrome, OMIM #530000	Emery-Dreifuss MD, OMIM #310300 (Xq28)
Myotonic dystrophy	Progressive familial heart block, OMIM #113900 (19q13.2-q13.3, 3p21)
Type 1, OMIM #160900 (19q13.2-13.3)	
Type 2, OMIM #602668 (3q13.3-q24)	
Inflammatory	
SLE	MCTD
Rheumatoid arthritis	Scleroderma
Infiltrative	
Amyloidosis	Hemochromatosis
Sarcoidosis	
Neoplastic/traumatic	
Lymphoma	Radiation
Mesothelioma	Catheter ablation
Melanoma	
Degenerative	
Lev disease	Lenègre disease
Coronary artery disease	
Acute MI	

Note: SLE, systemic lupus erythematosus; OMIM, Online Mendelian Inheritance in Man (database); MCTD, mixed connective tissue disease; MI, myocardial infarction.

fourth decade of life and may be accelerated by atherosclerosis, hypertension with arteriosclerosis, and diabetes mellitus. Accelerated forms of progressive familial heart block have been identified in families with mutations in the cardiac sodium channel gene (*SCN5A*) and a second locus that has been mapped to chromosome 19.

AV conduction block has been associated with heritable neuromuscular diseases, including the nucleotide repeat disease myotonic dystrophy, the mitochondrial myopathy Kearns-Sayre syndrome, and several of the monogenic muscular dystrophies. Congenital AV block may be observed in complex congenital cardiac anomalies

(Chap. 19), such as transposition of the great arteries, ostium primum atrial septal defects (ASD), ventricular septal defects (VSD), endocardial cushion defects, and some single ventricle defects. Congenital AV block in the setting of a structurally normal heart has been seen in children born to mothers with SLE. Iatrogenic AV block may occur during mitral or aortic valve surgery, rarely in the setting of thoracic radiation, and as a consequence catheter ablation. AV block is a decidedly rare complication of the surgical repair of VSDs or ASDs but may complicate Fontan or Mustard repairs of transposition of the great arteries.

CAD may produce transient or persistent AV block. In the setting of coronary spasm, ischemia, particularly in the right coronary artery distribution, may produce transient AV block. In acute MI, AV block transiently develops in 10–25% of patients; most commonly this is first- or second-degree AV block but complete heart block (CHB) may also occur. Second-degree and higher grade AV block tends to occur more often in inferior rather than anterior acute MI; however, the level of block in inferior MI tends to be in the AV node with more stable, narrow escape rhythms. In contrast, acute anterior MI is associated with block in the distal AV nodal complex, His bundle, or bundle branches and results in wide complex, unstable escape rhythms and a worse prognosis with high mortality.

Atrioventricular conduction block is typically diagnosed electrocardiographically which characterizes the severity of the conduction disturbance and allows one to draw inferences about the location of block. AV conduction block manifests as slow conduction in its mildest forms and failure to conduct, either intermittent or persistently, in more severe varieties. First-degree AV block (PR interval >200 ms) is a slowing of conduction through the AV junction (Fig. 15-5). The site of delay is typically in the AV node but may be in the atria, AV node bundle of His, or His-Purkinje system; a wide QRS complex favors distal conduction and narrow QRS complex delay in the node proper or, less commonly, in the bundle of His. In second-degree AV block there is an intermittent failure of electrical impulse conduction from atrium to ventricle. Second-degree AV block is subclassified as Mobitz type 1 or Wenckebach and Mobitz type 2. The periodic failure of conduction in Mobitz type 1 block is characterized by a progressively lengthening PR interval, shortening of the RR interval, and a pause that is less than two times the immediately preceding RR interval on the ECG. The ECG complex after the pause exhibits a shorter PR interval that immediately preceds the pause

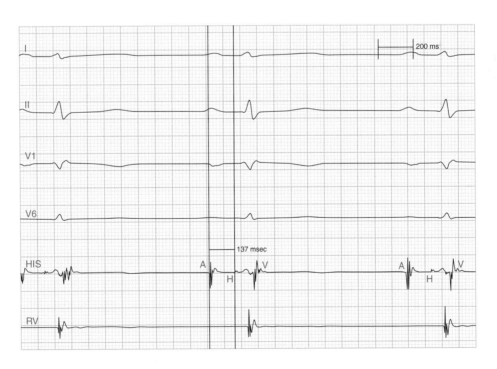

FIGURE 15-5

First-degree AV block with slowing of conduction in the AV node as indicated by the prolonged atrial-to-His bundle electrogram (AH) interval, in this case 157 ms. The His bundle-to-earliest ventricular activation on the surface ECG (HV) interval is normal. The normal HV interval suggests normal conduction below the AV node to the ventricle. I and V1 are surface ECG leads, HIS is the recording of the endocavitary electrogram at the His bundle position. A, H, and V are labels for the atrial, His bundle, and right ventricular electrograms respectively.

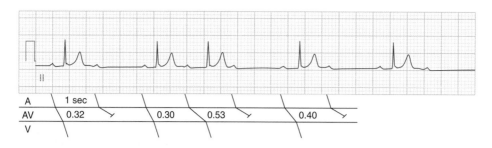

FIGURE 15-6

Mobitz type I second-degree AV block. The PR interval prolongs prior to the pause as shown in the ladder diagram.

The ECG pattern results from slowing of conduction in the AV node.

(Fig. 15-6). This ECG pattern most often arises because of decremental conduction of electrical impulses in the AV node.

It is important to distinguish type 1 from type 2 second-degree AV nodal block because the latter has more serious prognostic implications. Type 2 second-degree AV block is characterized by intermittent failure of conduction of the P wave without changes in the preceding PR or RR intervals. When AV block is 2:1 it may be difficult to distinguish type 1 from type 2 blocks. Type 2 second-degree AV block typically occurs in the distal or infra-His conduction system, is often associated with intraventricular conduction delays (e.g., bundle branch block), and is more likely to proceed to higher grades of AV block than is type 1 second-degree AV block. Second-degree AV block (particularly type 2) may be associated with a series of nonconducted P waves, referred to as *paroxysmal AV block* (Fig. 15-7), and implies significant conduction system disease and an indication for permanent pacing. Complete failure of conduction from atrium to ventricle is referred to as complete or third-degree AV block. AV block that is intermediate between

second and third degree is referred to as high-grade AV block, and, as with CHB, implies advanced AV conduction system disease. In both cases, block is most often distal to the AV node, and the duration of the QRS complex can be helpful in determining the level of block. In the absence of a preexisting bundle branch block, a wide QRS escape rhythm (Fig. 15-8B) implies block in the distal His or bundle branches; in contrast, a narrow QRS rhythm implies block in the AV node or proximal His and an escape rhythm originating in the AV junction (Fig. 15-8A). Narrow QRS escape rhythms are typically faster and more stable than wide QRS escape rhythms and originate more proximally in the AV conduction system.

Diagnostic Testing

Diagnostic testing in the evaluation of AV block is aimed at determining the level of conduction block, particularly in asymptomatic patients, since the prognosis and therapy depend upon whether block is in or below the AV node. Vagal maneuvers, carotid sinus massage,

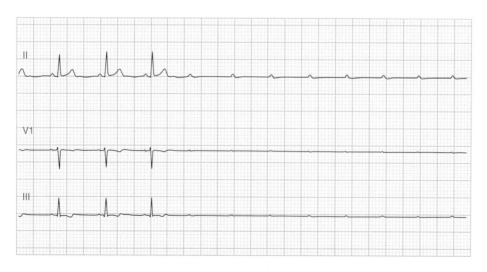

FIGURE 15-7

Paroxysmal AV block. Multiple nonconducted P waves following a period of sinus bradycardia with a normal PR

interval. This implies significant conduction system disease, requiring permanent pacemaker implantation.

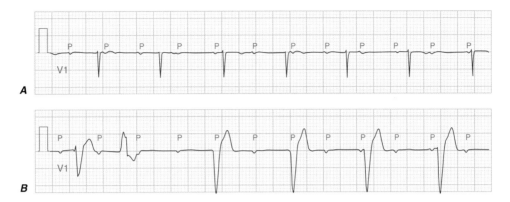

FIGURE 15-8

High-grade AV block. *A.* Multiple nonconducted P waves with a regular narrow complex QRS escape rhythm likely emanating from the AV junction. ***B.*** A wide complex QRS escape and a single PVC. In both cases there is no consistent temporal relationship between the P waves and QRS complexes.

exercise, and administration of drugs such as atropine or isoproterenol may be diagnostically informative. Owing to the differences in innervation of the AV node and infranodal conduction system, vagal stimulation and carotid sinus massage slow conduction in the AV node but have less of an effect on infranodal tissue and may even improve conduction due to a reduced rate of activation of distal tissues. Conversely, atropine, isoproterenol, and exercise improve conduction through the AV node and impair infranodal conduction. In patients with congenital CHB and a narrow QRS complex, exercise typically increases heart rate; by contrast, those with acquired CHB, particularly with wide QRS, do not respond to exercise with an increase in heart rate.

Additional diagnostic evaluation, including electrophysiologic testing, may be indicated in patients with syncope and suspected high-grade AV block. This is particularly relevant if noninvasive testing does not reveal the cause of syncope or if the patient has structural heart disease with ventricular tachyarrhythmias as a cause of symptoms. Electrophysiologic testing provides more precise information regarding the location of AV conduction block and permits studies of AV conduction under conditions of pharmacologic stress and exercise. Recording of the His bundle electrogram by a catheter positioned at the superior margin of the tricuspid valve annulus provides information about conduction at all levels of the AV conduction axis. A properly recorded His bundle electrogram reveals local atrial activity, the His electrogram, and local ventricular activation; when monitored simultaneously with recorded body surface electrocardiographic traces, intraatrial, AV nodal, and infranodal conduction times can be assessed (Fig. 15-5).

The *PA interval*, the time from the earliest onset of the P wave on the surface ECG to the onset of the atrial deflection on the His bundle catheter, is an index of intraatrial conduction time and should be ≤50 ms. The time from the most rapid deflection of the atrial electrogram in the His

bundle recording to the His electrogram (*AH interval*) represents conduction through the AV node and is normally <130 ms. Finally, the time from the His electrogram to the earliest onset of the QRS on the surface ECG (*HV interval*) represents the conduction time through the His-Purkinje system and is normally ≤55 ms. Rate stress produced by pacing can unveil abnormal AV conduction. Mobitz I second-degree AV block at short atrial paced cycle lengths is a normal response; however, when it occurs at atrial cycle lengths >500 ms (<120 beats/min) in the absence of high vagal tone, it is abnormal. Typically type I second-degree AV block is associated with prolongation of the AH interval representing conduction slowing and block in the AV node. Block below the node with prolongation of the HV interval or a His-bundle electrogram with no ventricular activation (**Fig. 15-9**) is abnormal unless it is elicited at fast pacing rates or short coupling intervals with extra stimulation.

First-degree AV block is classically intranodal and is associated with a prolonged AH interval. Often, AH prolongation is due to the effect of drugs (beta blockers, calcium channel blockers, digitalis), or increased vagal tone. Atropine can be used to reverse high vagal tone; however, if AH prolongation and AV block at long pacing cycle lengths persist, intrinsic AV node disease is likely. Mobitz type 1 second-degree AV block is usually intranodal and type 2 second-degree block is infranodal, frequently in the His-Purkinje system. It is often difficult to determine the type of second-degree AV block when 2:1 conduction is present; however, the finding of a His-bundle electrogram after every atrial electrogram indicates that block is occurring in the distal conduction system.

Intracardiac recording at electrophysiologic study that reveals the presence of His–Purkinje conduction block is associated with an increased risk of progression to higher grades of block and is generally an indication for pacing. In the setting of bundle branch block, the HV

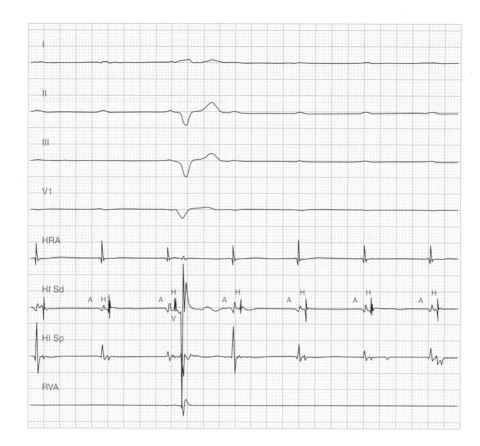

FIGURE 15-9

High-grade AV block below the His. The AH interval is normal and is not changing prior to block. Atrial and His bundle electrograms are recorded consistent with block below the distal AV junction. I, II, III, and V1 are surface ECG leads. HISp, HISd, RVA are the proximal HIS, distal HIS, and right ventricular apical electrical recordings. A, H, and V represent the atrial, His, and ventricular electrograms on the His bundle recording. *(Tracing courtesy of Dr. Joseph Marine; with permission.)*

interval may reveal the condition of the unblocked bundle and the prognosis for developing more advanced AV conduction block. Prolongation of the HV interval in patients with asymptomatic bundle branch block is associated with an increased risk of developing higher-grade AV block. The risk increases with greater prolongation of the HV interval such that in patients with an HV interval >100 ms, the annual incidence of complete AV block approaches 10%, indicating a need for pacing. In patients with acquired CHB, even if intermittent, there is little role for electrophysiologic testing, and pacemaker implantation is almost always indicated.

Treatment:
Rx ATRIOVENTRICULAR CONDUCTION BLOCK

Temporary or permanent artificial pacing is the most reliable treatment for patients with symptomatic AV conduction system disease. However, exclusion of reversible causes of AV block and the need for temporary heart rate support based on the hemodynamic condition of the patient are essential considerations in each patient.

Correction of electrolyte derangements and ischemia, inhibition of excessive vagal tone, and withholding drugs with AV nodal blocking properties may increase the heart rate. Adjunctive pharmacologic treatment with atropine or isoproterenol may be useful if block is in the AV node. Since most pharmacologic treatment may take some time to initiate and become effective, temporary pacing may be necessary. The most expeditious technique is the use of transcutaneous pacing, where pacing patches are placed anteriorly over the cardiac apex (cathode) and posteriorly between the spine and scapula or above the right nipple (anode). Acutely, transcutaneous pacing is highly effective, but its duration is limited by patient discomfort and longer-term failure to capture the ventricle owing to changes in lead impedance. If a patient requires more than a few minutes of pacemaker support, transvenous temporary pacing should be instituted. Temporary pacing leads can be placed from the jugular or subclavian venous system and advanced to the right ventricle, permitting stable temporary pacing for many days, if necessary. In most circumstances, in the absence of prompt resolution, conduction block distal to the AV node requires permanent pacemaking.

PERMANENT PACEMAKERS

Nomenclature and Complications

The main therapeutic intervention in SA node dysfunction and AV conduction block is permanent pacing. Since the first implementation of permanent pacing in the 1950s, many advances in technology have resulted in miniaturization, increased longevity of pulse generators, improvement in leads, and increased functionality. In order to better understand pacemaker therapy of bradycardias, it is important to be familiar with fundamentals of pacemaking. Pacemaker modes and function are named using a five-letter code. The first letter indicates the chamber(s) that is paced (O, none; A, atrium; V, ventricle; D, dual; S, single), the second letter is the chamber(s) in which sensing occurs (O, none; A, atrium; V, ventricle; D, dual; S, single), the third letter is the response to a sensed event (O, none; I, inhibition; T, triggered; D, inhibition + triggered), the fourth letter refers to the programmability or rate response (R, rate responsive), and the fifth letter refers to the existence of antitachycardia functions if present (O, none; P, antitachycardia pacing; S, shock; D, pace + shock). Almost all modern pacemakers are multiprogrammable and have the capability for rate responsiveness using one of several rate sensors: activity or motion, minute ventilation, or QT interval. The most commonly programmed modes of implanted single- and dual-chamber pacemakers are VVIR and DDDR, respectively, although multiple modes can be programmed in modern pacemakers.

Although pacemakers are highly reliable, they are subject to a number of complications related to implantation and electronic function. In adults, permanent pacemakers are most commonly implanted with access to the heart by way of the subclavian–superior vena cava venous system. Rare, but possible, acute complications of transvenous pacemaker implantation include infection, hematoma, pneumothorax, cardiac perforation, diaphragmatic/phrenic nerve stimulation, and lead dislodgment. Limitations of chronic pacemaker therapy include infection, erosion, lead failure, and abnormalities resulting from inappropriate programming or interaction with the patient's native electrical cardiac function. Rotation of the pacemaker pulse generator in its subcutaneous pocket, either intentionally or inadvertently, often referred to as "twiddler's syndrome," can wrap the leads around the generator and produce dislodgment with failure to sense or pace the heart. The small size and light weight of contemporary pacemakers makes this a rare complication.

A common problem is pacemaker syndrome; a constellation of signs and symptoms associated with any mode of pacing that does not maintain or restore AV synchrony. The symptoms include neck pulsation, fatigue, palpitations, cough, confusion, exertional dyspnea, dizziness, and syncope, and they may be associated with an elevation in jugular venous pressure, canon A waves, and

stigmata of congestive heart failure, including edema, rales, and a third heart sound. Often, there is a substantial drop in blood pressure with ventricular pacing. The management of pacemaker syndrome involves changing the pacing mode to restore AV synchrony.

Pacemaker Therapy in SA Node Dysfunction

Pacing in SA nodal disease is indicated to alleviate symptoms of bradycardia. Consensus guidelines published by the AHA/ACC/HRS outline the indications for the use of pacemakers, and categorize them by class based on levels of evidence. Class I conditions are those for which there is evidence or consensus of opinion that therapy is useful and effective. In class II conditions there is conflicting evidence or a divergence of opinion about the efficacy of a procedure or treatment; in class IIa conditions the weight of evidence or opinion favors treatment, and in class IIb conditions, efficacy is less well established by the evidence or opinion of experts. In class III conditions, the evidence or weight of opinion indicates that the therapy is not efficacious or useful, and may be harmful.

Class I indications for pacing in SA node dysfunction include documented symptomatic bradycardia, sinus node dysfunction–associated long-term drug therapy for which there is no alternative, or symptomatic chronotropic incompetence. Class IIa indications include those outlined previously in which sinus node dysfunction is suspected but not documented and for syncope of unexplained origin in the presence of major abnormalities of SA node dysfunction. Mildly symptomatic individuals with heart rates consistently <40 beats/min comprise a class IIb indication for pacing. Pacing is not indicated in patients with SA node dysfunction who do not have symptoms and in those in whom bradycardia is associated with the use of nonessential drugs (Table 15-3).

There is some controversy regarding the mode of pacing that should be employed in SA node disease. A number of randomized, single-blind trials of pacing mode have been performed. There are no trials that demonstrate an improvement in mortality with AV synchronous compared with single-chamber pacing in SA node disease. In some of these studies, the incidence of atrial fibrillation and thromboembolic events was reduced with AV synchronous pacing. In trials of patients with dual-chamber pacemakers designed to compare single-chamber with dual-chamber pacing by crossover design, the need for AV synchronous pacing due to pacemaker syndrome was common. Pacing modes that preserve AV synchrony appear to be associated with a reduction in the incidence of atrial fibrillation and improved quality of life. Because of the low but finite incidence of AV conduction disease, patients with SA node dysfunction will usually undergo dual-chamber pacemaker implantation.

TABLE 15-3

SUMMARY OF GUIDELINES FOR PACEMAKER IMPLANTATION IN SA NODE DYSFUNCTION

Class I
1. SA node dysfunction with symptomatic bradycardia or sinus pauses
2. Symptomatic SA node dysfunction as a result of essential long-term drug therapy with no acceptable alternatives
3. Symptomatic chronotropic incompetence

Class IIa
1. SA node dysfunction with heart rates <40 beats/min without a clear and consistent relationship between bradycardia and symptoms
2. SA node dysfunction with heart rates <40 beats/min on an essential long-term drug therapy with no acceptable alternatives, without a clear and consistent relationship between bradycardia and symptoms
3. Syncope of unknown origin when major abnormalities of SA node dysfunction are discovered or provoked by electrophysiologic testing

Class IIb
1. Mildly symptomatic patients with waking chronic heart rates <40 beats/min

Class III
1. SA node dysfunction in asymptomatic patients even those with heart rates <40 beats/min
2. SA node dysfunction in which symptoms suggestive of bradycardia are not associated with a slow heart rate
3. SA node dysfunction with symptomatic bradycardia due to nonessential drug therapy

Source: Modified from Gregoratos et al, 1997, and Gregoratos et al, 2002.

Pacemaker Therapy in Carotid Sinus Hypersensitivity and Vasovagal Syncope

Carotid sinus hypersensitivity, if accompanied by a significant cardioinhibitory component, responds well to pacing. In this circumstance, pacing is only required intermittently and single-chamber ventricular pacing is often sufficient. The mechanism of vasovagal syncope is incompletely understood but appears to involve activation of cardiac mechanoreceptors with consequent activation of neural centers that mediate vagal activation and withdrawal of sympathetic nervous system tone. Several randomized clinical trials have been performed in patients with drug-refractory vasovagal syncope, with a reduction in the frequency and the time to recurrent syncope in patients who were paced compared to those who were not.

Pacemakers in AV Conduction Disease

There are no randomized trials that evaluate the efficacy of pacing in patients with AV block as there are no reliable therapeutic alternatives for AV block and untreated

high-grade AV block is potentially lethal. The consensus guidelines for pacing in acquired AV conduction block in adults provide a general outline for situations in which pacing is indicated (Table 15-4). Pacemaker implantation should be performed in any patient with symptomatic bradycardia and irreversible second- or third-degree AV block, regardless of the cause or level of block in the conducting system. Symptoms may include those directly related to bradycardia and low cardiac output or to worsening heart failure, angina, or intolerance to an essential medication. Pacing in patients with

TABLE 15-4

GUIDELINE SUMMARY FOR PACEMAKER IMPLANTATION IN ACQUIRED AV BLOCK

Class I
1. Third-degree or high-grade AV block at any anatomic level associated with:
   a. Symptomatic bradycardia
   b. Essential drug therapy that produces symptomatic bradycardia
   c. Periods of asystole > 3 s or any escape rate <40 beats/min while awake
   d. Postoperative AV block not expected to resolve
   e. Catheter ablation of the AV junction
   f. Neuromuscular diseases such as myotonic dystrophy, Kearns-Sayre syndrome, Erb dystrophy, and peroneal muscular atrophy, regardless of the presence of symptoms
2. Second-degree AV block with symptomatic bradycardia
3. Type II second-degree AV block with a wide QRS complex with or without symptoms

Class IIa
1. Asymptomatic third-degree AV block regardless of level
2. Asymptomatic type II second-degree AV block with a narrow QRS complex
3. Asymptomatic type II second-degree AV block with block within or below the His at electrophysiologic study
4. First- or second-degree AV block with symptoms similar to pacemaker syndrome

Class IIb
1. Marked first-degree AV block (PR interval >300 ms) in patients with LV dysfunction in whom shortening the AV delay would improve hemodynamics
2. Neuromuscular diseases, such as myotonic dystrophy, Kearns-Sayre syndrome, Erb dystrophy, and peroneal muscular atrophy, with any degree of AV block regardless of the presence of symptoms

Class III
1. Asymptomatic first-degree AV block
2. Asymptomatic type I second-degree AV block at the AV node level
3. AV block that is expected to resolve or is unlikely to recur (Lyme disease, drug toxicity)

Source: Modified from Gregoratos et al, 1997, and Gregoratos et al, 2002.

asymptomatic AV block should be individualized; situations in which pacing should be considered are in those patients with acquired CHB, particularly in the setting of cardiac enlargement; left ventricular dysfunction; and waking heart rates of ≤40 beats/min. Patients who have asymptomatic second-degree AV block of either type should be considered for pacing if the block is demonstrated to be intra- or infraHis, or is associated with a wide QRS complex. Pacing may be indicated in asymptomatic patients under special circumstances; in patients with profound first-degree AV block and left ventricular dysfunction in whom a shorter AV interval produces hemodynamic improvement, and in the setting of milder forms of AV conduction delay (first-degree AV block, intraventricular conduction delay) in patients with neuromuscular diseases that have a predilection for the conduction system, such as myotonic dystrophy and other muscular dystrophies, and Kearns-Sayre syndrome.

Pacemaker Therapy in Myocardial Infarction

Atrioventricular block in acute MI is often transient, particularly in inferior infarction. The circumstances under which pacing is indicated in acute MI are persistent second- or third-degree AV block, particularly if symptomatic, and transient second- or third-degree AV block associated with bundle branch block (Table 15-5).

Pacing is generally not indicated in the setting of transient AV block in the absence of intraventricular conduction delays, or in the presence of fascicular block or first-degree AV block that develops in the setting of preexisting bundle branch block. Fascicular blocks that develop in acute MI in the absence of other forms of AV block also do not require pacing (Tables 15-5 and Table 15-6).

Distal forms of AV conduction block may require pacemaker implantation in certain clinical settings. In patients with bifascicular or trifascicular block and symptoms, particularly syncope that is not attributable to other causes, should undergo pacemaker implantation. Pacemaking is indicated in asymptomatic patients with bifascicular or trifascicular block who experience intermittent third-degree, type II second-degree AV block, or alternating bundle branch block. In patients with fascicular block who are undergoing electrophysiologic study, a markedly prolonged HV interval or block below the His at long cycle lengths may also constitute an indication for permanent pacing. In patients with fascicular block and the neuromuscular diseases previously described should also undergo pacemaker implantation (Table 15-6).

TABLE 15-5

GUIDELINE SUMMARY FOR PACEMAKER IMPLANTATION IN AV CONDUCTION BLOCK IN ACUTE MYOCARDIAL INFARCTION (AMI)

Class I
1. Persistent second-degree AV block in the His-Purkinje system with bilateral bundle branch block or third-degree block within or below the His after AMI
2. Transient advanced (second- or third-degree) infranodal AV block and associated bundle branch block. If the site of block is uncertain, an electrophysiologic study may be necessary
3. Persistent and symptomatic second- or third-degree AV block

Class IIb
1. Persistent second- or third-degree AV block at the AV node level

Class III
1. Transient AV block in the absence of intraventricular conduction defects
2. Transient AV block in the presence of isolated left anterior fascicular block
3. Acquired left anterior fascicular block in the absence of AV block
4. Persistent first-degree AV block in the presence of bundle branch block that is old or age-indeterminate

Source: Modified from Gregoratos et al, 1997.

TABLE 15-6

INDICATIONS FOR PACEMAKER IMPLANTATION IN CHRONIC BIFASCICULAR AND TRIFASCICULAR BLOCK

Class I
1. Intermittent third-degree AV block
2. Type II second-degree AV block
3. Alternating bundle branch block

Class IIa
1. Syncope not demonstrated to be due to AV block when other likely causes (e.g., ventricular tachycardia) have been excluded
2. Incidental finding at electrophysiologic study of a markedly prolonged HV interval (>100 ms) in asymptomatic patients
3. Incidental finding at electrophysiologic study of pacing-induced infra-His block that is not physiologic

Class IIb
1. Neuromuscular diseases, such as myotonic dystrophy, Kearns-Sayre syndrome, Erb dystrophy, and peroneal muscular atrophy, with any degree of fascicular block regardless of the presence of symptoms, because there may be unpredictable progression of AV conduction disease

Class III
1. Fascicular block without AV block or symptoms
2. Fascicular block with first-degree AV block without symptoms

Source: Modified from Gregoratos et al, 1997, and Gregoratos et al, 2002.

In general, a pacing mode that maintains AV synchrony reduces complications of pacing such as pacemaker syndrome and pacemaker-mediated tachycardia. This is particularly true in younger patients, but the importance of dual-chamber pacing, especially in the elderly, is not well established. Several studies have failed to demonstrate a difference in mortality in older patients with AV block treated with a single- (VVI) compared to a dual- (DDD) chamber pacing mode. In some of these studies that randomized pacing mode, the risk of chronic atrial fibrillation and stroke risk decreased with physiologic pacing. In patients with sinus rhythm and AV block, the very modest increase in risk with dual-chamber pacemaker implantation appears to be justified to avoid the possible complications of single-chamber pacing.

FURTHER READINGS

2008 Guidelines for device-based therapy of cardiac rhythm abnormalities, JACC 51:21, 2008

BHARATI S et al: Sinus node dysfunction, in *Electrophysiological Disorders of the Heart*, S Saksena, AJ Camm (eds). Philadelphia, Elsevier Churchill Livingstone, 2005, Chap. 12

GOLDSCHLAGER N et al: Atrioventricular block, in *Electrophysiological Disorders of the Heart*, S Saksena, AJ Camm (eds). Philadelphia, Elsevier Churchill Livingstone, 2005, Chap. 13

GREGORATOS G et al: ACC/AHA Guidelines for implantation of cardiac pacemakers and antiarrhythmia devices: Executive summary. Circulation 97:1325, 1997

——— et al: ACC/AHA/NASPE 2002 Guideline Update for implantation of cardiac pacemakers and antiarrhythmia devices: Summary article. Circulation 106:2145, 2002

JOSEPHSON ME: *Clinical Cardiac Electrophysiology: Techniques and Interpretations*, 3d ed. Philadelphia, Lippincott Williams & Wilkins, 2002

VIJAYARAMAN P, ELLENBOGEN KA: Bradyarrhythmias and pacemakers, in *Hurst's The Heart*, 12th ed, V Fuster et al (eds). New York, McGraw-Hill, 2008, Chap. 40

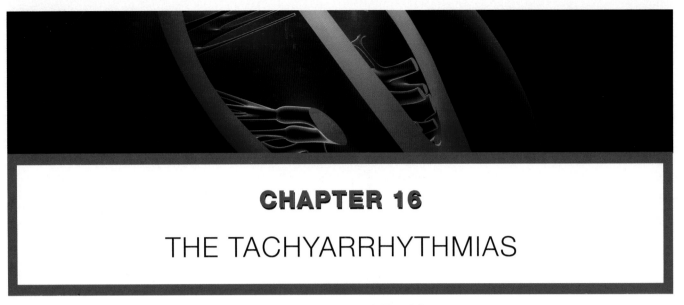

CHAPTER 16

THE TACHYARRHYTHMIAS

Francis Marchlinski

Tachyarrhythmias typically refer to isolated premature complexes (depolarizations) or to nonsustained and sustained forms of tachycardia originating from myocardial foci or reentrant circuits. The standard definition of tachycardia is rhythm that produces a ventricular rate >100 beats/min. This definition has some limitations in that atrial rates can exceed 100 beats/min despite a slow ventricular rate. Furthermore, ventricular rates may exceed the baseline sinus rate and be <100 beats/min but still represent an important "tachycardia" response, such as is observed with accelerated ventricular rhythms.

SYMPTOMS DUE TO TACHYARRHYTHMIAS

Tachyarrhythmias classically produce symptoms of palpitations or racing of the pulse. For premature beats, skipping of the pulse or a pause may be experienced, and patients may even sense slowing of the heart rate. A more dramatic irregularity of the pulse will be experienced with chaotic rapid rhythms or tachyarrhythmias that originate in the atrium and conduct variably to the ventricles. For very rapid tachyarrhythmias, hemodynamic compromise can occur, as can dizziness or syncope due to a decrease in cardiac output or breathlessness due to a marked increase in cardiac filling pressures. Occasionally, chest discomfort may be experienced that mimics symptoms of myocardial ischemia. The underlying cardiac condition typically dictates the severity of symptoms at any specific heart rate. Even patients with normal systolic left ventricular (LV) function may experience severe symptoms if diastolic compliance due to hypertrophy or valvular obstruction is present. Hemodynamic collapse with the development of ventricular fibrillation (VF) can lead to sudden cardiac death (SCD) (Chap. 29). SCD remains one of the principal causes of death in the adult population, thus emphasizing the importance of appropriate tachyarrhythmia prevention as well as management.

DIAGNOSTIC TESTS IN EVALUATING TACHYARRHYTHMIAS

In patients who present with non-life-threatening symptoms, such as palpitations or dizziness, electrocardiogram

(ECG) confirmation of an arrhythmia with the development of recurrent symptoms is essential. A 24-h Holter monitor should be considered only for patients with daily symptoms. For intermittent symptoms that are of a prolonged duration, a patient-activated event monitor can be used to obtain the ECG information without the need for continuous ECG lead attachment and recordings. A patient-activated monitor with a continuously recorded memory loop ("loop recorder") can be used to document short-lived episodes and the onset of the arrhythmia. This is the preferred monitoring technique for symptomatic patients with less frequent arrhythmia events but it requires continuous ECG recording. Patients with infrequent, severe symptoms that cannot be identified by intermittent ECG monitoring may receive an implanted loop ECG monitor that provides more extended periods of monitoring and automatic arrhythmia detection (Fig. 16-1).

In patients who present with more severe symptoms, such as syncope, outpatient monitoring may be insufficient. In patients with structural heart disease and syncope in whom there is suspicion of ventricular tachycardia (VT), hospitalization and diagnostic electrophysiologic testing are warranted, with strong consideration for an implantable cardioverter/defibrillator (ICD) device. The 12-lead ECG recorded in sinus rhythm should be carefully assessed in patients without structural heart disease for evidence of ST-segment elevation in leads V_1 and V_2 consistent with the Brugada syndrome, QT interval changes consistent with long or short QT syndromes, or a short PR interval and delta wave consistent with Wolff-Parkinson-White (WPW) syndrome. These ECG patterns identify an arrhythmogenic substrate that may cause intermittent life-threatening symptoms and warrant further evaluation and therapy. The individual syndromes are discussed in detail later in this chapter.

Monitoring for asymptomatic tachyarrhythmias is indicated in several specific situations. In patients with a suspected tachycardia-induced cardiomyopathy marked by chamber dilatation and depression in systolic function, the demonstration of arrhythmia control is essential.

Monitoring for asymptomatic ventricular premature complexes (VPCs) and nonsustained VT can be helpful in stratifying the risk of SCD in patients with depressed LV function after myocardial infarction. Finally, in patients with asymptomatic atrial fibrillation (AF), anticoagulation treatment strategies depend on an accurate assessment of the presence of this arrhythmia. The duration of monitoring for asymptomatic arrhythmias may vary. The transition from 24-h Holter monitoring to more extended periods of monitoring with technology capable of automatic arrhythmia detection improves the reliability of the monitoring information used in decision-making.

A 12-lead ECG recording during the tachycardia can be an important diagnostic tool in identifying the mechanism and the origin of a tachycardia not afforded by one- or two-lead ECG recordings. A 12-lead ECG of the tachyarrhythmia should be recorded and incorporated as a permanent part of the medical record whenever possible. For patients whose arrhythmias are provoked by exercise, an exercise test may provide the opportunity to obtain 12-lead ECG recordings of the arrhythmia and may obviate the need for more extended periods of monitoring.

Many paroxysmal supraventricular tachyarrhythmias are not associated with a significant risk of structural heart disease, and an evaluation for the presence of ischemic heart disease and cardiac function is uncommonly required unless dictated by the severity or characteristics of the symptoms. However in patients with focal or macroreentrant atrial tachycardias (ATs), atrial flutter (AFL), or AF, an evaluation of cardiac chamber size and function and of valve function is warranted. In patients with VT, an echocardiographic assessment of LV and right ventricular (RV) size and function should be the norm. VT occurring in the setting of depressed LV function should raise the suspicion of advanced coronary artery disease. Polymorphic VT in the absence of QT prolongation should always raise the concern for a potentially unstable ischemic process that may need to be corrected to effect VT control.

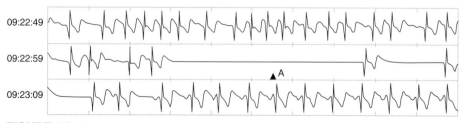

FIGURE 16-1

Spontaneous termination of atrial fibrillation at the time of a syncopal episode identified from implantable loop ECG recording.

MECHANISMS OF TACHYARRHYTHMIAS

Tachycardias are due to abnormalities of impulse formation and/or abnormalities of impulse propagation (Fig. 16-2).

Abnormalities in Impulse Formation

An increase in automaticity normally causes an increase in sinus rate and sinus tachycardia (Fig. 16-2*A*). Abnormal automaticity is due to an increase in the slope of phase 4 depolarization or a reduced threshold for action potential depolarization in myocardium other than the sinus node. Abnormal automaticity is thought to be responsible for most atrial premature complexes (APCs) and VPCs and some ATs. Pacing does not provoke automatic rhythms. Less commonly, abnormal impulse formation is due to the development of triggered activity. Triggered activity is related to cellular afterdepolarizations that occur at the end of the action potential, during phase 3, and are referred to as *early afterdepolarizations*, or they occur after the action potential, during phase 4, and are referred to as *late afterdepolarizations*. Afterdepolarizations are attributable to an increase in intracellular calcium accumulation. If sufficient afterdepolarization amplitude is achieved, repeated myocardial depolarization and a tachycardic response can occur. Early afterdepolarizations may be responsible for the VPCs that trigger the polymorphic ventricular arrhythmia known as *torsade de pointes* (TdP) (p. 165). Late afterdepolarizations are thought to be responsible for atrial, junctional, and

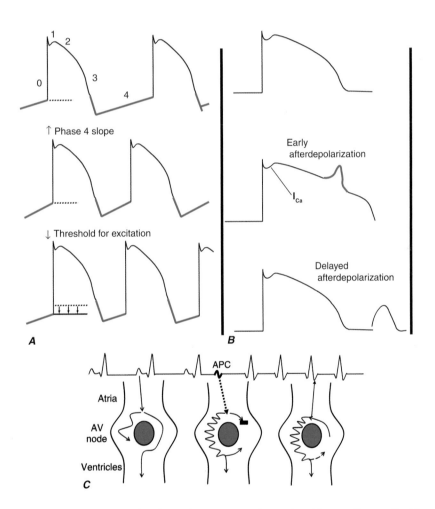

FIGURE 16-2

Schematic representation of the different mechanisms for arrhythmias. *A*. Abnormal automaticity due to an increased slope of phase 4 of the action potential or a decrease in the threshold for phase 0. ***B*.** Triggered activity due to early afterdepolarizations (EADs) during phase 3 of the action potential due to alteration of plateau currents, or delayed afterdepolarizations (DADs) during phase 4 of the action potential due to intracellular calcium accumulation. ***C*.** Reentry with basic requirements of two pathways that have heterogeneous electrophysiologic properties which allows conduction to block in one pathway and to propagate slowly in the other, allowing for sufficient delay so that the blocked site has time for recovery to allow for reentry or circus movement tachycardia. Shown is typical schema for reentry in the AV node. AV, atrioventricular; APC, atrial premature complex.

fascicular tachyarrhythmias caused by digoxin toxicity and also appear to be the basis for catecholamine-sensitive VT originating in the outflow tract. In contrast, to automatic tachycardias, tachycardias due to triggered activity (Fig. 16-2*B*) can frequently be provoked with pacing maneuvers.

Abnormalities in Impulse Propagation

Reentry is due to inhomogeneities in myocardial conduction and/or recovery properties. The presence of unidirectional block with slow conduction to allow for retrograde recovery of the blocked myocardium allows for a circuit to form that, if perpetuated, can sustain a tachycardia (Fig. 16-2*C*). These inhomogeneities are somewhat inherent but minimized in normal myocardial activation/recovery. The inhomogeneities can be exaggerated by the presence of extra pathways, such as occurs with the WPW syndrome; generalized genetically determined myocardial ion channel abnormalities, such as occurs with long QT syndrome (LQTS); or by the interruption of normal myocardial patterns of activation due to the development of fibrosis.

Reentry appears to be the basis for most abnormal sustained supraventricular tachycardias (SVTs) and VTs. In general, reentry can be anatomically driven (fixed) based on the presence of "extra" pathways, natural anatomic barriers of conduction such as the crista terminalis, the vertical crest on the interior wall of the right atrium that separates the sinus of the vena cava and nontrabeculated posterior right atrium from the rest of the trabeculated right atrium located lateral to the structure, and/or extensive fibrosis created by underlying myocardial disease. This form of reentry seems to be more stable and results in a tachycardia that has a uniform (often monomorphic), repetitive appearance. Other forms of reentry appear to be more functional and are more dependent on dynamic changes in electrophysiologic properties of the myocardium. These tachycardias tend to be more unstable and may result in tachycardias that have a polymorphic appearance. Two classic examples of reentry that is primarily functional include VF due to acute myocardial ischemia and polymorphic VT in patients with genetically determined ion channel abnormalities, such as the Brugada syndrome, LQTS, or catecholaminergic polymorphic VT (p. 174).

SUPRAVENTRICULAR TACHYARRHYTHMIAS

ATRIAL PREMATURE COMPLEXES

APCs are the most common arrhythmia identified during extended ECG monitoring. The incidence of APCs frequently increases with age and with the presence of structural heart diseases. APCs typically are asymptomatic, although some patients experience palpitations or an irregularity of the pulse.

ECG Diagnosis of APCs

The ECG diagnosis of premature atrial complexes is based on the identification of a P wave that occurs prior to the anticipated sinus beat (**Figs. 16-3***A* and **16-3***B*). The source of the APC appears to parallel the typical sites of origin for ATs. The orifices of the superior vena cava and pulmonary veins, the coronary sinus, the crista terminalis, mitral and tricuspid valve annuli, and left and right atrial appendages are common sites of origin of APCs. The P wave contour differs from that noted during sinus rhythm, although APCs from the right atrial appendage, superior vena cava (SVC), and superior aspect of the crista terminalis in the region of the sinus node may mimic the sinus P wave morphology. In response to an APC, the PR interval lengthens, although APCs that originate near the atrioventricular (AV) nodal

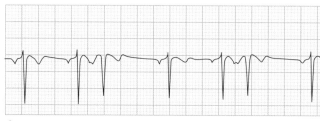

A

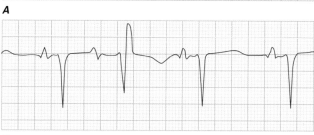

B

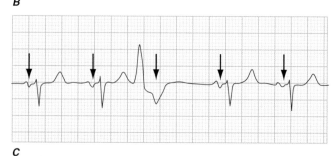

C

FIGURE 16-3

Atrial and ventricular premature complexes (APCs, VPCs). The APC resets the sinus node and no compensatory pause is present (**A**) even when conducted aberrantly in the ventricles with a bundle branch block type QRS pattern (**B**). VPCs tend not to reset the sinus activity (*arrows*) and will demonstrate a full compensatory pause (**C**).

region may actually have a shorter PR interval because the atrial conduction time to the junction is shortened. A very early APC may not conduct to the ventricle and can create a pulse irregularity that may be perceived as a pause or "dropped beat." If the APC conducts rapidly through the AV node, a partially recovered His-Purkinje system will be encountered and a QRS pattern consistent with a right or left bundle branch block may occur. This wide QRS pattern and the failure to recognize the preceding P wave may result in the misdiagnosis of VPCs. APCs characteristically reset the sinus node. The resulting sum of the pre- and post-APC RR interval is less than two sinus PP intervals.

Treatment:
℞ ATRIAL PREMATURE COMPLEXES

APCs uncommonly require intervention. For extremely symptomatic patients who do not respond to explanation and reassurance, an attempt can be made to suppress the APCs with pharmacologic agents. The repetitive focus can even be targeted for catheter ablation. Beta blockers are typical first-line therapy, but they may exacerbate symptoms if AV block occurs with the APC and irregularity of the pulse consequently becomes more profound. The use of class IC antiarrhythmic agents may eliminate the APCs but should be avoided if structural heart disease is present.

JUNCTIONAL PREMATURE COMPLEXES

Junctional premature complexes are extremely uncommon. The complexes originate from the AV node and His bundle region and may produce retrograde atrial activation with the P wave distorting the initial or terminal portions of the QRS complex producing pseudo Q or S waves in leads II, III, and aVF. Extrasystoles originating in the bundle of His that do not conduct to the ventricle and also block the atria can produce unexplained surface ECG PR prolongation that does not follow a typical Wenckebach periodicity, i.e., gradual PR prolongation culminating in atrial activity that fails to conduct to the ventricles. Intracardiac recordings can frequently identify a His depolarization, thus identifying the origin of the complex to the AV junction. Symptomatic patients may be typically treated with beta blockers or, if there is no structural heart disease, class IC antiarrhythmic agents.

SINUS TACHYCARDIA

Physiologic sinus tachycardia represents a normal or appropriate response to physiologic stress, such as occurs with exercise, anxiety, or fever. Pathologic conditions, such as thyrotoxicosis, anemia, or hypotension, may also produce sinus tachycardia. It is important to distinguish sinus tachycardia from other SVTs. Sinus tachycardia will produce a P wave contour consistent with its origin from the sinus node located in the superior-lateral and posterior aspect of the right atrium. The P wave is upright in leads II, III and aVF, and negative in lead aVR. The P wave morphology in lead V_1 characteristically has a biphasic, positive/negative contour. Onset of sinus tachycardia is gradual, and in response to carotid sinus pressure there may be some modest and transient slowing but no abrupt termination. Importantly, the diagnosis should not be based on the PR interval or the presence of a P wave before every QRS complex. The PR interval and the presence of 1:1 AV conduction properties are entirely determined by AV nodal and His-Purkinje conduction and, therefore, the PR interval can be dramatically prolonged while sinus tachycardia remains the mechanism of the atrial activity.

Treatment:
℞ PHYSIOLOGIC SINUS TACHYCARDIA

Treatment of physiologic sinus tachycardia is directed at the underlying condition causing the tachycardia response. Uncommonly, beta blockers are used to minimize the tachycardia response if it is determined to be potentially harmful, as may occur in a patient with ischemic heart disease and rate-related anginal symptoms.

Inappropriate sinus tachycardia represents an uncommon but important medical condition in which the heart rate increases either spontaneously or out of proportion to the degree of physiologic stress/exercise. Dizziness and even frank syncope can often accompany the sinus tachycardia and symptoms of palpitations. The syndrome can be quite disabling. Associated symptoms of chest pain, headaches, and gastrointestinal upset are common. In many patients, the syndrome occurs after a viral illness and may resolve spontaneously over the course of 3–12 months, suggesting a postviral dysautonomia.

Excluding the diagnosis of an automatic AT that originates in the region of the sinus node can be difficult and may require invasive electrophysiologic evaluation. Frequently, patients are misdiagnosed as having an anxiety disorder with physiologic sinus tachycardia.

℞ **Treatment:**
INAPPROPRIATE SINUS TACHYCARDIA

For symptomatic patients, maintaining an increased state of hydration, salt loading, and careful titration of beta blockers to the maximum tolerated dose, administered in divided doses, frequently minimizes symptoms. For severely symptomatic patients who are intolerant of or unresponsive to beta blockers, catheter ablation directed at modifying the sinus node may be effective. Because of the high recurrence rate after ablation and the frequent need for atrial pacing therapy, this intervention remains second-line treatment.

ATRIAL FIBRILLATION

(Fig. 16-4) AF is the most common sustained arrhythmia. It is marked by disorganized, rapid, and irregular atrial activation. The ventricular response to the rapid atrial activation is also irregular. In the untreated patient, the ventricular rate also tends to be rapid and is entirely dependent on the conduction properties of the AV junction. Although typically the rate will vary between 120 and 160 beats/min, in some patients it can be >200 beats/min. In other patients, because of heightened vagal tone or intrinsic AV nodal conduction properties,

the ventricular response is <100 beats/min and occasionally even profoundly slow. The mechanism for AF initiation and maintenance, although still debated, appears to represent a complex interaction between drivers responsible for the initiation and the complex anatomic atrial substrate that promotes the maintenance of multiple wavelets of (micro)reentry. The drivers appears to originate predominantly from the atrialized musculature that enters the pulmonary veins and either represent focal abnormal automaticity or triggered firing that is somewhat modulated by autonomic influences. Sustained forms of microreentry as drivers have also been documented around the orifice of pulmonary veins; nonpulmonary vein drivers have also been demonstrated. The role these drivers play in maintaining the tachycardias may also be significant and may explain the success of pulmonary vein isolation procedures in eliminating more chronic or persistent forms of AF.

Although AF is common in the adult population, it is extremely unusual in children unless structural heart disease is present or there is another arrhythmia that precipitates the AF, such as paroxysmal SVT in patients with WPW syndrome. The incidence of AF increases with age such that >5% of the adult population over 70 will experience the arrhythmia. As many patients are asymptomatic with AF, it is anticipated that the overall incidence, particularly that noted in the elderly, may be more than double previously reported rates. Occasionally AF

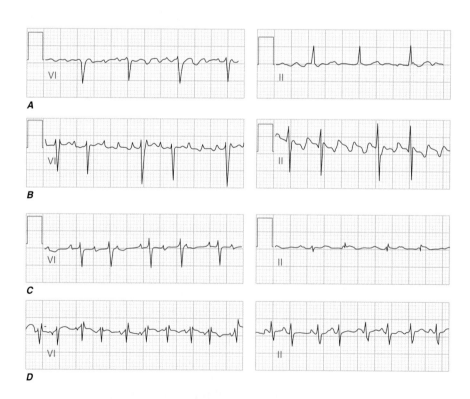

FIGURE 16-4

Supraventricular tachycardias with irregular ventricular rates. Atrial fibrillation (**A**), atrial flutter (**B**), atrial tachycardia (**C**), and multifocal atrial tachycardia (MAT; **D**) are shown.

The characteristics of the atrial activity with respect to the morphology and rate provide the clues to the diagnosis.

appears to have a well-defined etiology, such as acute hyperthyroidism, an acute vagotonic episode, or acute alcohol intoxication. Acute AF is particularly common during the acute or early recovery phase of major vascular, abdominal, and thoracic surgery where autonomic fluxes and/or direct mechanical irritation potentiate the arrhythmia. AF may also be triggered by other supraventricular tachycardias (p. 160), such as AV nodal reentrant tachycardia (AVNRT), and elimination of these arrhythmias may prevent AF recurrence.

AF has clinical importance related to (1) the loss of atrial contractility, (2) the inappropriate fast ventricular response, and (3) the loss of atrial appendage contractility and emptying leading to the risk of clot formation and subsequent thromboembolic events.

Symptoms from AF vary dramatically. Many patients are asymptomatic and have no apparent hemodynamic consequences to the development of AF. Other patients experience only minor palpitations or sense irregularity of their pulse. Many patients, however, experience severe palpitations. The hemodynamic effect in patients can be quite dramatic, depending on the need for normal atrial contractility and the ventricular response. Hypotension, pulmonary congestion, and anginal symptoms may be severe in some patients. In patients with the LV diastolic dysfunction that occurs with hypertension, hypertrophic cardiomyopathy, or obstructive aortic valvular disease, symptoms may be even more dramatic, especially if the ventricular rate does not permit adequate ventricular filling. Exercise intolerance and easy fatigability are the hallmarks of poor rate control with exertion. Occasionally, the only manifestation of AF is severe dizziness or syncope associated with the pause that occurs upon termination of AF before sinus rhythm resumes (Fig. 16–1).

The ECG in AF is characterized by the lack of organized atrial activity and the irregularly irregular ventricular response. Occasionally, one needs to record from multiple ECG leads simultaneously to identify the chaotic continuous atrial activation. Lead V_1 may frequently show the appearance of organized atrial activity that mimics AFL. This occurs because the crista terminalis serves as an effective anatomic barrier to electrical conduction, and the activation of the lateral right atrium may be represented by a more uniform activation wavefront that originates over the roof of the right atrium. ECG assessment of the PP interval (<200 ms) and the chaotic P wave morphology in the remaining ECG leads will confirm the presence of AF.

Evaluation of the patient with AF should include a search for reversible causes of the arrhythmia, such as hyperthyroidism or anemia. An echocardiogram should be performed to determine if there is structural heart disease. Persistent or labile hypertension should be identified and treated, and heart failure treatment should be optimized.

R_X Treatment:
ATRIAL FIBRILLATION

Treatment for AF must take into account the clinical situation in which the arrhythmia is encountered, the chronicity of the AF, the status of the patient's level of anticoagulation, risk factors for stroke, the patient's symptoms, the hemodynamic impact of the AF, and the ventricular rate.

ACUTE RATE CONTROL In the absence of hemodynamic compromise that might warrant emergent cardioversion to terminate the AF, the initial goals of therapy are (1) to establish control of the ventricular rate, and (2) to address anticoagulation status and begin IV heparin treatment if the duration of AF is >12 h and risk factors for stroke with AF are present (Table 16-1). Ventricular rate control for acute AF is best established with beta blockers and/or calcium channel-blocking agents, verapamil or diltiazem. The route of administration and dose will be dictated by the ventricular rate and clinical status. Digoxin may add to the rate-controlling benefit of the other agents but is uncommonly used as a stand-alone agent, especially in acute AF.

Anticoagulation is of particular importance in patients who have known risk factors for stroke associated with AF. Factors associated with the highest risk of stroke include a history of stroke, transient ischemic attack or systemic embolism, or the presence of rheumatic mitral stenosis. Other identified risk factors include age >65 years, history of congestive heart failure, diabetes mellitus, hypertension, LV dysfunction, and evidence of marked left atrial enlargement (>5.0 cm). Chronic anticoagulation with warfarin targeting an INR between 2.0 and 3.0 is recommended in patients with persistent or frequent and long-lived paroxysmal AF and risk factors. If patients have not been adequately anticoagulated and the AF is more than 24–48 h in duration, a transesophageal echocardiogram (TEE) can be performed to exclude the presence of a left atrial thrombus that might dislodge with the attempted restoration of sinus rhythm using either nonpharmacologic or pharmacologic therapy. Anticoagulation must be instituted coincident with the TEE and maintained for at least 1 month following restoration of sinus rhythm if the

TABLE 16-1

RISK FACTORS FOR STROKE IN ATRIAL FIBRILLATION	
History of stroke or transient ischemic attack	Age >75 years
	Congestive heart failure
	Left ventricular dysfunction
Mitral stenosis	Marked left atrial
Hypertension	enlargement (>5.0 cm)
Diabetes mellitus	Spontaneous echo contrast

duration of AF has been prolonged or is unknown. Heparin is maintained routinely until the INR is 1.8 with the administration of warfarin after the TEE. For patients who do not warrant early cardioversion of AF, anticoagulation should be maintained for at least 3 weeks with the INR confirmed to be >1.8 on at least two separate occasions prior to attempts at cardioversion.

Termination of AF acutely may be warranted based on clinical parameters and/or hemodynamic status. Confirmation of appropriate anticoagulation status as described above must be documented unless symptoms and clinical status warrant emergent intervention. Direct current transthoracic cardioversion during short-acting anesthesia is a reliable way to terminate AF. Conversion rates using a 200-J biphasic shock delivered synchronously with the QRS complex typically are >90%. Pharmacologic therapy to terminate AF is less reliable. Oral and/or IV administration of amiodarone or procainamide have only modest success. The acute IV administration of ibutilide appears to be somewhat more effective and may be used in selected patients to facilitate termination with direct current (DC) cardioversion (Tables 16-2 and 16-3).

Pharmacologic therapy to maintain sinus rhythm can be instituted once sinus rhythm has been established or in anticipation of cardioversion to attempt to maintain sinus rhythm (Table 16-3). A single episode of AF may not warrant any intervention or only a short course of beta blocker therapy. To prevent recurrent AF

unresponsive to beta blockade, a trial of antiarrhythmic therapy may be warranted, particularly if the AF is associated with rapid rates and/or significant symptoms. The selection of antiarrhythmic agents should be dictated primarily by the presence or absence of coronary artery disease, depressed LV function not attributable to a reversible tachycardia-induced cardiomyopathy, and/or severe hypertension with evidence of marked LV hypertrophy. The presence of any significant structural heart disease typically narrows treatment to the use of sotalol, amiodarone, or dofetilide. Severely depressed LV function may preclude sotalol therapy or require only low-dose therapy be considered. Owing to the risk of QT prolongation and polymorphic VT, sotalol and dofetilide need to be initiated in hospital in most cases.

In patients without evidence of structural heart disease or hypertensive heart disease without evidence of severe hypertrophy, the use of the class IC antiarrhythmic agents flecainide or propafenone appears to be well tolerated and does not have significant proarrhythmia risk. It is important to recognize that no drug is uniformly effective, and arrhythmia recurrence should be anticipated in over half the patients during long-term follow-up regardless of type and number of agents tried. It is also important to recognize that although the maintenance of sinus rhythm has been associated with improved long-term survival, the survival outcome of patients randomized to the pharmacologic maintenance of sinus rhythm was not superior to those treated

TABLE 16-2

COMMONLY USED ANTIARRHYTHMIC AGENTS—INTRAVENOUS DOSE RANGE/PRIMARY INDICATION

DRUG	LOADING	MAINTENANCE	PRIMARY INDICATION	CLASS[a]
Adenosine	6–18 mg (rapid bolus)	N/A	Terminate reentrant SVT involving AV node	—
Amiodarone	15 mg/min for 10 min, 1 mg/min for 6 h	0.5–1 mg/min	AF, AFL, SVT, VT/VF	III
Digoxin	0.25 mg q2h until 1.0 mg total	0.125–0.25 mg/d	AF/AFL rate control	—
Diltiazem	0.25 mg/kg over 3–5 min (max 20 mg)	5–15 mg/h	SVT, AF/AFL rate control	IV
Esmolol	500 µg/kg over 1 min	50 µg/kg per min	AF/AFL rate control	II
Ibutilide	1 mg over 10 min if over 60 kg	N/A	Terminate AF/AFL	III
Lidocaine	1–3 mg/kg at 20–50 mg/min	1–4 mg/min	VT	IB
Metoprolol	5 mg over 3–5 min times 3 doses	1.25–5 mg q6h	SVT, AF rate control; exercise-induced VT; long QT	II
Procainamide	15 mg/kg over 60 min	1–4 mg/min	Convert/prevent AF/VT	IA
Quinidine	6–10 mg/kg at 0.3–0.5 mg/kg per min	N/A	Convert/prevent AF/VT	IA
Verapamil	5–10 mg over 3–5 min	2.5–10 mg/h	SVT, AF rate control	IV

[a]Classification of antiarrhythmic drugs: Class I—agents that primarily block inward sodium current; class IA agents also prolong action potential duration; class II—antisympathetic agents; class III—agents that primarily prolong action potential duration; class IV—calcium channel-blocking agents.

Note: SVT, supraventricular tachycardia; AV, atrioventricular; AF, atrial fibrillation; AFL, atrial flutter; VT, ventricular tachycardia; VF, ventricular fibrillation.

TABLE 16-3

COMMONLY USED ANTIARRHYTHMIC AGENTS—CHRONIC ORAL DOSING/PRIMARY INDICATIONS

DRUG	DOSING ORAL, mg, MAINTENANCE	HALF-LIFE, h	PRIMARY ROUTE(S) OF METABOLISM/ELIMINATION	MOST COMMON INDICATION	CLASS[a]
Acebutolol	200–400 mg q12h	6–7	Renal/hepatic	AF rate control/SVT Long QT/RVOT VT	II
Amiodarone	100–400 qd	40–55 d	Hepatic	AF/VT prevention	III
Atenolol	25–100 mg/d	6–9	Renal	AF rate control/SVT Long QT/RVOT VT	II
Digoxin	0.125–0.5 qd	38–48	Renal	AF rate control	—
Diltiazem	30–60 q6h	3–4.5	Hepatic	AF rate control/SVT	IV
Disopyramide	100–300 q6–8h	4–10	Renal 50%/hepatic	AF/SVT prevention	Ia
Dofetilide	0.125–0.5 q12h	10	Renal	AF prevention	III
Flecainide	50–200 q12h	7–22	Hepatic 75%/renal	AF/SVT/VT prevention	Ic
Metoprolol	25–100 q6h	3–8	Hepatic	AF rate control/SVT Long QT/RVOT VT	II
Mexiletine	150–300 q8–12h	10–14	Hepatic	VT prevention	Ib
Moricizine	100–400 q8h	3–13	Hepatic 60%/renal	AF prevention	Ic
Nadolol	40–240 mg/d	10–24	Renal	Same as metoprolol	II
Procainamide	250–500 q3–6h	3–5	Hepatic/renal	AF/SVT/VT prevention	Ia
Propafenone	150–300 q8h	2–8	Hepatic	AF/SVT/VT prevention	Ic
Quinidine	300–600 q6h	6–8	Hepatic 75%/renal	AF/SVT/VT prevention	Ia
Sotalol	80–160 q12h	12	Renal	AF/VT prevention	III
Verapamil	80–120 q6–8h	4.5–12	Hepatic/renal	AF rate control/RVOT VT Idiopathic LV VT	IV

[a]Classification of antiarrhythmic drugs: Class I—agents that primarily block inward sodium current; class II—antisympathetic agents; class III—agents that primarily prolong action potential duration; class IV—calcium channel-blocking agents.
Note: AF, atrial fibrillation; SVT, supraventricular tachycardia; RVOT, right ventricular outflow tract; VT, ventricular tachycardia; LV, left ventriclar.

with rate control and anticoagulation in the AFFIRM and RACE trials. The AFFIRM and RACE trials compared outcome with respect to survival and thromboembolic events in patients with AF and risk factors for stroke using the two treatment strategies. It is believed that the poor outcome related to pharmacologic therapy used to maintain sinus rhythm was primarily due to frequent inefficacy of such drug therapy and an increased incidence of asymptomatic AF. Many of the drugs used for rhythm control, including sotalol, amiodarone, propafenone, and flecainide, enhance slowing of AV nodal conduction. The absence of symptoms frequently leads to stopping anticoagulant therapy, and asymptomatic AF without anticoagulation increases stroke risk. Any consideration for stopping anticoagulation must, therefore, be accompanied by a prolonged period of ECG monitoring to document asymptomatic AF. It is also recommended that patients participate in monitoring by learning to take their pulse on a twice-daily basis and to reliably identify its regularity if discontinuing anticoagulant therapy is seriously contemplated.

It is clear that to reduce the risk of drug-induced complications when treating AF, a thorough understanding of the drug planned to be used is critical— its dosing, metabolism, and common side effects and important drug-drug interactions. This information has been summarized in Tables 16-2, 16-3, 16-4, and 16-5 and serves as a starting point for a more complete review. When using antiarrhythmic agents that slow atrial conduction, strong consideration should be given to adding a beta blocker or a calcium channel blocker (verapamil or diltiazem) to the treatment regimen. This should help to avoid a rapid ventricular response if AF is converted to "slow" AF with the drug therapy (Fig. 16-5).

CHRONIC RATE CONTROL This is an option in patients who are asymptomatic or symptomatic due to the resulting tachycardia. Rate control is frequently difficult to achieve in patients who have paroxysmal AF. In patients with more persistent forms of AF, rate control with beta blockers, calcium channel blockers, diltiazem or verapamil, and/or digoxin can frequently be achieved. Using the drugs in combination may avoid some of the common side effects seen with high-dose monotherapy. An effort should be made to document the adequacy of rate control to reduce the risk of a tachycardia-induced cardiomyopathy. Heart rates >80 beats/min at rest or 100 beats/min with very modest physical activity are indications that rate control is inadequate in persistent AF. Extended periods of ECG monitoring and assessment of heart rate with exercise should be considered.

TABLE 16-4

DRUG	COMMON NONARRHYTHMIC TOXICITY
COMMON NONARRHYTHMIC TOXICITY OF MOST FREQUENTLY USED ANTIARRHYTHMIC AGENTS	
Amiodarone	Tremor, peripheral neuropathy, pulmonary inflammation, hypothyroidism and hyperthyroidism, photosensitivity
Adenosine	Cough, flushing
Digoxin	Anorexia, nausea, vomiting, visual changes
Disopyramide	Anticholinergic effects, decreased myocardial contractility
Dofetilide	Nausea
Flecainide	Dizziness, nausea, headache, decreased myocardial contractility
Ibutilide	Nausea
Lidocaine	Dizziness, confusion, delirium, seizures, coma
Mexiletine	Ataxia, tremor, gait disturbances, rash, nausea
Moricizine	Mood changes, tremor, loss of mental clarity, nausea,
Procainamide	Lupus erythematosus–like syndrome (more common in slow acetylators), anorexia, nausea, neutropenia
Propafenone	Taste disturbance, dyspepsia, nausea, vomiting
Quinidine	Diarrhea, nausea, vomiting, cinchonism, thrombocytopenia
Sotalol	Hypotension, bronchospasm

TABLE 16-5

DRUG	COMMON PROARRHYTHMIC TOXICITY
PROARRHYTHMIC MANIFESTATIONS OF MOST FREQUENTLY USED ANTIARRHYTHMIC AGENTS	
Amiodarone	Sinus bradycardia, AV block, increase in defibrillation threshold Rare: long QT and torsade de pointes, 1:1 ventricular conduction with atrial flutter
Adenosine	All arrhythmias potentiated by profound pauses, atrial fibrillation
Digoxin	High-grade AV block, fascicular tachycardia, accelerated junctional rhythm, atrial tachycardia
Disopyramide	Long QT and torsade de pointes, 1:1 ventricular response to atrial flutter; increased risk of some ventricular tachycardias in patients with structural heart disease
Dofetilide	Long QT and torsade de pointes
Flecainide	1:1 Ventricular response to atrial flutter; increased risk of some ventricular tachycardias in patients with structural heart disease; sinus bradycardia
Ibutilide	Long QT and torsade de pointes
Procainamide	Long QT and torsade de pointes, 1:1 ventricular response to atrial flutter; increased risk of some ventricular tachycardias in patients with structural heart disease
Propafenone	1:1 Ventricular response to atrial flutter; increased risk of some ventricular tachycardias in patients with structural heart disease; sinus bradycardia
Quinidine	Long QT and torsade de pointes, 1:1 ventricular response to atrial flutter; increased risk of some ventricular tachycardias in patients with structural heart disease
Sotalol	Long QT and torsade de pointes, sinus bradycardia

Note: AV, atrioventricular.

In patients with symptoms resulting from inadequate rate control with pharmacologic therapy or worsening LV function due to the persistent tachycardia, a His bundle/AV junction ablation can be performed. The ablation must be coupled with the implantation of an activity sensor pacemaker to maintain a physiologic range of heart rates. Recent evidence that RV pacing can occasionally modestly depress LV function should be taken into consideration in identifying which patients are appropriate candidates for the "ablate and pace" treatment strategy. Occasionally, biventricular pacing may be used to minimize the degree of dyssynchronization that can occur with RV apical pacing alone. Rate control treatment options must be coupled with chronic anticoagulation therapy in all cases. Trials evaluating the elimination of embolic risk by surgical elimination or isolation of the left atrial appendage or by endovascular insertion of a left atrial appendage–occluding device are ongoing and may provide other treatment options that can eliminate the need for chronic anticoagulation.

CATHETER AND SURGICAL ABLATIVE THERAPY TO PREVENT RECURRENT AF Although the optimum ablation strategy has not been defined, most ablation strategies incorporate techniques that isolate the atrial muscle sleeves entering the pulmonary veins; these muscle sleeves have been identified as the source of the majority of triggers responsible for the initiation of AF. Ablation therapy is currently considered an alternative to pharmacologic therapy in patients with recurrent symptomatic AF. Elimination of AF in 50–80% of patients with a catheter-based ablation procedure should be anticipated, depending on the chronicity of

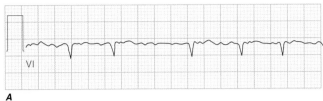

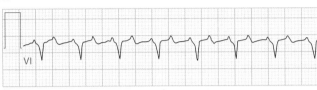

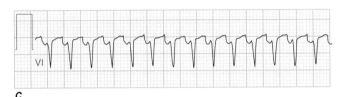

FIGURE 16-5

Atrial fibrillation (**A**) transitions to "slow" atrial flutter during antiarrhythmic drug therapy. (**B**) A rapid ventricular response with 1:1 atrioventricular conduction occurred with exercise, leading to (**C**) symptoms of dizziness.

the AF, with additional patients becoming responsive to previously ineffective medications.

Catheter ablative therapy also holds promise in patients with more persistent forms of AF and even those with severe atrial dilatation. If its efficacy is confirmed with additional study, it may also afford an important alternative to His bundle ablation and pacemaker insertion. Risks related to the left atrial ablation procedure, albeit low (overall 2–4%), include pulmonary vein stenosis, atrioesophageal fistula, systemic embolic events, and perforation/tamponade.

Surgical ablation of AF is typically performed at the time of other cardiac valve or coronary artery surgery and, less commonly, as a stand-alone procedure. The Cox surgical Maze procedure is designed to interrupt all macroreentrant circuits that might potentially develop in the atria, thereby precluding the ability of the atria to fibrillate. In an attempt to simplify the operation, the multiple incisions of the traditional Cox-Maze procedure have been replaced with linear lines of ablation and pulmonary vein isolation using a variety of energy sources.

Severity of AF symptoms and difficulties in rate and/or rhythm control with pharmacologic therapy will frequently dictate the optimum AF treatment strategy. Similar to the approach with pharmacologic rhythm control, a cautious approach to eliminating anticoagulant therapy is recommended after catheter or surgical ablation. Careful ECG monitoring for asymptomatic AF,

particularly in patients with multiple risk factors for stroke, should be considered until guidelines are firmly established. If the left atrial appendage has been removed surgically, then the threshold for stopping anticoagulation should be lowered. Antiarrhythmic therapy typically can be discontinued after catheter or surgical ablation of AF. However, in selected patients, satisfactory AF control may require maintenance of previously ineffective drug therapy after the ablation intervention.

ATRIAL FLUTTER AND MACROREENTRANT ATRIAL TACHYCARDIAS

Macroreentrant arrhythmias involving the atrial myocardium are collectively referred to as AFL. The terms *AFL* and *macroreentrant AT* are frequently used interchangeably, with both denoting a nonfocal source of an atrial arrhythmia. The typical or most common AFL circuit rotates in a clockwise or counterclockwise direction in the right atrium around the tricuspid valve annulus. The posterior boundary of the right AFL circuit is defined by the crista terminalis, the Eustachian ridge, and the inferior and superior vena cava. Counterclockwise right AFL represents ~80% of all AFL with superiorly directed activation of the interatrial septum, which produces the saw-toothed appearance of the P waves in ECG leads II, III, and aVF. Clockwise rotation of the same right atrial circuit produces predominantly positive P waves in leads II, III, and aVF (Fig. 16-4). Macroreentrant left AFL may also develop, albeit much less commonly. This type of arrhythmia may be the sequelae of surgical or catheter-based ablation procedures that create large anatomic barriers or promote slowing of conduction in the left atrium, especially around the mitral valve annulus. Atypical AFL or macroreentrant AT can also develop around incisions created during surgery for valvular or congenital heart disease or in and/or around large areas of atrial fibrosis.

Classic or typical right AFL has an atrial rate of 260–300 beats/min with a ventricular response that tends to be 2:1, or typically 130–150 beats/min. In the setting of severe atrial conduction disease and or antiarrhythmic drug therapy, the atrial rate can slow to <200 beats/min. In this setting, a 1:1 rapid ventricular response may occur, particularly with exertion, and produce adverse hemodynamic effects (Fig. 16-5). Atypical AFL or macroreentrant AT related to prior surgical incisions and atrial fibrosis demonstrates less predictability in terms of the atrial rate and is more likely to demonstrate slower rates that overlap with those identified with focal ATs (p. 159).

Because lead V_1 is frequently monitored in a hospitalized patient, coarse AF may be misdiagnosed as AFL. This occurs because in both typical right AFL and coarse

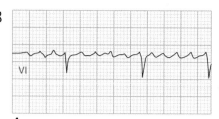
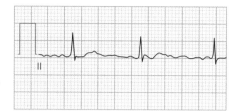
A

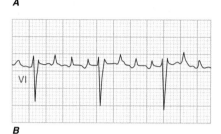
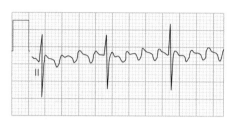
B

FIGURE 16-6
Atrial flutter/atrial fibrillation. Coarse atrial fibrillation (*A*) contrasted with organized atrial flutter (*B*).

SECTION III

Heart Rhythm Disturbances

AF the crista terminalis in the right atrium may serve as an effective anatomic barrier. The free wall of the right atrium, whose electrical depolarization is best reflected on the body surface by lead V_1, may demonstrate a uniform wavefront of atrial activation under both conditions. The timing of atrial activation is much more rapid in AF and always demonstrates variable atrial intervals with some intervals between defined P waves <200 ms (**Fig. 16-6**). A review of the other ECG leads demonstrates the disorganized atrial depolarization that is characteristic of AF. Frequently, an individual patient may alternate between AF and AFL or, less commonly, may manifest AF in one atria and AFL in the other, making the distinction more difficult.

℞ Treatment: ATRIAL FLUTTER

Because of the anticipated rapid regular ventricular rate associated with AFL and the failure to respond to pharmacologic therapy directed at slowing the ventricular rate, patients are frequently treated with DC cardioversion. The organized atrial flutter activity can frequently be terminated with low-energy external cardioversion of 50–100 J. The risk of thromboembolic events associated with typical AFL is high, and anticoagulation must be managed similarly to that described for patients with AF (p. 153).

Asymptomatic patients with AFL may develop heart failure symptoms with tachycardia-induced severe LV dysfunction. In all patients, an effort should be made to control the ventricular rate pharmacologically or restore sinus rhythm. Rate control with calcium antagonists (diltiazem or verapamil), beta blockers, and/or digoxin may be difficult. Even higher grade AV slowing, such as a 4:1 AV response, may only be transient and is easily overcome with activity or emotional stress. Because of the typically faster ventricular rate, AFL tends to be poorly tolerated in comparison with AF.

In selected patients with high anesthetic risk, an attempt at pharmacologic cardioversion with procainamide, amiodarone, or ibultilide is appropriate. Antiarrhythmic drug therapy may also enhance the efficacy of direct current cardioversion and the maintenance of sinus rhythm after cardioversion. Recurrence rates of AFL with pharmacologic attempts at rhythm control exceed 80% by 1 year.

Patients who manifest recurrent AFL appear to be effectively treated with catheter ablative therapy. For typical right AFL, an isthmus ablation line from the tricuspid annulus to the opening of the inferior vena cava can permanently eliminate flutter, with an anticipated success rate of >90% in most experienced centers. In patients with macroreentrant atrial tachycardia or AFL involving prior surgical incisions or in areas of atrial fibrosis, detailed mapping of the arrhythmia circuit is required to design the best ablation strategy to interrupt the circuit. In selected patient with AF and typical right AFL, pharmacologic therapy may help to prevent the AF but not the AFL. In this type of patient, hybrid therapy with antiarrhythmic agents coupled with a right atrial isthmus ablation may produce AF and AFL control.

MULTIFOCAL ATRIAL TACHYCARDIA

Multifocal AT (MAT) is the signature tachycardia of patients with significant pulmonary disease. The atrial rhythm is characterized by at least three distinct P wave morphologies and often at least three different PR intervals, and the associated atrial and ventricular rates are typically between 100 and 150 beats/min. The presence of an isoelectric baseline distinguishes this arrhythmia from AF (Fig. 16-4). The absence of any intervening sinus rhythm distinguishes MAT from normal sinus rhythm with frequent multifocal APCs, although this distinction may be moot as these processes define an electrophysiologic continuum.

℞ Treatment: MULTIFOCAL ATRIAL TACHYCARDIA

Therapy for MAT should be directed at improving the underlying medical condition, which is typically, although not invariably, chronic obstructive or restrictive lung disease. Treatment with the calcium channel blocker, verapamil, may also provide some benefit. The judicious use of flecainide or propafenone may also decrease atrial arrhythmias. Patients should be screened for the presence of significant ventricular dysfunction or coronary artery disease before starting these agents. Low-dose amiodarone therapy may also control the arrhythmia and minimize the risk of pulmonary toxicity noted with the drug.

FOCAL ATRIAL TACHYCARDIAS

The two general mechanisms for focal ATs can be distinguished by observations made at AT initiation and in response to adenosine. *Automatic ATs* start with a "warm-up" period over the first 3–10 complexes and, similarly, slow in rate prior to termination. They may respond to adenosine not only with evidence of AV block but also with gradual slowing of the atrial rhythm and termination. The initiation of automatic ATs can frequently be provoked by isoproterenol infusion. The first P wave of the tachycardia has the same morphology as the remaining waves. Some of the ATs may be triggered or provoked by burst atrial pacing but are not reliably initiated by programmed atrial stimulation.

In contrast, evidence supporting a focal reentrant AT includes the initiation of the tachycardia with programmed atrial stimulation or spontaneous premature beats. The P wave initiating the tachycardia will characteristically have a different morphology than the P wave during the sustained AT. In response to adenosine, reentrant ATs will demonstrate AV block but typically do not slow and/or terminate. Most focal ATs in the absence of structural heart disease originate from specific anatomic locations. These anatomic locations appear to be associated with anatomic ridges, such as the crista terminalis, the valve annuli, or the limbus of the fossa ovalis. ATs also appear to originate from the muscular sleeves associated with the cardiac thoracic veins, i.e., the SVC, the coronary sinus, and the pulmonary veins. As indicated, repetitive firing of these foci appears to serve as the triggering mechanism for AF in most patients.

It is important to distinguish focal ATs from reentrant tachycardias that incorporate the AV node in the circuit (Fig. 16-7). The primary distinction is related to the persistence of the AT in the presence of AV block that occurs spontaneously or is created by carotid sinus massage or the administration of adenosine (Fig. 16-4). Atrial activity drives the ventricles in AT and all changes in the PP interval accompanied by correlative changes in the RR intervals; in addition, the V–A relationship changes when the atrial rate changes. The P wave in AT is characteristically distinct from the sinus P wave morphology, and, unless there is significant AV nodal conduction delay, the PR interval is shorter than the measured RP interval when there is a 1:1 relationship between atria and ventricles (Fig. 16-7).

The P wave for ATs depends on the anatomic site of origin. In addition to attempting to create AV block to establish the diagnosis of AT, analysis of the P wave morphology on the 12-lead ECG may help to exclude AV nodal reentry, AV bypass tract–mediated reentrant tachycardias, and physiologic or inappropriate sinus tachycardia (Fig. 16-7).

The ECG distinction between focal automatic or microreentrant AT and macroreentrant AT or atypical AFL is not always possible. Although sustained focal ATs tend to be slower, the atrial rates will frequently overlap. Focal ATs, which are more common in the absence of structural heart disease, will tend to demonstrate an isoelectric baseline between P waves, whereas macroreentrant ATs represent atrial activation that is continuous and an isoelectric baseline between P waves may be frequently absent. In patients with a history of prior atrial surgery, one must suspect a macroreentrant mechanism. These distinctions are less important with respect to acute management but have importance related to ablation strategies and anticipated outcome (p. 156–157).

℞ Treatment: ATRIAL TACHYCARDIA

Pharmacologic treatment of AT is generally approached in a similar fashion to that of AF and AFL. AV nodal blocking agents are administered in the setting of rapid ventricular rates. Acute IV administration of procainamide or amiodarone may terminate the tachycardia. Tachycardias not responding to pharmacologic therapy may be terminated with electrical cardioversion. Typically, anticoagulation prior to treatment is not needed unless there is evidence of severe atrial dilatation, >5 cm left atrial diameter with a high risk of AF, and/or a history of coincident paroxysmal AF. Most focal ATs are readily amenable to catheter ablative therapy. In patients who fail to respond to medical therapy or who are reluctant to take chronic drug therapy, this option

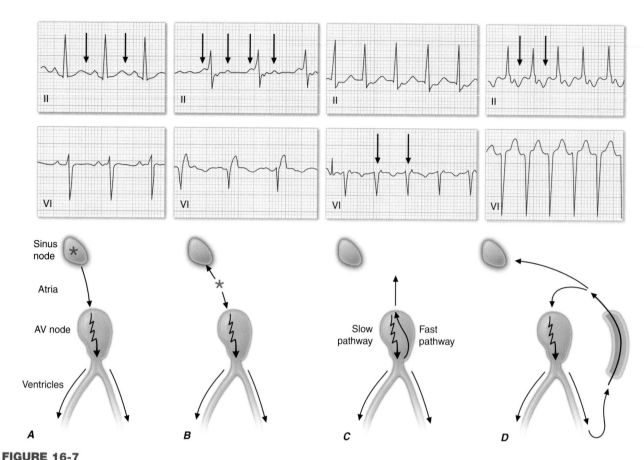

FIGURE 16-7

Pattern of atrial and ventricular activation and characteristic relationship of P wave and QRS complex as recorded in leads II and V₁ during regular supraventricular tachycardias.

A. Sinus tachycardia. *B.* Atrial tachycardia from top of the atria. *C.* Atrioventricular nodal reentry. *D.* Accessory pathway–mediated orthodromic supraventricular tachycardia.

should be considered, with an anticipated 90% cure rate. A para-Hisian location for the AT and/or focus that is located in the left atrium may modestly increase the risk related to the procedure, and, for this reason, every effort should be made to determine the likely origin of the AT based on an analysis of the P wave morphology on 12-lead ECG prior to the procedure.

AV NODAL TACHYCARDIAS

AV Nodal Reentrant Tachycardia

AVNRT is the most common paroxysmal regular SVT. It is more commonly observed in women than men and is typically manifest in the second to fourth decades of life. In general, because AVNRT tends to occur in the absence of structural heart disease, it is usually well tolerated. In the presence of hypertension or other forms of structural heart disease that limit ventricular filing, hypotension or syncope may occur.

AVNRT develops because of the presence of two electrophysiologically distinct pathways for conduction in the complex syncytium of muscle fibers that make up

the AV node. The fast pathway located in the more superior part of the node has a longer refractory period, while the pathway lower in the AV node region conducts more slowly but has a shorter refractory period. As a result of the inhomogeneities of conduction and refractoriness, a reentrant circuit can develop in response to premature stimulation. Although conduction occurs over both pathways during sinus rhythm, only the conduction over the fast pathway is manifest and, as a result, the PR interval is normal. APCs occurring at a critical coupling interval are blocked in the fast pathway because of the longer refractory period and are conducted slowly over the slow pathway. When sufficient conduction slowing occurs, the blocked fast pathway can recover excitability and atrial activation can occur over the fast pathway to complete the circuit. Repetitive activation down the slow and up the fast pathway results in typical AV nodal reentrant tachycardia (Fig. 16-7).

ECG Findings in AVNRT

The APC initiating AVNRT is characteristically followed by a long PR interval consistent with conduction via the slow pathway. AVNRT is manifest typically as a narrow QRS complex tachycardia at rates that range from 120–250 beats/min. The QRS-P wave pattern associated with typical AVNRT is quite characteristic, with simultaneous activation of the atria and ventricles from the reentrant AV nodal circuit. The P wave will frequently be buried inside the QRS complex and either not be visible or will distort the initial or terminal portion of the QRS complex (Fig. 16-7). Because, atrial activation originates in the region of the AV node, a negative deflection will be generated by retrograde atrial depolarization.

Occasionally, AVNRT occurs with activation in the reverse direction, conducting down the fast pathway and returning up the slow pathway. This form of AVNRT occurs much less commonly and produces a prolonged RP interval during the tachycardia with a negative P wave in leads 2, 3, and aVF. This atypical form of AVNRT is more easily precipitated by ventricular stimulation.

Treatment:
℞ ATRIOVENTRICULAR NODAL REENTRANT TACHYCARDIA

ACUTE TREATMENT Treatment is directed at altering conduction within the AV node. Vagal stimulation, such as occurs with the Valsalva maneuver or carotid sinus massage, can slow conduction in the AV node sufficiently to terminate AVNRT. In patients in whom physical maneuvers do not terminate the tachyarrhythmia, the administration of adenosine, 6–12 mg IV, frequently does so. Intravenous beta blockade or calcium channel therapy should be considered second-line agents. If hemodynamic compromise is present, R wave synchronous DC cardioversion using 100–200 J can terminate the tachyarrhythmia.

PREVENTION Prevention may be achieved with drugs that slow conduction in the antegrade slow pathway, such as digitalis, beta blockers, or calcium channel blockers. In patients who have a history of exercise-precipitated AVNRT, the use of beta blockers frequently eliminates symptoms. In patients who do not respond to drug therapy directed at the antegrade slow pathway, treatment with class IA or IC agents directed at altering conduction of the fast pathway may be considered.

Catheter ablation, directed at elimination or modification of slow pathway conduction, is very effective in permanently eliminating AVNRT. Patients with recurrent AVNRT that produces significant symptoms or heart rates >200 beats/min and patients reluctant to take chronic drug therapy should be considered for ablative therapy. Catheter ablation can cure AV nodal reentry in >95% of patients. The risk of AV block requiring a permanent pacemaker is ~1% with the ablation procedure. This risk may be further minimized with the use of cryoablation techniques when the slow pathway is in close proximity to the compact AV node.

These can also occur in the setting of enhanced normal automaticity, abnormal automaticity, or triggered activity. These tachycardias may or may not be associated with retrograde conduction to the atria, and the P waves may appear dissociated or produce intermittent conduction and early activation of the junction. These arrhythmias may occur as a manifestation of increased adrenergic tone or drug effect in patients with sinus node dysfunction or following surgical or catheter ablation. The arrhythmia may also be a manifestation of digoxin toxicity. The most common manifestation of digoxin intoxication is the sudden regularization of the response to AF. A junctional tachycardia due to digoxin toxicity typically does not manifest retrograde conduction. Sinus activity may appear dissociated or result in intermittent capture beats with a long PR interval. If the rate is >50 beats/min and <100 beats/min, the term *accelerated junctional rhythm* applies. Occasionally, automatic rhythms are mimicked by AVNRT that fails to conduct to the atrium. The triggering events associated with the onset of the tachycardia may provide a clue to the appropriate diagnosis. Initiation of the tachycardia without an atrial premature beat with a gradual acceleration in rate suggests an automatic focus.

Treatment:
℞ ATRIOVENTRICULAR JUNCTIONAL TACHYCARDIAS

Treatment of automatic/triggered junctional tachycardias is directed at decreasing adrenergic stimulation and reversing digoxin toxicity, if present. Digoxin therapy can be withheld if toxicity is suspected, and the administration of digoxin-specific antibody fragments can rapidly reverse digoxin toxicity if the tachycardia is producing significant symptoms and rapid termination is indicated. Junctional tachycardia due to abnormal automaticity can be treated pharmacologically with beta blockers. A trial of class IA or IC drugs may also be attempted. For incessant automatic junctional tachycardia, focal catheter ablation can be performed but is associated with an increased risk of AV block.

TACHYCARDIAS ASSOCIATED WITH ACCESSORY AV PATHWAYS

Tachycardias that involve accessory pathways (APs) between atria and ventricles commonly manifest a normal QRS complex with a short or long RP interval. They must be considered in the differential diagnosis of other narrow-complex tachycardias. Importantly, most tachycardias associated with APs involve a large macroreentrant circuit that includes the ventricles (Fig. 16-7). Thus, identifying these arrhythmias as "supraventricular" is actually a misnomer, and they deserve separate consideration.

APs are typically capable of conducting rapidly both in an antegrade and retrograde direction. In the absence of an AP, the sinus impulse normally activates the ventricles via the AV node and His-Purkinje system, resulting in a PR interval of 120–200 ms. When an antegradely conducting AP is present, the sinus impulse bypasses the AV node and can rapidly activate the ventricles, resulting in ventricular preexcitation. The resulting PR interval is shorter than anticipated. In addition, because the initial ventricular activation is due to muscle-to-muscle conduction, as opposed to rapid spread of activation via the His-Purkinje system, the initial portion of the QRS complex is slurred, creating the characteristic "delta wave." The remaining portion of the QRS complex in sinus rhythm is created by a fusion of the ventricular activation wavefront originating from the Purkinje network and the continued spread of activation from the site of insertion of the AP (Fig. 16-8). Evidence of ventricular preexcitation includes evidence in sinus rhythm of a short PR interval and a delta wave.

The most common AP connects the left atrium to the left ventricle, followed by posterior septal, right free wall, and anterior septal APs. APs typically insert from the atrium into the adjacent ventricular myocardium.

However, occasionally pathways, particularly those originating from the right atrium, can have a ventricular insertion at a site distant from the AV groove in the fascicles. These pathways tend to be long, conduct more slowly, and are referred to as *atriofascicular accessory pathways*. Atriofascicular APs are unique in their tendency to demonstrate decremental antegrade conduction.

Other accessory pathway connections from the AV node to the fascicles may also exist. These pathways are referred to as *Mahaim fibers* and typically manifest a normal PR interval with a delta wave.

Patients with manifest preexcitation and WPW syndrome are typically subject to both macroreentrant tachycardias and a rapid response to AF (Fig. 16-8). The most common macroreentrant tachycardia associated with the WPW syndrome is referred to as *orthodromic AV reentry*. Ventricular activation occurs via the AV node and the His-Purkinje system. Conduction then returns or reenters the atria via retrograde conduction over the AP. The reentrant circuit develops because of the inhomogeneity in conduction and refractoriness in the AP and normal AV node.

Characteristically, the AP has more rapid conduction but a longer refractory period when compared to that of the AV node. Typical APs do not show evidence of antegrade decremental conduction. An APC can block in the AP and conduct sufficiently slowly or with decrement via the AV node to allow for retrograde recovery of activation of the AP and, in turn, of the atria (Fig. 16-7). This retrograde activation of the atria via the AP is referred to as an *echo beat*. If the pattern repeats itself, a tachycardia develops. Uncommonly, the reentrant circuit can be reversed so that the impulse reaches the ventricle via the AP and conducts retrogradely through to the atria via the His-Purkinje system and the AV node; this is referred to as *antidromic AV reentry* and/or *preexcited macroreentry*, with the entire activation of the ventricle originating from the site of insertion of the AP. Although uncommon, it is important to recognize antidromic SVT. The ECG pattern during the tachycardia mimics VT originating from the site of ventricular insertion of the AP. The presence of a similar or lesser degree of manifest preexcitation in sinus rhythm provides a valuable clue to the diagnosis.

The second most common and potentially more serious arrhythmia associated with the WPW syndrome is rapidly conducting AF. Nearly 50% of patients with evidence of APs are predisposed to episodes of AF. In patients who have rapid antegrade conduction from the atria to the ventricles over the AP, the AP can conduct rapidly in response to AF, resulting in a faster ventricular rate than would occur normally via the AV node. The rapid ventricular rates can result in hemodynamic compromise and even precipitate VF. The QRS pattern during AF in patients with manifest preexcitation can appear quite bizarre and change on a beat-to-beat basis due to the variability in the degree of fusion from activation over the AV node (Fig. 16-8).

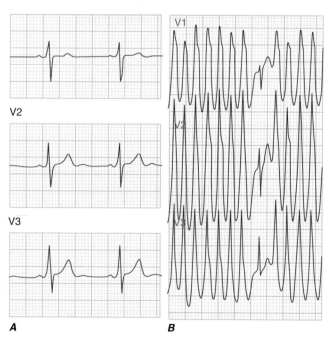

FIGURE 16-8

A. Sinus rhythm tracing of leads V$_1$–V$_3$ showing evidence of Wolff-Parkinson-White syndrome with short PR interval and delta wave. **B.** During atrial fibrillation, rapid conduction to the ventricles is observed producing a wide QRS complex tachycardia with marked irregularity of the ventricular response and morphology of the QRS complex.

Concealed APs

In ~50% of patients with APs, there is no antegrade conduction over the AP; however, retrograde conduction is preserved. As a result, the AP is not manifest in sinus rhythm and is only manifest during the sustained tachycardia. The presence of a concealed AP is suggested by the timing and pattern of atrial activation during the tachycardia: the P wave typically follows ventricular activation with a short RP wave interval (Fig. 16-7). Because, many APs connect the left ventricle to the left atrium, the pattern of atrial activation during the tachycardia frequently produces negative P waves in leads I and aVL. The tachycardia circuit, and, therefore, its ECG manifestation during orthodromic tachycardia, are identical both in patients with overt preexcitation in sinus rhythm and in those with concealed APs. Patients with concealed APs, although prone to episodes of AF, are not at risk for developing a rapid ventricular response to the AF.

Occasionally, APs conduct extremely slowly in a retrograde fashion, resulting in longer retrograde conduction and the development of a long RP interval during the tachycardia (*long RP tachycardia*). Because of the presence of this dramatically slowed conduction, additional conduction slowing created by premature atrial complexes is not required for tachycardia to ensue. These patients are more prone to frequent episodes of tachycardia and can present with "incessant" tachycardias and tachycardia-induced LV cardiomyopathy. The correct diagnosis of a long RP tachycardia may be suggested by the pattern of initiation and the P wave morphology. Frequently, however, an electrophysiologic evaluation is required to establish the diagnosis.

Treatment:
℞ ACCESSORY PATHWAY-MEDIATED TACHYCARDIAS

Acute treatment of AP-mediated macroreentrant orthodromic tachycardias is similar to that for AV nodal reentry and is directed at altering conduction in the AV node. Vagal stimulation with the Valsalva maneuver and carotid sinus pressure may create sufficient AV nodal slowing to terminate the atrioventricular reentrant tachycardia (AVRT). Intravenous administration of adenosine, 6–12 mg, is first-line pharmacologic therapy; IV calcium channel blockers, verapamil or diltiazem, or beta blockers may also be effective. In patients who demonstrate manifest preexcitation and AF, therapy should be aimed at preventing a rapid ventricular response. In life-threatening situations, DC cardioversion should be used to terminate the AF. In non-life-threatening situations, procainamide at a dose of 15 mg/kg

administered IV over 20–30 min will slow the ventricular response and may organize and terminate AF. Ibutilide can also be used to facilitate termination of AF. During AF there may be rapid conduction over the AV node as well as the AP. Caution should be used in attempting to slow AV nodal conduction with the use of digoxin or verapamil; when administered IV, these drugs may actually result in an acute increase in rate over the AP, placing the patient at risk for development of VF. Digoxin appears to shorten the refractory period of the AP directly and thus increases the ventricular rate. Verapamil appears to shorten the refractory period indirectly by causing vasodilatation and a reflex increase in sympathetic tone.

Chronic oral administration of beta blockers and/or verapamil or diltiazem may be used to prevent recurrent supraventricular reentrant tachycardias associated with APs. In patients with evidence of AF and a rapid ventricular response and in those with recurrences of SVT on AV nodal blocking drugs, strong consideration should be given to the administration of either a class IA or IC antiarrhythmic drug, such as quinidine, flecainide, or propafenone that slow conduction and increase refractoriness in the AP.

Patients with a history of recurrent symptomatic SVT episodes, incessant SVT, and heart rates >200 beats/min with SVT should be given strong consideration for undergoing catheter ablation. Patients who have demonstrated rapid antegrade conduction over their AP or the potential for rapid conduction should also be considered for catheter ablation. Catheter ablation therapy has been demonstrated to be successful in >95% of patients with documented WPW syndrome and appears effective regardless of age. The risk of catheter ablative therapy is low and is dictated primarily by the location of the AP. Ablation of para-Hisian APs is associated with a risk of heart block, and ablation in the left atrium is associated with a small but definite risk of thromboembolic phenomenon. These risks must be weighed against the potential serious complications associated with hemodynamic compromise, the risk of VF, and the severity of the patient's symptoms with AP-mediated tachycardias.

Patients who demonstrate evidence of ventricular preexcitation in the absence of any prior arrhythmia history deserve special consideration. The first arrhythmia manifestation can be a rapid SVT or, albeit of low risk (<1%), of a life-threatening rapid response to AF. Patients who demonstrate intermittent preexcitation during ECG monitoring or an abrupt loss of AP conduction during exercise testing are at low risk of a life-threatening rapid response to AF. All other patients should be advised of their risks and therapeutic options in advance of a documented arrhythmia event.

VENTRICULAR PREMATURE COMPLEXES (VPCS)

The origin of premature beats in the ventricle at sites remote from the Purkinje network produces slow ventricular activation and a wide QRS complex that is typically >140 ms in duration. VPCs are common and increase with age and the presence of structural heart disease. VPCs can occur with a certain degree of periodicity that has become incorporated into the lexicon of electrocardiography. VPCs may occur in patterns of *bigeminy*, in which every sinus beat is followed by a VPC, or *trigeminy*, in which two sinus beats are followed by a VPC. VPCs may have different morphologies and are thus referred to as *multiformed*. Two successive VPCs are termed *pairs* or *couplets*. Three or more consecutive VPCs are termed *VT* when the rate is >100 beats/min. If the repetitive VPCs terminate spontaneously and are more than three beats in duration, the arrhythmia is referred to as *nonsustained VT*.

APCs with aberrant ventricular conduction may also create a wide and early QRS complex. The premature P wave can occasionally be difficult to discern when it falls on the preceding T wave, and other clues must be used to make the diagnosis. The QRS pattern for a VPC does not appear to follow a typical right or left bundle branch block pattern as the QRS morphology is associated with aberrant atrial conduction and can be quite bizarre. On occasion, VPCs can arise from the Purkinje network of the ventricles, in which case the QRS pattern mimics aberration. The 12-lead ECG recording of the VPC may be required to identify subtle morphologic clues regarding the QRS complex to confirm its ventricular origin. Most commonly, VPCs are associated with a "fully compensatory pause"; i.e., the duration between the last QRS before the PVC and the next QRS complex is equal to twice the sinus rate (Fig. 16-3). The VPC typically does not conduct to the atrium. If the VPC does conduct to the atrium, it may not be sufficiently early to reset the sinus node. As a result, sinus activity will occur and the antegrade wavefront from the sinus node may encounter some delay in the AV node or His-Purkinje system from the blocked VPC wavefront, or it may collide with the retrograde atrial wavefront. Sinus activity will continue undisturbed, resulting in a delay to the next QRS complex (Fig. 16-3). Occasionally the VPC can occur early enough and conduct retrograde to the atrium to reset the sinus node; the pause that results will be less than compensatory. VPCs that fail to influence the oncoming sinus impulse are termed *interpolated VPCs*. A ventricular focus that fires repetitively at a fixed interval may produce variably coupled VPCs, depending on the sinus rate. This type of focus is referred to as a *parasystolic focus* because its firing

does not appear to be modulated by sinus activity and the conducted QRS complex. The ventricular ectopy will occur at a characteristic fixed integer or multiple of these intervals. The variability in coupling relative to the underlying QRS complex and a fixed interval between complexes of ventricular origin provide the diagnostic information necessary to identify a parasystolic focus.

Treatment:
℞ VENTRICULAR PREMATURE COMPLEXES

The threshold for treatment of VPCs is high, and the treatment is primarily directed at eliminating severe symptoms associated with palpitations. VPCs of sufficient frequency can cause a reversible cardiomyopathy. Depressed LV function in the setting of ventricular bigeminy and/or frequent nonsustained VT should raise the possibility of a cardiomyopathy that is reversible with control of the ventricular arrhythmia. In the absence of structural heart disease, VPCs do not appear to have prognostic significance. In patients with structural heart disease, frequent VPCs and runs of nonsustained VT have prognostic significance and may portend an increased risk of SCD. However, no study has documented that elimination of VPCs with antiarrhythmic drug therapy reduces the risk of arrhythmic death in patients with severe structural heart disease. Drug therapies that slow myocardial conduction and/or enhance dispersion of refractoriness can actually increase the risk of life-threatening arrhythmias (drug-induced QT prolongation and TdP) despite being effective at eliminating VPCs.

ACCELERATED IDIOVENTRICULAR RHYTHM (AIVR)

AIVR refers to a ventricular rhythm that is characterized by three or more complexes at a rate >40 beats/min and <120 beats/min. The arrhythmia mechanism causing AIVR is thought to be due to abnormal automaticity. By definition there is an overlap between AIVR and "slow" VT; both rhythms can manifest rates between 90 and 120 beats/min. Because AIVR tends to be a benign rhythm with different therapeutic implications, it is worthwhile to attempt to distinguish it from "slow" VT. AIVR has a characteristic gradual onset and offset and more variability in cycle length. It is typically a brief, self-limiting arrhythmia. AIVR can be seen in the absence of any structural heart disease, but it is frequently present in the setting of acute myocardial infarction, cocaine intoxication, acute myocarditis, digoxin intoxication, and postoperative cardiac surgery. Sustained forms of AIVR can exist, particularly in the setting of acute myocardial infarction and postoperatively. In the setting of sustained AIVR, hemodynamic compromise can occur because of the loss of AV synchrony. Patients with RV infarction associated with proximal right coronary artery occlusion are most susceptible to associated bradyarrhythmias and the hemodynamic consequences of AIVR. In these patients, acceleration of the atrial rate, either by the cautious administration of atropine or by atrial pacing, may be an important treatment consideration.

VENTRICULAR TACHYCARDIA

VT originates below the bundle of His at a rate >100 beats/min; most have rates >120 beats/min. Sustained VT at rates <120 beats/min and even <100 beats/min can be observed, particularly in association with the administration of antiarrhythmic agents that can slow the rate. Because of the overlap in rates with AIVR, the arrhythmia ECG characteristics and the clinical circumstance can sometimes be used to distinguish the two forms of tachycardia. Slow sustained VT is less likely to show a marked warm-up in rate and the marked cycle-length oscillations seen with AIVR, and it is more likely to occur in the setting of chronic infarction or cardiomyopathy and less likely with acute infarction or myocarditis. Obviously, significant overlap may exist. Typically, slow VT will be initiated with programmed stimulation and is found to represent a large macroreentrant circuit in chronically diseased myocardium capable of supporting markedly slow conduction.

The QRS complex during VT may be uniform (monomorphic) or may vary from beat to beat (polymorphic). Polymorphic VT in patients who demonstrate a long QT interval during their baseline rhythm is typically referred to as *TdP*. The polymorphic VT associated with QT prolongation dramatically oscillates around the baseline on most of the monitored ECG leads, mimicking the "turning of the points" stitching pattern (**Fig. 16-9**).

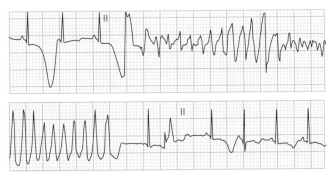

FIGURE 16-9

Sinus rhythm with long QT interval and the polymorphic ventricular arrhythmia torsade de pointes. Dramatic T wave alternans is present in sinus rhythm.

Monomorphic VT suggests a stable tachycardia focus in the absence of structural heart disease or a fixed anatomic substrate that can create the substrate for a stable reentrant VT circuit when structural disease is present. Monomorphic VT tends to be a reproducible and recurrent phenomenon and may be initiated with pacing and programmed ventricular stimulation. In contrast, polymorphic VT suggests a more dynamic and/or unstable process and, by its very nature, is less reproducible. Polymorphic VT may be produced by acute ischemia, myocarditis, or dynamic changes in the QT interval and enhanced dispersion of ventricular refractoriness. Polymorphic VTs are not reliably initiated with pacing or programmed stimulation.

A time duration of 30 s is frequently used to distinguish sustained from nonsustained VT. Hemodynamically unstable VT that requires termination before 30 s or VT that is terminated by therapy from an implantable defibrillator is also typically classified as sustained. Ventricular flutter appears as a sine wave on the ECG and has a rate of >250 beats/min. A rapid rate coupled with the sine wave nature of the arrhythmia makes it impossible to identify a discrete QRS morphology. When antiarrhythmic drugs are being administered, a sine wave appearance of the QRS complex can be observed, even at rates of 200 beats/min. VF is characterized by completely disorganized ventricular activation on the surface ECG. Polymorphic ventricular arrhythmias, ventricular flutter, and VF always produce hemodynamic collapse if allowed to continue. The hemodynamic stability of a unimorphic VT depends on the presence and severity of the underlying structural heart disease, the location of the site of origin of the arrhythmia, and the heart rate.

It is important to distinguish monomorphic VT from SVT with aberrant ventricular conduction due to right or left bundle branch block.

Importantly, the sinus or baseline 12-lead ECG tracing can provide important clues that help establish the correct diagnosis of a wide complex tachycardia. The presence of an aberrant QRS pattern that matches exactly that of the wide complex rhythm strongly supports the diagnosis of SVT. A right or left bundle branch block QRS pattern that does not match the QRS and/or that is wider in duration than the QRS during the wide complex tachycardia supports the diagnosis of VT. Most patients with VT have structural heart disease and show evidence of a prior Q wave myocardial infarction during sinus rhythm. Important exceptions to this rule are discussed (p. 168). Finally, the presence of a preexcited QRS pattern on the 12-lead ECG in sinus rhythm suggests that the wide complex rhythm represents an atrial arrhythmia, such as AFL or a focal AT, with rapid conduction over an AP or antidromic macroreentrant tachycardia (Fig. 16-8). If the arrhythmia is irregular with changing QRS complexes, then the diagnosis of AF with ventricular preexcitation should be considered.

With the exception of some idiopathic outflow tract tachycardias, most VTs do not respond to vagal stimulation provoked by carotid sinus massage, the Valsalva maneuver, or adenosine administration. The IV administration of verapamil and/or adenosine is not recommended as a diagnostic test. Verapamil has been associated with hemodynamic collapse when administered to patients with structural heart disease and VT.

Patients with VT frequently demonstrate AV disassociation. Findings on physical examination of intermittent cannon *a* waves and variability of the first heart sound are consistent with AV dissociation. The presence of AV dissociation is characteristically marked by the presence of sinus capture or fusion beats. The presence of 1:1 ventriculo-atrial conduction does not preclude a diagnosis of VT.

Additional characteristics of the 12-lead ECG during the tachycardia that suggest VT include (1) the presence of a QRS duration >140 ms in the absence of drug therapy, (2) a superior and rightward QRS frontal plane axis, (3) a bizarre QRS complex that does not mimic the characteristic QRS pattern associated with left or right bundle branch block, and (4) slurring of the initial portion of the QRS (**Fig. 16–10**). **Table 16–6** provides a useful summary of ECG criteria that have evolved based on the described characteristics of VT.

Treatment:
℞ **VENTRICULAR TACHYCARDIA/ FIBRILLATION**

Sustained polymorphic VT, ventricular flutter, and VF all lead to immediate hemodynamic collapse. Emergency asynchronous defibrillation is therefore required, with at least 200-J monophasic or 100-J biphasic shock. The shock should be delivered asynchronously to avoid delays related to sensing of the QRS complex. If the arrhythmia persists, repeated shocks with the maximum energy output of the defibrillator are essential to optimize the chance of successful resuscitation. Intravenous lidocaine and/or amiodarone should be administered but should not delay repeated attempts at defibrillation.

For any monomorphic wide complex rhythm that results in hemodynamic compromise, a prompt R wave synchronous shock is required. Conscious sedation should be provided if the hemodynamic status permits. For patients with a well-tolerated wide complex tachycardia, the appropriate diagnosis should be established based on strict ECG criteria (Table 16-6). Pharmacologic treatment to terminate monomorphic VT is not typically successful (<30%). Intravenous procainamide, lidocaine, or amiodarone can be utilized. If the arrhythmia persists,

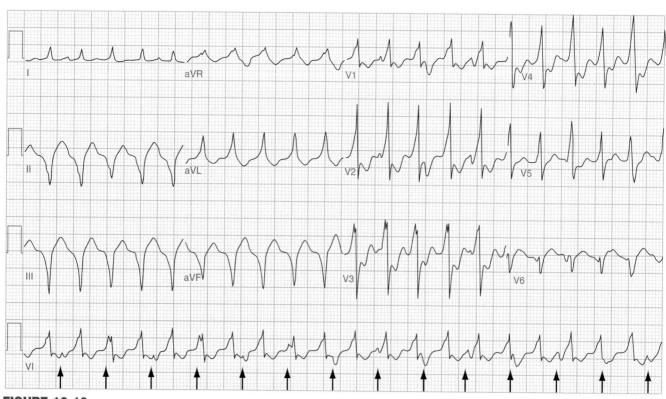

FIGURE 16-10

Ventricular tachycardia. ECG showing AV dissociation (arrows mark P waves), wide QRS >200 ms, superior frontal plane axis, slurring of the initial portion of the QRS, and large S wave in V₆—all clues to the diagnosis of ventricular tachycardia.

TABLE 16-6

ECG CLUES SUPPORTING THE DIAGNOSIS OF VENTRICULAR TACHYCARDIA

AV dissociation (atrial capture, fusion beats)

QRS duration >140 ms for RBBB type V_1 morphology; V_1 >160 ms for LBBB type V_1 morphology

Frontal plane axis –90° to 180°

Delayed activation during initial phase of the QRS complex

    LBBB pattern—R wave in V_1, V_2 >40 ms

    RBBB pattern—onset of R wave to nadir of S >100 ms

Bizarre QRS pattern that does not mimic typical RBBB or LBBB QRS complex

    Concordance of QRS complex in all precordial leads

    RS or dominant S in V_6 for RBBB VT

    Q wave in V_6 with LBBB QRS pattern

    Monophasic R or biphasic qR or R/S in V_1 with RBBB pattern

Note: AV, atrioventricular; RBBB/LBBB, right/left bundle branch block.

synchronous R wave cardioversion after the administration of conscious sedation is appropriate. Selected patients with focal outflow tract tachycardias (p. 169) who demonstrate triggered or automatic VT may respond to IV beta blocker administration. Idiopathic LV septal VT (see p. 169) appears to respond uniquely to IV verapamil administration.

VT in patients with structural heart disease is now almost always treated with the implantation of an ICD to manage anticipated VT recurrence. The ICD can provide rapid pacing and shock therapy to treat most VTs effectively (Fig. 16-11).

Prevention of VT remains important, and >50% of patients with a history of VT and an ICD may need to be treated with adjunctive antiarrhythmic drug therapy to prevent VT recurrences or to manage atrial arrhythmias. Because of the presence of an ICD, there is more flexibility with respect to antiarrhythmic drug therapy selection. The use of sotalol or amiodarone represents first-line therapy for patients with a history of structural heart disease and life-threatening monomorphic or polymorphic VT not due to long QT syndrome. Importantly, sotalol has been associated with a decrease in the defibrillation threshold, which reflects the amount of energy necessary to terminate VF. Amiodarone may be better tolerated in patients with a more marginal hemodynamic status and systolic blood pressure. The risk of end organ toxicity from amiodarone must be weighed against the ease of use and general efficacy. Antiarrhythmic drug therapy with agents such as quinidine, procainamide, or propafenone, which might not normally be used in patients with structural heart disease because of the risk of proarrhythmia, may be considered in patients with an ICD and recurrent VT.

Catheter ablative therapy for VT in patients without structural heart disease results in cure rates >90%. In patients with structural heart disease, catheter ablation that includes a strategy for eliminating unmappable/rapid VT and one that incorporates endocardial as well as epicardial mapping and ablation should be employed. In most patients, catheter ablation can reduce or eliminate

CHAPTER 16   The Tachyarrhythmias

Chart speed 25.0 mm/sec

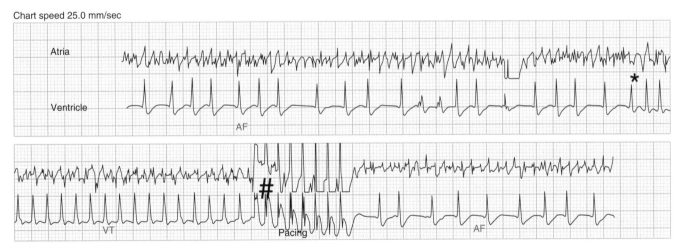

FIGURE 16-11

Ventricular tachycardia (VT) (*) during atrial fibrillation stopped by pacing (#) from an implantable cardioverter defibrillator (ICD) from recording stored by ICD. The atrial electrogram shows characteristic fibrillatory waves through the tracing. The ventricular electrogram shows an irregularly irregular response consistent with atrial fibrillation at the beginning of the tracing. The ventricular electrogram suddenly changes in morphology (*) and becomes regular, consistent with the diagnosis of VT. Pacing transiently accelerates the rate and interrupts the rapid VT. The patient was unaware of the life-threatening event.

the requirement for toxic drug therapy and should be considered in any patient with recurrent VT. The utilization of ablative therapy to reduce the incidence of ICD shocks for VT in patients who receive the ICD as part of primary prevention for VT is being actively investigated.

MANAGEMENT OF VT STORM Repeated VT episodes requiring external cardioversion/defibrillation or repeated appropriate ICD shock therapy is referred to as *VT storm*. While a definition of more than two episodes in 24 h is used, most patients with VT storm will experience many more episodes. In the extreme form of VT storm, the tachycardia becomes incessant and the baseline rhythm is unable to be restored for any extended period. In patients with recurrent polymorphic VT in the absence of the long QT interval, one should have a high suspicion of active ischemic disease or fulminant myocarditis. Intravenous lidocaine or amiodarone administration should be coupled with prompt assessment of the status of the coronary anatomy. Endomyocardial biopsy, if indicated by clinical circumstance, may be used to confirm the diagnosis of myocarditis, although the diagnostic yield is low. In patients who demonstrate QT prolongation and recurrent pause-dependent polymorphic VT (TdP), removal of an offending QT-prolonging drug, correction of potassium or magnesium deficiencies, and emergency pacing to prevent pauses should be considered. Intravenous beta blockade therapy should be considered for polymorphic VT storm. A targeted treatment strategy should be employed if the diagnosis of the polymorphic VT syndrome can be established. For example, quinidine or isoproterenol can be used in the treatment of Brugada's syndrome (p. 174). Intra-aortic balloon counterpulsation or acute coronary angioplasty may be needed to stop recurrent polymorphic VT precipitated by acute ischemia. In selected patients with a repeating VPC trigger for their polymorphic VT, the VPC can be targeted for ablation to prevent recurrent VT.

In patients with recurrent monomorphic VT, acute IV administration of lidocaine, procainamide, or amiodarone can prevent recurrences. The use of such therapy is empirical, and a clinical response is not certain. Procainamide and amiodarone are more likely to slow the tachycardia and make it hemodynamically tolerated. Unfortunately, antiarrhythmic drugs, especially those that slow conduction (e.g., amiodarone, procainamide), can also facilitate recurrent VT or even result in incessant VT. VT catheter ablation can eliminate frequent recurrent or incessant VT and frequent ICD shocks. Such therapy should be deployed earlier in the course of arrhythmia events to prevent adverse consequences of recurrent VT episodes and adverse effects from antiarrhythmic drugs.

UNIQUE VT SYNDROMES

Although most ventricular arrhythmias occur in the setting of coronary artery disease with prior myocardial infarction, a significant number of patients develop VT in other settings. A brief discussion of each unique VT syndrome is warranted. Information that illustrates a unique pathogenesis and enhances the ability to make the correct diagnosis and institute appropriate therapy will be highlighted.

Idiopathic Outflow Tract VT

VT in the absence of structural heart disease is referred to as *idiopathic VT*. There are two major varieties of these VTs. Outflow tachycardias originate in the RV and LV outflow tract regions. Approximately 80% of outflow tract VTs originate in the RV and ~20% in the LV outflow tract regions. Outflow tract VTs appear to originate from anatomic sites that form an arc beginning just above the tricuspid valve and extending along the roof of the outflow tract region to include the free wall and septal aspect of the right ventricle just beneath the pulmonic valve, the aortic valve region, and then the anterior/superior margin of the mitral valve annulus. These arrhythmias appear more commonly in women. Importantly, these ventricular arrhythmias are *not* associated with SCD. Patients manifest symptoms of palpitations with exercise, stress, and caffeine ingestion. In women, the arrhythmia is more commonly associated with hormonal triggers and can frequently be timed to the premenstrual period, gestation, and menopause. Uncommonly, the VPCs and VTs can be of sufficient frequency and duration to cause a tachycardia-induced cardiomyopathy.

The pathogenesis of outflow tract VT remains unknown, and there is no definite anatomic abnormality identified with these VTs. Vagal maneuvers, adenosine, and beta blockers tend to terminate the VTs, whereas catecholamine infusion, exercise, and stress tend to potentiate the outflow tract VTs. Based on these observations, the mechanism of the arrhythmia is most likely calcium-dependent triggered activity. Preliminary data suggest that at least in some patients, a somatic mutation of the inhibitory G protein (Gα I2) may serve as the genetic basis for the VT. In contrast to VT in patients with coronary artery disease, outflow tract VTs are uncommonly initiated with programmed stimulation but are able to be initiated by rapid-burst atrial or ventricular pacing, particularly when coupled with the infusion of isoproterenol.

Outflow tract VT typically produces large monophasic R waves in the inferior frontal plane leads II, III, and aVF, and typically occurs as nonsustained bursts of VT and/or frequent premature beats. Cycle length oscillations during the tachycardia are common. Since most VT originates in the RV outflow tract, the VT typically has a left bundle branch block pattern in lead V_1 (negative QRS vector) (**Fig. 16-12**). Outflow tract VT, originating in the left ventricle, particularly those associated with an origin from the mitral valve annulus, have a right bundle branch block pattern in lead V_1 (positive QRS vector).

Treatment:
Rx IDIOPATHIC OUTFLOW TRACT VENTRICULAR TACHYCARDIA

Acute medical therapy for idiopathic outflow tract VT is rarely required because the VT is hemodynamically tolerated and is typically nonsustained. Intravenous beta blockers frequently terminate the tachycardia. Chronic therapy with beta or calcium channel blockers frequently prevents recurrent episodes of the tachycardia. The arrhythmia also appears to respond to treatment with class IA or IC agents or with sotalol. In patients who are reluctant to take long-term drug therapy or who have persistent symptoms despite drug therapy, catheter ablative therapy has been utilized successfully to eliminate the tachycardia with success rates >90%. Because of the absence of structural heart disease and the focal nature of these arrhythmias, the 12-lead ECG pattern during VT can help localize the site of origin of the arrhythmia and help facilitate catheter ablation. Efficacy of therapy is assessed with treadmill testing and/or ECG monitoring, and electrophysiologic study is performed only when the diagnosis is in question or to perform catheter ablation.

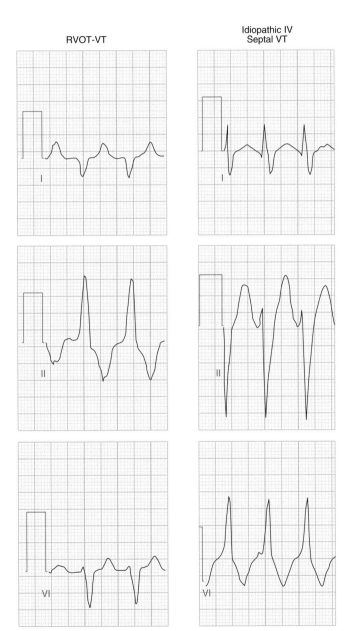

FIGURE 16-12
Common idiopathic ventricular tachycardia (VT) ECG patterns. Right ventricular outflow tract (RVOT) VT with typical left bundle QRS pattern in V_1 and inferiorly directed frontal plane axis, and left ventricular septal VT from the inferior septum with a narrow QRS right bundle branch block pattern in V_1 and superior and leftward front plane QRS axis.

Idiopathic LV Septal/Fascicular VT

The second most common idiopathic VT is linked anatomically to the Purkinje system in the left ventricle. The arrhythmia mechanism appears to be macroreentry involving calcium-dependent slow response fibers that are part of the Purkinje network, although automatic tachycardias have also been observed. A 12-lead ECG morphology of the VT shows a narrow right bundle branch block pattern and a superior leftward axis or an inferior rightward axis, depending upon whether the VT originates from the posterior or anterior fascicles (Fig. 16-12). Idiopathic LV septal VT is unique in its suppression with verapamil. Beta blockers have also been used with some success as primary or effective adjunctive therapy. Catheter ablation is very effective therapy for VT resistant to drug therapy or in patients reluctant to take daily therapy, with anticipated successful elimination of VT in >90% of patients.

VT Associated with LV Dilated Cardiomyopathy

Monomorphic and polymorphic VTs may occur in patients with nonischemic dilated cardiomyopathy (Chap. 21). Although the myopathic process may be diffuse, there appears to be a predilection for the development of fibrosis around the mitral and aortic valvular regions. Most uniform sustained VT can be mapped to these regions of fibrosis. Drug therapy is usually ineffective in preventing VT, and empirical trials of sotalol or amiodarone are usually initiated only for recurrent VT episodes after ICD implantation. VT associated with nonischemic dilated cardiomyopathy appears to be less amenable to catheter ablative therapy from the endocardium; frequently, the VT originates from epicardial areas of fibrosis and catheter access to the epicardium can be gained via a percutaneous pericardial puncture to improve the outcome of ablation techniques. In patients with a history of depressed myocardial dysfunction due to a nonischemic cardiomyopathy with an LV ejection fraction <30%, data now support the implantation of a prophylactic ICD device to reduce the risk of SCD from the first VT/VF episode effectively.

Bundle Branch Reentrant VT

Monomorphic VT in patients with idiopathic nonischemic cardiomyopathy or valvular cardiomyopathy is frequently due to a large macroreentrant circuit involving the various elements of the His-Purkinje network. The arrhythmia usually occurs in the presence of underlying His-Purkinje system disease. In sinus rhythm, an incomplete left bundle block is typically present and the time that it takes to traverse the His-Purkinje network is delayed; this slow conduction serves as the substrate for reentry. Characteristically, the VT circuit rotates in an antegrade direction down the right bundle and retrograde up the left posterior or anterior fascicles and left bundle branch. As a result, bundle branch reentrant VT typically has a QRS morphology that mimics RV apical pacing with a left bundle branch block type pattern and a leftward superior axis (Fig. 16–13). The circuit for bundle branch reentrant VT can occasionally rotate in the opposite direction, antegrade through the left bundle and retrograde through the right bundle, in which case a right bundle branch block pattern during VT will be manifest.

It is important to recognize bundle branch reentrant VT because it is readily amenable to ablative therapy that targets a component of the His-Purkinje system, typically the right bundle, to block the VT circuit. In most patients, because of the presence of severely depressed LV function and a high risk of SCD, ablative therapy is coupled with an ICD. Less commonly, bundle branch reentry may occur in the absence of structural heart disease or in the setting of coronary artery disease. The use of adjunctive ICD therapy is dictated by the ability to eliminate the VT successfully and the severity of the LV dysfunction.

VT Associated with Hypertrophic Cardiomyopathy

(See also Chap. 21) VT/VF have also been associated with hypertrophic cardiomyopathy. In patients with

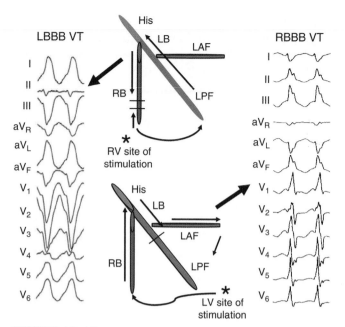

FIGURE 16-13

Bundle branch reentrant ventricular tachycardia (VT) showing typical QRS morphologies when ventricular tachycardia (VT) is initiated with stimulation from the right ventricle [left bundle branch block (LBBB) VT pattern] or left ventricle [right bundle branch block (RBBB) VT pattern] and schema for circuit involving the His-Purkinje network.

hypertrophic cardiomyopathy and a history of sustained VT/VF, unexplained syncope, a strong family history of SCD, LV septal thickness >30 mm, or nonsustained spontaneous VT, the risk of SCD is high and ICD implantation is usually indicated. Amiodarone, sotalol, and beta blockers have been used to control recurrent VT. Experience with ablative therapy is limited because of the infrequency with which the VT is tolerated hemodynamically. Ablation procedures that target the substrate for VT/VF and ablate areas of low voltage consistent with fibrosis appear to have promise in this setting. The WPW syndrome has been observed in patients with hypertrophic cardiomyopathy associated with *PRKAG2* mutations.

VT Associated with Other Infiltrative Cardiomyopathies and Neuromuscular Disorders

An increased arrhythmia risk has been identified when cardiac involvement occurs in a variety of infiltrative diseases and neuromuscular disorders (Table 16-7). Many patients manifest AV conduction disturbances and may require permanent pacemaker insertion. The decision to implant an ICD device should follow current established guidelines for patients with nonischemic cardiomyopathy, which include a history of syncope with depressed LV function, a history of severely depressed LV function,

TABLE 16-7

INFILTRATIVE/INFLAMMATORY AND NEUROMUSCULAR DISORDERS ASSOCIATED WITH AN INCREASED VENTRICULAR ARRHYTHMIA RISK

Sarcoidosis[a]	Emery-Dreyfuss muscular dystrophy[a]
Chagas disease[a]	Limb-girdle muscular dystrophy[a]
Amyloidosis[a]	Duchenne's muscular dystrophy
Fabry disease	Becker's muscular dystrophy
Hemochromatosis	Kearn-Sayre syndrome[a]
Myotonic muscular dystrophy[a]	Friedreich's ataxia

[a]High frequency of ventricular arrhythmias noted.

and LV ejection fraction <35% with class 2 or 3 heart failure symptoms. Additional study will be required to determine if patients with lesser degrees of LV dysfunction may also warrant primary ICD implantation. A potential proarrhythmic risk of antiarrhythmic drug therapy should be acknowledged, and drug therapy should be reserved for symptomatic arrhythmias and limited to amiodarone or sotalol if an ICD is not present.

Arrhythmogenic RV Cardiomyopathy/ Dysplasia (ARVCM/D)

(See also Chap. 21) ARVCM/D, due to a genetically determined dysplastic process or after a suspected viral myocarditis, is also associated with VT/VF. The sporadic nonfamilial/nondysplastic form of RV cardiomyopathy appears to be more common; however, this may vary based on ethnicity. In patients predisposed to VT, there appears to be a predominance of perivalvular fibrosis involving mostly the free wall of the right ventricle in proximity to the tricuspid and pulmonic valves. The surface ECG leads that reflect RV activation, including V_1–V_3, may show terminal notching of the QRS complex and inverted T waves in sinus rhythm. When the terminal notching is distinct and appears separated from the QRS complex, it is referred to as an *epsilon wave* (**Fig. 16-14**). Epsilon waves are consistent with markedly delayed ventricular activation in the region of the RV free wall near the base of the tricuspid and pulmonic valves in areas of extensive fibrosis.

In patients with ARVCM/D, echocardiography demonstrates RV enlargement with RV wall motion abnormalities and RV apical aneurysm formation. MRI may show fatty replacement of the ventricle, thinning of the RV free wall with increased fibrosis, and associated wall motion abnormalities. Because of the presence of extensive amounts of fat normally covering the epicardium in the region of the RV, caution must be used to not overinterpret the MRI in trying to determine the appropriate diagnosis. Patients tend to have multiple VT morphologies. The VT will typically have a left bundle branch block type QRS pattern in V_1 and tend to have poor R wave progression in V_1 through V_6, consistent with an RV free-wall origin. Areas of low electrogram voltage, identified during RV catheter endocardial sinus rhythm voltage mapping, may be helpful in confirming

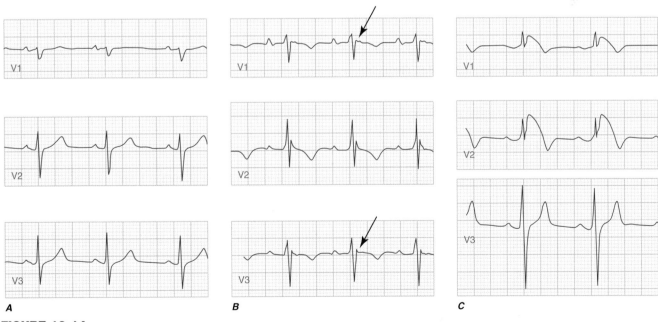

FIGURE 16-14

Leads V_1 to V_3 in sinus rhythm from a normal subject (**A**); from a patient with arrhythmogenic right ventricular cardiomyopathy showing epsilon waves (*arrow*) and T wave inversion (**B**); and from a patient with Brugada syndrome with ST-segment elevation in V_1 and V_2 (**C**).

the diagnosis. Importantly, endocardial biopsy may not identify the presence of fatty replacement or fibrosis unless directed to the basal RV free wall. The familial forms of this syndrome have been linked to a number of desmosomal protein mutations. A distinct genetic form of this syndrome, Naxos disease, consists of arrhythmogenic RV dysplasia coupled with palmar-plantar keratosis and woolly hair and is associated with a high risk of SCD in adolescents and young adults.

Treatment:
Rx **ARRHYTHMOGENIC RIGHT VENTRICULAR CARDIOMYOPATHY/ DYSPLASIA**

The threshold for ICD implantation in patients with an established diagnosis of ARVCM/D is low. An ICD will typically be implanted in patients deemed to have a persistent VT risk, those who have had spontaneous or inducible rapid VTs, and those patients who show concomitant LV cardiomyopathy. Treatment options for recurrent VT in patients with ARVCM/D include the use of the antiarrhythmic agent sotalol. Beta blockers serve as useful adjunctive therapy when coupled with other antiarrhythmic agents. Catheter ablative therapy directed at mappable sustained ventricular arrhythmias is also highly successful in controlling recurrent VT. In selected patients with multiple VT morphologies and unstable VT, linear ablation lesions directed at endocardial and, if required, epicardial scarring, defined by catheter-based bipolar voltage mapping, provide significant amelioration of the recurrent VT episodes.

VT After Operative Tetralogy of Fallot Repair

VT may also occur after surgical repair of tetralogy of Fallot. Patients typically develop VT many years after the surgery. VT tends to occur in patients with evidence of RV systolic dysfunction. The VT mechanism and location are typically a macroreentrant circuit around the right ventriculotomy scar to the valve annuli. Catheter ablation creating linear lesions that extend from either the pulmonic or tricuspid annuli to the ventriculotomy scar is typically effective in preventing arrhythmia recurrences. An ICD is usually implanted in patients who manifest rapid VT, have persistent inducible VT after ablation, or have concomitant LV dysfunction.

Fascicular Tachycardia Caused by Digoxin Toxicity

Digoxin toxicity can produce increased ventricular ectopy and, when coupled with bradyarrhythmias caused

by digoxin toxicity, may predispose to sustained polymorphic ventricular arrhythmias and VF. The signature VT associated with digoxin toxicity is bidirectional VT (**Fig. 16-15**). This unique VT is due to triggered activity associated with calcium overload resulting from the inhibition of sodium/potassium ATPase by digoxin. Bidirectional VT originates from the left anterior and posterior fascicles, creating a relatively narrow QRS right bundle branch configuration with beat-to-beat alternating right and left frontal plane QRS axis. This VT is uncommonly observed in the absence of digoxin toxicity. Treatment for bidirectional VT or other hemodynamically significant arrhythmias due to digoxin excess includes correction of electrolyte disorders and the IV infusion of digoxin-specific Fab fragments. The antibody fragments will, over the course of 1 h, bind digoxin and eliminate toxic effects. In the setting of normal renal function, the bound complex is secreted.

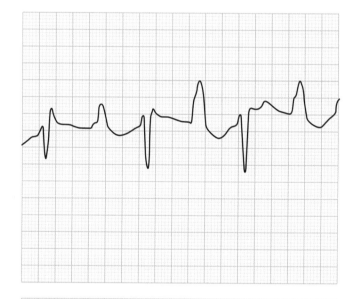

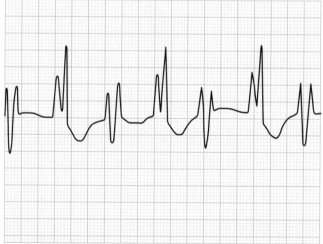

FIGURE 16-15

Digoxin toxic bidirectional fascicular tachycardia.

GENETICALLY DETERMINED ABNORMALITIES THAT PREDISPOSE TO POLYMORPHIC VENTRICULAR ARRHYTHMIAS

Ion channel defects that affect cardiac depolarization and repolarization may predispose to life-threatening polymorphic VT and SCD. These defects frequently produce unique ECG characteristics during sinus rhythm that facilitate the diagnosis.

Long QT Syndrome (LQTS)

The congenital form of the LQTS consists of defects in cardiac ion channels that are responsible for cardiac repolarization. Defects that enhance sodium or calcium inward currents or inhibit outward potassium currents during the plateau phase of the action potential lengthen action potential duration and, hence, the QT interval. Of the eight genetic mutations identified to date, five affect the α or β subunits of the three different potassium channels involved with repolarization (Table 16-8). Since many patients with QT prolongation do not have one of the defined mutations, it is anticipated that other genetic abnormalities affecting repolarization channel function will be identified.

The triggers for the ventricular arrhythmias are thought to be due to early afterdepolarizations potentiated by intracellular calcium accumulation from a prolonged action potential plateau. Heterogeneity of myocardial repolarization indexed by a longer QT interval predisposes to polymorphic ventricular arrhythmias in response to the triggers (Fig. 16-9).

In most patients with LQTS, the QT interval corrected for heart rate using Bazette's formula is 4–460 ms in men and 4–480 ms in women. Marked lengthening of the QT interval to >500 ms is clearly associated with a greater arrhythmia risk in patients with the LQTS. Many affected individuals may have QT intervals that intermittently measure within a normal range or that fail to shorten appropriately with exercise. Some individuals will only manifest the syndrome when exposed to a drug, such as sotalol, that alters channel function.

The genotype associated with the LQTS appears to influence prognosis, and identification of the genotype appears to help to optimize clinical management. The first three genotypic designations of the mutations identified, LQT1, LQT2, and LQT3, appear to account for >99% of patients with clinically relevant LQTSs. Surface ECG characteristics may be helpful in distinguishing the three most common genotypes, with genetic testing being definitive.

LQT1 represents the most common genotypic abnormality. Patients with LQT1 fail to shorten or actually prolong their QT interval with exercise. The T wave in patients with LQT1 tends to be broad and comprises the majority of the prolonged QT interval. The most common triggers for potentiating cardiac arrhythmias in patients with LQT1 are exercise followed by emotional stress.

More than 80% of male patients have their first cardiac event by 20 years, so competitive exercise should be restricted and swimming avoided for these patients. Patients tend to respond to beta blocker therapy. Patients with two LQT1 alleles have the Jervell and Lange-Neilsen

TABLE 16-8

INHERITED ARRHYTHMIA DISORDERS—"CHANNELOPATHIES" WITH HIGH RISK OF VENTRICULAR ARRHYTHMIAS

DISORDER	GENE	PROTEIN/CHANNEL AFFECTED
LQT1	*KCNQ1*	I_{Ks} channel α subunit
LQT2	*KCNH2 (HERG)*	I_{Kr} channel α subunit
LQT3	*SCN5A*	I_{Na} channel α subunit
LQT4	*ANK2*	Ankyrin-B
LQT5	*KCNE1*	I_{Ks} channel β subunit
LQT6	*KCNE2*	I_{Kr} channel β subunit
LQT7	*KCNJ2*	I_{K1} channel α subunit
LQT8	*CACNA1C*	I_{Ca} channel α subunit
Jervell LN1	*KCNQ1*	I_{Ks} channel β subunit
Jervell LN2	*KCNE1*	I_{Kr} channel β subunit
Brugada syndrome	*SCN5A*	I_{Na} channel
Catecholaminergic VT	*Ry R2*	Ryanodine receptor, calsequestron receptor
SQTS1	*KCNH2 (HERG)*	I_{Kr} channel α subunit
SQTS2	*KCNQ1 (KvLQT1)*	I_{Ks} channel α subunit
SQTS3	*KCNJ2*	I_{K1} channel

Note: LQT, long QT (interval); SQT, short QT (interval).

syndrome, with more dramatic QT prolongation and deafness and a worse arrhythmia prognosis.

LQT2 is the second most common genotypic abnormality. The T wave tends to be notched and bifid. In LQT2 patients, the most frequent precipitant is emotional stress, followed by sleep or auditory stimulation. Despite the occurrence during sleep, patients typically respond to beta blocker therapy.

LQT3 is due to a mutation in the gene that encodes the cardiac sodium channel located on chromosome 3. Prolongation of the action potential duration occurs because of failure to inactivate this channel. LQT3 patients either have late-onset peaked biphasic T waves or asymmetric peaked T waves. The arrhythmia events tend to be more life-threatening, and thus the prognosis for LQT3 is the poorest of all the LQTs. Male patients appear to have the worst prognosis in patients with LQT3. Most events in LQT3 patients occur during sleep, suggesting that they are at higher risk during slow heart rates. Beta blockers are not recommended, and exercise is not restricted in LQT3.

℞ Treatment: LONG QT SYNDROME

The institution of ICD therapy should be strongly considered in any patient with LQTS who has demonstrated any life-threatening arrhythmia. Patients with syncope with a confirmed diagnosis based on unequivocal ECG criteria or positive genetic testing should also be given the same strong consideration. Primary prevention with prophylactic ICD implantation should be considered in male patients with LQT3 and in all patients with marked QT prolongation (>500 ms), particularly when coupled with an immediate family history of SCD. Future epidemiologic investigation may provide firmer guidelines to sort patients further based on risks such as age, gender, arrhythmia history, and genetic characteristics. In all patients with documented or suspected LQTS, drugs that prolong the QT interval must be avoided. For an updated list of drugs, go to *www.qtdrugs.org*.

Acquired LQTS

Patients with a genetic predisposition related to what appear to be sporadic mutations and/or single nucleotide polymorphisms can develop marked QT prolongation in response to drugs that alter repolarization currents. The QT prolongation and associated polymorphic ventricular tachycardia (TdP) are more frequently seen in women and may be a manifestation of subclinical LQTS. Drug-induced long QT and TdP are frequently potentiated by the development of hypokalemia and bradycardia. The offending drugs typically block the potassium I_{Kr} channel (Table 16-5). Since most drug effects are dose-dependent, important drug-drug interactions that alter metabolism

and/or alterations in elimination kinetics because of hepatic or renal dysfunction frequently contribute to the arrhythmias.

℞ Treatment: ACQUIRED LONG QT SYNDROME

Acute therapy for acquired LQTS is directed at eliminating the offending drug therapy, reversing metabolic abnormalities by the infusion of magnesium and/or potassium, and preventing pause-dependent arrhythmias by temporary pacing or the cautious infusion of isoproterenol. Class IB antiarrhythmic agents (e.g., lidocaine), which do not cause QT prolongation, may also be used, though they are frequently ineffective. Supportive therapy to allay anxiety and prevent pain with required DC shock therapy for sustained arrhythmias as well as efforts to facilitate drug elimination are important.

Short QT Syndrome

A gain in function of repolarization currents can result in a shortening of atrial and ventricular refractoriness and marked QT shortening on the surface ECG (Table 16-8). The T wave tends to be tall and peaked. A QT interval <320 ms is required to establish the diagnosis of this uncommon syndrome. Mutations in the *HERG*, *KvLQT1*, and *KCNJ2* genes have been identified. Patients with the syndrome are predisposed to both AF and VF. ICD implantation is recommended. Double counting of QRS and T waves may lead to inappropriate ICD shocks. Drug therapy with quinidine has been used to lengthen the QT interval and reduce the amplitude of the T wave. This therapy is currently being evaluated to determine long-term efficacy in preventing arrhythmias in this syndrome.

Brugada Syndrome

Mutations of *SCN5A* genes resulting in diminished inward sodium current in the region of the RV outflow tract epicardium appear responsible for the Brugada syndrome (Table 16-8). A loss of the action potential dome in the RV epicardium due to unopposed I_{To} potassium outward current results in dramatic action potential shortening. The large potential difference between the normal endocardium and rapidly depolarized RV outflow epicardium gives rise to ST-segment elevation in V_1-V_3 in sinus rhythm and predisposes to local reentry and life-threatening ventricular arrhythmias in the absence of structural heart disease (Fig. 16-14). Although identified in both genders and all races, the arrhythmia syndrome is most common in young Asian male patients and is thought to be responsible for the sudden and unexpected nocturnal death syndrome (SUDS) previously described in Southeast Asian men.

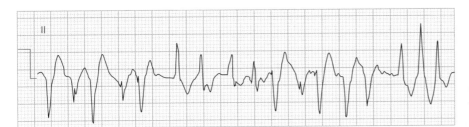

FIGURE 16-16
Catecholaminergic polymorphic ventricular tachycardia noted during an exercise stress test.

℞ Treatment:
BRUGADA SYNDROME

Patients do not benefit from beta blocker therapy. Sodium channel-blocking drugs, such as procainamide and flecainide, can exacerbate the syndrome and are used as a provocative test to identify the presence of the abnormality in family members with a more limited expression of the genetic abnormality. This drug challenge may also be important to establish more firmly the diagnosis and the probable cause of unexplained syncope when the surface ECG is equivocal. Acute management of recurrent VT has been reported to respond to isoproterenol administration or quinidine, although the efficacy of this treatment requires more extensive study. ICD treatment to manage recurrences is recommended for all patients who have had documented arrhythmia episodes. Family members should be screened for the presence of the abnormality. A history of syncope, spontaneous ST-segment elevation, and inducibility of VT with programmed stimulation may identify family members also at risk for SCD who warrant prophylactic ICD therapy.

Catecholaminergic Polymorphic VT

A mutation of the myocardial ryanodine release channel, which effectively creates a "leak" in calcium from the sarcoplasmic reticulum, has been identified in patients with catecholaminergic VT (Table 16-8). The accumulation of intracellular calcium potentiates delayed afterdepolarizations and triggered activity. Patients can manifest bidirectional VT, nonsustained polymorphic VT, or recurrent VF. Both an autosomal dominant familial and sporadic forms of the disease have been described. More recently, an autosomal recessive variant associated with a mutation in the sarcoplasmic reticulum calcium–buffering protein, calsequestrin, has also been identified. The arrhythmias are precipitated by exercise and emotional stress (**Fig. 16-16**). Exercise restriction is warranted. Treatment with beta blockers and ICD implantation has been recommended. Prevention of inappropriate or easily triggered ICD shocks by proper ICD programming are essential to prevent VT storm from endogenous catecholamine release.

FURTHER READINGS

CAPPATO R et al: Worldwide survey on the methods, efficacy, and safety of catheter ablation for human atrial fibrillation. Circulation 111(9):1100, 2005

DELACRETAZ E: Clinical practice. Supraventricular tachycardia. N Engl J Med 354(10):1039, 2006

FUSTER V et al: ACC/AHA/ESC 2006 guidelines for the management of patients with atrial fibrillation. Circulation 114:e257, 2006

HAISSAGUERRE M et al: Spontaneous initiation of atrial fibrillation by ectopic beats originating in the pulmonary veins. N Engl J Med 339(10):659, 1998

JOSEPHSON ME: *Clinical Cardiac Electrophysiology: Techniques and Interpretations*, 3d ed. Philadelphia, Lippincott Williams & Wilkins, 2002

———: *Clinical Cardiac Electrophysiology: Techniques and Interpretations*, 4th ed. Philadelphia, Lippincott Williams & Wilkins, 2008

KEATING MJ, SANGUINETTI MC: Molecular and cellular mechanisms of cardiac arrhythmia. Cell 104:569, 2001

MARCHLINSKI FE et al: Electroanatomic substrate and outcome of catheter ablative therapy for ventricular tachycardia in setting of right ventricular cardiomyopathy. Circulation 110(16):2293, 2004

——— et al: Ventricular tachycardia/ventricular fibrillation ablation in the setting of ischemic heart disease. J Cardiovasc Electrophysiol 16(1):59, 2005

MILLER JM, ZIPES DP: Therapy for cardiac arrhythmias, in *Braunwald's Heart Disease: A Textbook of Cardiovascular Medicine*, 7th ed. DP Zipes et al (eds). Philadelphia, Saunders, 2005, pp 712–756

PAGE RL: Medical management of atrial fibrillation: Future directions. Heart Rhythm 4:580, 2007

PRIORI SG et al: Clinical and molecular characterization of patients with the catecholaminergic polymorphic ventricular tachycardia. Circulation 106:69, 2002

——— et al: Risk stratification in the long QT syndrome. N Engl J Med 348:1866, 2003

RODEN DM: Drug-induced prolongation of the QT interval. N Engl J Med 350:1013, 2004

TAYLOR FC et al: Systematic review of long term anticoagulation or antiplatelet treatment in patients with non-rheumatic atrial fibrillation. BMJ 322:321, 2001

VAN GELDER IC et al: Rate Control versus Electrical Cardioversion for Persistent Atrial Fibrillation Study Group. A comparison of rate control and rhythm control in patients with recurrent persistent atrial fibrillation. N Engl J Med 347(23):1834, 2002

WELLENS HJ: Contemporary management of atrial flutter. Circulation 106:649, 2002

WYSE DG et al: AFFIRM: A comparison of rate control and rhythm control in patients with atrial fibrillation. N Engl J Med 347:1825, 2002

ZIPES DP et al: ACC/AHA/ESC 2006 guidelines for management of patients with ventricular arrhythmias and the prevention of sudden cardiac death. Circulation 114:e385, 2006

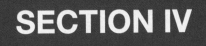

SECTION IV

DISORDERS OF THE HEART

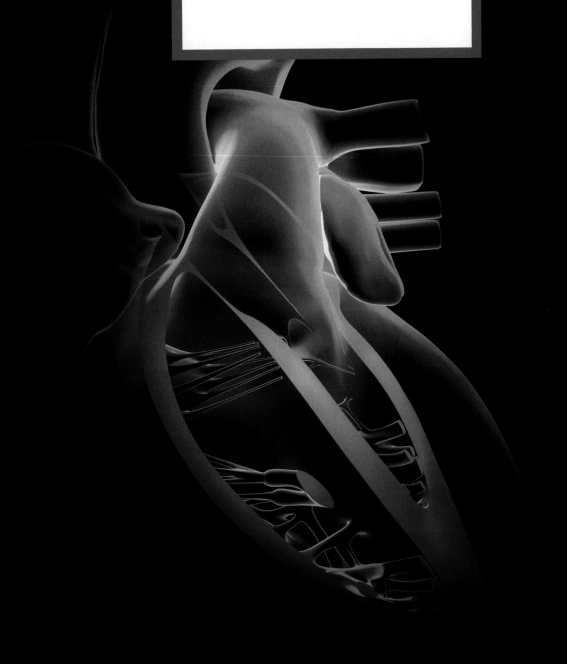

CHAPTER 17

HEART FAILURE AND COR PULMONALE

Douglas L. Mann

HEART FAILURE

DEFINITION

Heart failure (HF) is a clinical syndrome that occurs in patients who, because of an inherited or acquired abnormality of cardiac structure and/or function, develop a constellation of clinical symptoms (dyspnea and fatigue) and signs (edema and rales) that lead to frequent hospitalizations, a poor quality of life, and a shortened life expectancy.

EPIDEMIOLOGY

HF is a burgeoning problem worldwide, with more than 20 million people affected. The overall prevalence of HF in the adult population in developed countries is 2%. HF prevalence follows an exponential pattern, rising with age, and affects 6–10% of people older than 65 years. Although the relative incidence of HF is lower in women than in men, women constitute at least half of the cases of HF because of their longer life expectancy. In North America and Europe, the lifetime risk of developing HF is approximately one in five for a 40-year-old. The overall prevalence of HF is thought to be increasing, in part because current therapies of cardiac disorders, such as myocardial infarction (MI), valvular heart disease, and arrhythmias, are allowing patients to survive longer. Very little is known with respect to the prevalence or risk of developing HF in emerging nations because of the lack of population-based studies in these countries. Although HF was once thought to arise primarily in the setting of a depressed left ventricular (LV) ejection fraction (EF), epidemiological studies have shown that approximately one-half of patients who develop HF have a normal or preserved EF (EF ≥40–50%). Accordingly, HF patients are now broadly categorized into one of two groups: (1) HF with a depressed EF (commonly referred to as *systolic failure*) or (2) HF with a preserved EF (commonly referred to as *diastolic failure*).

ETIOLOGY

As shown in **Table 17-1**, a condition that leads to an alteration in LV structure or function can predispose a patient to developing HF. Although the etiology of HF in patients with a preserved EF differs from that of those with depressed EF, there is considerable overlap between the etiologies of these two conditions. In industrialized countries, coronary artery disease (CAD) has become the predominant cause in men and women and is responsible for 60–75% of cases of HF. Hypertension contributes to the development of HF in 75% of patients, including

TABLE 17-1

ETIOLOGIES OF HEART FAILURE

Depressed Ejection Fraction (<40%)

Coronary artery disease
   Myocardial infarction[a]
   Myocardial ischemia[a]
Chronic pressure overload
   Hypertension[a]
   Obstructive valvular disease[a]
Chronic volume overload
   Regurgitant valvular disease
   Intracardiac (left-to-right) shunting
   Extracardiac shunting
	Nonischemic dilated cardiomyopathy
	   Familial/genetic disorders
	   Infiltrative disorders[a]
	   Toxic/drug-induced damage
	   Metabolic disorder[a]
	   Viral
	   Chagas' disease
	Disorders of rate and rhythm
	   Chronic bradyarrhythmias
	   Chronic tachyarrhythmias

Preserved Ejection Fraction (>40–50%)

Pathological hypertrophy
   Primary (hypertrophic cardiomyopathies)
   Secondary (hypertension)
Aging
	Restrictive cardiomyopathy
	   Infiltrative disorders (amyloidosis, sarcoidosis)
	   Storage diseases (hemochromatosis)
	Fibrosis
	Endomyocardial disorders

Pulmonary Heart Disease

Cor pulmonale Pulmonary vascular disorders	

High-Output States

Metabolic disorders
   Thyrotoxicosis
   Nutritional disorders (beriberi)
	Excessive blood-flow requirements
	   Systemic arteriovenous shunting
	   Chronic anemia

[a]**Note:** Indicates conditions that can also lead to heart failure with a preserved ejection fraction.

most patients with CAD. Both CAD and hypertension interact to augment the risk of HF, as does diabetes mellitus.

In 20–30% of the cases of HF with a depressed EF, the exact etiologic basis is not known. These patients are referred to as having nonischemic, dilated, or idiopathic cardiomyopathy if the cause is unknown (Chap. 21). Prior viral infection or toxin exposure (e.g., alcoholic or chemotherapeutic) may also lead to a dilated cardiomyopathy. Moreover, it is becoming increasingly clear that a large number of the cases of dilated cardiomyopathy are secondary to specific genetic defects, most notably those in the cytoskeleton. Most of the forms of familial dilated cardiomyopathy are inherited in an autosomal dominant fashion. Mutations of genes encoding cytoskeletal proteins (desmin, cardiac myosin, vinculin) and nuclear membrane proteins (lamin) have been identified thus far. Dilated cardiomyopathy is also associated with Duchenne's, Becker's, and limb girdle muscular dystrophies. Conditions that lead to a high cardiac output (e.g., arteriovenous fistula, anemia) are seldom responsible for the development of HF in a normal heart. However, in the presence of underlying structural heart disease, these conditions can lead to overt HF.

GLOBAL CONSIDERATIONS

Rheumatic heart disease remains a major cause of HF in Africa and Asia, especially in the young. Hypertension is an important cause of HF in the African and African-American populations. Chagas' disease is still a major cause of HF in South America. Not surprisingly, anemia is a frequent concomitant factor in HF in many developing nations. As developing nations undergo socioeconomic development, the epidemiology of HF is becoming similar to that of Western Europe and North America, with CAD emerging as the single most common cause of HF. Although the contribution of diabetes mellitus to HF is not well understood, diabetes accelerates atherosclerosis and is often associated with hypertension.

PROGNOSIS

Despite many recent advances in the evaluation and management of HF, the development of symptomatic HF still carries a poor prognosis. Community-based studies indicate that 30–40% of patients die within 1 year of diagnosis and 60–70% die within 5 years, mainly from worsening HF or as a sudden event (probably because of a ventricular arrhythmia). Although it is difficult to predict prognosis in an individual, patients with symptoms at rest [New York Heart Association (NYHA) class IV] have a 30–70% annual mortality rate, whereas patients with symptoms with moderate activity (NYHA class II) have an annual mortality rate of 5–10%. Thus, functional status is an important predictor of patient outcome.

PATHOGENESIS

Figure 17-1 provides a general conceptual framework for considering the development and progression of HF with a depressed EF. As shown, HF may be viewed as a progressive disorder that is initiated after an *index event* either damages the heart muscle, with a resultant loss of functioning cardiac myocytes, or alternatively disrupts the ability of the myocardium to generate force, thereby preventing the heart from contracting normally. This index event may have an abrupt onset, as in the case of a MI; it may have a gradual or insidious onset, as in the case of hemodynamic pressure or volume overloading; or it may be hereditary, as in the case of many of the genetic cardiomyopathies. Regardless of the nature of the inciting event, the feature that is common to each of these index events is that they all, in some manner,

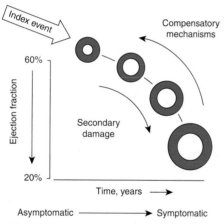

FIGURE 17-1

Pathogenesis of heart failure with a depressed ejection fraction. Heart failure begins after an index event produces an initial decline in the heart's pumping capacity. Following this initial decline in pumping capacity, a variety of compensatory mechanisms are activated, including the adrenergic nervous system, the renin-angiotensin-aldosterone system and the cytokine system. In the short term, these systems are able to restore cardiovascular function to a normal homeostatic range with the result that the patient remains asymptomatic. However, with time the sustained activation of these systems can lead to secondary end-organ damage within the ventricle, with worsening left-ventricular remodeling and subsequent cardiac decompensation. (*From D Mann: Circulation 100:999, 1999.*)

produce a decline in the pumping capacity of the heart. In most instances patients remain asymptomatic or minimally symptomatic following the initial decline in pumping capacity of the heart, or develop symptoms only after the dysfunction has been present for some time. Thus, when viewed within this conceptual framework, LV dysfunction is necessary, but not sufficient, for the development of the syndrome of HF.

Although the precise reasons why patients with LV dysfunction may remain asymptomatic is not certain, one potential explanation is that a number of compensatory mechanisms become activated in the presence of cardiac injury and/or LV dysfunction, and they appear to be able to sustain and modulate LV function for a period of months to years. The list of compensatory mechanisms that have been described thus far include (1) activation of the renin-angiotensin-aldosterone (RAA) and adrenergic nervous systems, which are responsible for maintaining cardiac output through increased retention of salt and water (**Fig. 17-2**), and (2) increased myocardial contractility. In addition, there is activation of a family of countervailing vasodilatory molecules, including the atrial and brain natriuretic peptides (ANP and BNP), prostaglandins (PGE_2 and PGI_2), and nitric oxide (NO), that offset the excessive peripheral vascular vasoconstriction. Genetic background, gender, age, or environment may influence these compensatory mechanisms, which are able to modulate LV function within a physiologic/homeostatic range, such that the functional capacity of the patient is preserved or is depressed only minimally. Thus, patients may remain asymptomatic or minimally symptomatic for a period of years. However, at some point patients become overtly symptomatic, with a resultant striking increase in morbidity and mortality. Although the exact mechanisms that are responsible for this transition are not known, as will be discussed below, the transition to symptomatic HF is accompanied by increasing activation of neurohormonal, adrenergic, and cytokine systems that lead to a series of adaptive changes within the myocardium, collectively referred to as *LV remodeling*.

In contrast to our understanding of the pathogenesis of HF with a depressed EF, our understanding of the mechanisms that contribute to the development of HF with a preserved EF is still evolving. That is, although diastolic dysfunction (see later) was thought to be the only mechanism responsible for the development of HF with a preserved EF, community-based studies suggest that additional mechanisms, such as increased vascular and ventricular (*ventricular-vascular*) stiffness, may also be important.

BASIC MECHANISMS OF HEART FAILURE

LV remodeling develops in response to a series of complex events that occur at the cellular and molecular levels. These changes include: (1) myocyte hypertrophy;

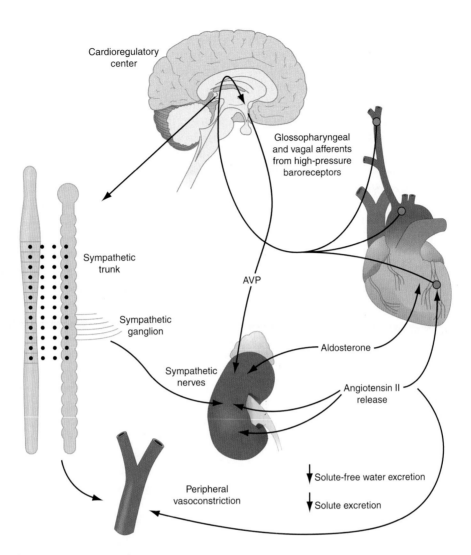

Cardioregulatory center

Glossopharyngeal and vagal afferents from high-pressure baroreceptors

Sympathetic trunk

AVP

Sympathetic ganglion

Sympathetic nerves

Aldosterone

Angiotensin II release

↓ Solute-free water excretion

↓ Solute excretion

Peripheral vasoconstriction

CHAPTER 17 Heart Failure and Cor Pulmonale

FIGURE 17-2

Activation of neurohormonal systems in heart failure. The decreased cardiac output in HF patients results in an "unloading" of high-pressure baroceptors (circles) in the left ventricle, carotid sinus, and aortic arch. This unloading leads to the generation of afferent signals to the central nervous system (CNS) that stimulate cardioregulatory centers in the brain which stimulate the release of arginine vasopression (AVP) from the posterior pituitary. AVP [or antidiuretic hormone (ADH)] is a powerful vasoconstrictor that increases the permeability of the renal collecting ducts, leading to the reabsorption of free water. These afferent signals to the CNS also activate efferent sympathetic nervous system pathways that innervate the heart, kidney, peripheral vasculature, and skeletal muscles. Sympathetic stimulation of the kidney leads to the release of renin, with a resultant increase in the circulating levels of angiotensin II and aldosterone. The activation of the renin-angiotensin-aldosterone system promotes salt and water retention and leads to vasoconstriction of the peripheral vasculature, myocyte hypertrophy, myocyte cell death, and myocardial fibrosis. While these neurohormonal mechanisms facilitate short-term adaptation by maintaining blood pressure, and hence perfusion to vital organs, these same neurohormonal mechanisms are believed to contribute to end-organ changes in the heart and the circulation, and to the excessive salt and water retention in advanced HF. *[From E Braunwald: Pathophysiology of heart failure, in Braunwald's Heart Disease, 7th ed, D Zipes et al (eds). Philadelphia, Elsevier Saunders, pp 509–538, 2005; and adapted from Schrier RW, Abraham WT: N Engl J Med 341:577, 1999.]*

(2) alterations in the contractile properties of the myocyte; (3) progressive loss of myocytes through necrosis, apoptosis, and autophagic cell death; (4) β-adrenergic desensitization; (5) abnormal myocardial energetics and metabolism; and (6) reorganization of the extracellular matrix with dissolution of the organized structural collagen weave surrounding myocytes and subsequent replacement by an interstitial collagen matrix that does not provide structural support to the myocytes. The biological stimuli for these profound changes include mechanical stretch of the myocyte, circulating neurohormones (e.g., norepinephrine, angiotensin II), inflammatory cytokines [e.g., tumor necrosis factor (TNF)], other peptides and growth factors (e.g., endothelin), and

reactive oxygen species (e.g., superoxide, NO). Although these molecules are collectively referred to as *neurohormones*, this historical terminology is somewhat misleading insofar as the classical neurohormones, such as norepinephrine and angiotensin II, may also be synthesized directly within the myocardium and thus may also act in an autocrine and paracrine manner. Nonetheless, the overarching concept is that the sustained overexpression of these biologically active molecules contributes to the progression of HF by virtue of the deleterious effects that they exert on the heart and the circulation. Indeed, this insight forms the clinical rationale for using pharmacologic agents that antagonize these systems [e.g., angiotensin-converting enzyme (ACE) inhibitors and beta blockers] in treating patients with HF.

Systolic Dysfunction

In order to understand how the changes that occur in the failing cardiac myocyte contribute to depressed LV systolic function in HF, it is instructive first to review the biology of the cardiac muscle cell (Chap. 1). Sustained neurohormonal activation results in transcriptional and posttranscriptional changes in the genes and proteins that regulate excitation–contraction coupling and cross-bridge interaction (Fig. 1-7). Collectively these changes impair the ability of the myocyte to contract and, therefore, contribute to the depressed LV systolic function observed in patients with HF.

Diastolic Dysfunction

Myocardial relaxation is an ATP-dependent process that is regulated by uptake of cytoplasmic calcium into the sarcoplasmic reticulum (SR) by sarcoplasmic reticulum Ca^{2+} adenosine triphosphatase (SERCA2A) and extrusion of calcium by sarcolemmal pumps (Fig. 1-7). Accordingly, reductions in ATP concentration, as occurs in ischemia, may interfere with these processes and lead to slowed myocardial relaxation. Alternatively, if LV filling is delayed because LV compliance is reduced (e.g., from hypertrophy or fibrosis), LV filling pressures will similarly remain elevated at end diastole (Fig. 1-11). An increase in heart rate disproportionately shortens the time for diastolic filling, which may lead to elevated LV filling pressures, particularly in noncompliant ventricles. Elevated LV end-diastolic filling pressures result in increases in pulmonary capillary pressures, which can contribute to the dyspnea experienced by patients with diastolic dysfunction. Importantly, diastolic dysfunction can occur alone or in combination with systolic dysfunction in patients with HF.

Left Ventricular Remodeling

Ventricular remodeling refers to the changes in LV mass, volume, shape, and composition of the heart that occur following cardiac injury and/or abnormal hemodynamic loading conditions. LV remodeling may contribute independently to the progression of HF by virtue of the mechanical burdens that are engendered by the changes in the geometry of the remodeled LV. For example, the change in LV shape from a prolate ellipsoid of revolution to a more spherical shape during LV remodeling results in an increase in meridional wall stress of the LV, which creates a de novo mechanical burden for the failing heart. In addition to the increase in LV end-diastolic volume, LV wall thinning also occurs as the left ventricle begins to dilate. The increase in wall thinning along with the increase in afterload created by LV dilation leads to a functional *afterload mismatch* that may contribute further to a decrease in stroke volume. Moreover, the high end-diastolic wall stress might be expected to lead to: (1) hypoperfusion of the subendocardium, with resultant worsening of LV function; (2) increased oxidative stress, with the resultant activation of families of genes that are sensitive to free radical generation (e.g., TNF and interleukin-1β); and (3) sustained expression of stretch-activated genes (angiotensin II, endothelin, and TNF) and/or stretch activation of hypertrophic signaling pathways.

A second important problem that results from increased sphericity of the ventricle is that the papillary muscles are pulled apart, resulting in incompetence of the mitral valve and the development of functional mitral regurgitation. In addition to the loss of forward blood flow, mitral regurgitation also results in further hemodynamic overloading of the ventricle. Taken together, the mechanical burdens that are engendered by LV remodeling can be expected to lead to decreased forward cardiac output, increased LV dilation (stretch), and increased hemodynamic overloading, all of which are sufficient to contribute to the progression of HF.

CLINICAL MANIFESTATIONS

Symptoms

The cardinal symptoms of HF are fatigue and shortness of breath. Although fatigue has been traditionally ascribed to the low cardiac output in HF, it is likely that skeletal-muscle abnormalities and other noncardiac comorbidities (e.g., anemia) also contribute to the symptom. In the early stages of HF, dyspnea is observed only during exertion; however, as the disease progresses, dyspnea occurs with less strenuous activity, and ultimately may occur even at rest. The origin of dyspnea in HF is likely multifactorial (Chap. 5). The most important mechanism is pulmonary congestion with accumulation of interstitial or intra-alveolar fluid, which activates juxtacapillary J receptors, which in turn stimulate rapid, shallow breathing characteristic of cardiac dyspnea. Other factors that contribute to dyspnea on exertion include reductions in pulmonary compliance, increased airway resistance, respiratory muscle and/or diaphragm fatigue, and anemia. Dyspnea may become less frequent with the onset of right ventricular (RV) failure and tricuspid regurgitation.

Orthopnea

Orthopnea, which is defined as dyspnea occurring in the recumbent position, is usually a later manifestation of HF than is exertional dyspnea. It results from the redistribution of fluid from the splanchnic circulation and lower extremities into the central circulation during recumbency, with a resultant increase in pulmonary capillary pressure. Nocturnal cough is a frequent manifestation of this process and a frequently overlooked symptom of HF. Orthopnea is generally relieved by sitting upright or by sleeping with additional pillows. Although orthopnea is a relatively specific symptom of HF, it may occur in patients with abdominal obesity or ascites and in patients with pulmonary disease whose lung mechanics favor an upright posture.

Paroxysmal nocturnal dyspnea (PND)

This term refers to acute episodes of severe shortness of breath and coughing that generally occur at night and awaken the patient from sleep, usually 1–3 h after the patient retires. PND may be manifest by coughing or wheezing, possibly because of increased pressure in the bronchial arteries leading to airway compression, along with interstitial pulmonary edema leading to increased airway resistance. Whereas orthopnea may be relieved by sitting upright at the side of the bed with the legs in a dependent position, patients with PND often have persistent coughing and wheezing even after they have assumed the upright position. *Cardiac asthma* is closely related to PND, is characterized by wheezing secondary to bronchospasm, and must be differentiated from primary asthma and pulmonary causes of wheezing.

Cheyne-Stokes Respiration

Also referred to as periodic respiration or cyclic respiration, Cheyne-Stokes respiration is common in advanced HF and is usually associated with low cardiac output. Cheyne-Stokes respiration is caused by a diminished sensitivity of the respiratory center to arterial P_{CO_2}. There is an apneic phase, during which the arterial P_{O_2} falls and the arterial P_{CO_2} rises. These changes in the arterial blood gas content stimulate the depressed respiratory center, resulting in hyperventilation and hypocapnia, followed in turn by recurrence of apnea. Cheyne-Stokes respirations may be perceived by the patient or the patient's family as severe dyspnea or as a transient cessation of breathing.

Acute Pulmonary Edema

See Chap. 28 for details on this topic.

Other Symptoms

Patients with HF may also present with gastrointestinal symptoms. Anorexia, nausea, and early satiety associated with abdominal pain and fullness are frequent complaints and may be related to edema of the bowel wall and/or a congested liver. Congestion of the liver and stretching of its capsule may lead to right-upper-quadrant pain. Cerebral symptoms, such as confusion, disorientation, and sleep and mood disturbances, may be observed in patients with severe HF, particularly elderly patients with cerebral arteriosclerosis and reduced cerebral perfusion. Nocturia is common in HF and may contribute to insomnia.

PHYSICAL EXAMINATION

A careful physical examination is always warranted in the evaluation of patients with HF. The purpose of the examination is to help determine the cause of HF, as well as to assess the severity of the syndrome. Obtaining additional information about the hemodynamic profile and the response to therapy and determining the prognosis are important additional goals of the physical examination.

General Appearance and Vital Signs

In mild or moderately severe HF, the patient appears in no distress at rest, except for feeling uncomfortable when lying flat for more than a few minutes. In more severe HF, the patient must sit upright, may have labored breathing, and may not be able to finish a sentence because of shortness of breath. Systolic blood pressure may be normal or high in early HF, but it is generally reduced in advanced HF because of severe LV dysfunction. The pulse pressure may be diminished, reflecting a reduction in stroke volume. Sinus tachycardia is a nonspecific sign caused by increased adrenergic activity. Peripheral vasoconstriction leading to cool peripheral extremities and cyanosis of the lips and nail beds is also caused by excessive adrenergic activity.

Jugular Veins

(See also Chap. 9) Examination of the jugular veins provides an estimation of right atrial pressure. The jugular venous pressure is best appreciated with the patient lying recumbent, with the head tilted at 45°. The jugular venous pressure should be quantified in centimeters of water (normal ≤8 cm) by estimating the height of the venous column of blood above the sternal angle in cm and then adding 5 cm. In the early stages of HF, the venous pressure may be normal at rest but may become abnormally elevated with sustained (~1 min) pressure on the abdomen (positive abdominojugular reflux). Giant *v* waves indicate the presence of tricuspid regurgitation.

Pulmonary Examination

Pulmonary crackles (rales or crepitations) result from the transudation of fluid from the intravascular space into the alveoli. In patients with pulmonary edema, rales may be heard widely over both lung fields and may be accompanied by expiratory wheezing (cardiac asthma). When present in patients without concomitant lung disease, rales are specific for HF. Importantly, rales are frequently absent in patients with chronic HF, even when LV filling pressures are elevated, because of increased lymphatic drainage of alveolar fluid. Pleural effusions result from the elevation of pleural capillary pressure and the resulting transudation of fluid into the pleural cavities. Since the pleural veins drain into both the systemic and pulmonary veins, pleural effusions occur most commonly with biventricular failure. Although pleural effusions are often bilateral in HF, when unilateral they occur more frequently in the right pleural space.

Cardiac Examination

Examination of the heart, although essential, frequently does not provide useful information about the severity of HF. If cardiomegaly is present, the point of maximal impulse (PMI) is usually displaced below the fifth intercostal space and/or lateral to the midclavicular line, and the impulse is palpable over two interspaces. Severe LV hypertrophy leads to a sustained PMI. In some patients, a third heart sound (S_3) is audible and palpable at the apex. Patients with enlarged or hypertrophied right ventricles may have a sustained and prolonged left parasternal impulse extending throughout systole. An S_3 (or *protodiastolic gallop*) is most commonly present in patients with volume overload who have tachycardia and tachypnea, and it often signifies severe hemodynamic compromise. A fourth heart sound (S_4) is not a specific indicator of HF but is usually present in patients with diastolic dysfunction. The murmurs of mitral and tricuspid regurgitation are frequently present in patients with advanced HF.

Abdomen and Extremities

Hepatomegaly is an important sign in patients with HF. When present, the enlarged liver is frequently tender and may pulsate during systole if tricuspid regurgitation is present. Ascites, a late sign, occurs as a consequence of increased pressure in the hepatic veins and the veins draining the peritoneum. Jaundice, also a late finding in HF, results from impairment of hepatic function secondary to hepatic congestion and hepatocellular hypoxia, and is associated with elevations of both direct and indirect bilirubin.

Peripheral edema is a cardinal manifestation of HF, but it is nonspecific and usually absent in patients who have been treated adequately with diuretics. Peripheral edema is usually symmetric and dependent in HF and occurs predominantly in the ankles and pretibial region in ambulatory patients. In bedridden patients, edema may be found in the sacral area (*presacral edema*) and the scrotum. Long-standing edema may be associated with indurated and pigmented skin.

Cardiac Cachexia

With severe chronic HF, there may be marked weight loss and cachexia. Although the mechanism of cachexia is not entirely understood, it is likely multifactorial and includes elevation of the resting metabolic rate; anorexia, nausea, and vomiting due to congestive hepatomegaly and abdominal fullness; elevation of circulating concentrations of cytokines such as TNF; and impairment of intestinal absorption due to congestion of the intestinal veins. When present, cachexia augers a poor overall prognosis.

DIAGNOSIS

The diagnosis of HF is relatively straightforward when the patient presents with classic signs and symptoms of HF; however, the signs and symptoms of HF are neither specific nor sensitive. Accordingly, the key to making the diagnosis is to have a high index of suspicion, particularly for high-risk patients. When these patients present with signs or symptoms of HF, additional laboratory testing should be performed.

Routine Laboratory Testing

Patients with new-onset HF and those with chronic HF and acute decompensation should have a complete blood count, a panel of electrolytes, blood urea nitrogen, serum creatinine, hepatic enzymes, and a urinalysis. Selected patients should have assessment for diabetes mellitus (fasting serum glucose or oral glucose tolerance test), dyslipidemia (fasting lipid panel), and thyroid abnormalities (thyroid-stimulating hormone level).

Electrocardiogram (ECG)

A routine 12-lead ECG is recommended. The major importance of the ECG is to assess cardiac rhythm, determine the presence of LV hypertrophy or a prior MI (presence or absence of Q waves), as well as to determine QRS width to ascertain whether the patient may benefit from resynchronization therapy (see later). A normal ECG virtually excludes LV systolic dysfunction.

Chest X-ray

This provides useful information about cardiac size and shape, as well as the state of the pulmonary vasculature, and may identify noncardiac causes of the patient's symptoms. Although patients with acute HF have evidence of pulmonary hypertension, interstitial edema, and/or pulmonary edema, the majority of patients with chronic HF do not. The absence of these findings in patients with chronic HF reflects the increased capacity of the lymphatics to remove interstitial and/or pulmonary fluid.

Assessment of LV Function

Noninvasive cardiac imaging (Chap. 12) is essential for the diagnosis, evaluation, and management of HF. The most useful test is the 2-D echocardiogram/Doppler, which can provide a semiquantitative assessment of LV size and function as well as the presence or absence of valvular and/or regional wall motion abnormalities (indicative of a prior MI). The presence of left atrial dilation and LV hypertrophy, together with abnormalities of LV diastolic filling provided by pulse-wave and tissue Doppler, are useful for the assessment of HF with a preserved EF. The 2-D echocardiogram/Doppler is also invaluable in assessing RV size and pulmonary pressures, which are critical in the evaluation and management of cor pulmonale (see later). MRI also provides a comprehensive analysis of cardiac anatomy and function and is now the gold standard for assessing LV mass and volumes.

The most useful index of LV function is the EF (stroke volume divided by end-diastolic volume). Because the EF is easy to measure by noninvasive testing and easy to conceptualize, it has gained wide acceptance among clinicians. Unfortunately, the EF has a number of limitations as a true measure of contractility, because it is influenced by alterations in afterload and/or preload. For example, the LV EF is increased in mitral regurgitation as a result of ejection of the blood into the low-pressure left atrium. Nonetheless, with the exceptions indicated above, when the EF is normal (≥50%), systolic function is usually adequate, and when the EF is significantly depressed (<30–40%), contractility is usually also depressed.

Biomarkers

Circulating levels of natriuretic peptides are useful adjunctive tools in the diagnosis of patients with HF. Both B-type natriuretic peptide (BNP) and N-terminal pro-BNP, which are released from the failing heart, are relatively sensitive markers for the presence of HF with depressed EF; they are also elevated in HF patients with a preserved HF, albeit to a lesser degree. However, it is important to recognize that natriuretic peptide levels increase with age and renal impairment, are more elevated in women, and can be elevated in right HF from any cause. Levels can be falsely low in obese patients and may normalize in some patients following appropriate treatment. A normal concentration of natriuretic peptides in an untreated patient is extremely useful for

excluding the diagnosis of HF. Other biomarkers, such as troponin T and I, C-reactive protein, TNF receptors, and uric acid, may be elevated in HF and provide important prognostic information. Serial measurements of one or more biomarkers may ultimately help to guide therapy in HF, but they are not currently recommended for this purpose.

Exercise Testing

Treadmill or bicycle exercise testing is not routinely advocated for patients with HF, but either is useful for assessing the need for cardiac transplantation in patients with advanced HF (Chap. 18). A peak oxygen uptake (VO_2) <14 mL/kg per min is associated with a relatively poor prognosis. Patients with a VO_2 <14 mL/kg per min have been shown, in general, to have better survival when transplanted than when treated medically.

DIFFERENTIAL DIAGNOSIS

HF resembles but should be distinguished from (1) conditions in which there is circulatory congestion secondary to abnormal salt and water retention but in which there is no disturbance of cardiac structure or function (e.g., renal failure) and (2) noncardiac causes of pulmonary edema (e.g., acute respiratory distress syndrome). In most patients who present with classic signs and symptoms of HF, the diagnosis is relatively straightforward. However, even experienced clinicians have difficulty in differentiating the dyspnea that arises from cardiac and pulmonary causes (Chap. 5). In this regard, noninvasive cardiac imaging, biomarkers, pulmonary function testing, and chest x-ray may be useful. A very low BNP or N-terminal pro-BNP may be helpful in excluding a cardiac cause of dyspnea in this setting. Ankle edema may arise secondary to varicose veins, obesity, renal disease, or gravitational effects. When HF develops in patients with a preserved EF, it may be difficult to determine the relative contribution of HF to the dyspnea that occurs in chronic lung disease and/or obesity.

℞ **Treatment:**
HEART FAILURE

HF should be viewed as a continuum that is comprised of four interrelated stages. *Stage A* includes patients who are at high risk for developing HF but without structural heart disease or symptoms of HF (e.g., patients with diabetes mellitus or hypertension). *Stage B* includes patients who have structural heart disease but without symptoms of HF (e.g., patients with a previous MI and asymptomatic LV dysfunction). *Stage C* includes patients who have structural heart disease and have developed symptoms of HF (e.g., patients with a previous MI with dyspnea and fatigue). *Stage D* includes patients with refractory HF requiring special interventions (e.g., patients with refractory HF who are awaiting cardiac transplantation). In this continuum, every effort should be made to prevent HF, not only by treating the preventable causes of HF (e.g., hypertension) but by treating the patient in Stages B and C with drugs that prevent disease progression (e.g., ACE inhibitors and beta blockers) and by symptomatic management of patients in stage D.

DEFINING AN APPROPRIATE THERAPEUTIC STRATEGY FOR CHRONIC HF

Once patients have developed structural heart disease, their therapy depends on their NYHA functional classification (Table 17-2). Although this classification system is notoriously subjective and has large interobserver variability, it has withstood the test of time and continues to be widely applied to patients with HF. For patients who have developed LV systolic dysfunction but remain asymptomatic (class I), the goal should be to slow disease progression by blocking neurohormonal systems that lead to cardiac remodeling (see later). For patients who have developed symptoms (class II–IV) the primary

goal, should be to alleviate fluid retention, lessen disability, and reduce the risk of further disease progression and death. These goals generally require a strategy that combines diuretics (to control salt and water retention) with neurohormonal interventions (to minimize cardiac remodeling).

MANAGEMENT OF HF WITH DEPRESSED EJECTION FRACTION (<40%)

General Measures Clinicians should aim to screen for and treat comorbidities such as hypertension, CAD, diabetes mellitus, anemia, and sleep-disordered breathing, as these conditions tend to exacerbate HF. HF patients should be advised to stop smoking and to limit alcohol consumption to two standard drinks per day in men or one per day in women. Patients suspected of having an alcohol-induced cardiomyopathy should be urged to abstain from alcohol consumption indefinitely. Extremes of temperature and heavy physical exertion should be avoided. Certain drugs are known to make HF worse and should also be avoided (Table 17-3). For example, nonsteroidal anti-inflammatory drugs (NSAIDs), including cyclooxygenase 2 inhibitors, are not recommended in patients with chronic HF because the risk of renal failure and fluid retention is markedly increased in the presence of reduced renal function or ACE inhibitor therapy. Patients should receive immunization with influenza and pneumococcal vaccines to prevent respiratory infections. It is equally important to educate the patient and family about HF, the importance of proper

TABLE 17-2

NEW YORK HEART ASSOCIATION CLASSIFICATION

FUNCTIONAL CAPACITY	OBJECTIVE ASSESSMENT
Class I	Patients with cardiac disease but without resulting limitation of physical activity. Ordinary physical activity does not cause undue fatigue, palpitations, dyspnea, or anginal pain.
Class II	Patients with cardiac disease resulting in slight limitation of physical activity. They are comfortable at rest. Ordinary physical activity results in fatigue, palpitation, dyspnea, or anginal pain.
Class III	Patients with cardiac disease resulting in marked limitation of physical activity. They are comfortable at rest. Less than ordinary activity causes fatigue, palpitation, dyspnea, or anginal pain.
Class IV	Patients with cardiac disease resulting in inability to carry on any physical activity without discomfort. Symptoms of heart failure or the anginal syndrome may be present even at rest. If any physical activity is undertaken, discomfort is increased.

Source: Adapted from New York Heart Association, Inc., *Diseases of the Heart and Blood Vessels: Nomenclature and Criteria for Diagnosis*, 6th ed. Boston, Little Brown, 1964, p. 114.

TABLE 17-3

FACTORS THAT MAY PRECIPITATE ACUTE DECOMPENSATION IN PATIENTS WITH CHRONIC HEART FAILURE

Dietary indiscretion
Myocardial ischemia/infarction
Arrhythmias (tachycardia or bradycardia)
Discontinuation of HF therapy
Infection
Anemia
Initiation of medications that worsen HF
  Calcium antagonists (verapamil, diltiazem)
  Beta blockers
  NSAIDs
  Antiarrhythmic agents [all class I agents, sotalol (class III)]
  Anti-TNF antibodies
Alcohol consumption
Pregnancy
Worsening hypertension
Acute valvular insufficiency

Note: HF, heart failure; NSAIDs, nonsteroidal anti-inflammatory drugs; TNF, tumor necrosis factor.

diet, as well the importance of compliance with the medical regimen. Supervision of outpatient care by a specially trained nurse or physician assistant and/or in specialized HF clinics have all been found to be helpful, particularly in patients with advanced disease.

Activity Although heavy physical labor is not recommended in HF, routine modest exercise has been shown to be beneficial in patients with NYHA class I–III HF. For euvolemic patients, regular isotonic exercise such as walking or riding a stationary bicycle ergometer, as tolerated, should be encouraged. Some trials of exercise training have led to encouraging results with reduced symptoms, increased exercise capacity, and improved quality and duration of life. The benefits of weight loss by restriction of caloric intake have not been clearly established.

Diet Dietary restriction of sodium (2–3 g daily) is recommended in all patients with HF and preserved or depressed EF. Further restriction (<2 g daily) may be considered in moderate to severe HF. Fluid restriction is generally unnecessary unless the patient develops hyponatremia (<130 meq/L), which may develop because of activation of the renin-angiotensin system, excessive secretion of antidiuretic hormone, or loss of salt in excess of water from diuretic use. Fluid restriction (<2 L/d) should be considered in hyponatremic patients or for those whose fluid retention is difficult to control despite high doses of diuretics and sodium restriction. Caloric supplementation is recommended for patients with advanced HF and unintentional weight loss or muscle wasting (cardiac cachexia); however, anabolic steroids are not recommended for these patients because of the potential problems with volume retention. The use of dietary supplements ("nutriceuticals") should be avoided in the management of symptomatic HF because of the lack of proven benefit and the potential for significant (adverse) interactions with proven HF therapies.

Diuretics Many of the clinical manifestations of moderate to severe HF result from excessive salt and water retention that leads to volume expansion and congestive symptoms. Diuretics (Table 17-4) are the only pharmacologic agents that can adequately control fluid retention in advanced HF, and they should be used to restore and maintain normal volume status in patients with congestive symptoms (dyspnea, orthopnea, edema) or signs of elevated filling pressures (rales, jugular venous distention, or peripheral edema). Furosemide, torsemide, and bumetanide act at the loop of Henle (*loop diuretics*) by reversibly inhibiting the reabsorption of Na^+, K^+, and Cl^- in the thick ascending limb of Henle's loop; thiazides and metolazone reduce the reabsorption of Na^+ and Cl^- in the first half of the distal convoluted tubule; and potassium-sparing diuretics such as spironolactone act at the level of the collecting duct.

Although all diuretics increase sodium excretion and urinary volume, they differ in their potency and pharmacologic properties. Whereas loop diuretics increase the fractional excretion of sodium by 20–25%, thiazide diuretics increase it by only 5–10% and tend to lose their effectiveness in patients with moderate or severe renal insufficiency (creatinine >2.5 mg/dL). Hence, loop diuretics are generally required to restore normal volume status in patients with HF. Diuretics should be initiated in low doses (Table 17-4) and then carefully titrated upward to relieve signs and symptoms of fluid overload in an attempt to obtain the patient's "dry weight." This typically requires multiple dose adjustments over many days and occasionally weeks in patients with severe fluid overload. Intravenous administration of diuretics may be necessary to relieve congestion acutely and can be done safely in the outpatient setting. Once the congestion has been relieved, treatment with diuretics should be continued to prevent the recurrence of salt and water retention.

Refractoriness to diuretic therapy may represent patient noncompliance, a direct effect of chronic diuretic use on the kidney or progression of underlying HF. The addition of thiazides or metolazone, once or twice daily, to loop diuretics may be considered in patients with persistent fluid retention despite high dose loop diuretic therapy. Metolazone is generally more potent and much longer-acting than the thiazides in this setting as well as in patients with chronic renal insufficiency. However, chronic daily use, especially of metolazone, should be avoided if possible because of the potential for electrolyte shifts and volume depletion. Ultrafiltration and dialysis may be used in cases of refractory fluid retention that are unresponsive to high doses of diuretics and have been shown to be helpful in the short term.

Adverse effects Diuretics have the potential to produce electrolyte and volume depletion, as well as worsening azotemia. In addition, they may lead to worsening neurohormonal activation and disease progression. One of the most important adverse consequences of diuresis is alterations in potassium homeostasis (hypokalemia or hyperkalemia), which increases the risk of life-threatening arrhythmias. In general, both loop- and thiazide-type diuretics lead to hypokalemia, whereas spironolactone, eplerenone, and triamterene lead to hyperkalemia.

PREVENTING DISEASE PROGRESSION (TABLE 17-4) Drugs that interfere with the excessive activation of the RAA system and the adrenergic nervous system can relieve the symptoms of HF with a depressed EF by stabilizing and/or reversing cardiac remodeling. In this regard, ACE inhibitors and beta blockers have emerged as the cornerstones of modern therapy for HF with a depressed EF.

TABLE 17-4

DRUGS FOR THE TREATMENT OF CHRONIC HEART FAILURE (EF <40%)

	INITIATING DOSE	MAXIMAL DOSE
Diuretics		
Furosemide	20–40 mg qd or bid	400 mg/d[a]
Torsemide	10–20 mg qd bid	200 mg/d[a]
Bumetanide	0.5–1.0 mg qd or bid	10 mg/d[a]
Hydrochlorthiazide	25 mg qd	100 mg/d[a]
Metolazone	2.5–5.0 mg qd or bid	20 mg/d[a]
Angiotensin-Converting Enzyme Inhibitors		
Captopril	6.25 mg tid	50 mg tid
Enalapril	2.5 mg bid	10 mg bid
Lisinopril	2.5–5.0 mg qd	20–35 mg qd
Ramipril	1.25–2.5 mg bid	2.5–5 mg bid
Trandolapril	0.5 mg qd	4 mg qd
Angiotensin Receptor Blockers		
Valsartan	40 mg bid	160 mg bid
Candesartan	4 mg qd	32 mg qd
Irbesartan	75 mg qd	300 mg qd[b]
Losartan	12.5 mg qd	50 mg qd
β-Receptor Blockers		
Carvedilol	3.125 mg bid	25–50 mg bid
Bisoprolol	1.25 mg qd	10 mg qd
Metoprolol succinate CR	12.5–25 mg qd	Target dose 200 mg qd
Additional Therapies		
Spironolactone	12.5–25 mg qd	25–50 mg qd
Eplerenone	25 mg qd	50 mg qd
Combination of hydralazine/isosorbide dinitrate	10–25 mg/10 mg tid	75 mg/40 mg tid
Fixed dose of hydralazine/ isosorbide dinitrate	37.5 mg/20 mg (one tablet) tid	75 mg/40 mg (two tablets) tid
Digoxin	0.125 mg qd	≤0.375 mg/d[b]

[a]Dose must be titrated to reduce the patient's congestive symptoms.
[b]Target dose not established.

ACE Inhibitors There is overwhelming evidence that ACE inhibitors should be used in symptomatic and asymptomatic patients (**Figs. 17-3** and **17-4**) with a depressed EF (<40%). ACE inhibitors interfere with the renin-angiotensin system by inhibiting the enzyme that is responsible for the conversion of angiotensin I to angiotensin II. However, because ACE inhibitors also inhibit kininase II, they may lead to the upregulation of bradykinin, which may further enhance the beneficial effects of angiotensin suppression. ACE inhibitors stabilize LV remodeling, improve symptoms, reduce hospitalization, and prolong life. Because fluid retention can attenuate the effects of ACE inhibitors, it is preferable to optimize the dose of diuretic before starting the ACE inhibitor. However, it may be necessary to reduce the dose of diuretic during the initiation of ACE inhibition in order to prevent symptomatic hypotension. ACE inhibitors should be initiated in low doses, followed by gradual increments if the lower doses have been well tolerated. The doses of ACE inhibitors should be increased until they are similar to those that have been shown to be effective in clinical trials (Table 17-4). Higher doses are more effective than lower doses in preventing hospitalization.

Adverse effects The majority of adverse effects are related to suppression of the renin-angiotensin system. The decreases in blood pressure and mild azotemia that may occur during the initiation of therapy are generally well tolerated and do not require a decrease in the dose of the ACE inhibitor. However, if hypotension is accompanied by dizziness or if the renal dysfunction becomes severe, it may be necessary to reduce the dose of the inhibitor. Potassium retention may also become

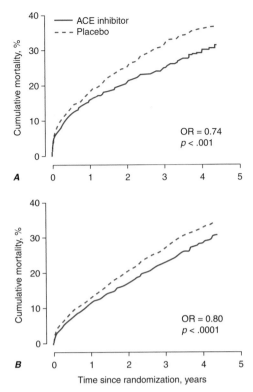

FIGURE 17-3

Meta-analysis of angiotensin-converting enzyme (ACE) inhibitors in heart failure patients with a depressed ejection fraction. *A*. The Kaplan-Meier curves for mortality for 5966 HF patients with a depressed EF treated with an ACE inhibitor following acute myocardial infarction (three trials). *B*. The Kaplan-Meier curves for mortality for 12,763 HF patients with a depressed EF treated with an ACE inhibitor in five clinical trials, including postinfarction trials. The benefits of ACE inhibitors were observed early and persisted long-term. *(Modified from Flather et al: Lancet 355:1575, 2000.)*

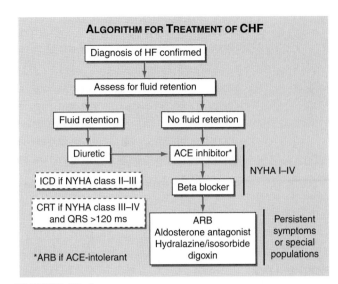

FIGURE 17-4

Treatment algorithm for chronic heart failure patients with a depressed ejection fraction. After the clinical diagnosis of HF is made, it is important to treat the patient's fluid retention before starting an ACE inhibitor (or an ARB if the patient is ACE-intolerant). Beta blockers should be started after the fluid retention has been treated and/or the ACE inhibitor has been uptitrated. If the patient remains symptomatic, an ARB, aldosterone antagonist, or digoxin can be added as "triple therapy." The fixed-dose combination of hydralazine/isosorbide dinitrate should be added to an ACE inhibitor and beta blocker in African-American patients with NYHA class II–IV HF. Device therapy should be considered in addition to pharmacological therapy in appropriate patients. HF, heart failure; ACE, angiotensin-converting enzyme; ARB, angiotensin receptor blocker; NYHA, New York Heart Association; CRT, cardiac resynchronization therapy; ICD, implantable cardiac defibrillator.

problematic if the patient is receiving potassium supplements or a potassium-sparing diuretic. Potassium retention that is not responsive to these measures may require a reduction in the dose of ACE inhibitor.

The side effects of ACE inhibitors related to kinin potentiation include a nonproductive cough (10–15% of patients) and angioedema (1% of patients). In patients who cannot tolerate ACE inhibitors because of cough or angioedema, angiotensin receptor blockers (ARBs) are the recommended first line of therapy (see later). Patients intolerant of ACE inhibitors because of hyperkalemia or renal insufficiency are likely to experience the same side effects with ARBs. In these cases, the combination of hydralazine and an oral nitrate should be considered (Table 17-4).

Angiotensin Receptor Blockers These drugs are well tolerated in patients who are intolerant of ACE inhibitors because of cough, skin rash, and angioedema. ARBs should be used in symptomatic

and asymptomatic patients with an EF <40% who are ACE-intolerant for reasons other than hyperkalemia or renal insufficiency (Table 17-4). Although ACE inhibitors and ARBs inhibit the renin-angiotensin system, they do so by different mechanisms. Whereas ACE inhibitors block the enzyme responsible for converting angiotensin I to angiotensin II, ARBs block the effects of angiotensin II on the angiotensin type 1 receptor. Some clinical trials have demonstrated a therapeutic benefit for the addition of ARB to an ACE inhibitor in patients with chronic HF. When given in concert with beta blockers, ARBs reverse the process of LV remodeling, improve patient symptoms, prevent hospitalization, and prolong life.

Adverse effects Both ACE inhibitors and ARBs have similar effects on blood pressure, renal function, and potassium. Therefore the problems of symptomatic hypotension, azotemia, and hyperkalemia are similar for both of these agents.

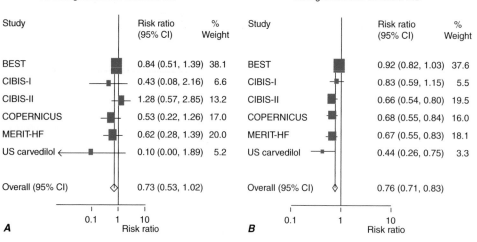

No background ACE-inhibitor/ARB

Study	Risk ratio (95% CI)	% Weight
BEST	0.84 (0.51, 1.39)	38.1
CIBIS-I	0.43 (0.08, 2.16)	6.6
CIBIS-II	1.28 (0.57, 2.85)	13.2
COPERNICUS	0.53 (0.22, 1.26)	17.0
MERIT-HF	0.62 (0.28, 1.39)	20.0
US carvedilol	0.10 (0.00, 1.89)	5.2
Overall (95% CI)	0.73 (0.53, 1.02)	

A

Background ACE-inhibitor/ARB

Study	Risk ratio (95% CI)	% Weight
BEST	0.92 (0.82, 1.03)	37.6
CIBIS-I	0.83 (0.59, 1.15)	5.5
CIBIS-II	0.66 (0.54, 0.80)	19.5
COPERNICUS	0.68 (0.55, 0.84)	16.0
MERIT-HF	0.67 (0.55, 0.83)	18.1
US carvedilol	0.44 (0.26, 0.75)	3.3
Overall (95% CI)	0.76 (0.71, 0.83)	

B

FIGURE 17-5

Meta-analysis of beta blockers on mortality in HF patients with a depressed EF. Effect of beta blockers vs. placebo in patients who were not (**A**) or who were (**B**) receiving an angiotensin-converting enzyme (ACE) inhibitor or an angiotensin receptor blocker (ARB) at baseline in six clinical trials. There was a similar impact of beta-blocker therapy on the endpoints of all-cause mortality as well as death and heart failure hospitalization in both the presence and absence of ACE inhibitor or ARB at baseline. BEST, Beta-blocker Evaluation of Survival Trial (bucindolol); CIBIS, Cardiac Insufficiency BIsoprolol Study (bisoprol); COPERNICUS, Carvedilol prOsPEctive RaNdomIzed Cumulative Survival (carvedilol); MERIT-HF, Metoprolol CR/XL Randomized Intervention Trial in Heart Failure (metoprolol CR/XL). *(Modified from Krum et al: Eur Heart J 26:2154, 2005.)*

β-Adrenergic Receptor Blockers Beta-blocker therapy represents a major advance in the treatment of patients with a depressed EF (**Fig. 17-5**). These drugs interfere with the harmful effects of sustained activation of the adrenergic nervous system by competitively antagonizing one or more adrenergic receptors (α_1, β_1, and β_2). Although there are a number of potential benefits to blocking all three receptors, most of the deleterious effects of adrenergic activation are mediated by the β_1 receptor. When given in concert with ACE inhibitors, beta blockers reverse the process of LV remodeling, improve patient symptoms, prevent hospitalization, and prolong life. Therefore beta blockers are indicated for patients with symptomatic or asymptomatic HF and a depressed EF <40%.

Analogous to the use of ACE inhibitors, beta blockers should be initiated in low doses (Table 17-4), followed by gradual increments in the dose if lower doses have been well tolerated. The dose of beta blocker should be increased until the doses used are similar to those that have been reported to be effective in clinical trials (Table 17-4). However, unlike ACE inhibitors, which may be titrated upward relatively rapidly, the titration of beta blockers should proceed no more rapidly than at 2-week intervals, because the initiation and/or increased dosing of these agents may lead to worsening fluid retention consequent to the withdrawal of adrenergic support to the heart and the circulation. Thus, it is important to optimize the dose of diuretic before starting therapy with beta blockers. If worsening fluid retention does occur, it is likely to do so within 3–5 days of initiating therapy, and it will be manifest as an increase in body weight and/or symptoms of worsening HF. The increased fluid retention can usually be managed by increasing the dose of diuretics. In some patients the dose of the beta blocker may have to be reduced.

Contrary to early reports, the aggregate results of clinical trials suggest that beta-blocker therapy is well tolerated by the great majority (≥85%) of HF patients, including patients with comorbid conditions such as diabetes mellitus, chronic obstructive lung disease, and peripheral vascular disease. Nonetheless, there is a subset of patients (10–15%) who remain intolerant to beta blockers because of worsening fluid retention or symptomatic hypotension or bradycardia.

Adverse effects The adverse effects of beta-blocker use are generally related to the predictable complications that arise from interfering with the adrenergic nervous system. These reactions generally occur within several days of initiating therapy and are generally responsive to adjusting concomitant medications, as described above. Therapy with beta blockers can lead to bradycardia and/or exacerbate heart block. Accordingly, the dose of beta blocker should be reduced if the heart rate decreases to <50 beats/min and/or second or third degree heart block or symptomatic hypotension develops. Beta blockers are not recommended for patients who have asthma with active bronchospasm. Beta blockers that also block the α_1 receptor can lead to vasodilatory side effects.

Aldosterone Antagonists Although classified as potassium-sparing diuretics, drugs that block the effects of aldosterone (spironolactone or eplerenone) have beneficial effects that are independent of the effects of these agents on sodium balance. Although ACE inhibition may transiently decrease aldosterone secretion, with chronic therapy there is a rapid return of aldosterone to levels similar to those before ACE inhibition. Accordingly, the administration of an aldosterone antagonist is recommended for patients with NYHA class IV or class III (previously class IV) HF who have a depressed EF (<35%) and who are receiving standard therapy, including diuretics, ACE inhibitors, and beta blockers. The dose of aldosterone antagonist should be increased until the doses used are similar to those that have been shown to be effective in clinical trials (Table 17-4).

Adverse effects The major problem with the use of aldosterone antagonists is the development of life-threatening hyperkalemia, which is more prone to occur in patients who are receiving potassium supplements or who have underlying renal insufficiency. Aldosterone antagonists are not recommended when the serum creatinine is >2.5 mg/dL (or creatinine clearance is <30 mL/min) or when the serum potassium is >5.0 mmol/L. Painful gynecomastia may develop in 10–15% of patients who use spironolactone, in which case eplerenone may be substituted.

SPECIAL POPULATIONS The combination of hydralazine and isosorbide dinitrate (Table 17-4) is recommended as part of standard therapy in addition to beta blockers and ACE inhibitors for African Americans with NYHA class II–IV HF. Although the exact mechanism for the effects of this combination is not known, it is believed to be secondary to the beneficial effects of NO on the peripheral circulation. Recent studies suggest that the combination of hydralazine and isosorbide dinitrate may be more effective for patients who have variant genotypic markers (polymorphisms) for the genes that encode for endothelial nitric oxide synthase (NOS3) and aldosterone synthase.

MANAGEMENT OF PATIENTS WHO REMAIN SYMPTOMATIC As noted above, an ACE inhibitor (or an ARB) plus a beta blocker should be standard background therapy for HF patients with a depressed LV EF. Additional pharmacologic therapy should be considered in patients who have persistent symptoms or progressive worsening despite optimized therapy with an ACE inhibitor and beta blocker. Agents that may be considered as part of additional therapy include an ARB, spironolactone, the combination of hydralazine and

isosorbide dinitrate, or digitalis. The optimal choice of additional drug therapy to further improve outcome has not been firmly established. Thus, the choice of specific agent will be influenced by clinical considerations, including renal function, serum potassium concentration, blood pressure, and race. The triple combination of an ACE inhibitor, an ARB, and an aldosterone antagonist should not be used because of the high risk of hyperkalemia.

Digoxin is recommended for patients with symptomatic LV systolic dysfunction who have concomitant atrial fibrillation, and it should be considered for patients who have signs or symptoms of HF while receiving standard therapy, including ACE inhibitors and beta blockers. Therapy with digoxin is commonly initiated and maintained at a dose of 0.125–0.25 mg daily. For the great majority of patients, the dose should be 0.125 mg daily, and the serum digoxin level should be <1.0 ng/mL, especially in elderly patients, patients with impaired renal function, and a low lean body mass. Higher doses (and serum concentrations) appear to be less beneficial. There is no indication for using loading doses of digoxin to initiate therapy in patients with HF.

ANTICOAGULATION AND ANTIPLATELET THERAPY Patients with HF have an increased risk for arterial or venous thromboembolic events. In clinical HF trials, the rate of stroke ranges from 1.3–2.4% per year. Depressed LV function is believed to promote relative stasis of blood in dilated cardiac chambers with increased risk of thrombus formation. Treatment with warfarin [goal international normalized ratio (INR) 2.0–3.0] is recommended for patients with HF and chronic or paroxysmal atrial fibrillation, or with a history of systemic or pulmonary emboli, including stroke or transient ischemic attack. Patients with symptomatic or asymptomatic ischemic cardiomyopathy and documented recent large anterior MI or recent MI with documented LV thrombus should be treated with warfarin (goal INR 2.0–3.0) for the initial 3 months after MI, unless there are contraindications to its use.

Aspirin is recommended in HF patients with ischemic heart disease for the prevention of MI and death. However, lower doses of aspirin (75 or 81 mg) may be preferable because of the concern of worsening of HF at higher doses.

MANAGEMENT OF CARDIAC ARRHYTHMIAS (See also Chap. 16) Atrial fibrillation occurs in 15–30% of patients with HF and is a frequent cause of cardiac decompensation. Most antiarrhythmic agents, with the exception of amiodarone and dofetilide, have negative inotropic effects and are proarrhythmic. Amiodarone is a class III antiarrhythmic that has little or no negative inotropic and/or proarrhythmic effects and is effective against most supraventricular arrhythmias. Amiodarone is the preferred drug for restoring and maintaining sinus rhythm, and it may improve the success of electrical cardioversion in patients with HF. Amiodarone increases the level of phenytoin and digoxin and prolongs the INR in patients taking warfarin. Therefore it is often necessary to reduce the dose of these drugs by as much as 50% when initiating therapy with amiodarone. The risk of adverse events, such as hyperthyroidism, hypothyroidism, pulmonary fibrosis, and hepatitis, are relatively low, particularly when lower doses of amiodarone are used (100–200 mg/d).

Implantable cardiac defibrillators (ICDs; see below) are highly effective in treating recurrences of sustained ventricular tachycardia and/or ventricular fibrillation in HF patients with recurrent arrhythmias and/or cardiac syncope, and they may be used as stand-alone therapy or in combination with amiodarone and/or a beta blocker (Chap. 16). There is no role for treating ventricular arrhythmias with an antiarrhythmic agent without an ICD.

DEVICE THERAPY

Cardiac Resynchronization Approximately one-third of patients with a depressed EF and symptomatic HF (NYHA class III–IV) manifest a QRS duration >120 ms. This ECG finding of abnormal inter- or intraventricular conduction has been used to identify patients with dyssynchronous ventricular contraction. The mechanical consequences of ventricular dyssynchrony include suboptimal ventricular filling, a reduction in LV contractility, prolonged duration (and therefore greater severity) of mitral regurgitation, and paradoxical septal wall motion. *Biventricular pacing,* also termed *cardiac resynchronization therapy* (CRT) stimulates both ventricles near simultaneously, thereby improving the coordination of ventricular contraction and reducing the severity of mitral regurgitation. When CRT is added to optimal medical therapy in patients in sinus rhythm, there is a significant decrease in patient mortality and hospitalization, a reversal of LV remodeling, as well as improved quality of life and exercise capacity. Accordingly, CRT is recommended for patients in sinus rhythm with an EF <35% and a QRS >120 ms and those who remain symptomatic (NYHA III–IV) despite optimal medical therapy. The benefits of CRT in patients with atrial fibrillation have not been established.

Implantable Cardiac Defibrillators (See also Chap. 16) The prophylactic implantation of ICDs in patients with mild to moderate HF (NYHA class II–III) has been shown to reduce the incidence of sudden cardiac death in patients with ischemic or nonischemic cardiomyopathy. Accordingly, implantation of an ICD should be considered for patients in NYHA class II–III HF with a depressed EF of <30–35% who are already on optimal background therapy, including an ACE inhibitor (or ARB), a beta blocker, and an aldosterone antagonist. An ICD may be combined with a biventricular pacemaker in appropriate patients.

MANAGEMENT OF HF WITH A PRESERVED EJECTION FRACTION (>40–50%) Despite the wealth of information with respect to the evaluation and management of HF with a depressed EF, there are no proven and/or approved pharmacologic or device therapies for the management of patients with HF and a preserved EF. Therefore, it is recommended that initial treatment efforts should be focused, wherever possible, on the underlying disease process (e.g., myocardial ischemia, hypertension) associated with HF with preserved EF. Precipitating factors, such as tachycardia or atrial fibrillation, should be treated as quickly as possible through rate control and restoration of sinus rhythm when appropriate. Dyspnea may be treated by reducing total blood volume (dietary sodium restriction and diuretics), decreasing central blood volume (nitrates), or blunting neurohormal activation with ACE inhibitors, ARBs, and/or beta blockers. Treatment with diuretics and nitrates should be initiated at low doses to avoid hypotension and fatigue.

ACUTE HF

Defining an Appropriate Therapeutic Strategy The therapeutic goals for the management of acute HF therapy are to (1) stabilize the hemodynamic derangements that provoked the symptoms responsible for the hospitalization, (2) identify and treat the reversible factors that precipitated decompensation, and (3) reestablish an effective outpatient medical regimen that will prevent disease progression and relapse. In most instances this will require hospitalization, often in an intensive care unit (ICU) setting. Every effort should be made to identify the precipitating causes, such as infection, arrhythmias, dietary indiscretion, pulmonary embolism, infective endocarditis, occult myocardial ischemia/infarction, environmental and/or emotional or environmental stress (Table 17-3), since removal of these precipitating events is critical to the success of treatment.

The two primary hemodynamic determinants of acute HF are elevated LV filling pressures and a depressed cardiac output. Frequently the depressed cardiac output is accompanied by an increase in systemic vascular resistance (SVR) as a result of excessive neurohormonal activation. Because these hemodynamic derangements may occur singly or together, patients with acute HF generally present with one of four basic hemodynamic profiles (Fig. 17-6): normal LV filling pressure with normal perfusion (Profile A), elevated LV filling pressure with normal perfusion (Profile B), elevated LV filling pressures with decreased perfusion (Profile C), and normal or low LV filling pressure with decreased tissue perfusion (Profile L).

Accordingly, the therapeutic approach to treating patients with acute HF should be tailored to reflect the patient's hemodynamic presentation. The goal should be, whenever possible, to restore the patient to a normal

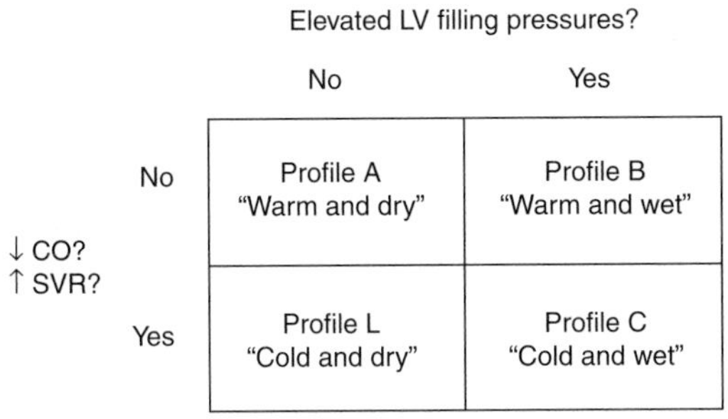

Elevated LV filling pressures?

	No	Yes
No	Profile A "Warm and dry"	Profile B "Warm and wet"
Yes	Profile L "Cold and dry"	Profile C "Cold and wet"

↓ CO?
↑ SVR?

FIGURE 17-6

Hemodynamic profiles in patients with acute heart failure. Most patients can be categorized into one of the four hemodynamic profiles by performing a brief bedside examination that includes examination of the neck veins, lungs, and peripheral extremities. More definitive hemodynamic information may be obtained by performing invasive hemodynamic monitoring, particularly if the patient is gravely ill or if the clinical presentation is unclear. This hemodynamic classification provides a useful guide for selecting the initial optimal therapies for the management of acute HF. LV, left ventricular; CO, cardiac output; SVR, systemic vascular resistance. *(Modified from Grady et al: Circulation102:2443, 2000.)*

hemodynamic profile (Profile A). In many instances the patient's hemodynamic presentation can be approximated from the clinical examination. For example, patients with elevated LV filling pressures may have signs of fluid retention (rales, elevated neck veins, peripheral edema) and are referred to as being "wet," whereas patients with a depressed cardiac output and an elevated SVR generally have poor tissue perfusion manifested by cool distal extremities and are referred to as being "cold." Nonetheless, it should be emphasized that patients with chronic heart failure may not have rales or evidence of peripheral edema at the time of the initial presentation with acute decompensation, which may lead to the underrecognition of elevated filling pressures. In these patients, it may be appropriate to perform invasive hemodynamic monitoring.

Patients who are not congested and have normal tissue perfusion are referred to as being "dry" and "warm," respectively. When acute HF patients present to the hospital with profile A, their symptoms are often due to conditions other than HF (e.g., pulmonary or hepatic disease, or transient myocardial ischemia). More commonly, however, acute HF patients present with congestive symptoms ["warm and wet" (profile B)], in which case treatment of the elevated filling pressures with diuretics and vasodilators is warranted to reduce LV filling pressures. Profile B includes most patients with acute pulmonary edema. The treatment of this life-threatening condition is described in Chap. 28.

Patients may also present with congestion and a significant elevated SVR and reduction of cardiac output ["cold and wet" (Profile C)]. In these patients, cardiac output can be increased and LV filling pressures reduced using intravenous vasodilators. Intravenous inotropic agents with vasodilating action [dobutamine, lowdose dopamine, milrinone (Table 17-5)] augment cardiac output by stimulating myocardial contractility as well as by functionally unloading the heart.

TABLE 17-5

DRUGS FOR THE TREATMENT FOR ACUTE HEART FAILURE

	INITIATING DOSE	MAXIMAL DOSE
Vasodilators		
Nitroglycerin	20 µg/min	40–400 µg/min
Nitroprusside	10 µg/min	30–350 µg/min
Nesiritide	Bolus 2 µg/kg	0.01–0.03 µg/kg per min[a]
Inotropes		
Dobutamine	1–2 µg/kg per min	2–10 µg/kg per min[b]
Milrinone	Bolus 50 µg/kg	0.1–0.75 µg/kg per min[b]
Dopamine	1–2 µg/kg per min	2–4 µg/kg per min[b]
Levosimendan	Bolus 12 µg/kg	0.1–0.2 µg/kg per min[c]
Vasoconstrictors		
Dopamine for hypotension	5 µg/kg per min	5–15 µg/kg per min
Epinephrine	0.5 µg/kg per min	50 µg/kg per min
Phenylephrine	0.3 µg/kg per min	3 µg/kg per min
Vasopression	0.05 units/min	0.1–0.4 units/min

[a]Usually <4 µg/kg per min.
[b]Inotropes will also have vasodilatory properties.
[c]Approved outside of the United States for the management of acute heart failure.

Patients who present with profile L ("cold and dry") should be carefully evaluated by right-heart catheterization for the presence of an occult elevation of LV filling pressures. If LV filling pressures are low [pulmonary capillary wedge pressure (PCWP) <12 mmHg] a cautious trial of fluid repletion may be considered. The goals of further therapy depend on the clinical situation. Therapy to reach the aforementioned goals may not be possible in some patients, particularly if they have disproportionate RV dysfunction or if they develop cardiorenal syndrome, in which renal function deteriorates during aggressive diuresis. Worsening renal dysfunction occurs in approximately 25% of patients hospitalized with HF and is associated with prolonged hospital stays and higher mortality after discharge.

Pharmacologic Management of Acute HF (Table 17-5)

Vasodilators After diuretics, intravenous vasodilators are the most useful medications for the management of acute HF. By stimulating guanylyl cyclase within smooth-muscle cells, nitroglycerin, nitroprusside, and nesiritide exert dilating effects on arterial resistance and venous capacitance vessels, which results in a lowering of LV filling pressure, a reduction in mitral regurgitation, and improved forward cardiac output, without increasing heart rate or causing arrhythmias.

Intravenous *nitroglycerin* is generally begun at 20 μg/min and is increased in 20 μg increments until patient symptoms are improved or PCWP is decreased to 16 mmHg without reducing systolic blood pressure <80 mmHg. The most common side effect of intravenous or oral nitrates is headache, which, if mild, can be treated with analgesics and often resolves during continued therapy.

Nitroprusside is generally initiated at 10 μg/min and increased by 10–20 μg every 10–20 min as tolerated, with the same hemodynamic goals as described above. The rapidity of onset and offset, with a half-life of approximately 2 min, facilitates early establishment of an individual patient's optimal level of vasodilation in the ICU. The major limitation of nitroprusside is side effects from cyanide, which manifests predominantly as gastrointestinal and central nervous system manifestations. Cyanide is most likely to accumulate in patients with severely reduced hepatic perfusion and decreased hepatic function from low cardiac output, and it is more likely to develop in patients receiving >250 μg/min for over 48 h. Suspected cyanide toxicity is treated by decreasing or discontinuing the nitroprusside infusion. Long-term (>48 h) use of both nitroprusside and nitroglycerin is associated with hemodynamic tolerance.

Nesiritide, the newest vasodilator, is a recombinant form of brain-type natriuretic peptide (BNP), which is an endogenous peptide secreted primarily from the LV in response to an increase in wall stress. Nesiritide is given as a bolus (2 μg/kg) followed by a fixed-dose infusion (0.01–0.03 μg/kg per min). Nesiritide effectively lowers LV filling pressures and improves symptoms during the treatment of acute HF. Headache is less common with nesiritide than with nitroglycerin. Although termed a *natriuretic peptide*, nesiritide has not been associated with major diuresis when used alone in clinical trials. It does, however, appear to potentiate the effect of concomitant diuretics such that the total required diuretic dose may be slightly lower.

Hypotension is the most common side effect of all three vasodilating agents, although less so with nesiritide. Hypotension is frequently associated with bradycardia, particularly when nitroglycerin is used. The three drugs can cause pulmonary artery vasodilation, which can lead to worsening hypoxia in patients with underlying ventilation-perfusion abnormalities.

Inotropic agents Positive inotropic agents produce direct hemodynamic benefits by stimulating cardiac contractility, as well as by producing peripheral vasodilation. Collectively, these hemodynamic effects result in an improvement in cardiac output and a fall in LV filling pressures.

Dobutamine, which is the most commonly used inotropic agent for the treatment of acute HF, exerts its effects by stimulating β_1 and β_2 receptors, with little effect on α_1 receptors. Dobutamine is given as a continuous infusion, at an initial infusion rate of 1–2 μg/kg per min. Higher doses (>5 μg/kg per min) are frequently necessary for severe hypoperfusion; however, there is little added benefit to increasing the dose above 10 μg/kg per min. Patients maintained on chronic infusions for >72 h generally develop tachyphylaxis and require increasing doses.

Milrinone is a phosphodiesterase III inhibitor that leads to increased cAMP by inhibiting its breakdown. Milrinone may act synergistically with β-adrenergic agonists to achieve further increase in cardiac output than either agent alone, and it may also be more effective than dobutamine in increasing cardiac output in the presence of beta blockers. Milrinone may be administered as a bolus dose of 0.5 μg/kg per min, followed by a continuous infusion rate of 0.1–0.75 μg/kg per min. Because milrinone is a more effective vasodilator than dobutamine, it produces a greater reduction in LV filling pressures, albeit with a greater risk of hypotension.

Although short-term use of inotropes provides hemodynamic benefits, these agents are more prone to cause tachyarrhythmias and ischemic events than vasodilators. Therefore inotropes are most appropriately used in clinical settings in which vasodilators and diuretics are not helpful, such as in patients with poor systemic perfusion and/or cardiogenic shock, in patients requiring short-term hemodynamic support after a MI or surgery, and in patients awaiting cardiac transplantation, or as palliative care in patients with advanced HF. If patients require sustained use of intravenous inotropes, strong consideration should be given to the use of an ICD to safeguard against the proarrhythmic effects of these agents.

Vasoconstrictors Vasoconstrictors are used to support systemic blood pressure in patients with HF. Of the three agents that are commonly used (Table 17-5), dopamine is generally the first choice for therapy in situations where modest inotropy and pressor support are required. Dopamine is an endogenous catecholamine that stimulates β_1, α_1 receptors, and dopaminergic receptors (DA$_1$ and DA$_2$) in the heart and circulation. The effects of dopamine are dose-dependent. Low doses of dopamine (<2 µg/kg per min) stimulate the DA$_1$ and DA$_2$ receptors and cause vasodilation of the splanchnic and renal vasculature. Moderate doses (2–4 µg/kg per min) stimulate the β_1 receptors and cause an increase in cardiac output with little or no change in heart rate or SVR. At higher doses ($\geq$5 µg/kg per min) the effects of dopamine on the α_1 receptors overwhelm the dopaminergic receptors, and vasoconstriction ensues, leading to an increase in SVR, LV filling pressures, and heart rate.

Dopamine also causes release of norepinephrine from nerve terminals, which itself stimulates α_1 and β_1 receptors, thus raising blood pressure. Dopamine is most useful in the treatment of HF patients who have depressed cardiac output with poor tissue perfusion (Profile C). Significant additional inotropic and blood pressure support can be provided by epinephrine, phenylephrine, and vasopressin (Table 17-5); however, prolonged use of these agents can lead to renal and hepatic failure and can cause gangrene of the limbs. Therefore, these agents should not be administered except in true emergency situations.

Mechanical and Surgical Interventions If pharmacologic interventions fail to stabilize the patient with refractory HF, mechanical and surgical interventions may provide effective circulatory support. These include intraaortic balloon counter pulsation, LV assist device, and cardiac transplantation (Chap. 18).

Planning for Hospital Discharge Patient education should take place during the entire hospitalization, with a specific focus on salt and fluid status and obtaining daily weights, in addition to medication schedules. Whereas the majority of patients hospitalized with HF can be stabilized and returned to a good level of function on an oral regimen designed to maintain stability, 30–50% of patients discharged with a diagnosis of HF are rehospitalized within 3–6 months.

Although there are multiple reasons for rehospitalization, failure to meet criteria for discharge is perhaps the most frequent. Criteria for discharge should include at least 24 h of stable fluid status, blood pressure, and renal function on the oral regimen planned for home. Patients should be free of dyspnea or symptomatic hypotension while at rest, washing, and walking on the ward.

COR PULMONALE

DEFINITION

Cor pulmonale, often referred to as *pulmonary heart disease*, is defined as dilation and hypertrophy of the right ventricle (RV) in response to diseases of the pulmonary vasculature and/or lung parenchyma. Historically, this definition has excluded congenital heart disease and those diseases in which the right heart fails secondary to dysfunction of the left side of the heart.

ETIOLOGY AND EPIDEMIOLOGY

Cor pulmonale develops in response to acute or chronic changes in the pulmonary vasculature and/or the lung parenchyma that are sufficient to cause pulmonary hypertension. The true prevalence of cor pulmonale is difficult to ascertain for two reasons. First, not all cases of chronic lung disease will develop cor pulmonale, and second, our ability to diagnose pulmonary hypertension and cor pulmonale by routine physical examination and laboratory testing is relatively insensitive. However, recent advances in 2-D echo/Doppler imaging and biomakers (BNP) make it easier to screen for and detect cor pulmonale.

Once patients with chronic pulmonary or pulmonary vascular disease develop cor pulmonale, their prognosis worsens. Although chronic obstructive pulmonary disease (COPD) and chronic bronchitis are responsible for approximately 50% percent of the cases of cor pulmonale in North America, any disease that affects the pulmonary vasculature (Chap. 40) or parenchyma can lead to cor pulmonale. Table 17-6 provides a list of common diseases that may lead to cor pulmonale. In contrast to COPD, the elevation in pulmonary artery pressure appears to be substantially higher in the interstitial lung diseases, in which there is an inverse correlation between pulmonary artery pressure and the diffusion capacity for carbon monoxide, as well as patient survival. Sleep-disordered breathing, once thought to be a major mechanism for cor pulmonale, is rarely the sole cause of pulmonary hypertension and RV failure. The combination of COPD and associated daytime hypoxemia is required to cause sustained pulmonary hypertension in obstructive sleep apnea.

TABLE 17-6

ETIOLOGY OF CHRONIC COR PULMONALE

Diseases Leading to Hypoxic Vasoconstriction

Chronic bronchitis
Chronic obstructive pulmonary disease
Cystic fibrosis
Chronic hypoventilation
  Obesity
  Neuromuscular disease
  Chest wall dysfunction
Living at high altitudes

Diseases That Cause Occlusion of the Pulmonary Vascular Bed

Recurrent pulmonary thromboembolism
Primary pulmonary hypertension
Venocclusive disease
Collagen vascular disease
Drug-induced lung disease

Diseases That Lead to Parenchymal Disease

Chronic bronchitis
Chronic obstructive pulmonary disease
Bronchiectasis
Cystic fibrosis
Pneumoconiosis
Sarcoid
Idiopathic pulmonary fibrosis

PATHOPHYSIOLOGY AND BASIC MECHANISMS

Although many conditions can lead to cor pulmonale, the common pathophysiologic mechanism in each case is pulmonary hypertension that is sufficient to lead to RV dilation, with or without the development of concomitant RV hypertrophy. The systemic consequences of cor pulmonale relate to alterations in cardiac output as well as salt and water homeostasis. Anatomically, the RV is a thin-walled, compliant chamber that is better suited to handle volume overload than pressure overload. Thus, the sustained pressure overload imposed by pulmonary hypertension and increased pulmonary vascular resistance eventually causes the RV to fail.

The response of the RV to pulmonary hypertension depends on the acuteness and severity of the pressure overload. Acute cor pulmonale occurs after a sudden and severe stimulus (e.g., massive pulmonary embolus), with RV dilatation and failure but no RV hypertrophy. Chronic cor pulmonale, however, is associated with a more slowly evolving and slowly progressive pulmonary hypertension that leads to RV dilation and hypertrophy. The severity of the pulmonary artery hypertension and the onset of RV failure are influenced by multiple factors that occur intermittently, including hypoxia secondary to alterations in gas exchange, hypercapnia, and

acidosis, as well as alterations in RV volume overload that are affected by exercise, heart rate, polycythemia, or increased salt and retention because of a fall in cardiac output (Fig. 17-2).

The most common mechanisms that lead to pulmonary hypertension, including vasoconstriction, activation of the clotting cascade, and obliteration of pulmonary arterial vessels, are discussed in Chap. 40.

CLINICAL MANIFESTATIONS

Symptoms

The symptoms of chronic cor pulmonale are generally related to the underlying pulmonary disorder. Dyspnea, the most common symptom, is usually the result of the increased work of breathing secondary to changes in elastic recoil of the lung (fibrosing lung diseases) or altered respiratory mechanics (e.g., overinflation with COPD), both of which may be aggravated by increased hypoxic respiratory drive. The hypoxia that occurs in lung disease is the result of reduced capillary membrane permeability, ventilation-perfusion mismatch, and occasionally intracardiac or intrapulmonary shunting.

Orthopnea and paroxysmal nocturnal dyspnea are rarely symptoms of isolated right HF. However, when present, these symptoms usually reflect the increased work of breathing in the supine position that results from compromised excursion of the diaphragm. Tussive or effort-related syncope may occur in patients with cor pulmonale with severe pulmonary hypertension because of the inability of the RV to deliver blood adequately to the left side of the heart. The abdominal pain and ascites that occur with cor pulmonale are similar to the right heart failure that ensues in chronic HF. Lower-extremity edema may occur secondary to neurohormonal activation, elevated RV filling pressures, or increased levels of carbon dioxide and hypoxia, which can lead to peripheral vasodilation and edema formation.

Signs

Many of the signs that are encountered in cor pulmonale are also present in HF patients with a depressed EF, including tachypnea, elevated jugular venous pressures, hepatomegaly, and lower-extremity edema. Patients may have prominent v waves in the jugular venous pulse as a result of tricuspid regurgitation. Other cardiovascular signs include an RV heave palpable along the left sternal border or in the epigastrium. A systolic pulmonary ejection click may be audible to the left of the upper sternum. The increase in intensity of the holosystolic murmur of tricuspid regurgitation with inspiration ("Carvallo's sign") may be eventually lost as RV failure worsens. Cyanosis is a late finding in cor pulmonale and is secondary to a low cardiac output with systemic vasoconstriction and ventilation-perfusion mismatches in the lung.

DIAGNOSIS

The most common cause of right heart failure is not pulmonary parenchymal or vascular disease, but left heart failure. Therefore, it is important to evaluate the patient for LV systolic and diastolic dysfunction. The ECG in severe pulmonary hypertension shows P pulmonale, right axis deviation, and RV hypertrophy. Radiographic examination of the chest may show enlargement of the main pulmonary artery, hilar vessels, and the descending right pulmonary artery. Spiral CT scans of the chest are useful in diagnosing acute thromboembolic disease; however, the ventilation-perfusion lung scan remains reliable in most centers for establishing the diagnosis of *chronic thromboembolic disease*. A high-resolution CT scan of the chest is the most accurate means of diagnosing emphysema and interstitial lung disease.

Two-dimensional echocardiography (2DE) is useful for measuring RV thickness and chamber dimensions as well as the anatomy of the pulmonary and tricuspid valves. The interventricular septum may move paradoxically during systole in the presence of pulmonary hypertension. As noted, Doppler echocardiography can be used to assess pulmonary artery pressures. MRI is also useful for assessing RV structure and function, particularly in patients who are difficult to image with 2DE because of severe lung disease. Right-heart catheterization is useful for confirming the diagnosis of pulmonary hypertension and for excluding elevated left-heart pressures (measured as the PCWP) as a cause for right heart failure. BNP and N-terminal BNP levels are elevated in patients with cor pulmonale secondary to RV stretch and may be dramatically elevated in acute pulmonary embolism.

℞ Treatment: COR PULMONALE

The primary treatment goal of cor pulmonale is to target the underlying pulmonary disease, since this will lead to a decrease in pulmonary vascular resistance and relieve the pressure overload on the RV. Most pulmonary diseases that lead to chronic cor pulmonale are far advanced and are, therefore, less amenable to treatment. General principles of treatment include decreasing the work of breathing using noninvasive mechanical ventilation, bronchodilation, and steroids, as well as

treating any underlying infection. Adequate oxygenation (oxygen saturation ≥90–92%) will also decrease pulmonary vascular resistance and reduce the demands on the RV. Patients should be transfused if they are anemic, and a phlebotomy should be performed to reduce pulmonary artery pressure if the hematocrit exceeds 65%.

Diuretics are effective in the treatment of RV failure, and the indications for their use are similar to those for chronic HF. One caveat of chronic diuretic use is that they may lead to contraction alkalosis and worsening hypercapnea. Digoxin is of uncertain benefit in the treatment of cor pulmonale and may lead to arrhythmias in the setting of tissue hypoxia and acidosis. Therefore, if digoxin is administered, it should be given at low doses and monitored carefully. The treatment of pulmonary hypertension is discussed in Chap. 40.

FURTHER READINGS

Ashrafian H et al: Metabolic mechanisms in heart failure. Circulation 116:434, 2007

Bardy GH et al: Amiodarone or an implantable cardioverter-defibrillator for congestive heart failure. N Engl J Med 352:225, 2005

Chapman HA: Disorders of lung matrix remodeling. J Clin Invest 113:148, 2004

Cleland JG et al: The effect of cardiac resynchronization on morbidity and mortality in heart failure. N Engl J Med 352:1539, 2005

Friedrich EB, Bohm M: Management of end stage heart failure. Heart 93:626, 2007

Hunt SA et al: 2009 focused update incorporated into the ACC/AHA 2005 Guidelines for the Diagnosis and Management of Heart Failure in Adults: a report of the American College of Cardiology Foundation/American Heart Association Task Force on Practice Guidelines. Developed in collaboration with the International Society for Heart and Lung Transplantation. Circulation 119:e391, 2009

Kessler R et al: "Natural history" of pulmonary hypertension in a series of 131 patients with chronic obstructive lung disease. Am J Respir Crit Care Med 164:219, 2001

Mann DL, Bristow MR: Mechanisms and models in heart failure: The biomechanical model and beyond. Circulation 111:2837, 2005

Mazhari R, Hare JM: Advances in cell-based therapy for structural heart disease. Prog Cardiovasc Dis 49:387, 2007

Mosterd A, Hoes AW: Clinical epidemiology of heart failure. Heart 93:1137, 2007

Pengo V et al: Incidence of chronic thromboembolic pulmonary hypertension after pulmonary embolism. N Engl J Med 350:2257, 2004

CHAPTER 18

CARDIAC TRANSPLANTATION AND PROLONGED ASSISTED CIRCULATION

Sharon A. Hunt

Advanced or end-stage heart failure is an increasingly frequent sequela as progressively more effective palliation for the earlier stages of heart disease and prevention of sudden death associated with heart disease become more widely recognized and employed (Chap. 17). When patients with end-stage or refractory heart failure are identified, the physician is faced with the decision of advising compassionate end-of-life care or choosing to recommend extraordinary life-extending measures. For the occasional patient who is relatively young and without serious comorbidities, the latter may represent a reasonable option. Current therapeutic options are limited to cardiac transplantation (with the option of mechanical cardiac assistance as a "bridge" to transplantation) or (at least in theory) the option of permanent mechanical assistance of the circulation.

CARDIAC TRANSPLANTATION

Surgical techniques for orthotopic transplantation of the heart were devised in the 1960s and taken into the clinical arena in 1967. The procedure did not gain widespread clinical acceptance until the introduction of "modern" and more effective immunosuppression in the early 1980s. By the 1990s the demand for transplantable hearts met, and then exceeded, the available donor supply and leveled off at about 4000 heart transplants annually

worldwide, according to data from the Registry of the International Society for Heart and Lung Transplantation (ISHLT). Subsequently heart transplant activity in the United States has remained stable at ~2200/year, but worldwide activity reported to this Registry has decreased some. The apparent decline in numbers may be a result of the fact that reporting is legally mandated in the United States, but not elsewhere, and several countries have started their own databases.

SURGICAL TECHNIQUE

Donor and recipient hearts are excised in virtually identical operations with incisions made across the atria and atrial septum at the midatrial level (leaving the posterior walls of the atria in place) and across the great vessels just above the semilunar valves. The donor heart is generally "harvested" in an anatomically identical manner by a separate surgical team and transported from the donor hospital in a bag of iced saline solution and then is reanastomosed into the waiting recipient in the orthotopic or normal anatomic position. The only change in surgical technique since this method was first described has been a movement in recent years to move the right atrial anastamosis back to the level of the superior and inferior vena cavae in order to better preserve right atrial geometry and prevent atrial arrhythmias. Both methods of implantation leave the recipient with a surgically denervated heart that does not respond to any direct sympathetic or parasympathetic stimuli but does respond to circulating catecholamines. The physiologic responses of the denervated heart to the demands of exercise are atypical but quite adequate to carry on normal physical activity.

DONOR ALLOCATION SYSTEM

In the United States the allocation of donor organs is accomplished under the supervision of the United Network for Organ Sharing (UNOS), a private organization under contract to the federal government. The United States is divided geographically into 11 regions for donor heart allocation. Allocation of donor hearts within a region is decided according to a system of priority that takes into account (1) the severity of illness, (2) geographic distance from the donor, and (3) patient time on the waiting list. A physiologic limit of ~3 h of "ischemic" (out of body) time for hearts precludes a national sharing of hearts. The allocation system design is reissued annually and is responsive to input from a variety of constituencies, including donor families and transplant professionals.

At the current time, highest priority according to severity of illness is assigned to patients requiring hospitalization at the transplant center for IV inotropic support with a pulmonary artery catheter in place for hemodynamic monitoring or to patients requiring mechanical circulatory support [i.e., intra-aortic balloon pump (IABP), right or left ventricular assist device (RVAD, LVAD), extracorporeal membrane oxygenation (ECMO), or mechanical ventilation]. Second highest priority is given to patients requiring ongoing inotropic support, but without a pulmonary artery catheter in place. All other patients have priority according to their time on the waiting list, and matching is achieved only according to ABO blood group compatibility and gross body size compatibility, although some patients who are "presensitized" and have preexisting anti-HLA antibodies (commonly multiparous women or patients previously multiply transfused) undergo prospective cross-matching with the donor.

INDICATIONS/CONTRAINDICATIONS

Heart failure is an increasingly common cause of death, particularly in the elderly. Most patients who reach what has recently been categorized as stage D, or refractory end-stage heart failure, are appropriately treated with compassionate end-of-life care. A subset of such patients who are younger and without significant comorbidities can be considered as candidates for heart transplantation. Exact criteria vary in different centers but generally take into consideration the patient's physiologic age and the existence of comorbidities such as peripheral or cerebrovascular disease, obesity, diabetes, cancer, or chronic infection.

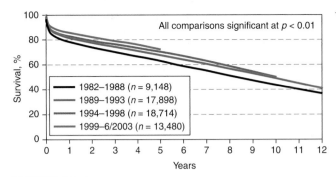

FIGURE 18-1

Adult heart transplantation. Kaplan-Meier. Actuarial survival for heart transplants performed between 1982 and 2003 by era of transplantation. (*J Heart Lung Transplant 24:945, 2005. Data by permission from International Society for Heart and Lung Transplantation.*)

RESULTS

A registry organized by the ISHLT has tracked worldwide and U.S. survival rates after heart transplantation since 1982. The most recent update reveals 83% and 76% survival 1 and 3 years posttransplant, or a posttransplant "half-life" of 9.3 years (**Fig. 18-1**). The quality of life in these patients is generally excellent, with well above 90% of patients in the registry returning to normal and unrestricted function following transplantation.

IMMUNOSUPPRESSION

Medical regimens employed to provide suppression of the normal immune response to a solid organ allograft vary from center to center and are in a constant state of evolution as more effective agents with improved side-effect profiles and less toxicity are introduced. All currently used regimens are nonspecific, providing general hyporeactivity to foreign antigens rather than donor-specific hyporeactivity as well as the attendant, and unwanted, susceptibility to infections and malignancy. Most cardiac transplant programs currently use a three-drug regimen including a calcineurin inhibitor (cyclosporine or tacrolimus), an inhibitor of T cell proliferation or differentiation (azathioprine, mycophenolate mofetil, or sirolimus), and at least a short initial course of glucocorticoids. Many programs also include an initial "induction" course of polyclonal or monoclonal anti-T cell antibodies in the perioperative period to decrease the frequency or severity of early posttransplant rejection. Most recently introduced have been monoclonal antibodies (daclizumab and basiliximab), which block the interleukin-2 receptor and may provide prevention of allograft rejection without additional global immunosuppression.

Diagnosis of cardiac allograft rejection is usually made with the use of endomyocardial biopsy, either done on a surveillance basis or in response to clinical deterioration.

Biopsy surveillance is performed on a regular basis in most programs for the first year postoperatively and for the first 5 years in many programs. Therapy consists of augmentation of immunosuppression, the intensity and duration of which is dictated by the severity of the rejection.

LATE POSTTRANSPLANT MANAGEMENT ISSUES

Increasing numbers of heart transplant patients are surviving for years following transplantation and constitute a population of patients with a number of long-term management issues.

Allograft Coronary Artery Disease

Despite usually having young donor hearts, cardiac allograft recipients are prone to develop coronary artery disease (CAD). This CAD is generally a diffuse, concentric, and longitudinal process that is quite different from "ordinary" atherosclerotic CAD, which is more focal and often eccentric. The underlying etiology is most likely primarily immunologic injury of the vascular endothelium, but a variety of risk factors influence its existence and progression and include nonimmunologic factors such as dyslipidemia, diabetes, and cytomegalovirus (CMV) infection. It is hoped that newer and improved immunosuppressive modalities will reduce the incidence and impact of these devastating complications, which currently account for the majority of late posttransplant deaths. Thus far the newer immunosuppressive agents mycophenolate mofetil and the mammalian target of rapamycin (mTOR) inhibitors sirolimus and everolimus have been shown to be associated with short-term lesser incidence and extent of coronary intimal thickening; in anecdotal reports institution of sirolimus was associated with some reversal of the disease. The use of statins has also been shown to be associated with a reduced incidence of this vasculopathy, and these drugs are now almost universally used in transplant recipients unless contraindicated. Palliation of the disease with percutaneous interventions is probably safe and effective in the short term, although the disease often advances relentlessly. Because of the denervated status of the organ, patients rarely experience angina pectoris, even with advanced stages of the disease.

Retransplantation is the only definitive form of therapy for advanced allograft CAD, but the scarcity of donor hearts make the decision to pursue retransplantation a difficult one in an individual patient, as well as a difficult ethical issue.

Malignancy

The occurrence of an increased incidence of malignancy is a well-recognized sequela of any program of chronic immunosuppression, and organ transplantation is no exception. Lymphoproliferative disorders are among the most frequent posttransplant complications and, in most cases, seem to be driven by the Epstein-Barr virus. Effective therapy includes reduction of immunosuppression (a clear "double-edged sword" in the setting of a life-sustaining organ), antiviral agents, and traditional chemo- and radiotherapy. Most recently, specific antilymphocyte (CD20) therapy has shown great promise. Cutaneous malignancies (both basal cell and squamous cell carcinomas) also occur with increased frequency in transplant recipients and can pursue very aggressive courses. The role of decreasing immunosuppression for treatment of these cancers is much less clear.

Infections

The use of currently available nonspecific immunosuppressive modalities to prevent allograft rejection naturally results in an increased susceptibility to infectious complications in transplant recipients. Although their incidence has decreased since the introduction of cyclosporine, infections with unusual and opportunistic organisms remain the major cause of death during the first postoperative year and remain a threat to the chronically immunosuppressed patient throughout life. Effective therapy depends on careful surveillance for early signs and symptoms of opportunistic infection and an extremely aggressive approach to obtaining a specific diagnosis as well as expertise in recognizing the more common clinical presentations of CMV, *Aspergillus*, and other opportunistic infectious agents.

PROLONGED ASSISTED CIRCULATION

The modern era of mechanical circulatory support can be traced back to 1953 when cardiopulmonary bypass was first used in a clinical setting and ushered in the possibility of brief periods of circulatory support to permit open-heart surgery. There have subsequently been developed a variety of extracorporeal pumps to provide circulatory support for brief periods of time. The use of a mechanical device to support the circulation for more than a few hours got off to a slow start in the 1980s when the first artificial hearts were introduced with much publicity but failed to produce the hoped-for treatment of end-stage heart disease. Subsequently, technology evolved to provide mechanical assistance to (rather than replacement of) the failing ventricle, although newer versions of the total artificial heart are now once again in preliminary clinical trials.

Although conceived of initially as alternatives to biologic replacement of the heart, LVADs were introduced as, and are still employed primarily as, temporary "bridges" to heart transplantation in candidates who begin to fail medical therapy before a donor heart becomes available.

Several devices are approved by the U.S. Food and Drug Administration (FDA) and are currently in widespread use. Those that are implantable within the body are compatible with hospital discharge and offer the patient chance for life at home while waiting for a donor heart. However successful such "bridging" is for the individual patient, it does nothing to alleviate the scarcity of donor hearts, and the ultimate goal in the field remains that of providing a reasonable alternative to biologic replacement of the heart—one that is widely and easily available and cost effective.

AVAILABLE DEVICES

In the United States there are currently three FDA-approved devices that are used as bridges to transplantation. There are a number of other devices that are approved only for short-term support for postcardiac surgery shock and these will not be considered here. None of the long-term devices as yet are totally implantable, and, because of this need for transcutaneous connections, all share a common problem with infectious complications. Likewise, all share some tendency to thromboembolic complications as well as the expected possibility of mechanical device failure common to any man-made machine.

The Thoratec LVAD (Thoratec Corp., Pleasanton, CA) is an extracorporeal pump that takes blood from a large cannula placed in the left ventricular apex and propels it forward through an outflow cannula inserted into the ascending aorta. The pump itself sits in the paracorporeal position on the abdomen and is attached to a device console cart with wheels, allowing for limited ambulation. The extracorporeal nature of this pump allows it to be used for small adults for whom the intracorporeal pumps would be too large.

The Novacor LVAD (WorldHeart Inc., Oakland, CA) also takes blood from the left ventricular apex through a cannula and propels it into the ascending aorta through a second cannula. With this device the pump itself is placed in a surgically created pocket in the preperitoneal fascia in the abdomen. A drive line that connects to the power source is tunneled subcutaneously and usually exits in the right upper quadrant of the abdomen.

The HeartMate LVAD (Thoratec Corp., Pleasanton, CA) uses a configuration identical to that of the Novacor device (Fig. 18-2). Differences between the two have to do with the materials used and the tendency for thromboembolic complications. Both commonly lead to hospital discharge and an outpatient wait for a donor heart. Newer devices, currently in clinical trials, include several axial-flow pumps that have basically the same connections to the circulatory system but are considerably smaller, have fewer moving parts than previous devices, and provide non-pulsatile blood flow. All current axial-flow pumps continue to require transcutaneous connections.

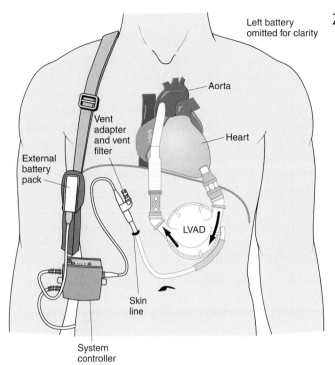

FIGURE 18-2

Diagram of HeartMate left ventricular assist device (LVAD). *(Reprinted with permission from Thoratec Corp., Pleasanton, CA.)*

RESULTS

The use of these devices in the United States is limited mainly to patients with postcardiac surgery shock and to those who are "bridged" to transplantation. The results of bridging to transplantation with the available devices are quite good, with nearly 75% of younger patients receiving a transplant by 1 year and those having excellent posttransplant survival rates.

Publication of the REMATCH (Randomized Evaluation of Mechanical Assistance in the Treatment of Heart Failure) trial in 2001 documented a somewhat improved survival in nontransplant candidates with end-stage heart disease randomized to a HeartMate LVAD (albeit with a high rate of complications, especially neurologic ones) as opposed to continued medical therapy; this led to renewed interest in also using the devices as non-biologic permanent replacement of heart function as well as to FDA approval of one device for this indication. This, in turn, led the ISHLT to initiate a Mechanical Circulatory Support database in 2002. This database collects voluntary data from 60 international centers and contained data from 655 patients in its most recent publication. Only 12% of these had the device placed with the intention of permanent, or "destination," use, with survival rates of only 65% at 6 months and 34% at 1 year.

Future developments in this field can be expected in two directions. First, newer generations of the pumps will likely be smaller and mechanically simpler and, most important, totally implantable. Second, increased use of the newer generations of pumps as "permanent" (destination) therapy in patients with end-stage heart failure who are not considered eligible for transplantation will likely happen in the near future. Eventually it is hoped that improved assist devices will be accepted as valid alternatives to biologic replacement of the heart even in transplant-eligible patients and help to modify the supply/demand mismatch for cardiac replacement therapy.

FURTHER READINGS

DENG MC et al: Mechanical circulatory support device database of the International Society for Heart and Lung Transplantation: Third annual report—2005. J Heart Lung Transplant 24:1182, 2005

GARNIER JL et al: Treatment of post-transplant lymphomas with anti-B-cell monoclonal antibodies. Recent Results Cancer Res 159:113, 2002

GRAY NA JR, SELZMAN CH: Current status of the total artificial heart. Am Heart J 152:4, 2006

HUNT SA et al: ACC/AHA 2005 guideline update for the diagnosis and management of chronic heart failure in the adult: A report of the American College of Cardiology/American Heart Association Task Force on Practice Guidelines (Writing committee to update the 2001 guidelines for the evaluation and management of heart failure). Available at *http://www.acc.org/clinical/guidelines/failure//index.pdf*

KIRKLIN JK et al: INTERMACS Database for Durable Devices for Circulatory Support: First Annual Report. J Heart Lung Transplant 27:1065, 2008

MANCINI D et al: Use of rapamycin slows progression of cardiac transplantation vasculopathy. Circulation 108:48, 2003

TAYLOR DO et al: Registry of the International Society for Heart and Lung Transplantation: Twenty-second official adult heart transplant report—2005. J Heart Lung Transplant 224:945, 2005

CHAPTER 19

CONGENITAL HEART DISEASE IN THE ADULT

John S. Child

Congenital heart disease (CHD) complicates ~1% of all live births in the general population but occurs in 4% of offspring of women with CHD. Substantial numbers of affected infants and children, estimated at >85% currently, reach adulthood because of successful medical and surgical management or because they have successfully adapted to their particular cardiovascular physiology. More than 800,000 adults with operated or unoperated CHD exist in the United States today; as such, adults now outnumber children with CHD.

ETIOLOGY

CHD is generally the result of aberrant embryonic development of a normal structure or failure of such a structure to progress beyond an early stage of embryonic or fetal development. Malformations are due to complex multifactorial genetic and environmental causes. Recognized chromosomal aberrations and mutations of single genes account for <10% of all cardiac malformations.

The presence of a cardiac malformation as a component of the multiple system involvement in Down syndrome, Turner syndrome, and the trisomy 13-15(D1) and 17-18(E) syndromes may be anticipated in occasional pregnancies by detection of abnormal chromosomes in fetal cells obtained from amniotic fluid or chorionic villus biopsy. Identification in such cells of the enzyme disorders characteristic of Hurler's syndrome, homocystinuria, or type II glycogen storage disease may also allow one to predict cardiac disease.

PATHOPHYSIOLOGY

The anatomic and physiologic changes in the heart and circulation due to any specific CHD lesion are not static but, rather, progress from prenatal life to adulthood. Malformations that are benign or escape detection in childhood may become clinically significant in the adult. For example, a functionally normal congenitally bicuspid aortic valve may thicken and calcify with time, resulting in significant aortic stenosis; or a well-tolerated left-to-right shunt of an atrial septal defect (ASD) may result in cardiac decompensation or pulmonary hypertension only after the fourth to fifth decade.

Pulmonary Hypertension

The status of the pulmonary vascular bed is often a principal determinant of the clinical manifestations and course of a given lesion and of the feasibility of surgical repair. Increased pulmonary arterial pressure results from increased pulmonary blood flow and/or resistance, the latter usually the result of obstructive, obliterative structural changes within the pulmonary vascular bed. It is important to quantitate and compare pulmonary to systemic flows and resistances in patients with severe pulmonary hypertension. The causes of pulmonary vascular obstructive disease are unknown, although increased pulmonary blood flow, increased pulmonary arterial blood pressure, elevated pulmonary venous pressure, erythrocytosis, systemic hypoxemia, acidosis, and the bronchial circulation have been implicated. The term *Eisenmenger syndrome* is applied to patients with a large communication between the two circulations at the aortopulmonary, ventricular, or atrial levels and bidirectional or predominantly right-to-left shunts because of high-resistance and obstructive pulmonary hypertension. Pulmonary arterial vasodilators and both single lung transplantation with intracardiac defect repair and total heart-lung transplantation show promise for improvement in symptoms (Chap. 18).

Erythrocytosis

Chronic hypoxemia in cyanotic CHD results in secondary *erythrocytosis* due to increased erythropoietin production (Chap. 6). The commonly used term *polycythemia* is a misnomer because white cell counts are normal and platelet counts are normal to decreased. Cyanotic patients with erythrocytosis may have compensated or decompensated hematocrits. Compensated erythrocytosis with iron-replete equilibrium hematocrits rarely result in symptoms of hyperviscosity at hematocrits <65% and occasionally not even with hematocrits ≥70%. Therapeutic phlebotomy is rarely required in compensated erythrocytosis. In contrast, patients with decompensated erythrocytosis fail to establish equilibrium with unstable, rising hematocrits and recurrent hyperviscosity symptoms. Therapeutic phlebotomy, a two-edged sword, allows temporary relief of symptoms but limits oxygen delivery, begets instability of the hematocrit, and compounds the problem by iron depletion. Iron-deficiency symptoms are usually indistinguishable from those of hyperviscosity; progressive symptoms after recurrent phlebotomy are usually due to iron depletion with hypochromic microcytosis. Iron depletion results in a larger number of smaller (microcytic) hypochromic red cells that are less capable of carrying oxygen. Because these microcytes are less deformable in the microcirculation and there are more of them relative to the plasma volume, the viscosity is greater than for an equivalent hematocrit with fewer, larger, iron-replete, deformable cells. As such, iron-depleted erythrocytosis results in increasing symptoms due to decreased oxygen delivery to the tissues.

Hemostasis is abnormal in cyanotic CHD, due in part to the increased blood volume and engorged capillaries, abnormalities in platelet function and sensitivity to aspirin or nonsteroidal anti-inflammatory agents, and abnormalities of the extrinsic and intrinsic coagulation

system. Oral contraceptives are often contraindicated for cyanotic women because of the enhanced risk of vascular thrombosis.

The risk of stroke is greatest in children <4 years with cyanotic heart disease and iron deficiency, often with dehydration as an aggravating cause. Adults with cyanotic CHD do not appear to be at increased risk for stroke, unless there are excessive injudicious phlebotomies, inappropriate use of aspirin or anticoagulants, or the presence of atrial arrhythmias or infective endocarditis.

Symptoms of hyperviscosity can be produced in any cyanotic patient with erythrocytosis if dehydration reduces plasma volume. Phlebotomy for symptoms of hyperviscosity not due to dehydration or iron deficiency is a simple outpatient removal of 500 mL of blood over 45 min with isovolumetric replacement with isotonic saline. Acute phlebotomy without volume replacement is contraindicated. Iron repletion in decompensated iron-depleted erythrocytosis reduces iron-deficiency symptoms but must be done gradually to avoid an excessive rise in hematocrit and resultant hyperviscosity.

Pregnancy

The physiologic alterations during normal gestation can create symptoms and physical findings that may be attributed erroneously to heart disease. The mother's health is most at risk if she has a cardiovascular lesion associated with pulmonary vascular disease and pulmonary hypertension (e.g., Eisenmenger physiology or mitral stenosis) or left ventricular (LV) outflow tract obstruction (e.g., aortic stenosis), but she is also at risk of death with any malformation that may cause heart failure or a hemodynamically important arrhythmia. The fetus is most at risk with maternal cyanosis, heart failure, or pulmonary hypertension. Women with aortic coarctation or Marfan syndrome risk aortic dissection. Patients with cyanotic heart disease, pulmonary hypertension, or Marfan syndrome with a dilated aortic root should not become pregnant; those with correctable lesions should be counseled about the risks of pregnancy with an uncorrected malformation versus repair and later pregnancy. The effect of pregnancy in postoperative patients depends on the outcome of the repair, including the presence and severity of residua, sequelae, or complications. Contraception is an important topic with such patients. Tubal ligation should be considered in those in whom pregnancy is strictly contraindicated.

INFECTIVE ENDOCARDITIS

(See also Chap. 25) Routine antimicrobial prophylaxis is recommended for most patients with CHD, whether operated on or not, for all dental procedures, gastrointestinal and genitourinary surgery, and some diagnostic procedures, e.g., sigmoidoscopy and cystoscopy. The clinical and bacteriologic profile of infective endocarditis in patients with CHD has changed with the advent of intracardiac surgery and of prosthetic devices. Two major predisposing causes of infective endocarditis are a susceptible cardiovascular substrate and a source of bacteremia. Prophylaxis includes both antimicrobial and hygienic measures. Meticulous dental and skin care is required.

EXERCISE

Advice on athletics and exercise is governed by the nature of the exercise and by the type and severity of the congenital cardiovascular lesion. Patients with LV outflow tract obstruction, if more than moderate, or pulmonary vascular disease risk syncope or sudden death. In unrepaired tetralogy of Fallot, isotonic exercise–induced decrease in systemic vascular resistance relative to the right ventricular (RV) outflow obstruction augments the right-to-left shunt, increases hypoxemia, and causes an increase in subjective breathlessness owing to the response of the respiratory center to the changes in blood gases and pH.

SPECIFIC CARDIAC DEFECTS

Tables 19-1, 19-2, and 19-3 list CHD malformations as complex, intermediate, or simple. The goal of these tables is to suggest when cardiology consultation or advanced CHD specialty care is needed. Patients with complex CHD (which includes most "named" surgeries that usually involve complex CHD) should virtually always be managed in conjunction with an experienced specialty adult CHD center. Intermediate lesions should have initial consultation and subsequent occasional intermittent follow-up with a cardiologist. Simple lesions may be managed by a well-informed internist, though consultation with a cardiologist is occasionally advisable.

ACYANOTIC CONGENITAL HEART DISEASE WITH A LEFT-TO-RIGHT SHUNT

Atrial Septal Defect

ASD is a common cardiac anomaly that may be first encountered in the adult and occurs more frequently in

TABLE 19-1

COMPLEX ADULT CONGENITAL HEART DISEASE
Cyanotic congenital heart diseases (all forms)
Eisenmenger syndrome
Ebstein anomaly
Tetralogy of Fallot or pulmonary atresia (all forms)
Transposition of the great arteries
Single ventricle; tricuspid or mitral atresia
Double-outlet ventricle
Truncus arteriosus
Fontan or Rastelli procedures

TABLE 19-2

INTERMEDIATE COMPLEXITY CONGENITAL HEART DISEASE
Ostium primum or sinus venosus ASD
Anomalous pulmonary venous drainage, partial or total
Atrioventricular canal defects (partial or complete)
VSD, complicated (e.g., absent or abnormal valves or with associated obstructive lesions, aortic regurgitation)
Coarctation of the aorta
Pulmonic valve stenosis (moderate to severe)
Infundibular right ventricular outflow obstruction of significance
Pulmonary valve regurgitation (moderate to severe)
Patent ductus arteriosus (non-closed)—moderate to large
Sinus of Valsalva fistula/aneurysm
Subvalvular or supravalvular aortic stenosis

Note: ASD, atrial septal defect; VSD, ventricular septal defect.

TABLE 19-3

SIMPLE ADULT CONGENITAL HEART DISEASE
Native disease
Uncomplicated congenital aortic valve disease
Mild congenital mitral valve disease (e.g., except parachute valve, cleft leaflet)
Uncomplicated small ASD
Uncomplicated small VSD
Mild pulmonic stenosis
Repaired conditions
Previously ligated or occluded ductus arteriosus
Repaired secundum or sinus venosus ASD without residua
Repaired VSD without residua

Note: ASD, atrial septal defect; VSD, ventricular septal defect.

females. The *sinus venosus* type occurs high in the atrial septum near the entry of the superior vena cava into the right atrium and is associated frequently with anomalous pulmonary venous connection from the right lung to the superior vena cava or right atrium. *Ostium primum* anomalies lie adjacent to the atrioventricular valves, either of which may be deformed and regurgitant. Ostium primum defects are common in Down syndrome; the more complex atrioventricular septal defects with a common atrioventricular valve and a posterior defect of the basal portion of the interventricular septum are more typical of this chromosomal defect. The most common *ostium secundum* type ASD involves the fossa ovalis and is midseptal in location. This type of defect should not be confused with a *patent foramen ovale*. Anatomic obliteration of the foramen ovale ordinarily follows its functional closure soon after birth, but residual "probe patency" is a normal variant; ASD denotes a true deficiency of the atrial septum and implies functional and anatomic patency.

The magnitude of the left-to-right shunt depends on the ASD size, ventricular diastolic properties, and the relative impedance in the pulmonary and systemic circulations. The left-to-right shunt causes diastolic overloading of the right ventricle and increased pulmonary blood flow.

Patients with ASD are usually asymptomatic in early life, although there may be some physical underdevelopment and an increased tendency for respiratory infections; cardiorespiratory symptoms occur in many older patients. Beyond the fourth decade, a significant number of patients develop atrial arrhythmias, pulmonary arterial hypertension, bidirectional and then right-to-left shunting of blood, and cardiac failure. Patients exposed to the chronic environmental hypoxia of high altitude tend to develop pulmonary hypertension at younger ages. In some older patients, left-to-right shunting across the defect increases as progressive systemic hypertension and/or coronary artery disease result in reduced compliance of the left ventricle.

Physical Examination

Examination usually reveals a prominent RV impulse and palpable pulmonary artery pulsation. The first heart sound is normal or split, with accentuation of the tricuspid valve closure sound. Increased flow across the pulmonic valve is responsible for a midsystolic pulmonary outflow murmur. The second heart sound is widely split and is relatively fixed in relation to respiration. A mid-diastolic rumbling murmur, loudest at the fourth intercostal space and along the left sternal border, reflects increased flow across the tricuspid valve. In patients with ostium primum defects, an apical thrill and holosystolic murmur indicate associated mitral or tricuspid regurgitation or a ventricular septal defect (VSD).

The physical findings are altered when an increase in the pulmonary vascular resistance results in diminution of the left-to-right shunt. Both the pulmonary outflow and tricuspid inflow murmurs decrease in intensity, the pulmonic component of the second heart sound and a systolic ejection sound are accentuated, the two components of the second heart sound may fuse, and a diastolic murmur of pulmonic regurgitation appears. Cyanosis and clubbing accompany the development of a right-to-left shunt.

In adults with an ASD and atrial fibrillation, the physical findings may be confused with the findings of mitral stenosis with pulmonary hypertension because the tricuspid diastolic flow murmur and widely split second heart sound may be mistakenly thought to represent the diastolic murmur of mitral stenosis and the mitral "opening snap," respectively.

Electrocardiogram (ECG)

In patients with an ostium secundum defect, the ECG usually shows right-axis deviation and an rSr′ pattern in the right precordial leads representing enlargement of the RV outflow tract. An ectopic atrial pacemaker or first-degree heart block may occur with defects of the sinus venous type. In ostium primum defect, the RV conduction defect is accompanied by left superior axis deviation and counterclockwise rotation of the frontal plane QRS loop. Varying degrees of RV and right atrial (RA) hypertrophy may occur with each type of defect, depending on the height of the pulmonary artery pressure. *Chest x-ray* reveals enlargement of the right atrium and right ventricle, dilatation of the pulmonary artery and its branches, and increased pulmonary vascular markings.

Echocardiogram

Echocardiography reveals pulmonary arterial and RV and RA dilatation with abnormal (paradoxical) ventricular septal motion in the presence of a significant right heart volume overload. The ASD may be visualized directly by two-dimensional imaging, color flow imaging, or echocontrast. In most institutions, two-dimensional echocardiography (2DE) plus color Doppler flow examination has supplanted cardiac catheterization. Transesophageal echocardiography (TEE) is indicated if the transthoracic echocardiogram is ambiguous, which is often the case with sinus venosus defects, or during catheter device closure (**Fig. 19-1**). Cardiac catheterization is performed if inconsistencies exist in the clinical data, if significant pulmonary hypertension or associated malformations are suspected, or if coronary artery disease is a possibility.

℞ **Treatment:**
ATRIAL SEPTAL DEFECT

Operative repair, usually with a patch of pericardium or of prosthetic material, or percutaneous transcatheter device closure, if the defect is of an appropriate size and shape, should be advised for all patients with uncomplicated secundum ASDs with significant left-to-right shunting, i.e., pulmonary-to-systemic flow ratios ≥2.0:1.0. Excellent results may be anticipated, at low risk, even in patients >40 years, in the absence of severe pulmonary hypertension. In ostium primum defects, cleft mitral valves may require repair in addition to patch closure of the atrial defect. Closure should not be carried out in patients with small defects and trivial left-to-right shunts or in those with severe pulmonary vascular disease without a significant left-to-right shunt.

Patients with ASD of the sinus venosus or ostium secundum types rarely die before the fifth decade. During the fifth and sixth decades, the incidence of progressive symptoms, often leading to severe disability, increases substantially. Medical management should include prompt treatment of respiratory tract infections,

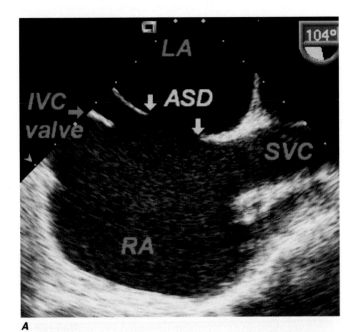

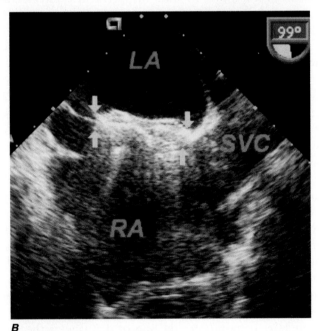

FIGURE 19-1

Secundum atrial septal defect. Transesophageal echocardiogram of secundum ASD and device closure. **A.** The atrial septal defect (ASD) between the left atrium (LA) and right atrium (RA) is shown. **B.** A percutaneous catheter–delivered device has occluded the defect. IVC, inferior vena cava; SVC, superior vena cava.

antiarrhythmic medications for atrial fibrillation or supraventricular tachycardia, and the usual measures for hypertension, coronary disease, or heart failure (Chap. 17), if these complications occur. The risk of infective endocarditis is quite low unless the defect is complicated by valvular regurgitation or has recently been repaired with a patch or device (Chap. 25).

Ventricular Septal Defect

Defects of the ventricular septum are common as isolated defects or as a component of a combination of anomalies. The opening is usually single and situated in the membranous portion of the septum. The functional disturbance depends on its size and on the status of the pulmonary vascular bed. Only small or moderate-size defects are usually seen initially in adulthood as most patients with isolated large defects come to medical and, often, surgical attention early in life.

A wide spectrum exists in the natural history of VSD, ranging from spontaneous closure to congestive cardiac failure and death in early infancy. Within this spectrum is the possible development of pulmonary vascular obstruction, RV outflow tract obstruction, aortic regurgitation, and infective endocarditis. Spontaneous closure is more common in patients born with a small ventricular septal defect and occurs in early childhood in most patients.

Patients with large VSDs and pulmonary hypertension are those at greatest risk for developing pulmonary vascular obstruction. Thus, large defects should be corrected surgically early in life when pulmonary vascular disease is still reversible or not yet developed. In patients with severe pulmonary vascular obstruction (Eisenmenger syndrome), symptoms in adult life consist of exertional dyspnea, chest pain, syncope, and hemoptysis. The right-to-left shunt leads to cyanosis, clubbing, and erythrocytosis. In all patients, the degree to which pulmonary vascular resistance is elevated before operation is a critical factor determining prognosis. If the pulmonary vascular resistance is one-third or less of the systemic value, progression of pulmonary vascular disease after operation is unusual. However, if a moderate to severe increase in pulmonary vascular resistance exists preoperatively, either no change or a progression of pulmonary vascular disease is common postoperatively.

RV outflow tract obstruction develops in ~5–10% of patients who present in infancy with a moderate to large left-to-right shunt. With time, as subvalvular RV outflow tract obstruction progresses, the findings in these patients whose VSD remains sizeable begin to resemble more closely those of the cyanotic tetralogy of Fallot.

In ~5% of patients, aortic valve regurgitation results from insufficient cusp tissue or prolapse of the cusp through the interventricular defect; the aortic regurgitation then complicates and dominates the clinical course.

2DE with spectral and color Doppler examination defines the number and location of defects in the ventricular septum and associated anomalies and the hemodynamic physiology of the defect(s). Hemodynamic and angiographic study may be occasionally required to assess the status of the pulmonary vascular bed and clarify details of the altered anatomy.

CHAPTER 19

Congenital Heart Disease in the Adult

Rx Treatment:
VENTRICULAR SEPTAL DEFECT

Surgery is not recommended for patients with normal pulmonary arterial pressures with small shunts (pulmonary-to-systemic flow ratios of <1.5 to 2.0:1.0). Operative correction or transcatheter closure is indicated when there is a moderate to large left-to-right shunt with a pulmonary-to-systemic flow ratio >1.5:1.0 or 2.0:1.0, in the absence of prohibitively high levels of pulmonary vascular resistance.

Patent Ductus Arteriosus

The ductus arteriosus is a vessel leading from the bifurcation of the pulmonary artery to the aorta just distal to the left subclavian artery. Normally, the vascular channel is open in the fetus but closes immediately after birth. The flow across the ductus is determined by the pressure and resistance relationships between the systemic and pulmonary circulations and by the cross-sectional area and length of the ductus. In most adults with this anomaly, pulmonary pressures are normal and a gradient and shunt from aorta to pulmonary artery persist throughout the cardiac cycle, resulting in a characteristic thrill and a continuous "machinery" murmur with late systolic accentuation at the upper left sternal edge. In adults who were born with a large left-to-right shunt through the ductus arteriosus, pulmonary vascular obstruction (Eisenmenger syndrome) with pulmonary hypertension, right-to-left shunting, and cyanosis have usually developed. Severe pulmonary vascular disease results in reversal of flow through the ductus; unoxygenated blood is shunted to the descending aorta; and the toes, but not the fingers, become cyanotic and clubbed, a finding termed *differential cyanosis*. The leading causes of death in adults with patent ductus are cardiac failure and infective endocarditis; occasionally severe pulmonary vascular obstruction may cause aneurysmal dilatation, calcification, and rupture of the ductus.

Rx Treatment:
PATENT DUCTUS ARTERIOSUS

In the absence of severe pulmonary vascular disease and predominant left-to-right shunting of blood, the patent ductus should be surgically ligated or divided. Transcatheter closure using coils, buttons, plugs, and umbrellas has become commonplace for appropriately shaped defects. Thoracoscopic surgical approaches are considered experimental. Operation should be deferred for several months in patients treated successfully for infective endocarditis because the ductus may remain somewhat edematous and friable.

Aortic Root to Right Heart Shunts

The three most common causes of aortic root to right heart shunts are congenital aneurysm of an aortic sinus of Valsalva with fistula, coronary arteriovenous fistula, and anomalous origin of the left coronary artery from the pulmonary trunk. *Aneurysm of an aortic sinus of Valsalva* consists of a separation or lack of fusion between the media of the aorta and the annulus of the aortic valve. Rupture usually occurs in the third or fourth decade of life; most often the aorticocardiac fistula is between the right coronary cusp and the right ventricle, but occasionally, when the noncoronary cusp is involved, the fistula drains into the right atrium. Abrupt rupture causes chest pain, bounding pulses, a continuous murmur accentuated in diastole, and volume overload of the heart. Diagnosis is confirmed by 2DE and Doppler echocardiographic studies; cardiac catheterization quantitates the left-to-right shunt, and thoracic aortography visualizes the fistula. Medical management is directed at cardiac failure, arrhythmias, or endocarditis. At operation, the aneurysm is closed and amputated, and the aortic wall is reunited with the heart, either by direct suture or with a patch or prosthesis.

Coronary arteriovenous fistula, an unusual anomaly, consists of a communication between a coronary artery and another cardiac chamber, usually the coronary sinus, right atrium, or right ventricle. The shunt is usually of small magnitude and myocardial blood flow is not usually compromised; if the shunt is large, there may be a coronary "steal" syndrome with myocardial ischemia and possible angina or ventricular arrhythmias. Potential complications include infective endocarditis, thrombus formation with occlusion or distal embolization with myocardial infarction, rupture of an aneurysmal fistula, and, rarely, pulmonary hypertension and congestive failure. A loud, superficial, continuous murmur at the lower or midsternal border usually prompts a further evaluation of asymptomatic patients. Doppler echocardiography demonstrates the site of drainage; if the site of origin is proximal, it may be detectable by two-dimensional echocardiography. Angiography (classic catheterization, CT, or magnetic resonance angiography) permits identification of the size and anatomic features of the fistulous tract, which may be closed by suture or transcatheter obliteration.

The third anomaly causing a shunt from the aortic root to the right heart is *anomalous origin of the left coronary artery from the pulmonary artery*. Myocardial infarction and fibrosis commonly lead to death within the first year, although up to 20% of patients survive to adolescence and beyond without surgical correction. The diagnosis is supported by the ECG findings of an anterolateral myocardial infarction and LVH. Operative management of adults consists of coronary artery bypass with an internal mammary artery graft or saphenous vein–coronary artery graft.

ACYANOTIC CONGENITAL HEART DISEASE WITHOUT A SHUNT

Congenital Aortic Stenosis

Malformations that cause obstruction to LV outflow include congenital valvular aortic stenosis, discrete subaortic stenosis, supravalvular aortic stenosis, and hypertrophic obstructive cardiomyopathy (Chap. 21).

Valvular Aortic Stenosis

Bicuspid aortic valves are more common in males than in females. The congenital bicuspid aortic valve, which may initially be functionally normal, is one of the most common congenital malformations of the heart and may go undetected in early life. Because bicuspid valves may develop stenosis or regurgitation with time or be the site of infective endocarditis, the lesion may be difficult to distinguish in older adults from acquired rheumatic or degenerative calcific aortic valve disease. The dynamics of blood flow associated with a congenitally deformed, rigid aortic valve commonly lead to thickening of the cusps and, in later life, to calcification. Hemodynamically significant obstruction causes concentric hypertrophy of the LV wall. The ascending aorta is often dilated, misnamed "poststenotic" dilatation; this is due to histologic abnormalities of the aortic media similar to those in Marfan syndrome, and may result in aortic dissection. Diagnosis is best made by echocardiography, which can reveal the morphology of the aortic valve and aortic root and quantitate the degree of stenosis or regurgitation. The clinical manifestations and hemodynamic abnormalities are discussed in Chap. 20.

℞ **Treatment:**
VALVULAR AORTIC STENOSIS

The medical management of congenital valvular aortic stenosis includes prophylaxis against infective endocarditis and, in patients with diminished cardiac reserve, the administration of digoxin and diuretics and sodium restriction while awaiting operation. A dilated aortic root may require beta blockers. If severe aortic stenosis is present, strenuous physical activity should be avoided even when the patient is asymptomatic, and participation in competitive sports should probably be restricted in patients with milder degrees of obstruction. Aortic valve replacement is indicated in adults with critical obstruction, i.e., with an aortic valve area <0.45 cm^2/m^2, with symptoms secondary to LV dysfunction or myocardial ischemia, or with hemodynamic evidence of LV dysfunction. In asymptomatic children or adolescents or young adults with critical aortic stenosis without valvular calcification or these features, aortic balloon valvuloplasty is often useful (Chap. 36). If surgery is contraindicated in older patients because of a complicating medical problem such as malignancy or renal or hepatic failure, balloon valvuloplasty may provide short-term improvement. This procedure may serve as a bridge to aortic valve replacement in patients with severe heart failure.

Subaortic Stenosis

The most common form of subaortic stenosis is the *idiopathic hypertrophic* variety, also termed *hypertrophic cardiomyopathy*, which is present at birth in about one-third of the patients and is discussed in Chap. 21. The *discrete* form of subaortic stenosis consists of a membranous diaphragm or fibromuscular ring encircling the LV outflow tract just beneath the base of the aortic valve. The jet impact from the subaortic stenotic jet on the underside of the aortic valve often begets progressive aortic valve fibrosis and valvular regurgitation. Echocardiography demonstrates the anatomy of the subaortic obstruction; Doppler studies show turbulence proximal to the aortic valve and can quantitate the pressure gradient and severity of aortic regurgitation. Treatment consists of complete excision of the membrane or fibromuscular ring.

Supravalvular Aortic Stenosis

This anomaly consists of a localized or diffuse narrowing of the ascending aorta originating just above the level of the coronary arteries at the superior margin of the sinuses of Valsalva. In contrast to other forms of aortic stenosis, the coronary arteries are subjected to elevated systolic pressures from the left ventricle, are often dilated and tortuous, and are susceptible to premature atherosclerosis. In most patients, a genetic defect for the anomaly is located in the same chromosomal region as elastin on chromosome 7.

Coarctation of the Aorta

Narrowing or constriction of the lumen of the aorta may occur anywhere along its length but is most common distal to the origin of the left subclavian artery near the insertion of the ligamentum arteriosum. Coarctation occurs in ~7% of patients with congenital heart disease, is more common in males than females, and is particularly frequent in patients with gonadal dysgenesis (e.g., Turner syndrome). Clinical manifestations depend on the site and extent of obstruction and the presence of associated cardiac anomalies, most commonly a bicuspid aortic valve. Circle of Willis aneurysms may occur in up to 10% and pose a high risk of sudden rupture and death.

Most children and young adults with isolated, discrete coarctation are asymptomatic. Headache, epistaxis, cold extremities, and claudication with exercise may occur, and attention is usually directed to the cardiovascular system when a heart murmur or hypertension in the upper extremities and absence, marked diminution, or delayed pulsations in the femoral arteries are detected on physical examination. Enlarged and pulsatile collateral vessels may be palpated in the intercostal spaces anteriorly, in the axillae, or posteriorly in the interscapular area. The upper extremities and thorax may be more developed than the lower extremities. A midsystolic murmur over the left interscapular space may become continuous if the lumen is narrowed sufficiently to result in a high-velocity jet across the lesion throughout the cardiac cycle. Additional systolic and continuous murmurs over the lateral thoracic wall may reflect increased flow through dilated and tortuous collateral vessels. The ECG usually reveals LV hypertrophy. Chest x-ray may show a dilated left subclavian artery high on the left mediastinal border and a dilated ascending aorta. Indentation of the aorta at the site of coarctation and pre- and poststenotic dilatation (the "3" sign) along the left paramediastinal shadow are almost pathognomonic. Notching of the third–ninth ribs, an important radiographic sign, is due to inferior rib erosion by dilated collateral vessels (**Figs. 19-2** and **19-3**). 2DE from para- or suprasternal windows identifies the site and length of coarctation, whereas Doppler quantitates the pressure gradient. TEE and MRI or three-dimensional CT allows visualization of the length and severity of the obstruction and the associated collateral arteries (Figs. 19-2 and 19-3). In adults, cardiac catheterization is indicated primarily to evaluate the coronary arteries or to perform catheter based intervention (angioplasty and stent of the coarctation).

The chief hazards of proximal aortic severe hypertension include cerebral aneurysms and hemorrhage, aortic dissection and rupture, premature coronary arteriosclerosis, and LV failure; infective endarteritis may occur on the coarctation site or endocarditis may settle on an associated bicuspid aortic valve.

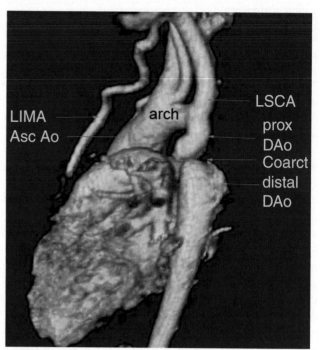

FIGURE 19-3

Aortic coarctation. The coarctation (Coarct) of the aorta is shown in the typical "adult" location in the descending aorta (DAo) just distal to the dilated left subclavian artery (LSCA) in this three-dimensional reconstruction of an MR angiogram. There is a post-coarct aneurysm that is in part due to intrinsic aortic medial tissue weakness. The left internal mammary artery (LIMA) is dilated. AscAo, ascending aorta; prox, proximal.

℞ Treatment:
COARCTATION OF THE AORTA

Treatment is usually surgical, although percutaneous catheter balloon with stent dilatation is now a viable option for many patients. Late postoperative systemic hypertension in the absence of residual coarctation appears to be related to the duration of preoperative hypertension. Follow-up of rest and exercise blood pressures is important; in many only excessive systolic hypertension is seen during exercise, in part due to a diffuse vasculopathy. All operated or stented coarctation patients deserve a high-quality MRI or CT imaging procedure in follow-up.

Pulmonary Stenosis with Intact Ventricular Septum

Obstruction to RV outflow may be localized to the supravalvular, valvular, or subvalvular levels or occur at a combination of these sites. Multiple sites of narrowing of the peripheral pulmonary arteries are a feature of *rubella embryopathy* and may occur with both the familial

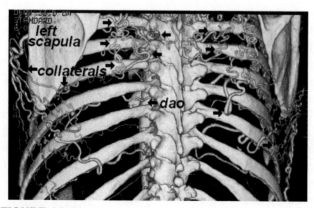

FIGURE 19-2

Aortic coarctation. The extensive collaterals (*left*) underneath the ribs and in the periscapular region are shown on a posterior view of a three-dimensional CT angiogram, which are responsible for rib notching on chest x-ray. dao, descending aorta.

and sporadic forms of supravalvular aortic stenosis. Valvular pulmonic stenosis is the most common form of isolated RV obstruction.

The severity of the obstructing lesion, rather than the site of narrowing, is the most important determinant of the clinical course. In the presence of a normal cardiac output, a peak systolic transvalvular pressure gradient between 50 and 80 mmHg is considered to be moderate stenosis; levels below and above that range are classified as mild and severe, respectively. Patients with mild pulmonic stenosis are generally asymptomatic and demonstrate little or no progression in the severity of obstruction with age. In patients with more significant stenosis, the severity may increase with time. Symptoms vary with the degree of obstruction. Fatigue, dyspnea, RV failure, and syncope may limit the activity of older patients, in whom moderate or severe obstruction may prevent an augmentation of cardiac output with exercise. In patients with severe obstruction, the systolic pressure in the right ventricle may exceed that in the left ventricle, since the ventricular septum is intact. RV ejection is prolonged with moderate or severe stenosis, and the sound of pulmonary valve closure is delayed and soft. RV hypertrophy reduces the compliance of that chamber, and a forceful RA contraction is necessary to augment RV filling.

A fourth heart sound, prominent *a* waves in the jugular venous pulse, and, occasionally, presystolic pulsations of the liver reflect vigorous atrial contraction. The clinical diagnosis is supported by a left parasternal lift and harsh systolic crescendo-decrescendo murmur and thrill at the upper left sternal border, typically preceded by a systolic ejection sound if the obstruction is due to a mobile nondysplastic pulmonary valve. The holosystolic murmur of tricuspid regurgitation may accompany severe pulmonic stenosis, especially in the presence of congestive heart failure. Cyanosis usually reflects right-to-left shunting through a patent foramen ovale or ASD. In patients with supravalvular or peripheral pulmonary arterial stenosis, the murmur is systolic or continuous and is best heard over the area of narrowing, with radiation to the peripheral lung fields.

In mild cases, the ECG is normal, whereas moderate and severe stenoses are associated with RV hypertrophy. The chest x-ray with mild or moderate pulmonic stenosis shows a heart of normal size with normal lung vascularity. In pulmonary valvular stenosis, dilatation of the main and left pulmonary arteries occurs in part due to the direction of the PS jet and in part due to intrinsic tissue weakness. With severe obstruction, RV hypertrophy is generally evident. The pulmonary vascularity may be reduced with severe stenosis, RV failure, and/or a right-to-left shunt at the atrial level. 2DE visualizes pulmonary valve morphology; the outflow tract pressure gradient can be quantitated by Doppler echocardiography.

℞ **Treatment:
PULMONARY STENOSIS**

The cardiac catheter technique of balloon valvuloplasty (Chap. 13) is usually effective. Direct surgical relief of moderate and severe obstruction may be accomplished at a low risk. Multiple stenoses of the peripheral pulmonary arteries are usually inoperable, but narrowing of a proximal branch or at the bifurcation of the main pulmonary trunk may be surgically corrected or undergo balloon dilatation and stenting.

COMPLEX CONGENITAL HEART LESIONS
Tetralogy of Fallot

The four components of the tetralogy of Fallot are malaligned VSD, obstruction to RV outflow, aortic override of the VSD, and RV hypertrophy due to the RV "seeing" aortic pressure via the large VSD (**Fig. 19-4**).

The severity of RV outflow obstruction determines the clinical presentation. The severity of hypoplasia of the RV outflow tract varies from mild to complete (pulmonary atresia). Pulmonary valve stenosis and supravalvular and peripheral pulmonary arterial obstruction may coexist; rarely there is unilateral absence of a pulmonary artery (usually the left). A right-sided aortic arch and descending thoracic aorta occur in ~25% of patients with tetralogy.

The relationship between the resistance of blood flow from the ventricles into the aorta and into the pulmonary vessels plays a major role in determining the hemodynamic and clinical picture. When the obstruction is severe, the pulmonary blood flow is reduced markedly, and a large volume of desaturated systemic

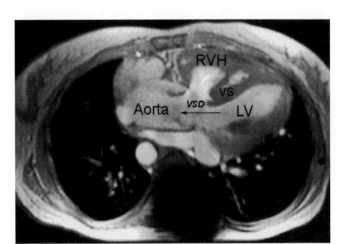

FIGURE 19-4
Tetralogy of Fallot. Magnetic resonance imaging angiogram. A mid-systolic frame showing the malaligned ventricular septal defect (VSD) with the aorta overriding the ventricular septal defect. LV, left ventricle; RVH, RV hypertrophy; VS, ventricular septum.

venous blood is shunted from right to left across the VSD. Severe cyanosis and erythrocytosis occur, and symptoms of systemic hypoxemia are prominent. In many infants and children the obstruction is mild but progressive.

The ECG shows RV hypertrophy. Chest x-ray shows a normal-sized, boot-shaped heart (*coeur en sabot*) with a prominent right ventricle and a concavity in the region of the pulmonary conus. Pulmonary vascular markings are typically diminished, and the aortic arch and knob may be on the right side. 2DE demonstrates the malaligned VSD with the overriding aorta and the site and severity of pulmonary stenosis, which may be subpulmonic (fixed or dynamic), at the pulmonary valve or in the main or branch pulmonary arteries. Classic contrast angiography may provide details regarding the RV outflow tract, pulmonary valve and annulus, and caliber of the main branches of the pulmonary artery as well of possible associated aortopulmonary collaterals. Coronary arteriography identifies the anatomy and course of the coronary arteries. In experienced centers, these issues are often well demonstrated in adults by MR (Fig. 19-4) or CT angiography with three-dimensional reconstruction.

℞ Treatment: TETRALOGY OF FALLOT

For a variety of reasons, only a few adults with tetralogy of Fallot have not had some form of previous surgical intervention. Reoperation in adults is most commonly for severe pulmonary regurgitation. Long-term concerns about ventricular function persist. Ventricular and atrial arrhythmias may require medical treatment or electrophysiologic study and ablation. Interventional catheterization may be needed in selected patients (i.e., angioplasty and stenting of branch pulmonary stenosis). The aortic root has a medial tissue defect; it is commonly enlarged and associated with aortic regurgitation. Endocarditis remains a risk despite surgical repair.

Complete Transposition of the Great Arteries

This condition is commonly called *dextrotransposition* or D-*transposition of the great arteries*. The aorta arises rightward anteriorly from the right ventricle, and the pulmonary artery emerges leftward and posteriorly from the left ventricle, which results in two separate parallel circulations; some communication between them must exist after birth to sustain life. Most patients have an interatrial communication, two-thirds have a patent ductus arteriosus, and about one-third have an associated VSD. Transposition is more common in males and accounts for ~10% of cyanotic heart disease.

The course is determined by the degree of tissue hypoxia, the ability of each ventricle to sustain an increased work load in the presence of reduced coronary arterial oxygenation, the nature of the associated cardiovascular anomalies, and the status of the pulmonary vascular bed. By the third decade of life, ~30% of patients will have developed decreased RV function and progressive tricuspid regurgitation, which may lead to congestive heart failure. Pulmonary vascular obstruction develops by 1–2 years of age in patients with an associated large ventricular septal defect or large patent ductus arteriosus in the absence of obstruction to LV outflow.

℞ Treatment: TRANSPOSITION OF THE GREAT ARTERIES

The balloon or blade catheter or surgical creation or enlargement of an interatrial communication in the neonate is the simplest procedure for providing increased intracardiac mixing of systemic and pulmonary venous blood. Systemic–pulmonary artery anastomosis may be indicated in the patient with severe obstruction to LV outflow and diminished pulmonary blood flow. Intracardiac repair may be accomplished by rearranging the venous returns (intraatrial switch, i.e., Mustard or Senning operation) so that the systemic venous blood is directed to the mitral valve and hence to the left ventricle and pulmonary artery, while the pulmonary venous blood is diverted through the tricuspid valve and right ventricle to the aorta. The late survival after these repairs is good, but arrhythmias (e.g., atrial flutter) or conduction defects (e.g., sick sinus syndrome) occur in ~50% of such patients by 30 years after the intraatrial switch surgery. Progressive dysfunction of the systemic subaortic right ventricle, tricuspid regurgitation, ventricular arrhythmias or cardiac arrest and late sudden death are worrisome features. Preferably, this malformation is corrected in infancy by transposing both coronary arteries to the posterior artery and transecting, contraposing, and anastomosing the aorta and pulmonary arteries (arterial switch operation). For those patients with a VSD in whom it is necessary to bypass a severely obstructed LV outflow tract, corrective operation employs an intracardiac ventricular baffle and extracardiac prosthetic conduit to replace the pulmonary artery (Rastelli procedure).

Single Ventricle

This is a family of complex lesions with both atrioventricular valves or a common atrioventricular valve opening to a single ventricular chamber. Associated anomalies include abnormal great artery positional relationships, pulmonic valvular or subvalvular stenosis, and subaortic stenosis.

Survival to adulthood depends on a relatively normal pulmonary blood flow, yet normal pulmonary resistance, and good ventricular function. Modifications of the Fontan approach are generally applied to carefully selected patients with creation of a pathway(s) from the systemic veins to the pulmonary arteries.

Tricuspid Atresia

This malformation is characterized by atresia of the tricuspid valve, an interatrial communication, and, frequently, hypoplasia of the right ventricle and pulmonary artery. The clinical picture is usually dominated by severe cyanosis due to obligatory admixture of systemic and pulmonary venous blood in the left ventricle. The ECG characteristically shows RA enlargement, left-axis deviation, and LV hypertrophy.

Atrial septostomy and palliative operations to increase pulmonary blood flow, often by anastomosis of a systemic artery or vein to a pulmonary artery, may allow survival to the second or third decade. A Fontan atriopulmonary or total cavopulmonary connection may then allow functional correction in those patients with normal or low pulmonary arterial resistance pressure and good LV function.

Ebstein Anomaly

Characterized by a downward displacement of the tricuspid valve into the right ventricle, due to anomalous attachment of the tricuspid leaflets, the Ebstein tricuspid valve tissue is dysplastic and results in tricuspid regurgitation. The abnormally situated tricuspid orifice produces an "atrialized" portion of the right ventricle lying between the atrioventricular ring and the origin of the valve, which is continuous with the RA chamber. Often the right ventricle is hypoplastic. Although the clinical manifestations are variable, some patients come to initial attention because of (1) progressive cyanosis from right-to-left atrial shunting, (2) symptoms due to tricuspid regurgitation and RV dysfunction, or (3) paroxysmal atrial tachyarrhythmias with or without atrioventricular bypass tracts (WPW syndrome). Diagnostic findings by 2DE include the abnormal positional relation between the tricuspid and mitral valves with abnormally increased apical displacement of the septal tricuspid leaflet. Tricuspid regurgitation is quantitated by Doppler examination. Surgical approaches include prosthetic replacement of the tricuspid valve when the leaflets are tethered or repair of the native valve.

Congenitally Corrected Transposition

The two fundamental anatomic abnormalities in this malformation are transposition of the ascending aorta and pulmonary trunk and inversion of the ventricles. This arrangement results in desaturated systemic venous blood passing from the right atrium through the mitral valve to the left ventricle and into the pulmonary trunk, whereas oxygenated pulmonary venous blood flows from the left atrium through the tricuspid valve to the right ventricle and into the aorta. Thus, the circulation is corrected functionally. The clinical presentation, course, and prognosis of patients with congenitally corrected transposition vary depending on the nature and severity of any complicating intracardiac anomalies and of development of dysfunction of the systemic subaortic RV. Progressive RV dysfunction and tricuspid regurgitation may also develop in a third of patients by age 30; Ebstein-type anomalies of the left-side tricuspid atrioventricular valve are common. Ventricular septal defect or "pulmonary stenosis" due to obstruction to outflow from the right-sided subpulmonary (anatomic left) ventricle may coexist. Complete heart block occurs at a rate of 2–10% per decade. The diagnosis of the malformation and associated lesions can be established by comprehensive 2DE and Doppler examination.

Malpositions of the Heart

Positional anomalies refer to conditions in which the cardiac apex is in the right side of the chest (*dextrocardia*), or at the midline (*mesocardia*), or in which there is a normal location of the heart in the left side of the chest but abnormal position of the viscera (*isolated levocardia*). Knowledge of the position of the abdominal organs and of the branching pattern of the main stem bronchi is important in categorizing these malpositions. When dextrocardia occurs without situs inversus, when the visceral situs is indeterminate, or if isolated levocardia is present, associated, often complex, multiple cardiac anomalies are usually present. In contrast, mirror-image dextrocardia is usually observed with complete situs inversus, which occurs most frequently in individuals whose hearts are otherwise normal.

SURGICALLY MODIFIED CONGENITAL HEART DISEASE

Because of the enormous strides in cardiovascular surgical techniques that have occurred in the past 50 years, a large number of long-term survivors of corrective operations in infancy and childhood have reached adulthood. These patients are often challenging because of the diversity of anatomic, hemodynamic, and electrophysiologic residua and sequelae of cardiac operations.

The proper care of the survivor of operation for CHD requires that the clinician understand the details of the malformation before operation; pay meticulous attention to the details of the operative procedure; and recognize the postoperative residua (conditions left totally or partially uncorrected), the sequelae (conditions caused by surgery), and the complications that may have resulted from the operation. With the exception of ligation and division of an uncomplicated patent ductus arteriosus, almost every other surgical repair of an anomaly leaves behind or causes some abnormality of the heart and circulation that may range from trivial to serious. Intraoperative TEE assists in detecting unsuspected lesions, in monitoring the repair, and in verifying a satisfactory result or directing further repair. Thus, even with results that are considered clinically to be good to excellent, continued long-term postoperative follow-up is advisable.

Cardiac operations importantly involving the atria, such as closure of ASD, repair of total or partial anomalous pulmonary venous return, or venous switch corrections of complete transposition of the great arteries (the Mustard or Senning operations), may be followed years later by sinus node or atrioventricular node dysfunction or by atrial arrhythmias (especially atrial flutter). Intraventricular surgery may also result in electrophysiologic consequences, including complete heart block necessitating pacemaker insertion to avoid sudden death. In addition, valvular problems may arise late after initial cardiac operation. An example is the progressive stenosis of an initially nonobstructive bicuspid aortic valve in the patient who underwent aortic coarctation repair. Such aortic valves may also be the site of infective endocarditis. After repair of the ostium primum ASD, the cleft mitral valve may become progressively regurgitant. Tricuspid regurgitation may also be progressive in the postoperative patient with tetralogy of Fallot if RV outflow tract obstruction was not relieved adequately at initial surgery. In many patients with surgically modified CHD, inadequate relief of an obstructive lesion, or a residual regurgitant lesion, or a residual shunt will cause or hasten the onset of clinical signs and symptoms of myocardial dysfunction. Despite a good hemodynamic repair, many patients with a subaortic right ventricle develop RV decompensation and signs of "left heart failure." In many patients, particularly those who were cyanotic for many years before operation, a preexisting compromise in ventricular performance is due to the original underlying malformation.

A final category of postoperative problems involves the use of prosthetic valves, patches, or conduits in the operative repair. The special risks include infective endocarditis, thrombus formation, and premature degeneration and calcification of the prosthetic materials. There are many patients in whom extracardiac conduits are required to correct the circulation functionally and often to carry blood to the lungs from the right atrium or right ventricle. These conduits may develop intraluminal obstruction, and, if they include a prosthetic valve, it may show progressive calcification and thickening.

FURTHER READINGS

ABOULHOSN J AND CHILD JS: *Congenital Heart Disease in Adults* in V Fuster, RA O'Rourke, RA Walsh, et al (eds): Hurst's The Heart 12th ed., New York, McGraw Medical 1922—1948: 2008

————: *Congenital Heart Disease in Adults* in RA O'Rourke, RA Walsh, and V Fuster (eds): Hurst's The Heart Manual of Cardiology 12th ed, New York, McGraw Medical 546-556: 2009

ATTIE F et al: Surgical treatment for secundum atrial septal defects in patients >40 years old. A randomized clinical trial. J Am Coll Cardiol 38:2035, 2001

BASHORE T: Adult congenital heart disease: Right ventricular outflow tract lesions. Circulation 115:1933, 2007

CHILD JS: Transthoracic and transesophageal echocardiographic imaging: Anatomic and hemodynamic assessment, in *Congenital Heart Disease in Adults*, 2d ed, JK Perloff, JS Child (eds), Philadelphia, Saunders, 1998

FEDAK PWM et al: Clinical and pathophysiological implications of a bicuspid aortic valve. Circulation 106:900, 2002

LEWIN MB, OTTO CM: The bicuspid aortic valve: Adverse outcomes from infancy to old age. Circulation 111:832, 2005

MARSHALL AC, LOCK JE: Leaving neverland: A randomized trial for coarctation shows pediatric interventional cardiology is growing up. Circulation 111:3347, 2005

PERLOFF JK et al: *Congenital Heart Disease in Adults*. 3d Ed., Philadelphia, Saunders Elsevier 1—488: 2009

SALEHIAN O et al: Improvements in cardiac form and function after transcatheter closure of secundum atrial septal defects. J Am Coll Cardiol 45:499, 2005

WARNES CA: The adult with congenital heart disease: born to be bad? J Am Coll Cardiol 46:1, 2005

————: Bicuspid aortic valve and coarctation: Two villains part of a diffuse problem. Heart 89:965, 2003

———— et al: ACC/AHA 2008 Guidelines for the Management of Adults with Congenital Heart Disease. Circulation 118:e714, 2008

WEBB G et al: Congenital heart disease, in: *Braunwald's Heart Disease: A Textbook of Cardiovascular Medicine*, 7th ed, Zipes D et al (eds), Philadelphia, Elsevier Saunders, 2005

WU JC, CHILD JS: Common congenital heart disorders in adults. Curr Probl Cardiol 29:641, 2004

CHAPTER 20

VALVULAR HEART DISEASE

Patrick O'Gara ■ Eugene Braunwald

The role of the physical examination in the evaluation of patients with valvular heart disease is also considered in Chaps. 9 and 10; of electrocardiography (ECG) in Chap. 11; of echocardiography and other noninvasive imaging techniques in Chap. 12; and of cardiac catheterization and angiography in Chap. 13.

MITRAL STENOSIS

ETIOLOGY AND PATHOLOGY

Rheumatic fever is the leading cause of mitral stenosis (MS) (Table 20-1). Other less common etiologies of obstruction to left atrial outflow include congenital mitral valve stenosis, cor triatriatum, mitral annular calcification with extension onto the leaflets, systemic lupus erythematosus, rheumatoid arthritis, left atrial myxoma, and infective endocarditis with large vegetations. Pure or predominant MS occurs in approximately 40% of all patients with rheumatic heart disease and a history of rheumatic fever (Chap. 26). In other patients with rheumatic heart disease, lesser degrees of MS may accompany mitral regurgitation (MR) and aortic valve disease. With reductions in the incidence of acute rheumatic fever, particularly in temperate climates and developed countries, the incidence of MS has declined considerably over the past few decades. However, it remains a major problem in developing nations, especially in tropical and semitropical climates).

In rheumatic MS, the valve leaflets are diffusely thickened by fibrous tissue and/or calcific deposits. The mitral commissures fuse, the chordae tendineae fuse and shorten, the valvular cusps become rigid, and these changes, in turn, lead to narrowing at the apex of the funnel-shaped ("fish-mouth") valve. Although the initial insult to the mitral valve is rheumatic, the later changes may be a nonspecific process resulting from trauma to the valve caused by altered flow patterns due to the initial

TABLE 20-1

MAJOR CAUSES OF VALVULAR HEART DISEASES

VALVE LESION	ETIOLOGIES
Mitral stenosis	Rheumatic fever
	Congenital
	Severe mitral annular calcification
	SLE, RA
Mitral regurgitation	Acute
	Endocarditis
	Papillary muscle rupture
	(post-MI)
	Trauma
	Chordal rupture/Leaflet flail
	(MVP, IE)
	Chronic
	Myxomatous (MVP)
	Rheumatic fever
	Endocarditis (healed)
	Mitral annular calcification
	Congenital (cleft, AV canal)
	HOCM with SAM
	Ischemic (LV remodeling)
	Dilated cardiomyopathy
Aortic atenosis	Congenital (bicuspid, unicuspid)
	Degenerative calcific
	Rheumatic fever
Aortic regurgitation	Valvular
	Congenital (bicuspid)
	Endocarditis
	Rheumatic fever
	Myxomatous (prolapse)
	Traumatic
	Syphilis
	Ankylosing spondylitis
	Root disease
	Aortic dissection
	Cystic medial degeneration
	Marfan syndrome
	Bicuspid aortic valve
	Nonsyndromic familial
	aneurysm
	Aortitis
	Hypertension
Tricuspid stenosis	Rheumatic
	Congenital
Tricuspid regurgitation	Primary
	Rheumatic
	Endocarditis
	Myxomatous (TVP)
	Carcinoid
	Congenital (Ebstein's)
	Trauma
	Papillary muscle injury
	(post-MI)
	Secondary
	RV and tricuspid annular
	dilatation
	Multiple causes of RV
	enlargement (e.g., long-
	standing pulmonary HTN)
	Chronic RV apical pacing

TABLE 20-1 (CONTINUED)

MAJOR CAUSES OF VALVULAR HEART DISEASES

VALVE LESION	ETIOLOGIES
Pulmonic stenosis	Congenital
	Carcinoid
Pulmonic regurgitation	Valve disease
	Congenital
	Postvalvotomy
	Endocarditis
	Annular enlargement
	Pulmonary hypertension
	Idiopathic dilatation
	Marfan syndrome

Note: AV, atrioventricular; HOCM, hypertrophic obstructive cardiomyopathy; HTN, hypertension; IE, infective endocarditis; LV, left ventricular; MI, myocardial infarction; MVP, mitral valve prolapse; RA, rheumatoid arthritis; RV, right ventricular; SAM, systolic anterior motion of the anterior mitral valve leaflet; SLE, systemic lupus erythematosus; TVP, tricuspid valve prolapse.

deformity. Calcification of the stenotic mitral valve immobilizes the leaflets and narrows the orifice further. Thrombus formation and arterial embolization may arise from the calcific valve itself, but in patients with atrial fibrillation (AF), thrombi arise more frequently from the dilated left atrium (LA), particularly the left atrial appendage.

PATHOPHYSIOLOGY

In normal adults, the area of the mitral valve orifice is 4–6 cm². In the presence of significant obstruction, i.e., when the orifice area is reduced to <~2 cm², blood can flow from the LA to the left ventricle (LV) only if propelled by an abnormally elevated left atrioventricular pressure gradient (see Fig. 13-2), the hemodynamic hallmark of MS. When the mitral valve opening is reduced to <1 cm², often referred to as "severe" MS, a LA pressure of ~25 mmHg is required to maintain a normal cardiac output (CO). The elevated pulmonary venous and pulmonary arterial (PA) wedge pressures reduce pulmonary compliance, contributing to exertional dyspnea. The first bouts of dyspnea are usually precipitated by clinical events that increase the rate of blood flow across the mitral orifice, resulting in further elevation of the LA pressure (see later).

To assess the severity of obstruction hemodynamically, both the transvalvular pressure gradient and the flow rate must be measured (Chap. 13). The latter depends not only on the CO but on the heart rate as well. An increase in heart rate shortens diastole proportionately more than systole and diminishes the time available for flow across the mitral valve. Therefore, at any given level of CO, tachycardia including that associated with AF augments the transvalvular pressure gradient and elevates further the LA pressure. Similar considerations apply to the pathophysiology of tricuspid stenosis.

The LV diastolic pressure and ejection fraction (EF) are normal in isolated MS. In MS and sinus rhythm, the elevated LA and PA wedge pressures exhibit a prominent atrial contraction (*a* wave) and a gradual pressure decline after mitral valve opening (*y* descent) (see Fig. 13-2). In severe MS and whenever pulmonary vascular resistance is significantly increased, the pulmonary arterial pressure (PAP) is elevated at rest and rises further during exercise, often causing secondary elevations of right ventricular (RV) end-diastolic pressure and volume.

Cardiac Output

In patients with moderate MS (mitral valve orifice 1.0 cm^2–1.5 cm^2), the CO is normal or almost so at rest but rises subnormally during exertion. In patients with severe MS (valve area <1.0 cm^2), particularly those in whom pulmonary vascular resistance is markedly elevated, the CO is subnormal at rest and may fail to rise or may even decline during activity.

Pulmonary Hypertension

The clinical and hemodynamic features of MS are influenced importantly by the level of the PAP. Pulmonary hypertension results from: (1) passive backward transmission of the elevated LA pressure; (2) pulmonary arteriolar constriction, which presumably is triggered by LA and pulmonary venous hypertension (reactive pulmonary hypertension); (3) interstitial edema in the walls of the small pulmonary vessels; and (4) organic obliterative changes in the pulmonary vascular bed. Severe pulmonary hypertension results in RV enlargement, secondary tricuspid regurgitation (TR) and pulmonic regurgitation (PR), as well as right-sided heart failure.

SYMPTOMS

In temperate climates, the latent period between the initial attack of rheumatic carditis (in the increasingly rare circumstances in which a history of one can be elicited) and the development of symptoms due to MS is generally about two decades; most patients begin to experience disability in the fourth decade of life. Studies carried out before the development of mitral valvotomy revealed that once a patient with MS became seriously symptomatic, the disease progressed continuously to death within 2–5 years.

In patients whose mitral orifices are large enough to accommodate a normal blood flow with only mild elevations of LA pressure, marked elevations of the pressure leading to dyspnea and cough may be precipitated by sudden changes in the heart rate, volume status, or CO, as for example with severe exertion, excitement, fever, severe anemia, paroxysmal AF and other tachycardias, sexual intercourse, pregnancy, and thyrotoxicosis. As MS progresses, lesser stresses precipitate dyspnea, and the

patient becomes limited in daily activities, and orthopnea and paroxysmal nocturnal dyspnea develop. The development of permanent AF often marks a turning point in the patient's course and is generally associated with acceleration of the rate at which symptoms progress.

Hemoptysis results from rupture of pulmonary-bronchial venous connections secondary to pulmonary venous hypertension. It occurs most frequently in patients who have elevated LA pressures without markedly elevated pulmonary vascular resistances and is almost never fatal. *Recurrent pulmonary emboli*, sometimes with infarction, are an important cause of morbidity and mortality late in the course of MS. *Pulmonary infections*, i.e., bronchitis, bronchopneumonia, and lobar pneumonia, commonly complicates untreated MS, especially during the winter months. *Infective endocarditis* (Chap. 25) is rare in isolated MS.

Pulmonary Changes

In addition to the aforementioned changes in the pulmonary vascular bed, fibrous thickening of the walls of the alveoli and pulmonary capillaries occurs commonly in MS. The vital capacity, total lung capacity, maximal breathing capacity, and oxygen uptake per unit of ventilation are reduced. Pulmonary compliance falls further as pulmonary capillary pressure rises during exercise.

Thrombi and Emboli

Thrombi may form in the left atria, particularly in the enlarged atrial appendages of patients with MS. Systemic embolization, the incidence of which is 10–20%, occurs more frequently in patients with AF, in older patients, and in those with a reduced CO. However, systemic embolization may be the presenting feature in otherwise asymptomatic patients with only mild MS.

PHYSICAL FINDINGS

(See also Chaps. 10 and 9)

Inspection and Palpation

In patients with severe MS, there may be a malar flush with pinched and blue facies. In patients with sinus rhythm and severe pulmonary hypertension or associated tricuspid stenosis (TS), the jugular venous pulse reveals prominent *a* waves due to vigorous right atrial systole. The systemic arterial pressure is usually normal or slightly low. An RV tap along the left sternal border signifies an enlarged RV. A diastolic thrill may be present at the cardiac apex, with the patient in the left lateral recumbent position.

Auscultation

The first heart sound (S$_1$) is usually accentuated and slightly delayed. The pulmonic component of the second heart sound (P_2) also is often accentuated, and the two components of the second heart sound (S_2) are closely split. The opening snap (OS) of the mitral valve is most readily audible in expiration at, or just medial to the cardiac apex. This sound generally follows the sound of aortic valve closure (A_2) by 0.05–0.12 s. The time interval between A_2 and OS varies inversely with the severity of the MS. The OS is followed by a low-pitched, rumbling, diastolic murmur; heard best at the apex with the patient in the left lateral recumbent position (see Fig. 9-4B). It is accentuated by mild exercise (e.g., a few rapid sit-ups) carried out just before auscultation. In general, the duration of this murmur correlates with the severity of the stenosis in patients with preserved CO. In patients with sinus rhythm, the murmur often reappears or becomes louder during atrial systole (presystolic accentuation). Soft grade I or II/VI systolic murmurs are commonly heard at the apex or along the left sternal border in patients with pure MS and do not necessarily signify the presence of MR. Hepatomegaly, ankle edema, ascites, and pleural effusion, particularly in the right pleural cavity, may occur in patients with MS and RV failure.

Associated Lesions

With severe pulmonary hypertension, a pansystolic murmur produced by functional TR may be audible along the left sternal border. This murmur is usually louder during inspiration and diminishes during forced expiration (Carvallo's sign). When the CO is markedly reduced in MS, the typical auscultatory findings, including the diastolic rumbling murmur, may not be detectable (silent MS), but they may reappear as compensation is restored. The *Graham Steell murmur* of PR, a high-pitched, diastolic, decrescendo blowing murmur along the left sternal border, results from dilatation of the pulmonary valve ring and occurs in patients with mitral valve disease and severe pulmonary hypertension. This murmur may be indistinguishable from the more common murmur produced by aortic regurgitation (AR), though it may increase in intensity with inspiration and is accompanied by a loud P_2.

LABORATORY EXAMINATION

Electrocardiogram

In MS and sinus rhythm, the P wave usually suggests LA enlargement (see Fig. 11-8). It may become tall and peaked in lead II and upright in lead V_1 when severe pulmonary hypertension or TS complicates MS and right atrial (RA) enlargement occurs. The QRS complex is usually normal. However, with severe pulmonary hypertension, right axis deviation and RV hypertrophy are often present.

Echocardiogram

(See also Chap. 12) Transthoracic two-dimensional echocardiography (TTE) with color flow Doppler imaging provides critical information, including an estimate of the transvalvular peak and mean gradients and of mitral orifice size, the presence and severity of accompanying MR, the extent of restriction of valve leaflets and their thickness, the degree of distortion of the subvalvular apparatus, and the anatomic suitability for percutaneous mitral balloon valvotomy [(PMBV); see later]. In addition, TTE provides an assessment of the size of the cardiac chambers, an estimation of LV function, an estimation of the pulmonary artery pressure (PAP), and an indication of the presence and severity of associated valvular lesions. Transesophageal echocardiography (TEE) provides superior images and should be employed when TTE is inadequate for guiding therapy. TEE is especially indicated to exclude the presence of left atrial thrombi prior to PMBV.

Chest X-ray

The earliest changes are straightening of the upper left border of the cardiac silhouette, prominence of the main pulmonary arteries, dilatation of the upper lobe pulmonary veins, and posterior displacement of the esophagus by an enlarged LA. Kerley B lines are fine, dense, opaque, horizontal lines that are most prominent in the lower and mid-lung fields and that result from distention of interlobular septae and lymphatics with edema when the resting mean LA pressure exceeds ~20 mmHg.

DIFFERENTIAL DIAGNOSIS

Like MS, significant MR may also be associated with a prominent diastolic murmur at the apex due to increased flow, but in MR this diastolic murmur commences slightly later than in patients with MS, and there is often clear-cut evidence of LV enlargement. An apical pansystolic murmur of at least grade III/VI intensity as well as an S_3 suggests significant associated MR. Similarly, the apical mid-diastolic murmur associated with severe AR (*Austin Flint murmur*) may be mistaken for MS but can be differentiated from it because it is not intensified in presystole. TS, which occurs rarely in the absence of MS, may mask many of the clinical features of MS or be clinically silent.

Atrial septal defect [(ASD); Chap. 19] may be mistaken for MS; in both conditions there is often clinical, ECG, and chest x-ray evidence of RV enlargement and accentuation of pulmonary vascularity. However, the absence of LA enlargement and of Kerley B lines and the demonstration of fixed splitting of S_2 all favor ASD over MS.

Left atrial myxoma (Chap. 23) may obstruct LA emptying, causing dyspnea, a diastolic murmur, and hemodynamic changes resembling those of MS. However, patients with an LA myxoma often have features suggestive of a systemic disease, such as weight loss, fever, anemia, systemic emboli, and elevated serum IgG and interleukin-6 (IL-6) concentrations. The auscultatory findings may change markedly with body position. The diagnosis can be established by the demonstration of a characteristic echo-producing mass in the LA with TTE.

CARDIAC CATHETERIZATION

Left and right heart catheterization is useful when there is a discrepancy between the clinical and TTE findings that cannot be resolved with either TEE or cardiac magnetic resonance (CMR) imaging. The growing experience with cardiac MRI for the assessment of patients with valvular heart disease may decrease the need for invasive catheterization. Catheterization is helpful in assessing associated lesions such as aortic stenosis (AS) and AR. Catheterization and coronary arteriography are not usually necessary to aid in the decision about surgery in younger patients, with typical findings of severe obstruction on clinical examination and TTE. In males older than 45 years, females older than 55 years, and younger persons with coronary risk factors, especially those with positive noninvasive stress tests for myocardial ischemia, coronary angiography is advisable preoperatively to identify patients with critical coronary obstructions that should be bypassed at the time of operation. Computed tomographic angiography (CTA) (Chap. 12) is now used in some centers to screen preoperatively for the presence of coronary artery disease (CAD) in patients with valvular heart disease. Catheterization and left ventriculography are also indicated in most patients who have undergone PMBV or previous mitral valve surgery and who have redeveloped serious symptoms, if questions remain after both TTE and TEE.

℞ Treatment:
MITRAL STENOSIS

(Fig. 20-1)

Penicillin prophylaxis of Group A β-hemolytic streptococcal infections (Chap. 26) to prevent rheumatic fever is important for at-risk patients with MS (**Table 20-2**). Recommendations for infective endocarditis prophylaxis have recently changed. In symptomatic patients, some improvement usually occurs with restriction of sodium intake and maintenance doses of oral diuretics. Digitalis glycosides usually do not benefit patients with MS and sinus rhythm, but they are helpful in slowing the ventricular rate of patients with AF. Beta blockers and nondihydropyridine calcium channel blockers (e.g., verapamil or diltiazem) are also useful in this regard.

Warfarin to an international normalized ratio (INR) of 2–3 should be administered indefinitely to patients with MS who have AF or a history of thromboembolism. The routine use of warfarin in patients in sinus rhythm with LA enlargement (maximal dimension >5.5 cm) with or without spontaneous echo contrast is more controversial.

If AF is of relatively recent onset in a patient whose MS is not severe enough to warrant PMBV or surgical commissurotomy, reversion to sinus rhythm pharmacologically or by means of electrical countershock is indicated. Usually, cardioversion should be undertaken after the patient has had at least 3 consecutive weeks of anticoagulant treatment to a therapeutic INR. If cardioversion is indicated more urgently, then intravenous heparin should be provided and a TEE performed to exclude the presence of left atrial thrombus before the procedure. Conversion to sinus rhythm is rarely successful or sustained in patients with severe MS, particularly those in whom the LA is especially enlarged or in whom AF has been present for more than 1 year.

MITRAL VALVOTOMY   Unless there is a contraindication, mitral valvotomy is indicated in symptomatic [New York Heart Association (NYHA) Functional Class II–IV] patients with isolated MS whose effective orifice (valve area) is <~1.0 cm^2/m^2 body surface area, or <1.5 cm^2 in normal-sized adults. Mitral valvotomy can be carried out by two techniques: PMBV and surgical valvotomy. In PMBV (**Figs. 20-2** and **20-3**), a catheter is directed into the LA after transseptal puncture, and a single balloon is directed across the valve and inflated in the valvular orifice. Ideal patients have relatively pliable leaflets with little or no commissural calcium. In addition, the subvalvular structures should not be significantly scarred or thickened and there should be no left atrial thrombus. The short- and long-term results of this procedure in appropriate patients are similar to those of surgical valvotomy, but with less morbidity and a lower periprocedural mortality rate. Event-free survival in younger (<45 years) patients with pliable valves is excellent, with rates as high as 80–90% over 3–7 years. Therefore, PMBV has become the procedure of choice for such patients when it can be performed by a skilled operator in a high-volume center.

Transthoracic echocardiography is helpful in identifying patients for the percutaneous procedure, and TEE is performed routinely to exclude left atrial thrombus. An "echo score" has been developed to help guide decision-making. The score accounts for the degree of leaflet thickening, calcification, and mobility, and for the extent of subvalvular thickening. A lower score predicts a higher likelihood of successful PMBV.

In patients in whom PMBV is not possible or unsuccessful, or in many patients with restenosis, an "open" valvotomy using cardiopulmonary bypass is necessary.

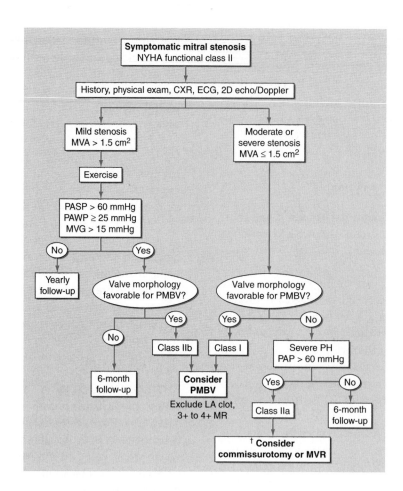

FIGURE 20-1

Management strategy for patients with mitral stenosis (MS) and mild symptoms. †There is controversy as to whether patients with severe MS (MVA <1.0 cm²) and severe pulmonary hypertension (PH) (PASP >60 mmHg) should undergo percutaneous mitral balloon valvotomy (PMBV) or mitral valve replacement (MVR) to prevent right ventricular failure. CXR, chest x-ray; ECG, electrocardiogram; echo, echocardiography; LA, left atrial; MR, mitral regurgitation; MVA, mitral valve area; MVG, mean mitral valve pressure gradient; NYHA, New York Heart Association; PASP, pulmonary arterial systolic pressure; PAWP, pulmonary arterial wedge pressure; 2D, two-dimensional. *(From Bonow et al.)*

TABLE 20-2

MEDICAL THERAPY OF VALVULAR HEART DISEASE

LESION	SYMPTOM CONTROL	NATURAL HISTORY
Mitral stenosis	Beta blockers, nondihydropyridine calcium channel blockers, or digoxin for rate control of AF; cardioversion for new-onset AF and HF; diuretics for HF	Warfarin for AF or thromboembolism; PCN for RF prophylaxis
Mitral regurgitation	Diuretics for HF Vasodilators for acute MR	Warfarin for AF or thromboembolism Vasodilators for HTN
Aortic stenosis	Diuretics for HF	No proven therapy
Aortic regurgitation	Diuretics and vasodilators for HF	Vasodilators for HTN

Note: Antibiotic prophylaxis is recommended according to current American Heart Association guidelines. For patients with these forms of valvular heart disease, prophylaxis is indicated for a prior history of endocarditis. HF is an indication for surgical or percutaneous treatment, and the recommendations here pertain to short-term therapy prior to definitive correction of the valve lesion. For patients whose comorbidities prohibit surgery, the medical therapies listed can be continued according to available guidelines for the management of HF. See text.

AF, atrial fibrillation; HF, heart failure; HTN, systemic hypertension; PCN, penicillin; RF, rheumatic fever.

Source: Adapted from NA Boon, P Bloomfield: The medical management of valvular heart disease. Heart 87:395, 2002, with permission.

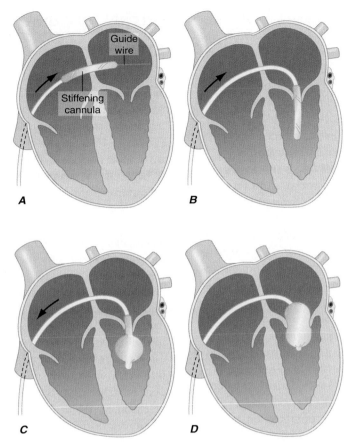

FIGURE 20-2

Inoue balloon technique for mitral balloon valvotomy. A. After transseptal puncture, the deflated balloon catheter is advanced across the inter-atrial septum, then across the mitral valve and into the left ventricle. **B.** The balloon is then inflated stepwise within the mitral orifice.

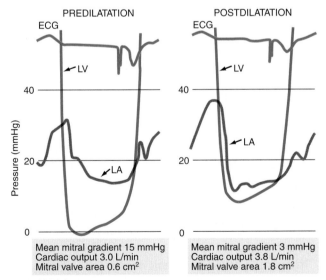

FIGURE 20-3

Simultaneous left atrial (LA) and left ventricular (LV) pressure before and after percutaneous mitral balloon valvuloplasty (PMBV) in a patient with severe mitral stenosis. *(Courtesy of Raymond G. McKay, MD; with permission.)*

In addition to opening the valve commissures, it is important to loosen any subvalvular fusion of papillary muscles and chordae tendineae and to remove large deposits of calcium, thereby improving valvular function, as well as to remove atrial thrombi. The perioperative mortality rate is ~2%.

Successful valvotomy is defined by a 50% reduction in the mean mitral valve gradient and a doubling of the mitral valve area. Successful valvotomy, whether balloon or surgical, usually results in striking symptomatic and hemodynamic improvement and prolongs survival. However, there is no evidence that the procedure improves the prognosis of patients with slight or no functional impairment. Therefore, unless recurrent systemic embolization or severe pulmonary hypertension has occurred (PA systolic pressures >50 mmHg at rest or >60 mmHg with exercise), valvotomy is *not* recommended for patients who are entirely asymptomatic and/or who have mild stenosis (mitral valve area >1/5 cm²). When there is little symptomatic improvement after valvotomy, it is likely that the procedure was ineffective, that it induced MR, or that associated valvular or myocardial disease was present. About half of all patients undergoing surgical mitral valvotomy require reoperation by 10 years. In the pregnant patient with MS, valvotomy should be carried out if pulmonary congestion occurs despite intensive medical treatment. PMBV is the preferred strategy in this setting and is performed with TEE and no or minimal x-ray exposure.

Mitral valve replacement (MVR) is necessary in patients with MS and significant associated MR, those in whom the valve has been severely distorted by previous transcatheter or operative manipulation, or those in whom the surgeon does not find it possible to improve valve function significantly. MVR is now routinely performed with preservation of the chordal attachments to optimize LV functional recovery. Perioperative mortality rates with MVR vary with age, LV function, the presence of CAD, and associated comorbidities. They average 5% overall but are lower in young patients and may be twice as high in older patients with comorbidities (Table 20-3). Because there are also long-term complications of valve replacement (p. 1480), patients in whom preoperative evaluation suggests the possibility that MVR may be required should be operated on only if they have severe MS—i.e., an orifice area ≤1 cm²—and are in NYHA Class III, i.e., symptomatic with ordinary activity despite optimal medical therapy. The overall 10-year survival of surgical survivors is ~70%. Long-term prognosis is worse in older patients and those with marked disability and marked depression of the CO preoperatively. Pulmonary hypertension and RV dysfunction are additional risk factors for poor outcome.

TABLE 20-3

MORTALITY RATES AFTER VALVE SURGERY[a]

OPERATION	NUMBER	OPERATIVE MORTALITY (%)
AVR (isolated)	12,501	2.8
MVR (isolated)	3788	5.3
AVR + CAB	12,748	5.2
MVR + CAB	2683	10.3
AVR + MVR	1018	8.8
MVP	3982	1.0
MVP + CAB	4293	7.0
TV surgery	4358	9.6
PV surgery	432	5.2

[a]Data are for calendar year 2004, in which 594 sites reported a total of 232,050 procedures. Data are available from the Society of Thoracic Surgeons at http://www.sts.org/sections/stsnationaldatabase/publications/executive/article.html

Note: AVR, aortic valve replacement; CAB, coronary artery bypass; MVR, mitral valve replacement; MVP, mitral valve repair; TV surgery, tricuspid valve repair and replacement; PV surgery, pulmonic valve repair and replacement.

MITRAL REGURGITATION

ETIOLOGY

MR may result from an abnormality or disease process that affects any one or more of the five functional components of the mitral valve apparatus (leaflets, annulus, chordae tendineae, papillary muscles, and subjacent myocardium) (Table 20-1). Acute MR can occur in the setting of acute myocardial infarction (MI) with papillary muscle rupture (Chap. 35), following blunt chest wall trauma, or during the course of infective endocarditis. With acute MI, the posteromedial papillary muscle is involved much more frequently than the anterolateral papillary muscle because of its singular blood supply. Transient, acute MR can occur during periods of active ischemia and bouts of angina pectoris. Rupture of chordae tendineae can result in "acute or chronic MR" in patients with myxomatous degeneration of the valve apparatus.

Chronic MR can result from rheumatic disease, mitral valve prolapse (MVP) extensive mitral annular calcification, congenital valve defects, hypertrophic obstructive cardiomyopathy (HOCM), and dilated cardiomyopathy (Chap. 21). Rheumatic heart disease is the cause of chronic MR in only about one-third of patients and occurs more frequently in males. The rheumatic process produces rigidity, deformity, and retraction of the valve cusps and commissural fusion, as well as shortening, contraction, and fusion of the chordae tendineae. The MR associated with both MVP and HOCM is usually dynamic in nature. MR in HOCM occurs as a consequence of anterior papillary muscle displacement and systolic anterior motion of the anterior mitral valve leaflet into the narrowed LV outflow tract. Annular calcification is especially prevalent among patients with advanced renal disease and is commonly observed in elderly women with hypertension and diabetes. MR may occur as a congenital anomaly (Chap. 19), most commonly as a defect of the endocardial cushions (atrioventricular cushion defects). A cleft anterior mitral valve leaflet accompanies primum ASD. Chronic MR is frequently secondary to ischemia and may occur as a consequence of ventricular remodeling, papillary muscle displacement, and leaflet tethering, or with fibrosis of a papillary muscle, in patients with healed MI(s) and ischemic cardiomyopathy. Similar mechanisms of annular dilatation and ventricular remodeling contribute to the MR that occurs universally among patients with nonischemic forms of dilated cardiomyopathy once the left ventricular end-diastolic dimension reaches 6.0 cm.

Irrespective of cause, chronic severe MR is often progressive, since enlargement of the LA places tension on the posterior mitral leaflet, pulling it away from the mitral orifice and thereby aggravating the valvular dysfunction. Similarly, LV dilatation increases the regurgitation, which in turn enlarges the LA and LV further, causing chordal rupture and resulting in a vicious circle; hence the aphorism "mitral regurgitation begets mitral regurgitation."

PATHOPHYSIOLOGY

The resistance to LV emptying (LV afterload) is reduced in patients with MR. As a consequence, the LV is decompressed into the LA during ejection, and with the reduction in LV size during systole, there is a rapid decline in LV tension. The initial compensation to MR is more complete LV emptying. However, LV volume increases progressively with time as the severity of the regurgitation increases and as LV contractile function deteriorates. This increase in LV volume is often accompanied by a reduced forward CO, though LV compliance is often increased and thus LV diastolic pressure does not elevate until late in the course. The regurgitant volume varies directly with the LV systolic pressure and the size of the regurgitant orifice; as mentioned above, the latter, in turn, is influenced profoundly by the extent of LV and mitral annular dilatation. Since EF rises in severe MR in the presence of normal LV function, even a modest reduction in this parameter (<60%) reflects significant dysfunction.

During early diastole, as the distended LA empties, there is a particularly rapid y descent in the absence of accompanying MS. A brief, early diastolic LA-LV pressure gradient [often generating a rapid filling sound (S_3) and mid-diastolic murmur masquerading as MS] may occur in patients with pure MR as a result of the very rapid flow of blood across a normal-sized mitral orifice.

Quantitative estimates of left ventricular ejection fraction (LVEF), CO, PA pressure, regurgitant volume, regurgitant fraction (RF), and the effective regurgitant orifice area can be obtained during a careful Doppler echocardiographic examination. These measurements can also be obtained with CMR. Left and right heart catheterization with contrast ventriculography is utilized less frequently. Severe MR is defined by a regurgitant volume ≥60 mL/beat, RF ≥50%, and effective regurgitant orifice area ≥0.40 cm².

LA Compliance

In acute severe MR, the regurgitant volume is delivered into a normal-sized LA having normal or reduced compliance. As a result, LA pressures rise markedly for any increase in LA volume. The v wave in the LA pressure pulse is usually prominent (Fig. 13-3), LA and pulmonary venous pressures are markedly elevated, and pulmonary edema is common. Because of the rapid rise in LA pressures during ventricular systole, the murmur of acute MR is early in timing and decrescendo in configuration, as a reflection of the progressive diminution in the LV-LA pressure gradient. LV systolic function in acute MR may be normal, hyperdynamic, or reduced, depending on the clinical context.

Patients with chronic severe MR, on the other hand, develop marked LA enlargement and *increased* LA compliance with little if any increase in LA and pulmonary venous pressures for any increase in LA volume. The LA v wave is relatively less prominent. The murmur of chronic MR is classically holosystolic in timing and plateau in configuration, as a reflection of the near–constant LV-LA pressure gradient. These patients usually complain of severe fatigue and exhaustion secondary to a low CO, while symptoms resulting from pulmonary congestion are less prominent initially; AF is almost invariably present once the LA dilates significantly.

Most common are patients whose clinical and hemodynamic features are intermediate between those in the two aforementioned groups.

SYMPTOMS

Patients with chronic mild-to-moderate isolated MR are usually asymptomatic. This form of LV volume overload is well tolerated. Fatigue, exertional dyspnea, and orthopnea are the most prominent complaints in patients with chronic severe MR. Palpitations are common and may signify the onset of AF. Right-sided heart failure, with painful hepatic congestion, ankle edema, distended neck veins, ascites, and secondary TR, occurs in patients with MR who have associated pulmonary vascular disease and marked pulmonary hypertension. On the other hand, acute pulmonary edema is common in patients with acute severe MR.

PHYSICAL FINDINGS

In patients with chronic severe MR, the arterial pressure is usually normal, though the arterial pulse may show a sharp upstroke. A systolic thrill is often palpable at the cardiac apex, the LV is hyperdynamic with a brisk systolic impulse and a palpable rapid-filling wave (S_3), and the apex beat is often displaced laterally.

In patients with acute severe MR, the arterial pressure may be reduced with a narrow pulse pressure, the jugular venous pressure and wave forms may be normal or increased and exaggerated, the apical impulse is not displaced, and signs of pulmonary congestion are prominent.

Auscultation

The S_1 is generally absent, soft, or buried in the holosystolic murmur of chronic MR. In patients with severe MR, the aortic valve may close prematurely, resulting in wide but physiologic splitting of S_2. A low-pitched S_3 occurring 0.12–0.17 s after the aortic valve closure sound, i.e., at the completion of the rapid-filling phase of the LV, is believed to be caused by the sudden tensing of the papillary muscles, chordae tendineae, and valve

CHAPTER 20 Valvular Heart Disease

leaflets. It may be followed by a short, rumbling, mid-diastolic murmur, even in the absence of MS. A fourth heart sound is often audible in patients with *acute* severe MR who are in sinus rhythm. A presystolic murmur is not ordinarily heard with isolated MR.

A systolic murmur of at least grade III/VI intensity is the most characteristic auscultatory finding in chronic severe MR. It is usually holosystolic (see Fig. 9-4), but as previously noted it is decrescendo and ceases in mid- to late systole in patients with acute severe MR. The systolic murmur of chronic MR is usually most prominent at the apex and radiates to the axilla. However, in patients with ruptured chordae tendineae or primary involvement of the posterior mitral leaflet with prolapse or flail, the regurgitant jet is eccentric, directed anteriorly, and strikes the LA wall adjacent to the aortic root. In this situation, the systolic murmur is transmitted to the base of the heart and therefore may be confused with the murmur of AS. In patients with ruptured chordae tendineae, the systolic murmur may have a cooing or "sea gull" quality, while a flail leaflet may cause a murmur with a musical quality. The systolic murmur of chronic MR not due to MVP is intensified by isometric exercise (handgrip) but is reduced during the strain phase of the Valsalva maneuver.

LABORATORY EXAMINATION
ECG

In patients with sinus rhythm, there is evidence of LA enlargement, but RA enlargement also may be present when pulmonary hypertension is severe. Chronic severe MR is generally associated with AF. In many patients there is no clear-cut ECG evidence of enlargement of either ventricle. In others, the signs of LV hypertrophy are present.

Echocardiogram

TTE with Doppler imaging is indicated to assess the mechanism of the MR and its hemodynamic severity. LV function can be assessed from LV end-diastolic and end-systolic volumes and EF. Observations can be made regarding leaflet structure and function, chordal integrity, LA and LV size, annular calcification, and regional and global LV systolic function. Doppler imaging should demonstrate the width or area of the color flow MR jet within the LA, the intensity of the continuous wave Doppler signal, the pulmonary venous flow contour, the early peak mitral inflow velocity, and the quantitative measures of regurgitant volume, RF, and effective regurgitant orifice area. In addition, the PA pressures can be estimated from the TR jet velocity. TTE is also indicated to follow the course of patients with chronic MR and to provide rapid assessment for any clinical change.

The echocardiogram in patients with MVP is described in the next section. TEE provides greater detail than TTE (Fig. 12-3).

Chest X-ray

The LA and LV are the dominant chambers in chronic MR; late in the course of the disease, the former may be massively enlarged and forms the right border of the cardiac silhouette. Pulmonary venous congestion, interstitial edema, and Kerley B lines are sometimes noted. Marked calcification of the mitral leaflets occurs commonly in patients with longstanding combined MR and MS. Calcification of the mitral annulus may be visualized, particularly on the lateral view of the chest. Patients with acute severe MR may have asymmetric pulmonary edema if the regurgitant jet is directed predominantly to the orifice of an upper lobe pulmonary vein.

℞ Treatment: MITRAL REGURGITATION

(Fig. 20-4)

MEDICAL (Table 20-2) The management of chronic severe MR depends to some degree on its cause. Warfarin should be provided once AF intervenes with a target INR of 2–3. Cardioversion should be considered depending on the clinical context and left atrial size. In contrast to the acute setting, there are no large, long-term prospective studies to substantiate the use of vasodilators for the treatment of chronic, isolated severe MR *in the absence of systemic hypertension*. The severity of MR in the setting of an ischemic or nonischemic dilated cardiomyopathy may diminish with aggressive, evidence-based treatment of heart failure, including the use of diuretics, beta blockers, ACE inhibitors, and digitalis. Asymptomatic patients with severe MR in sinus rhythm with normal LV size and systolic function should avoid isometric forms of exercise.

Patients with acute severe MR require urgent stabilization and preparation for surgery. Diuretics, intravenous vasodilators (particularly sodium nitroprusside), and even intra-aortic balloon counterpulsation may be needed for patients with post-MI papillary muscle rupture or other forms of acute severe MR.

Surgical In the selection of patients with chronic severe MR for surgical treatment, the often slowly progressive nature of the condition must be balanced against the immediate and long-term risks associated with operation. These risks are significantly lower for primary valve repair than for valve replacement (Table 20-3). Repair usually consists of valve reconstruction utilizing a variety of valvuloplasty techniques and

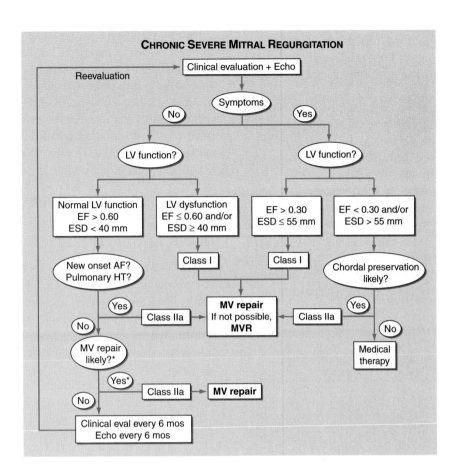

FIGURE 20-4

Management strategy for patients with chronic severe mitral regurgitation. *Mitral valve (MV) repair may be performed in asymptomatic patients with normal left ventricular (LV) function if performed by an experienced surgical team and if the likelihood of successful MV repair is >90%. AF, atrial fibrillation; Echo, echocardiography; EF, ejection fraction; ESD, end-systolic dimension; eval, evaluation; HT, hypertension; MVR, mitral valve replacement. *(From Bonow et al.)*

insertion of an annuloplasty ring. Repair spares the patient the long-term adverse consequences of valve replacement, i.e., thromboembolic and hemorrhagic complications in the case of mechanical prostheses and late valve failure necessitating repeat valve replacement in the case of bioprostheses (p. 1480). In addition, by preserving the integrity of the papillary muscles, subvalvular apparatus, and chordae tendineae, mitral repair and valvuloplasty maintain LV function to a relatively greater degree.

Surgery for chronic severe MR is indicated once symptoms occur, especially if valve repair is feasible (Fig. 20-4). Other indications for early consideration of mitral valve repair include recent-onset AF and pulmonary hypertension, defined as a PA pressure ≥50 mmHg at rest or ≥60 mmHg with exercise. Surgical treatment of chronic severe MR is indicated for asymptomatic patients when LV dysfunction is progressive, with LVEF declining below 60% and/or end-systolic cavity dimension on echocardiography rising above 40 mm. These aggressive recommendations for surgery are predicated on the outstanding results achieved with mitral valve repair, particularly when applied to patients with myxomatous disease. Indeed, primary valvuloplasty repair of patients younger than 75 years with normal LV systolic function and no CAD can now be performed by experienced surgeons with <1% perioperative mortality risk. Repair is feasible in up to 95% of patients with myxomatous disease. Long-term durability is excellent; the incidence of reoperative surgery for failed primary repair is ~1% per year for 10 years after surgery. For patients with AF, a left atrial Maze procedure or radiofrequency ablation of the pulmonary vein ostia is often performed to reduce the risk of recurrent AF.

In patients with significantly impaired LV function (EF <30%), the risk of surgery rises, the recovery of LV performance is incomplete, and the long-term survival is reduced. However, conservative management has little to offer these patients, so operative treatment may be indicated, and the clinical and hemodynamic improvement that follows surgical treatment of patients with advanced disease is occasionally dramatic, especially when severe CAD is also present and bypass grafting can be performed. Though most patients who survive surgery appear to be greatly improved, some degree of myocardial dysfunction often persists, as indicated by a further fall in LVEF.

Patients with acute severe MR can often be stabilized temporarily with appropriate medical therapy, but surgical correction will be necessary, emergently in the case of papillary muscle rupture and within days to weeks in most other settings.

When surgical treatment is contemplated, left and right heart catheterization and left ventriculography *may* be helpful in confirming the presence of severe MR in patients in whom there is a discrepancy between the clinical and TTE findings that cannot be resolved with TEE or CMR. Coronary arteriography identifies patients who require concomitant coronary revascularization.

MITRAL VALVE PROLAPSE

MVP, also variously termed the *systolic click-murmur syndrome*, *Barlow's syndrome*, *floppy-valve syndrome*, and *billowing mitral leaflet syndrome*, is a relatively common but highly variable clinical syndrome resulting from diverse pathogenic mechanisms of the mitral valve apparatus. Among these are excessive or redundant mitral leaflet tissues, which is commonly associated with myxomatous degeneration and greatly increased concentrations of acid mucopolysaccharide.

In most patients with MVP, the cause is unknown, but in some it appears to be a genetically determined collagen disorder. A reduction in the production of type III collagen has been incriminated, and electron microscopy has revealed fragmentation of collagen fibrils.

MVP is a frequent finding in patients with heritable disorders of connective tissue, including Marfan syndrome, osteogenesis imperfecta, and Ehler-Danlos syndrome.

MVP may be associated with thoracic skeletal deformities similar to but not as severe as those in Marfan syndrome, encompassing a high-arched palate and alterations of the chest and thoracic spine, including the so-called straight back syndrome.

In most patients with MVP, myxomatous degeneration is confined to the mitral (or, less commonly, the tricuspid or aortic) valves without other clinical or pathologic manifestations of disease. The posterior leaflet is usually more affected than the anterior, and the mitral valve annulus is often greatly dilated. In many patients, elongated, redundant, or ruptured chordae tendineae cause or contribute to the regurgitation.

MVP also may occur rarely as a sequel to acute rheumatic fever, in ischemic heart disease, and in various cardiomyopathies, as well as in 20% of patients with ostium secundum ASD.

MVP may lead to excessive stress on the papillary muscles, which in turn leads to dysfunction and ischemia of the papillary muscles and the subjacent ventricular myocardium. Rupture of chordae tendineae and progressive annular dilatation and calcification also contribute to valvular regurgitation, which then places more stress on the diseased mitral valve apparatus, thereby creating a vicious circle. The ECG changes (see later) and ventricular arrhythmias appear to result from regional ventricular dysfunction related to increased stress placed on the papillary muscles.

CLINICAL FEATURES

MVP is more common in females and occurs most commonly between the ages of 15 and 30 years; the clinical course is often benign. MVP may also be observed in older (>50 years) patients, often males, in whom MR is often more severe and requires surgical treatment. There is an increased familial incidence for some patients, suggesting an autosomal dominant form of inheritance. MVP encompasses a broad spectrum of severities, ranging from only a systolic click and murmur and mild prolapse of the posterior leaflet of the mitral valve to severe MR due to chordal rupture and massive prolapse of both leaflets. In many patients this condition progresses over years or decades. In others it worsens rapidly as a result of chordal rupture or endocarditis.

Most patients are asymptomatic and remain so for their entire lives. However, in North America MVP is now the most common cause of isolated severe MR requiring surgical treatment. Arrhythmias, most commonly ventricular premature contractions and paroxysmal supraventricular and ventricular tachycardia, as well as AF, have been reported and may cause palpitations, light-headedness, and syncope. Sudden death is a very rare complication and occurs most often in patients with severe MR and depressed LV systolic function. There may be an excess risk of sudden death among patients with a flail leaflet. Many patients have chest pain that is difficult to evaluate. It is often substernal, prolonged, and poorly related to exertion, and it rarely resembles angina pectoris. Transient cerebral ischemic attacks secondary to emboli from the mitral valve due to endothelial disruption have been reported, though a causal relationship has not been established. Infective endocarditis may occur in patients with MR and/or leaflet thickening.

Auscultation

The most important finding is the mid- or late (nonejection) systolic click, which occurs 0.14 s or more after the S_1 and is thought to be generated by the sudden tensing of slack, elongated chordae tendineae or by the prolapsing mitral leaflet when it reaches its maximum excursion. Systolic clicks may be multiple and may be followed by a high-pitched, late systolic crescendo-decrescendo murmur, which occasionally is "whooping" or "honking" and is heard best at the apex. The click and murmur occur earlier with standing, during the strain of the Valsalva maneuver, and with any intervention that decreases LV volume, exaggerating the propensity of mitral leaflet prolapse. Conversely, squatting and isometric exercises, which increase LV volume, diminish MVP, and the click-murmur complex is delayed, moves away from S_1, and may even disappear. Some patients have a midsystolic click without the murmur; others have the murmur without a click. Still others have both sounds at different times.

LABORATORY EXAMINATION

The ECG most commonly is normal but may show biphasic or inverted T waves in leads II, III, and aVF, and occasionally supraventricular or ventricular premature beats. *TTE* is particularly effective in identifying the abnormal position and prolapse of the mitral valve leaflets. A useful echocardiographic definition of MVP is systolic displacement (in the parasternal long axis view) of the mitral valve leaflets by at least 2 mm into the LA superior to the plane of the mitral annulus. Color flow and continuous wave Doppler imaging is helpful in revealing and evaluating associated MR. TEE is indicated when more accurate information is required and is performed routinely for intraoperative guidance for valve repair. Invasive left ventriculography is rarely necessary but can also show prolapse of the posterior and sometimes of both mitral valve leaflets.

℞ **Treatment:**
MITRAL VALVE PROLAPSE

Infective endocarditis prophylaxis is indicated only for patients with a prior history of endocarditis. Beta blockers sometimes relieve chest pain and control palpitations. If the patient is symptomatic from severe MR, mitral valve repair (or rarely, replacement) is indicated (Fig. 20-4). Antiplatelet agents such as aspirin should be given to patients with transient ischemic attacks, and if these are not effective, anticoagulants such as warfarin should be considered.

AORTIC STENOSIS

AS occurs in about one-fourth of all patients with chronic valvular heart disease; approximately 80% of adult patients with symptomatic valvular AS are male.

(Table 20-1) AS in adults may be due to degenerative calcification of the aortic cusps. It may be congenital in origin or it may be secondary to rheumatic inflammation. *Age-related degenerative calcific AS* (also known as senile or sclerocalcific AS) is now the most common cause of AS in adults in North America and Western Europe. About 30% of persons older than 65 years exhibit aortic valve sclerosis; many of these have a systolic murmur of AS but without obstruction, while 2% exhibit frank stenosis. Aortic sclerosis is defined echocardiographically as focal thickening or calcification of the valve cusps with a peak Doppler transaortic velocity of ≤2.5 m/s. Aortic sclerosis appears to be a marker for an increased risk of coronary heart disease events. On histologic examination these valves frequently exhibit changes similar to those seen with atherosclerosis and vascular inflammation. Interestingly, risk factors for atherosclerosis, such as age, male sex, smoking, diabetes mellitus, hypertension, chronic kidney disease, increased LDL, reduced HDL cholesterol, and elevated C-reactive protein are all risk factors for aortic valve calcification.

The *congenitally affected valve* may be stenotic at birth (Chap. 19) and may become progressively more fibrotic, calcified, and stenotic. In other cases the valve may be congenitally deformed, usually bicuspid [bicuspid aortic valve (BAV)], without serious narrowing of the aortic orifice during childhood; its abnormal architecture makes its leaflets susceptible to otherwise ordinary hemodynamic stresses, which ultimately lead to valvular thickening, calcification, increased rigidity, and narrowing of the aortic orifice.

Rheumatic disease of the aortic leaflets produces commissural fusion, sometimes resulting in a bicuspid-appearing valve. This condition in turn makes the leaflets more susceptible to trauma and ultimately leads to fibrosis, calcification, and further narrowing. By the time the obstruction to LV outflow causes serious clinical disability, the valve is usually a rigid calcified mass, and careful examination may make it difficult or even impossible to determine the etiology of the underlying process. Rheumatic AS is almost always associated with involvement of the mitral valve and with AR.

OTHER FORMS OF OBSTRUCTION TO LEFT VENTRICULAR OUTFLOW

Besides valvular AS, three other lesions may be responsible for obstruction to LV outflow: *hypertrophic obstructive cardiomyopathy* (Chap. 21), *discrete congenital subvalvular AS*, and *supravalvular AS* (Chap. 19). The causes of left ventricular outflow obstruction can be differentiated on the basis of the cardiac examination and Doppler echocardiographic findings.

PATHOPHYSIOLOGY

The obstruction to LV outflow produces a systolic pressure gradient between the LV and aorta. When severe obstruction is suddenly produced experimentally, the LV responds by dilatation and reduction of stroke volume. However, in some patients the obstruction may be present at birth and/or increase gradually over the course of many years, and LV output is maintained by the presence of concentric LV hypertrophy. Initially, this serves as an adaptive mechanism because it reduces toward normal the systolic stress developed by the myocardium, as predicted by the Laplace relation ($S = Pr/h$, where S = systolic wall stress, P = pressure, r = radius, and h = wall thickness). A large transaortic valvular pressure gradient may exist for many years without a reduction in CO or LV dilatation; ultimately, however, excessive hypertrophy becomes maladaptive, and LV function declines.

A mean systolic pressure gradient >40 mmHg with a normal CO or an effective aortic orifice area <~1.0 cm² (or ~<0.6 cm²/m² body surface area in a normal-sized adult)—i.e., less than approximately one-third of the normal orifice—is generally considered to represent severe obstruction to LV outflow (Fig. 13-4). The elevated LV end-diastolic pressure observed in many patients with severe AS signifies the presence of LV dilatation and/or diminished compliance of the hypertrophied LV wall. Although the CO at rest is within normal limits in most patients with severe AS, it usually fails to rise normally during exercise. Loss of an appropriately timed, vigorous atrial contraction, as occurs in AF or atrioventricular dissociation, may cause rapid progression of symptoms. Late in the course, the CO and LV–aortic pressure gradient decline, and the mean LA, PA, and RV pressures rise.

The hypertrophied LV elevates myocardial oxygen requirements. In addition, even in the absence of obstructive CAD, there may be interference with coronary blood flow. This is because the pressure compressing the coronary arteries exceeds the coronary perfusion pressure, often causing ischemia (especially in the subendocardium), both in the presence and in the absence of coronary arterial narrowing.

SYMPTOMS

AS is rarely of clinical importance until the valve orifice has narrowed to ~1.0 cm². Even severe AS may exist for many years without producing any symptoms because of the ability of the hypertrophied LV to generate the elevated intraventricular pressures required for a normal stroke volume.

Most patients with pure or predominant AS have gradually increasing obstruction for years but do not become symptomatic until the sixth to eighth decades. Exertional dyspnea, angina pectoris, and syncope are the three cardinal symptoms. Often there is a history of insidious progression of fatigue and dyspnea associated with gradual curtailment of activities. *Dyspnea* results primarily from elevation of the pulmonary capillary pressure caused by elevations of LV diastolic pressures secondary to reduced left ventricular compliance. *Angina pectoris* usually develops somewhat later and reflects an imbalance between the augmented myocardial oxygen requirements and reduced oxygen availability; the former results from the increased myocardial mass and intraventricular pressure, while the latter may result from accompanying CAD, which is not uncommon in patients with AS, as well as from compression of the coronary vessels by the hypertrophied myocardium. Therefore, angina may occur in severe AS even without obstructive epicardial CAD. *Exertional syncope* may result from a decline in arterial pressure caused by vasodilatation in the exercising muscles and inadequate vasoconstriction in nonexercising muscles in the face of a fixed CO, or from a sudden fall in CO produced by an arrhythmia.

Since the CO at rest is usually well maintained until late in the course, marked fatigability, weakness, peripheral cyanosis, cachexia, and other clinical manifestations of a low CO are usually not prominent until this stage is reached. Orthopnea, paroxysmal nocturnal dyspnea, and pulmonary edema, i.e., symptoms of LV failure, also occur only in the advanced stages of the disease. Severe pulmonary hypertension leading to RV failure and systemic venous hypertension, hepatomegaly, AF, and TR are usually late findings in patients with isolated severe AS.

When AS and MS coexist, the reduction in CO induced by MS lowers the pressure gradient across the aortic valve and thereby masks many of the clinical findings produced by AS.

PHYSICAL FINDINGS

The rhythm is generally regular until late in the course; at other times, AF should suggest the possibility of associated mitral valve disease. The systemic arterial pressure is usually within normal limits. In the late stages, however, when stroke volume declines, the systolic pressure may fall and the pulse pressure narrow. The peripheral arterial pulse rises slowly to a delayed sustained peak (pulsus parvus et tardus; see Fig. 9-2). In the elderly, the stiffening of the arterial wall may mask this important physical sign. In many patients the *a* wave in the jugular venous pulse is accentuated. This results from the diminished distensibility of the RV cavity caused by the bulging, hypertrophied interventricular septum.

The LV impulse is usually displaced laterally. A double apical impulse may be recognized, particularly with the patient in the left lateral recumbent position. A systolic thrill is generally present at the base of the heart, in the suprasternal notch, and along the carotid arteries.

Auscultation

An early systolic ejection sound is frequently audible in children and adolescents with congenital noncalcific valvular AS. This sound usually disappears when the valve becomes calcified and rigid. As AS increases in severity, LV systole may become prolonged so that the aortic valve closure sound no longer precedes the pulmonic valve closure sound, and the two components may become synchronous, or aortic valve closure may even follow pulmonic valve closure, causing paradoxic splitting of S_2 (Chap. 9). The sound of aortic valve closure can be heard most frequently in patients with AS who have pliable valves, and calcification diminishes the intensity of this sound. Frequently, an S_4 is audible at the apex and reflects the presence of LV hypertrophy and an elevated LV end-diastolic pressure; an S_3 generally occurs late in the course, when the LV dilates.

The murmur of AS is characteristically an ejection (mid) systolic murmur that commences shortly after the S_1, increases in intensity to reach a peak toward the middle of ejection, and ends just before aortic valve closure (Fig. 9-4). It is characteristically low-pitched, rough and rasping in character, and loudest at the base of the heart, most commonly in the second right intercostal space. It is transmitted upward along the carotid arteries. Occasionally it is transmitted downward and to the apex, where it may be confused with the systolic murmur of MR (Gallavardin effect). In almost all patients with severe obstruction and preserved CO, the murmur is at least grade III/VI. In patients with mild degrees of obstruction or in those with severe stenosis with heart failure in whom the stroke volume and therefore the transvalvular flow rate are reduced, the murmur may be relatively soft and brief.

LABORATORY EXAMINATION

ECG

In most patients with severe AS there is LV hypertrophy (see Fig. 11-9). In advanced cases, ST-segment depression and T-wave inversion (LV "strain") in standard leads I and aVL and in the left precordial leads are evident. However, there is no close correlation between the ECG and the hemodynamic severity of obstruction, and the absence of ECG signs of LV hypertrophy does not exclude severe obstruction.

Echocardiogram

The key findings are LV hypertrophy and, in patients with valvular calcification (i.e., most adult patients with symptomatic AS), multiple, bright, thick, echoes from the valve (see Fig. 12-2). Eccentricity of the aortic valve cusps is characteristic of congenitally bicuspid valves. TEE imaging usually displays the obstructed orifice extremely

well, but it is not routinely required for adequate characterization. The valve gradient and aortic valve area can be estimated by Doppler measurement of the transaortic velocity. Severe AS is defined by a valve area <1.0 cm^2, whereas moderate AS is defined by a valve area of $1.0–1.5$ cm^2 and mild AS by a valve area of $1.5–2.0$ cm^2. LV dilatation and reduced systolic shortening reflect impairment of LV function.

Echocardiography is useful for identifying coexisting valvular abnormalities such as MS and AR, which sometimes accompany AS; for differentiating valvular AS from other forms of outflow obstruction; and for measurement of the aortic root. Aneurysmal enlargement (maximal dimension >4.5 cm) of the root or ascending aorta can occur in up to 20% of patients with bicuspid aortic valve disease, independent of the severity of the valve lesion. Dobutamine stress echocardiography is useful for the evaluation of patients with severe AS and severe LV systolic dysfunction (EF <0.35).

Chest X-Ray

The chest x-ray may show no or little overall cardiac enlargement for many years. Hypertrophy without dilatation may produce some rounding of the cardiac apex in the frontal projection and slight backward displacement in the lateral view; severe AS is often associated with poststenotic dilatation of the ascending aorta. As noted above, however, aortic enlargement may be an independent process and mediated by the same type of structural changes that occur in patients with Marfan syndrome. Aortic calcification is usually readily apparent on fluoroscopic examination or by echocardiography; the absence of valvular calcification in an adult suggests that severe valvular AS is *not* present. In later stages of the disease, as the LV dilates there is increasing roentgenographic evidence of LV enlargement, pulmonary congestion, and enlargement of the LA, PA, and right side of the heart.

Catheterization

Right and left heart catheterization for invasive assessment of AS is performed infrequently but can be useful when there is a discrepancy between the clinical and echocardiographic findings. Concerns have been raised that attempts to cross the aortic valve for measurement of left ventricular pressures are associated with a risk of cerebral embolization. Catheterization is also useful in three distinct categories of patients: (1) *patients with multivalvular disease*, in whom the role played by each valvular deformity should be defined to aid in the planning of definitive operative treatment; (2) *young, asymptomatic patients with noncalcific congenital AS*, to define with precision the severity of obstruction to LV outflow, since operation [which does not usually require aortic valve replacement (AVR)] or PABV may be indicated if severe

AS is present, even in the absence of symptoms; balloon valvotomy may follow left heart catheterization immediately; and (3) *patients in whom it is suspected that the obstruction to LV outflow may not be at the aortic valve* but rather in the sub- or supravalvular regions.

Coronary angiography is indicated to detect or exclude CAD in patients >45 years old with severe AS who are being considered for operative treatment. The incidence of significant CAD for which bypass grafting is indicated at the time of AVR exceeds 50% among adult patients.

NATURAL HISTORY

Death in patients with severe AS occurs most commonly in the seventh and eighth decades. Based on data obtained at postmortem examination in patients before surgical treatment became widely available, the average time to death after the onset of various symptoms was as follows: angina pectoris, 3 years; syncope, 3 years; dyspnea, 2 years; congestive heart failure, 1.5–2 years. Moreover, in >80% of patients who died with AS, symptoms had existed for <4 years. Among adults dying with valvular AS, sudden death, which presumably resulted from an arrhythmia, occurred in 10–20%. However, most sudden deaths occurred in patients who had previously been symptomatic; thus, sudden death is very uncommon

(<1% per year) in asymptomatic adult patients with severe AS. Obstructive calcific AS is a progressive disease, with an annual reduction in valve area averaging 0.1 cm²/year and an annual increase in mean gradient averaging 7 mmHg/year.

℞ Treatment: AORTIC STENOSIS

(Table 20-2, **Fig. 20-5**)

MEDICAL TREATMENT In patients with severe AS (<1.0 cm²), strenuous physical activity should be avoided, even in the asymptomatic stage. Care must be taken to avoid dehydration and hypovolemia to protect against a significant reduction in CO. Medications used for the treatment of hypertension or CAD, including beta blockers and ACE inhibitors, are generally safe for asymptomatic patients with preserved left ventricular systolic function. Nitroglycerin is helpful in relieving angina pectoris. Retrospective studies have shown that patients with degenerative calcific AS who receive HMG-CoA reductase inhibitors ("statins") exhibit slower progression of leaflet calcification and aortic valve area reduction than those who do not. One prospective randomized clinical trial using high-dose atorvastatin failed

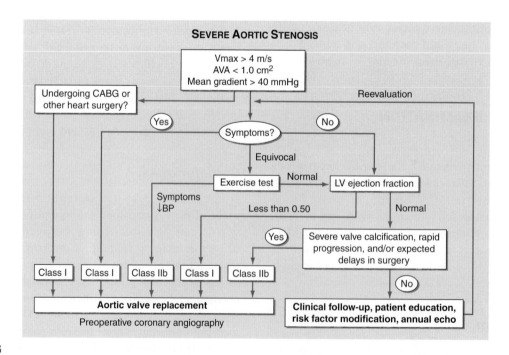

FIGURE 20-5

Management strategy for patients with severe aortic stenosis. Preoperative coronary angiography should be performed routinely as determined by age, symptoms, and coronary risk factors. Cardiac catheterization and angiography may also be helpful when there is discordance between clinical findings and echocardiography. AVA, aortic valve area; BP, blood pressure; CABG, coronary artery bypass graft surgery; echo, echocardiography; LV, left ventricle; Vmax, maximal velocity across aortic valve by Doppler echocardiography. *(From Bonow et al. Modified from CM Otto: J Am Coll Cardiol 47:2141, 2006.)*

to show a measurable benefit, although a more recent trial using rosuvastatin did show a beneficial effect. The role of statin medications may be more clearly defined with further study.

SURGICAL TREATMENT Asymptomatic patients with calcific AS and severe obstruction should be followed carefully for the development of symptoms and by serial echocardiograms for evidence of deteriorating LV function. Operation is indicated in patients with severe AS (valve area <1.0 cm² or 0.6 cm²/m² body surface area) who are symptomatic, those who exhibit LV dysfunction (EF <50%), as well as those with an aneurysmal or expanding aortic root (maximal dimension >4.5 cm or annual increase in size >0.5 cm/year), even if they are asymptomatic. In patients without heart failure, the operative risk of AVR is ~3% (Table 20-3). It is prudent to postpone operation in patients with severe calcific AS who are truly asymptomatic and who exhibit normal LV function, i.e., EF >50%, since they may continue to do well for years. However, some advocate AVR in patients with severe valve calcification and rapid progression of obstruction. The risk of surgical mortality exceeds that of sudden death in asymptomatic patients. Exercise testing is employed in many centers to assess objectively the functional capacity of asymptomatic patients for whom the history is ambiguous. As many as one-third of patients will show signs of functional impairment during exercise for which AVR should be considered. AVR is carried out in asymptomatic patients with severe or moderately severe stenosis who undergo coronary artery bypass grafting. AVR is also routinely performed in patients with moderate AS who are undergoing coronary bypass grafting or aortic root reconstruction.

Operation should, if possible, be carried out before frank LV failure develops; at this late stage, the aortic valve pressure gradient declines as the CO, stroke volume, and EF decline (low gradient, low output AS). In such patients the perioperative risk is high (15–20%), and evidence of myocardial disease may persist even when the operation is technically successful. Furthermore, long-term postoperative survival also correlates inversely with preoperative LV dysfunction. Nonetheless, in view of the even worse prognosis of such patients when they are treated medically, there is usually little choice but to advise surgical treatment, especially in patients in whom contractile reserve can be demonstrated by dobutamine echocardiography (defined by a ≥20% in stroke volume after dobutamine challenge). In patients in whom severe AS and CAD coexist, relief of the AS and revascularization of the myocardium by means of aortocoronary bypass grafting may result in striking clinical and hemodynamic improvement (Table 20-3).

Because many patients with calcific AS are elderly, particular attention must be directed to the adequacy of hepatic, renal, and pulmonary function before AVR is recommended. Age alone is not a contraindication to AVR for AS. The mortality rate depends to a substantial extent on the patient's preoperative clinical and hemodynamic state. The 10-year survival rate of patients with AVR is ~60%. Approximately 30% of bioprosthetic valves evidence primary valve failure in 10 years, requiring re-replacement, and an approximately equal percentage of patients with mechanical prostheses develop significant hemorrhagic complications as a consequence of treatment with anticoagulants.

PERCUTANEOUS BALLOON AORTIC VALVU-LOPLASTY This procedure is preferable to operation in children and young adults with congenital, noncalcific AS (Chap. 19). It is not commonly used in adults with severe calcific AS because of a very high restenosis rate and the risk of procedural complications, but on occasion it has been used successfully as a "bridge to operation" in patients with severe LV dysfunction and shock who are too ill to tolerate surgery.

AORTIC REGURGITATION

ETIOLOGY

(Table 20-1) AR may be caused by primary valve disease or by primary aortic root disease.

Primary Valve Disease

In approximately two-thirds of patients with valvular AR, the disease is rheumatic in origin, resulting in thickening, deformity, and shortening of the individual aortic valve cusps, changes that prevent their proper opening during systole and closure during diastole. A rheumatic origin is much less common in patients with isolated AR who do not have associated mitral valve disease. Patients with congenital BAV disease may develop predominant AR. Congenital fenestrations of the aortic valve occasionally produce mild AR. Membranous subaortic stenosis often leads to thickening and scarring of the aortic valve leaflets with secondary AR. Prolapse of an aortic cusp, resulting in progressive chronic AR, occurs in approximately 15% of patients with VSD (Chap. 19) but may also occur as an isolated phenomenon or as a consequence of myxomatous degeneration sometimes associated with mitral (p. 226) and/or tricuspid valve involvement.

AR may result from infective endocarditis, which can develop on a valve previously affected by rheumatic disease, a congenitally deformed valve, or, rarely, on a normal aortic valve, and may lead to perforation or erosion of one or more leaflets. The aortic valve leaflets may become scarred and retracted during the course of syphilis or ankylosing spondylitis and contribute further to the AR that derives primarily from the associated root disease. Although traumatic rupture or avulsion of the aortic valve is an uncommon cause of acute AR, it does represent the most frequent serious lesion in patients surviving nonpenetrating cardiac injuries. The coexistence of hemodynamically significant AS with AR usually excludes all the rarer forms of AR because it occurs almost exclusively in patients with rheumatic or congenital AR. In patients with AR due to primary valvular disease, dilatation of the aortic annulus may occur secondarily and intensify the regurgitation.

Primary Aortic Root Disease

AR may also be due entirely to marked aortic dilatation, i.e., aortic root disease, without primary involvement of the valve leaflets; widening of the aortic annulus and separation of the aortic leaflets are responsible for the AR (Chap. 38). Cystic medial degeneration of the ascending aorta, which may or may not be associated with other manifestations of Marfan syndrome; idiopathic dilatation of the aorta; annulo-aortic ectasia; osteogenesis imperfecta; and severe hypertension, may all widen the aortic annulus and lead to progressive AR. Occasionally AR is caused by retrograde dissection of the aorta involving the aortic annulus. Syphilis and ankylosing spondylitis, both of which may affect aortic valves, may also be associated with cellular infiltration and scarring of the media of the thoracic aorta, leading to aortic dilatation, aneurysm formation, and severe regurgitation. In syphilis of the aorta, now a very rare condition, the involvement of the intima may narrow the coronary ostia, which in turn may be responsible for myocardial ischemia.

PATHOPHYSIOLOGY

The total stroke volume ejected by the LV (i.e., the sum of the effective forward stroke volume and the volume of blood that regurgitates back into the LV) is increased in patients with AR. In patients with wide-open (free) AR, the volume of regurgitant flow may equal the effective forward stroke volume. In contrast to MR, in which a fraction of the LV stroke volume is delivered into the low-pressure LA, in AR the entire LV stroke volume is ejected into a high-pressure zone, the aorta. An increase in the LV end-diastolic volume (increased preload) constitutes the major hemodynamic compensation for AR. The dilatation and eccentric hypertrophy of the LV allow this chamber to eject a larger stroke volume without requiring any increase in the relative shortening of each myofibril. Therefore, severe AR may occur with a normal effective forward stroke volume and a normal left ventricular EF [total (forward plus regurgitant) stroke volume/end-diastolic volume], together with an elevated LV end-diastolic pressure and volume. However, through the operation of Laplace's law, LV dilatation increases the LV systolic tension required to develop any given level of systolic pressure. Chronic AR is thus a state in which LV preload and afterload are both increased. Ultimately, these adaptive measures fail. As LV function deteriorates, the end-diastolic volume rises further and the forward stroke volume and EF decline. Deterioration of LV function often precedes the development of symptoms. Considerable thickening of the LV wall also occurs with chronic AR, and at autopsy the hearts of these patients may be among the largest encountered, sometimes weighing >1000 g.

The reverse pressure gradient from aorta to LV, which drives the AR flow, falls progressively during diastole (Fig. 13-5), accounting for the decrescendo nature of the diastolic murmur. Equilibration between aortic and LV pressures may occur toward the end of diastole in patients with chronic severe AR, particularly when the heart rate is slow. In patients with acute severe AR, the LV is unprepared for the regurgitant volume load. LV compliance is normal or reduced, and LV diastolic pressures rise rapidly, occasionally to levels >40 mmHg. The LV pressure may exceed the LA pressure toward the end of diastole, and this reversed pressure gradient closes the mitral valve prematurely.

In patients with chronic severe AR, the effective forward CO usually is normal or only slightly reduced at rest, but often it fails to rise normally during exertion. Early signs of LV dysfunction include reduction in the EF. In advanced stages there may be considerable elevation of the LA, PA wedge, PA, and RV pressures and lowering of the forward CO at rest.

Myocardial ischemia may occur in patients with AR because myocardial oxygen requirements are elevated by LV dilatation, hypertrophy, and elevated LV systolic tension. However, a large fraction of coronary blood flow occurs during diastole, when arterial pressure is subnormal, thereby reducing coronary perfusion pressure. This combination of increased oxygen demand and reduced supply may cause myocardial ischemia, particularly of the subendocardium, even in the absence of concomitant CAD.

HISTORY

Approximately three-fourths of patients with pure or predominant valvular AR are males; females predominate among patients with primary valvular AR who have associated mitral valve disease. A history compatible with infective endocarditis may sometimes be elicited from patients with rheumatic or congenital involvement of the aortic valve, and the infection often precipitates or seriously aggravates preexisting symptoms.

In patients with *acute severe AR*, as may occur in infective endocarditis, aortic dissection, or trauma, the LV cannot dilate sufficiently to maintain stroke volume, and LV diastolic pressure rises rapidly with associated marked elevations of LA and PA wedge pressures. Pulmonary edema and/or cardiogenic shock may develop rapidly.

Chronic severe AR may have a long latent period, and patients may remain relatively asymptomatic for as long as 10–15 years. However, uncomfortable awareness of the heartbeat, especially on lying down, may be an early complaint. Sinus tachycardia, during exertion or with emotion, or premature ventricular contractions may produce particularly uncomfortable palpitations as well as head pounding. These complaints may persist for many years before the development of exertional dyspnea, usually the first symptom of diminished cardiac reserve. The dyspnea is followed by orthopnea, paroxysmal nocturnal dyspnea, and excessive diaphoresis. Anginal chest pain occurs frequently in patients with severe AR, even in younger patients, and it is not necessary to invoke the presence of CAD to explain this symptom in patients with severe AR. Anginal pain may develop at rest as well as during exertion. Nocturnal angina may be a particularly troublesome symptom, and it may be accompanied by marked diaphoresis. The anginal episodes can be prolonged and often do not respond satisfactorily to sublingual nitroglycerin. Systemic fluid accumulation, including congestive hepatomegaly and ankle edema, may develop late in the course of the disease.

PHYSICAL FINDINGS

In chronic severe AR, the jarring of the entire body and the bobbing motion of the head with each systole can be appreciated, and the abrupt distention and collapse of the larger arteries are easily visible. The examination should be directed toward the detection of conditions predisposing to AR, such as Marfan syndrome, ankylosing spondylitis, and VSD.

Arterial Pulse

A rapidly rising "water-hammer" pulse, which collapses suddenly as arterial pressure falls rapidly during late systole and diastole (Corrigan's pulse), and capillary pulsations, an alternate flushing and paling of the skin at the root of the nail while pressure is applied to the tip of the nail (Quincke's pulse), are characteristic of free AR. A booming "pistol-shot" sound can be heard over the femoral arteries (Traube's sign), and a to-and-fro murmur (Duroziez's sign) is audible if the femoral artery is lightly compressed with a stethoscope.

The arterial pulse pressure is widened, and there is an elevation of the systolic pressure, sometimes to as high as 300 mmHg, and a depression of the diastolic pressure. The measurement of arterial diastolic pressure with a sphygmomanometer may be complicated by the fact that systolic sounds are frequently heard with the cuff

completely deflated. However, the level of cuff pressure at the time of muffling of the Korotkoff sounds (phase IV) generally corresponds fairly closely to the true intraarterial diastolic pressure. As the disease progresses and the LV end-diastolic pressure rises, the arterial diastolic pressure may actually rise as well, since the aortic diastolic pressure cannot fall below the LV end-diastolic pressure. For the same reason, acute severe AR may also be accompanied by only a slight widening of the pulse pressure. Such patients are invariably tachycardic as the heart rate increases in an attempt to preserve the CO.

Palpation

In patients with chronic severe AR, the LV impulse is heaving and displaced laterally and inferiorly. The systolic expansion and diastolic retraction of the apex are prominent. A diastolic thrill is often palpable along the left sternal border, and a prominent systolic thrill may be palpable in the suprasternal notch and transmitted upward along the carotid arteries. This systolic thrill and the accompanying murmur do not necessarily signify the coexistence of AS. In many patients with pure AR or with combined AS and AR, the carotid arterial pulse is bisferiens, i.e., with two systolic waves separated by a trough (Fig. 9-2D).

Auscultation

In patients with severe AR, the aortic valve closure sound (A_2) is usually absent. An S_3 and systolic ejection sound are frequently audible, and occasionally an S_4 also may be heard. The murmur of chronic AR is typically a high-pitched, blowing, decrescendo diastolic murmur, heard best in the third intercostal space along the left sternal border (Fig. 9-4B). In patients with mild AR, this murmur is brief but, as the severity increases, generally becomes louder and longer, indeed holodiastolic. When the murmur is soft, it can be heard best with the diaphragm of the stethoscope and with the patient sitting up, leaning forward, and with the breath held in forced expiration. In patients in whom the AR is caused by primary valvular disease, the diastolic murmur is usually louder along the left than the right sternal border. However, when the murmur is heard best along the right sternal border, it suggests that the AR is caused by aneurysmal dilatation of the aortic root. "Cooing" or musical diastolic murmurs suggest eversion of an aortic cusp vibrating in the regurgitant stream.

A midsystolic ejection murmur is frequently audible in isolated AR. It is generally heard best at the base of the heart and is transmitted along the carotid vessels. This murmur may be quite loud without signifying aortic obstruction. A third murmur frequently heard in patients with severe AR is the *Austin Flint murmur*, a soft, low-pitched, rumbling mid-diastolic murmur. It is probably produced by the diastolic displacement of the anterior leaflet of the mitral valve by the AR stream but does not appear to be associated with hemodynamically significant mitral obstruction. The auscultatory features of AR are intensified by strenuous handgrip, which augments systemic resistance.

In acute severe AR, the elevation of LV end-diastolic pressure may lead to early closure of the mitral valve, an associated mid-diastolic sound, a soft or absent S_1, a pulse pressure that is not particularly wide, and a soft, short diastolic murmur of AR.

LABORATORY EXAMINATION

ECG

In patients with chronic severe AR, the ECG signs of LV hypertrophy become manifest (Chap. 11). In addition, these patients frequently exhibit ST-segment depression and T-wave inversion in leads I, aVL, V_5, and V_6 ("LV strain"). Left axis deviation and/or QRS prolongation denote diffuse myocardial disease, generally associated with patchy fibrosis, and usually signify a poor prognosis.

Echocardiogram

The extent and velocity of wall motion are normal or even supernormal, until myocardial contractility declines. A rapid, high-frequency fluttering of the anterior mitral leaflet produced by the impact of the regurgitant jet is a characteristic finding. The echocardiogram is also useful in determining the cause of AR, by detecting dilatation of the aortic annulus and root or aortic dissection (Fig. 12-3). Thickening and failure of coaptation of the leaflets also may be noted. Color flow Doppler echocardiographic imaging is very sensitive in the detection of AR, and Doppler echocardiography is helpful in assessing its severity. With severe AR, the central jet width exceeds 65% of the left ventricular outflow tract, the regurgitant volume is ≥60 mL/beat, the regurgitant fraction is ≥50%, and there is diastolic flow reversal in the proximal descending thoracic aorta. The continuous wave Doppler profile shows a rapid deceleration time in patients with acute severe AR, due to the rapid increase in LV diastolic pressure. Serial two-dimensional echocardiography is valuable in assessing LV performance and in detecting progressive myocardial dysfunction.

Chest X-ray

In chronic severe AR, the apex is displaced downward and to the left in the frontal projection. In the left anterior oblique and lateral projections, the LV is displaced posteriorly and encroaches on the spine. When AR is caused by primary disease of the aortic root, aneurysmal dilatation of the aorta may be noted, and the aorta may fill the retrosternal space in the lateral view. Echocardiography and CT angiography are more sensitive than the chest x-ray for the detection of aortic root enlargement.

Cardiac Catheterization and Angiography

When needed, right and left heart catheterization with contrast aortography can provide accurate confirmation of the magnitude of regurgitation and the status of LV function. Coronary angiography is performed routinely in appropriate patients prior to surgery.

℞ Treatment: AORTIC REGURGITATION

(Fig. 20-6)

ACUTE AORTIC REGURGITATION Patients with acute severe AR may respond to intravenous diuretics and vasodilators (such as sodium nitroprusside), but stabilization is usually short-lived and operation is indicated urgently. Intra-aortic balloon counterpulsation is contraindicated. Beta-blockers are also best avoided so as not to reduce the CO further or slow the heart rate, which might allow proportionately more time in diastole for regurgitation to occur. Surgery is the treatment of choice.

CHRONIC AORTIC REGURGITATION Early symptoms of dyspnea and effort intolerance respond to treatment with diuretics and vasodilators (ACE inhibitors, dihydropyridine calcium channel blockers, or hydralazine) may be useful as well. Surgery can then be performed in more controlled circumstances. The use of vasodilators to extend the compensated phase of chronic severe AR before the onset of symptoms or the development of LV dysfunction is more controversial. Expert consensus is strong regarding the need to control systolic blood pressure (goal <140 mmHg) in patients with chronic AR, and vasodilators are an excellent first choice as antihypertensive agents. It is often difficult to achieve adequate control in such patients because of the increased stroke volume. Cardiac arrhythmias and systemic infections are poorly tolerated in patients with severe AR and must be treated promptly and vigorously. Although nitroglycerin and long-acting nitrates are not as helpful in relieving anginal pain as they are in patients with ischemic heart disease, they are worth a trial. Patients with syphilitic aortitis should receive a full course of penicillin therapy. Beta blockers may be useful to retard the rate of aortic root enlargement in young patients with Marfan syndrome and aortic root dilatation with no or only mild AR. Patients with severe AR should avoid isometric exercises.

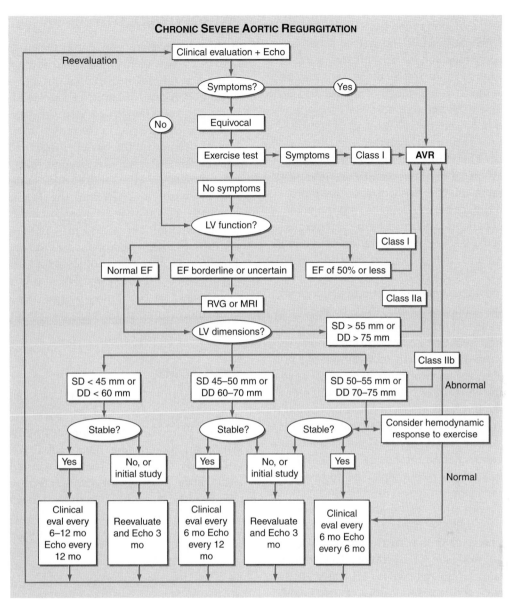

FIGURE 20-6

Management strategy for patients with chronic severe aortic regurgitation. Preoperative coronary angiography should be performed routinely, as determined by age, symptoms, and coronary risk factors. Cardiac catheterization and angiography may also be helpful when there is discordance between clinical findings and echocardiography. "Stable" refers to stable echocardiographic measurements. In some centers, serial follow-up may be performed with radionuclide ventriculography (RVG) or magnetic resonance imaging (MRI) rather than echocardiography (echo) to assess left ventricular (LV) volume and systolic function. AVR, aortic valve replacement; DD, end-diastolic dimension; EF, ejection fraction; eval, evaluation; SD, end-systolic dimension. *(Modified from Bonow et al.)*

SURGICAL TREATMENT In deciding on the advisability and proper timing of surgical treatment, two points should be kept in mind: (1) patients with chronic severe AR usually do not become symptomatic until *after* the development of myocardial dysfunction; and (2) when delayed too long (defined as >1 year from onset of symptoms or LV dysfunction), surgical treatment often does not restore normal LV function. Therefore, in patients with chronic severe AR, careful clinical follow-up and noninvasive testing with echocardiography at ~6-month intervals are necessary if operation is to be undertaken at the optimal time, i.e., *after* the onset of LV dysfunction but *prior* to the development of severe symptoms. Operation can be deferred as long as the patient both remains asymptomatic and retains normal LV function.

AVR is indicated for the treatment of severe AR in symptomatic patients irrespective of LV function. In general, operation should be carried out in asymptomatic patients with severe AR and progressive LV dysfunction defined by an LVEF <50%, an LV end-systolic dimension >55 mm or end-systolic volume >55 mL/m², or an LV diastolic dimension >75 mm. Smaller dimensions may be appropriate thresholds in individuals of smaller stature. Patients with severe AR without indications for operation should be followed by clinical and echocardiographic examination every 3–12 months.

Surgical options for management of aortic valve and root disease have expanded considerably over the past decade. AVR with a suitable mechanical or tissue prosthesis is generally necessary in patients with rheumatic AR and in many patients with other forms of regurgitation. Rarely, when a leaflet has been perforated during infective endocarditis or torn from its attachments to the aortic annulus by thoracic trauma, primary surgical repair may be possible. When AR is due to aneurysmal dilatation of the annulus and ascending aorta rather than to primary valvular involvement, it may be possible to reduce the regurgitation by narrowing the annulus or by excising a portion of the aortic root without replacing the valve. Resuspension of the native aortic valve leaflets is possible in ~50% of patients with acute AR in the setting of Type A aortic dissection. In other conditions, however, regurgitation can be eliminated only by replacing the aortic valve, excising the dilated or aneurysmal ascending aorta responsible for the regurgitation, and replacing it with a graft. This formidable procedure entails a higher risk than isolated AVR.

As in patients with other valvular abnormalities, both the operative risk and the late mortality are largely dependent on the stage of the disease and on myocardial function at the time of operation. The overall operative mortality for isolated AVR is ~3% (Table 20-3). However, patients with marked cardiac enlargement and prolonged LV dysfunction experience an operative mortality rate of ~10% and a late mortality rate of ~5% per year due to LV failure despite a technically satisfactory operation. Nonetheless, because of the very poor prognosis with medical management, even patients with LV failure should be considered for operation.

Patients with acute severe AR require prompt surgical treatment, which may be lifesaving.

TRICUSPID STENOSIS

TS, much less prevalent than MS in North America and Western Europe, is generally rheumatic in origin and is more common in females than in males. It does not occur as an isolated lesion and is usually associated with MS. Hemodynamically significant TS occurs in 5–10% of patients with severe MS; rheumatic TS is commonly associated with some degree of TR. Nonrheumatic causes of TS are rare.

PATHOPHYSIOLOGY

A diastolic pressure gradient between the RA and RV defines TS. It is augmented when the transvalvular blood flow increases during inspiration and declines during expiration. A mean diastolic pressure gradient of 4 mmHg is usually sufficient to elevate the mean RA pressure to levels that result in systemic venous congestion. Unless sodium intake has been restricted and diuretics administered, this venous congestion is associated with hepatomegaly, ascites, and edema, sometimes severe. In patients with sinus rhythm, the RA *a* wave may be extremely tall and may even approach the level of the RV systolic pressure. The *y* descent is prolonged. The CO at rest is usually depressed, and it fails to rise during exercise. The low CO is responsible for the normal or only slightly elevated LA, PA, and RV systolic pressures despite the presence of MS. Thus, the presence of TS can mask the hemodynamic and clinical features of the MS, which usually accompanies it.

SYMPTOMS

Since the development of MS generally precedes that of TS, many patients initially have symptoms of pulmonary congestion. Spontaneous improvement of these symptoms should raise the possibility that TS may be developing. Characteristically, patients complain of relatively little dyspnea for the degree of hepatomegaly, ascites, and edema that they have. However, fatigue secondary to a low CO and discomfort due to refractory edema, ascites, and marked hepatomegaly are common in patients with TS and/or TR. In some patients, TS may be suspected for the first time when symptoms of right-sided failure persist after an adequate mitral valvotomy.

PHYSICAL FINDINGS

Since TS usually occurs in the presence of other obvious valvular disease, the diagnosis may be missed unless it is considered and searched for. Severe TS is associated with marked hepatic congestion, often resulting in cirrhosis, jaundice, serious malnutrition, anasarca, and ascites. Congestive hepatomegaly and, in cases of severe tricuspid valve disease, splenomegaly are present. The jugular veins are distended, and in patients with sinus rhythm there may be giant *a* waves. The *v* waves are less conspicuous, and since tricuspid obstruction impedes RA emptying during diastole, there is a slow *y* descent. In patients with sinus rhythm there may be prominent presystolic pulsations of the enlarged liver as well.

On auscultation, an OS of the tricuspid valve may occasionally be heard ~0.06 s after pulmonic valve closure. The diastolic murmur of TS has many of the qualities of the diastolic murmur of MS, and since TS almost always occurs in the presence of MS, the less-common valvular lesion may be missed. However, the tricuspid murmur is generally heard best along the left lower sternal margin and over the xiphoid process, and it is most prominent during presystole in patients with sinus rhythm. The murmur of TS is augmented during inspiration, and it is reduced during expiration and particularly during the strain phase of the Valsalva maneuver, when tricuspid blood flow is reduced.

LABORATORY EXAMINATION

The ECG features of RA enlargement (Fig. 11-8) include tall, peaked P waves in lead II, as well as prominent, upright P waves in lead V_1. The *absence* of ECG evidence of right ventricular hypertrophy (RVH) in a patient with right-sided heart failure who is believed to have MS should suggest associated tricuspid valve disease. The chest x-ray in patients with combined TS and MS shows particular prominence of the RA and superior vena cava without much enlargement of the PA and with less evidence of pulmonary vascular congestion than occurs in patients with isolated MS. On echocardiographic examination, the tricuspid valve is usually thickened and domes in diastole; the transvalvular gradient can be estimated by Doppler echocardiography. TTE provides additional information regarding mitral valve structure and function, LV and RV size and function, and PA pressure.

℞ **Treatment:**
TRICUSPID STENOSIS

Patients with TS generally exhibit marked systemic venous congestion; intensive salt restriction, bed rest, and diuretic therapy are required during the preoperative period. Such a preparatory period may diminish hepatic congestion and thereby improve hepatic function sufficiently so that the risks of operation, particularly bleeding, are diminished. Surgical relief of the TS should be carried out, preferably at the time of surgical mitral valvotomy or MVR, in patients with moderate or severe TS who have mean diastolic pressure gradients exceeding ~4 mmHg and tricuspid orifice areas <1.5–2.0 cm². TS is almost always accompanied by significant TR. Operative repair may permit substantial improvement of tricuspid valve function. If repair cannot be accomplished, the tricuspid valve may have to be replaced with a prosthesis, preferably a large bioprosthetic valve. Mechanical valves in the tricuspid position are more prone to thromboembolic complications than in other positions.

Most commonly, TR is functional and secondary to marked dilatation of the tricuspid annulus. Functional TR may complicate RV enlargement of any cause, including inferior wall infarcts that involve the RV. It is commonly seen in the late stages of heart failure due to rheumatic or congenital heart disease with severe pulmonary hypertension (pulmonary artery systolic pressure >55 mmHg), as well as in ischemic heart disease and dilated cardiomyopathy. It is reversible in part if pulmonary hypertension is relieved. Rheumatic fever may produce organic (primary) TR, often associated with TS. Infarction of RV papillary muscles, tricuspid valve prolapse, carcinoid heart disease, endomyocardial fibrosis, infective endocarditis, and trauma all may produce TR. Less commonly, TR results from congenitally deformed tricuspid valves, and it occurs with defects of the atrioventricular canal, as well as with Ebstein's malformation of the tricuspid valve (Chap. 19). TR also develops eventually in patients with chronic RV apical pacing.

As is the case for TS, the clinical features of TR result primarily from systemic venous congestion and reduction of CO. With the onset of TR in patients with pulmonary hypertension, symptoms of pulmonary congestion diminish, but the clinical manifestations of right-sided heart failure become intensified. The neck veins are distended with prominent *v* waves and rapid *y* descents, marked hepatomegaly, ascites, pleural effusions, edema, systolic pulsations of the liver, and a positive hepatojugular reflux. A prominent RV pulsation along the left parasternal region and a blowing holosystolic murmur along the lower left sternal margin, which may be intensified during inspiration and reduced during expiration or the strain of the Valsalva maneuver (Carvallo's sign), are characteristic findings; AF is usually present.

The ECG usually shows changes characteristic of the lesion responsible for the enlargement of the RV that leads to TR, e.g., inferior wall MI or severe RVH. Echocardiography may be helpful by demonstrating RV dilatation and prolapsing, flail, scarred, or displaced tricuspid leaflets; the diagnosis of TR can be made by color flow Doppler echocardiography, and its severity can be estimated by Doppler examination (Fig. 12-4). Severe TR is accompanied by hepatic vein systolic flow reversal. Continuous wave Doppler is also useful in estimating PA pressure. Roentgenographic examination usually reveals enlargement of both the RA and RV.

In patients with severe TR, the CO is usually markedly reduced, and the RA pressure pulse may exhibit no *x* descent during early systole but a prominent *c-v* wave with a rapid *y* descent. The mean RA and the RV end-diastolic pressures are often elevated.

CHAPTER 20

Valvular Heart Disease

℞ **Treatment:**
TRICUSPID REGURGITATION

Isolated TR, in the absence of pulmonary hypertension, such as that occurring as a consequence of infective endocarditis or trauma, is usually well tolerated and does not require operation. Indeed, even total excision of an infected tricuspid valve may be well tolerated for several years if the PA pressure is normal. Treatment of the underlying cause of heart failure usually reduces the severity of functional TR, by reducing the size of the tricuspid annulus. In patients with mitral valve disease and TR secondary to pulmonary hypertension and massive RV enlargement, effective surgical correction of the mitral valvular abnormality results in lowering of the PA pressures and gradual reduction or disappearance of the TR without direct treatment of the tricuspid valve. However, recovery may be much more rapid in patients with severe secondary TR if, at the time of mitral valve surgery, and especially when there is measurable enlargement of the tricuspid valve annulus, tricuspid annuloplasty (generally with the insertion of a plastic ring), open tricuspid valve repair, or, in the rare instance of severe organic tricuspid valve disease, tricuspid valve replacement is performed (Table 20-3). Tricuspid annuloplasty or replacement may be required for severe TR with primary involvement of the valve.

PULMONIC VALVE DISEASE

The pulmonic valve is affected by rheumatic fever far less frequently than are the other valves, and it is uncommonly the seat of infective endocarditis. The most common *acquired* abnormality affecting the pulmonic valve is regurgitation secondary to dilatation of the pulmonic valve ring as a consequence of severe pulmonary hypertension. This produces the *Graham Steell murmur*, a high-pitched, decrescendo, diastolic blowing murmur along the left sternal border, which is difficult to differentiate from the far more common murmur produced by AR. Pulmonic regurgitation is usually of little hemodynamic significance; indeed, surgical removal or destruction of the pulmonic valve by infective endocarditis does not produce heart failure unless serious pulmonary hypertension is also present.

The *carcinoid syndrome* may cause pulmonic stenosis and/or regurgitation. Pulmonic regurgitation occurs universally among patients who have undergone childhood repair of Tetralogy of Fallot with reconstruction of the RV outflow tract. Congenital pulmonic stenosis is discussed in Chap. 19.

VALVE REPLACEMENT

The results of replacement of any valve are dependent primarily on (1) the patient's myocardial function and general medical condition at the time of operation; (2) the technical abilities of the operative team and the quality of the postoperative care; and (3) the durability, hemodynamic characteristics, and thrombogenicity of the prosthesis. Increased perioperative mortality is associated with advanced age and comorbidity (e.g., pulmonary or renal disease, the need for nonvalvular cardiovascular surgery, diabetes mellitus) as well as with greater levels of preoperative functional disability and pulmonary hypertension. Late complications of valve replacement include paravalvular leakage, thromboemboli, bleeding due to anticoagulants, structural deterioration of the prosthesis, and infective endocarditis.

The considerations involved in the choice between a bioprosthetic (tissue) and artificial mechanical valve are similar in the mitral and aortic positions and in the treatment of stenotic, regurgitant, or mixed lesions. All patients who have undergone replacement of any valve with a mechanical prosthesis are at risk of thromboembolic complications and must be maintained permanently on anticoagulants, a treatment that imposes a hazard of hemorrhage. The primary advantage of bioprostheses over mechanical prostheses is the virtual absence of thromboembolic complications 3 months after implantation, and except for patients with chronic AF, few such instances have been associated with their use. The major disadvantage of bioprosthetic valves is their structural deterioration, the incidence of which is inversely proportional to the patient's age. This deterioration results in the need to replace the prosthesis in up to 30% of patients by 10 years and in 50% by 15 years. Rates of structural valve deterioration are higher for mitral than for aortic bioprostheses. This phenomenon may be due in part to the greater closing pressure to which a mitral prosthesis is exposed.

Traditionally, a mechanical prosthesis was considered preferable for a patient younger than 65 years who could take anticoagulation reliably. Bioprostheses were recommended for older (>65 years) patients who did not otherwise have an indication for anticoagulation (e.g.,, AF). However, more recent surveys of cardiac surgery in the United States, as reflected in the Society of Thoracic Surgeons database, show a clear and progressive trend favoring the implantation of bioprosthetic valves in younger (<65 years) patients. Reasons for this development include improved durability of newer generation bioprostheses, decreased risk at time of reoperation, the aggregate risks of long-term anticoagulation, and patient preference to avoid anticoagulation. Patient preference should be factored into any decision regarding the type of valve replacement. A mechanical prosthesis is reasonable for aortic or mitral valve replacement in patients <65 years without a contraindication to anticoagulation. A bioprosthesis is equally reasonable for aortic or mitral valve replacement in patients <65 years who elect this strategy for lifestyle reasons with full knowledge of the likely need for reoperation over time.

Bioprostheses remain the preferred valve choice for patients >65 years, in both the aortic and mitral position. Bioprosthetic valves are also indicated for women who expect to become pregnant, as well as for others who refuse to take anticoagulation or for whom anticoagulation may be contraindicated. Types of bioprostheses include xenografts (i.e., porcine aortic valves; cryopreserved, mounted bovine pericardium), homograft (allograft) aortic valves obtained from cadavers, as well as pulmonary autografts transplanted into the aortic position. Homograft replacement may be preferred for the management of complicated aortic valve infective endocarditis.

In patients without contraindications to anticoagulants, particularly those younger than 65 years, a mechanical prosthesis is reasonable. Many surgeons now select the St. Jude prosthesis, a double-disk tilting prosthesis, for replacement of both aortic and mitral valves because of favorable hemodynamic characteristics and possible association with lower thrombogenicity.

GLOBAL BURDEN OF VALVULAR HEART DISEASE

Primary valvular heart disease ranks well below coronary heart disease, stroke, hypertension, obesity, and diabetes as major threats to the public health. Nevertheless, it is the source of significant morbidity and mortality. Rheumatic fever (Chap. 26) is the dominant cause of valvular heart disease in developing countries. Its prevalence has been estimated to range from as low as 1.0 per 100,000 school-age children in Costa Rica to as high as 150 per 100,000 in China. Rheumatic heart disease accounts for 12–65% of hospital admissions related to cardiovascular disease and 2–10% of hospital discharges in some developing countries. Prevalence and mortality rates vary among communities even within the same country as a function of crowding and the availability of medical resources and population-wide programs for detection and treatment of Group A streptococcal pharyngitis. In economically deprived areas, tropical and subtropical climates (particularly on the Indian subcontinent), Central America, and the Middle East, rheumatic valvular disease progresses more rapidly than in more-developed nations and frequently causes serious symptoms in patients <20 years. This accelerated natural history may be due to repeated infections with more virulent strains of rheumatogenic streptococci.

TS, a relatively uncommon valvular lesion in North America and Western Europe, is more common in tropical and subtropical climates, especially in southern Asia and in Latin America.

As of the year 2000, worldwide death rates for rheumatic heart disease approximated 5.5 per 100,000 population ($n = 332,000$), with the highest rates reported from Southeast Asia. Although there have been reports of recent isolated outbreaks of streptococcal infection in North America, valve disease in developed countries is now dominated by degenerative or inflammatory processes that lead to valve thickening, calcification, and dysfunction. The prevalence of valvular heart disease increases with age. Important left-sided valve disease may affect as much as 12–13% of adults older than 75 years.

The incidence of infective endocarditis (Chap. 25) has increased with the aging of the population, the more widespread prevalence of vascular grafts and intracardiac devices, the emergence of more virulent multidrug-resistant microorganisms, and the growing epidemic of diabetes. Infective endocarditis has become a more frequent cause of acute valvular regurgitation.

Bicuspid aortic valve disease affects as much as 1–2% of the population, and an increasing number of childhood survivors of congenital heart disease present later in life with valvular dysfunction. The past several years have witnessed significant improvements in surgical outcomes with progressive refinement of relatively less-invasive techniques. Percutaneous heart valve replacement or repair is under active clinical investigation.

FURTHER READINGS

BONOW RO et al: ACC/AHA 2006 Guidelines for the management of patients with valvular heart disease: Executive summary. Circulation 114:450, 2006

COATS L, BONHOEFFER P: New percutaneous treatments for valve disease. Heart 93:639, 2007

ENRIQUEZ-SARANO M, TAJIK AJ: Aortic regurgitation. N Engl J Med 351:1539, 2004

HARA H et al: Percutaneous balloon aortic valvuloplasty revisited: Time for a renaissance? Circulation 115:e334, 2007

NKOMO VT et al: Burden of valvular heart diseases: A population-based study. Lancet 368:1005, 2006

OTTO CM (ed): Valvular Heart Disease, 2d ed. Philadelphia, Saunders, 2003

———, BONOW RO: Valvular heart disease, in P Libby et al (eds): Braunwald's Heart Disease, 8th ed. Philadelphia, Saunders, 2008

PELLIKKA PA et al: Outcome of 622 adults with asymptomatic, hemodynamically significant aortic stenosis during prolonged follow-up. Circulation 111:3290, 2005

QUERE JP et al: Influence of left ventricular preoperative contractile reserve on postoperative ejection fraction in low-gradient aortic stenosis. Circulation 113:1738, 2006

ROSENHEK R et al: Outcome of watchful waiting in asymptomatic severe mitral regurgitation. Circulation 113:2238, 2006

240 SOCIETY OF THORACIC SURGEONS: STS Adult Cardiovascular National Surgery Database—Fall 2005 executive summary. Available at *http://www.sts.org/documents/pdf/STS-ExecutiveSummaryFall2005.pdf*

———: STS national database risk calculator. Available at *http://www.sts.org/sections/stsnationaldatabase/riskcalculator/*

WILSON W et al: Prevention of infective endocarditis. Guidelines from the American Heart Association Rheumatic Fever, Endocarditis, and Kawasaki Disease Committee, Council on Cardiovascular Disease in the Young, and the Council on Clinical Cardiology, Council on Cardiovascular Surgery and Anesthesia and the Quality of Care and Outcomes Research Interdisciplinary Working Group. Published April 2007, at *http://circ.ahajournals.org*

WORLD HEALTH ORGANIZATION: WHO expert consultation on rheumatic fever and rheumatic heart disease. Geneva, Switzerland, WHO technical report series: 923, 2001

CHAPTER 21

CARDIOMYOPATHY AND MYOCARDITIS

Joshua Wynne ■ Eugene Braunwald

The cardiomyopathies are a group of diseases that primarily affect the heart muscle and are *not* the result of congenital, acquired valvular, hypertensive, coronary arterial, or pericardial abnormalities. The diffuse myocardial fibrosis that accompanies multiple myocardial scars produced by myocardial infarctions can impair left ventricular (LV) function and is frequently referred to as *ischemic cardiomyopathy*. The colloquial use of the term *cardiomyopathy* should be avoided; instead, the term should be restricted to a condition *primarily* involving the myocardium.

Two fundamental forms of cardiomyopathy are recognized: (1) a primary type, consisting of heart muscle disease predominantly involving the myocardium and/or of unknown cause; and (2) a secondary type, consisting of myocardial disease of known cause or associated with a systemic disease such as amyloidosis or chronic alcohol use (Table 21-1). In many cases it is not possible to arrive at a specific etiologic diagnosis, and thus it is often more desirable to classify the cardiomyopathies into one of three morphologic types (dilated, restrictive, and hypertrophic) on the basis of differences in their pathophysiology and clinical presentation (Fig. 21-1; Tables 21-2 and 21-3). In some patients, two of these types may be present simultaneously or sequentially. An important additional consideration is whether or not the particular cardiomyopathy in question (whether primary or secondary) has a genetic basis.

DILATED CARDIOMYOPATHY

About one in three cases of congestive heart failure (CHF; Chap. 17) is due to dilated cardiomyopathy (DCM). LV and/or right ventricular (RV) systolic pump function is impaired, leading to progressive cardiac dilatation (remodeling). Symptoms of heart failure (HF) typically appear only after remodeling has been ongoing for some time (months or even years).

Although no cause is apparent in many cases, DCM is either familial or the end result of myocardial damage produced by a variety of known or unknown infectious, metabolic, or toxic agents. DCM may be the late

TABLE 21-1

CLASSIFICATION OF CARDIOMYOPATHIES

Primary Myocardial Involvement

Idiopathic (D,R,H)
Familial (D,R,H)
Eosinophilic endomyocardial disease (R)
Endomyocardial fibrosis (R)

Secondary Myocardial Involvement

Infective (D)
  Viral myocarditis
  Bacterial myocarditis
  Fungal myocarditis
  Protozoal myocarditis
  Metazoal myocarditis
  Spirochetal
  Rickettsial
Metabolic (D)
Familial storage disease (D,R)
  Glycogen storage disease
  Mucopolysaccharidoses
  Hemochromatosis
  Fabry's disease
Deficiency (D)
  Electrolytes
  Nutritional

Connective tissue disorders (D)
  Systemic lupus erythematosus
  Polyarteritis nodosa
  Rheumatoid arthritis
  Progressive systemic sclerosis
  Dermatomyositis
Infiltrations and granulomas (R,D)
  Amyloidosis
  Sarcoidosis
  Malignancy
Neuromuscular (D)
  Muscular dystrophy
  Myotonic dystrophy
  Friedreich's ataxia (H,D)
Sensitivity and toxic reactions (D)
  Alcohol
  Radiation
  Drugs
Peripartum heart disease (D)

Note: The principal clinical manifestation(s) of each etiologic grouping is denoted by D (dilated), R (restrictive), or H (hypertrophic) cardiomyopathy.

Source: Adapted from the WHO/ISFC task force report on the definition and classification of cardiomyopathies, 1980 and 1995.

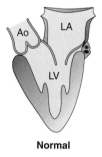

Normal

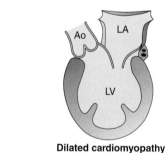

Dilated cardiomyopathy

Hypertrophic cardiomyopathy

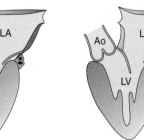

Restrictive cardiomyopathy

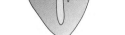

FIGURE 21-1

Drawing comparing the morphologic classes of cardiomyopathies. Ao, aorta; LA, left atrium; LV, left ventricle. *(From BF Waller: J Am Soc Echocardiogr 1:4, 1988.)*

TABLE 21-2

CLINICAL CLASSIFICATION OF CARDIOMYOPATHIES

1. Dilated: Left and/or right ventricular enlargement, impaired systolic function, congestive heart failure, arrhythmias, emboli
2. Restrictive: Endomyocardial scarring or myocardial infiltration resulting in restriction to left and/or right ventricular filling
3. Hypertrophic: Disproportionate left ventricular hypertrophy, typically involving septum more than free wall, with or without an intraventricular systolic pressure gradient; usually of a nondilated left ventricular cavity

consequence of acute viral myocarditis (see later), possibly mediated in part through an immunologic mechanism. Although DCM may occur at any age, it most commonly becomes apparent clinically in the third or fourth decades. A reversible form of DCM may be found with alcohol abuse (see later), pregnancy (see later), thyroid disease, cocaine use (see later), and chronic uncontrolled tachycardia.

TABLE 21-3 243

	DILATED	RESTRICTIVE	HYPERTROPHIC
LABORATORY EVALUATION OF THE CARDIOMYOPATHIES			
Chest roentgenogram	Moderate to marked cardiac silhouette enlargement Pulmonary venous hypertension	Mild cardiac silhouette enlargement	Mild to moderate cardiac silhouette enlargement
Electrocardiogram	ST-segment and T-wave abnormalities	Low voltage, conduction defects	ST-segment and T-wave abnormalities Left ventricular hypertrophy Abnormal Q waves
Echocardiogram	Left ventricular dilatation and dysfunction	Increased left ventricular wall thickness Normal or mildly reduced systolic function	Asymmetric septal hypertrophy (ASH) Systolic anterior motion (SAM) of the mitral valve
Radionuclide studies	Left ventricular dilatation and dysfunction (RVG)	Normal or mildly reduced systolic function (RVG)	Vigorous systolic function (RVG) Perfusion defect (^{201}TI or technetium sestamibi)
Cardiac catheterization	Left ventricular dilatation and dysfunction Elevated left- and often right-sided filling pressures Diminished cardiac output	Normal or mildly reduced systolic function Elevated left- and right-sided filling pressures	Vigorous systolic function Dynamic left ventricular outflow obstruction Elevated left- and right-sided filling pressures

Note: RVG, radionuclide ventriculogram; ^{201}TI, thallium 201.

GENETIC CONSIDERATIONS

One-fifth to one-third of patients have familial forms of DCM. Mutations in >20 genes that are transmitted in an autosomal dominant fashion have been described. Most common are mutations in genes encoding sarcomeric proteins, such as α–cardiac actin; β- and α-myosin; heavy chain α-tropomyosin; and troponins T, I, and C. It is believed that the abnormal proteins cause contractile dysfunction by impairing the production and/or transmission of force.

Patients with genetic DCM may also exhibit skeletal myopathies, particularly Duchenne's and Emery-Dreifuss muscular dystrophy (see later). Mutations in the gene encoding the nuclear envelope protein lamin A/C are also inherited in an autosomal dominant manner; they are responsible for the development of DCM associated with atrioventricular (AV) conduction disorder and other electrophysiologic disturbances that may cause sudden cardiac death (SCD). An X-linked autosomal recessive disorder caused by the dystrophin gene occurs in young males and is associated with a rapid downhill course; mutations in mitochondrial genes have also been reported in DCM.

CLINICAL FEATURES

Symptoms of left- and right-sided CHF usually develop gradually (Chap. 17). Some patients have LV dilatation for months or even years before becoming symptomatic.

Although vague chest pain may be present, typical angina pectoris is unusual and suggests the presence of ischemic heart disease. Syncope due to arrhythmias and systemic embolism (often emanating from a ventricular thrombus) may occur.

PHYSICAL EXAMINATION

Variable degrees of cardiac enlargement and findings of CHF (Chap. 17) are noted. In patients with advanced disease, the pulse pressure is narrow and the jugular venous pressure is elevated. Third and fourth heart sounds are common, and mitral or tricuspid regurgitation may occur.

LABORATORY EXAMINATIONS

The chest roentgenogram demonstrates enlargement of the cardiac silhouette due to LV dilatation, although generalized cardiomegaly is often seen. The lung fields may demonstrate pulmonary vascular redistribution and interstitial or, in advanced cases, alveolar edema. The electrocardiogram (ECG) often shows sinus tachycardia or atrial fibrillation, ventricular arrhythmias, left atrial abnormality, low voltage, diffuse nonspecific ST-T-wave abnormalities, and sometimes intraventricular and/or AV conduction defects. Echocardiography, computed tomographic imaging (CTI), and cardiac magnetic resonance imaging (MRI) show LV dilatation, with normal, minimally thickened, or thinned walls, and systolic dysfunction. Circulating levels of brain natriuretic peptide are usually elevated.

Cardiac catheterization and coronary angiography are often performed to exclude ischemic heart disease, and bedside hemodynamic monitoring may be helpful in the management of selected acutely decompensated patients. Angiography reveals a dilated, diffusely hypokinetic left ventricle, often with some degree of mitral regurgitation. Cardiac CTI may distinguish between DCM and proximal coronary artery disease and, thereby, reduce the need for invasive procedures. Transvenous endomyocardial biopsy is usually not necessary in idiopathic or familial DCM; however, it may be helpful in the recognition of secondary cardiomyopathies, such as amyloidosis and acute myocarditis (see later).

Rx Treatment: DILATED CARDIOMYOPATHY

Most patients pursue an inexorably downhill course, and the majority, particularly those >55 years, die within 4 years of the onset of symptoms. Patients of African ancestry are more likely to suffer more rapidly progressive CHF and death than Caucasians. Spontaneous improvement or stabilization occurs in about one-quarter of patients. Death is due to either progressive HF or ventricular tachy- or bradyarrhythmia; SCD is a constant threat. Systemic embolization is a concern, and patients should be considered for chronic anticoagulation. Standard therapy of HF, as described in Chap. 17, is indicated. Alcohol should be avoided because of its cardiotoxic effects (see later), as should calcium channel blockers and nonsteroidal anti-inflammatory drugs. Antiarrhythmic agents are best avoided owing to the risk of proarrhythmia. Cardiac resynchronization therapy and insertion of an implantable cardioverter defibrillator (ICD) should be employed in DCM as in HF of other etiologies. In patients with advanced disease who are refractory to other therapies, cardiac transplantation should be considered (Chap. 18).

ALCOHOLIC CARDIOMYOPATHY

Individuals who consume large quantities (>90 g/d) of alcohol over many years may develop a clinical picture resembling idiopathic or familial DCM. The risk of developing cardiomyopathy is partially determined genetically. A polymorphism of the gene encoding the alcohol metabolizing enzyme, alcohol dehydrogenase (*ALDH2*2*), as well as the DD form of the angiotensin-converting enzyme (*ACE*) gene increase the predilection for the development of alcoholic cardiomyopathy. Patients with advanced alcoholic cardiomyopathy and severe CHF have a poor prognosis, particularly if they continue to drink; fewer than one-quarter of such patients survive 3 years. Management consists of abstention, which may halt the progression or even reverse the course of this disease.

A second presentation of alcoholic cardiotoxicity may be found in individuals without overt HF and consists of recurrent supraventricular or ventricular tachyarrhythmias. Termed the *holiday heart syndrome*, it typically appears after a drinking binge; atrial fibrillation is seen most frequently, followed by atrial flutter and frequent ventricular premature depolarizations.

In contrast to the adverse cardiac effects of excessive alcohol consumption, moderate consumption (20–30 g/d) appears to be cardioprotective; it raises high-density lipoprotein (HDL) cholesterol and is associated with a reduced incidence of ischemic heart disease, ischemic stroke, and metabolic syndrome.

PERIPARTUM CARDIOMYOPATHY

Cardiac dilatation and CHF may develop during the last trimester of pregnancy or within 6 months of delivery. The cause is unknown, although inflammatory myocarditis, immune activation, and gestational hypertension have all been incriminated. The patient who develops peripartum cardiomyopathy typically is multiparous, of African ancestry, and >30 years, although the disease may be found in a wide spectrum of patients. The symptoms, signs, and treatment are similar to those in patients with idiopathic DCM, the latter including implantation of an ICD or cardiac transplantation if the criteria for these therapies are satisfied. The mortality rate of this disorder is around 10%.

The prognosis is related to whether the heart size returns to normal after the first episode of CHF. If it does, subsequent pregnancies may sometimes be tolerated, albeit with an increased risk of recurrent CHF; if the heart remains enlarged, and/or the LV ejection fraction (EF) remains depressed after 6 months, the prognosis is poor, and further pregnancies frequently produce additional myocardial damage, ultimately leading to refractory CHF. Patients who recover from peripartum cardiomyopathy should be encouraged to avoid further pregnancies, particularly if LV dysfunction persists.

NEUROMUSCULAR DISEASE

Cardiac involvement is common in many of the muscular dystrophies. In *Duchenne's progressive muscular dystrophy*, mutations in a gene that encodes a cardiac structural protein (*dystrophin*) lead to myocyte death. Myocardial involvement is most frequently indicated by a distinctive and unique ECG pattern consisting of tall R waves in the right precordial leads with an R/S ratio >1.0, often associated with deep Q waves in the limb and lateral precordial leads. A variety of supraventricular and ventricular arrhythmias is frequently found. Rapidly progressive HF may develop despite extended periods of apparent circulatory stability.

Myotonic dystrophy is characterized by a variety of ECG abnormalities, especially disorders of impulse formation and AV conduction, but other overt clinical evidence of heart disease is uncommon. Because of these abnormalities, syncope and sudden death are major hazards. In appropriate patients, insertion of an ICD and/or permanent pacemaker may be effective.

DRUGS

A variety of pharmacologic agents may damage the myocardium acutely, producing a pattern of inflammation (myocarditis, see later), or they may lead to chronic damage of the type seen with DCM. Certain drugs produce only ECG abnormalities, while others may precipitate fulminant CHF and death.

The anthracycline derivatives, particularly doxorubicin (Adriamycin), are powerful antineoplastic agents. Systolic dysfunction and ventricular arrhythmias occur in a dose-dependent manner with a dose >450 mg/m^2 and are frequent with doses >550 mg/m^2. The development of these complications appears to be related to damage to the inner mitochondrial membrane and interference with the synthesis of adenosine triphosphate. This development is related not only to the dose of the drug but also to the presence or absence of several risk factors, which include cardiac irradiation, underlying heart disease, hypertension, and concurrent treatment with cyclophosphamide. At any dose of doxorubicin, patients with these risk factors have a greater frequency of developing HF than do patients lacking them. Doxorubicin cardiotoxicity may occur acutely but more commonly develops a median of 3 months after the last dose. In others, late contractile dysfunction may develop years after doxorubicin administration.

By measuring cardiac-specific troponin and monitoring LV function with radionuclide ventriculography or echocardiography, usually combined with exercise stress, it is possible to document preclinical deterioration of LV function and allow appropriate dose adjustments. Also, monitoring may make it possible to continue doxorubicin even in patients at high risk for developing HF. Efforts to modify the dose schedule by giving the drug more slowly, along with the selective use of potentially cardioprotective agents such as the iron-chelator dexrazoxone, have reduced the risk of cardiotoxicity. Some patients have demonstrated recovery of cardiac function with aggressive management using ACE inhibitors.

Trastuzumab (*Herceptin*), used in the treatment of breast cancer, causes cardiomyopathy in 7% of patients when used as monotherapy and four times as frequently when combined with doxorubicin. High-dose *cyclophosphamide* may produce CHF acutely or within 2 weeks of administration; a characteristic histopathologic feature is myocardial edema and hemorrhagic necrosis. LV dysfunction has also been reported with the administration of the nonreceptor tyrosine kinase inhibitor *imatinib mesylate* (Gleevec), used in the treatment of chronic myeloid leukemia.

ECG changes and arrhythmias may result from treatment with tricyclic antidepressants, the phenothiazines, emetine, lithium, and various aerosol propellants. *Cocaine abuse* is associated with a variety of life-threatening cardiac complications, including SCD, myocarditis, DCM, and acute myocardial infarction (resulting from coronary spasm and/or thrombosis with or without underlying coronary artery disease). Nitrates, calcium channel blockers, antiplatelet agents, and benzodiazepines have been used to treat cocaine-induced cardiotoxicities.

ARRHYTHMOGENIC RIGHT VENTRICULAR CARDIOMYOPATHY/DYSPLASIA (ARVCM/D)

ARVCM/D is a familial cardiomyopathy characterized by progressive fibrofatty replacement of the right ventricle and, to a much lesser degree, of the LV myocardium. It is most commonly inherited in an autosomal dominant manner and is caused by multiple mutations of several genes encoding proteins that constitute desmosomes, structures that maintain normal contacts between cells. It has been suggested that abnormalities in the desmosomes cause detachment of myocytes with consequent myocyte apoptosis and fibrofatty replacement. Among the desmosomal protein genes, the most common gene mutation occurs in plakophilin-2 (*PKP-2*). Mutations in the cardiac ryanodine receptor gene (*RyR2*) and other genes have also been described.

On clinical examination, patients may manifest RV failure with jugular venous distention, hepatomegaly, and edema. Clinical manifestations usually develop during the second decade and include ventricular tachyarrhythmias as well as varying degrees of RV failure; both of these complications may be fatal.

The ECG typically shows QRS prolongation localized to the right precordial leads and left bundle branch block–type ventricular tachycardia. CTI and CMRI typically show RV dilatation, RV aneurysm, and fatty replacement (**Fig. 21-2**).

Restriction from competitive sports and antiarrhythmic therapy with beta blockers or amiodarone may be useful. Implantation of an ICD may be required (Chap. 16). If RV failure becomes intractable, cardiac transplantation (Chap. 18) may be necessary.

TAKO-TSUBO (STRESS) CARDIOMYOPATHY

Also known as *apical ballooning syndrome*, this uncommon cardiac syndrome is characterized by the abrupt onset of severe chest discomfort preceded by a very stressful

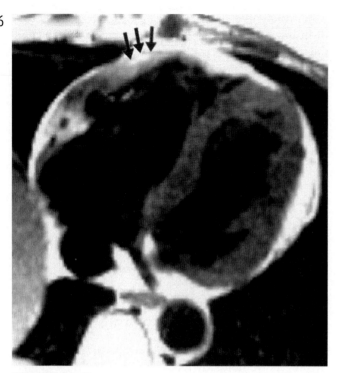

FIGURE 21-2

Cardiac MRI showing right ventricular (RV) enlargement (*left*) and fatty replacement of the RV myocardium (*black arrows*) of a patient with arrhythmogenic RV dysplasia. (*From S Sen-Chowdhry et al: Am J Med 117:685, 2004; with permission.*)

emotional or physical event. It occurs most commonly in women >50 years and is accompanied by ST-segment elevations and/or deep T-wave inversions in the precordial leads. No obstruction in the epicardial coronary arteries is noted on angiography. There is severe akinesia of the distal portion of the left ventricle with reduction of the EF. Troponins are usually mildly elevated. Cardiac imaging typically shows "ballooning" of the left ventricle in end-systole, especially of the LV apex. All of these changes, which are often quite dramatic, are reversible within 3–7 days and do not cause long-term cardiac dysfunction or disability.

The mechanism responsible for Tako-tsubo cardiomyopathy is not clear, although it is likely that an adrenergic surge that includes circulating catecholamines, acting on the epicardial coronary vessels and/or coronary microcirculation, is involved. Although beta blockers are used in therapy, there is no definitive evidence that they are beneficial.

LEFT VENTRICULAR NONCOMPACTION

Left ventricular noncompaction (LVNC) is a recently characterized uncommon congenital cardiomyopathy that may present at any age with symptoms of CHF, thromboembolism, or ventricular arrhythmias. It results from the arrest of normal embryogenesis, with the persistence of the deep recesses and sinusoids in the myocardium that characterize the embryonic heart. These sinusoids and associated spongy network of myocardial fibers ordinarily undergo organization and "compaction" early in embryonic life; when this fails to occur, LVNC results. This condition is diagnosed on echocardiography by the demonstration of multiple deep trabeculations into the myocardium, all of which communicate with the ventricular cavity, associated with LV contractile dysfunction. Standard therapy for CHF is routinely employed, typically along with chronic anticoagulation.

HYPERTROPHIC CARDIOMYOPATHY

Hypertrophic cardiomyopathy (HCM) is characterized by LV hypertrophy, typically of a nondilated chamber, without obvious cause, such as hypertension or aortic stenosis. It is found in about 1 in 500 of the general population. Two features of HCM have attracted the greatest attention: (1) asymmetric LV hypertrophy, often with preferential hypertrophy of the interventricular septum; and (2) a dynamic LV outflow tract pressure gradient, related to narrowing of the subaortic area. About one-third of patients with HCM demonstrate an outflow tract pressure gradient at rest and a similar fraction develop one with provocation. The ubiquitous pathophysiologic abnormality is *diastolic* dysfunction, which can be detected by Doppler tissue imaging and results in elevated LV end-diastolic pressures; the latter may be present despite a hyperdynamic, nondilated LV.

The pattern of hypertrophy is distinctive in HCM and usually differs from that seen in secondary hypertrophy (as in hypertension or aortic stenosis). Most patients have striking regional variations in the extent of hypertrophy in different portions of the left ventricle, and the majority demonstrate a ventricular septum whose thickness is disproportionately increased when compared with the free wall. Other patients may demonstrate symmetric hypertrophy, while others have mid-ventricular cavity obstruction or disproportionate involvement of the apex or LV free wall. In the disproportionately hypertrophied portions of the left ventricle, there is a bizarre and disorganized arrangement of myocytes, with disorganization of the myofibrillar architecture, along with a variable degree of myocardial fibrosis and thickening of the small intramural coronary arteries.

GENETIC CONSIDERATIONS

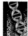 About one-half of all patients with HCM have a positive family history compatible with autosomal dominant transmission. More than 400 mutations of 11 different genes that encode sarcomeric proteins have been identified; these account for ~60% of cases. The most common are mutations of the cardiac β-myosin

heavy chain gene on chromosome 14. Others involve α-myosin heavy chains; cardiac troponins C, I, and T; cardiac myosin-binding protein C; actin; myosin light chains; and titin. Certain mutations are associated with more malignant prognoses. Many sporadic cases of HCM probably represent spontaneous mutations. Echocardiographic studies have confirmed that by the age of 20, when full expression has usually occurred, about one-half of the first-degree relatives of patients with familial HCM have evidence of the disease. However, in many of these relatives the extent of hypertrophy is mild, no outflow tract pressure gradient is present, and symptoms are not prominent. Since the hypertrophic characteristics may not be apparent in childhood, a single normal echocardiogram in a child does not exclude the presence of the disease. Screening by echocardiography of first-degree relatives between 12 and 20 years should be carried out every 12–24 months, unless the diagnosis is established or excluded by genetic testing.

Genetic Testing

Although not yet routinely available, genetic testing may allow a definitive diagnosis of HCM with a genetic cause to be established by identifying a mutation in a gene encoding a sarcomeric protein. Genetic testing can identify family members who are at risk for developing HCM and who, therefore, require echocardiographic screening and follow-up. It can also exclude the disease in family members.

CLINICAL FEATURES

The clinical course of HCM is highly variable. Many patients are asymptomatic or mildly symptomatic and may be relatives of patients with known disease. Unfortunately, the first clinical manifestation may be SCD, frequently occurring in children and young adults during or after physical exertion. Indeed, HCM is the most common cause of SCD in young competitive athletes. In symptomatic patients, the most common complaint is dyspnea, largely due to diastolic ventricular dysfunction, which impairs ventricular filling and leads to elevated LV diastolic, left atrial, and pulmonary capillary pressures. Other symptoms include syncope, angina pectoris, and fatigue. Symptoms are not closely related to the presence or severity of an outflow pressure gradient.

PHYSICAL EXAMINATION

Most patients demonstrate a double or triple apical precordial impulse and a fourth heart sound. Those with intraventricular pressure gradients may have a rapidly rising arterial pulse. The hallmark of obstructive HCM is a systolic murmur, which is typically harsh, diamond-shaped, and usually begins well after the first heart sound.

The murmur is best heard at the lower left sternal border as well as at the apex, where it is often more holosystolic and blowing in quality, no doubt due to the mitral regurgitation that usually accompanies obstructive HCM.

HEMODYNAMICS

In contrast to the obstruction produced by a fixed narrowed orifice, such as valvular aortic stenosis, the pressure gradient in HCM, when present, is dynamic and may change between examinations and even from beat to beat. Obstruction appears to result from narrowing of the LV outflow tract by systolic anterior movement (SAM) of the mitral valve against the hypertrophied septum.

Three basic mechanisms are involved in the production and intensification of the dynamic intraventricular obstruction: (1) increased LV contractility; (2) decreased ventricular preload; and (3) decreased aortic impedance and pressure (afterload). Interventions that increase myocardial contractility, such as exercise and sympathomimetic amines, and those that reduce ventricular preload, such as the strain phase of the Valsalva maneuver, sudden standing, or nitroglycerin, reduce LV end-diastolic volume and, thereby, may cause an increase in the gradient and the murmur. Conversely, elevation of arterial pressure by squatting, sustained handgrip, augmentation of venous return by passive leg raising, and expansion of the blood volume (as during pregnancy) all increase ventricular volume and ameliorate the gradient and murmur.

LABORATORY EVALUATION

The ECG commonly shows LV hypertrophy and widespread deep, broad Q waves. The latter suggest an old myocardial infarction but actually reflect severe septal hypertrophy. Many patients demonstrate arrhythmias, both atrial (supraventricular tachycardia or atrial fibrillation) and ventricular (ventricular tachycardia), during ambulatory (Holter) monitoring. *Chest roentgenography* may be normal, although a mild to moderate increase in the cardiac silhouette is common.

The mainstay of the diagnosis of HCM is the *echocardiogram*, which demonstrates LV hypertrophy, often with the septum ≥1.3 times the thickness of the posterior LV free wall. The septum may demonstrate an unusual "ground-glass" appearance, probably related to its myocardial fibrosis. SAM of the mitral valve, often accompanied by mitral regurgitation, is found in patients with pressure gradients. The LV cavity typically is small in HCM, with vigorous motion of the posterior wall but with reduced septal excursion. An uncommon form of cardiomyopathy, characterized by apical hypertrophy, is associated with giant negative T waves on the ECG and a "spade-shaped" LV cavity; it usually has a benign clinical course. CMRI is superior to echocardiography in providing accurate measurements of regional hypertrophy and in identifying sites of regional fibrosis.

Although cardiac catheterization is not required to diagnose HCM, the two typical *hemodynamic* features are an elevated LV diastolic pressure due to diminished compliance and, in some patients, a systolic pressure gradient, usually between the body of the left ventricle and the subaortic region. When a gradient is not present, it can be induced in some patients by provocative maneuvers, such as infusion of isoproterenol, inhalation of amyl nitrite, the Valsalva maneuver, or a premature ventricular contraction.

℞ Treatment: HYPERTROPHIC CARDIOMYOPATHY

Because SCD often occurs during or just after physical exertion, competitive sports and very strenuous activities should be proscribed. Dehydration should be avoided, and diuretics used with caution. β-Adrenergic blockers ameliorate angina pectoris and syncope in one-third to one-half of patients. Although resting intraventricular pressure gradients are usually unchanged, these drugs may limit the increase in the gradient that occurs during exercise. It does not appear that β-adrenergic blockers offer any protection against SCD. Amiodarone appears to be effective in reducing the frequency of supraventricular as well as of life-threatening ventricular arrhythmias, and anecdotal data suggest that it may reduce the risk of SCD. Nondihydropyridine calcium channel blockers (verapamil and diltiazem) may reduce the stiffness of the left ventricle, reduce the elevated diastolic pressures, increase exercise tolerance, and, in some instances, reduce the severity of outflow tract pressure gradients. Disopyramide has been used in some patients to reduce LV contractility and the outflow pressure gradient; it may reduce symptoms as well.

Digitalis, diuretics, nitrates, dihydropyridine calcium blockers, vasodilators, and β-adrenergic agonists are best avoided, particularly in patients with known LV outflow tract pressure gradients. Alcohol ingestion may produce sufficient vasodilatation to exacerbate an outflow pressure gradient.

Atrial fibrillation is poorly tolerated, and a strong effort should be made to restore and then maintain sinus rhythm. Slowing of the heart rate with a β-adrenergic blocker or ablation of the AV node and insertion of a pacemaker may be indicated when sinus rhythm cannot be sustained.

Surgical myotomy/myectomy of the hypertrophied septum usually abolishes intraventricular obstruction and provides lasting symptomatic improvement in about three-quarters of severely symptomatic patients with large pressure gradients who are unresponsive to medical management. Infarction of the interventricular septum induced by ethanol injections into the septal artery (alcohol septal ablation) can also reduce obstruction and improve symptoms. However, it should be carried out only by experts.

The insertion of an ICD should be considered in patients with a high-risk profile for SCD (see later).

PROGNOSIS

The natural history of HCM is variable, although many patients never exhibit any clinical manifestations. Atrial fibrillation is common late in the course of the disease; its onset often leads to the development of or an increase in symptoms. Infective endocarditis occurs in <10% of patients. However, endocarditis prophylaxis is currently recommended only in HCM patients with a prior episode of infective endocarditis. Progression of HCM to left ventricular dilatation and dysfunction (DCM) with wall thinning and disappearance of a preexisting outflow pressure gradient (so-called burnt out HCM) occurs in 5–10% of patients and may be associated with nonresponsive CHF requiring cardiac transplantation.

The major cause of mortality in HCM is SCD, which may occur in asymptomatic patients or interrupt an otherwise stable course in symptomatic ones. Patients at increased risk of SCD include those with a history of resuscitation, recurrent syncope, ventricular tachycardia on ambulatory monitoring or at electrophysiologic testing, marked ventricular hypertrophy (ventricular septal thickness >30 mm), failure of blood pressure to rise during exercise, a family history of SCD, and certain genetic mutations.

INHERITED METABOLIC CARDIOMYOPATHIES WITH LEFT VENTRICULAR HYPERTROPHY

Cardiac Danon Disease

This condition is caused by mutations in an X-linked lysosome-associated membrane protein (LAMP2). It is characterized by enlarged ventricular myocytes with periodic acid Schiff (PAS)–positive inclusions. Patients present in childhood with CHF and serious arrhythmias. The ECG shows severe LV hypertrophy and ventricular preexcitation.

Glycogen Storage Cardiomyopathy

This recently characterized condition is caused by a mutation in the γ_2 regulatory subunit (*PRKAG2*) of adenosine monophosphate–activated protein kinase (AMPK). It is characterized by ventricular hypertrophy resembling that observed in hypertrophic cardiomyopathies and enlarged myocytes with vacuoles in the myocytes that stain for glycogen.

Fabry Disease

This X-linked recessive lysosomal storage disorder is caused by deficiency of lysosomal α-galactoside A and can lead to the accumulation of glycosphingolipids in the heart, with ventricular hypertrophy resembling HCM. Because of severe impairment in ventricular filling, it is sometimes classified as a restrictive cardiomyopathy (see later). It may be associated with AV conduction abnormalities and ventricular tachyarrhythmias. CMRI is helpful in establishing the diagnosis. Treatment consists of enzyme replacement therapy with agalsidase β.

Friedreich's Ataxia

This is an autosomal recessive spinocerebellar degenerative disease caused by inadequate levels of frataxin, a protein involved in mitochondrial iron metabolism. Approximately one-half of the patients develop cardiac symptoms. The ECG most commonly demonstrates ST-segment and T-wave abnormalities. Echocardiography and other imaging studies (CTI, CMRI) usually show symmetric LV hypertrophy or asymmetric hypertrophy of the interventricular septum compared with the free wall. Although the gross morphologic appearance of the heart in Friedreich's ataxia may be similar to that in HCM (see earlier), cellular disarray is lacking.

RESTRICTIVE CARDIOMYOPATHY

The hallmark of the restrictive cardiomyopathies (RCMs) is abnormal diastolic function (Chap. 1); the ventricular walls are excessively rigid and impede ventricular filling. In late stages systolic function is also impaired. Myocardial fibrosis, hypertrophy, or infiltration due to a variety of causes is responsible. Myocardial involvement with *amyloid* is a common cause of secondary restrictive cardiomyopathy, although restriction is also seen in the transplanted heart, in hemochromatosis, glycogen deposition, endomyocardial fibrosis, sarcoidosis, hypereosinophilic disease, and scleroderma; following mediastinal irradiation; and in neoplastic infiltration and myocardial fibrosis of diverse causes. In many of these conditions, particularly those with substantial concomitant endocardial involvement, partial obliteration of the ventricular cavity by fibrous tissue and thrombus contributes to the abnormally increased resistance to ventricular filling. Thromboembolic complications are frequent in such patients.

CLINICAL FEATURES

The inability of the ventricles to fill limits cardiac output and raises filling pressures; thus, exercise intolerance and dyspnea are usually prominent. As a result of persistently elevated systemic venous pressure, these patients commonly have dependent edema, ascites, and an enlarged, tender, and often pulsatile liver. The jugular venous pressure is elevated and does not fall normally (or may rise) with inspiration (Kussmaul's sign). The heart sounds may be distant, and third and fourth heart sounds are common. In contrast to constrictive pericarditis (Chap. 22), which RCM resembles in many respects, the apex impulse is usually easily palpable, and mitral regurgitation is more common.

LABORATORY EXAMINATIONS

In patients with infiltrative cardiomyopathies, the ECG often shows low-voltage, nonspecific ST-T-wave abnormalities and various arrhythmias. Pericardial calcification on x-ray, which occurs in constrictive pericarditis, is absent. Echocardiography, CTI, and cardiac MRI typically reveal symmetrically thickened LV walls and normal or slightly reduced ventricular volumes and systolic function; the atria are usually dilated. Doppler echocardiography typically shows diastolic dysfunction. Cardiac catheterization shows a reduced cardiac output, elevation of the RV and LV end-diastolic pressures, and a dip-and-plateau configuration of the diastolic portion of the ventricular pressure pulses resembling constrictive pericarditis.

Differentiation of RCM from constrictive pericarditis (Chap. 22) is of importance because the latter is often curable by surgery. Helpful in the differentiation of these two conditions are RV transvenous endomyocardial biopsy (by revealing myocardial infiltration or fibrosis in RCM) and CTI or CMRI (by demonstrating a thickened pericardium in constrictive pericarditis but not in RCM).

℞ **Treatment:**
RESTRICTIVE CARDIOMYOPATHY

Management is usually disappointing, except for hemochromatosis (see later) and Fabry's disease (see earlier). Chronic anticoagulation is often recommended to reduce the risk of embolization from the heart.

EOSINOPHILIC ENDOMYOCARDIAL DISEASE

Also called *Loeffler's endocarditis* and *fibroplastic endocarditis*, this condition occurs in temperate climates. It appears to be a subcategory of the hypereosinophilic syndrome in which the heart is predominantly involved, with cardiac damage the apparent result of the toxic effects of eosinophilic proteins. Typically, the endocardium of either or both ventricles is thickened markedly, with involvement of the underlying myocardium. Cardiac imaging typically reveals ventricular thickening, especially of the posterobasal LV wall. Mitral regurgitation is frequently present on Doppler echocardiography. Large mural thrombi may develop in either ventricle, thereby compromising the size of the ventricular cavity and serving as a source of pulmonary and systemic emboli. Hepatosplenomegaly and localized eosinophilic infiltration of other organs are usually present. Management usually includes diuretics, afterload-reducing agents, and anticoagulation. The use of glucocorticoids and hydroxyurea appears to improve survival. Surgical treatment with resection of fibrotic tissue and mitral valve repair or replacement may be helpful in selected patients.

CARDIAC AMYLOIDOSIS

Involvement of the heart is the most frequent cause of death in *primary amyloidosis* (AL) and *hereditary amyloidosis* (ATTR), with deposition of amyloid in the cardiac interstitium. On gross pathologic examination, the heart is firm, rubbery, and noncompliant and has a waxy appearance. Clinically significant cardiac involvement is uncommon in the secondary form.

Focal deposits of amyloid in the hearts of elderly persons (*senile cardiac amyloidosis*), although common, are usually clinically insignificant.

Four clinical presentations (alone or in combination) are seen: (1) diastolic dysfunction, (2) systolic dysfunction, (3) arrhythmias and conduction disturbances, and (4) orthostatic hypotension. The two-dimensional echocardiogram may be helpful in establishing the diagnosis of amyloidosis and may show a thickened myocardial wall with a diffuse, hyperrefractile "speckled" appearance. Cardiac MRI typically shows late gadolinium enhancement of the subendocardium. Aspiration of abdominal fat or biopsy of the myocardium or other organs permits the ante mortem diagnosis to be established in over three-quarters of cases.

Chemotherapy, often with alkylating agents such as melphalan, together with glucocorticoids, appears to have improved survival in individual cases. Heart transplantation (often combined with bone marrow transplantation or liver or kidney transplantation for hereditary amyloidosis) may help selected patients. However, the overall prognosis is poor, especially in the primary form with advanced cardiac involvement.

OTHER RESTRICTIVE CARDIOMYOPATHIES

Iron-overload cardiomyopathy (hemochromatosis) is often the result of multiple transfusions or a hemoglobinopathy, most frequently β-thalassemia; the familial (autosomal recessive) form should be suspected if cardiomyopathy occurs in the presence of diabetes mellitus, hepatic

cirrhosis, and increased skin pigmentation. The diagnosis may be confirmed by endomyocardial biopsy. Cardiac MRI shows a reduced $T2^*$ signal as iron levels rise. Phlebotomy may be of some benefit if employed early in the course of the disease. Continuous subcutaneous administration of deferoxamine or other iron chelators may reduce body iron stores and result in clinical improvement.

Myocardial *sarcoidosis* is generally associated with other manifestations of systemic disease. It may cause restrictive as well as congestive features, since cardiac infiltration by sarcoid granulomas results not only in increased stiffness of the myocardium but also in diminished systolic contractile function. A variety of arrhythmias, including high-grade AV block, have been noted. A common cardiac manifestation of systemic sarcoidosis is RV overload due to pulmonary hypertension as a result of parenchymal pulmonary involvement. Many patients are treated empirically with glucocorticoids.

The *carcinoid syndrome* (Chap. 20) results in endocardial fibrosis and stenosis and/or regurgitation of the tricuspid and/or pulmonary valve; morphologically similar lesions have been seen with the use of the anorexic agents fenfluramine and phentermine.

MYOCARDITIS

Myocarditis, i.e., cardiac inflammation, is most commonly the result of an infectious process, frequently complicated by autoimmunity. Myocarditis may also result from hypersensitivity to drugs (most commonly tricyclic antidepressants, antibiotics, and antipsychotics) or it may be caused by irradiation, chemicals, or physical agents. While almost every infective agent is capable of producing myocarditis (Table 21-1), clinically significant acute myocarditis in the United States is caused most commonly by viruses, especially Coxsackievirus B, adenovirus, hepatitis C virus, and HIV. Symptomatic viral myocarditis may be secondary to continued viral replication and/or autoimmune activation following viral infection.

CLINICAL FEATURES

Patients with viral myocarditis may give a history of a preceding upper respiratory febrile illness or a flulike syndrome, and viral nasopharyngitis or tonsillitis may be evident. The clinical spectrum ranges from an asymptomatic state, with the presence of myocarditis inferred only by the finding of transient electrocardiographic ST-T-wave abnormalities, to a fulminant condition with arrhythmias, acute CHF, and early death. In some patients, myocarditis simulates an acute coronary syndrome (Chap. 34), with chest pain, ECG changes, and elevated serum levels of troponin, but it typically occurs in patients younger than those with coronary atherosclerosis.

The *physical examination* is often normal, although more severe cases may show a muffled first heart sound, along with a third heart sound and a murmur of mitral regurgitation. A pericardial friction rub may be audible in patients with associated pericarditis. The isolation of virus from the stool, pharyngeal washings, or other body fluids and changes in specific antibody titers may be helpful clinically. Endomyocardial biopsy, carried out early in the illness, may show round-cell infiltration and necrosis of adjacent myocytes. CMRI frequently exhibits contrast enhancement (Chap. 12) and is valuable in identifying sites likely to exhibit typical histologic changes on biopsy, as well as in monitoring the activity of the disease.

Although viral myocarditis is most often self-limited and without sequelae, severe involvement may recur. Acute viral myocarditis, especially when accompanied by severe LV dysfunction (LVEF <35%), may progress to a chronic form and to DCM.

R℞ Treatment:
MYOCARDITIS

Exercise may be deleterious in patients with acute myocarditis, and strenuous activity should be proscribed until the ECG and LV function have returned to normal. Patients who develop CHF should be treated with the usual measures (Chap. 17). Arrhythmias are common and are occasionally difficult to manage. Deaths attributed to CHF, tachyarrhythmias, and AV block have been reported; the ECG should be monitored during the acute illness and in patients with arrhythmias.

Patients with fulminant myocarditis may require mechanical cardiopulmonary support or cardiac transplantation; however, the majority of these patients survive, and many demonstrate substantial recovery of LV function.

MYOCARDITIS IN PATIENTS WITH HIV

Many HIV-infected patients have subclinical cardiac involvement, including pericardial effusion, right-sided chamber enlargement, arrhythmias, and neoplastic involvement. Overt clinical manifestations are seen in 10% of HIV patients. The most common finding is LV dysfunction that in some cases appears to be due to infection of the myocardium by the virus itself. In other patients, the heart is affected by one of the various opportunistic infections common in HIV-AIDS, such as toxoplasmosis; by cardiac involvement by neoplastic disorders; or by toxicity from anti-HIV drugs. CHF in HIV myocarditis may respond, at least transiently, to standard anti-HIV therapy.

BACTERIAL MYOCARDITIS

Bacterial involvement of the heart is uncommon, but when it does occur, it is usually as a complication of infective endocarditis (Chap. 25) in which abscess formation involves the valve rings and interventricular septum.

Diphtheritic myocarditis develops in over one-quarter of patients with diphtheria; it is one of the more serious complications and the most common cause of death in this infection. Cardiac damage is due to the liberation of a toxin that inhibits protein synthesis and leads to a dilated, flabby, hypocontractile heart. The conduction system is frequently involved, as well. Cardiomegaly and severe CHF typically appear after the first week of illness. Prompt therapy with antitoxin is critical; antibiotic therapy is also indicated but is of less urgency.

GIANT CELL MYOCARDITIS

This rare myocarditis of unknown cause is characterized by rapidly progressive CHF and ventricular tachyarrhythmia and occurs most commonly in the third or fourth decades; approximately two-thirds of patients die within 1 year. At necropsy, the distinctive features include cardiac enlargement, ventricular thrombi, grossly visible serpiginous areas of necrosis in both ventricles, and microscopic evidence of giant cells within an extensive inflammatory infiltrate. The etiology of giant cell myocarditis has not been identified, although an autoimmune cause appears to be likely. While treatment with immunosuppressive therapy may help some patients, cardiac transplantation is often necessary.

LYME CARDITIS

Lyme disease is caused by a tick-borne spirochete and is most common in the Northeast, upper Midwest, and Pacific Coastal regions of the United States during the summer months. About 10% of patients develop symptomatic cardiac involvement during the acute phase of the disease. AV conduction abnormalities are the most common manifestations of involvement and may lead to syncope. Concomitant myopericarditis is not uncommon, and mild, asymptomatic LV dysfunction may occur.

Intravenous ceftriaxone or penicillin is indicated in all but the mildest forms of Lyme carditis, in which case oral amoxicillin or doxycycline is employed. Hospitalization with ECG monitoring is indicated in patients with second- or third-degree AV block. A temporary pacemaker may be needed for symptomatic AV block, but permanent pacing is rarely required. Although glucocorticoids are often given, their effectiveness in reversing AV block is uncertain. Long-term cardiac manifestations of Lyme disease are uncommon.

Chagas Heart Disease

(See also Chap. 27) Chagas disease, caused by the protozoan *Trypanosoma cruzi* and transmitted by an insect vector, the reduviid bug, produces an extensive myocarditis that typically becomes evident years after the initial infection. It is one of the more common causes of heart disease encountered in Central and South America; in rural endemic areas, 20–75% of the population may be affected. It has been estimated that ~18 million persons are affected, with 200,000 new cases each year. An increasing number of cases are found in the United States as patients migrate from endemic areas; in rare cases, it has been transmitted by transfusion and organ donation.

About 1% of infected individuals have an acute illness, which may include acute myocarditis that usually resolves in 2–3 months. After a quiescent, asymptomatic period, the so-called *indeterminate phase*, approximately one-third of infected persons develop chronic myocardial damage. A combination of infection by the parasite as well as autoimmune reactions are responsible for the cardiac manifestations. Cardiac involvement in chronic Chagasic heart disease varies widely, from asymptomatic to severe cardiac failure involving the left ventricle, and sometimes the right ventricle, and/or AV block. This condition, which is more frequent in males, is characterized by dilatation of several cardiac chambers, fibrosis and thinning of the ventricular wall, aneurysm formation in the left ventricle (**Fig. 21-3**), and mural thrombi.

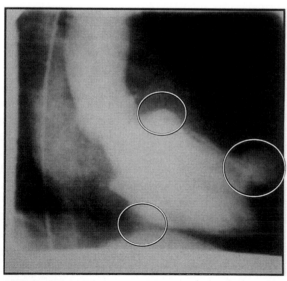

FIGURE 21-3

Left ventriculogram of a 55-year-old woman with chronic Chagas disease. Multiple left ventricular aneurysms are noted in inferobasal, anterior, and inferior aspects of left ventricle (circled). *(From P Venegoni, HS Bhatia: Circulation 96:1363, 1997.)*

Survival is poor in patients who develop overt CHF. The cause of death is either intractable CHF or SCD secondary to an arrhythmia, with a minority of patients dying from embolic phenomena.

The ECG is abnormal in most patients and typically shows low voltage, along with right bundle branch block and left anterior hemiblock, and may progress to complete AV block. The chest roentgenogram may show LV enlargement. Echocardiography may reveal hypokinesis of the posterior LV wall and relatively preserved septal motion. Ventricular arrhythmias are common and are seen on Holter monitoring, especially during and after exertion.

> ℞ **Treatment:**
> **CHAGAS HEART DISEASE**
>
> Therapy is directed toward amelioration of the CHF and ventricular tachyarrhythmias; oral amiodarone appears to be particularly effective in treating the latter. Progressive conduction system disease and AV block may require implantation of a pacemaker. Anticoagulation reduces the risk of thromboembolism. Medical therapy is often unsatisfactory or unavailable (especially in poor rural areas); however, a more promising tactic in endemic areas is the use of insecticides to eliminate the vector.

CARDIOMYOPATHY IN AFRICA

Endomyocardial Fibrosis

This is a progressive disease that presents as a RCM. It occurs most commonly in children and young adults residing in tropical and subtropical Africa, particularly Uganda and Nigeria, as well as in tropical Asia and South America. It is related and similar to hypereosinophilic endomyocardial disease (see earlier), although the eosinophilia is less severe and the course more chronic in endomyocardial fibrosis. Endomyocardial fibrosis is a frequent cause of CHF in Africa, accounting for up to one-quarter of deaths due to heart disease. The condition is characterized by severe fibrosis of the endocardium, with involvement of the inflow portion of the right or left ventricle (or both). Endomyocardial fibrosis often involves the AV valves, producing valvular regurgitation. The apex of the ventricles may be obliterated by a mass of thrombus and fibrous tissue.

The clinical picture depends on which ventricle and AV valve shows predominant involvement; left-sided involvement results in symptoms of pulmonary congestion, whereas predominant right-sided disease presents features of systemic venous congestion. Medical treatment is often disappointing, and surgical excision of the fibrotic endocardium and replacement of the involved

AV valve have led to substantial symptomatic improvement in some patients.

Dilated Cardiomyopathy

DCM is a common cause of heart failure in Africa and has been reported in up to one-half of patients hospitalized with CHF. The etiology of DCM in Africa is multifactorial. Infection with *Toxoplasma gondii* and *Coxsackievirus B* has been reported to be common in DCM patients in Nigeria, whereas *African trypanosomiasis* appears to be a common cause in Cameroon. Excess alcohol ingestion is considered to be causal or an important contributory factor in almost one-half of cases of DCM; severe thiamine deficiency may be present in some of these patients as well.

Peripartum cardiomyopathy is far more common in Africa than in North America or Europe; the incidence has been reported to be especially high in Nigeria. Pathogenetic factors that may be operative include low socioeconomic status, high parity, prolonged lactation, excessive dietary salt intake, and selenium deficiency.

CARDIOMYOPATHY IN ASIA

Thiamine (vitamin B_1) deficiency occurs in Asian countries, especially China, where polished rice, deficient in thiamine, is a major component of the diet and flour is not enriched with thiamine, as it is in the West. However, thiamine deficiency in the West may occur in patients with severe alcoholism.

So-called *wet beri-beri heart disease* is an important clinical manifestation of serious thiamine deficiency. It is characterized by cardiac failure secondary to a high cardiac output state caused by arteriolar vasodilation; it is associated with tachycardia, wide pulse pressure, a third heart sound, and warm extremities. ECG findings include reduced voltage, diffuse T-wave abnormalities and prolongation of the QT interval. On chest x-ray, the heart appears diffusely enlarged with pulmonary congestion. The response to thiamine is usually dramatic, but it should be accompanied by diuretics.

Selenium deficiency is also most common in China. It may cause *Keshan's disease*, a dilated cardiomyopathy with cardiomegaly, ventricular arrhythmias, and heart failure.

FURTHER READINGS

BAUGHMAN KL et al: *Braunwald's Heart Disease*. Elsevier, Philadelphia, Pennsylvania, 2005

CORRADO D, THIENE G: Arrhythmogenic right ventricular cardiomyopathy/dysplasia: Clinical impact of molecular genetic studies. Circulation 113:1634, 2006

DUTRA WO et al: The clinical immunology of human Chagas disease. Trends Parasitol 21:581, 2005

FALK RH: Diagnosis and management of the cardiac amyloidoses. Circulation 112:2047, 2005

HO CY, SEIDMAN CE: A contemporary approach to hypertrophic cardiomyopathy. Circulation 113:e858, 2006

HUNT SA et al: ACC/AHA 2005 Guideline Update for the Diagnosis and Management of Chronic Heart Failure in the Adult. Circulation 112:e154, 2005

LUCAS DL et al: Alcohol and the cardiovascular system. J Am Coll Cardiol 45:1916, 2005

MAGNANI JW, DEC GW: Myocarditis: Current trends in diagnosis and treatment. Circulation 113:876, 2006

MARON BJ et al: American College of Cardiology/European Society of Cardiology Clinical Expert Consensus Document on Hypertrophic Cardiomyopathy. J Am Coll Cardiol 42:1688, 2003

——— et al: Contemporary definitions and classification of the cardiomyopathies: An American Heart Association Scientific Statement. Circulation 113:1807, 2006

MCCROHON JA et al: Differentiation of heart failure related to dilated cardiomyopathy and coronary artery disease using gadolinium-enhanced cardiovascular magnetic resonance. Circulation 108:54, 2003

RASSI A JR et al: Development and validation of a risk score for predicting death in Chagas' heart disease. N Engl J Med 355:799, 2006

——— et al: Challenges and opportunities for primary, secondary, and tertiary prevention of Chagas' disease. Heart 95:524, 2009

SEIDMAN CE et al: Genetic factors in myocardial disease, in *Braunwald's Heart Disease*, 8th ed, P Libby et al (eds). Philadelphia, Saunders, 2008

SLIWA K et al: Epidemiology and etiology of cardiomyopathy in Africa. Circulation 112:3577, 2005

——— et al: Peripartum cardiomyopathy. Lancet 368:687, 2006

SUDANO I et al: Cardiovascular disease in HIV infection. Am Heart J 151:1147, 2006

TOWBIN JA and VATTA M: Genetics and genomics of dilated cardiomyopathy. In D Roden (ed). *Cardiovascular Genetics and Genomics*. American Heart Association Clinical Series. Wiley Blackwell; Oxford England 118—135, 2009

WEIFORD BC et al: Noncompaction of the ventricular myocardium. Circulation 109:2965, 2004

YEH ET, BICKFORD CL: Cardiovascular complications of cancer therapy: incidence, pathogenesis, diagnosis, and management. J Am Coll Cardiol, 53:2231, 2009.

CHAPTER 22

PERICARDIAL DISEASE

Eugene Braunwald

NORMAL FUNCTIONS OF THE PERICARDIUM

The normal pericardium is a double-layered sac; the visceral pericardium is a serous membrane that is separated by a small quantity (15–50 mL) of fluid, an ultrafiltrate of plasma, from the fibrous parietal pericardium. The normal pericardium, by exerting a restraining force, prevents sudden dilation of the cardiac chambers, especially of the right atrium and ventricle, during exercise and with hypervolemia. It also restricts the anatomic position of the heart, minimizes friction between the heart and surrounding structures, prevents displacement of the heart and kinking of the great vessels, and probably retards the spread of infections from the lungs and pleural cavities to the heart. Notwithstanding the foregoing, total absence of the pericardium, either congenital or following surgery, does not produce obvious clinical disease. In partial left pericardial defects, the main pulmonary artery and left atrium may bulge through the defect; very rarely, herniation and subsequent strangulation of the left atrium may cause sudden death.

ACUTE PERICARDITIS

Acute pericarditis, by far the most common pathologic process involving the pericardium, may be classified both clinically and etiologically (Table 22-1). Pain, a pericardial friction rub, electrocardiographic changes, and pericardial effusion with cardiac tamponade and paradoxical pulse are cardinal manifestations of many forms of acute pericarditis.

Chest pain is an important but not invariable symptom in various forms of acute pericarditis (Chap. 4); it is usually present in the acute infectious types and in many of the forms presumed to be related to hypersensitivity or autoimmunity. Pain is often absent in slowly developing tuberculous, postirradiation, neoplastic, or uremic pericarditis. The pain of acute pericarditis is often severe, retrosternal and left precordial, and referred to the neck, arms, or the left shoulder. Often the pain is pleuritic, consequent to accompanying pleural inflammation, i.e., sharp and aggravated by inspiration, coughing, and changes in body position, but sometimes it is a steady, constricting pain that radiates into either arm or both arms and resembles that of myocardial ischemia; therefore, confusion with acute myocardial infarction (AMI) is common. Characteristically, however, pericardial pain may be relieved by sitting up and leaning forward and is intensified by lying supine. The differentiation of AMI from acute pericarditis becomes perplexing when, with acute pericarditis, serum biomarkers of myocardial damage such as creatine kinase and troponin rise, presumably because of concomitant involvement of the epicardium in the inflammatory process (an epi-myocarditis) with resulting myocyte necrosis. However, these elevations, if they occur, are quite modest, given the extensive electrocardiographic ST-segment elevation in pericarditis.

TABLE 22-1

CLASSIFICATION OF PERICARDITIS

Clinical Classification

I. Acute pericarditis (<6 weeks)
  a. Fibrinous
  b. Effusive (serous or sanguineous)
II. Subacute pericarditis (6 weeks to 6 months)
  a. Effusive-constrictive
  b. Constrictive
III. Chronic pericarditis (>6 months)
  a. Constrictive
  b. Effusive
  c. Adhesive (nonconstrictive)

Etiologic Classification

I. Infectious pericarditis
  a. Viral (coxsackievirus A and B, echovirus, mumps, adenovirus, hepatitis, HIV)
  b. Pyogenic (pneumococcus, streptococcus, staphylococcus, *Neisseria, Legionella*)
  c. Tuberculous
  d. Fungal (histoplasmosis, coccidioidomycosis, *Candida*, blastomycosis)
  e. Other infections (syphilitic, protozoal, parasitic)
II. Noninfectious pericarditis
  a. Acute myocardial infarction
  b. Uremia
  c. Neoplasia
    1. Primary tumors (benign or malignant, mesothelioma)
    2. Tumors metastatic to pericardium (lung and breast cancer, lymphoma, leukemia)
  d. Myxedema
  e. Cholesterol
  f. Chylopericardium
  g. Trauma
    1. Penetrating chest wall
    2. Nonpenetrating
  h. Aortic dissection (with leakage into pericardial sac)
  i. Postirradiation
  j. Familial Mediterranean fever
  k. Familial pericarditis
    1. Mulibrey nanism[a]
  l. Acute idiopathic
  m. Whipple's disease
  n. Sarcoidosis
III. Pericarditis presumably related to hypersensitivity or autoimmunity
  a. Rheumatic fever
  b. Collagen vascular disease (SLE, rheumatoid arthritis, ankylosing spondylitis, scleroderma, acute rheumatic fever, Wegener's granulomatosis)
  c. Drug-induced (e.g., procainamide, hydralazine, phenytoin, isoniazide, minoxidil, anticoagulants, methysergide)
  d. Post-cardiac injury
    1. Postmyocardial infarction (Dressler's syndrome)
    2. Postpericardiotomy
    3. Posttraumatic

[a]An autosomal recessive syndrome, characterized by growth failure, muscle hypotonia, hepatomegaly, ocular changes, enlarged cerebral ventricles, mental retardation, ventricular hypertrophy, and chronic constrictive pericarditis.

This dissociation is useful in the differentiation between these conditions.

The *pericardial friction rub,* audible in about 85% of patients, may have up to three components per cardiac cycle, is high-pitched, and is described as rasping, scratching, or grating (Chap. 9); it can be elicited sometimes only when the diaphragm of the stethoscope is applied firmly to the chest wall at the left lower sternal border. It is heard most frequently at end-expiration with the patient upright and leaning forward. The rub is often inconstant, and the loud to-and-fro leathery sound may disappear within a few hours, possibly to reappear on the following day. A pericardial rub is heard throughout the respiratory cycle, while a pleural rub disappears when respiration is suspended.

The *electrocardiogram* (ECG) in acute pericarditis without massive effusion usually displays changes secondary to acute subepicardial inflammation (**Fig. 22-1**). It typically evolves through four stages. In stage 1, there is widespread elevation of the ST segments, often with upward concavity, involving two or three standard limb leads and V_2 to V_6, with reciprocal depressions only in aVR and sometimes V_1, as well as PR-segment depression. Usually there are no significant changes in QRS complexes. In stage 2, after several days, the ST segments return to normal, and only then, or even later, do the T waves become inverted (stage 3). Ultimately, weeks or months after the onset of acute pericarditis, the ECG returns to normal in stage 4. In contrast, in AMI, ST elevations are convex, and reciprocal depression is usually more prominent; QRS changes occur, particularly the development of Q waves, as well as notching and loss of R-wave amplitude; and T-wave inversions are usually seen within hours *before* the ST segments have become isoelectric. Sequential ECGs are useful in distinguishing acute pericarditis from AMI. In the latter, elevated ST segments return to normal within hours.

Early repolarization is a normal variant and may also be associated with widespread ST-segment elevation, most prominent in left precordial leads. However, in this condition the T waves are usually tall and the ST/T ratio is <0.25; importantly, this ratio is higher in acute pericarditis. Depression of the PR segment (below the TP segment) is also common and reflects atrial involvement.

PERICARDIAL EFFUSION

In acute pericarditis, effusion is usually associated with pain and/or the above-mentioned ECG changes, as well as with an enlargement of the cardiac silhouette. Pericardial effusion is especially important clinically when it develops within a relatively short time as it may lead to cardiac tamponade (see later). Differentiation from cardiac enlargement may be difficult on physical examination, but heart sounds may be fainter with pericardial

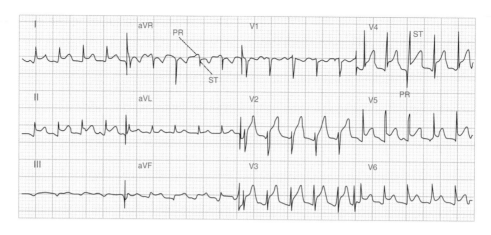

FIGURE 22-1

Acute pericarditis often produces diffuse ST-segment elevations (in this case in leads I, II, aVF, and V_2–V_6) due to a ventricular current of injury. Note also the characteristic PR-segment deviation (opposite in polarity to the ST segment) due to a concomitant atrial injury current.

effusion. The friction rub may disappear, and the apex impulse may vanish, but sometimes it remains palpable, albeit medial to the left border of cardiac dullness. The base of the left lung may be compressed by pericardial fluid, producing *Ewart's sign*, a patch of dullness and increased fremitus (and egophony) beneath the angle of the left scapula. The chest roentgenogram may show a "water bottle" configuration of the cardiac silhouette (Fig. 22-2) but may also be normal.

Diagnosis

Echocardiography (Chap. 12) is the most effective imaging technique available since it is sensitive, specific, simple, noninvasive, may be performed at the bedside, and can identify accompanying cardiac tamponade (see later) (Fig. 22-3). The presence of pericardial fluid is recorded

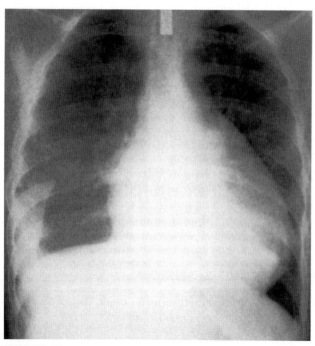

FIGURE 22-2

Chest radiogram from a patient with a pericardial effusion showing typical "water bottle" heart. There is also a right pleural effusion. *[From SS Kabbani, M LeWinter, in MH Crawford et al (eds): Cardiology. London, Mosby, 2001.]*

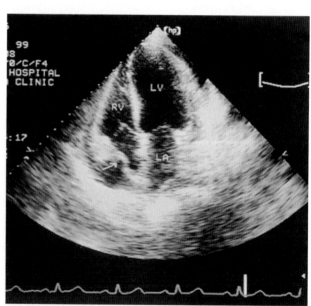

FIGURE 22-3

Apical four-chamber echocardiogram recorded in a patient with a moderate pericardial effusion and evidence of hemodynamic compromise. The frame is recorded in early ventricular systole, immediately after atrial contraction. Note that the right atrial wall is indented inward and its curvature is frankly reversed (*arrow*), implying elevated intrapericardial pressure above right atrial pressure. LA, left atrium; LV, left ventricle; RV, right ventricle. *[From WF Armstrong: Echocardiography, in DP Zipes et al (eds): Braunwald's Heart Disease, 7th ed. Philadelphia, Elsevier, 2005.]*

by two-dimensional transthoracic echocardiography as a relatively echo-free space between the posterior pericardium and left ventricular epicardium in patients with small effusions, and as a space between the anterior right ventricle and the parietal pericardium just beneath the anterior chest wall in those with larger effusions. In the latter the heart may swing freely within the pericardial sac. When severe, the extent of this motion alternates and may be associated with electrical alternans. Echocardiography allows localization and estimation of the quantity of pericardial fluid.

The diagnosis of pericardial fluid or thickening may be confirmed by a CT or MRI (**Fig. 22-4**). These techniques may be superior to echocardiography in detecting loculated pericardial effusions, pericardial thickening, and the presence of pericardial masses.

CARDIAC TAMPONADE

The accumulation of fluid in the pericardial space in a quantity sufficient to cause serious obstruction to the inflow of blood to the ventricles results in cardiac tamponade. This complication may be fatal if it is not recognized and treated promptly. The three most common causes of tamponade are neoplastic disease, idiopathic pericarditis, and pericardial effusion secondary to renal failure.

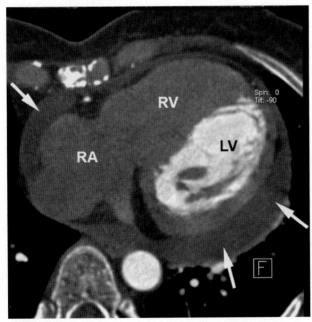

FIGURE 22-4
Chronic pericardial effusion in a 54-year-old female patient with Hodgkin's disease seen in contrast-enhanced 64-slice CT. The arrows point at the pericardial effusion (LV, left ventricle; RV, right ventricle; RA, right atrium). Due to the timing of the scan relative to contrast injection, only the blood in the left ventricle is contrast-enhanced, hence the low attenuation in the right-sided chambers. (*Courtesy of Stephan Achenbach, MD; with permission.*)

Tamponade may also result from bleeding into the pericardial space either following cardiac operations and trauma (including cardiac perforation during cardiac catheterization, percutaneous coronary intervention, or insertion of pacemaker wires) or from tuberculosis and hemopericardium. The latter may occur when a patient with any form of acute pericarditis is treated with anticoagulants.

The three principal features of tamponade (*Beck's triad*) are hypotension, soft or absent heart sounds, and jugular venous distention with a prominent *x* descent but an absent *y* descent. There are both limitation of ventricular filling and reduction of cardiac output. The quantity of fluid necessary to produce this critical state may be as little as 200 mL when the fluid develops rapidly or >2000 mL in slowly developing effusions when the pericardium has had the opportunity to stretch and adapt to an increasing volume. The volume of fluid required to produce tamponade also varies directly with the thickness of the ventricular myocardium and inversely with the thickness of the parietal pericardium.

Tamponade may also develop more slowly, and under these circumstances the clinical manifestations may resemble those of heart failure, including dyspnea, orthopnea, and hepatic engorgement. A high index of suspicion for cardiac tamponade is required since, in many instances, no obvious cause for pericardial disease is apparent, and it should be considered in any patient with hypotension and elevation of jugular venous pressure. Otherwise unexplained enlargement of the cardiac silhouette (especially in subacute or chronic tamponade), reduction in amplitude of the QRS complexes, and *electrical alternans* of the P, QRS, or T waves each should raise the suspicion of cardiac tamponade.

Table 22-2 lists the features that distinguish acute cardiac tamponade from constrictive pericarditis.

Paradoxical Pulse

This important clue to the presence of cardiac tamponade consists of a greater than normal (10 mmHg) inspiratory decline in systolic arterial pressure. When severe, it may be detected by palpating weakness or disappearance of the arterial pulse during inspiration, but usually sphygmomanometric measurement of systolic pressure during slow respiration is required.

Since both ventricles share a tight incompressible covering, i.e., the pericardial sac, the inspiratory enlargement of the right ventricle in cardiac tamponade compresses and reduces left ventricular volume; leftward bulging of the interventricular septum further reduces the left ventricular cavity as the right ventricle enlarges during inspiration. Thus, in cardiac tamponade the normal inspiratory augmentation of right ventricular volume causes an exaggerated reciprocal reduction in left ventricular volume. Also, respiratory distress increases the fluctuations in intrathoracic pressure, which exaggerates the

TABLE 22-2

FEATURES THAT DISTINGUISH CARDIAC TAMPONADE FROM CONSTRICTIVE PERICARDITIS AND SIMILAR CLINICAL DISORDERS

CHARACTERISTIC	TAMPONADE	CONSTRICTIVE PERICARDITIS	RESTRICTIVE CARDIOMYOPATHY	RVMI
Clinical				
Pulsus paradoxus	Common	Usually absent	Rare	Rare
Jugular veins				
Prominent y descent	Absent	Usually present	Rare	Rare
Prominent x descent	Present	Usually present	Present	Rare
Kussmaul's sign	Absent	Present	Absent	Present
Third heart sound	Absent	Absent	Rare	May be present
Pericardial knock	Absent	Often present	Absent	Absent
Electrocardiogram				
Low ECG voltage	May be present	May be present	May be present	Absent
Electrical alternans	May be present	Absent	Absent	Absent
Echocardiography				
Thickened pericardium	Absent	Present	Absent	Absent
Pericardial calcification	Absent	Often present	Absent	Absent
Pericardial effusion	Present	Absent	Absent	Absent
RV size	Usually small	Usually normal	Usually normal	Enlarged
Myocardial thickness	Normal	Normal	Usually increased	Normal
Right atrial collapse and RVDC	Present	Absent	Absent	Absent
Increased early filling, ↑ mitral flow velocity	Absent	Present	Present	May be present
Exaggerated respiratory variation in flow velocity	Present	Present	Absent	Absent
CT/MRI				
Thickened/calcific pericardium	Absent	Present	Absent	Absent
Cardiac catheterization				
Equalization of diastolic pressures	Usually present	Usually present	Usually absent	Absent or present
Cardiac biopsy helpful?	No	No	Sometimes	No

Note: RV, right ventricle; RVMI, right ventricular myocardial infarction; RVDC, right ventricular diastolic collapse; ECG, electrocardiograph.
Source: From GM Brockington et al, Cardiol Clin 8:645, 1990, with permission.

mechanism just described. Right ventricular infarction (Chap. 35) may resemble cardiac tamponade with hypotension, elevated jugular venous pressure, an absent y descent in the jugular venous pulse, and, occasionally, pulsus paradoxus. The differences between these two conditions are shown in Table 22-2.

Paradoxical pulse occurs not only in cardiac tamponade but also in approximately one-third of patients with constrictive pericarditis (see later). This physical finding is not pathognomonic of pericardial disease because it may be observed in some cases of hypovolemic shock, acute and chronic obstructive airways disease, and pulmonary embolus.

Low-pressure tamponade refers to mild tamponade in which the intrapericardial pressure is increased from its slightly subatmospheric levels from +5 to +10 mmHg; in some instances, hypovolemia coexists. As a consequence, the central venous pressure is normal or only slightly elevated, while arterial pressure is unaffected and there is no paradoxical pulse. The patients are asymptomatic or complain of mild weakness and dyspnea. The diagnosis is aided by echocardiography, and both hemodynamic and clinical manifestations improve following pericardiocentesis.

Diagnosis

Since immediate treatment of cardiac tamponade may be lifesaving, prompt measures to establish the diagnosis by echocardiography should be undertaken (Fig. 22-2). When pericardial effusion causes tamponade, Doppler ultrasound shows that tricuspid and pulmonic valve flow velocities increase markedly during inspiration, while pulmonic vein, mitral, and aortic flow velocities diminish. Often the right ventricular cavity is reduced in diameter, and there is late diastolic inward motion (collapse) of the right ventricular free wall and of the right atrium. Transesophageal echocardiography may be necessary to diagnose a loculated or hemorrhagic effusion responsible for cardiac tamponade.

℞ Treatment: CARDIAC TAMPONADE

Patients with acute pericarditis should be observed frequently for the development of an effusion; if a large effusion is present, the patient should be hospitalized and watched closely for signs of tamponade. Arterial and venous pressures and heart rate should be monitored or followed carefully and serial echocardiograms obtained.

PERICARDIOCENTESIS If manifestations of tamponade appear, echocardiographically guided pericardiocentesis using an apical, parasternal, or, most commonly, a subxiphoid approach must be carried out at once as reduction of the elevated intrapericardial pressure may be lifesaving. Intravenous saline may be administered as the patient is being readied for the procedure. Intrapericardial pressure should be measured before fluid is withdrawn, and the pericardial cavity should be drained as completely as possible. A small, multiholed catheter advanced over the needle inserted into the pericardial cavity may be left in place to allow draining of the pericardial space if fluid reaccumulates. Surgical drainage through a limited (subxiphoid) thoracotomy may be required in recurrent tamponade, when it is necessary to remove loculated effusions, and/or when it is necessary to obtain tissue for diagnosis.

Pericardial fluid obtained from an effusion often has the physical characteristics of an exudate. Bloody fluid is most commonly due to neoplasm in the United States and tuberculosis in developing nations but may also be found in the effusion of rheumatic fever, post-cardiac injury, and post-myocardial infarction, as well as in the pericarditis associated with renal failure or dialysis. Transudative pericardial effusions may occur in heart failure.

The pericardial fluid should be analyzed for red and white blood cells, and cytologic studies for cancer, microscopic studies, and cultures should be obtained. The presence of DNA of *Mycobacterium tuberculosis* determined by polymerase chain reaction or an elevated adenosine deaminase activity (>30 U/L) strongly supports the diagnosis of tuberculous pericarditis.

VIRAL OR IDIOPATHIC FORM OF ACUTE PERICARDITIS

In some cases of this common disorder, coxsackievirus A or B or the virus of influenza, echovirus, mumps, herpes simplex, chickenpox, adenovirus, cytomegalovirus, Epstein-Barr virus, or HIV has been isolated from pericardial fluid and/or appropriate elevations in viral antibody titers have been noted. In many instances, acute pericarditis occurs in association with illnesses of known viral origin and, presumably, are caused by the same agent. Commonly, there is an antecedent infection of the respiratory tract, but in many patients such an association is not evident, and viral isolation and serologic studies are negative. Pericardial effusion is a common cardiac manifestation of HIV; it is usually secondary to infection (often mycobacterial) or neoplasm, most frequently lymphoma. In full-blown AIDS, pericardial effusion is associated with a shortened survival.

Most frequently, a viral causation cannot be established; the term *idiopathic acute pericarditis* is then appropriate. Viral or idiopathic acute pericarditis occurs at all ages but is more frequent in young adults, and is often associated with pleural effusions and pneumonitis. The almost simultaneous development of fever and precordial pain, often 10–12 days after a presumed viral illness, constitutes an important feature in the differentiation of acute pericarditis from AMI, in which pain precedes fever. The constitutional symptoms are usually mild to moderate, and a pericardial friction rub is often audible. The disease ordinarily runs its course in a few days to 4 weeks. The ST-segment alterations in the ECG usually disappear after 1 or more weeks, but the abnormal T waves may persist for several years and be a source of confusion in persons without a clear history of pericarditis.

Pleuritis and pneumonitis frequently accompany pericarditis. Accumulation of some pericardial fluid is common, and both tamponade and constrictive pericarditis are possible complications. Recurrent (relapsing) pericarditis occurs in about one-fourth of patients with acute idiopathic pericarditis. In a smaller number, there are multiple recurrences.

℞ Treatment: IDIOPATHIC ACUTE PERICARDITIS

Hyperimmune globulin has been reported to be beneficial in cytomegalovirus, adenovirus, and parvovirus pericarditis, while interferon α has been reported to be so in coxsackie B pericarditis. In acute idiopathic pericarditis there is no specific therapy, but bed rest and anti-inflammatory treatment with aspirin (2–4 g/d) may be given. If this is ineffective, one of the nonsteroidal anti-inflammatory drugs (NSAIDs), such as ibuprofen (400–800 mg qid) or colchicine (0.6 mg bid), is often effective. Glucocorticoids (e.g., prednisone, 40–80 mg daily) usually suppress the clinical manifestations of the acute illness and may be useful in patients in whom purulent bacterial pericarditis has been excluded and in patients with pericarditis secondary to connective tissue disorders and renal failure (see later). Anticoagulants should be avoided since their use could cause bleeding into the pericardial cavity and tamponade.

After the patient has been asymptomatic and afebrile for about a week, the dose of the NSAID may be tapered gradually. Colchicine may prevent recurrences, but when recurrences are multiple, frequent, disabling, continue beyond 2 years, and are not controlled by pulses of high doses of glucocorticoids, pericardiectomy may be carried out in an attempt to terminate the illness.

Post-cardiac Injury Syndrome

Acute pericarditis may appear under a variety of circumstances that have one common feature: previous injury to the myocardium with blood in the pericardial cavity. The syndrome may develop after a cardiac surgery (postpericardiotomy syndrome); after cardiac trauma, blunt or penetrating (Chap. 23); or after perforation of the heart with a catheter. Rarely, it follows AMI.

The clinical picture mimics acute viral or idiopathic pericarditis. The principal symptom is the pain of acute pericarditis, which usually develops 1–4 weeks following the cardiac injury (1–3 days following AMI) but sometimes appears only after an interval of months. Recurrences are common and may occur up to 2 years or more after the injury. Fever with temperature up to 40°C, pericarditis, pleuritis, and pneumonitis are the outstanding features, and the bout of illness usually subsides in 1 or 2 weeks. The pericarditis may be of the fibrinous variety or it may be a pericardial effusion, which is often serosanguineous, but rarely causes tamponade. Leukocytosis, an increased sedimentation rate, and electrocardiographic changes typical of acute pericarditis may also occur.

The mechanisms responsible for this syndrome have not been identified, but they are probably the result of a hypersensitivity reaction to antigen which originates from injured myocardial tissue and/or pericardium. Circulating myocardial antisarcolemmal and antifibrillar autoantibodies occur frequently, but their precise role has not been defined. Viral infection may also play an etiologic role, since antiviral antibodies are often elevated in patients who develop this syndrome following cardiac surgery.

Often no treatment is necessary aside from aspirin and analgesics. The management of pericardial effusion and tamponade is discussed above. When the illness is followed by a series of disabling recurrences, therapy with an NSAID, colchicine, or a glucocorticoid is usually effective.

DIFFERENTIAL DIAGNOSIS

Because there is no specific test for *acute idiopathic pericarditis*, the diagnosis is one of exclusion. Consequently, all other disorders that may be associated with acute fibrinous pericarditis must be considered. A common diagnostic error is mistaking acute viral or idiopathic pericarditis for AMI and vice versa. When acute fibrinous pericarditis is associated with AMI (Chap. 35), it is characterized by fever, pain, and a friction rub in the first 4 days following the development of the infarct. ECG abnormalities (such as the appearance of Q waves, brief ST-segment elevations with reciprocal changes, and earlier T-wave changes in AMI) and the extent of the elevations of myocardial enzymes are helpful in differentiating pericarditis from AMI.

Pericarditis secondary to post-cardiac injury is differentiated from acute idiopathic pericarditis chiefly by timing. If it occurs within a few days or weeks of an AMI, a chest blow, a cardiac perforation, or cardiac operation, it may be justified to conclude that the two are probably related. If the infarct has been silent or the chest blow forgotten, the relationship to the pericarditis may not be recognized.

It is important to distinguish *pericarditis due to collagen vascular disease* from acute idiopathic pericarditis. Most important in the differential diagnosis is the pericarditis due to systemic lupus erythematosus (SLE) or drug-induced (procainamide or hydralazine) lupus. Pain is often present in pericarditis due to collagen vascular disease. Sometimes in SLE the pericarditis appears as an asymptomatic effusion and, rarely, tamponade develops. When pericarditis occurs in the absence of any obvious underlying disorder, the diagnosis of SLE may be suggested by a rise in the titer of antinuclear antibodies. Acute pericarditis is an occasional complication of *rheumatoid arthritis*, *scleroderma*, and *polyarteritis nodosa*, and other evidence of these diseases is usually obvious. Asymptomatic pericardial effusion is also frequent in these disorders. It is important to question every patient with acute pericarditis about the ingestion of procainamide, hydralazine, isoniazid, cromolyn, and minoxidil, since these drugs can cause this syndrome. The pericarditis of *acute rheumatic fever* is generally associated with evidence of severe pancarditis and with cardiac murmurs (Chap. 26).

Pyogenic (purulent) pericarditis is usually secondary to cardiothoracic operations, by extension of infection from the lungs or pleural cavities, from rupture of the esophagus into the pericardial sac, or rupture of a ring abscess in a patient with infective endocarditis, or can occur if septicemia complicates aseptic pericarditis. It is accompanied by fever, chills, septicemia, and evidence of infection elsewhere and generally has a poor prognosis. The diagnosis is made by examination of the pericardial fluid. Acute pericarditis may also complicate the viral, pyogenic, mycobacterial, and fungal infections that occur with HIV infection.

Pericarditis of renal failure occurs in up to one-third of patients with chronic uremia (*uremic pericarditis*), is also seen in patients undergoing chronic dialysis with normal levels of blood urea and creatinine, and is termed *dialysis-associated pericarditis*. These two forms of pericarditis may be fibrinous and are generally associated with an effusion that may be sanguineous. A friction rub is common, but pain is usually absent or mild. Treatment with an NSAID and intensification of dialysis are usually adequate. Occasionally, tamponade occurs and pericardiocentesis is required. When the pericarditis of renal failure is recurrent or persistent, a pericardial window should be created or pericardiectomy may be necessary.

Pericarditis due to *neoplastic diseases* results from extension or invasion of metastatic tumors (most commonly carcinoma of the lung and breast, malignant melanoma, lymphoma, and leukemia) to the pericardium; pain, atrial arrhythmias, and tamponade are complications that occur occasionally. Diagnosis is made by pericardial fluid cytology or pericardial biopsy. *Mediastinal irradiation* for neoplasm may cause acute pericarditis and/or chronic constrictive pericarditis after eradication of the tumor. Unusual causes of acute pericarditis include syphilis, fungal infection (histoplasmosis, blastomycosis, aspergillosis, and candidiasis), and parasitic infestation (amebiasis, toxoplasmosis, echinococcosis, trichinosis).

CHRONIC PERICARDIAL EFFUSIONS

Chronic pericardial effusions are sometimes encountered in patients without an antecedent history of acute pericarditis. They may cause few symptoms per se, and their presence may be detected by finding an enlarged cardiac silhouette on chest roentgenogram. Tuberculosis is a common cause.

Other Causes

Myxedema may be responsible for chronic pericardial effusion that is sometimes massive but rarely, if ever, causes cardiac tamponade. The cardiac silhouette is markedly enlarged, and an echocardiogram distinguishes cardiomegaly from pericardial effusion. The diagnosis of myxedema can be confirmed by tests for thyroid function. Myxedematous pericardial effusion responds to thyroid hormone replacement.

Neoplasms, SLE, rheumatoid arthritis, mycotic infections, radiation therapy to the chest, pyogenic infections, and chylopericardium may also cause chronic pericardial effusion and should be considered and specifically sought in such patients.

Aspiration and analysis of the pericardial fluid are often helpful in diagnosis. Pericardial fluid should be analyzed as described earlier. Grossly sanguineous pericardial fluid results most commonly from a neoplasm, tuberculosis, renal failure, or slow leakage from an aortic aneurysm. Pericardiocentesis may resolve large effusions, but pericardiectomy may be required with recurrence. Intrapericardial instillation of sclerosing agents or antineoplastic agents (e.g., bleomycin) may be used to prevent reaccumulation of fluid.

CHRONIC CONSTRICTIVE PERICARDITIS

This disorder results when the healing of an acute fibrinous or serofibrinous pericarditis or the resorption of a chronic pericardial effusion is followed by obliteration of the pericardial cavity with the formation of granulation tissue. The latter gradually contracts and forms a firm scar, encasing the heart and interfering with filling of the ventricles. In developing nations where the condition is prevalent, a high percentage of cases is of tuberculous origin, but in North America this is now an infrequent cause. Chronic constrictive pericarditis may follow acute or relapsing viral or idiopathic pericarditis, trauma with organized blood clot, cardiac surgery of any type, mediastinal irradiation, purulent infection, histoplasmosis, neoplastic disease (especially breast cancer, lung cancer, and lymphoma), rheumatoid arthritis, SLE, and chronic renal failure with uremia treated by chronic dialysis. In many patients the cause of the pericardial disease is undetermined, and in them an asymptomatic or forgotten bout of viral pericarditis, acute or idiopathic, may have been the inciting event.

The basic physiologic abnormality in patients with chronic constrictive pericarditis is the inability of the ventricles to fill because of the limitations imposed by the rigid, thickened pericardium or the tense pericardial fluid. In constrictive pericarditis, ventricular filling is unimpeded during early diastole but it is reduced abruptly when the elastic limit of the pericardium is reached, while in cardiac tamponade, ventricular filling is impeded throughout diastole. In both conditions, ventricular end-diastolic and stroke volumes are reduced and the end-diastolic pressures in both ventricles and the mean pressures in the atria, pulmonary veins, and systemic veins are all elevated to similar levels, i.e., within 5 mmHg of one another. Despite these hemodynamic changes, myocardial function may be normal or only slightly impaired in chronic constrictive pericarditis. However, the fibrotic process may extend into the myocardium and cause myocardial scarring, and atrophy, and venous congestion may then be due to the combined effects of the pericardial and myocardial lesions.

In constrictive pericarditis, the right and left atrial pressure pulses display an M-shaped contour, with prominent *x* and *y* descents; the *y* descent, which is absent or diminished in cardiac tamponade, is the most prominent deflection in constrictive pericarditis; it reflects rapid early filling of the ventricles. The *y* descent is interrupted by a rapid rise in atrial pressure during early diastole, when ventricular filling is impeded by the constricting pericardium. These characteristic changes are transmitted to the jugular veins, where they may be recognized by inspection. In constrictive pericarditis, the ventricular pressure pulses in both ventricles exhibit characteristic "square root" signs during diastole. These hemodynamic changes, although characteristic, are not pathognomonic of constrictive pericarditis and may also be observed in cardiomyopathies characterized by restriction of ventricular filling (Chap. 21) (Table 22-2).

CLINICAL AND LABORATORY FINDINGS

Weakness, fatigue, weight gain, increased abdominal girth, abdominal discomfort, a protuberant abdomen, and edema are common. The patient often appears chronically ill, and in advanced cases there are anasarca, skeletal muscle wasting, and cachexia. Exertional dyspnea is common, and orthopnea may occur, although it is usually not severe. Acute left ventricular failure (acute pulmonary edema) is very uncommon. The cervical veins are distended and may remain so even after intensive diuretic treatment, and venous pressure may fail to decline during inspiration (*Kussmaul's sign*). The latter is frequent in chronic pericarditis but may also occur in tricuspid stenosis, right ventricular infarction, and restrictive cardiomyopathy.

The pulse pressure is normal or reduced. In about one-third of the cases, a paradoxical pulse (p. 257) can be detected. Congestive hepatomegaly is pronounced and may impair hepatic function and cause jaundice; ascites is common and is usually more prominent than dependent edema. The apical pulse is reduced and may retract in systole (*Broadbent's sign*). The heart sounds may be distant; an early third heart sound, i.e., a pericardial knock, occurring 0.09–0.12 s after aortic valve closure at the cardiac apex, is often conspicuous; it occurs with the abrupt cessation of ventricular filling. A systolic murmur of tricuspid regurgitation may be present.

The *ECG* frequently displays low voltage of the QRS complexes and diffuse flattening or inversion of the T waves. Atrial fibrillation is present in about one-third of patients. The *chest roentgenogram* shows a normal or slightly enlarged heart; pericardial calcification is most common in tuberculous pericarditis.

Inasmuch as the usual physical signs of cardiac disease (murmurs, cardiac enlargement) may be inconspicuous or absent in chronic constrictive pericarditis, hepatic enlargement and dysfunction associated with jaundice and intractable ascites may lead to a mistaken diagnosis of hepatic cirrhosis. This error can be avoided if the neck veins are inspected carefully in patients with ascites and hepatomegaly. Given a clinical picture resembling hepatic cirrhosis, but with the added feature of distended neck veins, careful search for thickening of the pericardium by CT (Fig. 12-8) or MRI should be carried out and may disclose this curable or remediable form of heart disease.

The two-dimensional transthoracic *echocardiogram* typically shows pericardial thickening, dilatation of the inferior vena cava and hepatic veins, and a sharp halt in ventricular filling in early diastole, with normal ventricular systolic function and flattening of the left ventricular posterior wall. Atrial enlargement may be seen, especially in patients with long-standing constrictive physiology. There is a distinctive pattern of transvalvular flow velocity on Doppler flow-velocity echocardiography. During inspiration there is an exaggerated reduction in blood flow velocity in the pulmonary veins and across the mitral valve and a leftward shift of the ventricular septum; the opposite occurs during expiration. Diastolic flow velocity in the vena cavae into the right atrium and across the tricuspid valve increases in an exaggerated manner during inspiration and declines during expiration (**Fig. 22-5**). However, echocardiography cannot definitively exclude the diagnosis of constrictive pericarditis. MRI and CT scanning (**Fig. 22-6**) are more accurate than echocardiography in establishing or excluding the presence of a thickened pericardium. Pericardial thickening and even pericardial calcification, however, are not synonymous with constrictive pericarditis since they may occur without seriously impairing ventricular filling.

DIFFERENTIAL DIAGNOSIS

Like chronic constrictive pericarditis, cor pulmonale (Chap. 17) may be associated with severe systemic venous hypertension but little pulmonary congestion; the heart is usually not enlarged, and a paradoxical pulse may be present. However, in cor pulmonale, advanced parenchymal pulmonary disease is usually obvious and venous pressure *falls* during inspiration, i.e., Kussmaul's sign is negative. *Tricuspid stenosis* (Chap. 20) may also simulate chronic constrictive pericarditis; congestive hepatomegaly,

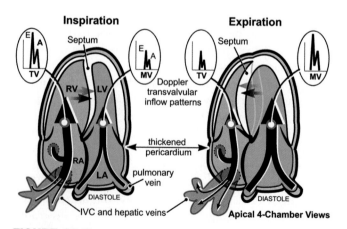

FIGURE 22-5

Constrictive pericarditis Doppler schema of respirophasic changes in mitral and tricuspid inflow. Reciprocal patterns of ventricular filling are assessed on pulsed Doppler examination of mitral (MV) and tricuspid (TV) inflow. (*Courtesy of Bernard E. Bulwer, MD; with permission.*)

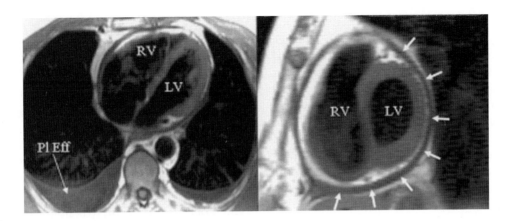

FIGURE 22-6

Cardiovascular magnetic resonance in a patient with constrictive pericarditis. On the right is a basal short-axis view of the ventricles showing a thickened pericardium encasing the heart (arrows). On the left is a transaxial view, again showing the thickened pericardium, particularly over the right heart, but also a pleural effusion (Pl Eff). LV, left ventricle; RV, right ventricle. [*From D Pennell: Cardiovascular magnetic resonance, in DP Zipes et al (eds): Braunwald's Heart Disease, 7th ed. Philadelphia, Elsevier, 2005.*]

splenomegaly, ascites, and venous distention may be equally prominent. However, in tricuspid stenosis, a characteristic murmur as well as the murmur of accompanying mitral stenosis are usually present. In tricuspid stenosis, a paradoxical pulse and a steep, deep *y* descent in the jugular venous pulse do *not* occur, serving to differentiate it from chronic constrictive pericarditis.

Because constrictive pericarditis can be corrected surgically, it is important to distinguish chronic constrictive pericarditis from restrictive cardiomyopathy (Chap. 21), which has a similar physiologic abnormality, i.e., restriction of ventricular filling. In many of these patients the ventricular wall is thickened on echocardiographic examination (Table 22-2). The features favoring the diagnosis of restrictive cardiomyopathy over chronic constrictive pericarditis include a well-defined apex beat, cardiac enlargement, and pronounced orthopnea with attacks of acute left ventricular failure, left ventricular hypertrophy, gallop sounds (in place of a pericardial knock), bundle branch block, and in some cases abnormal Q waves on the ECG. The typical echocardiographic features of constrictive pericarditis (see earlier) are useful in the differential diagnosis in chronic constrictive pericarditis (Fig. 22-5). CT scanning (usually with contrast) and MRI are key in distinguishing between restrictive cardiomyopathy and chronic constrictive pericarditis. In the former, the ventricular walls are hypertrophied, while in the latter the pericardium is thickened and sometimes calcified. When a patient has progressive, disabling, and unresponsive congestive heart failure and displays any of the features of constrictive heart disease, Doppler echocardiography to record respiratory effects on transvalvular flow, and an MRI or CT scan should be obtained to detect or exclude constrictive pericarditis, since the latter is usually curable.

℞ Treatment:
CONSTRICTIVE PERICARDITIS

Pericardial resection is the only definitive treatment of constrictive pericarditis, but dietary sodium restriction and diuretics are useful during preoperative preparation. Coronary arteriography should be carried out preoperatively in patients older than 50 years to exclude unsuspected coronary disease. The benefits derived from cardiac decortication are usually progressive over a period of months. The risk of this operation depends on the extent of penetration of the myocardium by the calcific process, by the severity of myocardial atrophy, by the extent of secondary impairment of hepatic and/or renal function, and by the patient's general condition. Operative mortality is in the range of 5–10%; the patients with the most severe disease are at highest risk. Therefore, surgical treatment should be carried out relatively early in the course.

Subacute Effusive-Constrictive Pericarditis

This form of pericardial disease is characterized by the combination of a tense effusion in the pericardial space and constriction of the heart by thickened pericardium. It shares a number of features both with chronic pericardial effusion producing cardiac compression and with pericardial constriction. It may be caused by tuberculosis (see later), multiple attacks of acute idiopathic pericarditis, radiation, traumatic pericarditis, renal failure, scleroderma, and neoplasms. The heart is generally enlarged, and a paradoxical pulse and a prominent *x* descent (without a prominent *y* descent) are present in the atrial and jugular venous pressure pulses. Following pericardiocentesis, the physiologic findings may change from those of cardiac tamponade to those of pericardial constriction, with a "square root" sign in the ventricular pressure pulse and a prominent γ descent in the atrial and jugular venous pressure pulses. Furthermore, the intrapericardial pressure and the central venous pressure may decline, but not to normal. The diagnosis can be established by pericardiocentesis followed by pericardial biopsy. In many patients the condition progresses to the chronic constrictive form of the disease. Wide excision of both the visceral and parietal pericardium is usually effective therapy.

TUBERCULOUS PERICARDIAL DISEASE

This chronic infection is a common cause of chronic pericardial effusion, although less so in the United States than in Africa, Asia, the Middle East, and other parts of the developing world where active tuberculosis is endemic. The clinical picture is that of a chronic, systemic illness in a patient with pericardial effusion. It is important to consider this diagnosis in a patient with known tuberculosis, with HIV, and with fever, chest pain, weight loss, and enlargement of the cardiac silhouette of undetermined origin. Inasmuch as treatment is quite effective, overlooking a tuberculous pericardial effusion may have serious consequences. If the etiology of chronic pericardial effusion remains obscure, despite detailed analysis of the pericardial fluid (see earlier), a pericardial biopsy, preferably by a limited thoracotomy, should be performed. If definitive evidence is then still lacking but the specimen shows granulomata with caseation, antituberculous chemotherapy is indicated.

If the biopsy specimen shows a thickened pericardium, pericardiectomy should be carried out to prevent the development of constriction, a serious complication of tuberculosis that occurs in about one-half of patients with tuberculous pericardial effusion despite treatment with chemotherapy and glucocorticoids. Tubercular cardiac constriction should be treated surgically while the patient is receiving antituberculous chemotherapy. In many patients, subacute effusive-constrictive pericarditis develops.

OTHER DISORDERS OF THE PERICARDIUM

Pericardial cysts appear as rounded or lobulated deformities of the cardiac silhouette, most commonly at the right cardiophrenic angle. They do not cause symptoms, and their major clinical significance lies in the possibility of confusion with a tumor, ventricular aneurysm, or massive cardiomegaly. *Tumors* involving the pericardium are most commonly secondary to malignant neoplasms originating in or invading the mediastinum, including carcinoma of the bronchus and breast, lymphoma, and melanoma. The most common *primary* malignant tumor is the mesothelioma. The usual clinical picture of malignant pericardial tumor is an insidiously developing, often bloody, pericardial effusion. Surgical exploration is required to establish a definitive diagnosis and to carry out definitive or, more commonly, palliative treatment.

FURTHER READINGS

Axel L: Assessment of pericardial disease by magnetic resonance and computed tomography. J Magn Reson Imaging 19:816, 2004

Hoit BD: Management of effusive and constrictive pericardial heart disease. Circulation 105:2939, 2002

Imazio M et al: Diagnosis an management of pericardial diseases. Nat Rev Cardiol 6:743, 2009

Lange RA, Hillis LD: Acute pericarditis. N Engl J Med 351:2195, 2004

LeWinter M, Kabbani S: Pericardial diseases, in *Braunwald's Heart Disease*, 8th ed, P. Libby et al (eds). Philadelphia, Saunders, 2008

Maisch B et al: Guidelines on the diagnosis and management of pericardial diseases executive summary: the Task Force on the Diagnosis and Management of Pericardial Diseases of the European Society of Cardiology. Eur Heart J 25:587, 2004

Mayosi BM et al: Tuberculous pericarditis. Circulation 112:3608, 2005

————: Contemporary trends in the epidemiology and management of cardiomyopathy and pericarditis in Sub-Saharan Africa. Heart 93:1176, 2007

Rajagopalan N et al: Comparison of new Doppler echocardiographic methods to differentiate constrictive pericardial heart disease and restrictive cardiomyopathy. Am J Cardiol 87:86, 2001

CHAPTER 23

TUMORS AND TRAUMA OF THE HEART

Eric H. Awtry ■ Wilson S. Colucci

TUMORS OF THE HEART

PRIMARY TUMORS

Primary tumors of the heart are rare. Approximately three-quarters are histologically benign, more than one-half of which are myxomas. Malignant tumors, almost all of which are sarcomas, account for 25% of primary cardiac tumors (Table 23–1). All cardiac tumors, regardless of pathologic type, have the potential to cause life-threatening complications. Many tumors are now curable by surgery; thus, early diagnosis is imperative.

Clinical Presentation

Cardiac tumors may present with a wide array of cardiac and noncardiac manifestations, which depend in large part on the location and size of the tumor. Many of the manifestations are nonspecific features of more common forms of heart disease, such as chest pain, syncope, heart failure, murmurs, arrhythmias, conduction disturbances, and pericardial effusion with or without tamponade. Additionally, embolic phenomena and constitutional symptoms may occur.

Myxoma

Myxomas are the most common type of primary cardiac tumor in all age groups, accounting for one-third to one-half of all cases at postmortem and for about three-quarters of the tumors treated surgically. They occur at all ages, most commonly in the third through sixth decades, with a female predilection. Approximately 90% of myxomas are sporadic; the remainder are familial with autosomal dominant transmission. The familial variety often occurs as part of a syndrome complex (Carney complex) that comprises (1) myxomas (cardiac, skin, and/or breast), (2) lentigines and/or pigmented nevi, and (3) endocrine overactivity (primary nodular adrenal cortical disease with or without Cushing's syndrome, testicular tumors, and/or pituitary adenomas with gigantism or acromegaly). Certain constellations of findings have been referred to as the *NAME* syndrome (nevi, atrial myxoma, myxoid neurofibroma, and ephelides) or the *LAMB* syndrome (lentigines, atrial myxoma, and blue nevi), although these likely represent subsets of the Carney complex. The genetic basis of this complex has not been completely elucidated; however, patients frequently have mutations in the tumor-suppressor gene *PRKAR1A*, which encodes the protein kinase A type I-α regulatory subunit.

Pathologically, myxomas are gelatinous structures consisting of myxoma cells embedded in a stroma rich in glycosaminoglycans. Most are pedunculated on a fibrovascular stalk and average 4–8 cm in diameter. Most are solitary and located in the atria, particularly the left atrium, where they usually arise from the interatrial septum in the vicinity of the fossa ovalis. In contrast to sporadic tumors, familial or myxoma syndrome tumors tend to occur in younger individuals, are often multiple, may be ventricular in location, and are more likely to recur after initial resection.

TABLE 23-1

RELATIVE INCIDENCE OF PRIMARY TUMORS OF THE HEART

TYPE	NUMBER	PERCENT
Benign	199	58.0
Myxoma	114	33.2
Rhabdomyoma	20	5.8
Fibroma	20	5.8
Hemangioma	17	5.0
Atrioventricular nodal	10	2.9
Granular cell	4	1.2
Lipoma	2	0.6
Paraganglioma	2	0.6
Myocytic hamartoma	2	0.6
Histiocytoid cardiomyopathy	2	0.6
Inflammatory pseudotumor	2	0.6
Other benign tumors	4	1.2
Malignant	144	42.0
Sarcoma	137	39.9
Lymphoma	7	2.1

Source: Modified from A Burke, R Virmani: *Atlas of Tumor Pathology. Tumors of the Heart and Great Vessels.* Washington, DC, Armed Forces Institute of Pathology 1996, p. 231; with permission.

Myxomas commonly present with obstructive signs and symptoms. The most common clinical presentation mimics that of mitral valve disease—either stenosis owing to tumor prolapse into the mitral orifice or regurgitation resulting from tumor-induced valvular trauma. Ventricular myxomas may cause outflow obstruction similar to that caused by subaortic or subpulmonic stenosis. The symptoms and signs of myxoma may be sudden in onset or positional in nature, owing to the effects of gravity on tumor position. A characteristic low-pitched sound, referred to as a "tumor plop," may be appreciated on auscultation during early or mid-diastole and is thought to result from the impact of the tumor against the mitral valve or ventricular wall. Myxomas may also present with peripheral or pulmonary emboli or with constitutional signs and symptoms, including fever, weight loss, cachexia, malaise, arthralgias, rash, digital clubbing, Raynaud's phenomenon, hypergammaglobulinemia, anemia, polycythemia, leukocytosis, elevated erythrocyte sedimentation rate, thrombocytopenia, or thrombocytosis. Not surprisingly, patients with myxomas are frequently misdiagnosed as having endocarditis, collagen vascular disease, or a paraneoplastic syndrome.

Two-dimensional transthoracic or omniplane transesophageal echocardiography is useful in the diagnosis of cardiac myxoma and allows assessment of tumor size and determination of the site of tumor attachment, both important considerations in the planning of surgical excision (**Fig. 23-1**). CT and MRI may provide important information regarding size, shape, composition, and surface characteristics of the tumor (**Fig. 23-2**).

Although cardiac catheterization and angiography were previously performed routinely prior to tumor resection, they are no longer considered mandatory when adequate noninvasive information is available and other cardiac disorders (e.g., coronary artery disease) are not considered likely. Additionally, catheterization of the chamber from which the tumor arises carries the risk of tumor embolization. Because myxomas may be familial, echocardiographic screening of first-degree relatives is appropriate, particularly if the patient is young and has multiple tumors or evidence of myxoma syndrome.

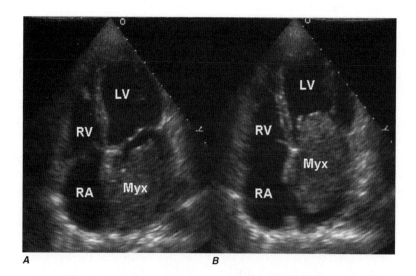

FIGURE 23-1

Transthoracic echocardiogram demonstrating a large atrial myxoma. The myxoma (Myx) fills the entire left atrium in systole (*panel **A***) and prolapses across the mitral valve and into the left ventricle (LV) during diastole (*panel **B***). RA, right atrium; RV, right ventricle. (*Courtesy of Dr. Michael Tsang; with permission.*)

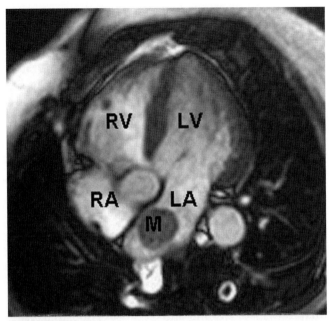

FIGURE 23-2
Cardiac MRI demonstrating a rounded mass (M) within the left atrium (LA). Pathologic evaluation at the time of surgery revealed it to be an atrial myxoma. LV, left ventricle; RA, right atrium; RV, right ventricle.

℞ **Treatment:**
PRIMARY TUMOR

Surgical excision utilizing cardiopulmonary bypass is indicated, regardless of tumor size, and is generally curative. Myxomas recur in ~12–22% of familial cases but in only 1–2% of sporadic cases. Tumor recurrence is most likely due to multifocal lesions in the former and inadequate resection in the latter.

Other Benign Tumors

Cardiac *lipomas*, although relatively common, are usually incidental findings at postmortem examination; however, they may grow as large as 15 cm and may present with symptoms owing to mechanical interference with cardiac function, arrhythmias, or conduction disturbances, or as an abnormality of the cardiac silhouette on chest x-ray. *Papillary fibroelastomas* are the most common tumors of the cardiac valves. Although usually clinically silent, they can cause valve dysfunction and may embolize distally, resulting in transient ischemic attacks, stroke, or myocardial infarction. Therefore, these tumors should be resected even when asymptomatic. *Rhabdomyomas* and *fibromas* are the most common cardiac tumors in infants and children and usually occur in the ventricles where they may produce mechanical obstruction to blood flow, thereby mimicking valvular stenosis, congestive heart

failure (CHF), restrictive or hypertrophic cardiomyopathy, or pericardial constriction. Rhabdomyomas are probably hamartomatous growths, are multiple in 90% of cases, and are strongly associated with tuberous sclerosis. These tumors have a tendency to regress completely or partially; only those tumors that cause obstruction require surgical resection. Fibromas are usually single, are often calcified, tend to grow and cause obstructive symptoms, and should be resected. *Hemangiomas* and *mesotheliomas* are generally small tumors, most often intramyocardial in location, and may cause atrioventricular (AV) conduction disturbances and even sudden death as a result of their propensity to develop in the region of the AV node. Other benign tumors arising from the heart include *teratoma*, *chemodectoma*, *neurilemoma*, *granular cell myoblastoma*, and *bronchogenic cysts*.

Sarcoma

Almost all primary cardiac malignancies are sarcomas, which may be of several histologic types. In general, the tumors are characterized by rapid progression culminating in the patient's death within weeks to months from the time of presentation, as a result of hemodynamic compromise, local invasion, or distant metastases. Sarcomas commonly involve the right side of the heart, are characterized by rapid growth, frequently invade the pericardial space, and may obstruct the cardiac chambers or vena cavae. Sarcomas may also occur on the left side of the heart and may be mistaken for myxomas.

℞ **Treatment:**
SARCOMA

At the time of presentation sarcomas have often spread too extensively to allow for surgical excision. Although scattered reports exist of palliation with surgery, radiotherapy, and/or chemotherapy, the response of cardiac sarcomas to these therapies is generally poor. The one exception appears to be cardiac lymphosarcomas, which may respond to a combination of chemotherapy and radiotherapy.

TUMORS METASTATIC TO THE HEART

Tumors metastatic to the heart are much more common than primary tumors, and their incidence is likely to increase as the life expectancy of patients with various forms of malignant neoplasms is extended by more effective therapy. Although cardiac metastases occur in 1–20% of all tumor types, the relative incidence is especially high in malignant melanoma and, to a somewhat lesser extent, in leukemia and lymphoma. In absolute terms, the most common primary originating sites of cardiac metastases are carcinoma of the breast and lung, reflecting the high incidence of these cancers. Cardiac metastases almost always occur in the setting of widespread primary disease, and most often either primary or metastatic disease exists elsewhere in the thoracic cavity. Nevertheless, cardiac metastasis may occasionally be the initial presentation of an extrathoracic tumor.

Cardiac metastases may occur via hematogenous or lymphangitic spread or by direct tumor invasion. They generally manifest as small, firm nodules; diffuse infiltration may also occur, especially with sarcomas or hematologic neoplasms. The pericardium is most often involved, followed by myocardial involvement of any chamber, and, rarely, by involvement of the endocardium or cardiac valves.

Cardiac metastases are clinically apparent only ~10% of the time, are usually not the cause of the patient's presentation, and rarely are the cause of death. The vast majority occur in the setting of a previously recognized malignant neoplasm. When symptomatic, cardiac metastases may result in a variety of clinical features, including dyspnea, acute pericarditis, cardiac tamponade, ectopic tachyarrhythmias, heart block, CHF, and rapid enlargement of the cardiac silhouette on chest x-ray. As with primary cardiac tumors, the clinical presentation reflects more the location and size of the tumor rather than its histologic type. Many of these signs and symptoms may also result from myocarditis, pericarditis, or cardiomyopathy induced by radiotherapy or chemotherapy.

Electrocardiographic (ECG) findings are nonspecific. On chest x-ray, the cardiac silhouette is most often normal but may be enlarged or exhibit a bizarre contour. Echocardiography is useful for identifying pericardial effusions and for visualizing larger metastases, although CT and radionuclide imaging with gallium or thallium may more clearly define the tumor burden. Cardiac MRI offers superb image quality and plays a central role in the diagnostic evaluation of cardiac metastases and cardiac tumors in general. Pericardiocentesis may allow for a specific cytologic diagnosis in patients with malignant pericardial effusions. Angiography is rarely necessary but may delineate discrete lesions.

℞ Treatment:
TUMORS METASTATIC TO THE HEART

Most patients with cardiac metastases have advanced malignant disease; thus, therapy is generally palliative and consists of treatment of the primary tumor. Symptomatic malignant pericardial effusions should be drained by pericardiocentesis. Concomitant instillation of a sclerosing agent (e.g., tetracycline) may delay or prevent reaccumulation of the effusion, while creation of a pericardial window allows drainage of the effusion to the pleural space.

TRAUMATIC CARDIAC INJURY

Traumatic cardiac injury may be caused by either penetrating or nonpenetrating trauma. *Penetrating injuries* most often result from gunshot or knife wounds, and the site of entry is usually obvious. *Nonpenetrating injuries* most often occur during motor vehicle accidents, either from a rapid deceleration injury or from impact of the chest against the steering wheel, and may be associated with significant cardiac injury even in the absence of external signs of thoracic trauma.

Myocardial contusions are the most common form of nonpenetrating cardiac injury and may initially be overlooked in trauma patients as the clinical focus is directed toward other more obvious injuries. Myocardial necrosis may occur as a direct result of the blunt injury or as a result of traumatic coronary laceration or thrombosis. The contused myocardium is pathologically similar to infarcted myocardium and may be associated with atrial or ventricular arrhythmias, conduction disturbances including bundle branch block, or ECG abnormalities resembling those of infarction or pericarditis. Thus, it is important to consider contusion as a cause of otherwise unexplained ECG changes in a trauma patient. Serum creatine kinase (CK-MB) isoenzyme levels are increased in ~20% of patients suffering blunt chest trauma but may be falsely elevated in the presence of massive skeletal muscle injury. Cardiac troponin levels are more specific for identifying cardiac injury in this setting. Echocardiography is useful in detecting structural and functional sequelae of contusion, including wall motion abnormalities, pericardial effusion, valvular dysfunction, and ventricular rupture. Although radionuclide scanning can detect myocardial contusion, its role is limited, given the ease and availability of echocardiography.

Rupture of the cardiac valves or their supporting structures, most commonly of the tricuspid or mitral valve, leads to acute valvular incompetence. This complication is usually heralded by the development of a loud murmur, may be associated with rapidly progressive heart failure, and can be diagnosed by either transthoracic or transesophageal echocardiography.

The most serious consequence of nonpenetrating injury is myocardial rupture, which may result in hemopericardium and tamponade (free wall rupture) or intracardiac shunting (ventricular septal rupture). Although generally fatal, up to 40% of patients with cardiac rupture have been reported to survive long enough to reach a specialized trauma center. Hemopericardium may also result from traumatic rupture of a pericardial vessel or a coronary artery. Additionally, a pericardial effusion may develop weeks or even months after blunt chest trauma as a manifestation of the post-cardiac injury syndrome, which resembles the post-pericardiotomy syndrome (Chap. 22).

Blunt, nonpenetrating, often innocent-appearing injuries to the chest may trigger ventricular fibrillation even in absence of overt signs of injury. This syndrome, referred to as *commotio cordis*, occurs most often in adolescents during sporting events (e.g., baseball, hockey, football, and lacrosse) and likely results from an impact to the chest wall overlying the heart during the susceptible phase of repolarization just prior to the peak of the T wave. Survival depends on prompt defibrillation.

Sudden emotional or physiologic trauma may precipitate a transient cardiomyopathy that is characterized by dysfunction of the mid-portion and apex of the left ventricle with hyperdynamic function at the ventricular base. This syndrome, referred to as *Tako-Tsubo syndrome* or the *apical ballooning syndrome*, is more common in women and usually presents with chest pain, anterior ST-segment elevation, and mildly elevated cardiac enzymes despite the absence of significant epicardial coronary artery disease. The pathophysiology of this syndrome likely relates to catecholamine excess, and possibly to coronary vasospasm. The prognosis is favorable, and complete and spontaneous resolution of the ventricular dysfunction usually occurs within several weeks.

Rupture of the aorta, usually just above the aortic valve or at the site of the ligamentum arteriosum, is a common consequence of nonpenetrating chest trauma and is the most common vascular deceleration injury. The clinical presentation is similar to that of aortic dissection (Chap. 38). The arterial pressure and pulse amplitude may be increased in the upper extremities and decreased in the lower extremities, and chest x-ray may reveal mediastinal widening. Occasionally, aortic rupture is contained by the aortic adventitia, resulting in a false, or *pseudo-*, aneurysm that may be discovered months or years after the initial injury.

Penetrating injuries of the heart produced by knife or bullet wounds usually result in rapid clinical deterioration and frequently in death as a result of hemopericardium/pericardial tamponade or massive hemorrhage. Nonetheless, up to 50% of such patients may survive long enough to reach a specialized trauma center if immediate resuscitation is performed. Prognosis in these patients relates to the mechanism of injury, their clinical condition at presentation, and the specific cardiac chamber(s) involved. Iatrogenic cardiac or coronary arterial perforation may occur as a complication during placement of central venous or intracardiac catheters, pacemaker leads, or intracoronary stents and is associated with a better prognosis than other forms of penetrating cardiac trauma.

Traumatic rupture of a great vessel from penetrating injury is usually associated with hemothorax and, less often, hemopericardium. Local hematoma formation may compress major vessels and produce ischemic symptoms, and AV fistulae may develop, occasionally resulting in high-output CHF.

Occasionally, patients who survive penetrating cardiac injuries may subsequently present with a new cardiac murmur or CHF as a result of mitral regurgitation or an intracardiac shunt (i.e., ventricular or atrial septal defect, aortopulmonary fistula, or coronary AV fistula) that was undetected at the time of their initial injury or developed subsequently. Therefore, trauma patients should be carefully examined several weeks after their injury. If a mechanical complication is suspected, it can be confirmed by echocardiography or cardiac catheterization.

℞ **Treatment:**
TRAUMATIC CARDIAC INJURY

The treatment of an uncomplicated myocardial contusion is similar to that for a myocardial infarction, except that anticoagulation is contraindicated, and should include monitoring for the development of arrhythmias and mechanical complications such as cardiac rupture (Chap. 35). Acute myocardial failure resulting from traumatic valve rupture usually requires urgent operative correction. Immediate thoracotomy should be carried out for most cases of penetrating injury or if there is evidence of cardiac tamponade and/or shock regardless of the type of trauma. Pericardiocentesis may be lifesaving in patients with tamponade but is usually only a temporizing maneuver while they await definitive surgical therapy. Pericardial hemorrhage often leads to constriction (Chap. 22), which must be treated by decortication.

FURTHER READINGS

BURKE A et al: Cardiac tumors: an update. Heart 94:117, 2008

KALRA MK, ABBARA S: Imaging cardiac tumors. Cancer Treat Res 143:177, 2008

MATTOX KL: Traumatic heart disease, in *Braunwald's Heart Disease*, 7th ed, DP Zipes et al (eds). Philadelphia, Saunders, 2005

PRETRE R, CHILCOTT M: Blunt trauma to the heart and great vessels. N Engl J Med 336:626, 1997

REYMAN K: Cardiac myxomas. N Engl J Med 333:1610, 1995

RHEE PM et al: Penetrating cardiac injuries: A population-based study. J Trauma 45:366, 1998

SABATINE M, SCHOEN F: Primary tumors of the heart, in *Braunwald's Heart Disease*, 7th ed, DP Zipes et al (eds). Philadelphia, Saunders, 2005

SIMMERS TA et al: Traumatic papillary muscle rupture. Ann Thorac Surg 72:257, 2001

SYBRANDY KC et al: Diagnosing cardiac contusion: Old wisdom and new insights. Heart 89:485, 2003

TYBURSKI JG et al: Factors affecting prognosis with penetrating wounds of the heart. J Trauma 48:587, 2000

VAUGHAN CJ et al: Tumors and the heart: Molecular genetic advances. Curr Opin Cardiol 16:195, 2001

CHAPTER 24

CARDIAC MANIFESTATIONS OF SYSTEMIC DISEASE

Eric H. Awtry ■ Wilson S. Colucci

The common systemic disorders that have associated cardiac manifestations are summarized in Table 24-1.

DIABETES MELLITUS

Diabetes mellitus, both insulin- and non–insulin-dependent, is an independent risk factor for coronary artery disease [(CAD); Chap. 30], accounting for 14–50% of new cases of cardiovascular disease. Furthermore, CAD is the most common cause of death in adults with diabetes mellitus. In the diabetic population the incidence of CAD relates to the duration of diabetes and the level of glycemic control, and its pathogenesis involves endothelial dysfunction, increased lipoprotein peroxidation, increased inflammation, a prothrombotic state, and associated metabolic abnormalities.

Diabetic patients are more likely to suffer a myocardial infarction (MI), have a greater burden of CAD, have larger infarct size, and suffer more postinfarct complications, including heart failure, shock, and death, than nondiabetics. Importantly, diabetic patients are more likely to have atypical ischemic symptoms; nausea, dyspnea, pulmonary edema, arrhythmias, heart block, or syncope may be their anginal equivalent. Additionally, "silent ischemia," resulting from autonomic nervous system dysfunction, is more common in diabetics, accounting for up to 90% of their ischemic episodes. Thus, one must have a low threshold for suspecting CAD in diabetic patients. The treatment of diabetics with CAD must include aggressive risk factor management. Pharmacologic therapy and revascularization are similar in diabetics and nondiabetics, excepting that diabetics have greater morbidity and mortality associated with revascularization, have an increased risk of restenosis after percutaneous coronary intervention (PCI), and likely have improved survival when treated with surgical bypass compared with PCI for multivessel CAD.

Patients with diabetes mellitus may also have abnormal left ventricular systolic and diastolic function, reflecting concomitant epicardial CAD and hypertension, coronary microvascular disease, endothelial dysfunction, ventricular hypertrophy, and autonomic dysfunction. A restrictive cardiomyopathy may be present with abnormal myocardial relaxation and elevated ventricular filling pressures. Histologically, interstitial fibrosis is seen, and intramural arteries may demonstrate intimal thickening, hyaline deposition, and inflammatory changes. Diabetic patients have an increased risk of developing clinical heart failure, which likely contributes to their excessive cardiovascular morbidity and mortality. There is some evidence that insulin therapy may ameliorate diabetes-related myocardial dysfunction.

TABLE 24-1

COMMON SYSTEMIC DISORDERS AND THEIR ASSOCIATED CARDIAC MANIFESTATIONS

SYSTEMIC DISORDER	COMMON CARDIAC MANIFESTATIONS
Diabetes mellitus	CAD, atypical angina, CMP, systolic or diastolic CHF
Protein-calorie malnutrition	Dilated CMP, CHF
Thiamine deficiency	High-output failure, dilated CMP
Hyperhomocysteinemia	Premature atherosclerosis
Obesity	CMP, systolic or diastolic CHF
Hyperthyroidism	Palpitations, SVT, atrial fibrillation, hypertension
Hypothyroidism	Hypotension, bradycardia, dilated CMP, CHF, pericardial effusion
Malignant carcinoid	Tricuspid and pulmonary valve disease, right heart failure
Pheochromocytoma	Hypertension, palpitations, CHF
Acromegaly	Systolic or diastolic heart failure
Rheumatoid arthritis	Pericarditis, pericardial effusions, coronary arteritis, myocarditis, valvulitis
Seronegative arthropathies	Aortitis, aortic and mitral insufficiency, conduction abnormalities
Systemic lupus erythematosus	Pericarditis, Libman-Sacks endocarditis, myocarditis, arterial and venous thrombosis
HIV	Myocarditis, dilated CMP, pericardial effusion
Amyloidosis	CHF, restrictive CMP, valvular regurgitation, pericardial effusion
Sarcoidosis	CHF, dilated or restrictive CMP, ventricular arrhythmias, heart block
Hemochromatosis	CHF, arrhythmias, heart block
Marfan syndrome	Aortic aneurysm and dissection, aortic insufficiency, mitral valve prolapse
Ehlers-Danlos syndrome	Aortic and coronary aneurysms, mitral and tricuspid valve prolapse

Note: CAD, coronary artery disease; CHF, congestive heart failure; CMP, cardiomyopathy; SVT, supraventricular tachycardia.

MALNUTRITION AND VITAMIN DEFICIENCY

Malnutrition

In patients whose intake of protein, calories, or both is severely deficient, the heart may become thin, pale, and hypokinetic with myofibrillar atrophy and interstitial edema. The systolic pressure and cardiac output fall, and the pulse pressure narrows. Generalized edema is common and relates to a variety of factors, including reduced serum oncotic pressure and myocardial dysfunction. Such profound states of protein and calorie malnutrition, termed *kwashiorkor* and *marasmus,* respectively, are most common in underdeveloped countries. However, significant nutritional heart disease may also occur in developed nations, particularly in patients with chronic diseases such as AIDS, in patients with anorexia nervosa, and in patients with severe cardiac failure in whom gastrointestinal hypoperfusion and venous congestion may lead to anorexia and malabsorption. Open-heart surgery poses increased risk in malnourished patients, and they may benefit from preoperative hyperalimentation.

Thiamine Deficiency (Beriberi)

Generalized malnutrition is often accompanied by thiamine deficiency, although this hypovitaminosis may also occur in the presence of an adequate protein and caloric intake, particularly in the Far East where polished rice deficient in thiamine may be a major dietary component. In Western nations where the use of thiamine-enriched flour is widespread, clinical thiamine deficiency is limited primarily to alcoholics, food faddists, and patients receiving chemotherapy. Nonetheless, when thiamine stores are measured using the thiamine-pyrophosphate effect (TPPE), thiamine deficiency has been found in 20–90% of patients with chronic heart failure. This deficiency appears to result from both reduced dietary intake and a diuretic-induced increase in the urinary excretion of thiamine. The acute administration of thiamine to these patients increases the left ventricular ejection fraction and the excretion of salt and water.

Clinically, patients with thiamine deficiency usually have evidence of generalized malnutrition, peripheral neuropathy, glossitis, and anemia. The classic cardiovascular syndrome is characterized by high-output heart failure, tachycardia, and often elevated left and right ventricular filling pressures. The major cause of the high-output state is vasomotor depression leading to reduced systemic vascular resistance, the precise mechanism of which is not understood. The cardiac examination reveals a wide pulse pressure, tachycardia, a third heart sound, and, frequently, an apical systolic murmur. The ECG may reveal decreased voltage, a prolonged QT interval, and T-wave abnormalities. The chest x-ray generally reveals cardiomegaly and signs of congestive heart failure (CHF). The response to thiamine is often dramatic, with an increase in systemic vascular resistance, a decrease in cardiac output, clearing of pulmonary congestion, and a reduction in heart size often occurring in 12–48 h. Although the response to inotropes and diuretics may be poor before thiamine therapy, these agents may be important *after* thiamine is given, since the left ventricle may not be able to handle the increased work load presented by the return of vascular tone.

Vitamin B$_6$, B$_{12}$, and Folate Deficiency

Vitamins B$_6$, B$_{12}$, and folate are cofactors in the metabolism of homocysteine. Their deficiency probably contributes to the majority of cases of hyperhomocysteinemia, a disorder associated with increased atherosclerotic risk. Supplementation of these vitamins has reduced the incidence of hyperhomocysteinemia in the United States; however, the clinical cardiovascular benefit of normalizing elevated homocysteine levels remains unproven.

OBESITY

Severe obesity, especially abdominal obesity, is associated with an increase in cardiovascular morbidity and mortality. Although obesity itself is not considered a disease, it is associated with an increased prevalence of hypertension, glucose intolerance, and atherosclerotic CAD. In addition, obese patients have a distinct cardiovascular abnormality characterized by increased total and central blood volumes, cardiac output, and left ventricular filling pressure. The elevated cardiac output appears to be required to support the metabolic needs of the excess adipose tissue. Left ventricular filling pressure is often at the upper limits of normal at rest and rises excessively with exercise. As a result of chronic volume overload, eccentric cardiac hypertrophy with cardiac dilatation and ventricular dysfunction may develop. Pathologically, there are left and, in some cases, right ventricular hypertrophy and generalized cardiac dilatation. Pulmonary congestion, peripheral edema, and exercise intolerance may all ensue; however, the recognition of these findings may be difficult in massively obese patients.

Weight reduction is the most effective therapy and results in reduction in blood volume and in the return of cardiac output toward normal. However, rapid weight reduction may be dangerous, as cardiac arrhythmias and sudden death owing to electrolyte imbalance have been described. Treatment with angiotensin-converting enzyme inhibitors, sodium restriction, and diuretics may be useful to control heart failure symptoms. This form of heart disease should be distinguished from the Pickwickian syndrome, which may share several of the cardiovascular features of heart disease secondary to severe obesity but, in addition, frequently has components of central apnea, hypoxemia, pulmonary hypertension, and cor pulmonale.

THYROID DISEASE

Thyroid hormone exerts a major influence on the cardiovascular system by a number of direct and indirect mechanisms and, not surprisingly, cardiovascular effects are prominent in both hypo- and hyperthyroidism. Thyroid hormone causes increases in total-body metabolism and oxygen consumption that indirectly increase the cardiac workload. In addition, thyroid hormone exerts direct inotropic, chronotropic, and dromotropic effects that are similar to those seen with adrenergic stimulation (e.g., tachycardia, increased cardiac output); they are mediated at least partly by both transcriptional and non-transcriptional effects of thyroid hormone on myosin, calcium-activated ATPase, Na$^+$,K$^+$-ATPase, and myocardial β-adrenergic receptors.

Hyperthyroidism

Common cardiovascular manifestations of hyperthyroidism include palpitations, systolic hypertension, and fatigue. Sinus tachycardia is present in ~40% of patients and atrial fibrillation in ~15%. Physical examination may reveal a hyperdynamic precordium, a widened pulse pressure, increases in the intensity of the first heart sound and the pulmonic component of the second heart sound, and a third heart sound. An increased incidence of mitral valve prolapse has been described in hyperthyroid patients, in which case a midsystolic murmur may be heard at the left sternal border with or without a systolic ejection click. A systolic pleuropericardial friction rub (*Means-Lerman scratch*) may be heard at the left second intercostal space during expiration and is thought to result from the hyperdynamic cardiac motion.

Elderly patients with hyperthyroidism may present with only cardiovascular manifestations of thyrotoxicosis, such as sinus tachycardia, atrial fibrillation, and hypertension, all of which may be resistant to therapy until the hyperthyroidism is controlled. Angina pectoris and CHF are unusual with hyperthyroidism unless there is coexistent heart disease; in such cases, symptoms often resolve with treatment of the hyperthyroidism.

Hypothyroidism

Cardiac manifestations of hypothyroidism include a reduction in cardiac output, stroke volume, heart rate, blood pressure, and pulse pressure. Pericardial effusions are present in about one-third of patients, rarely progress to tamponade, and likely result from increased capillary permeability. Other clinical signs include cardiomegaly, bradycardia, weak arterial pulses, distant heart sounds, and pleural effusions. Although the signs and symptoms of myxedema may mimic those of CHF, in the absence of other cardiac disease, myocardial failure is uncommon. The ECG generally reveals sinus bradycardia and low voltage, and may show prolongation of the QT interval, decreased P-wave voltage, prolonged AV conduction time, intraventricular conduction disturbances, and nonspecific ST-T wave abnormalities. Chest x-ray may show cardiomegaly, often with a "water bottle" configuration, pleural effusions, and, in some cases, evidence of CHF. Pathologically, the heart is pale and dilated, and often demonstrates myofibrillar swelling, loss of striations, and interstitial fibrosis.

Patients with hypothyroidism frequently have elevations of cholesterol and triglycerides, resulting in premature atherosclerotic CAD. Before treatment with thyroid hormone, patients with hypothyroidism frequently do not have angina pectoris, presumably because of the low metabolic demands caused by their condition. However, angina and MI may be precipitated during initiation of thyroid hormone replacement, especially in elderly patients with underlying heart disease. Therefore, replacement should be done with care, starting with low doses that are increased gradually.

MALIGNANT CARCINOID

Carcinoid tumors most often originate in the small bowel and elaborate a variety of vasoactive amines (e.g., serotonin), kinins, indoles, and prostaglandins that are believed to be responsible for the diarrhea, flushing, and labile blood pressure that characterize the carcinoid syndrome. Some 50% of patients with carcinoid syndrome have cardiac involvement, usually manifesting as abnormalities of the right-sided cardiac structures. These patients invariably have hepatic metastases allowing vasoactive substances to circumvent hepatic metabolism. Left-sided cardiac involvement is rare and indicates either pulmonary carcinoid or an intracardiac shunt. Pathologically, carcinoid lesions are fibrous plaques that consist of smooth-muscle cells embedded in a stroma of glycosaminoglycans and collagen. They occur on the cardiac valves where they cause valvular dysfunction, as well as on the endothelium of the cardiac chambers and great vessels.

Carcinoid heart disease most often presents as tricuspid regurgitation, pulmonic stenosis, or both. In some cases a high cardiac output state may occur, presumably as a result of a decrease in systemic vascular resistance resulting from vasoactive substances released by the tumor. Treatment with somatostatin analogues (e.g., octreotide) or interferon-α improves symptoms and survival in patients with carcinoid heart disease but does not appear to improve valvular abnormalities. In some severely symptomatic patients, valve replacement is indicated. Coronary artery spasm, presumably due to a circulating vasoactive substance, may occur in patients with carcinoid syndrome.

PHEOCHROMOCYTOMA

In addition to causing labile or sustained hypertension, the high circulating levels of catecholamines resulting from a pheochromocytoma may also cause direct myocardial injury. Focal myocardial necrosis and inflammatory cell infiltration are present in ~50% of patients who die with pheochromocytoma and may contribute to clinically significant left ventricular failure and pulmonary edema. In addition, associated hypertension results in left ventricular hypertrophy. Left ventricular dysfunction and CHF may resolve after removal of the tumor.

ACROMEGALY

Exposure of the heart to excessive growth hormone may cause CHF as a result of high cardiac output, diastolic dysfunction owing to ventricular hypertrophy (with increased left ventricular chamber size or wall thickness), or global systolic dysfunction. Hypertension occurs in up to one-third of patients with acromegaly and is characterized by suppression of the renin-angiotensin-aldosterone axis and increases in total-body sodium and plasma volume. Some form of cardiac disease occurs in about one-third of patients with acromegaly and is associated with a doubling of the risk of cardiac death.

RHEUMATOID ARTHRITIS AND THE COLLAGEN VASCULAR DISEASES

Rheumatoid Arthritis

Rheumatoid arthritis may be associated with inflammatory changes in any or all cardiac structures, although pericarditis is the most common clinical entity. Pericardial effusions may be found echocardiographically in 10–50% of patients with rheumatoid arthritis, particularly those with subcutaneous nodules. Nonetheless, only a small percentage of these patients have symptomatic pericarditis and, when present, it usually follows a benign course, only occasionally progressing to cardiac tamponade or constrictive pericarditis. The pericardial fluid is generally exudative, with decreased concentrations of complement and glucose and elevated cholesterol. Coronary arteritis with intimal inflammation and edema is present in ~20% of cases but only rarely results in angina pectoris or MI. Inflammation and granuloma formation may affect the cardiac valves, most often the mitral and aortic, and may cause clinically significant regurgitation owing to valve deformity. Myocarditis is uncommon and rarely results in cardiac dysfunction.

Treatment is directed at the underlying rheumatoid arthritis and may include glucocorticoids. Urgent pericardiocentesis should be performed in patients with tamponade, whereas pericardiectomy is usually required in cases of pericardial constriction.

Seronegative Arthropathies

The seronegative arthropathies, including ankylosing spondylitis, reactive arthritis, psoriatic arthritis, and the arthritides associated with ulcerative colitis and regional enteritis, are all strongly associated with the HLA-B27 histocompatibility antigen and may be accompanied by a pancarditis and proximal aortitis. The aortic inflammation is usually limited to the aortic root but may extend to involve the aortic valve, mitral valve, and ventricular myocardium, resulting in aortic and mitral regurgitation, conduction abnormalities, and ventricular dysfunction. One-tenth of patients have significant aortic insufficiency and one-third have conduction disturbances; both are more common in patients with peripheral joint involvement and long-standing disease. Treatment with aortic valve replacement and permanent pacemaker placement may be required. Occasionally, aortic regurgitation precedes the onset of arthritis, and, therefore, the diagnosis of a seronegative arthritis should be considered in young males with isolated aortic regurgitation.

Systemic Lupus Erythematosus (SLE)

A significant percentage of patients with SLE have cardiac involvement. Pericarditis is common, occurring in about two-thirds of patients, and generally follows a benign course, although rarely tamponade or constriction may result. The characteristic endocardial lesions of SLE are verrucous valvular abnormalities, known as *Libman Sacks endocarditis*. They are most often located on the left-sided cardiac valves, particularly on the ventricular surface of the posterior mitral leaflet, and are made up almost entirely of fibrin. The lesions may embolize or become infected but rarely cause hemodynamically important valvular regurgitation. Myocarditis generally parallels the activity of the disease and, although common histologically, seldom results in clinical heart failure unless associated with hypertension. While arteritis of epicardial coronary arteries may occur, it rarely results in myocardial ischemia. There is, however, an increased incidence of coronary atherosclerosis that likely is related more to associated risk factors and glucocorticoid use than to SLE itself. Patients with the antiphospholipid antibody syndrome may have a higher incidence of cardiovascular abnormalities, including valvular regurgitation, venous and arterial thrombosis, premature stroke, MI, pulmonary hypertension, and cardiomyopathy.

FURTHER READINGS

BRUCE IN: "Not only . . . but also": Factors that contribute to accelerated atherosclerosis and premature coronary artery disease in systemic lupus erythematosus. Rheumatology 44:1492, 2005

FOX DJ, KHATTAR RS: Carcinoid heart disease: Presentation, diagnosis, and management. Heart 90:1224, 2004

GRUNDY SM et al: Prevention Conference VI: Diabetes and cardiovascular disease, executive summary. Circulation 105:2231, 2002

HOFFMAN GS: Rheumatic diseases and the heart, in *Braunwald's Heart Disease*, 7th ed, DP Zipes et al (eds). Philadelphia, Saunders, 2005

KENCHAIAH S et al: Obesity and the risk of heart failure. N Engl J Med 347:305, 2002

KLEIN I, OJAMAA K: Thyroid hormone and the cardiovascular system. N Engl J Med 344:501, 2001

CHAPTER 25

INFECTIVE ENDOCARDITIS

Adolf W. Karchmer

The prototypic lesion of infective endocarditis, the *vegetation* (Fig. 25-1), is a mass of platelets, fibrin, microcolonies of microorganisms, and scant inflammatory cells. Infection most commonly involves heart valves (either native or prosthetic) but may also occur on the low-pressure side of the ventricular septum at the site of a defect, on the mural endocardium where it is damaged by aberrant jets of blood or foreign bodies, or on intracardiac devices themselves. The analogous process involving arteriovenous shunts, arterioarterial shunts (patent ductus arteriosus), or a coarctation of the aorta is called *infective endarteritis*.

Endocarditis may be classified according to the temporal evolution of disease, the site of infection, the cause of infection, or a predisposing risk factor such as injection drug use. Although each classification criterion provides therapeutic and prognostic insight, none is sufficient alone. *Acute endocarditis* is a hectically febrile illness that rapidly damages cardiac structures, hematogenously seeds extracardiac sites, and, if untreated, progresses to death within weeks. *Subacute endocarditis* follows an indolent course; causes structural cardiac damage only slowly, if at all; rarely metastasizes; and is gradually progressive unless complicated by a major embolic event or ruptured mycotic aneurysm.

In developed countries, the incidence of endocarditis ranges from 2.6–7.0 cases per 100,000 population per year and remained relatively stable from 1950–2000. While rates of congenital heart diseases remain constant, other predisposing conditions in developed countries have shifted from chronic rheumatic heart disease to illicit IV drug use, degenerative valve disease, intracardiac devices, and health care–associated infection. The incidence of endocarditis is notably increased among the elderly. In reported series, 10–30% of endocarditis cases involve prosthetic valves. The risk of prosthesis infection is greatest during the first 6 months after valve replacement; gradually declines to a low, stable rate thereafter; and is similar for mechanical and bioprosthetic devices.

ETIOLOGY

Although many species of bacteria and fungi cause sporadic episodes of endocarditis, only a few bacterial species cause the majority of cases (Table 25-1). The pathogens vary somewhat with the clinical types of endocarditis, in part because of different portals of entry. The oral cavity, skin, and upper respiratory tract are the respective primary portals for the viridans streptococci, staphylococci, and HACEK organisms (*Haemophilus*, *Actinobacillus*, *Cardiobacterium*, *Eikenella*, and *Kingella*) causing community-acquired native valve endocarditis. *Streptococcus bovis* originates from the gastrointestinal tract, where it is associated with polyps and colonic tumors, and enterococci enter the bloodstream from the genitourinary tract. Health care–associated native valve endocarditis is the consequence of bacteremia arising from intravascular catheter infections, nosocomial wound and urinary tract infections, and chronic invasive procedures such as hemodialysis. Endocarditis complicates

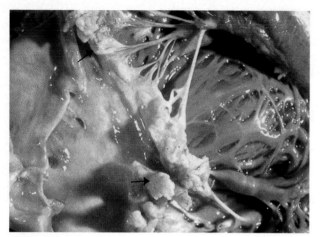

FIGURE 25-1

Vegetations (*arrows*) due to viridans streptococcal endocarditis involving the mitral valve.

6–25% of episodes of catheter-associated *Staphylococcus aureus* bacteremia; the higher rates are detected by careful transesophageal echocardiography (TEE) screening (see Echocardiography later in the chapter).

Prosthetic valve endocarditis arising within 2 months of valve surgery is generally the result of intraoperative contamination of the prosthesis or a bacteremic postoperative complication. The nosocomial nature of these infections is reflected in their primary microbial causes: coagulase-negative staphylococci (CoNS), *S. aureus*, facultative gram-negative bacilli, diphtheroids, and fungi. The portals of entry and organisms causing cases beginning >12 months after surgery are similar to those in community-acquired native valve endocarditis. Epidemiologic evidence suggests that prosthetic valve endocarditis due to CoNS that presents 2–12 months after surgery often represents delayed-onset nosocomial infection. At least 85% of CoNS strains that cause prosthetic valve endocarditis within 12 months of surgery are methicillin-resistant; the rate of methicillin resistance decreases to 25% among CoNS strains causing prosthetic valve endocarditis that presents >1 year after valve surgery.

Transvenous pacemaker lead– and/or implanted defibrillator–associated endocarditis is usually nosocomial. The majority of episodes occur within weeks of implantation or generator change and are caused by *S. aureus* or CoNS.

TABLE 25-1

ORGANISMS CAUSING MAJOR CLINICAL FORMS OF ENDOCARDITIS

	PERCENT OF CASES							
	NATIVE VALVE ENDOCARDITIS		PROSTHETIC VALVE ENDOCARDITIS AT INDICATED TIME OF ONSET (MONTHS) AFTER VALVE SURGERY			ENDOCARDITIS IN INJECTION DRUG USERS		
ORGANISM	COMMUNITY-ACQUIRED (*n* = 683)	HEALTH CARE–ASSOCIATED (*n* = 128)	<2 (*n* = 144)	2–12 (*n* = 31)	>12 (*n* = 194)	RIGHT-SIDED (*n* = 346)	LEFT-SIDED (*n* = 204)	TOTAL (*n* = 675)[a]
Streptococci[b]	32	8	1	9	31	5	15	12
Pneumococci	1	—	—	—	—	—	—	—
Enterococci	8	16	8	12	11	2	24	9
Staphylococcus aureus	35	44[c]	22	12	18	77	23	57
Coagulase-negative staphylococci	4	15	33	32	11	—	—	—
Fastidious gram-negative coccobacilli (HACEK group)[d]	3	—	—	—	6	—	—	—
Gram-negative bacilli	3	5	13	3	6	5	13	7
Candida spp.	1	6	8	12	1	—	12	4
Polymicrobial/ miscellaneous	6	1	3	6	5	8	10	7
Diphtheroids	—	—	6	—	3	—	—	0.1
Culture-negative	5	5	5	6	8	3	3	3

[a]The total number of cases is larger than the sum of right- and left-sided cases because the location of infection was not specified in some cases.
[b]Includes viridans streptococci; *Streptococcus bovis;* other non–group A, groupable streptococci; and *Abiotrophia* spp. (nutritionally variant, pyridoxal-requiring streptococci).
[c]Methicillin resistance is common among these *S. aureus* strains.
[d]Includes *Haemophilus* spp., *Actinobacillus actinomycetemcomitans, Cardiobacterium hominis, Eikenella* spp., and *Kingella* spp.
Source: Data are compiled from multiple studies.

Endocarditis occurring among injection drug users, especially when infection involves the tricuspid valve, is commonly caused by *S. aureus* strains, many of which are methicillin-resistant. Left-sided valve infections in addicts have a more varied etiology and involve abnormal valves, often ones damaged by prior episodes of endocarditis. A number of these cases are caused by *Pseudomonas aeruginosa* and *Candida* species, and sporadic cases are due to unusual organisms such as *Bacillus*, *Lactobacillus*, and *Corynebacterium* species. Polymicrobial endocarditis is more common among injection drug users than among patients who do not inject drugs. The presence of HIV in the former population does not significantly influence the causes of endocarditis.

From 5–15% of patients with endocarditis have negative blood cultures; in one-third to one-half of these cases, cultures are negative because of prior antibiotic exposure. The remainder of these patients are infected by fastidious organisms, such as nutritionally variant organisms (now designated *Granulicatella* and *Abiotrophia* species), HACEK organisms, and *Bartonella* species. Some fastidious organisms that cause endocarditis do so in characteristic epidemiologic settings (e.g., *Coxiella burnetii* in Europe, *Brucella* species in the Middle East). *Tropheryma whipplei* causes an indolent, culture-negative, afebrile form of endocarditis.

PATHOGENESIS

Unless it is injured, the endothelium is resistant to infection by most bacteria and to thrombus formation. Endothelial injury (e.g., at the site of impact of high-velocity blood jets or on the low-pressure side of a cardiac structural lesion) causes aberrant flow and allows either direct infection by virulent organisms or the development of an uninfected platelet-fibrin thrombus—a condition called *nonbacterial thrombotic endocarditis* (NBTE). The thrombus subsequently serves as a site of bacterial attachment during transient bacteremia. The cardiac conditions most commonly resulting in NBTE are mitral regurgitation, aortic stenosis, aortic regurgitation, ventricular septal defects, and complex congenital heart disease. These conditions result from rheumatic heart disease (particularly in the developing world, where rheumatic fever remains prevalent), mitral valve prolapse, degenerative heart disease, and congenital malformations. NBTE also arises as a result of a hypercoagulable state; this phenomenon gives rise to the clinical entity of *marantic endocarditis* (uninfected vegetations seen in patients with malignancy and chronic diseases) and to bland vegetations complicating systemic lupus erythematosus and the antiphospholipid antibody syndrome.

Organisms that cause endocarditis generally enter the bloodstream from mucosal surfaces, the skin, or sites of focal infection. Except for more virulent bacteria (e.g., *S. aureus*) that can adhere directly to intact endothelium or exposed subendothelial tissue, microorganisms in the blood adhere to sites at NBTE. If resistant to the bactericidal activity of serum and the microbicidal peptides released locally by platelets, the organisms proliferate and induce a procoagulant state at the site by eliciting tissue factor from adherent monocytes or, in the case of *S. aureus*, from monocytes and from intact endothelium. Fibrin deposition combines with platelet aggregation, stimulated by tissue factor and independently by proliferating microorganisms, to generate an infected vegetation. The organisms that commonly cause endocarditis have surface adhesin molecules, collectively called microbial surface components recognizing adhesin matrix molecules (MSCRAMMs) that mediate adherence to NBTE sites or injured endothelium. Fibronectin-binding proteins present on many gram-positive bacteria, clumping factor (a fibrinogen- and fibrin-binding surface protein) on *S. aureus*, and glucans or FimA (a member of the family of oral mucosal adhesins) on streptococci facilitate adherence. Fibronectin-binding proteins are required for *S. aureus* invasion of intact endothelium; thus these surface proteins may facilitate infection of previously normal valves. In the absence of host defenses, organisms enmeshed in the growing platelet-fibrin vegetation proliferate to form dense microcolonies. Organisms deep in vegetations are metabolically inactive (nongrowing) and relatively resistant to killing by antimicrobial agents. Proliferating surface organisms are shed into the bloodstream continuously.

The pathophysiologic consequences and clinical manifestations of endocarditis—other than constitutional symptoms, which probably result from cytokine production—arise from damage to intracardiac structures; embolization of vegetation fragments, leading to infection or infarction of remote tissues; hematogenous infection of sites during bacteremia; and tissue injury due to the deposition of circulating immune complexes or immune responses to deposited bacterial antigens.

CLINICAL MANIFESTATIONS

The clinical syndrome of infective endocarditis is highly variable and spans a continuum between acute and subacute presentations. Native valve endocarditis (whether acquired in the community or in association with health care), prosthetic valve endocarditis, and endocarditis due to injection drug use share clinical and laboratory manifestations (Table 25-2). The causative microorganism is primarily responsible for the temporal course of endocarditis. β-Hemolytic streptococci, *S. aureus*, and pneumococci typically result in an acute course, although *S. aureus* occasionally causes subacute disease. Endocarditis caused by *Staphylococcus lugdunensis* (a coagulase-negative species) or by enterococci may present acutely. Subacute endocarditis is typically caused by viridans streptococci, enterococci, CoNS, and the HACEK group. Endocarditis

TABLE 25-2

CLINICAL AND LABORATORY FEATURES OF INFECTIVE ENDOCARDITIS

FEATURE	FREQUENCY, %
Fever	80–90
Chills and sweats	40–75
Anorexia, weight loss, malaise	25–50
Myalgias, arthralgias	15–30
Back pain	7–15
Heart murmur	80–85
New/worsened regurgitant murmur	10–40
Arterial emboli	20–50
Splenomegaly	15–50
Clubbing	10–20
Neurologic manifestations	20–40
Peripheral manifestations (Osler's nodes, subungual hemorrhages, Janeway lesions, Roth's spots)	2–15
Petechiae	10–40
Laboratory manifestations	
Anemia	70–90
Leukocytosis	20–30
Microscopic hematuria	30–50
Elevated erythrocyte sedimentation rate	>90
Elevated C-reactive protein level	>90
Rheumatoid factor	50
Circulating immune complexes	65–100
Decreased serum complement	5–40

caused by *Bartonella* species and the agent of Q fever, *C. burnetii*, is exceptionally indolent.

The clinical features of endocarditis are nonspecific. However, these symptoms in a febrile patient with valvular abnormalities or a behavior pattern that predisposes to endocarditis (e.g., injection drug use) suggest the diagnosis, as do bacteremia with organisms that frequently cause endocarditis, otherwise-unexplained arterial emboli, and progressive cardiac valvular incompetence. In patients with subacute presentations, fever is typically low-grade and rarely exceeds 39.4°C (103°F); in contrast, temperatures of 39.4°–40°C (103°–104°F) are often noted in acute endocarditis. Fever may be blunted or absent in patients who are elderly or severely debilitated or who have marked cardiac or renal failure.

Cardiac Manifestations

Although heart murmurs are usually indicative of the predisposing cardiac pathology rather than of endocarditis, valvular damage and ruptured chordae may result in new regurgitant murmurs. In acute endocarditis involving a normal valve, murmurs are heard on presentation in only 30–45% of patients but ultimately are detected in 85%. Congestive heart failure develops in 30–40% of patients; it is usually a consequence of valvular dysfunction

but occasionally is due to endocarditis-associated myocarditis or an intracardiac fistula. Heart failure due to aortic valve dysfunction progresses more rapidly than does that due to mitral valve dysfunction. Extension of infection beyond valve leaflets into adjacent annular or myocardial tissue results in perivalvular abscesses, which in turn may cause fistulae (from the root of the aorta into cardiac chambers or between cardiac chambers) with new murmurs. Abscesses may burrow from the aortic valve annulus through the epicardium, causing pericarditis. Extension of infection into paravalvular tissue adjacent to either the right or the noncoronary cusp of the aortic valve may interrupt the conduction system in the upper interventricular septum, leading to varying degrees of heart block. Although perivalvular abscesses arising from the mitral valve may potentially interrupt conduction pathways near the atrioventricular node or in the proximal bundle of His, such interruption occurs infrequently. Emboli to a coronary artery may result in myocardial infarction; nevertheless, embolic transmural infarcts are rare.

Noncardiac Manifestations

The classic nonsuppurative peripheral manifestations of subacute endocarditis are related to the duration of infection and, with early diagnosis and treatment, have become infrequent. In contrast, septic embolization mimicking some of these lesions (subungual hemorrhage, Osler's nodes) is common in patients with acute *S. aureus* endocarditis (Fig. 25-2). Musculoskeletal symptoms, including nonspecific inflammatory arthritis and back pain, usually remit promptly with treatment but must be distinguished from focal metastatic infection. Hematogenously seeded focal infection may involve any organ but most often is

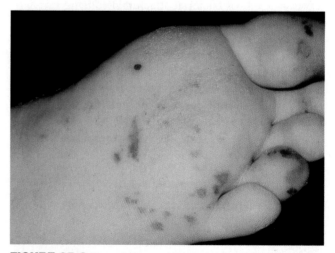

FIGURE 25-2

Septic emboli with hemorrhage and infarction due to acute *Staphylococcus aureus* endocarditis. *(Used with permission of L. Baden.)*

clinically evident in the skin, spleen, kidneys, skeletal system, and meninges. Arterial emboli are clinically apparent in up to 50% of patients. Vegetations >10 mm in diameter (as measured by echocardiography) and those located on the mitral valve are more likely to embolize than are smaller or nonmitral vegetations. Embolic events—often with infarction—involving the extremities, spleen, kidneys, bowel, or brain are often noted at presentation. With effective antibiotic treatment, the frequency of embolic events decreases from 13 per 1000 patient-days during the initial week to 1.2 per 1000 patient-days after the third week. Emboli occurring late during or after effective therapy do not in themselves constitute evidence of failed antimicrobial treatment. Neurologic symptoms, most often resulting from embolic strokes, occur in up to 40% of patients. Other neurologic complications include aseptic or purulent meningitis, intracranial hemorrhage due to hemorrhagic infarcts or ruptured mycotic aneurysms, seizures, and encephalopathy. (*Mycotic aneurysms* are focal dilations of arteries occurring at points in the artery wall that have been weakened by infection in the vasa vasorum or where septic emboli have lodged.) Microabscesses in brain and meninges occur commonly in *S. aureus* endocarditis; surgically drainable intracerebral abscesses are infrequent.

Immune complex deposition on the glomerular basement membrane causes diffuse hypocomplementemic glomerulonephritis and renal dysfunction, which typically improve with effective antimicrobial therapy. Embolic renal infarcts cause flank pain and hematuria but rarely cause renal dysfunction.

Manifestations of Specific Predisposing Conditions

In almost 50% of patients who have endocarditis associated with injection drug use, infection is limited to the tricuspid valve. These patients present with fever, faint or no murmur, and (in 75% of cases) prominent pulmonary findings related to septic emboli, including cough, pleuritic chest pain, nodular pulmonary infiltrates, and occasionally pyopneumothorax. Infection involving valves on the left side of the heart presents with the typical clinical features of endocarditis.

Health care–associated endocarditis (defined as that which is nosocomial, arises after recent hospitalization, or is a direct consequence of long-term indwelling devices) has typical manifestations if it is not associated with a retained intracardiac device. Endocarditis associated with flow-directed pulmonary artery catheters is often cryptic, with symptoms masked by comorbid critical illness, and is commonly diagnosed at autopsy. Transvenous pacemaker lead– and/or implanted defibrillator–associated endocarditis may be associated with obvious or cryptic generator pocket infection and results in fever, minimal murmur, and pulmonary symptoms due to septic emboli.

Late-onset prosthetic valve endocarditis presents with typical clinical features. Cases arising within 60 days of valve surgery (early onset) lack peripheral vascular manifestations, and typical symptoms may be obscured by comorbidity associated with recent surgery. In both early-onset and more delayed presentations, paravalvular infection is common and often results in partial valve dehiscence, regurgitant murmurs, congestive heart failure, or disruption of the conduction system.

DIAGNOSIS

The Duke Criteria

The diagnosis of infective endocarditis is established with certainty only when vegetations obtained at cardiac surgery, at autopsy, or from an artery (an embolus) are examined histologically and microbiologically. Nevertheless, a highly sensitive and specific diagnostic schema— known as the *Duke criteria*—has been developed on the basis of clinical, laboratory, and echocardiographic findings (**Table 25-3**). Documentation of two major criteria, of one major and three minor criteria, or of five minor criteria allows a clinical diagnosis of definite endocarditis. The diagnosis of endocarditis is rejected if an alternative diagnosis is established, if symptoms resolve and do not recur with ≤4 days of antibiotic therapy, or if surgery or autopsy after ≤4 days of antimicrobial therapy yields no histologic evidence of endocarditis. Illnesses not classified as definite endocarditis or rejected are considered cases of possible infective endocarditis when either one major and one minor criterion or three minor criteria are identified. Requiring the identification of clinical features of endocarditis for classification as possible infective endocarditis increases the specificity of the schema without significantly reducing its sensitivity.

The roles of bacteremia and echocardiographic findings in the diagnosis of endocarditis are appropriately emphasized in the Duke criteria. The requirement for multiple positive blood cultures over time is consistent with the continuous low-density bacteremia characteristic of endocarditis (≤100 organisms/mL). Among patients with untreated endocarditis who ultimately have a positive blood culture, 95% of all blood cultures are positive; in 98% of these cases, one of the initial two sets of cultures yields the microorganism. The diagnostic criteria attach significance to the species of organism isolated from blood cultures. To fulfill a major criterion, the isolation of an organism that causes both endocarditis and bacteremia in the absence of endocarditis (e.g., *S. aureus*, enterococci) must take place repeatedly (i.e., persistent bacteremia) and in the absence of a primary focus of infection. Organisms that rarely cause endocarditis but commonly contaminate blood cultures (e.g., diphtheroids, CoNS) must be isolated repeatedly if their isolation is to serve as a major criterion.

TABLE 25-3

THE DUKE CRITERIA FOR THE CLINICAL DIAGNOSIS OF INFECTIVE ENDOCARDITIS

Major Criteria

1. Positive blood culture
   Typical microorganism for infective endocarditis from two separate blood cultures
   Viridans streptococci, *Streptococcus bovis*, HACEK group, *Staphylococcus aureus*, or
   Community-acquired enterococci in the absence of a primary focus, *or*
   Persistently positive blood culture, defined as recovery of a microorganism consistent with infective endocarditis from:
   Blood cultures drawn >12 h apart; *or*
   All of three or a majority of four or more separate blood cultures, with first and last drawn at least 1 h apart
   Single positive blood culture for *Coxiella burnetii* or phase I IgG antibody titer of >1:800
2. Evidence of endocardial involvement
   Positive echocardiogram[a]
   Oscillating intracardiac mass on valve or supporting structures or in the path of regurgitant jets or in implanted material, in the absence of an alternative anatomic explanation, *or*
   Abscess, *or*
   New partial dehiscence of prosthetic valve, *or*
   New valvular regurgitation (increase or change in preexisting murmur not sufficient)

Minor Criteria

1. Predisposition: predisposing heart condition or injection drug use
2. Fever ≥38.0°C (≥100.4°F)
3. Vascular phenomena: major arterial emboli, septic pulmonary infarcts, mycotic aneurysm, intracranial hemorrhage, conjunctival hemorrhages, Janeway lesions
4. Immunologic phenomena: glomerulonephritis, Osler's nodes, Roth's spots, rheumatoid factor
5. Microbiologic evidence: positive blood culture but not meeting major criterion as noted previously[b] or serologic evidence of active infection with organism consistent with infective endocarditis

[a]Transesophageal echocardiography is recommended for assessing possible prosthetic valve endocarditis or complicated endocarditis.
[b]Excluding single positive cultures for coagulase-negative staphylococci and diphtheroids, which are common culture contaminants, and organisms that do not cause endocarditis frequently, such as gram-negative bacilli.
Note: HACEK, *Haemophilus* spp., *Actinobacillus actinomycetemcomitans, Cardiobacterium hominis, Eikenella corrodens, Kingella* species.
Source: Adapted from Li et al., with permission from the University of Chicago Press.

Blood Cultures

Isolation of the causative microorganism from blood cultures is critical not only for diagnosis but also for determination of antimicrobial susceptibility and planning of treatment. In the absence of prior antibiotic therapy, three blood culture sets (with two bottles per set), separated from each other by at least 1 h, should be obtained from different venipuncture sites over 24 h. If the cultures remain negative after 48–72 h, two or three additional blood culture sets should be obtained, and the laboratory should be consulted for advice regarding optimal culture techniques. Empirical antimicrobial therapy should not be administered initially to hemodynamically stable patients with subacute endocarditis, especially those who have received antibiotics within the preceding 2 weeks; thus, if necessary, additional blood culture sets can be obtained without the confounding effect of empirical treatment. Patients with acute endocarditis or with deteriorating hemodynamics who may require urgent surgery should be treated empirically immediately after three sets of blood cultures are obtained over several hours.

Non-Blood-Culture Tests

Serologic tests can be used to implicate causally some organisms that are difficult to recover by blood culture: *Brucella, Bartonella, Legionella,* and *C. burnetii.* Pathogens can also be identified in surgically recovered vegetations or emboli by culture, by microscopic examination with special stains (i.e., the periodic acid–Schiff stain for *T. whipplei*), and by use of polymerase chain reaction (PCR) to recover unique microbial DNA or 16S rRNA that, when sequenced, allows identification of organisms.

Echocardiography

Imaging with echocardiography allows anatomic confirmation of infective endocarditis, sizing of vegetations, detection of intracardiac complications, and assessment of cardiac function (**Fig. 25-3**). Transthoracic echocardiography (TTE) is noninvasive and exceptionally specific; however, it cannot image vegetations <2 mm in diameter, and in 20% of patients it is technically inadequate because of emphysema or body habitus. Thus, TTE detects vegetations in only 65% of patients with definite clinical endocarditis; i.e., it has a sensitivity of 65%. Moreover, TTE is not adequate for evaluating prosthetic valves or detecting intracardiac complications. TEE is safe and significantly more sensitive than TTE. It detects vegetations in >90% of patients with definite endocarditis; nevertheless, false-negative studies are noted in 6–18% of endocarditis patients. TEE is the optimal method for the diagnosis of prosthetic endocarditis or the detection of myocardial abscess, valve perforation, or intracardiac fistulae.

Experts favor echocardiographic evaluation of all patients with a clinical diagnosis of endocarditis; however, the test should not be used to screen patients with a low probability of endocarditis (e.g., patients with unexplained fever). An American Heart Association approach to the use of echocardiography for evaluation of patients with suspected endocarditis is illustrated in **Fig. 25-4**. A negative TEE when endocarditis is likely does not exclude the diagnosis but rather warrants repetition of the study in 7–10 days.

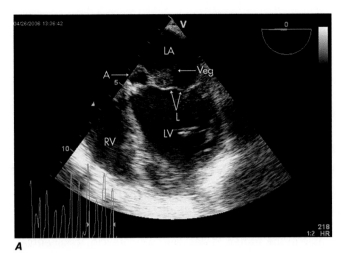

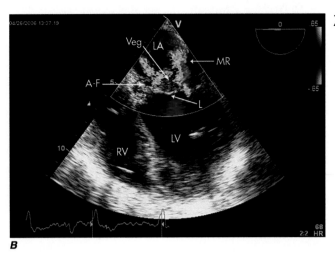

A

B

FIGURE 25-3

Imaging of a mitral valve infected with *Staphylococcus aureus* by low-esophageal four-chamber-view transesophageal echocardiography (TEE). **A.** Two-dimensional echocardiogram showing a large vegetation with an adjacent echolucent abscess cavity. **B.** Color-flow Doppler image showing severe mitral regurgitation through both the abscess-fistula and the central valve orifice. A, abscess; A-F, abscess-fistula; L, valve leaflets; LA, left atrium; LV, left ventricle; MR, mitral central valve regurgitation; RV, right ventricle; veg, vegetation. *(With permission of Andrew Burger, M.D.)*

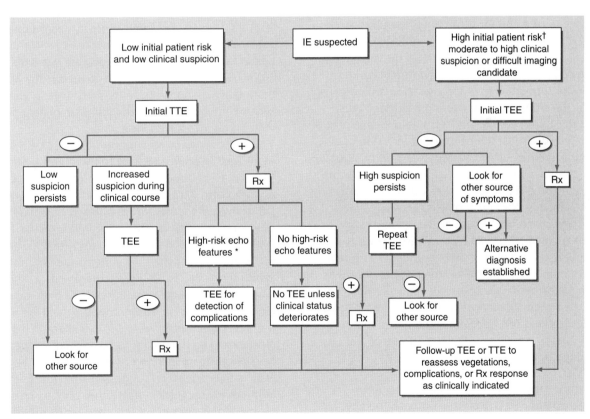

FIGURE 25-4

The diagnostic use of transesophageal and transtracheal echocardiography (TEE and TTE, respectively). †High initial patient risk for endocarditis as listed in Table 25-8 or evidence of intracardiac complications (new regurgitant murmur, new electrocardiographic conduction changes, or congestive heart failure). *High-risk echocardiographic features include large vegetations, valve insufficiency, paravalvular infection, or ventricular dysfunction. Rx indicates initiation of antibiotic therapy. *[Reproduced with permission from Diagnosis and Management of Infective Endocarditis and Its Complications (Circulation 1998; 98:2936-2948. © 1998 American Heart Association.)]*

Many laboratory studies that are not diagnostic—i.e., complete blood count, creatinine determination, liver function tests, chest radiography, and electrocardiography—are nevertheless important in the management of patients with endocarditis. The erythrocyte sedimentation rate, C-reactive protein level, and circulating immune complex titer are commonly increased in endocarditis (Table 25-2). Cardiac catheterization is useful primarily to assess coronary artery patency in older individuals who are to undergo surgery for endocarditis.

℞ Treatment: INFECTIVE ENDOCARDITIS

ANTIMICROBIAL THERAPY It is difficult to eradicate bacteria from the avascular vegetation in infective endocarditis because this site is relatively deficient in host defenses and because the largely nongrowing, metabolically inactive bacteria are less easily killed by antibiotics. To cure endocarditis, all bacteria in the vegetation must be killed; therefore, therapy must be bactericidal and prolonged. Antibiotics are generally given parenterally and must reach high serum concentrations that will, through passive diffusion, lead to effective concentrations in the depths of the vegetation. The choice of effective therapy requires precise knowledge of the susceptibility of the causative microorganisms. The decision to initiate treatment before a cause is defined must balance the need to establish a microbiologic diagnosis against the potential progression of disease or the need for urgent surgery (see Blood Cultures, earlier in the chapter). The individual vulnerabilities of the patient should be weighed in the selection of therapy—e.g., simultaneous infection at other sites (such as meningitis), allergies, end-organ dysfunction, interactions with concomitant medications, and risks of adverse events.

Although given for several weeks longer, the regimens recommended for the treatment of endocarditis involving prosthetic valves (except for staphylococcal infections) are similar to those used to treat native valve infection (Table 25-4). Recommended doses and durations of therapy should be adhered to unless alterations are required by adverse events.

Organism-Specific Therapies
Streptococci To select the optimal therapy for streptococcal endocarditis, the minimum inhibitory concentration (MIC) of penicillin for the causative isolate must be determined (Table 25-4). The 2-week penicillin/gentamicin or ceftriaxone/gentamicin regimens should not be used to treat complicated native valve infection or prosthetic valve endocarditis. The regimen

recommended for relatively penicillin-resistant streptococci is advocated for treatment of endocarditis caused by organisms of group B, C, or G. Endocarditis caused by nutritionally variant organisms (*Granulicatella* or *Abiotrophia* species) and *Gemella morbillorum* is treated with the regimen for moderately penicillin-resistant streptococci, as is prosthetic valve endocarditis caused by these organisms or by streptococci with a penicillin MIC of >0.1 μg/mL (Table 25-4).

Enterococci Enterococci are resistant to oxacillin, nafcillin, and the cephalosporins and are only inhibited—not killed—by penicillin, ampicillin, teicoplanin (not available in the United States), and vancomycin. To kill enterococci requires the synergistic interaction of a cell wall–active antibiotic (penicillin, ampicillin, vancomycin, or teicoplanin) that is effective at achievable serum concentrations and an aminoglycoside (gentamicin or streptomycin) to which the isolate does not exhibit high-level resistance. An isolate's resistance to cell wall–active agents or its ability to replicate in the presence of gentamicin at ≥500 μg/mL or streptomycin at 1000–2000 μg/mL—a phenomenon called *high-level aminoglycoside resistance*—indicates that the ineffective antimicrobial agent cannot participate in the interaction to produce killing. High-level resistance to gentamicin predicts that tobramycin, netilmicin, amikacin, and kanamycin also will be ineffective. In fact, even when enterococci are not highly resistant to gentamicin, it is difficult to predict the ability of these other aminoglycosides to participate in synergistic killing; consequently, they should not in general be used to treat enterococcal endocarditis.

Enterococci causing endocarditis must be tested for high-level resistance to streptomycin and gentamicin, β-lactamase production, and susceptibility to penicillin and ampicillin (MIC ≤16 μg/mL) and to vancomycin (MIC ≤8 μg/mL). If the isolate produces β-lactamase, ampicillin/sulbactam or vancomycin can be used as the cell wall–active component; if the penicillin/ampicillin MIC is >16 μg/mL, vancomycin can be considered; and if the vancomycin MIC is >8 μg/mL, penicillin or ampicillin may be considered. In the absence of high-level resistance, gentamicin or streptomycin should be used as the aminoglycoside (Table 25-4). If there is high-level resistance to both these drugs, no aminoglycoside should be given; instead, an 8- to 12-week course of a single cell wall–active agent is suggested—or, for *E. faecalis*, high doses of ampicillin plus either ceftriaxone or cefotaxime. If this alternative therapy fails or the isolate is resistant to all of the commonly used agents, surgical treatment is advised. The role of newer agents potentially active against multidrug-resistant enterococci [quinupristin/dalfopristin (*E. faecium* only), linezolid, and daptomycin] in the treatment of endocarditis has not been established. Although the dose of gentamicin

TABLE 25-4   283

ANTIBIOTIC TREATMENT FOR INFECTIVE ENDOCARDITIS CAUSED BY COMMON ORGANISMS[a]

ORGANISM	DRUG (DOSE, DURATION)	COMMENTS
Streptococci		
Penicillin-susceptible[b] streptococci, S. bovis	• Penicillin G (2–3 mU IV q4h for 4 weeks) • Ceftriaxone (2 g/d IV as a single dose for 4 weeks)	— Can use ceftriaxone in patients with nonimmediate penicillin allergy
	• Vancomycin[c] (15 mg/kg IV q12h for 4 weeks)	Use vancomycin in patients with severe or immediate β-lactam allergy
	• Penicillin G (2–3 mU IV q4h) or ceftriaxone (2 g IV qd) for 2 weeks plus gentamicin[d] (3 mg/kg qd IV or IM, as a single dose[e] or divided into equal doses q8h for 2 weeks)	Avoid 2-week regimen when risk of aminoglycoside toxicity is increased and in prosthetic valve or complicated endocarditis
Relatively penicillin-resistant[f] streptococci	• Penicillin G (4 mU IV q4h) or ceftriaxone(2 g IV qd) for 4 weeks plus gentamicin[d] (3 mg/kg qd IV or IM, as a single dose[e] or divided into equal doses q8h for 2 weeks)	Penicillin alone at this dose for 6 weeks or with gentamicin during initial 2 weeks preferred for prosthetic valve endocarditis caused by streptococci with penicillin MIC ≤ 0.1 µg/mL
	Vancomycin[c] as noted above for 4 weeks	—
Moderately penicillin-resistant[g] streptococci, nutritionally variant organisms, or Gemella morbillorum	• Penicillin G (4–5 mU IV q4h) or ceftriaxone (2 g IV qd) for 6 weeks plus gentamicin[d] (3 mg/kg qd IV or IM as a single dose[e] or divided into equal doses q8h for 6 weeks)	Preferred for prosthetic valve endocarditis caused by streptococci with penicillin MICs of >0.1 µg/mL
	• Vancomycin[c] as noted above for 4 weeks	—
Enterococci[h]		
	• Penicillin G (4–5 mU IV q4h) plus gentamicin[d] (1 mg/kg IV q8h), both for 4–6 weeks	Can use streptomycin (7.5 mg/kg q12h) in lieu of gentamicin if there is not high-level resistance to streptomycin
	• Ampicillin (2 g IV q4h) plus gentamicin[d] (1 mg/kg IV q8h), both for 4–6 weeks	—
	• Vancomycin[c] (15 mg/kg IVq12h) plus gentamicin[d] (1 mg/kg IV q8h), both for 4–6 weeks	Use vancomycin plus gentamicin for penicillin-allergic patients, or desensitize to penicillin
Staphylococci		
Methicillin-susceptible, infecting native valves (no foreign devices)	• Nafcillin or oxacillin (2 g IV q4h for 4–6 weeks) plus (optional) gentamicin[d] (1 mg/kg IM or IV q8h for 3–5 days)	Can use penicillin (4 mU q4h) if isolate is penicillin-susceptible (does not produce β-lactamase)
	• Cefazolin (2 g IV q8h for 4–6 weeks) plus (optional) gentamicin[d] (1 mg/kg IM or IV q8h for 3–5 days)	Can use cefazolin regimen for patients with nonimmediate penicillin allergy
	• Vancomycin[c] (15 mg/kg IV q12h for 4–6 weeks)	Use vancomycin for patients with immediate (urticarial) or severe penicillin allergy

CHAPTER 25 Infective Endocarditis

(Continued)

TABLE 25-4 (*CONTINUED*)

ANTIBIOTIC TREATMENT FOR INFECTIVE ENDOCARDITIS CAUSED BY COMMON ORGANISMS[a]

ORGANISM	DRUG (DOSE, DURATION)	COMMENTS
Streptococci		
Methicillin-resistant, infecting native valves (no foreign devices) Methicillin-susceptible, infecting prosthetic valves	• Vancomycin[c] (15 mg/kg IV q12h for 4–6 weeks) • Nafcillin or oxacillin (2 g IV q4h for 6–8 weeks) *plus* gentamicin[d] (1 mg/kg IM or IV q8h for 2 weeks) *plus* rifampin[i] (300 mg PO q8h for 6–8 weeks)	No role for routine use of rifampin Use gentamicin during initial 2 weeks; determine susceptibility to gentamicin before initiating rifampin (see text); if patient is highly allergic to penicillin, use regimen for methicillin-resistant staphylococci; if β-lactam allergy is of the minor, nonimmediate type, can substitute cefazolin for oxacillin/nafcillin
Methicillin-resistant, infecting prosthetic valves	• Vancomycin[c] (15 mg/kg IV q12h for 6–8 weeks) *plus* gentamicin[d] (1 mg/kg IM or IV q8h for 2 weeks) *plus* rifampin[i] (300 mg PO q8h for 6–8 weeks)	Use gentamicin during initial 2 weeks; determine gentamicin susceptibility before initiating rifampin (see text)
HACEK Organisms		
	• Ceftriaxone (2 g/d IV as a single dose for 4 weeks)	Can use another third-generation cephalosporin at comparable dosage
	• Ampicillin/sulbactam (3 g IV q6h for 4 weeks)	—

[a]Doses are for adults with normal renal function. Doses of gentamicin, streptomycin, and vancomycin must be adjusted for reduced renal function. Ideal body weight is used to calculate doses of gentamicin and streptomycin per kilogram (men = 50 kg + 2.3 kg per inch over 5 feet; women = 45.5 kg + 2.3 kg per inch over 5 feet).
[b]MIC, ≤0.1 g/mL.
[c]Desirable peak vancomycin level 1 h after completion of a 1-h infusion is 30–45 μg/mL.
[d]Aminoglycosides should not be administered as single daily doses for enterococcal endocarditis and should be introduced as part of the initial treatment. Target peak and trough serum concentrations of divided-dose gentamicin 1 h after a 20- to 30-min infusion or IM injection are ~3.5 μg/mL and ≤1 μg/mL, respectively; target peak and trough serum concentrations of streptomycin (timing as with gentamicin) are 20–35 μg/mL and <10 μg/mL, respectively.
[e]Netilmicin (4 mg/kg qd, as a single dose) can be used in lieu of gentamicin.
[f]MIC, >0.1 μg/mL and <0.5 μg/mL.
[g]MIC, >0.5 μg/mL and <8.0 μg/mL.
[h]Antimicrobial susceptibility must be evaluated; see text.
[i]Rifampin increases warfarin and dicumarol requirements for anticoagulation.

used to achieve bactericidal synergy in treating enterococcal endocarditis is smaller than that used in standard therapy, nephrotoxicity is not uncommon during treatment for 4–6 weeks. Regimens wherein the aminoglycoside component of treatment has been truncated at 2–3 weeks because of toxicity have been curative. Thus, discontinuation of the aminoglycoside

is recommended when toxicity develops in patients with enterococcal endocarditis who have responded satisfactorily to therapy.

Staphylococci The regimens used to treat staphylococcal endocarditis (Table 25-4) are based not on coagulase production but rather on the presence or absence of a prosthetic valve or foreign device, the native valve(s) involved, and the resistance of the isolate to penicillin and methicillin. Penicillinase is produced by 95% of staphylococci; thus, all isolates should be considered penicillin-resistant until shown not to produce this enzyme. Similarly, methicillin resistance has become so prevalent among staphylococci, including *S. aureus*, that therapy should be initiated with a regimen for methicillin-resistant organisms and subsequently revised if the strain proves to be susceptible to methicillin. The addition of gentamicin (if the isolate is susceptible) to a β-lactam antibiotic to enhance therapy for native mitral or aortic valve endocarditis is optional. Its addition hastens eradication of bacteremia but does not improve survival rates. If added, gentamicin should be limited to the initial 3–5 days of therapy to minimize nephrotoxicity. Gentamicin generally is not added to the vancomycin regimen in this setting. The efficacy of linezolid or daptomycin as an alternative to vancomycin for left-sided, methicillin-resistant *S. aureus* (MRSA) endocarditis has not been established.

Methicillin-susceptible *S. aureus* endocarditis that is uncomplicated and limited to the tricuspid or pulmonic valve—a condition occurring almost exclusively in injection drug users—can often be treated with a 2-week course that combines oxacillin or nafcillin (but not vancomycin) with gentamicin. Prolonged fevers (≥5 days) during therapy suggest that these patients should receive standard therapy. Right-sided endocarditis caused by MRSA is treated for 4 weeks with standard doses of vancomycin or daptomycin (6 mg/kg as a single daily dose).

Staphylococcal prosthetic valve endocarditis is treated for 6–8 weeks with a multidrug regimen. Rifampin is an essential component because it kills staphylococci that are adherent to foreign material. Two other agents (selected on the basis of susceptibility testing) are combined with rifampin to prevent in vivo emergence of resistance. Because many staphylococci (particularly MRSA and *S. epidermidis*) are resistant to gentamicin, the utility of gentamicin or an alternative agent should be established before rifampin treatment is begun. If the isolate is resistant to gentamicin, another aminoglycoside or a fluoroquinolone (chosen in light of susceptibility results) or another active agent should be substituted for gentamicin.

Other organisms In the absence of meningitis, endocarditis caused by *Streptococcus pneumoniae* with a penicillin MIC of ≤1.0 can be treated with IV penicillin (4 million units every 4 h), ceftriaxone (2 g/d as a single dose), or cefotaxime (at a comparable dosage). Infection caused by pneumococcal strains with a penicillin MIC of ≥2.0 should be treated with vancomycin. Until the strain's susceptibility to penicillin is established, therapy should consist of vancomycin plus ceftriaxone, especially if concurrent meningitis is suspected. *P. aeruginosa* endocarditis is treated with an antipseudomonal penicillin (ticarcillin or piperacillin) and high doses of tobramycin (8 mg/kg per day in three divided doses). Endocarditis caused by Enterobacteriaceae is treated with a potent β-lactam antibiotic plus an aminoglycoside. Corynebacterial endocarditis is treated with penicillin plus an aminoglycoside (if the organism is susceptible to the aminoglycoside) or with vancomycin, which is highly bactericidal for most strains. Therapy for *Candida* endocarditis consists of amphotericin B plus flucytosine and early surgery; long-term (if not indefinite) suppression with an oral azole is advised. Caspofungin treatment of *Candida* endocarditis has been effective in sporadic cases; nevertheless, the role of echinocandins in this setting has not been established.

Empirical Therapy In designing and executing therapy without culture data (i.e., before culture results are known or when cultures are negative), clinical and epidemiologic clues to etiology must be weighed, and both the pathogens associated with the specific endocarditis syndrome and the hazards of suboptimal therapy must be considered. Thus, empirical therapy for acute endocarditis in an injection drug user should cover MRSA and gram-negative bacilli. The initiation of treatment with vancomycin plus gentamicin immediately after blood is obtained for cultures covers these as well as many other potential causes. In the treatment of culture-negative episodes, marantic endocarditis must be excluded and fastidious organisms sought serologically. In the absence of confounding prior antibiotic therapy, it is unlikely that *S. aureus*, CoNS, or enterococcal infection will present with negative blood cultures. Thus, in this situation, these organisms are not the determinants of therapy for subacute endocarditis. Pending the availability of diagnostic data, blood culture–negative subacute native valve endocarditis is treated with ceftriaxone plus gentamicin; these two antimicrobial agents plus vancomycin should be used if prosthetic valves are involved.

Outpatient Antimicrobial Therapy Fully compliant patients who have sterile blood cultures, are afebrile during therapy, and have no clinical or echocardiographic findings that suggest an impending complication may complete therapy as outpatients. Careful follow-up and a stable home setting are necessary, as are predictable IV access and use of antimicrobial agents that are stable in solution.

Monitoring Antimicrobial Therapy The serum bactericidal titer—the highest dilution of the patient's serum during therapy that kills 99.9% of the standard inoculum of the infecting organism—is no longer recommended for assessment of standard regimens. However, in the treatment of endocarditis caused by unusual organisms, this measurement, although not standardized and difficult to interpret, may provide a patient-specific assessment of in vivo antibiotic effect. Serum concentrations of aminoglycosides and vancomycin should be monitored.

Antibiotic toxicities, including allergic reactions, occur in 25–40% of patients and commonly arise during the third week of therapy. Blood tests to detect renal, hepatic, and hematologic toxicity should be performed periodically.

In most patients, effective antibiotic therapy results in subjective improvement and resolution of fever within 5–7 days. Blood cultures should be repeated daily until sterile, rechecked if there is recrudescent fever, and performed again 4–6 weeks after therapy to document cure. Blood cultures become sterile within 2 days after the start of appropriate therapy when infection is caused by viridans streptococci, enterococci, or HACEK organisms. In S. aureus endocarditis, β-lactam therapy results in sterile cultures in 3–5 days, whereas positive cultures may persist for 7–9 days with vancomycin treatment. When fever persists for 7 days despite appropriate antibiotic therapy, patients should be evaluated for paravalvular abscess and for extracardiac abscesses (spleen, kidney) or complications (embolic events). Recrudescent fever raises the question of these complications but also of drug reactions or complications of hospitalization. Serologic abnormalities (e.g., in C-reactive protein level, erythrocyte sedimentation rate, rheumatoid factor) resolve slowly and do not reflect response to treatment. Vegetations become smaller with effective therapy, but at 3 months after cure half are unchanged and 25% are slightly larger.

SURGICAL TREATMENT Intracardiac and central nervous system complications of endocarditis are important causes of morbidity and death associated with this infection. In some cases, effective treatment for these complications requires surgery. Most of the clinical indications for surgical treatment of endocarditis are not absolute (Table 25-5). The risks and benefits as well as the timing of surgical treatment must therefore be individualized (Table 25-6).

Intracardiac Surgical Indications Most surgical interventions are warranted by intracardiac findings, detected most reliably by TEE. Because of the highly invasive nature of prosthetic valve endocarditis, up to 40% of affected patients merit surgical treatment. In many patients, coincident rather than single intracardiac events necessitate surgery.

Congestive heart failure Moderate to severe refractory congestive heart failure caused by new or

TABLE 25-5

INDICATIONS FOR CARDIAC SURGICAL INTERVENTION IN PATIENTS WITH ENDOCARDITIS

Surgery required for optimal outcome

Moderate to severe congestive heart failure due to valve dysfunction
Partially dehisced unstable prosthetic valve
Persistent bacteremia despite optimal antimicrobial therapy
Lack of effective microbicidal therapy (e.g., fungal or *Brucella* endocarditis)
S. aureus prosthetic valve endocarditis with an intracardiac complication
Relapse of prosthetic valve endocarditis after optimal antimicrobial therapy

Surgery to be strongly considered for improved outcome[a]

Perivalvular extension of infection
Poorly responsive *S. aureus* endocarditis involving the aortic or mitral valve
Large (>10-mm diameter) hypermobile vegetations with increased risk of embolism
Persistent unexplained fever (≥10 days) in culture-negative native valve endocarditis
Poorly responsive or relapsed endocarditis due to highly antibiotic-resistant enterococci or gram-negative bacilli

[a]Surgery must be carefully considered; findings are often combined with other indications to prompt surgery.

worsening valve dysfunction is the major indication for cardiac surgical treatment of endocarditis. Of patients with moderate to severe heart failure due to valve dysfunction who are treated medically, 60–90% die within 6 months. In this setting, surgical treatment improves outcome, with mortality rates of 20% in native valve endocarditis and 35–55% in prosthetic valve infection. Surgery can relieve functional stenosis due to large vegetations or restore competence to damaged regurgitant valves.

Perivalvular infection This complication, which occurs in 10–15% of native valve and 45–60% of prosthetic valve infections, is suggested by persistent unexplained fever during appropriate therapy, new electrocardiographic conduction disturbances, and pericarditis. Extension can occur from any valve but is most common with aortic valve infection. TEE with color Doppler is the test of choice to detect perivalvular abscesses (sensitivity, ≥85%). Although occasional perivalvular infections are cured medically, surgery is warranted when fever persists, fistulae develop, prostheses are dehisced and unstable, and invasive infection relapses after appropriate treatment. Cardiac rhythm

TABLE 25-6

TIMING OF CARDIAC SURGICAL INTERVENTION IN PATIENTS WITH ENDOCARDITIS

	INDICATION FOR SURGICAL INTERVENTION	
TIMING	STRONG SUPPORTING EVIDENCE	CONFLICTING EVIDENCE, BUT MAJORITY OF OPINIONS FAVOR SURGERY
Emergent (same day)	Acute aortic regurgitation plus preclosure of mitral valve Sinus of Valsalva abscess ruptured into right heart Rupture into pericardial sac	
Urgent (within 1–2 days)	Valve obstruction by vegetation Unstable (dehisced) prosthesis Acute aortic or mitral regurgitation with heart failure (New York Heart Association class III or IV) Septal perforation Perivalvular extension of infection with/without new electrocardiographic conduction system changes Lack of effective antibiotic therapy	Major embolus plus persisting large vegetation (>10 mm in diameter)
Elective (earlier usually preferred)	Progressive paravalvular prosthetic regurgitation Valve dysfunction plus persisting infection after ≥7–10 days of antimicrobial therapy Fungal (mold) endocarditis	Staphylococcal PVE Early PVE (≤2 months after valve surgery) Fungal endocarditis (*Candida* spp.) Antibiotic-resistant organisms

Note: PVE, prosthetic valve endocarditis.
Source: Adapted from L Olaison, G Pettersson: Infect Dis Clin North Am 16:453, 2002.

must be monitored since high-grade heart block may require insertion of a pacemaker.

Uncontrolled infection Continued positive blood cultures or otherwise-unexplained persistent fevers (in patients with either blood culture–positive or –negative endocarditis) despite optimal antibiotic therapy may reflect uncontrolled infection and may warrant surgery. Surgical treatment is also advised for endocarditis caused by organisms against which clinical experience indicates that effective antimicrobial therapy is lacking. This category includes infections caused by yeasts, fungi, *P. aeruginosa*, other highly resistant gram-negative bacilli, *Brucella* species, and probably *C. burnetii*.

S. aureus endocarditis Mortality rates for *S. aureus* prosthetic valve endocarditis exceed 70% with medical treatment but are reduced to 25% with surgical treatment. In patients with intracardiac complications associated with *S. aureus* prosthetic valve infection, surgical treatment reduces the mortality rate twentyfold. Surgical treatment should be considered for patients with *S. aureus* native aortic or mitral valve infection who have TTE-demonstrable vegetations and remain septic during the initial week of therapy. Isolated tricuspid valve endocarditis, even with persistent fever, rarely requires surgery.

Prevention of systemic emboli Death and persisting morbidity due to emboli are largely limited to patients suffering occlusion of cerebral or coronary arteries. Echocardiographic determination of vegetation size and anatomy, although predictive of patients at high risk of systemic emboli, does not identify those patients in whom the benefits of surgery to prevent emboli clearly exceed the risks of the surgical procedure and an implanted prosthetic valve. Net benefits favoring surgery are most likely when the risk of embolism is high and other surgical benefits can be achieved simultaneously—e.g., repair of a moderately dysfunctional valve or debridement of a paravalvular abscess. Reduced overall risks of surgical intervention (e.g., use of vegetation resection and valve repair to avoid insertion of a prosthesis) make the benefit-to-risk ratio more favorable and this intervention more attractive.

Timing of Cardiac Surgery In general, when indications for surgical treatment of infective endocarditis are identified, surgery should not be delayed simply to permit additional antibiotic therapy, since this course of action increases the risk of death (Table 25-6). Delay is justified only when infection is controlled and congestive heart failure is fully compensated with medical therapy. After 14 days of recommended antibiotic therapy, excised valves are culture-negative in 99% and 50% of patients with streptococcal and *S. aureus* endocarditis, respectively. Recrudescent endocarditis involving a new implanted prosthetic valve follows surgery in 2% of patients with culture-positive native valve endocarditis and in 6–15% of patients with active prosthetic valve endocarditis. These risks are more acceptable than the high mortality rates that result when surgery is inappropriately delayed or not performed.

Among patients who have experienced a neurologic complication of endocarditis, further neurologic deterioration can occur as a consequence of cardiac surgery. The risk of significant neurologic exacerbation is related to the interval between the complication and the surgery. Whenever feasible, cardiac surgery should be delayed for 2–3 weeks after a nonhemorrhagic embolic stroke and for 4 weeks after a hemorrhagic embolic stroke. A ruptured mycotic aneurysm should be clipped and cerebral edema allowed to resolve before cardiac surgery.

Antibiotic Therapy after Cardiac Surgery

Bacteria visible in Gram-stained preparations of excised valves do not necessarily indicate a failure of antibiotic therapy. Organisms have been detected on Gram's stain—or their DNA has been detected by PCR—in excised valves from 45% of patients who have successfully completed the recommended therapy for endocarditis. In only 7% of these patients are the organisms, most of which are unusual and antibiotic resistant, cultured from the valve. Despite the detection of organisms or their DNA, relapse of endocarditis after surgery is uncommon. Thus, for uncomplicated native valve infection caused by susceptible organisms in conjunction with negative valve cultures, the duration of preoperative plus postoperative treatment should equal the total duration of recommended therapy, with ~2 weeks of treatment administered after surgery. For endocarditis complicated by paravalvular abscess, partially treated prosthetic valve infection, or cases with culture-positive valves, a full course of therapy should be given postoperatively.

Extracardiac Complications

Splenic abscess develops in 3–5% of patients with endocarditis. Effective therapy requires either image-guided percutaneous drainage or splenectomy. Mycotic aneurysms occur in 2–15% of endocarditis patients; half of these cases involve the cerebral arteries and present as headaches, focal neurologic symptoms, or hemorrhage. Cerebral aneurysms should be monitored by angiography. Some will resolve with effective antimicrobial therapy, but those that persist, enlarge, or leak should be treated surgically if possible. Extracerebral aneurysms present as local pain, a mass, local ischemia, or bleeding; these aneurysms are treated by resection.

OUTCOME

Older age, severe comorbid conditions, delayed diagnosis, involvement of prosthetic valves or the aortic valve, an invasive (*S. aureus*) or antibiotic-resistant (*P. aeruginosa*, yeast) pathogen, intracardiac complications, and major neurologic complications adversely impact outcome. Death and poor outcome often are related not to failure of antibiotic therapy but rather to the interactions of comorbidities and endocarditis-related end-organ complications. Overall survival rates for patients with native valve endocarditis caused by viridans streptococci, HACEK organisms, or enterococci (susceptible to synergistic therapy) are 85–90%. For *S. aureus* native valve endocarditis in patients who do not inject drugs, survival rates are 55–70%, whereas 85–90% of injection drug users survive this infection. Prosthetic valve endocarditis beginning within 2 months of valve replacement results in mortality rates of 40–50%, whereas rates are only 10–20% in later-onset cases.

PREVENTION

Antibiotic prophylaxis has been recommended by the American Heart Association in conjunction with selected procedures considered to entail a risk for bacteremia and endocarditis. The benefits of prophylaxis, however, are not established and in fact may be modest: only 50% of patients presenting with native valve endocarditis know that they have a predisposing valve lesion, most endocarditis cases do not follow a procedure, and 35% of cases are caused by organisms not targeted by prophylaxis. Dental treatments, the procedures most widely accepted as predisposing to endocarditis, are no more frequent during the 3 months preceding endocarditis than in uninfected matched controls. Furthermore, the frequency and magnitude of bacteremia associated with dental procedures and routine daily activities (e.g., tooth brushing and flossing) are similar. Because patients undergo dental procedures infrequently, exposure of endocarditis-vulnerable cardiac structures to bacteremia–causing oral cavity organisms is notably greater from routine daily activities than from dental care. It is estimated that annual exposure of heart valves to bacteremia–causing organisms may be 5.6 million times greater from routine daily activity than from a tooth extraction. The relation of gastrointestinal and genitourinary procedures to subsequent endocarditis is more tenuous than that of dental procedures.

Antibiotic prophylaxis, if 100% effective, likely prevents only a small number of cases of endocarditis; nevertheless, it is possible that rare cases are prevented. Weighing the potential benefits, potential adverse events, and costs associated with antibiotic prophylaxis, the expert committee of the American Heart Association has dramatically restricted the recommendations for antibiotic prophylaxis.

SECTION IV

Disorders of the Heart

TABLE 25-7

ANTIBIOTIC REGIMENS FOR PROPHYLAXIS OF ENDOCARDITIS IN ADULTS WITH HIGH-RISK CARDIAC LESIONS [a,b]

A. Standard oral regimen
   1. Amoxicillin 2.0 g PO 1 h before procedure
B. Inability to take oral medication
   1. Ampicillin 2.0 g IV or IM within 1 h before procedure
C. Penicillin allergy
   1. Clarithromycin or azithromycin 500 mg PO 1 h before procedure
   2. Cephalexin[c] 2.0 g PO 1 h before procedure
   3. Clindamycin 600 mg PO 1 h before procedure
D. Penicillin allergy, inability to take oral medication
   1. Cefazolin[c] or ceftriaxone[c] 1.0 g IV or IM 30 min before procedure
   2. Clindamycin 600 mg IV or IM 1 h before procedure

[a]Dosing for children: for amoxicillin, ampicillin, cephalexin, or cefadroxil, use 50 mg/kg PO; cefazolin, 25 mg/kg IV; clindamycin, 20 mg/kg PO, 25 mg/kg IV; clarithromycin, 15 mg/kg PO; and vancomycin, 20 mg/kg IV.
[b]For high-risk lesions, see Table 25-8. Prophylaxis is not advised for other lesions.
[c]Do not use cephalosporins in patients with immediate hypersensitivity (urticaria, angioedema, anaphylaxis) to penicillin.
Source: W Wilson et al: Circulation, published online 4/19/07.

Prophylactic antibiotics (Table 25-7) are advised only for those patients at highest risk for severe morbidity or death from endocarditis (Table 25-8). Prophylaxis is recommended only for dental procedures wherein there is manipulation of gingival tissue or the periapical region of the teeth or perforation of the oral mucosa (including surgery on the respiratory tract). Although prophylaxis is not advised for patients undergoing gastrointestinal or genitourinary tract procedures, it is recommended that effective treatment be given to these high-risk patients before or when they undergo procedures on an infected genitourinary tract or on infected skin and related soft tissue. Maintaining good dental hygiene is also advised. (W Wilson et al.)

TABLE 25-8

HIGH-RISK CARDIAC LESIONS FOR WHICH ENDOCARDITIS PROPHYLAXIS IS ADVISED BEFORE DENTAL PROCEDURES

Prosthetic heart valves
Prior endocarditis
Unrepaired cyanotic congenital heart disease, including palliative shunts or conduits
Completely repaired congenital heart defects during the 6 months after repair
Incompletely repaired congenital heart disease with residual defects adjacent to prosthetic material
Valvulopathy developing after cardiac transplantation

Source: W Wilson et al: Circulation, published online 4/19/07.

FURTHER READINGS

BADDOUR LM et al: Diagnosis, antimicrobial therapy, and management of complications. A statement for healthcare professionals from the Committee on Rheumatic Fever, Endocarditis, and Kawasaki Disease, Council on Cardiovascular Disease in the Young, and the Councils on Clinical Cardiology, Stroke, and Cardiovascular Surgery and Anesthesia, American Heart Association. Circulation 111:e394, 2005

DURACK DT (ed): Infective endocarditis. Infect Dis Clin North Am 16:255, 2002

FOWLER VG JR et al: Endocarditis and intravascular infections, in *Principles and Practice of Infectious Diseases*, 6th ed, GL Mandell et al (eds). Philadelphia, Elsevier Churchill Livingstone, 2005, pp 975–1021

HORSTKOTTE D et al: Guidelines on prevention, diagnosis and treatment of infective endocarditis. Executive summary, The Task Force on Infective Endocarditis of the European Society of Cardiology. Eur Heart J 25:267, 2004

KARCHMER AW: Infective endocarditis, in *Heart Disease*, 8th ed, E Braunwald et al (eds). Philadelphia, Elsevier Saunders, 2008

————, LONGWORTH DL: Infections of intracardiac devices. Cardiol Clin 21:253, 2003

LI JS et al: Proposed modifications to the Duke criteria for the diagnosis of infective endocarditis. Clin Infect Dis 30:633, 2000

MOREILLON P, QUE YA: Infective endocarditis. Lancet 363:139, 2004

MORRIS AJ et al: Bacteriological outcome after valve surgery for active infective endocarditis: Implications for duration of treatment after surgery (abstract). Clin Infect Dis 41:187, 2005

VIKRAM HR et al: Impact of valve surgery on 6-month mortality in adults with complicated, left-sided native valve endocarditis: A propensity analysis. JAMA 290:3207, 2003

WILSON W et al: Prevention of infective endocarditis. Guidelines from the American Heart Association. A guideline from the American Heart Association Rheumatic Fever, Endocarditis, and Kawasaki Disease Committee, Council on Cardiovascular Disease in the Young, and the Council on Clinical Cardiology, Council on Cardiovascular Surgery and Anesthesia, and the Quality of Care and Outcomes Research Interdisciplinary Working Group. Circulation 116:1736, 2007

CHAPTER 25 Infective Endocarditis

CHAPTER 26

ACUTE RHEUMATIC FEVER

Jonathan R. Carapetis

Acute rheumatic fever (ARF) is a multisystem disease resulting from an autoimmune reaction to infection with group A streptococci. Although many parts of the body may be affected, almost all of the manifestations resolve completely. The exception is cardiac valvular damage [rheumatic heart disease (RHD)], which may persist after the other features have disappeared.

ARF and RHD are diseases of poverty. They were common in all countries until the early twentieth century, when their incidence began to decline in industrialized nations. This decline was largely attributable to improved living conditions—particularly less crowded housing and better hygiene—which resulted in reduced transmission of group A streptococci. The introduction of antibiotics and improved systems of medical care had a supplemental effect. Recurrent outbreaks of ARF began in the 1980s in the Rocky Mountain states of the United States, where elevated rates persist.

The virtual disappearance of ARF and reduction in the incidence of RHD in industrialized countries during the twentieth century unfortunately was not replicated in developing countries, where these diseases continue unabated. RHD is the most common cause of heart disease in children in developing countries and is a major cause of mortality and morbidity in adults as well. It was recently estimated that between 15 and 19 million people worldwide are affected by RHD, with approximately one-quarter of a million deaths occurring each year. Some 95% of ARF cases and RHD deaths now occur in developing countries.

Although ARF and RHD are relatively common in all developing countries, they occur at particularly elevated rates in certain regions. The "hot spots" are sub-Saharan Africa, Pacific nations, Australasia, and the Indian subcontinent (**Fig. 26-1**).

EPIDEMIOLOGY

ARF is mainly a disease of children aged 5–14 years. Initial episodes become less common in older adolescents and young adults and are rare in persons older than 30 years. By contrast, recurrent episodes of ARF remain relatively common in adolescents and young adults. This pattern contrasts with the prevalence of RHD, which peaks between 25 and 40 years. There is no clear gender association for ARF, but RHD more commonly affects females, sometimes up to twice as frequently as males.

PATHOGENESIS

Organism Factors

Based on currently available evidence, ARF is exclusively caused by infection of the upper respiratory tract with group A streptococci. It is now thought that any strain of group A streptococcus has the potential to cause ARF. Potential role of skin infection and of groups C and G streptococci are currently being investigated. It has been postulated that a series of preceding streptococcal infections is needed to "prime" the immune system prior to the final infection that directly causes disease.

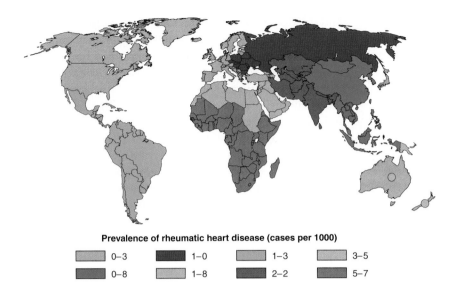

Prevalence of rheumatic heart disease (cases per 1000)

- 0–3
- 0–8
- 1–0
- 1–8
- 1–3
- 2–2
- 3–5
- 5–7

FIGURE 26-1

Prevalence of rheumatic heart disease in children aged 5–14 years. Circles within Australia and New Zealand represent indigenous populations, and also Pacific Islanders in New Zealand. *(Reprinted with permission from JR Carapetis et al: Lancet Infect Dis.)*

Host Factors

Approximately 3–6% of any population may be susceptible to ARF, and this proportion does not vary dramatically between populations. Findings of familial clustering of cases and concordance in monozygotic twins—particularly for chorea—confirm that susceptibility to ARF is an inherited characteristic. Particular HLA class II alleles appear to be strongly associated with susceptibility. Associations have also been described with high levels of circulating mannose-binding lectin and polymorphisms of transforming growth factor β_1 gene and immunoglobulin genes. High-level expression of a particular alloantigen present on B cells, D8-17, has been found in patients with a history of ARF in many populations, with intermediate-level expression in first-degree family members, suggesting that this may be a marker of inherited susceptibility.

The Immune Response

When a susceptible host encounters a group A streptococcus, an autoimmune reaction results which leads to damage to the human tissues as a result of cross-reactivity between epitopes on the organism and the host (Fig. 26-2).

Epitopes present in the cell wall, cell membrane, and the A, B, and C repeat regions of the streptococcal M protein are immunologically similar to molecules in human myosin, tropomyosin, keratin, actin, laminin, vimentin, and N-acetylglucosamine. This molecular mimicry is the basis for the autoimmune response that leads to ARF. It has been hypothesized that human molecules—particularly epitopes in cardiac myosin—result in T cell sensitization. These T cells are then recalled following subsequent exposure to group A streptococci bearing immunologically similar epitopes.

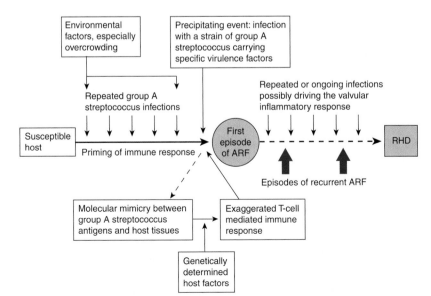

FIGURE 26-2

Pathogenetic pathway for acute rheumatic fever and rheumatic heart disease. *(Reprinted with permission from Lancet 366:155, 2005.)*

However, myosin cross-reactivity with M protein does not explain the valvular damage that is the hallmark of rheumatic carditis, given that myosin is not present in valvular tissue. The link may be laminin, another α-helical coiled-coil protein like myosin and M protein, which is found in cardiac endothelium and is recognized by anti-myosin, anti-M protein T cells. Moreover, antibodies to cardiac valve tissue cross-react with the N-acetylglucosamine of group A streptococcal carbohydrate, and there is some evidence that these antibodies may be responsible for valvular damage.

CLINICAL FEATURES

There is a latent period of ~3 weeks (1–5 weeks) between the precipitating group A streptococcal infection and the appearance of the clinical features of ARF. The exceptions are chorea and indolent carditis, which may follow prolonged latent periods lasting up to 6 months. Although many patients report a prior sore throat, the preceding group A streptococcal infection is commonly subclinical; in these cases it can only be confirmed using streptococcal antibody testing. The most common clinical presentation of ARF is polyarthritis and fever. Polyarthritis is present in 60–75% of cases and carditis in 50–60%. The prevalence of chorea in ARF varies substantially between populations, ranging from <2 to 30%. Erythema marginatum and subcutaneous nodules are now rare, being found in <5% of cases.

Heart Involvement

Up to 60% of patients with ARF progress to RHD. The endocardium, pericardium, or myocardium may be affected. Valvular damage is the hallmark of rheumatic carditis. The mitral valve is almost always affected, sometimes together with the aortic valve; isolated aortic valve involvement is rare. Early valvular damage leads to regurgitation. Over ensuing years, usually as a result of recurrent episodes, leaflet thickening, scarring, calcification, and valvular stenosis may develop. Pericarditis most commonly causes a friction rub or a small effusion on echocardiography and may occasionally cause pleuritic central chest pain. Myocardial involvement is almost never responsible in itself for cardiac failure. Therefore, the characteristic manifestation of carditis in previously unaffected individuals is mitral regurgitation, sometimes accompanied by aortic regurgitation. Myocardial inflammation may affect electrical conduction pathways, leading to P-R interval prolongation (first-degree AV block or rarely higher-level block) and softening of the first heart sound.

Joint Involvement

To qualify as a major manifestation, joint involvement in ARF must be arthritic, i.e., objective evidence of inflammation, with hot, swollen, red and/or tender joints and involvement of more than one joint (i.e., polyarthritis). The typical arthritis is migratory, moving from one joint to another over a period of hours. ARF almost always affects the large joints—most commonly the knees, ankles, hip, and elbows—and is asymmetric. The pain is severe and usually disabling until anti-inflammatory medication is commenced.

Less severe joint involvement is also relatively common but qualifies only as a minor manifestation. Arthralgia without objective joint inflammation usually affects large joints in the same migratory pattern as polyarthritis. In some populations, aseptic monoarthritis may be a presenting feature of ARF. This may occur because of early commencement of anti-inflammatory medication before the typical migratory pattern is established.

The joint manifestations of ARF are highly responsive to salicylates and other nonsteroidal anti-inflammatory drugs (NSAIDs). Indeed, joint involvement that persists more than 1 or 2 days after starting salicylates is unlikely to be due to ARF. Conversely, if salicylates are commenced early in the illness, before fever and migratory polyarthritis have become manifest, it may be difficult to make a diagnosis of ARF. For this reason, salicylates and other NSAIDs should be withheld—and pain managed with acetaminophen or codeine—until the diagnosis is confirmed.

Chorea

Sydenham's chorea commonly occurs in the absence of other manifestations, follows a prolonged latent period after group A streptococcal infection, and is found mainly in females. The choreiform movements affect particularly the head (causing characteristic darting movements of the tongue) and the upper limbs. They may be generalized or restricted to one side of the body (hemi-chorea). The chorea varies in severity. In mild cases it may be evident only on careful examination, while in the most severe cases the affected individuals are unable to perform activities of daily living and are at risk of injuring themselves. Chorea eventually resolves completely, usually within 6 weeks.

Skin Manifestations

The classic rash of ARF is *erythema marginatum*, which begins as pink macules that clear centrally, leaving a serpiginous, spreading edge. The rash is evanescent, appearing and disappearing before the examiner's eyes. It occurs usually on the trunk, sometimes on the limbs, but almost never on the face.

Subcutaneous nodules occur as painless, small (0.5–2 cm), mobile lumps beneath the skin overlying bony prominences, particularly of the hands, feet, elbows, occiput, and occasionally the vertebrae. They are a delayed manifestation, appearing 2–3 weeks after the onset of disease, last for just a few days up to 3 weeks, and are commonly associated with carditis.

Other Features

Fever occurs in most cases of ARF, although rarely in cases of pure chorea. Although high-grade fever (≥39°C) is the rule, lower grade temperature elevations are not uncommon. Elevated acute-phase reactants are also present in most cases. C-reactive protein (CRP) and erythrocyte sedimentation rate (ESR) are often dramatically elevated. Occasionally the peripheral leukocyte count is mildly elevated.

Evidence of a Preceding Group A Streptococcal Infection

With the exception of chorea and low-grade carditis, both of which may become manifest many months later, evidence of a preceding group A streptococcal infection is essential in making the diagnosis of ARF. As most cases do not have a positive throat swab culture or rapid antigen test, serologic evidence is usually needed. The most common serologic tests are the anti-streptolysin O (ASO) and anti-DNase B (ADB) titers. Where possible, age-specific reference ranges should be determined in a local population of healthy people without a recent group A streptococcal infection.

Other Post-Streptococcal Syndromes That May Be Confused with Rheumatic Fever

Post-streptococcal reactive arthritis (PSRA) is differentiated from ARF on the basis of: (1) small-joint involvement that is often symmetric; (2) a short latent period following streptococcal infection (usually <1 week); (3) occasional causation by non–group A β-hemolytic streptococcal infection; (4) slower responsiveness to salicylates; and (5) the absence of other features of ARF, particularly carditis.

Pediatric Autoimmune Neuropsychiatric Disorders Associated with Streptococcal infection (PANDAS) is a term that links a range of tic disorders and obsessive-compulsive symptoms with group A streptococcal infections. People with PANDAS are said not to be at risk of carditis, unlike patients with Sydenham's chorea. The diagnoses of PANDAS and PSRA should rarely be made in populations with a high incidence of ARF.

Confirming the Diagnosis

Because there is no definitive test, the diagnosis of ARF relies on the presence of a combination of typical clinical features together with evidence of the precipitating group A streptococcal infection, and the exclusion of other diagnoses. This uncertainty led Dr. T. Duckett Jones in 1944 to develop a set of criteria (subsequently known as the *Jones criteria*) to aid in the diagnosis. An

expert panel convened by the World Health Organization (WHO) clarified the use of the Jones criteria in ARF recurrences (Table 26-1). These criteria include a preceding streptococcal type A infection as well as some combination of major and minor manifestations.

℞ Treatment: ACUTE RHEUMATIC FEVER

Patients with possible ARF should be followed closely to ensure that the diagnosis is confirmed, treatment of heart failure and other symptoms is undertaken, and preventive measures including commencement of secondary prophylaxis, inclusion on an ARF registry, and health education are commenced. Echocardiography should be performed on all possible cases to aid in making the diagnosis and to determine the severity at baseline of any carditis. Other tests that should be performed are listed in Table 26-2.

There is no treatment for ARF that has been proven to alter the likelihood of developing, or the severity of, RHD. With the exception of treatment of heart failure, which may be life-saving in cases of severe carditis, the treatment of ARF is symptomatic.

ANTIBIOTICS All patients with ARF should receive antibiotics sufficient to treat the precipitating group A streptococcal infection. Penicillin is the drug of choice and can be given orally (as penicillin, 500 mg PO twice daily for 10 days) or as a single dose of 1.2 million units IM benzathine penicillin G. Erythromycin, 250 mg bid, may be used for patients with penicillin allergy. Because long-term secondary prophylaxis will be needed—and penicillin is the drug of choice for this—reported penicillin allergy should be confirmed, preferably in consultation with an allergist.

SALICYLATES AND NSAIDS These may be used for the treatment of arthritis, arthralgia, and fever, once the diagnosis is confirmed. They are of no value in the treatment of carditis or chorea. Aspirin is the drug of choice. An initial dose of 80–100 mg/kg per day in children (4–8 g/d in adults) in 4–5 divided doses is often needed for the first few days up to 2 weeks. A lower dose should be used if symptoms of salicylate toxicity emerge, such as nausea, vomiting, or tinnitus. When the acute symptoms are substantially resolved, the dose can be reduced to 60–70 mg/kg per day for a further 2–4 weeks. Fever, joint manifestations, and elevated acute-phase reactants sometimes recur up to 3 weeks after the medication is discontinued. This does not indicate a recurrence and can be managed by recommencing salicylates for a brief period. Although less well studied, naproxen at a dose of 10–20 mg/kg per day has been reported to lead to good symptomatic response.

TABLE 26-1

2002–2003 WORLD HEALTH ORGANIZATION CRITERIA FOR THE DIAGNOSIS OF RHEUMATIC FEVER AND RHEUMATIC HEART DISEASE (BASED ON THE 1992 REVISED JONES CRITERIA)

DIAGNOSTIC CATEGORIES	CRITERIA
Primary episode of rheumatic fever[a]	Two major or one major and two minor manifestations plus evidence of preceding group A streptococcal infection
Recurrent attack of rheumatic fever in a patient without established rheumatic heart disease	Two major or one major and two minor manifestations plus evidence of preceding group A streptococcal infection
Recurrent attack of rheumatic fever in a patient with established rheumatic heart disease[b]	Two minor manifestations plus evidence of preceding group A streptococcal infection[c]
Rheumatic chorea	Other major manifestations or evidence of group
Insidious onset rheumatic carditis[b]	A streptococcal infection not required
Chronic valve lesions of rheumatic heart disease (patients presenting for the first time with pure mitral stenosis or mixed mitral valve disease and/or aortic valve disease)[d]	Do not require any other criteria to be diagnosed as having rheumatic heart disease
Major manifestations	Carditis
	Polyarthritis
	Chorea
	Erythema marginatum
	Subcutaneous nodules
Minor manifestations	Clinical: fever, polyarthralgia
	Laboratory: elevated erythrocyte sedimentation rate or leukocyte count[e]
	Electrocardiogram: prolonged P-R interval
Supporting evidence of a preceding streptococcal infection within the last 45 days	Elevated or rising anti-streptolysin O or other streptococcal antibody, or
	A positive throat culture, or
	Rapid antigen test for group A streptococcus, or
	Recent scarlet fever[e]

[a]Patients may present with polyarthritis (or with only polyarthralgia or monoarthritis) and with several (3 or more) other minor manifestations, together with evidence of recent group A streptococcal infection. Some of these cases may later turn out to be rheumatic fever. It is prudent to consider them as cases of "probable rheumatic fever" (once other diagnoses are excluded) and advise regular secondary prophylaxis. Such patients require close follow up and regular examination of the heart. This cautious approach is particularly suitable for patients in vulnerable age groups in high incidence settings.
[b]Infective endocarditis should be excluded.
[c]Some patients with recurrent attacks may not fulfill these criteria.
[d]Congenital heart disease should be excluded.
[e]1992 Revised Jones criteria do not include elevated leukocyte count as a laboratory minor manifestation (but do include elevated C-reactive protein), and do not include recent scarlet fever as supporting evidence of a recent streptococcal infection.
Source: Reprinted with permission from WHO Expert Consultation on Rheumatic Fever and Rheumatic Heart Disease (2001: Geneva, Switzerland): *Rheumatic Fever and Rheumatic Heart Disease: Report of a WHO Expert Consultation* (WHO Tech Rep Ser, 923). Geneva, World Health Organization, 2004.

CONGESTIVE HEART FAILURE

Glucocorticoids The use of glucocorticoids in ARF remains controversial. Two meta-analyses have failed to demonstrate a benefit of glucocorticoids compared to placebo or salicylates in improving the short- or longer term outcome of carditis. However, the studies included in these meta-analyses all took place >40 years ago and did not use medications in common usage today. Many clinicians treat cases of severe carditis (causing heart failure) with glucocorticoids in the belief that they may reduce the acute inflammation and result in more rapid resolution of failure. However, the potential benefits of this treatment should be balanced against the possible adverse effects, including gastrointestinal bleeding and fluid retention. If used, prednisone or prednisolone is recommended at doses of 1–2 mg/kg per day (maximum, 80 mg). Intravenous methylprednisolone may be used in very severe carditis. Glucocorticoids are often only required for a few days or up to a maximum of 3 weeks.

MANAGEMENT OF HEART FAILURE See Chap. 17.

BED REST Traditional recommendations for long-term bed rest, once the cornerstone of management, are no longer widely practiced. Instead, bed rest should be prescribed as needed while arthritis and arthralgia are present, and for patients with heart failure. Once symptoms are well controlled, gradual mobilization can commence as tolerated.

TABLE 26-2

RECOMMENDED TESTS IN CASES OF POSSIBLE ACUTE RHEUMATIC FEVER

Recommended for all cases

White blood cell count
Erythrocyte sedimentation rate
C-reactive protein
Blood cultures if febrile
Electrocardiogram (repeat in 2 weeks and 2 months if prolonged P-R interval or other rhythm abnormality)
Chest x-ray if clinical or echocardiographic evidence of carditis
Echocardiogram (consider repeating after 1 month if negative)
Throat swab (preferably before giving antibiotics)—culture for group A streptococcus
Anti-streptococcal serology: both anti-streptolysin O and anti-DNase B titres, if available (repeat 10–14 days later if 1st test not confirmatory)

Tests for alternative diagnoses, depending on clinical features

Repeated blood cultures if possible endocarditis
Joint aspirate (microscopy and culture) for possible septic arthritis
Copper, ceruloplasmin, anti-nuclear antibody, drug screen for choreiform movements
Serology and auto-immune markers for arboviral, auto-immune or reactive arthritis

Source: Reprinted with permission from National Heart Foundation of Australia.

CHOREA Medications to control the abnormal movements do not alter the duration or outcome of chorea. Milder cases can usually be managed by providing a calm environment. In patients with severe chorea, carbamazepine or sodium valproate is preferred to haloperidol. A response may not be seen for 1–2 weeks, and a successful response may only be to reduce rather than resolve the abnormal movements. Medication should be continued for 1–2 weeks after symptoms subside.

INTRAVENOUS IMMUNOGLOBULIN (IVIg) Small studies have suggested that IVIg may lead to more rapid resolution of chorea but has shown no benefit on the short- or long-term outcome of carditis in ARF without chorea. In the absence of better data, IVIg is *not* recommended except in cases of severe chorea refractory to other treatments.

PROGNOSIS

Untreated, ARF lasts on average 12 weeks. With treatment, patients are usually discharged from hospital within 1–2 weeks. Inflammatory markers should be monitored every 1–2 weeks until they have normalized (usually within 4–6 weeks), and an echocardiogram should be performed after 1 month to determine if there has been progression of carditis. Cases with more severe carditis need close clinical and echocardiographic monitoring in the longer term.

Once the acute episode has resolved, the priority in management is to ensure long-term clinical follow-up and adherence to a regimen of secondary prophylaxis. Patients should be entered onto the local ARF registry (if present) and contact made with primary care practitioners to ensure a plan for follow-up and administration of secondary prophylaxis before the patient is discharged. Patients and their families should also be educated about their disease, emphasizing the importance of adherence to secondary prophylaxis. If carditis is present, they should also be informed of the need for antibiotic prophylaxis against endocarditis for dental and surgical procedures.

PREVENTION

Primary Prevention

Ideally, primary prevention would entail elimination of the major risk factors for streptococcal infection, particularly overcrowded housing and inadequate hygiene infrastructure. This is difficult to achieve in most places where ARF is common.

Therefore, the mainstay of primary prevention for ARF remains primary prophylaxis, i.e., the timely and complete treatment of group A streptococcal sore throat with antibiotics. If commenced within 9 days of sore throat onset, a course of 10 days of penicillin V (500 mg bid PO in adults) or a single IM injection of 1.2 million units of benzathine penicillin G will prevent almost all cases of ARF that would otherwise have developed. This important strategy relies on individuals presenting for medical care when they have a sore throat, the availability of trained health and microbiology staff along with the materials and infrastructure to take throat swabs, and a reliable supply of penicillin. Unfortunately, many of these elements are not available in developing countries. Moreover, the majority of cases of ARF do not follow a sore throat sufficiently severe for the patient to seek medical attention.

Secondary Prevention

The mainstay of controlling ARF and RHD is secondary prevention. Because patients with ARF are at dramatically higher risk than the general population of developing a further episode of ARF after a group A streptococcal infection, they should receive long-term penicillin prophylaxis to prevent recurrences. The best antibiotic for secondary prophylaxis is benzathine penicillin G (1.2 million units, or 600,000 units if <30 kg) delivered every 4 weeks or more frequently (e.g., every 3 weeks

CHAPTER 26 Acute Rheumatic Fever

or even every 2 weeks) to persons considered to be at particularly high risk. Oral penicillin V (250 mg) can be given twice-daily instead but is somewhat less effective than benzathine penicillin G. Penicillin allergic patients can receive erythromycin (250 mg) twice daily.

The duration of secondary prophylaxis is determined by many factors, in particular the duration since the last episode of ARF (recurrences become less likely with increasing time), age (recurrences are less likely with increasing age), and the severity of RHD (if severe, it may be prudent to avoid even a very small risk of recurrence because of the potentially serious consequences) (Table 26-3). Secondary prophylaxis is best delivered

as part of a coordinated RHD control program, based around a registry of patients. Registries improve the ability to follow patients and identify those who default from prophylaxis and institute strategies to improve adherence.

TABLE 26-3

SUGGESTED DURATION OF SECONDARY PROPHYLAXIS[a]

CATEGORY OF PATIENT	DURATION OF PROPHYLAXIS
Patient without proven carditis	For 5 years after the last attack or 18 years of age (whichever is longer)
Patient with carditis (mild mitral regurgitation or healed carditis)	For 10 years after the last attack, or 25 years of age (whichever is longer)
More severe valvular disease	Lifelong
Valvular surgery	Lifelong

[a]These are recommendations only and must be modified by individual circumstances as warranted.
Source: Reprinted with permission from WHO Expert Consultation on Rheumatic Fever and Rheumatic Heart Disease (2001: Geneva, Switzerland): *Rheumatic Fever and Rheumatic Heart Disease: Report of a WHO Expert Consultation* (WHO Tech Rep Ser, 923). Geneva, World Health Organization, 2004.

FURTHER READINGS

CARAPETIS JR et al: Acute rheumatic fever. Lancet 366:155, 2005
——— et al: The global burden of group A streptococcal diseases. Lancet Infect Dis 5:685, 2005
CILLIERS AM: Rheumatic fever and its management. BMJ 333:1153, 2006
GERBER MA et al: Prevention of rheumatic fever and diagnosis and treatment of acute Streptococcal pharyngitis: A scientific statement from the American Heart Association Rheumatic Fever, Endocarditis, and Kawasaki Disease Committee of the Council on Cardiovascular Disease in the Young, the Interdisciplinary Council on Functional Genomics and Translational Biology, and the Interdisciplinary Council on Quality of Care and Outcomes Research: endorsed by the American Academy of Pediatrics. Circulation 119:541, 2009
GUILHERME L et al: Molecular mimicry in the autoimmune pathogenesis of rheumatic heart disease. Autoimmunity 39:31, 2006
NATIONAL HEART FOUNDATION OF AUSTRALIA: *Diagnosis and Management of Acute Rheumatic Fever and Rheumatic Heart Disease in Australia: Complete Evidence-Based Review and Guideline.* Melbourne, National Heart Foundation of Australia, 2006
SPECIAL WRITING GROUP OF THE COMMITTEE ON RHEUMATIC FEVER, ENDOCARDITIS AND KAWASAKI DISEASE OF THE AMERICAN HEART ASSOCIATION: Guidelines for the diagnosis of acute rheumatic fever: Jones criteria, 1992 update. JAMA 268:2069, 1992
STEER A et al: Prevention and treatment of rheumatic heart disease in the developing world. Nat Rev Cardiol 6:689, 2009
——— et al: Group A streptococcal vaccines: facts versus fantasy. Curr Opin Infect Dis 22:544, 2009

CHAPTER 27

CHAGAS' DISEASE

Louis V. Kirchhoff

The genus *Trypanosoma* contains many species of protozoans. *Trypanosoma cruzi*, the cause of Chagas' disease in the Americas, and the two trypanosome subspecies that cause human African trypanosomiasis, *Trypanosoma brucei gambiense* and *T. brucei rhodesiense*, are the only members of the genus that cause disease in humans.

CHAGAS' DISEASE

DEFINITION

Chagas' disease, or American trypanosomiasis, is a zoonosis caused by the protozoan parasite *T. cruzi*. Acute Chagas' disease is usually a mild febrile illness that results from initial infection with the organism. After spontaneous resolution of the acute illness, most infected persons remain for life in the indeterminate phase of chronic Chagas' disease, which is characterized by subpatent parasitemia, easily detectable antibodies to *T. cruzi*, and an absence of symptoms. In a minority of chronically infected patients, cardiac and gastrointestinal lesions develop that can result in serious morbidity and even death.

LIFE CYCLE AND TRANSMISSION

T. cruzi is transmitted among its mammalian hosts by hematophagous triatomine insects, often called *reduviid bugs*. The insects become infected by sucking blood from animals or humans who have circulating parasites. Ingested organisms multiply in the gut of the triatomines, and infective forms are discharged with the feces at the time of subsequent blood meals. Transmission to a second vertebrate host occurs when breaks in the skin, mucous membranes, or conjunctivae become contaminated with bug feces that contain infective parasites. *T. cruzi* can also be transmitted by the transfusion of blood donated by infected persons, by organ transplantation, from mother to fetus, and in laboratory accidents.

PATHOLOGY

An indurated inflammatory lesion called a *chagoma* often appears at the parasites' portal of entry. Local histologic changes include the presence of parasites within leukocytes and cells of subcutaneous tissues and the development of interstitial edema, lymphocytic infiltration, and reactive hyperplasia of adjacent lymph nodes. After dissemination of the organisms through the lymphatics and the bloodstream, muscles (including the myocardium), may become heavily parasitized (**Fig. 27-1**). The characteristic pseudocysts present in sections of infected tissues are intracellular aggregates of multiplying parasites.

In the minority of persons with chronic *T. cruzi* infections who develop related clinical manifestations, the heart is the organ most commonly affected. Changes include thinning of the ventricular walls, biventricular

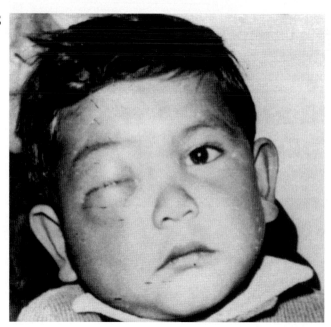

FIGURE 27-1

Trypanosoma cruzi in the heart muscle of a child who died of acute Chagas' myocarditis. An infected myocyte containing several dozen *T. cruzi* amastigotes is in the center of the field (hematoxylin and eosin, ×900).

enlargement, apical aneurysms, and mural thrombi. Widespread lymphocytic infiltration, diffuse interstitial fibrosis, and atrophy of myocardial cells are often apparent, but parasites are difficult to find in myocardial tissue. Conduction-system involvement often affects the right branch and the left anterior branch of the bundle of His. In chronic Chagas' disease of the gastrointestinal tract (megadisease), the esophagus and colon may exhibit varying degrees of dilatation. On microscopic examination, focal inflammatory lesions with lymphocytic infiltration are seen, and the number of neurons in the myenteric plexus may be markedly reduced. Accumulating experimental evidence implicates the persistence of parasites and the accompanying chronic inflammation—rather than autoimmune mechanisms—as the basis for the pathology in patients with chronic *T. cruzi* infection.

EPIDEMIOLOGY

T. cruzi is found only in the Americas. Wild and domestic mammals harboring *T. cruzi* and infected triatomines are found in spotty distributions from the southern United States to southern Argentina. Humans become involved in the cycle of transmission when infected vectors take up residence in the primitive wood, adobe, and stone houses common in much of Latin America. Thus human *T. cruzi* infection is a health problem primarily among the poor in rural areas of Mexico and Central and South America. Most new *T. cruzi*

infections in rural settings occur in children, but the incidence is unknown because most cases go undiagnosed. Historically, transfusion-associated transmission of *T. cruzi* has been a serious public health problem in many endemic countries. However, with some notable exceptions, transmission by this route has been markedly reduced as effective programs for the screening of donated blood have been implemented. Several dozen patients with HIV and chronic *T. cruzi* infections who underwent acute recrudescence of the latter have been described. These patients generally presented with *T. cruzi* brain abscesses, a manifestation of the illness that does not occur in immunocompetent persons. Currently, it is estimated that 12 million people are chronically infected with *T. cruzi* and that 25,000 deaths due to the illness occur each year. Of chronically infected persons, 10–30% eventually develop symptomatic cardiac lesions or gastrointestinal disease. The resulting morbidity and mortality make Chagas' disease the most important parasitic disease burden in Latin America.

In recent years, the rate of *T. cruzi* transmission has decreased markedly in several endemic countries as a result of successful programs involving vector control, blood-bank screening, and education of at-risk populations. A major program begun in 1991 in the "southern cone" nations of South America (Uruguay, Paraguay, Bolivia, Brazil, Chile, and Argentina) has provided the framework for much of this progress. Uruguay and Chile were certified transmission-free in the late 1990s, and Brazil was declared free of transmission in 2006. Transmission has been reduced markedly in Argentina as well. Similar control programs have been initiated in the countries of northern South America and in the Central American nations.

Acute Chagas' disease is rare in the United States. Five cases of autochthonous transmission and five instances of transmission by blood transfusion have been reported. Moreover, *T. cruzi* was transmitted to five recipients of organs from three *T. cruzi*–infected donors. Two of these recipients became infected through cardiac transplants. Acute Chagas' disease has not been reported in tourists returning to the United States from Latin America, although two such instances have been reported in Europe. In contrast, the prevalence of chronic *T. cruzi* infections in the United States has increased considerably in recent years. Data from the 2000 census indicate that >12 million immigrants from Chagas'-endemic countries currently live in the United States, ~8 million of whom are Mexicans. The prevalence of *T. cruzi* infection in Mexico is 0.5–1.0%, and most of the 4 million immigrants from Chagas'-endemic nations who are not Mexicans come from countries in which the prevalence of *T. cruzi* infection is greater than it is in Mexico. The total number of *T. cruzi*–infected persons living in the United States can be estimated reasonably to be 80,000–120,000. The number of instances of transfusion-associated transmission in this country is likely to be considerably greater than the number reported. Screening of the U.S. blood supply for evidence of *T. cruzi* infection has recently begun (see Diagnosis, later in the chapter).

CLINICAL COURSE

The first signs of acute Chagas' disease develop at least 1 week after invasion by the parasites. When the organisms enter through a break in the skin, an indurated area of erythema and swelling (the chagoma), accompanied by local lymphadenopathy, may appear. *Romaña's sign*—the classic finding in acute Chagas' disease, which consists of unilateral painless edema of the palpebrae and periocular tissues—can result when the conjunctiva is the portal of entry (**Fig. 27-2**). The initial local signs may be followed by malaise, fever, anorexia, and edema of the face and lower extremities. A morbilliform rash may also appear. Generalized lymphadenopathy and hepatosplenomegaly may develop. Severe myocarditis develops rarely; most deaths in acute Chagas' disease are due to heart failure. Neurologic signs are not common, but meningoencephalitis occurs occasionally. The acute symptoms resolve spontaneously in virtually all patients, who then enter the asymptomatic or indeterminate phase of chronic *T. cruzi* infection.

Symptomatic chronic Chagas' disease becomes apparent years or even decades after the initial infection. The heart is commonly involved, and symptoms are caused by rhythm disturbances, dilated cardiomyopathy, and thromboembolism. Right bundle-branch block is a common electrocardiographic abnormality, but other types of atrioventricular block, premature ventricular contractions, and tachy- and bradyarrhythmias occur frequently. Cardiomyopathy often results in right-sided or biventricular heart failure. Embolization of mural thrombi to the

brain or other areas may take place. Patients with megaesophagus suffer from dysphagia, odynophagia, chest pain, and regurgitation. Aspiration can occur (especially during sleep) in patients with severe esophageal dysfunction, and repeated episodes of aspiration pneumonitis are common. Weight loss, cachexia, and pulmonary infection can result in death. Patients with megacolon are plagued by abdominal pain and chronic constipation, and advanced megacolon can cause obstruction, volvulus, septicemia, and death.

DIAGNOSIS

The diagnosis of acute Chagas' disease requires the detection of parasites. Microscopic examination of fresh anticoagulated blood or of the buffy coat is the simplest way to see the motile organisms. Parasites also can be seen in Giemsa-stained thin and thick blood smears. Microhematocrit tubes containing acridine orange as a stain can be used for the same purpose. When repeated attempts to visualize the organisms are unsuccessful, polymerase chain reaction (PCR) or hemoculture in special media can be performed. When used by experienced personnel, all of these methods yield positive results in a high proportion of cases of acute Chagas' disease. Hemoculture has the disadvantage of taking several weeks to give positive results. Serologic testing plays no role in diagnosing acute Chagas' disease.

Chronic Chagas' disease is diagnosed by the detection of specific antibodies that bind to *T. cruzi* antigens. Demonstration of the parasite is not of primary importance. In Latin America, ~20 assays are commercially available, including several based on recombinant antigens. Unfortunately, these tests have varying levels of sensitivity and specificity, and false-positive reactions are a particular problem—typically with samples from patients who have other infectious and parasitic diseases or autoimmune disorders. In addition, confirmatory testing has presented a persistent challenge. For these reasons, it is generally recommended that specimens be tested in at least two assays and that well-characterized positive and negative comparison samples be included in each run. The radioimmune precipitation assay (Chagas' RIPA) is a highly sensitive and specific confirmatory method for detecting antibodies to *T. cruzi* [approved under the Clinical Laboratory Improvement Amendment (CLIA) and available in the author's laboratory]. In December 2006, the U.S. Food and Drug Administration (FDA) approved a test to screen blood and organ donors for *T. cruzi* infection (Ortho *T. cruzi* ELISA Test System, Ortho-Clinical Diagnostics, Raritan, NJ). In late January 2007, the American Red Cross and Blood Systems, Inc.—blood-collection agencies that together account for ~65% of the U.S. blood supply—initiated screening of all the donations they process for *T. cruzi*. The Chagas' RIPA is being used as the confirmatory assay. Data

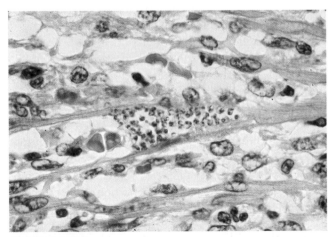

FIGURE 27-2

Romaña's sign in an Argentinean patient with acute *T. cruzi* infection. *(Courtesy of Dr. Humberto Lugones, Centro de Chagas, Santiago del Estero, Argentina; with permission.)*

generated during the first 2 months of screening suggest that if 65% of the blood supply continues to be tested, ~1500 Ortho-reactive donors will be identified annually, ~350 of whom will be RIPA-positive; these figures reflect an overall prevalence of ~1 in 30,000 donors. The use of PCR assays to detect *T. cruzi* DNA in chronically infected persons has been studied extensively. The sensitivity of this approach has not been shown to be reliably greater than that of serology, and no PCR assays are commercially available.

℞ Treatment: CHAGAS' DISEASE

Therapy for Chagas' disease is unsatisfactory. For many years, only two drugs—nifurtimox and benznidazole—have been available for this purpose. Unfortunately, both drugs lack efficacy and often cause severe side effects.

In acute Chagas' disease, nifurtimox markedly reduces the duration of symptoms and parasitemia and decreases the mortality rate. Nevertheless, limited studies have shown that only ~70% of acute infections are cured parasitologically by a full course of treatment. Despite its limitations, treatment with nifurtimox should be initiated as early as possible in acute Chagas' disease. Common adverse effects of nifurtimox include abdominal pain, anorexia, nausea, vomiting, and weight loss. Neurologic reactions to the drug may include restlessness, disorientation, insomnia, twitching, paresthesia, polyneuritis, and seizures. These symptoms usually disappear when the dosage is reduced or treatment is discontinued. The recommended daily dosage is 8–10 mg/kg for adults, 12.5–15 mg/kg for adolescents, and 15–20 mg/kg for children 1–10 years of age. The drug should be given orally in four divided doses each day, and therapy should be continued for 90–120 days. Nifurtimox is available from the Drug Service of the Centers for Disease Control and Prevention (CDC) in Atlanta (telephone number, 770-639-3670).

The efficacy of benznidazole is similar to that of nifurtimox; a cure rate of 90% among congenitally infected infants treated before their first birthday has been reported. Adverse effects include peripheral neuropathy, rash, and granulocytopenia. The recommended oral dosage is 5 mg/kg per day for 60 days. Benznidazole is generally considered the drug of choice in Latin America.

The question of whether patients in the indeterminate or chronic symptomatic phase of Chagas' disease should be treated with nifurtimox or benznidazole has been debated for years. The fact that parasitologic cure rates in chronically infected persons may be <10% is central to this controversy. There is no convincing evidence from properly controlled trials that treatment of adults with long-standing *T. cruzi* infections with either of the drugs is beneficial. The current consensus of Latin American authorities is that all *T. cruzi*–infected persons up to 18 years of age should be given benznidazole or nifurtimox.

The usefulness of allopurinol, fluconazole, and itraconazole for the treatment of acute Chagas' disease has been studied in laboratory animals and to a lesser extent in humans. None of these drugs has exhibited a level of anti–*T. cruzi* activity that warrants its use in patients. Several newer antifungal azoles have shown promise in animal studies but have not yet been tested in humans.

Patients who develop cardiac and/or gastrointestinal disease in association with *T. cruzi* infection should be referred to appropriate subspecialists for further evaluation and treatment. Cardiac transplantation is an option for patients with end-stage chagasic cardiopathies, and >100 such transplantations have been done in Brazil and the United States. The survival rate among Chagas' disease cardiac transplant recipients is higher than that among persons receiving cardiac transplants for other reasons. This better outcome may be due to the fact that lesions are limited to the heart in most patients with symptomatic chronic Chagas' disease.

PREVENTION

Since drug therapy is unsatisfactory and vaccines are not available, the control of *T. cruzi* transmission in endemic countries must depend on reduction of domiciliary vector populations by spraying of insecticides, improvements in housing, and education of at-risk persons. As noted earlier, these measures, coupled with serologic screening of blood donors, have markedly reduced transmission of the parasite in many endemic countries. Tourists would be wise to avoid sleeping in dilapidated houses in rural areas of endemic countries. Mosquito nets and insect repellent provide additional protection.

In view of the possibly serious consequences of chronic *T. cruzi* infection, it would be prudent for all immigrants from endemic regions living in the United States to be tested for evidence of infection. Identification of persons harboring the parasite would permit periodic electrocardiographic monitoring, which can be important because pacemakers benefit some patients who develop ominous rhythm disturbances. The possibility of congenital transmission is yet another justification for screening. Guidance for the evaluation and long-term monitoring of *T. cruzi*–infected persons is being developed by staff at the CDC.

Laboratory personnel should wear gloves and eye protection when working with *T. cruzi* and infected vectors.

FURTHER READINGS

CHANG CD et al: Evaluation of a prototype *Trypanosoma cruzi* antibody assay with recombinant antigens on a fully automated chemiluminescence analyzer for blood donor screening. Transfusion 46:1737, 2006

FIORELLI AI et al: Later evolution after cardiac transplantation in Chagas' disease. Transplant Proc 37:2793, 2005

KIRCHHOFF LV et al: Transfusion-associated Chagas' disease (American trypanosomiasis) in Mexico: Implications for transfusion medicine in the United States. Transfusion 46:298, 2006

LAMBERT N et al: Chagasic encephalitis as the initial manifestation of AIDS. Ann Intern Med 144:941, 2006

MASCOLA L et al: Chagas disease after organ transplantation—Los Angeles, California, 2006. MMWR 55:798, 2006

RASSI A JR et al: Development and validation of a risk score for predicting death in Chagas' heart disease. N Engl J Med 355:799, 2006

SARTORI AM et al: Exacerbation of HIV viral load simultaneous with asymptomatic reactivation of chronic Chagas' disease. Am J Trop Med Hyg 67:521, 2002

SCHMUNIS GA, CRUZ JR: Safety of the blood supply in Latin America. Clin Microbiol Rev 18:12, 2005

CHAPTER 27

Chagas' Disease

CHAPTER 28

CARDIOGENIC SHOCK AND PULMONARY EDEMA

Judith S. Hochman ■ David H. Ingbar

Cardiogenic shock and pulmonary edema are life-threatening conditions that should be treated as medical emergencies. The most common etiology for both is severe left ventricular (LV) dysfunction, leading to pulmonary congestion and/or systemic hypoperfusion (**Fig. 28-1**).

The pathophysiology of pulmonary edema is discussed in Chap. 5.

CARDIOGENIC SHOCK

Cardiogenic shock (CS) is characterized by systemic hypoperfusion due to severe depression of the cardiac index [<2.2 (L/min)/m^2] and sustained systolic arterial hypotension (<90 mmHg), despite an elevated filling pressure [pulmonary capillary wedge pressure (PCWP) >18 mmHg]. It is associated with in-hospital mortality rates >50%. The major causes of CS are listed in **Table 28-1**. Circulatory failure based on cardiac dysfunction may be caused by primary myocardial failure, most commonly secondary to acute myocardial infarction (MI) (Chap. 35), and less frequently by cardiomyopathy or myocarditis (Chap. 21) or cardiac tamponade (Chap. 22).

Incidence

CS is the leading cause of death of patients hospitalized with MI. Early reperfusion therapy for acute MI decreases the incidence of CS. The rate of CS complicating acute MI fell from 20% in the 1960s but has plateaued at ~8% for >20 years. Shock is typically associated with ST elevation MI (STEMI) and is less common with non-ST elevation MI (Chap. 35).

LV failure accounts for ~80% of the cases of CS complicating acute MI. Acute severe mitral regurgitation (MR), ventricular septal rupture (VSR), predominant right ventricular (RV) failure, and free wall rupture or tamponade account for the remainder.

Pathophysiology

CS is characterized by a vicious circle in which depression of myocardial contractility, usually due to ischemia, results in reduced cardiac output and arterial pressure (BP), which result in hypoperfusion of the myocardium and further ischemia and depression of the cardiac output (Fig. 28-1). Systolic myocardial dysfunction reduces stroke volume and, together with diastolic dysfunction, leads to elevated LV end-diastolic pressure and PCWP as well as to pulmonary congestion. Reduced coronary perfusion leads to worsening ischemia and progressive myocardial dysfunction and a rapid downward spiral, which, if uninterrupted, is often fatal. A systemic inflammatory response syndrome may accompany large infarctions and shock. Inflammatory cytokines, inducible nitric

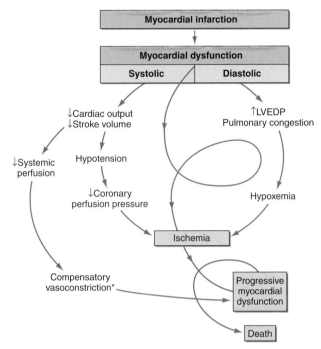

FIGURE 28-1

Pathophysiology of cardiogenic shock. Systolic and diastolic myocardial dysfunction result in a reduction in cardiac output and often pulmonary congestion. Systemic and coronary hypoperfusion occur, resulting in progressive ischemia. Although a number of compensatory mechanisms are activated in an attempt to support the circulation, these compensatory mechanisms may become maladaptive and produce a worsening of hemodynamics. *Release of inflammatory cytokines after myocardial infarction may lead to inducible nitrous oxide expression, excess NO, and inappropriate vasodilation. This causes further reduction in systemic and coronary perfusion. A vicious spiral of progressive myocardial dysfunction occurs that ultimately results in death if it is not interrupted. LVEDP, left ventricular end-diastolic pressure. *(From SM Hollenberg et al: Ann Intern Med 131:47, 1999.)*

oxide synthase, and excess nitric oxide and peroxynitrite may contribute to the genesis of CS as they do to other forms of shock. Lactic acidosis from poor tissue perfusion and hypoxemia from pulmonary edema may result from pump failure and then contribute to the vicious circle by worsening myocardial ischemia and hypotension. Severe acidosis (pH <7.25) reduces the efficacy of endogenous and exogenously administered catecholamines. Refractory sustained ventricular or atrial tachyarrhythmias can cause or exacerbate CS.

Autopsy specimens often reflect the stuttering course and piecemeal necrosis of the LV, showing varying stages of infarction. Reinfarction is apparent as new areas of necrosis contiguous with or remote from a slightly older infarct. Infarctions that extend through the full myocardial thickness and result in rupture of the interventricular septum, papillary muscle, or ventricular free wall may result in shock (Chap. 35).

TABLE 28-1

ETIOLOGIES OF CARDIOGENIC SHOCK (CS)[a] AND CARDIOGENIC PULMONARY EDEMA

Etiologies of Cardiogenic Shock or Pulmonary Edema

Acute myocardial infarction/ischemia
  LV failure
  VSR
  Papillary muscle/chordal rupture—severe MR
  Ventricular free wall rupture with subacute tamponade
  Other conditions complicating large MIs
    Hemorrhage
    Infection
    Excess negative inotropic or vasodilator medications
    Prior valvular heart disease
    Hyperglycemia/ketoacidosis
Post-cardiac arrest
Post-cardiotomy
Refractory sustained tachyarrhythmias
Acute fulminant myocarditis
End-stage cardiomyopathy
Left ventricular apical ballooning
Tako-tsubo cardiomyopathy
Hypertrophic cardiomyopathy with severe outflow obstruction
Aortic dissection with aortic insufficiency or tamponade
Pulmonary embolus
Severe valvular heart disease
  Critical aortic or mitral stenosis
  Acute severe aortic or MR
Toxic-metabolic
  Beta-blocker or calcium channel antagonist overdose

Other Etiologies of Cardiogenic Shock[b]

RV failure due to:
  Acute myocardial infarction
  Acute coronary pulmonale
Refractory sustained bradyarrhythmias
Pericardial tamponade
Toxic/metabolic
  Severe acidosis, severe hypoxemia

[a]The etiologies of CS are listed. Most of these can cause pulmonary edema instead of shock or pulmonary edema with CS.
[b]These cause CS but not pulmonary edema.
Note: LV, left ventricular; VSR, ventricular septal rupture; MR, mitral regurgitation; RV, right ventricular.

Patient Profile

In patients with acute MI, older age, female sex, prior MI, diabetes, and anterior MI location are all associated with increased risk of CS. Shock associated with a first inferior MI should prompt a search for a mechanical cause. Reinfarction soon after MI increases the risk of CS. Two-thirds of patients with CS have flow-limiting stenoses in all three major coronary arteries, and 20% have left main coronary artery stenosis. CS may rarely occur in the absence of significant stenosis, as seen in LV apical ballooning/Tako-tsubo cardiomyopathy, often in response to sudden severe emotional stress.

Shock is present on admission in only one-quarter of patients who develop CS complicating MI; one-quarter develop it rapidly thereafter, within 6 h of MI onset. Another quarter develops shock later on the first day. Subsequent onset of CS may be due to reinfarction, marked infarct expansion, or a mechanical complication.

Diagnosis

Due to the unstable condition of these patients, supportive therapy must be initiated simultaneously with diagnostic evaluation (Fig. 28-2). A focused history and physical examination should be performed, blood specimens sent to the laboratory, and an electrocardiogram (ECG) and chest x-ray obtained.

Echocardiography is an invaluable diagnostic tool in patients suspected of CS.

Clinical Findings

Most patients have continuing chest pain and dyspnea and appear pale, apprehensive, and diaphoretic. Mentation may be altered, with somnolence, confusion, and agitation. The pulse is typically weak and rapid, often in the range of 90–110 beats/min, or severe bradycardia due to high-grade heart block may be present. Systolic blood pressure (BP) is reduced (<90 mmHg) with a narrow pulse pressure (<30 mmHg), but occasionally BP may be maintained by very high systemic vascular resistance. Tachypnea,

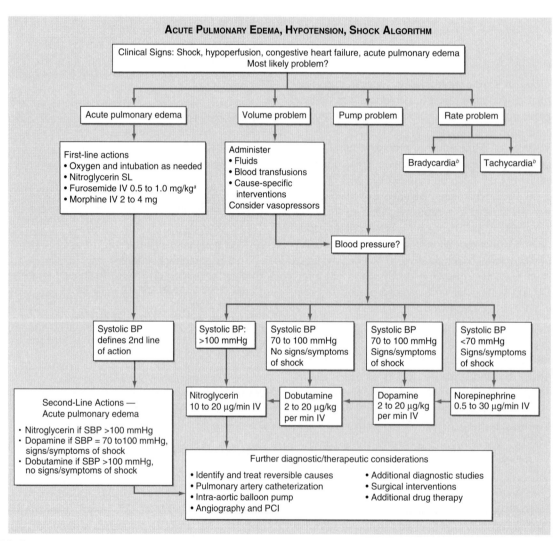

FIGURE 28-2

The emergency management of patients with cardiogenic shock, acute pulmonary edema, or both is outlined. [a]Furosemide: <0.5 mg/kg for new-onset acute pulmonary edema without hypervolemia; 1 mg/kg for acute on chronic volume overload, renal insufficiency. [b]For management of bradycardia and tachycardia, see Chaps. 15 and 16. ACE, angiotensin-converting enzyme; BP, blood pressure; MI, myocardial infarction. [From J Fields et al (eds): Handbook of Emergency Cardiovascular Care for Healthcare Providers. Copyright 2006, American Heart Association, Inc. Reprinted with permission.]

Cheyne-Stokes respirations, and jugular venous distention may be present. The precordium is typically quiet, with a weak apical pulse. S_1 is usually soft, and an S_3 gallop may be audible. Acute, severe MR and VSR are usually associated with characteristic systolic murmurs (Chap. 35). Rales are audible in most patients with LV failure causing CS. Oliguria (urine output <30 mL/h) is common.

Laboratory Findings
The white blood cell count is typically elevated with a left shift. In the absence of prior renal insufficiency, renal function is initially normal, but blood urea nitrogen and creatinine rise progressively. Hepatic transaminases may be markedly elevated due to liver hypoperfusion. Poor tissue perfusion may result in an anion gap acidosis and elevation of lactic acid level. Prior to support with supplemental O_2, arterial blood gases usually demonstrate hypoxemia and metabolic acidosis, which may be compensated by respiratory alkalosis. Cardiac markers, creatine phosphokinase and its MB fraction, are markedly elevated, as are troponins I and T.

Electrocardiogram
In CS due to acute MI with LV failure, Q waves and/or >2-mm ST elevation in multiple leads or left bundle branch block are usually present. More than one-half of all infarcts associated with shock are anterior. Global ischemia due to severe left main stenosis is usually accompanied by severe (e.g., >3 mm) ST depressions in multiple leads.

Chest Roentgenogram
The chest x-ray typically shows pulmonary vascular congestion and often pulmonary edema, but these findings may be absent in up to a third of patients. The heart size is usually normal when CS results from a first MI but is enlarged when it occurs in a patient with a previous MI.

Echocardiogram
A two-dimensional echocardiogram with color flow Doppler (Chap. 12) should be obtained promptly in patients with suspected CS to help define its etiology. Doppler mapping demonstrates a left-to-right shunt in patients with VSR and the severity of MR when the latter is present. Proximal aortic dissection with aortic regurgitation or tamponade may be visualized or evidence for pulmonary embolism obtained.

Pulmonary Artery Catheterization
There is controversy regarding the use of pulmonary artery (Swan-Ganz) catheters in patients with established or suspected CS (Chap. 13). However, their use is generally recommended for measurement of filling pressures and cardiac output to confirm the diagnosis and optimize use of IV fluids, inotropic agents, and vasopressors (Table 28-2). Blood samples for O_2 saturation

CHAPTER 28 Cardiogenic Shock and Pulmonary Edema

TABLE 28-2

HEMODYNAMIC PATTERNS[a]

	RA, mmHg	RVS, mmHg	RVD, mmHg	PAS, mmHg	PAD, mmHg	PCW, mmHg	CI, (L/min)/m²	SVR, (dyn · s)/ cm⁵
Normal values	<6	<25	0–12	<25	0–12	<6–12	≥2.5	(800–1600)
MI without pulmonary edema[b]	—	—	—	—	—	~13 (5–18)	~2.7 (2.2–4.3)	—
Pulmonary edema	↔↑	↔↑	↔↑	↑	↑	↑	↔↓	↑
Cardiogenic shock								
LV failure	↔↑	↔↑	↔↑	↔↑	↑	↑	↓	↔↑
RV failure[c]	↑	↓↔↑[d]	↑	↓↔↑[d]	↔↓↑[d]	↓↔↑[d]	↓	↑
Cardiac tamponade	↑	↔↑	↑	↔↑	↔↑	↔↑	↓	↑
Acute mitral regurgitation	↔↑	↑	↔↑	↑	↑	↑	↔↓	↔↑
Ventricular septal rupture	↑	↔↑	↑	↔↑	↔↑	↔↑	↑ PBF ↓ SBF	↔↑
Hypovolemic shock	↓	↔↓	↔↓	↓	↓	↓	↓	↑
Septic shock	↓	↔↓	↔↓	↓	↓	↓	↑	↓

[a]There is significant patient-to-patient variation. Pressure may be normalized if cardiac output is low.

[b]Forrester et al classified non-reperfused MI patients into four hemodynamic subsets. (From Forrester JS et al: N Engl J Med 295:1356, 1976.) PCWP and CI in clinically stable subset 1 patients are shown. Values in parentheses represent range.

[c]"Isolated" or predominant RV failure.

[d]PCW and PA pressures may rise in RV failure after volume loading due to RV dilation, right-to-left shift of the interventricular septum, resulting in impaired LV filling. When biventricular failure is present, the patterns are similar to those shown for LV failure.

Note: RA, right atrium; RVS/D, right ventricular systolic/diastolic; PAS/D, pulmonary artery systolic/diastolic; PCW, pulmonary capillary wedge; CI, cardiac index; SVR, systemic vascular resistance; MI, myocardial infarction; P/SBF, pulmonary/systemic blood flow.

Source: Table prepared with the assistance of Krishnan Ramanathan, MD.

measurement should be obtained from the right atrium, right ventricle, and pulmonary artery to rule out a left-to-right shunt. Mixed venous O_2 saturations are low and arterial-venous O_2 differences are elevated, reflecting low cardiac index and high fractional O_2 extraction. The PCWP is elevated. However, use of sympathomimetic amines may return these measurements and the systemic BP toward normal. Systemic vascular resistance may be low, normal, or elevated in CS. Equalization of right- and left-sided filling pressures (right atrial and PCWP) suggests cardiac tamponade as the cause of CS (Chap. 22).

Left Heart Catheterization and Coronary Angiography

Measurement of LV pressure, definition of the coronary anatomy, and left ventriculography provide useful information and are indicated in most patients with CS complicating MI. Because of the procedural risk in this critically ill population, cardiac catheterization should be performed when there is a plan and capability for immediate coronary intervention (see later) or when a definitive diagnosis has not been made by other tests.

℞ Treatment:
ACUTE MYOCARDIAL INFARCTION

GENERAL MEASURES (Fig. 28-2) In addition to the usual treatment of acute MI (Chap. 35), initial therapy is aimed at maintaining adequate systemic and coronary perfusion by raising systemic BP with vasopressors and adjusting volume status to a level that ensures optimum LV filling pressure. There is inter-patient variability, but the values that are generally associated with adequate perfusion are systolic BP of ~90 mmHg or mean BP >60 mmHg and PCWP of ~20 mmHg. Hypoxemia and acidosis must be corrected; most patients require ventilatory support with either endotracheal intubation or bilevel positive airway pressure (Bi-PAP) to correct these abnormalities and reduce the work of breathing (see Pulmonary Edema, later in this chapter). Negative inotropic agents should be discontinued and the doses of renally cleared medications adjusted. Hyperglycemia should be corrected with continuous infusion of insulin. Bradyarrhythmias may require transvenous pacing. Recurrent ventricular tachycardia or rapid atrial fibrillation may require immediate treatment (Chap. 16).

VASOPRESSORS Various IV drugs may be used to augment BP and cardiac output in patients with CS. All have important disadvantages, and none has been shown to change the outcome in patients with established shock. *Norepinephrine* is a potent vasoconstrictor and inotropic stimulant that increases myocardial O_2 consumption; it should be reserved for patients with CS and refractory hypotension, in particular those without

elevated systemic vascular resistance. It should be started at a dosage of 2–4 µg/min and titrated upward as necessary. If systemic perfusion or systolic pressure cannot be maintained at >90 mmHg with a dosage of 15 µg/min, it is unlikely that a further increase will be beneficial.

Dopamine is useful in many patients; at low doses (≤2 µg/kg per min), it dilates the renal vascular bed; at moderate doses (2–10 µg/kg per min), it has positive chronotropic and inotropic effects as a consequence of β-adrenergic receptor stimulation. At higher doses, a vasoconstrictor effect results from α-receptor stimulation. It is started at an infusion rate of 2–5 µg/kg per min, and the dosage is increased every 2–5 min to a maximum of 20–50 µg/kg per min. *Dobutamine* is a synthetic sympathomimetic amine with positive inotropic action and minimal positive chronotropic activity at low doses (2.5 µg/kg per min), but moderate chronotropic activity at higher doses. Although the usual dosage is up to 10 µg/kg per min, its vasodilating activity precludes its use when a vasoconstrictor effect is required.

AORTIC COUNTERPULSATION In CS, mechanical assistance with an intra-aortic balloon pumping (IABP) system capable of augmenting both arterial diastolic pressure and cardiac output is helpful in rapidly stabilizing patients. A sausage-shaped balloon is introduced percutaneously into the aorta via the femoral artery; the balloon is automatically inflated during early diastole, augmenting coronary blood flow. The balloon collapses in early systole, reducing the afterload against which the LV ejects. IABP improves hemodynamic status temporarily in most patients. In contrast to vasopressors and inotropic agents, myocardial O_2 consumption is reduced, ameliorating ischemia. IABP is useful as a stabilizing measure in patients with CS prior to and during cardiac catheterization and percutaneous coronary intervention (PCI) or prior to urgent surgery. IABP is contraindicated if aortic regurgitation is present or aortic dissection is suspected. Ventricular assist devices may be considered for eligible young patients with refractory shock as a bridge to cardiac transplantation (Chap. 18).

REPERFUSION-REVASCULARIZATION The rapid establishment of blood flow in the infarct-related artery is essential in the management of CS and forms the centerpiece of management. The randomized SHOCK Trial demonstrated 132 lives saved per 1000 patients treated with early revascularization with PCI or coronary artery bypass graft (CABG) compared to initial medical therapy including IABP with fibrinolytics followed by delayed revascularization (Fig. 28-3). The benefit is seen across the risk strata and is sustained up to 11 years post MI. Early revascularization with PCI or CABG is a class I recommendation for patients age <75 years with ST elevation or left bundle branch block

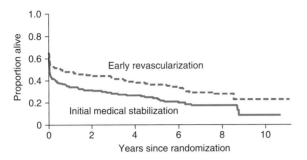

FIGURE 28-3

Early revascularization (ERV) (percutaneous intervention or coronary artery bypass graft) for cardiogenic shock complicating acute myocardial infarction resulted in substantially improved 1-year and long-term survival compared to initial mechanical stabilization (IMS), including intra-aortic balloon pumping and fibrinolytic agents, followed by selective delayed revascularization in the SHOCK Trial (SHould we emergently revascularize Occluded coronaries for Cardiogenic shocK?). *(From JS Hochman et al: JAMA 295:2511–2515, 2006; reprinted with permission from JAMA.)*

MI who develop CS within 36 h of MI and who can be revascularized within 18 h of development of CS. When mechanical revascularization is not possible, IABP and fibrinolytic therapy are recommended. Older patients who are suitable candidates for aggressive care should also be offered early revascularization.

Prognosis

Within this high-risk condition, there is a wide range of expected death rates based on age, severity of hemodynamic abnormalities, severity of the clinical manifestations of hypoperfusion, and the performance of early revascularization. Independent risk factors are advanced age; depressed cardiac index, ejection fraction, and BP; more extensive coronary artery disease; and renal insufficiency.

SHOCK SECONDARY TO RIGHT VENTRICULAR INFARCTION

Although transient hypotension is common in patients with RV infarction and inferior MI (Chap. 35), persistent CS due to RV failure accounts for only 3% of CS complicating MI. The salient features of RV shock are absence of pulmonary congestion, high right atrial pressure (which may be seen only after volume loading), RV dilatation and dysfunction, only mildly or moderately depressed LV function, and predominance of single-vessel proximal right coronary artery occlusion. Management includes IV fluid administration to optimize right atrial pressure (10–15 mmHg); avoidance of excess fluids, which cause a shift of the interventricular septum

into the LV; sympathomimetic amines; IABP; and the early reestablishment of infarct-artery flow.

MITRAL REGURGITATION

(See also Chap. 35) Acute severe MR due to papillary muscle dysfunction and/or rupture may complicate MI and result in CS and/or pulmonary edema. This complication most often occurs on the first day, with a second peak several days later. The diagnosis is confirmed by echo-Doppler. Rapid stabilization with IABP is recommended, with administration of dobutamine as needed to raise cardiac output. Reducing the load against which the LV pumps (afterload) reduces the volume of regurgitant flow of blood into the left atrium. Mitral valve surgery is the definitive therapy and should be performed early in the course in suitable candidates.

VENTRICULAR SEPTAL RUPTURE

(See also Chap. 35) Echo-Doppler demonstrates shunting of blood from the left to the right ventricle and may visualize the opening in the interventricular septum. Timing and management are similar to that for MR with IABP support and surgical correction for suitable candidates.

FREE WALL RUPTURE

Myocardial rupture is a dramatic complication of STEMI that is most likely to occur during the first week after the onset of symptoms; its frequency increases with the age of the patient. First infarction, a history of hypertension, no history of angina pectoris, and a relatively large Q-wave infarct are associated with a higher incidence of cardiac rupture. The clinical presentation typically is a sudden loss of pulse, blood pressure, and consciousness but sinus rhythm on ECG (pulseless electrical activity). The myocardium continues to contract, but forward flow is not maintained as blood escapes into the pericardium. Cardiac tamponade (Chap. 22) ensues, and closed-chest massage is ineffective. This condition is almost universally fatal, although dramatic cases of urgent pericardiotensis followed by successful surgical repair have been reported. Free wall rupture may also result in subacute tamponade when the pericardium temporarily seals the rupture sites. Definitive surgical repair is required.

ACUTE FULMINANT MYOCARDITIS

(See also Chap. 21) Myocarditis can mimic acute MI with ST deviation or bundle branch block on the ECG and marked elevation of cardiac markers. Acute myocarditis causes CS in ~15% of cases. These patients are typically younger than those with CS due to acute MI and often do not have typical ischemic chest pain. Echocardiography usually shows global LV dysfunction.

Initial management is the same as for CS complicating acute MI (Fig. 28-2) but of course does not involve coronary revascularization.

PULMONARY EDEMA

The etiologies and pathophysiology of pulmonary edema are discussed in Chap. 5.

Diagnosis

Acute pulmonary edema usually presents with the rapid onset of dyspnea at rest, tachypnea, tachycardia, and severe hypoxemia. Rales and wheezing due to airway compression from peribronchial cuffing may be audible. Hypertension is usually present due to release of endogenous catecholamines.

It is often difficult to distinguish cardiogenic and noncardiogenic causes of acute pulmonary edema. *Echocardiography* may identify systolic and diastolic ventricular dysfunction and valvular lesions. Pulmonary edema associated with electrocardiographic ST elevation and evolving Q waves is usually diagnostic of acute MI and should prompt immediate institution of MI protocols and coronary artery reperfusion therapy (Chap. 35). Brain natriuretic peptide levels, when substantially elevated, support heart failure as the etiology of acute dyspnea with pulmonary edema (Chap. 17).

The use of a *Swan-Ganz catheter* permits measurement of PCWP and helps differentiate high pressure (cardiogenic) and normal pressure (noncardiogenic) causes of pulmonary edema. Pulmonary artery catheterization is indicated when the etiology of the pulmonary edema is uncertain, when it is refractory to therapy, or when it is accompanied by hypotension. Data derived from use of a catheter often alters the treatment plan, but impact on mortality has not been demonstrated.

℞ Treatment:
PULMONARY EDEMA

The treatment of pulmonary edema depends upon the specific etiology. Given the acute, life-threatening nature of the condition, a number of measures must be applied immediately to support the circulation, gas exchange, and lung mechanics. In addition, conditions that frequently complicate pulmonary edema, such as infection, acidemia, anemia, and renal failure, must be corrected.

SUPPORT OF OXYGENATION AND VENTILATION Patients with acute cardiogenic pulmonary edema generally have an identifiable cause of acute LV failure such as arrhythmia, ischemia/infarction, or myocardial decompensation (Chap. 17) that can be rapidly treated, with improvement in gas exchange. In contrast, noncardiogenic edema usually resolves much less quickly, and most patients require mechanical ventilation.

Oxygen Therapy Support of oxygenation is essential to ensure adequate O_2 delivery to peripheral tissues, including the heart.

Positive-Pressure Ventilation Pulmonary edema increases the work of breathing and the O_2 requirements of this work and may pose a significant physiologic stress on the heart. For patients with inadequate oxygenation or ventilation in spite of supplemental O_2, assisted ventilation by face or nasal mask or by endotracheal intubation should be initiated. Continuous or bilevel positive airway pressure can rest the respiratory muscles, improve oxygenation and cardiac function, and reduce the need for intubation. In refractory cases, mechanical ventilation can relieve the work of breathing more completely than noninvasive ventilation. Mechanical ventilation with positive end-expiratory pressure can have multiple beneficial effects on pulmonary edema: (1) it can decrease both preload and afterload, thereby improving cardiac function; (2) it can redistribute lung water from the intraalveolar to the extraalveolar space where the fluid does not interfere as much with gas exchange; and (3) it can increase lung volume to avoid atelectasis.

REDUCTION OF PRELOAD In most forms of pulmonary edema, the quantity of extravascular lung water is related to both the PCWP and the intravascular volume status.

Diuretics The "loop diuretics" furosemide, bumetanide, and torsemide are effective in most forms of pulmonary edema, even in the presence of hypoalbuminemia, hyponatremia, or hypochloremia. Furosemide is also a venodilator that can reduce preload rapidly, prior to any diuresis, and is the diuretic of choice. The initial dose of furosemide should be ≤0.5 mg/kg, but a higher dose (1 mg/kg) is required in patients with renal insufficiency, chronic diuretic use, or hypervolemia or after failure of a lower dose.

Nitrates Nitroglycerin and isosorbide dinitrate act predominantly as venodilators, with coronary vasodilating properties as well. They are rapid in onset and effective when administered by a variety of routes. Sublingual nitroglycerin (0.4 mg × 3 every 5 min) is first-line therapy for acute cardiogenic pulmonary edema. If pulmonary edema persists in the absence of hypotension, sublingual may be followed by IV nitroglycerin, commencing at 5–10 µg/min. IV nitroprusside (0.1–5 µg/kg per min) is a potent venous and arterial vasodilator. It is useful for patients with pulmonary edema and hypertension, but is not recommended in states of reduced coronary artery perfusion. It requires close monitoring and titration, including the use of an arterial catheter for continuous BP measurement in the intensive care unit.

Morphine Given in 2- to 4-mg IV boluses, morphine is a transient venodilator that reduces preload while relieving dyspnea and anxiety. These effects can diminish stress, catecholamine levels, tachycardia, and ventricular afterload in patients with pulmonary edema and systemic hypertension.

Angiotensin-Converting Enzyme (ACE) Inhibitors ACE inhibitors reduce both afterload and preload and are recommended in hypertensive patients. A low dose of a short-acting agent may be initiated and followed by increasing oral doses. In acute MI with heart failure, ACE inhibitors reduce short- and long-term mortality.

Other Preload-Reducing Agents IV recombinant brain natriuretic peptide (nesiritide) is a potent vasodilator with diuretic properties and is effective in the treatment of cardiogenic pulmonary edema. It should be reserved for refractory patients and is not recommended in the setting of ischemia or MI.

Physical Methods Reduction of venous return reduces preload. Patients without hypotension should be maintained in the sitting position with the legs dangling along the side of the bed.

Inotropic and Inodilator Drugs The sympathomimetic amines dopamine and dobutamine (see earlier) are potent inotropic agents. The bipyridine phosphodiesterase-3 inhibitors (inodilators), such as milrinone (50 μg/kg followed by 0.25–0.75 μg/kg per min), stimulate myocardial contractility while promoting peripheral and pulmonary vasodilation. Such agents are indicated in patients with cardiogenic pulmonary edema and severe LV dysfunction.

Digitalis Glycosides Once a mainstay of treatment because of their positive inotropic action (Chap. 17), digitalis glycosides are rarely used at present. However, they may be useful for control of ventricular rate in patients with rapid atrial fibrillation or flutter and LV dysfunction, since they do not have the negative inotropic effects of other drugs that inhibit atrioventricular nodal conduction.

Intra-aortic Counterpulsation IABP may help to relieve cardiogenic pulmonary edema. It is indicated as a stabilizing measure when acute severe mitral regurgitation or ventricular septal rupture causes refractory pulmonary edema, especially in preparation for surgical repair. IABP or LV-assist devices (Chap. 18) are useful as bridging therapy to cardiac transplantation in patients with refractory pulmonary edema secondary to myocarditis or cardiomyopathy.

Treatment of Tachyarrhythmias and Atrial-Ventricular Resynchronization (See also Chap. 16) Sinus tachycardia or atrial fibrillation can result from elevated left atrial pressure and sympathetic stimulation. Tachycardia itself can also limit LV filling time and raise left atrial pressure further. While relief of pulmonary congestion will slow the sinus rate or ventricular response in atrial fibrillation, a primary tachyarrhythmia may require cardioversion. In patients with reduced LV function and without atrial contraction or with lack of synchronized atrioventricular contraction, placement of an atrioventricular sequential pacemaker should be considered (Chap. 15).

Stimulation of Alveolar Fluid Clearance Recent mechanistic studies on alveolar epithelial ion transport have defined a variety of ways to upregulate the clearance of solute and water from the alveolar space. In patients with acute lung injury (noncardiogenic pulmonary edema), IV β-adrenergic agonist treatment decreases extravascular lung water.

SPECIAL CONSIDERATIONS

The Risk of Iatrogenic Cardiogenic Shock In the treatment of pulmonary edema vasodilators lower BP, and, particularly when used in combination, their use may lead to hypotension, coronary artery hypoperfusion, and shock (Fig. 28-1). In general, patients with a *hypertensive* response to pulmonary edema tolerate and are benefited by these medications. In normotensive patients, low doses of single agents should be instituted sequentially, as needed.

Acute Coronary Syndromes (See also Chap. 35) Acute STEMI complicated by pulmonary edema is associated with in-hospital mortality rates of 20–40%. After immediate stabilization, coronary artery blood flow must be reestablished rapidly. When available, primary PCI is preferable; alternatively, a fibrinolytic agent should be administered. Early coronary angiography and revascularization by PCI or CABG are also indicated for patients with non-ST elevation acute coronary syndrome. IABP use may be required to stabilize patients for coronary angiography if hypotension develops or for refractory pulmonary edema in patients with LV failure who are candidates for revascularization.

Unusual Types of Edema Specific etiologies of pulmonary edema may require particular therapy. Reexpansion pulmonary edema can develop after removal of air or fluid that has been in the pleural space for some time. These patients may develop hypotension or oliguria resulting from rapid fluid shifts into the lung. In contrast to cardiogenic edema, diuretics and preload reduction are contraindicated, and intravascular volume repletion is often needed while supporting oxygenation and gas exchange.

High-altitude pulmonary edema can often be prevented by use of dexamethasone, calcium channel-blocking drugs, or long-acting inhaled β_2-adrenergic agonists. Treatment includes descent from altitude, bed rest, oxygen, and, if feasible, inhaled nitric oxide; nifedipine may also be effective.

For pulmonary edema resulting from upper airway obstruction, recognition of the obstructing cause is key, since treatment then is to relieve or bypass the obstruction.

FURTHER READINGS

ANTMAN EM: Treatment of ST elevation myocardial infarction, in *Braunwald's Heart Disease*, 8th ed, P Libby et al (eds). Philadelphia, Saunders, 2008

——— et al: ACC/AHA Guidelines for the management of patients with acute myocardial infarction. A report of the American College Of Cardiology/American Heart Association task force on practice guidelines (Committee on Management of Acute Myocardial Infarction). J Am Coll Cardiol 44:671, 2004

BABAEV A et al for the NRMI Investigators: National guidelines and trends in management of patients with acute myocardial infarction complicated by cardiogenic shock: Observations from the National Registry of Myocardial Infarction. J Am Med Assoc 294:448, 2005

GOLDBERG RJ et al: Thirty-year trends (1975 to 2005) in the magnitude of, management of, and hospital death rates associated with cardiogenic shock in patients with acute myocardial infarction: a population-based perspective. Circulation 119:1211, 2009

HOCHMAN JS: Cardiogenic shock complicating acute myocardial infarction: Expanding the paradigm. Circulation 107:2998, 2003

——— et al: Early revascularization and long-term survival in cardiogenic shock complicating acute myocardial infarction. JAMA 295:2511, 2006

HOCHMAN JS and OHMAN EM: Cardiogenic Shock, American Heart Association Clinical Series (E. Antman, Ed). New York, Wiley, Blackwell, 2008

MATTHAY MA, INGBAR DH (eds): *Pulmonary Edema. Lung Biology in Health and Disease*, vol 116. New York, Marcel Dekker, 1998

OKUDA M: A multidisciplinary overview of cardiogenic shock. 25:557, 2006

REYNOLDS HR and HOCHMAN JS: Cardiogenic shock: current concepts and improving outcomes. Circulation 117:686, 2008

WARE LB, MATTHAY MA: Clinical practice: Acute pulmonary edema. N Engl J Med 353(26):2788, 2005

CHAPTER 29

CARDIOVASCULAR COLLAPSE, CARDIAC ARREST, AND SUDDEN CARDIAC DEATH

Robert J. Myerburg ■ Agustin Castellanos

OVERVIEW AND DEFINITIONS

The vast majority of naturally occurring sudden deaths are caused by cardiac disorders. The magnitude of sudden *cardiac* death (SCD) as a public health problem is highlighted by the estimate that ~50% of all cardiac deaths are sudden and unexpected, at least two-thirds of which are first cardiac events or occur among population subsets with previously known heart disease considered to be relatively low risk. The total SCD burden is estimated to range from <200,000 to >450,000 deaths each year in the United States. SCD is a direct consequence of cardiac arrest, which may be reversible if responded to promptly. Since resuscitation techniques and emergency rescue systems are available to respond to victims of out-of-hospital cardiac arrest, which was uniformly fatal in the past, understanding the SCD problem has practical importance.

SCD must be defined carefully. In the context of time, "sudden" is defined, for most clinical and epidemiologic purposes, as 1 h or less between a change in clinical status heralding the onset of the terminal clinical event and the cardiac arrest itself. An exception is unwitnessed deaths in which pathologists may expand the definition of time to 24 h after the victim was last seen to be alive and stable.

Because of community-based interventions, victims may remain biologically alive for days or even weeks after a cardiac arrest that has resulted in irreversible central nervous system damage. Confusion in terms can be avoided by adhering strictly to definitions of cardiovascular collapse, cardiac arrest, and death (Table 29-1). Death is biologically, legally, and literally an absolute and irreversible event. Death may be delayed in a survivor of cardiac arrest, but "survival after sudden death" is an irrational term. A generally accepted definition of SCD is *natural death due to cardiac causes*, heralded by abrupt loss of consciousness within *1 h* of the onset of acute symptoms, in an individual who may have known *preexisting* heart disease but in whom the *time* and *mode* of death are *unexpected*. When biologic death of the cardiac arrest victim is delayed because of interventions, the relevant pathophysiologic event remains the sudden and unexpected cardiac arrest that leads ultimately to death, even though delayed by artificial methods. The language used should reflect the fact that the index event was a cardiac arrest and that death was due to its delayed consequences. Accordingly, for statistical purposes, deaths that

TABLE 29-1

	DISTINCTION BETWEEN CARDIOVASCULAR COLLAPSE, CARDIAC ARREST, AND DEATH	
TERM	**DEFINITION**	**QUALIFIERS OR EXCEPTIONS**
Cardiovascular collapse	A sudden loss of effective blood flow due to cardiac and/or peripheral vascular factors which may reverse spontaneously (e.g., neurocardiogenic syncope; vasovagal syncope) or only with interventions (e.g., cardiac arrest)	Nonspecific term that includes cardiac arrest and its consequences and also events that characteristically revert spontaneously
Cardiac arrest	Abrupt cessation of cardiac pump function which may be reversible by a prompt intervention but will lead to death in its absence	Rare spontaneous reversions; likelihood of successful interventions relates to mechanism of arrest, clinical setting, and prompt return of circulation
Death	Irreversible cessation of all biologic functions	None

occur during hospitalization or within 30 days after resuscitated cardiac arrest are counted as sudden deaths.

CLINICAL DEFINITION OF FORMS OF CARDIOVASCULAR COLLAPSE

Cardiovascular collapse is a general term connoting loss of effective blood flow due to acute dysfunction of the heart and/or peripheral vasculature. Cardiovascular collapse may be caused by vasodepressor syncope (vasovagal syncope, postural hypotension with syncope, neurocardiogenic syncope), a transient severe bradycardia, or cardiac arrest. Cardiac arrest is distinguished from the transient forms of cardiovascular collapse in that it usually requires an intervention to achieve resuscitation. In contrast, vasodepressor syncope and other primary bradyarrhythmic syncopal events are transient and non-life-threatening, with spontaneous return of consciousness.

The most common electrical mechanism for cardiac arrest is ventricular fibrillation (VF), which is responsible for 50–80% of cardiac arrests. Severe persistent bradyarrhythmias, asystole, and pulseless electrical activity [(PEA) an organized electrical activity without mechanical response, formerly called electromechanical dissociation] cause another 20–30%. Pulseless sustained ventricular tachycardia (VT) is a less-common mechanism. Acute low cardiac output states, having precipitous onset, may also present clinically as a cardiac arrest. These hemodynamic causes include massive acute pulmonary emboli, internal blood loss from ruptured aortic aneurysm, intense anaphylaxis, and cardiac rupture with tamponade after myocardial infarction (MI).

ETIOLOGY, INITIATING EVENTS, AND CLINICAL EPIDEMIOLOGY

Clinical and epidemiologic studies have identified population subgroups at high risk for SCD. In addition, a large body of pathologic data provides information on the underlying *structural abnormalities* in victims of SCD, and studies of clinical physiology have begun to identify a group of *transient functional factors* that may convert a long-standing underlying structural abnormality from a stable to an unstable state (Table 29-2).

Cardiac disorders constitute the most common causes of sudden *natural* death. After an initial peak incidence of sudden death between birth and 6 months of age (the sudden infant death syndrome), the incidence of sudden death declines sharply and remains low through childhood and adolescence. Among adolescents and young adults, the incidence of SCD is approximately 1 per 100,000 population per year. The incidence begins to increase in adults older than 30 years, reaching a second peak in the age range of 45–75 years, when the incidence approximates 1–2 per 1000 per year among the unselected adult population. Increasing age within this range is associated with increasing risk for sudden *cardiac* death (Fig. 29-1A). From 1–13 years of age, only one of five sudden *natural* deaths is due to cardiac causes. Between 14 and 21 years of age, the proportion increases to 30%, and then to 88% in the middle aged and elderly.

Young and middle aged men and women have different susceptibilities to SCD, but the gender differences decrease with advancing age. The difference in risk for SCD parallels the differences in age-related risks for other manifestations of coronary heart disease (CHD) between men and women. As the gender gap for manifestations of CHD closes in the sixth to eighth decades of life, the excess risk of SCD in males progressively narrows. Despite the lower incidence among younger women, coronary risk factors such as cigarette smoking, diabetes, hyperlipidemia, and hypertension are highly influential, and SCD remains an important clinical and epidemiologic problem. The incidence of SCD among the African-American population appears to be higher than among the white population; the reasons remain uncertain.

Genetic factors contribute to the risk of SCD. In one sense, they contribute to familial predisposition to CHD

TABLE 29-2

CARDIAC ARREST AND SUDDEN CARDIAC DEATH

Structural Causes

I. Coronary heart disease
   A. Coronary artery abnormalities
     1. Chronic atherosclerotic lesions
     2. Acute (active) lesions (plaque fissuring, platelet aggregation, acute thrombosis)
     3. Anomalous coronary artery anatomy
   B. Myocardial infarction
     1. Healed
     2. Acute
II. Myocardial hypertrophy
   A. Secondary
   B. Hypertrophic cardiomyopathy
     1. Obstructive
     2. Nonobstructive
III. Dilated cardiomyopathy—primary muscle disease
IV. Inflammatory and infiltrative disorders
   A. Myocarditis
   B. Noninfectious inflammatory diseases
   C. Infiltrative diseases
   D. Right ventricular dysplasia
V. Valvular heart disease
VI. Electrophysiologic abnormalities, structural
   A. Anomalous pathways in Wolff-Parkinson-White syndrome
   B. Conducting system disease
VII. Inherited disorders of molecular structure associated with electrophysiologic abnormalities (e.g., congenital long QT syndromes, Brugada syndrome)

Functional Contributing Factors

I. Alterations of coronary blood flow
   A. Transient ischemia
   B. Reperfusion after ischemia
II. Low cardiac output states
   A. Heart failure
     1. Chronic
     2. Acute decompensation
   B. Shock
III. Systemic metabolic abnormalities
   A. Electrolyte imbalance (e.g., hypokalemia)
   B. Hypoxemia, acidosis
IV. Neurophysiologic disturbances
   A. Autonomic fluctuations: central, neural, humoral
   B. Receptor function
V. Toxic responses
   A. Proarrhythmic drug effects
   B. Cardiac toxins (e.g., cocaine, digitalis intoxication)
   C. Drug interactions

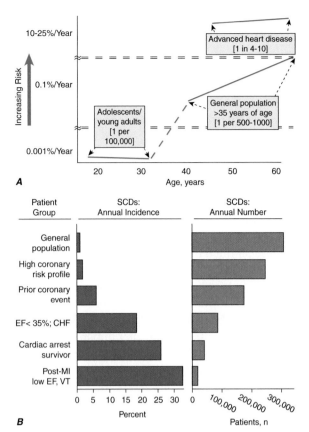

FIGURE 29-1

***Panel A* demonstrates age-related risk for SCD.** For the general population 35 years and older, SCD risk is 0.1–0.2% per year (1 per 500–1,000 population). Among the general population of adolescents and adults younger than 30 years, the overall risk of SCD is 1 per 100,000 population, or 0.001% per year. The risk of SCD increases dramatically after 35 years. The greatest rate of increase is between 40 and 65 years (vertical axis is discontinuous). Among patients older than 30 years, with advanced structural heart disease and markers of high risk for cardiac arrest, the event rate may exceed 25% per year, and age-related risk attenuates. ***Panel B* demonstrates the incidence of SCD in population subgroups** and the relation of total number of events per year to incidence figures. Approximations of subgroup incidence figures and the related population pool from which they are derived are presented. Approximately 50% of all cardiac deaths are sudden and unexpected. The incidence triangle on the left ("Percent/Year") indicates the approximate percentage of sudden and nonsudden deaths in each of the population subgroups indicated, ranging from the lowest percentage in unselected adult populations (0.1–2% per year) to the highest percentage in patients with VT or VF during convalescence after an MI (~50% per year). The triangle on the right indicates the total number of events per year in each of these groups, to reflect incidence in context with the size of the population subgroups. The highest risk categories identify the smallest number of total annual events, and the lowest incidence category accounts for the largest number of events per year. EF, ejection fraction; VT, ventricular tachycardia; VF, ventricular fibrillation; MI, myocardial infarction. *[From RJ Myerburg et al, Circulation 85(Suppl 1):2, 1992. Reproduced with permission of the American Heart Association.]*

and its expression as acute coronary syndromes. In addition, however, there are data suggesting a familial predisposition to SCD as a specific form of expression of CHD. A strong parental history of SCD as an initial coronary event increases the probability of a similar expression in the offspring. In a few syndromes, such as hypertrophic cardiomyopathy, congenital long QT interval syndromes, right ventricular dysplasia, and the syndrome of right bundle branch block and nonischemic ST-segment elevations (Brugada syndrome), there is a specific inherited risk of SCD (Chap. 16).

The structural causes of and functional factors contributing to the SCD syndrome are listed in Table 29-2. Worldwide, and especially in Western cultures, coronary atherosclerotic heart disease is the most common structural abnormality associated with SCD in middle-aged and older adults. Up to 80% of all SCDs in the United States are due to the consequences of coronary atherosclerosis. The cardiomyopathies (dilated and hypertrophic, collectively; Chap. 21) account for another 10–15% of SCDs, and all the remaining diverse etiologies cause only 5–10% of all SCDs. The inherited arrhythmia syndromes (see earlier and Table 29-2) are more common causes in adolescents and young adults. For some of these syndromes, such as hypertrophic cardiomyopathy (Chap. 21), risk of SCD begins to increase after puberty.

Transient ischemia in the previously scarred or hypertrophied heart, hemodynamic and fluid and electrolyte disturbances, fluctuations in autonomic nervous system activity, and transient electrophysiologic changes caused by drugs or other chemicals (e.g., proarrhythmia) have all been implicated as mechanisms responsible for the transition from electrophysiologic stability to instability. In addition, reperfusion of ischemic myocardium may cause transient electrophysiologic instability and arrhythmias.

PATHOLOGY

Data from postmortem examinations of SCD victims parallel the clinical observations on the prevalence of CHD as the major structural etiologic factor. More than 80% of SCD victims have pathologic findings of CHD. The pathologic description often includes a combination of longstanding, extensive atherosclerosis of the epicardial coronary arteries and unstable coronary artery lesions, which include various permutations of fissured or ruptured plaques, platelet aggregates, hemorrhage, and/or thrombosis. As much as 70–75% of males who die suddenly have preexisting healed MIs, whereas only 20–30% have recent acute MIs, despite the prevalence of unstable plaques and thrombi. The latter suggests transient ischemia as the mechanism of onset. Regional or global left ventricular (LV) hypertrophy often coexists with prior MIs.

PREDICTION AND PREVENTION OF CARDIAC ARREST AND SUDDEN CARDIAC DEATH

SCD accounts for approximately one-half the total cardiovascular mortality rate. As shown in Fig. 29-1B, the very-high-risk subgroups provide more focused populations ("percent per year") for predicting cardiac arrest or

SCD; but the impact of such subgroups on the overall problem of SCD, indicated by the absolute number of events ("events per year"), is relatively small. The requirements for achieving a major population impact are effective prevention of underlying diseases and/or new epidemiologic probes that will allow better resolution of subgroups at specific risk within the large general populations.

Strategies for predicting and preventing SCD are categorized as primary and secondary, in addition to responses intended to abort cardiac arrests. *Primary prevention*, as defined in various implantable defibrillator trials, refers to the attempt to identify individual patients at specific risk for SCD and institute preventive strategies. *Secondary prevention* refers to measures taken to prevent recurrent cardiac arrest or death in individuals who have survived a previous cardiac arrest. The primary prevention strategies currently used depend upon magnitude of risk among the various population subgroups. Because the annual incidence of SCD among the unselected adult population is limited to 1–2 per 1000 population per year (Fig. 29-1), and more than 30% of all SCDs due to coronary artery disease occur as the first clinical manifestation of the disease (Fig. 29-2A), the only practical strategies are profiling for risk of developing CHD and risk factor control (Fig. 29-2B). The most powerful long-term risk factors include age, cigarette smoking, elevated serum cholesterol, diabetes mellitus, elevated blood pressure, LV hypertrophy, and nonspecific electrocardiographic (ECG) abnormalities. Markers of inflammation (e.g., C-reactive protein levels) that may predict plaque destabilization, have been added to risk classifications. The presence of multiple risk factors progressively increases incidence, but not sufficiently or specifically enough to warrant therapies targeted to potentially fatal arrhythmias (Fig. 29-1A). However, recent studies offer the hope that genetic markers for specific risk may become available. These studies suggest that a family history of SCD associated with acute coronary syndromes predicts a higher likelihood of cardiac arrest as the initial manifestation of coronary artery disease in first-degree family members.

After coronary artery disease has been identified in a patient, additional strategies for risk profiling become available (Fig. 29-2B), but the majority of SCDs occur among the large unselected groups rather than in the specific high-risk subgroups that become evident among populations with established disease (compare events per year with percent per year in Fig. 29-1B). Under most conditions of higher level of risk, particularly those indexed to a major recent cardiovascular event (e.g., MI, recent onset of heart failure, survival after out-of-hospital cardiac arrest), the highest risk of death occurs during the initial 6–18 months and then plateaus toward the baseline risk of the underlying disease. However, many of the early deaths are nonsudden, diluting the potential benefit of strategies targeted specifically to SCD.

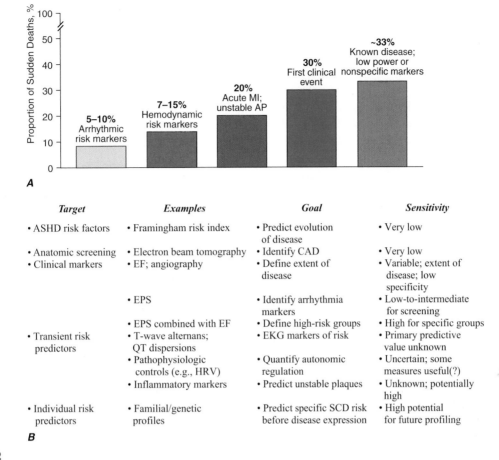

FIGURE 29-2

Population subsets, risk predictors, and distribution of sudden cardiac deaths (SCDs) according to clinical circumstances. A. The population subset with high-risk arrhythmia markers in conjunction with low ejection fraction (EF) is a group at high risk of SCD but accounts for <10% of the total SCD burden attributable to coronary artery disease. In contrast, nearly two-thirds of all SCD victims present with SCD as the first and only manifestation of underlying disease or have known disease but are considered relatively low-risk because of the absence of high-risk markers. **B.** Risk profile for prediction and prevention of SCD is difficult. The highest absolute numbers of events occur among the general population who may have risk factors for coronary heart disease or expressions of disease that do not predict high risk. This results in a low sensitivity for predicting and preventing SCD. New approaches that include epidemiologic modeling of transient risk factors and methods of predicting individual patient risk offer hope for greater sensitivity in the future. AP, angina pectoris; ASHD, arteriosclerotic heart disease; CAD, coronary artery disease; EPS, electrophysiologic study; HRV, heart rate variability. *(From Myerburg, reproduced with permission.)*

Thus, even though post-MI beta-blocker therapy has an identifiable benefit for both early SCD and nonsudden mortality risk, a total mortality benefit for ICD therapy early after MI has not been observed.

Among patients in the acute, convalescent, and chronic phases of MI (Chap. 35), subgroups at high absolute risk of SCD can be identified. During the acute phase, the potential risk of cardiac arrest from onset through the first 48 hours may be as high as 15%, emphasizing the importance for patients to respond promptly to the onset of symptoms. Those who survive acute-phase VF, however, are not at continuing risk for recurrent cardiac arrest indexed to that event. During the convalescent phase after MI (3 days to ~6 weeks), an episode of sustained VT or VF, associated with a large infarct, predicts a natural history mortality risk of up to 50% at 12 months. At least 50% of the deaths are sudden. Aggressive intervention techniques may reduce this incidence.

After passage into the chronic phase of MI, the longer-term risk for total and SCD mortality is predicted by a number of factors (Fig. 29-2B). The most important factor for both SCD and nonsudden death is the extent of myocardial damage sustained as a result of the acute MI. This is measured by the magnitude of reduction of the ejection fraction (EF), functional capacity, and/or the occurrence of heart failure. Various studies have demonstrated that ventricular arrhythmias identified by ambulatory monitoring contribute significantly to this risk, especially in patients with an EF <40%. In addition, inducibility of VT or VF during electrophysiologic

CHAPTER 29

Cardiovascular Collapse, Cardiac Arrest, and Sudden Cardiac Death testing of patients who have ambient ventricular arrhythmias [premature ventricular contractions (PVCs) and nonsustained VT] and an EF <35 or 40% is a strong predictor of SCD risk. Patients in this subgroup are now considered candidates for implantable cardioverter defibrillators (ICDs) (see later). Risk falls off sharply with EFs >40% after MI and the absence of ambient arrhythmias, and conversely is high with EFs <30% even without the ambient arrhythmia markers.

The cardiomyopathies (dilated and hypertrophic, Chap. 21) are the second most common category of diseases associated with risk of SCD, following CHD (Table 29-2). Some risk factors have been identified, largely related to extent of disease, documented ventricular arrhythmias, and symptoms of arrhythmias (e.g., unexplained syncope). The less common causes of SCD include valvular heart disease (primarily aortic), and inflammatory and infiltrative disorders of the myocardium. The latter include viral myocarditis, sarcoidosis, and amyloidosis.

Among adolescents and young adults, rare inherited disorders, such as hypertrophic cardiomyopathy, the long QT interval syndromes, right ventricular dysplasia, and the Brugada syndrome, have received attention as important causes of SCD because of advances in genetics and the ability to identify some of those at risk before a fatal event. The subgroup of young competitive athletes has received special attention. The incidence of SCD among athletes appears to be higher than the general adolescent and young adult population, perhaps up to 1 in 75,000. Hypertrophic cardiomyopathy (Chap. 21) is the most common cause in the United States, in contrast to Italy, where more comprehensive screening programs remove potential victims from the population of athletes.

Secondary prevention strategies should be applied to surviving victims of a cardiac arrest that was not associated with an acute MI or a transient risk of SCD (e.g., drug exposures, correctable electrolyte imbalances). Multivessel coronary artery disease or dilated cardiomyopathy with left ventricular EF <40% or the presences of life-threatening arrhythmias with long QT syndromes or right ventricular dysplasia predict a 1–2-year risk of recurrence of a SCD or cardiac arrest of up to 30% in the absence of specific interventions (see below).

CLINICAL CHARACTERISTICS OF CARDIAC ARREST

PRODROME, ONSET, ARREST, DEATH

SCD may be presaged by days, weeks, or months of increasing angina, dyspnea, palpitations, easy fatigability, and other nonspecific complaints. However, these *prodromal complaints* are generally predictive of any major cardiac event; they are not specific for predicting SCD.

The *onset of the clinical transition*, leading to cardiac arrest, is defined as an acute change in cardiovascular status preceding cardiac arrest by up to 1 h. When the onset is instantaneous or abrupt, the probability that the arrest is cardiac in origin is >95%. Continuous ECG recordings, fortuitously obtained at the onset of a cardiac arrest, commonly demonstrate changes in cardiac electrical activity during the minutes or hours before the event. There is a tendency for the heart rate to increase and for advanced grades of PVCs to evolve. Most cardiac arrests that are caused by VF begin with a run of sustained or nonsustained VT, which then degenerates into VF.

The probability of achieving successful resuscitation from cardiac arrest is related to the interval from onset to institution of resuscitative efforts, the setting in which the event occurs, the mechanism (VF, VT, pulseless electrical activity, asystole), and the clinical status of the patient prior to the cardiac arrest. Return of circulation and survival rates as a result of defibrillation decrease linearly from the first minute to 10 min. By 5 min, survival rates are no greater than 25–30% in out-of-hospital settings. Those settings in which it is possible to institute prompt cardiopulmonary resuscitation (CPR) with rapid defibrillation of VF provide a better chance of a successful outcome. However, the outcome in intensive care units and other in-hospital environments is heavily influenced by the patient's preceding clinical status. The immediate outcome is good for cardiac arrest occurring in the intensive care unit in the presence of an acute cardiac event or transient metabolic disturbance, but survival among patients with far-advanced chronic cardiac disease or advanced noncardiac diseases (e.g., renal failure, pneumonia, sepsis, diabetes, cancer) is low, and not much more successful in the in-hospital than in the out-of-hospital setting.

The success rate for initial resuscitation and survival to hospital discharge after an out-of-hospital cardiac arrest depends heavily on the mechanism of the event. When the mechanism is VT, the outcome is best; VF is the next most successful; and asystole and PEA generate dismal outcome statistics. Advanced age also adversely influences the chances of successful resuscitation.

Progression to biologic death is a function of the mechanism of cardiac arrest and the length of the delay before interventions. VF or asystole without CPR within the first 4–6 min has a poor outcome even if defibrillation is successful, because of superimposed brain damage; there are few survivors among patients who had no life support activities for the first 8 min after onset. Outcome statistics are improved by lay bystander intervention (basic life support—see later) prior to definitive interventions (advanced life support), and even more by early defibrillation. In regard to the latter, evaluations of deployment of automated external defibrillators (AEDs) in communities (e.g., police vehicles, large buildings, airports, and stadiums) are beginning to generate encouraging data. Increased deployment is to be encouraged.

Death during the hospitalization after a successfully resuscitated cardiac arrest relates closely to the severity of central nervous system injury. Anoxic encephalopathy and infections subsequent to prolonged respirator dependence account for 60% of the deaths. Another 30% occur as a consequence of low cardiac output states that fail to respond to interventions. Recurrent arrhythmias are the least common cause of death, accounting for only 10% of in-hospital deaths.

In the setting of acute MI (Chap. 35), it is important to distinguish between primary and secondary cardiac arrests. *Primary cardiac arrests* refer to those that occur in the absence of hemodynamic instability, and *secondary cardiac arrests* are those that occur in patients in whom abnormal hemodynamics dominate the clinical picture before cardiac arrest. The success rate for immediate resuscitation in primary cardiac arrest during acute MI in a monitored setting should approach 100%. In contrast, as much as 70% of patients with secondary cardiac arrest succumb immediately or during the same hospitalization.

℞ Treatment:
CARDIAC ARREST

The individual who collapses suddenly is managed in five stages: (1) the initial response and basic life support, (2) public access defibrillation (if available), (3) advanced life support, (4) postresuscitation care, and (5) long-term management. The initial response, including basic life support and public access defibrillation, can be carried out by physicians, nurses, paramedical personnel, and trained lay persons. There is a requirement for increasingly specialized skills as the patient moves through the stages of advanced life support, postresuscitation care, and long-term management.

INITIAL RESPONSE AND BASIC LIFE SUPPORT The initial evaluation will confirm whether a sudden collapse is indeed due to a cardiac arrest. Observations of the state of consciousness, respiratory movements, skin color, and the presence or absence of pulses in the carotid or femoral arteries can promptly determine whether a life-threatening cardiac arrest has occurred. For lay responders, the pulse check is no longer recommended. As soon as a cardiac arrest is suspected, confirmed, or even considered to be impending, calling an emergency rescue system (e.g., 911) is the immediate priority. With the development of AEDs that are easily used by nonconventional emergency responders, an additional layer for response has evolved (see later).

Agonal respiratory movements may persist for a short time after the onset of cardiac arrest, but it is important to observe for severe stridor with a persistent pulse as a clue to aspiration of a foreign body or food. If this is suspected, a Heimlich maneuver (see below) may dislodge the obstructing body. A precordial blow, or "thump," delivered firmly by the clenched fist to the junction of the middle and lower third of the sternum may occasionally revert VT or VF, but there is concern about converting VT to VF. Therefore, it is recommended to use precordial thumps as an advanced life support technique when monitoring and defibrillation are available. This conservative application of the technique remains controversial.

The third action during the initial response is to clear the airway. The head is tilted back and chin lifted so that the oropharynx can be explored to clear the airway. Dentures or foreign bodies are removed, and the Heimlich maneuver is performed if there is reason to suspect that a foreign body is lodged in the oropharynx. If respiratory arrest precipitating cardiac arrest is suspected, a second precordial thump is delivered after the airway is cleared.

Basic life support, more popularly known as CPR, is intended to maintain organ perfusion until definitive interventions can be instituted. The elements of CPR are the maintenance of ventilation of the lungs and compression of the chest. Mouth-to-mouth respiration may be used if no specific rescue equipment is immediately available (e.g., plastic oropharyngeal airways, esophageal obturators, masked Ambu bag). Conventional ventilation techniques during single-responder CPR require the lungs to be inflated twice in succession every 30 chest compressions.

Chest compression is based on the assumption that cardiac compression allows the heart to maintain a pump function by sequential filling and emptying of its chambers, with competent valves maintaining forward direction of flow. The palm of one hand is placed over the lower sternum, with the heel of the other hand resting on the dorsum of the lower hand. The sternum is depressed, with the arms remaining straight, at a rate of ~100 per minute. Sufficient force is applied to depress the sternum 4–5 cm, and relaxation is abrupt.

AUTOMATED EXTERNAL DEFIBRILLATION (AED) AEDs have been developed that are easily used by nonconventional responders, such as nonparamedic firemen, police, ambulance drivers, trained security guards, and minimally trained or untrained lay persons. This advance has inserted another level of response into the cardiac arrest paradigm. A number of studies have demonstrated that AED use by nonconventional and lay responders in strategic response systems can improve cardiac arrest survival rates. This strategy is based on shortening the time to first defibrillation attempt while awaiting arrival of advanced life support.

ADVANCED LIFE SUPPORT This is intended to achieve adequate ventilation, control cardiac arrhythmias, stabilize blood pressure and cardiac output, and restore organ perfusion. The activities carried out to achieve these goals include (1) defibrillation/cardioversion and/or pacing, (2) intubation with an endotracheal tube, and (3) insertion of an intravenous line. The speed with which defibrillation/cardioversion is carried out is an important element for successful resuscitation, both for restoration of spontaneous circulation and protection of the central nervous system. Immediate defibrillation should precede intubation and insertion of an intravenous line; CPR should be carried out while the defibrillator is being charged. As soon as a diagnosis of VF or VT is established, a shock of at least 300 J should be delivered. Additional shocks, up to a maximum of 360 J, are tried if the initial shock does not successfully abolish VT or VF, but it is now recommended that 60–90 s of CPR be carried out before repeated shocks, if the first shock fails to restore an organized rhythm, or before the first shock if 5 min has elapsed between the onset

of cardiac arrest and ability to deliver a shock. Epinephrine, 1 mg intravenously, is given after failed defibrillation, and attempts to defibrillate are repeated. The dose of epinephrine may be repeated after intervals of 3–5 min (**Fig. 29-3A**). Vasopressin (a single 40-unit dose given IV) has been suggested as an alternative to epinephrine.

If the patient is less than fully conscious upon reversion, or if two or three attempts fail, prompt intubation, ventilation, and arterial blood gas analysis should be carried out. Ventilation with O_2 (room air if O_2 is not immediately available) may promptly reverse hypoxemia and acidosis. The patient who is persistently acidotic after successful defibrillation and intubation should be given 1 meq/kg $NaHCO_3$ initially and an additional 50% of the dose repeated every 10–15 min. However, it should not be used routinely.

After initial unsuccessful defibrillation attempts, or with persistent/recurrent electrical instability, antiarrhythmic therapy should be instituted. Intravenous amiodarone has emerged as the initial treatment of choice (150 mg over 10 min, followed by 1 mg/min for up to 6 h and 0.5 mg/min thereafter) (Fig. 29-3A). For cardiac arrest due to VF in the early phase of an acute coronary syndrome, a bolus of 1 mg/kg of lidocaine may

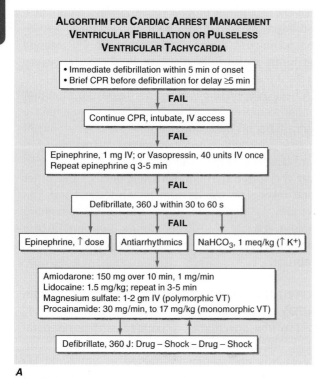

A

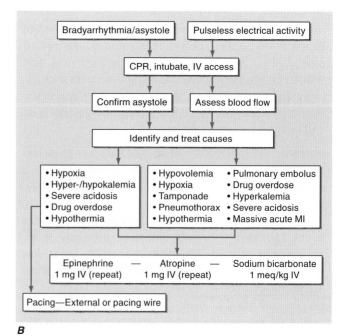

B

FIGURE 29-3

A. The algorithm of ventricular fibrillation or pulseless ventricular tachycardia begins with defibrillation attempts. If that fails, it is followed by epinephrine and then antiarrhythmic drugs. See text for details. **B. The algorithms for bradyarrhythmia/asystole** (left) or pulseless electrical activity

(right) is dominated first by continued life support and a search for reversible causes. Subsequent therapy is nonspecific and accompanied by a low success rate. See text for details. CPR, cardiopulmonary resuscitation; MI, myocardial infarction.

be given intravenously as an alternative, and the dose may be repeated in 2 min. It also may be tried in those patients in whom amiodarone is unsuccessful. Intravenous procainamide (loading infusion of 100 mg/5 min to a total dose of 500–800 mg, followed by continuous infusion at 2–5 mg/min) is now rarely used in this setting but may be tried for persisting, hemodynamically stable arrhythmias. Intravenous calcium gluconate is no longer considered safe or necessary for routine administration. It is used only in patients in whom acute hyperkalemia is known to be the triggering event for resistant VF, in the presence of known hypocalcemia, or in patients who have received toxic doses of calcium channel antagonists.

Cardiac arrest secondary to bradyarrhythmias or asystole is managed differently (Fig. 29-3B). The patient is promptly intubated, CPR is continued, and an attempt is made to control hypoxemia and acidosis. Epinephrine and/or atropine are given intravenously or by an intracardiac route. External pacing devices are now available to attempt to establish a regular rhythm, but the prognosis is generally very poor in this form of cardiac arrest, even with successful electrical pacing. PEA is treated similarly to bradyarrhythmias, but its outcome is also dismal. The one exception is bradyarrhythmic/asystolic cardiac arrest secondary to airway obstruction. This form of cardiac arrest may respond promptly to removal of foreign bodies by the Heimlich maneuver or, in hospitalized patients, by intubation and suctioning of obstructing secretions in the airway.

POSTRESUSCITATION CARE This phase of management is determined by the clinical setting of the cardiac arrest. Primary VF in acute MI (Chap. 35) is generally very responsive to life-support techniques and easily controlled after the initial event. In the in-hospital setting, respirator support is usually not necessary or is needed for only a short time, and hemodynamics stabilize promptly after defibrillation or cardioversion. In secondary VF in acute MI (those events in which hemodynamic abnormalities predispose to the potentially fatal arrhythmia), resuscitative efforts are less often successful; and in those patients who are successfully resuscitated, the recurrence rate is high. The clinical picture and outcome are dominated by hemodynamic instability and the ability to control hemodynamic dysfunction. Bradyarrhythmias, asystole, and PEA are commonly secondary events in hemodynamically unstable patients. The in-hospital phase of care of the out-of-hospital cardiac arrest survivor is dictated by specific clinical circumstances. The most difficult is the presence of anoxic encephalopathy, which is a strong predictor of in-hospital death. A recent addition to the management of this condition is induced hypothermia to reduce metabolic demands and cerebral edema.

The outcome after in-hospital cardiac arrest associated with noncardiac diseases is poor, and in the few successfully resuscitated patients, the postresuscitation course is dominated by the nature of the underlying disease. Patients with end-stage cancer, renal failure, acute central nervous system disease, and uncontrolled infections, as a group, have a survival rate of <10% after in-hospital cardiac arrest. Some major exceptions are patients with transient airway obstruction, electrolyte disturbances, proarrhythmic effects of drugs, and severe metabolic abnormalities, most of whom may have an excellent chance of survival if they can be resuscitated promptly and maintained while the transient abnormalities are being corrected.

LONG-TERM MANAGEMENT AFTER SURVIVAL OF OUT-OF-HOSPITAL CARDIAC ARREST Patients who survive cardiac arrest without irreversible damage to the central nervous system, and who achieve hemodynamic stability, should have extensive diagnostic testing and appropriate therapeutic interventions for their long-term management. This aggressive approach is driven by the fact that survival after out-of-hospital cardiac arrest was followed by a 25–30% mortality rate during the first 2 years after the event, and there are data suggesting that significant reductions in risk can be achieved by use of the implantable cardioverter defibrillator (ICD).

Among patients in whom an acute transmural MI is identified as the specific mechanism triggering an out-of-hospital cardiac arrest, the management is dictated in part by the transient nature of life-threatening arrhythmia risk in the acute phase of MI, and in part by the extent of permanent myocardial damage that results. Several clinical trials have now documented an improved survival among cardiac arrest survivors who have EFs <40% and receive ICDs.

For patients with cardiac arrest thought to be due to a transient ischemic mechanism, particularly with higher EFs, anti-ischemic therapy by pharmacologic or interventional methods is generally accepted as appropriate management. However, despite the absence of supportive clinical trial evidence, some adopt a more aggressive attitude about the use of ICDs in this group of cardiac arrest survivors as well, given the unpredictability of recurrent ischemia.

The principles guiding therapy for patients with coronary artery disease who survive a cardiac arrest generally apply to the other cardiac disorders as well, with the exception that there is less focus on the extent of disease in certain disorders. Generally, cardiac arrest survivors from other categories of disease, such as the hypertrophic or dilated cardiomyopathies and various rare inherited disorders (e.g., RV dysplasia, long QT syndrome, Brugada syndrome, arrhythmic VF) are all considered ICD candidates.

PREVENTION OF SCD IN HIGH-RISK INDIVIDUALS WITHOUT PRIOR CARDIAC ARREST

Post-MI patients have been the subject of clinical trials for ICD benefit. It is now established that for post-MI patients with EFs <40%, ambient ventricular arrhythmias, and inducible ventricular tachyarrhythmias in the electrophysiology laboratory, ICDs provide a significant reduction in relative risk of SCD and total mortality. Total mortality benefits in the range of a 20–30% reduction over 2–3 years have been observed, and ICD has emerged as preferred therapy for such patients. One study suggests that when the EF <30%, electrophysiologic testing is not necessary to identify ICD benefit, and another demonstrates benefit for patients with functional class II or III heart failure and EFs ≤35%, regardless of etiology (ischemic or nonischemic) or ambient or induced arrhythmias (see Chaps. 16 and 17).

Decision-making for primary prevention in disorders other than coronary artery disease and dilated cardiomyopathy is generally driven by observational data and judgment based on clinical observations. Controlled clinical trials providing evidence-based indicators for ICDs are lacking for these smaller population subgroups. In general, for the rare disorders listed above, indicators of arrhythmic risk such as syncope, documented ventricular tachyarrhythmias, aborted cardiac arrest or perhaps a family history of premature SCD, and a number of other clinical or ECG markers, may be used as indicators for ICDs.

FURTHER READINGS

GOLDBERGER Z, LAMPERT R: Implantable cardioverter-defibrillators: Expanding indications and technologies. JAMA 295:809, 2006

HUIKURI H et al: Sudden death due to cardiac arrhythmias. N Engl J Med 345:1473, 2001

INTERNATIONAL LIAISON COMMITTEE ON RESUSCITATION: 2005 International Consensus on Cardiopulmonary Resuscitation and Emergency Cardiovascular Care Science with Treatment Recommendations. Circulation 112(Suppl III):III-1–III-136, 2005

KOKOLIS S et al: Ventricular arrhythmias and sudden cardiac death. Prog Cardiovasc Dis 48:426, 2006

MARENCO JP et al: Improving survival from sudden cardiac arrest: The role of the automated external defibrillator. JAMA 285:1193, 2001

MARON BJ, PELLICCIA A: The heart of trained athletes: Cardiac remodeling and the risks of sports, including sudden death. Circulation 114:1633, 2006

MYERBURG RJ, CASTELLANOS A: Cardiac arrest and sudden cardiac death, in *Braunwald's Heart Disease*, 8th ed, P Libby et al (eds). Philadelphia, Saunders, 2008

———— et al: Indications for implantable cardioverter-defibrillators based on evidence and judgment. J Am Coll Cardiol 54:747, 2009

NOSEWORTHY PA and NEWTON-CHEH C: Genetic determinants of sudden cardiac death. Circulation 118:1854, 2008

ROBERTS R: Genomics and cardiac arrhythmias. J Am Coll Cardiol 47:9, 2006

WIK L et al: Delaying defibrillation to give basic cardiopulmonary resuscitation to patients with out-of-hospital ventricular fibrillation: a randomized trial. JAMA 289:1389, 2003 http://circ.ahajournals.org/content/vol112/24_suppl/

SECTION V

DISORDERS OF THE VASCULATURE

CHAPTER 30

THE PATHOGENESIS, PREVENTION, AND TREATMENT OF ATHEROSCLEROSIS

Peter Libby

PATHOGENESIS

Atherosclerosis remains the major cause of death and premature disability in developed societies. Moreover, current predictions estimate that by the year 2020 cardiovascular diseases, notably atherosclerosis, will become the leading global cause of total disease burden. Although many generalized or systemic risk factors predispose to its development, atherosclerosis affects various regions of the circulation preferentially and yields distinct clinical manifestations depending on the particular circulatory bed affected. Atherosclerosis of the coronary arteries commonly causes myocardial infarction (MI) (Chap. 35) and angina pectoris (Chap. 33). Atherosclerosis of the arteries supplying the central nervous system frequently provokes strokes and transient cerebral ischemia. In the peripheral circulation, atherosclerosis causes intermittent claudication and gangrene and can jeopardize limb viability. Involvement of the splanchnic circulation can cause mesenteric ischemia. Atherosclerosis can affect the kidneys either directly (e.g., renal artery stenosis) or as a frequent site of atheroembolic disease (Chap. 38).

Even within a given arterial bed, stenoses due to atherosclerosis tend to occur focally, typically in certain predisposed regions. In the coronary circulation, for example, the proximal left anterior descending coronary artery exhibits a particular predilection for developing atherosclerotic disease. Likewise, atherosclerosis preferentially affects the proximal portions of the renal arteries and, in the extracranial circulation to the brain, the carotid bifurcation. Indeed, atherosclerotic lesions often form at branching points of arteries, regions of disturbed blood flow. Not all manifestations of atherosclerosis result from stenotic, occlusive disease. Ectasia and development of aneurysmal disease, for example, frequently occur in the aorta (Chap. 38). In addition to focal, flow-limiting stenoses, nonocclusive intimal atherosclerosis also occurs diffusely in affected arteries, as shown by intravascular ultrasound and postmortem studies.

Atherogenesis in humans typically occurs over a period of many years, usually many decades. Growth of atherosclerotic plaques probably does not occur in a smooth, linear fashion, but rather discontinuously, with periods of relative quiescence punctuated by periods of rapid evolution. After a generally prolonged "silent" period, atherosclerosis may become clinically manifest. The clinical expressions of atherosclerosis may be *chronic*, as in the development of stable, effort-induced angina pectoris or of predictable and reproducible intermittent claudication. Alternatively, a dramatic *acute* clinical event, such as MI, a stroke, or sudden cardiac death, may first herald the presence of atherosclerosis. Other individuals may never experience clinical manifestations of arterial disease despite the presence of widespread atherosclerosis demonstrated post-mortem.

INITIATION OF ATHEROSCLEROSIS

An integrated view of experimental results in animals and studies of human atherosclerosis suggests that the "fatty streak" represents the initial lesion of atherosclerosis. These early lesions most often seem to arise from focal increases in the content of lipoproteins within regions of the intima. This accumulation of lipoprotein particles may not result simply from an increased permeability, or "leakiness," of the overlying endothelium (Fig. 30-1). Rather, these lipoproteins may collect in the intima of arteries because they bind to constituents of the extracellular matrix, increasing the residence time of the lipid-rich particles within the arterial wall. Lipoproteins that accumulate in the extracellular space of the intima of arteries often associate with glycosaminoglycans of the arterial extracellular matrix, an interaction that may slow the egress of these lipid-rich particles from the intima. Lipoprotein particles in the extracellular space of the intima, particularly those retained by binding to matrix macromolecules, may undergo oxidative modifications. Considerable evidence supports a pathogenic role for products of oxidized lipoproteins in atherogenesis. Lipoproteins sequestered from plasma antioxidants in the extracellular space of the intima become particularly susceptible to oxidative modification, giving rise to hydroperoxides, lysophospholipids, oxysterols, and aldehydic breakdown products of fatty acids and phospholipids. Modifications of the apoprotein moieties may include breaks in the peptide backbone as well as derivatization of certain amino acid residues. Local production of hypochlorous acid by myeloperoxidase associated with inflammatory cells within the plaque yields chlorinated species such as chlorotyrosyl moieties. Considerable evidence supports the presence of such oxidation products in atherosclerotic lesions.

Leukocyte Recruitment

Accumulation of leukocytes characterizes the formation of early atherosclerotic lesions (Fig. 30-1). Thus, from its very inception, atherogenesis involves elements of inflammation, a process that now provides a unifying theme in the pathogenesis of this disease. The inflammatory cell types typically found in the evolving atheroma include monocyte-derived macrophages and lymphocytes. A number of adhesion molecules or receptors for leukocytes expressed on the surface of the arterial endothelial cell likely participate in the recruitment of leukocytes to the nascent atheroma. Constituents of oxidatively modified

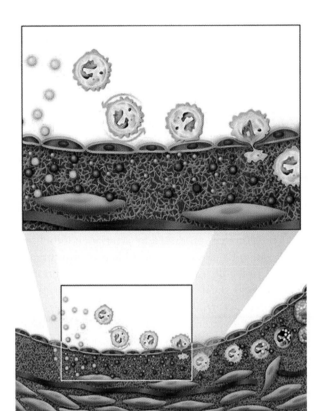

FIGURE 30-1

Cross-sectional view of an artery depicting steps in development of an atheroma, from left to right. The *upper panel* shows a detail of the boxed area below. The endothelial monolayer overlying the intima contacts blood. Hypercholesterolemia promotes accumulation of LDL particles (light spheres) in the intima. The lipoprotein particles often associate with constituents of the extracellular matrix, notably proteoglycans. Sequestration within the intima separates lipoproteins from some plasma antioxidants and favors oxidative modification. Such modified lipoprotein particles (darker spheres) may trigger a local inflammatory response responsible for signaling subsequent steps in lesion formation. The augmented expression of various adhesion molecules for leukocytes recruits monocytes to the site of a nascent arterial lesion.

Once adherent, some white blood cells will migrate into the intima. The directed migration of leukocytes probably depends on chemoattractant factors including modified lipoprotein particles themselves and chemoattractant cytokines depicted by the smaller spheres, such as the chemokine macrophage chemoattractant protein-1 produced by vascular wall cells in response to modified lipoproteins. Leukocytes in the evolving fatty streak can divide and exhibit augmented expression of receptors for modified lipoproteins (scavenger receptors). These mononuclear phagocytes ingest lipids and become foam cells, represented by a cytoplasm filled with lipid droplets. As the fatty streak evolves into a more complicated atherosclerotic lesion, smooth-muscle cells migrate from the media (*bottom of lower panel*), through the internal elastic membrane (*solid wavy line*), and accumulate within the expanding intima where they lay down extracellular matrix that forms the bulk of the advanced lesion (*bottom panel, right-hand side*).

low-density lipoprotein (LDL) can augment expression of leukocyte adhesion molecules. This example illustrates how the accumulation of lipoproteins in the arterial intima may link mechanistically with leukocyte recruitment, a key event in lesion formation.

Laminar shear forces such as those encountered in most regions of normal arteries can also suppress the expression of leukocyte adhesion molecules. Sites of predilection for atherosclerotic lesions (e.g., branch points) often have disturbed laminar flow. Ordered, pulsatile laminar shear of normal blood flow augments the production of nitric oxide by endothelial cells. This molecule, in addition to its vasodilator properties, can act at the low levels constitutively produced by arterial endothelium as a local anti-inflammatory autacoid, e.g., limiting local adhesion molecule expression. Exposure of endothelial cells to laminar shear stress increases the transcription of Kruppel-like factor 2 (KLF2) and reduces the expression of a thioredoxin-interacting protein (Txnip) that inhibits the activity of thioredoxin. KLF2 augments the activity of endothelial nitric oxide synthase, and reduced Txnip levels boost the function of the endogenous antioxidant thioredoxin. Laminar shear stress also stimulates endothelial cells to produce superoxide dismutase, an antioxidant enzyme. These examples indicate how hemodynamic forces may influence the cellular events that underlie atherosclerotic lesion initiation and provide a potential explanation for the favored localization of atherosclerotic lesions at sites that experience disturbance to laminar shear stress.

Once captured on the surface of the arterial endothelial cell by adhesion receptors, the monocytes and lymphocytes penetrate the endothelial layer and take up residence in the intima. In addition to products of modified lipoproteins, cytokines (protein mediators of inflammation) can regulate the expression of adhesion molecules involved in leukocyte recruitment. For example, interleukin 1 (IL-1) or tumor necrosis factor α (TNF-α) induces or augments the expression of leukocyte adhesion molecules on endothelial cells. Because products of lipoprotein oxidation can induce cytokine release from vascular wall cells, this pathway may provide an additional link between arterial accumulation of lipoproteins and leukocyte recruitment. Chemoattractant cytokines such as monocyte chemoattractant protein-1 appear to direct the migration of leukocytes into the arterial wall.

Foam Cell Formation

Once resident within the intima, the mononuclear phagocytes mature into macrophages and become lipid-laden foam cells, a conversion that requires the uptake of lipoprotein particles by receptor-mediated endocytosis. One might suppose that the well-recognized "classical" receptor for LDL mediates this lipid uptake; however, patients or animals lacking effective LDL receptors due to genetic alterations (e.g., familial hypercholesterolemia) have abundant arterial lesions and extraarterial xanthomata rich in macrophage-derived foam cells. In addition, the exogenous cholesterol suppresses expression of the LDL receptor; thus, the level of this cell-surface receptor for LDL decreases under conditions of cholesterol excess. Candidates for alternative receptors that can mediate lipid-loading of foam cells include a growing number of macrophage "scavenger" receptors, which preferentially endocytose modified lipoproteins, and other receptors for oxidized LDL or beta very low density lipoprotein (β-VLDL). Monocyte attachment to the endothelium, migration into the intima, and maturation to form lipid-laden macrophages thus represent key steps in the formation of the fatty streak, the precursor of fully formed atherosclerotic plaques.

ATHEROMA EVOLUTION AND COMPLICATIONS

Although the fatty streak commonly precedes the development of a more advanced atherosclerotic plaque, not all fatty streaks progress to form complex atheromata. By ingesting lipids from the extracellular space, the mononuclear phagocytes bearing such scavenger receptors may remove lipoproteins from the developing lesion. Some lipid-laden macrophages may leave the artery wall, exporting lipid in the process. Lipid accumulation, and hence propensity to form atheroma, ensues if the amount of lipid entering the artery wall exceeds that removed by mononuclear phagocytes or other pathways.

Export by phagocytes may constitute one response to local lipid overload in the evolving lesion. Another mechanism, reverse cholesterol transport mediated by high-density lipoproteins (HDL), probably provides an independent pathway for lipid removal from atheroma. The transfer of cholesterol from the cell to the HDL particle involves specialized cell surface molecules such as the ATP binding cassette (ABC) transporters. *ABCA1*, the gene mutated in Tangier disease, a condition characterized by very low HDL levels, transfers cholesterol from cells to nascent HDL particles and ABCG1 to mature HDL particles. "Reverse cholesterol transport" mediated by these ABC transporters allows HDL loaded with cholesterol to deliver it to hepatocytes by binding to scavenger receptor B 1 or other receptors. The liver cell can metabolize the sterol to bile acids that can be excreted. This export pathway from macrophage foam cells to peripheral cells such as hepatocytes explains part of HDL's antiatherogenic action. (Anti-inflammatory and antioxidant properties may also contribute to HDL's atheroprotective effects.) Thus, macrophages may play a vital role in the dynamic economy of lipid accumulation in the arterial wall during atherogenesis.

Some lipid-laden foam cells within the expanding intimal lesion perish. Some foam cells may die as a result of programmed cell death, or *apoptosis*. The death of mononuclear phagocytes results in formation of the lipid-rich center, often called the *necrotic core*, in established atherosclerotic plaques. Macrophages loaded with modified lipoproteins may elaborate cytokines and growth factors that can further signal some of the cellular events in lesion complication. While accumulation of lipid-laden macrophages characterizes the fatty streak, build-up of fibrous tissue formed by extracellular matrix typifies the more advanced atherosclerotic lesion. The smooth-muscle cell synthesizes the bulk of the extracellular matrix of the complex atherosclerotic lesion. A number of growth factors or cytokines elaborated by mononuclear phagocytes can stimulate smooth-muscle cell proliferation and production of extracellular matrix. Cytokines found in the plaque, including IL-1 or TNF-α, can induce local production of growth factors, including forms of platelet-derived growth factor (PDGF), fibroblast growth factors, and others that may contribute to plaque evolution and complication. Other cytokines, notably interferon γ (IFN-γ) derived from activated T cells within lesions, can limit the synthesis of interstitial forms of collagen by smooth-muscle cells. These examples illustrate how atherogenesis involves a complex mix of mediators that in the balance determines the characteristics of particular lesions.

The arrival of smooth-muscle cells and their elaboration of extracellular matrix probably provides a critical transition, yielding a fibrofatty lesion in place of a simple accumulation of macrophage-derived foam cells. For example, PDGF elaborated by activated platelets, macrophages, and endothelial cells can stimulate the migration of smooth-muscle cells normally resident in the tunica media into the intima. Such growth factors and cytokines produced locally can stimulate the proliferation of resident smooth-muscle cells in the intima as well as those that have migrated from the media. Transforming growth factor β (TGF-β), among other mediators, potently stimulates interstitial collagen production by smooth-muscle cells. These mediators may arise not only from neighboring vascular cells or leukocytes (a "paracrine" pathway) but also, in some instances, from the same cell that responds to the factor (an "autocrine" pathway). Together, these alterations in smooth-muscle cells, signaled by these mediators acting at short distances, can hasten transformation of the fatty streak into a more fibrous smooth-muscle cell and extracellular matrix-rich lesion.

In addition to locally produced mediators, products of blood coagulation and thrombosis likely contribute to atheroma evolution and complication. This involvement justifies the use of the term *atherothrombosis* to convey the inextricable links between atherosclerosis and thrombosis. Fatty streak formation begins beneath a morphologically intact endothelium. In advanced fatty streaks, however, microscopic breaches in endothelial integrity

may occur. Microthrombi rich in platelets can form at such sites of limited endothelial denudation owing to exposure of the thrombogenic extracellular matrix of the underlying basement membrane. Activated platelets release numerous factors that can promote the fibrotic response, including PDGF and TGF-β. Thrombin itself generates fibrin, not only during coagulation but also through protease-activated receptors that can signal smooth-muscle migration, proliferation, and extracellular matrix production. Many arterial mural microthrombi resolve without clinical manifestation by a process of local fibrinolysis, resorption, and endothelial repair, yet can lead to lesion progression by stimulating these pro-fibrotic functions of smooth-muscle cells (Fig. 30-2D).

Microvessels

As atherosclerotic lesions advance, abundant plexuses of microvessels develop in connection with the artery's vasa vasorum. Newly developing microvascular networks may contribute to lesion complications in several ways. These blood vessels provide an abundant surface area for leukocyte trafficking and may serve as the portal of entry and exit of white blood cells from the established atheroma. Microvessels in the plaques may also furnish foci for intraplaque hemorrhage. Like the neovessels in the diabetic retina, microvessels in the atheroma may be friable and prone to rupture and can produce focal hemorrhage. Such a vascular leak leads to thrombosis in situ and thrombin generation from prothrombin. In addition to its role in blood coagulation, thrombin can modulate many aspects of vascular cell function, as described earlier. Atherosclerotic plaques often contain fibrin and hemosiderin, an indication that episodes of intraplaque hemorrhage contribute to plaque complications.

Calcification

As they advance, atherosclerotic plaques also accumulate *calcium*. Proteins usually found in bone also localize in atherosclerotic lesions, e.g., osteocalcin, osteopontin, and bone morphogenetic proteins. Mineralization of the atherosclerotic plaque recapitulates many aspects of bone formation.

Plaque Evolution

Although atherosclerosis research has focused much attention on proliferation of smooth-muscle cells, as in the case of macrophages, smooth-muscle cells can also undergo apoptosis in the atherosclerotic plaque. Indeed, complex atheromata often have a mostly fibrous character and lack the hypercellularity of less advanced lesions. The relative paucity of smooth-muscle cells in advanced atheromata may result from the predominance of cytostatic mediators such as TGF-β or IFN-γ (which can inhibit smooth-muscle cell proliferation) and also from smooth-muscle cell apoptosis. Some of the same pro-inflammatory cytokines that activate atherogenic functions of vascular wall cells can also sensitize these cells to undergo apoptosis.

Thus, during the evolution of the atherosclerotic plaque, a complex balance between entry and egress of lipoproteins and leukocytes, cell proliferation and cell death, extracellular matrix production and remodeling as well as calcification and neovascularization contribute to lesion formation. Multiple and often competing signals regulate these various cellular events. Increasingly, we appreciate links between atherogenic risk factors, inflammation, and the altered behavior of intrinsic vascular wall cells and infiltrating leukocytes that underlie the complex pathogenesis of these lesions.

CLINICAL SYNDROMES OF ATHEROSCLEROSIS

Atherosclerotic lesions occur ubiquitously in Western societies. Most atheromata produce no symptoms, and many never cause clinical manifestations. Numerous patients with diffuse atherosclerosis may succumb to unrelated illnesses without ever having experienced a clinically significant manifestation of atherosclerosis. What accounts for this variability in the clinical expression of atherosclerotic disease?

Arterial remodeling during atheroma formation (Fig. 30-2A) represents a frequently overlooked but clinically important feature of lesion evolution. During the initial phases of atheroma development, the plaque usually grows outward, in an abluminal direction. Vessels affected by atherogenesis tend to increase in diameter, a phenomenon known as *compensatory enlargement*, in a type of vascular remodeling. The growing atheroma does not encroach upon the arterial lumen until the burden of atherosclerotic plaque exceeds ~40% of the area encompassed by the internal elastic lamina. Thus, during much of its life history, an atheroma will not cause stenosis that can limit tissue perfusion.

Flow-limiting stenoses commonly form later in the history of the plaque. Many such plaques cause stable syndromes such as demand-induced angina pectoris or intermittent claudication in the extremities. In the coronary and other circulations, even total vascular occlusion by atheroma does not invariably lead to infarction. The hypoxic stimulus of repeated bouts of ischemia characteristically induces formation of collateral vessels in the myocardium, mitigating the consequences of an acute occlusion of an epicardial coronary artery. By contrast, we now appreciate that many lesions that cause acute or unstable atherosclerotic syndromes, particularly in the coronary circulation, may arise from atherosclerotic plaques that do not produce a flow-limiting stenosis. Such lesions may produce only minimal luminal irregularities on traditional angiograms and often do not meet the traditional criteria for "significance" by arteriography. Instability of such nonocclusive stenoses may explain the frequency of MI as an initial manifestation of coronary artery disease (in at least one-third of cases) in patients who report no prior history of angina pectoris, a syndrome usually caused by flow-limiting stenoses.

Plaque Instability and Rupture

Postmortem studies afford considerable insight into the microanatomic substrate underlying the "instability" of plaques that do not cause critical stenoses. A superficial erosion of the endothelium or a frank plaque rupture or fissure usually produces the thrombus that causes episodes of unstable angina pectoris or the occlusive and relatively persistent thrombus that causes acute MI (Fig. 30-2B). In the case of carotid atheromata, a deeper ulceration that provides a nidus for formation of platelet thrombi may cause transient cerebral ischemic attacks.

Rupture of the plaque's fibrous cap (Fig. 30-2C) permits contact between coagulation factors in the blood with highly thrombogenic tissue factor expressed by macrophage foam cells in the plaque's lipid-rich core. If the ensuing thrombus is nonocclusive or transient, the episode of plaque disruption may not cause symptoms or may result in episodic ischemic symptoms such as rest angina. Occlusive thrombi that endure will often cause acute MI, particularly in the absence of a well-developed collateral circulation supplying the affected territory. Repetitive episodes of plaque disruption and healing provide one likely mechanism of transition of the fatty streak to a more complex fibrous lesion (Fig. 30-2D). The healing process in arteries, as in skin wounds, involves the laying down of new extracellular matrix and fibrosis.

Not all atheromata exhibit the same propensity to rupture. Pathologic studies of culprit lesions that have caused acute MI reveal several characteristic features. Plaques that have caused fatal thromboses tend to have thin fibrous caps, relatively large lipid cores, and a high content of macrophages. Morphometric studies of such culprit lesions show that at sites of plaque rupture macrophages and T lymphocytes predominate and contain relatively few smooth-muscle cells. The cells that concentrate at sites of plaque rupture bear markers of inflammatory activation. The presence of the transplantation, or histocompatibility, antigen HLA-DR provides one convenient gauge of the degree of inflammation in cells in atheroma. Resting cells in normal arteries seldom express this transplantation antigen. However, macrophages and smooth-muscle cells at sites of human coronary artery plaque disruption do bear this inducible cell-surface marker. Therefore, the presence of HLA-DR-positive macrophages and T cells indicates an ongoing inflammatory response at sites of plaque rupture. In addition, patients with active atherosclerosis and acute coronary syndromes display signs of disseminated inflammation.

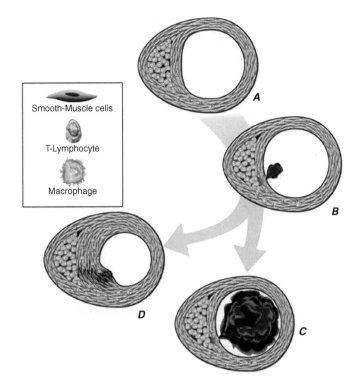

FIGURE 30-2

Plaque rupture, thrombosis, and healing. A. Arterial remodeling during atherogenesis. During the initial part of the life history of an atheroma, growth is often outward, preserving the caliber of lumen. This phenomenon of "compensatory enlargement" accounts in part for the tendency of coronary arteriography to underestimate the degree of atherosclerosis. **B.** Rupture of the plaque's fibrous cap causes thrombosis. Physical disruption of the atherosclerotic plaque commonly causes arterial thrombosis by allowing blood coagulant factors to contact thrombogenic collagen found in the arterial extracellular matrix and tissue factor produced by macrophage-derived foam cells in the lipid core of lesions. In this manner, sites of plaque rupture form the nidus for thrombi. The normal artery wall possesses several fibrinolytic or antithrombotic mechanisms that tend to resist thrombosis and lyse clots that begin to form in situ. Such antithrombotic or thrombolytic molecules include thrombomodulin, tissue and urokinase-type plasminogen activators, heparan sulfate proteoglycans, prostacyclin, and nitric oxide. **C.** When the clot overwhelms the endogenous fibrinolytic mechanisms, it may propagate and lead to arterial occlusion. The consequences of this occlusion depend on the degree of existing collateral vessels. In a patient with chronic multivessel, occlusive coronary artery disease, collateral channels have often

formed. In such circumstances, even a total arterial occlusion may not lead to MI, or it may produce an unexpectedly modest or a non-ST-segment elevation infarct because of collateral flow. In the patient with less advanced disease and without substantial stenotic lesions to provide a stimulus to collateral vessel formation, sudden plaque rupture and arterial occlusion commonly produces ST-segment elevation infarction. These are the types of patients who may present with MI or sudden death as a first manifestation of coronary atherosclerosis. In some cases, the thrombus may lyse or organize into a mural thrombus without occluding the vessel. Such instances may be clinically silent. **D.** The subsequent thrombin-induced fibrosis and healing causes a fibroproliferative response that can lead to a more fibrous lesion, one that can produce an eccentric plaque that causes a hemodynamically significant stenosis. In this way, a nonocclusive mural thrombus, even if clinically silent or causing unstable angina rather than infarction, can provoke a healing response that can promote lesion fibrosis and luminal encroachment. Such a sequence of events may convert a "vulnerable" atheroma with a thin fibrous cap prone to rupture into a more "stable" fibrous plaque with a reinforced cap. Angioplasty of unstable coronary lesions may "stabilize" the lesions by a similar mechanism, producing a wound followed by healing.

For example, atherosclerotic plaques and even microvascular endothelial cells at sites remote from the "culprit" lesion of an acute coronary syndrome can exhibit markers of activation such as HLA-DR.

Inflammatory mediators regulate processes that govern the integrity of the plaque's fibrous cap and hence its propensity to rupture. For example, the T cell–derived

cytokine IFN-γ, found in atherosclerotic plaques and required to induce the HLA-DR present at sites of rupture, can inhibit growth and collagen synthesis of smooth-muscle cells, as noted above. Cytokines derived from activated macrophages and lesional T cells can elicit the expression of genes encoding proteolytic enzymes that can degrade the extracellular matrix of the plaque's fibrous cap. Thus, inflammatory mediators can impair collagen synthesis required for maintenance and repair of the fibrous cap and trigger degradation of extracellular matrix macromolecules, processes that weaken the plaque's fibrous cap and enhance its vulnerability to rupture. In contrast to plaques with these features of vulnerability, those with a dense extracellular matrix and relatively thick fibrous cap without substantial tissue factor-rich lipid cores seem generally resistant to rupture and unlikely to provoke thrombosis.

Features of the biology of the atheromatous plaque in addition to its degree of luminal encroachment influence the clinical manifestations of this disease. This enhanced understanding of plaque biology provides insight into the diverse ways in which atherosclerosis can present clinically and why the disease may remain silent or stable for prolonged periods, punctuated by acute complications at certain times. Increased understanding of atherogenesis provides new insight into the mechanisms linking it to the risk factors discussed below, indicates the ways in which current therapies may improve outcomes, and also suggests new targets for future intervention.

PREVENTION AND TREATMENT

THE CONCEPT OF ATHEROSCLEROTIC RISK FACTORS

The systematic study of risk factors for atherosclerosis emerged from a coalescence of experimental results as well as cross-sectional and ultimately longitudinal studies in humans. The prospective, community-based Framingham Heart Study provided rigorous support for the concept that hypercholesterolemia, hypertension, and other factors correlated with cardiovascular risk. Similar observational studies performed worldwide bolstered the concept of "risk factors" for cardiovascular disease.

From a practical viewpoint, the cardiovascular risk factors that have emerged from such studies fall into two categories: those modifiable by lifestyle and/or pharmacotherapy and those such as age and gender that are immutable. The weight of evidence supporting various risk factors differs. For example, hypercholesterolemia and hypertension certainly predict coronary risk, but other so-called nontraditional risk factors, such as levels of homocysteine, lipoprotein (a) [Lp(a)], or infection, remain controversial. Moreover, the causality of some biomarkers that predict cardiovascular risk, such as C-reactive protein (CRP), remains uncertain. Table 30-1 lists the risk factors recognized by the current National Cholesterol Education Project Adult Treatment Panel III (ATP III). The following sections consider some of these risk factors and approaches to their modification.

TABLE 30-1

MAJOR RISK FACTORS (EXCLUSIVE OF LDL CHOLESTEROL) THAT MODIFY LDL GOALS
Cigarette smoking
Hypertension (BP ≥140/90 mmHg or on antihypertensive medication)
Low HDL cholesterol[a] [<1.0 mmol/L (<40 mg/dL)]
Diabetes mellitus
Family history of premature CHD
CHD in male first-degree relative <55 years
CHD in female first-degree relative <65 years
Age (men ≥45 years; women ≥55 years)
Lifestyle risk factors
Obesity (BMI ≥30 kg/m^2)
Physical inactivity
Atherogenic diet
Emerging risk factors
Lipoprotein(a)
Homocysteine
Prothrombotic factors
Proinflammatory factors
Impaired fasting glucose
Subclinical atherogenesis

[a]HDL cholesterol ≥1.6 mmol/L (≥60 mg/dL) counts as a "negative" risk factor; its presence removes one risk factor from the total count.
Note: LDL, low-density lipoprotein; BP, blood pressure; HDL, high-density lipoprotein; CHD, coronary heart disease; BMI, body-mass index.
Source: Modified from Expert Panel on Detection, Evaluation, and Treatment of High Blood Cholesterol in Adults (Adult Treatment Panel III). JAMA 285:2486, 2001.

Lipid Disorders

Abnormalities in plasma lipoproteins and derangements in lipid metabolism rank among the most firmly established and best understood risk factors for atherosclerosis. Chapter 31 describes the lipoprotein classes and provides a detailed discussion of lipoprotein metabolism. Current ATP III guidelines recommend lipid screening in all adults >20 years. The screen should include a fasting lipid profile (total cholesterol, triglycerides, LDL cholesterol, and HDL cholesterol) repeated every 5 years.

ATP III guidelines strive to match the intensity of treatment to an individual's risk. A quantitative estimate of risk places individuals in one of three treatment strata (Table 30-2). The first step in applying these guidelines involves counting an individual's risk factors (Table 30-1). Individuals with fewer than two risk factors fall into the lowest treatment intensity stratum [LDL goal <4.1 mmol/L (<160 mg/dL)]. In those with two or more risk factors, the next step involves a simple calculation that estimates the 10-year risk of developing coronary heart disease (CHD) (Table 30-2); see also *http://www.nhlbi.nih.gov/guidelines/cholesterol/* for the algorithm and a downloadable risk calculator. Those with

TABLE 30-2

LDL CHOLESTEROL GOALS AND CUTPOINTS FOR THERAPEUTIC LIFESTYLE CHANGES (TLC) AND DRUG THERAPY IN DIFFERENT RISK CATEGORIES

RISK CATEGORY	LDL LEVEL, mmol/L (mg/dL)		
	GOAL	INITIATE TLC	CONSIDER DRUG THERAPY
Very high ACS, or CHD w/DM, or mult CRF	<1.8 (<70)	≥1.8 (≥70)	≥1.8 (≥70)
High CHD or CHD risk equivalents (10-year risk >20%)	<2.6 (<100) [optional goal: <1.8 (<70)]	≥2.6 (≥100)	≥2.6 (≥100) [<2.6 (<100): consider drug Rx]
If LDL <2.6 (<100)	<1.8 (<70)		
Moderately high 2+ risk factors (10-year risk, 10–20%)	<2.6 (<100)	≥3.4 (≥130)	≥3.4 (≥130) [2.6–3.3 (100–129): consider drug Rx]
Moderate 2+ risk factors (risk <10%)	<3.4 (<130)	≥3.4 (≥130)	≥4.1 (≥160)
Lower 0–1 risk factor	<4.1 (<160)	≥4.1 (≥160)	≥4.9 (≥190)

Note: LDL, low-density lipoprotein; ACS, acute coronary syndrome; CHD, coronary heart disease; DM, diabetes mellitus; CRF, coronary risk factors.
Source: Adapted from S Grundy et al: Circulation 110:227, 2004.

a 10-year risk ≤20% fall into the intermediate stratum [LDL goal <3.4 mmol/L (<130 mg/dL)]. Those with a calculated 10-year CHD risk of >20%, any evidence of established atherosclerosis, or diabetes (now considered a CHD risk-equivalent) fall into the most intensive treatment group [LDL goal <2.6 mmol/L (<100 mg/dL)]. Members of the ATP III panel have recently suggested 1.8 mmol/L (70 mg/dL) as a goal for very high risk and as an optional goal for high-risk patients based on recent clinical trial data (Table 30-2).

The first maneuver to achieve the LDL goal involves therapeutic lifestyle changes (TLC), including specific diet and exercise recommendations established by the guidelines. According to ATP III criteria, those with LDL levels exceeding goal for their risk group by >0.8 mmol/L (>30 mg/dL) merit consideration for drug therapy. In patients with triglycerides >2.6 mmol/L (>200 mg/dL), ATP III guidelines specify a secondary goal for therapy, "non-HDL cholesterol" (simply, the HDL cholesterol level subtracted from the total cholesterol). Cutpoints for therapeutic decision for non-HDL cholesterol are 0.8 mmol/L (30 mg/dL) more than those for LDL.

An extensive and growing body of rigorous evidence now supports the effectiveness of aggressive management of dyslipidemia. Addition of drug therapy to dietary and other nonpharmacologic measures reduces cardiovascular risk in patients with established coronary atherosclerosis and also in individuals who have not previously suffered CHD events (Fig. 30-3). As guidelines often lag the emerging clinical trial evidence base, the practitioner may elect to exercise clinical judgment in making therapeutic decisions in individual patients.

LDL-lowering therapies do not appear to exert their beneficial effect on cardiovascular events by causing a marked "regression" of obstructive coronary lesions. Angiographically monitored studies of lipid lowering have shown at best a modest reduction in coronary

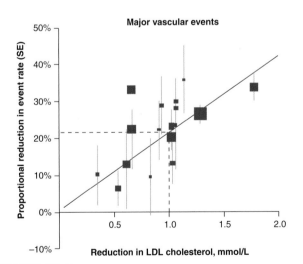

FIGURE 30-3

Lipid lowering reduces coronary events, as reflected on this graph showing the reduction in major cardiovascular events as a function of LDL level in a compendium of clinical trials with statins. *(Adapted from CTT Collaborators, Lancet 366:1267, 2005.)* The Management of Elevated Cholesterol in the Primary Prevention Group of Adult Japanese (MEGA), Treating to New Targets (TNT), and Incremental Decrease in Endpoints through Aggressive Lipid Lowering (IDEAL) studies have been added.

artery stenoses over the duration of study. Yet these same studies consistently show substantial decreases in coronary events. These results suggest that the beneficial mechanism of lipid lowering does not require a substantial reduction in the fixed stenoses. Rather, the benefit may derive from "stabilization" of atherosclerotic lesions without decreased stenosis. Such stabilization of atherosclerotic lesions and the attendant decrease in coronary events may result from the egress of lipids or by favorably influencing aspects of the biology of atherogenesis discussed earlier. In addition, as sizeable lesions may protrude abluminally rather than into the lumen due to complementary enlargement, shrinkage of such plaques might not be apparent on angiograms. The consistent benefit of LDL lowering by 3-hydroxy-3-methylgluatryl coenzyme A (HMG-CoA) reductase inhibitors (statins) observed in many risk groups may depend not only on their salutary effects on the lipid profile but also on direct modulation of plaque biology independent of lipid lowering.

A new class of LDL-lowering medications reduces cholesterol absorption from the proximal small bowel by targeting an enterocyte cholesterol transporter with the unwieldy name Niemann-Pick C1-like 1 protein (NPC1L1). The NPC1L1 inhibitor ezetimibe provides a useful adjunct to current therapies to achieve LDL goals; however, no clinical trial evidence yet demonstrates that ezetimibe benefits CHD outcomes.

As the mechanism by which elevated LDL levels promote atherogenesis likely involves oxidative modification, several trials have tested the possibility that antioxidant vitamin therapy might reduce CHD events. Rigorous and well-controlled clinical trials have failed to demonstrate that antioxidant vitamin therapy improves CHD outcomes. Therefore, the current evidence base does *not* support the use of antioxidant vitamins for this indication.

The clinical use of effective pharmacologic strategies for lowering LDL has markedly reduced cardiovascular events, but even their optimal utilization in clinical trials prevents only a minority of these endpoints. Hence other aspects of the lipid profile have become tempting targets for addressing the residual burden of cardiovascular disease that persists despite aggressive LDL lowering. Indeed, in the "post-statin" era, patients with LDL levels at or below target not infrequently present with acute coronary syndromes. Low levels of HDL remain a prevalent problem in patients with coronary artery disease. Blood HDL levels vary inversely with those of triglycerides, and the independent role of triglycerides as a cardiovascular risk factor remains unsettled. For these reasons, approaches to raising HDL have emerged as a prominent next hurdle in the management of dyslipidemia. Weight loss and physical activity can raise HDL. Nicotinic acid, particularly in combination with statins, can robustly raise HDL. Some clinical trial data support the effectiveness of nicotinic acid in cardiovascular

risk reduction. However, flushing and pruritus remain a challenge to patient acceptance, even with improved dosage forms of nicotinic acid. The identification of a cell-surface receptor for nicotinic acid may speed understanding of its mechanism of action and spur the development of new approaches to raising HDL.

Agonists of nuclear receptors that raise HDL levels provide another potential avenue to cardiovascular risk reduction. Peroxisome proliferator–activated receptor alpha (PPAR-α) agonists effectively raise HDL (by increasing transcription of its major apolipoprotein, AI) and lower triglyceride levels (by decreasing transcription of apolipoprotein CIII, an inhibitor of lipoprotein lipase, hence augmenting catabolism of triglyceride-rich lipoproteins). Cardiovascular outcome trials with PPAR-α and -γ agonists have yielded mixed results to date. Other agents in clinical development raise HDL levels by inhibiting cholesteryl ester transfer protein. Clinical studies currently underway will assess the effectiveness of this strategy to increase HDL in improvement of patient outcomes.

Hypertension

(See also Chap. 37) A wealth of epidemiologic data support a relationship between hypertension and atherosclerotic risk, and extensive clinical trial evidence has established that pharmacologic treatment of hypertension can reduce the risk of stroke, heart failure, and CHD events.

Diabetes Mellitus, Insulin Resistance, and the Metabolic Syndrome

Most patients with diabetes mellitus die of atherosclerosis and its complications. Aging and rampant obesity in the U.S. population underlie a current epidemic of type 2 diabetes mellitus. The abnormal lipoprotein profile associated with insulin resistance, known as *diabetic dyslipidemia*, accounts for part of the elevated cardiovascular risk in patients with type 2 diabetes. While diabetic patients often have LDL cholesterol levels near average, the LDL particles tend to be smaller and denser, and, therefore, more atherogenic. Other features of diabetic dyslipidemia include low HDL and elevated triglyceride levels. Hypertension also frequently accompanies obesity, insulin resistance, and dyslipidemia. Indeed, the ATP III guidelines now recognize this cluster of risk factors and provide criteria for diagnosis of the "metabolic syndrome" (Table 30-3). Despite legitimate concerns regarding whether clustered components confer more risk than an individual component, the metabolic syndrome concept has considerable clinical utility.

Therapeutic objectives for intervention in these patients include addressing the underlying causes, including obesity and low physical activity, by initiating TLC.

TABLE 30-3

CLINICAL IDENTIFICATION OF THE METABOLIC SYNDROME—ANY THREE RISK FACTORS

RISK FACTOR	DEFINING LEVEL
Abdominal obesity[a]	
Men (waist circumference)[b]	>102 cm (>40 in.)
Women	>88 cm (>35 in.)
Triglycerides	>1.7 mmol/L (>150 mg/dL)
HDL cholesterol	
Men	<1.0 mmol/L (<40 mg/dL)
Women	<1.3 mmol/L (<50 mg/dL)
Blood pressure	≥130/≥85 mmHg
Fasting glucose	>6.1 mmol/L (>110 mg/dL)

[a]Overweight and obesity are associated with insulin resistance and the metabolic syndrome. However, the presence of abdominal obesity is more highly correlated with the metabolic risk factors than is an elevated body-mass index (BMI). Therefore, the simple measure of waist circumference is recommended to identify the BMI component of the metabolic syndrome.

[b]Some male patients can develop multiple metabolic risk factors when the waist circumference is only marginally increased, e.g., 94–102 cm (37–39 in.). Such patients may have a strong genetic contribution to insulin resistance. They should benefit from lifestyle changes, similarly to men with categorical increases in waist circumference.

The ATP III guidelines provide an explicit step-by-step plan for implementing TLC, and treatment of the component risk factors should accompany TLC. Establishing that strict glycemic control reduces the risk of macrovascular complications of diabetes has proven much more elusive than the established beneficial effects on microvascular complications such as retinopathy or renal disease. In the absence of clear-cut evidence that tight glycemic control reduces coronary risk in patients with type 2, attention to other aspects of risk in this patient population assumes even greater importance. In this regard, multiple clinical trials, including the recent Collaborative Atorvastatin Diabetes Study (CARDS) that addressed specifically the diabetic population, have demonstrated unequivocal benefit of HMG-CoA reductase inhibitor therapy in diabetic patients over all ranges of LDL cholesterol levels. The Veterans Affairs HDL Intervention Trial (VA-HIT) showed that gemfibrozil, a PPAR-α agonist, reduced CHD and stroke in a population of men, many of whom had features of the metabolic syndrome. The recent Fenofibrate Intervention and Event Lowering in Diabetes (FIELD) trial did not meet its primary endpoint of reduced CHD death or nonfatal MI but did show a significant reduction in a composite endpoint of total cardiovascular events. A cardiovascular endpoint study in diabetic patients with the PPAR-γ agonist pioglitazone likewise did not meet its multipartite primary endpoint but did show a significant reduction in a secondary composite endpoint of all-cause mortality, nonfatal MI, and stroke. In view of the consistent benefit for diabetic populations of statin treatment, and the thus far equivocal results with PPAR agonists, the current stance of the American Diabetic Association that statins be considered for persons with diabetes older than 40 years who have a total cholesterol level ≥135 appears amply justified. Among the oral hypoglycemic agents, metformin possesses the best evidence base for cardiovascular event reduction.

Diabetic populations appear to derive particular benefit from antihypertensive strategies that block the action of angiotensin II. Thus, the antihypertensive regimen for patients with the metabolic syndrome should include angiotensin-converting enzyme inhibitors or angiotensin receptor blockers when possible. Most of these individuals will require more than one antihypertensive agent to achieve the recently updated American Diabetes Association blood pressure goal of 130/80 mmHg.

Male Gender/Postmenopausal State

Decades of observational studies have verified excess coronary risk in men compared with premenopausal women. After menopause, however, coronary risk accelerates in women. At least part of the apparent protection against CHD in premenopausal women derives from their relatively higher HDL levels compared with those of men. After menopause, HDL values fall in concert with increased coronary risk. Estrogen therapy lowers LDL cholesterol and raises HDL cholesterol, changes that should decrease coronary risk.

Multiple observational and experimental studies suggested that estrogen therapy reduces coronary risk. However, a spate of recent clinical trials has failed to demonstrate a net benefit of estrogen with or without progestins on CHD outcomes. In the Heart and Estrogen/Progestin Replacement Study (HERS), postmenopausal female survivors of acute MI were randomized to an estrogen/progestin combination or to placebo. This study showed no overall reduction in recurrent coronary events in the active treatment arm. Indeed, early in the 5-year course of this trial, there was a trend toward an actual increase in vascular events in the treated women. Extended follow-up of this cohort did not disclose an accrual of benefit in the treatment group. The Women's Health Initiative (WHI) study arm using a similar estrogen plus progesterone regimen was halted due to a small but significant hazard of cardiovascular events, stroke, and breast cancer. The estrogen without progestin arm of WHI (conducted in women without a uterus) ceased early due to an increase in strokes, and failed to afford protection from MI or CHD death during observation over 7 years. The excess cardiovascular events in these trials may result from an increase in thromboembolism. Physicians should work with women to provide information and help weigh the small but evident CHD risk of estrogen ± progestin vs. the benefits on postmenopausal symptoms and osteoporosis, taking personal preferences into account. Post hoc analyses of observational studies suggest that estrogen therapy in women younger than or closer to menopause than the women enrolled in WHI might confer cardiovascular benefit. Thus, the timing in relation to menopause or age at which estrogen therapy begins may influence its risk/benefit balance.

The lack of efficacy of estrogen therapy in cardiovascular risk reduction highlights the need for redoubled attention to known modifiable risk factors in women. In the recent clinical trials with HMG-CoA reductase inhibitors, women, when included, have derived benefits at least commensurate with those seen in men.

Dysregulated Coagulation or Fibrinolysis

Thrombosis ultimately causes the gravest complications of atherosclerosis. The propensity to form thrombi and/or to lyse clots once they form clearly influences the manifestations of atherosclerosis. Thrombosis provoked by atheroma rupture and subsequent healing may promote plaque growth. Certain individual characteristics can influence thrombosis or fibrinolysis and have received attention as potential coronary risk factors. For example, fibrinogen levels correlate with coronary risk and provide information regarding coronary risk independent of the lipoprotein profile. Elevated fibrinogen levels might promote thrombosis. As an acute-phase reactant, fibrinogen may also serve as a marker of inflammation.

The stability of an arterial thrombus depends on the balance between fibrinolytic factors, such as plasmin, and inhibitors of the fibrinolytic system, such as plasminogen activator inhibitor 1 (PAI-1). However, the levels of tissue plasminogen activator and PAI-1 in plasma have not proved to add considerable information beyond the lipid profile to the assessment of cardiovascular risk. Lp(a) (Chap. 31) may modulate fibrinolysis, and although individuals with elevated Lp(a) levels have increased CHD risk, Lp(a) levels do not potently predict risk in the population at large.

Aspirin reduces CHD events in several contexts. Chapter 33 discusses aspirin therapy in stable ischemic heart disease, Chap. 34 reviews recommendations for aspirin treatment in acute coronary syndromes. In primary prevention, pooled trial data show that low-dose aspirin treatment (81 mg qd to 325 mg alternate days) can reduce risk of first MI in men. Although the recent Women's Health Study (WHS) showed that aspirin (100 mg alternate days) reduced strokes by 17%, it did not prevent MI in women. Current American Heart Association (AHA) guidelines recommend the use of low-dose aspirin (75–160 mg/d) in women with high cardiovascular risk (≥20% 10-year risk), for men with a ≥10% 10-year risk of CHD, and for all aspirin-tolerant patients with established cardiovascular disease who lack contraindications.

Homocysteine

A large body of literature suggests a relationship between hyperhomocysteinemia and coronary events. Several mutations in the enzymes involved in homocysteine accumulation correlate with thrombosis and, in some studies, coronary risk. Prospective studies have not shown a robust utility of hyperhomocysteinemia in CHD risk stratification. Clinical trials have not shown that intervention to lower homocysteine levels reduces CHD events. Fortification of the U.S. diet with folic acid to reduce neural tube defects has lowered homocysteine levels in the population at large. Measurement of homocysteine levels should be reserved for individuals with atherosclerosis at a young age or out of proportion to established risk factors. Physicians who advise consumption of supplements containing folic acid should consider that this treatment might mask pernicious anemia.

Inflammation

An accumulation of clinical evidence shows that markers of inflammation correlate with coronary risk. For example, plasma levels of CRP, as measured by a high-sensitivity assay, prospectively predict risk of MI. CRP levels also correlate with outcome of patients with acute coronary syndromes. In contrast to several other novel risk factors, CRP adds predictive information to that derived from established risk factors, such as those included in the Framingham score (**Fig. 30-4**). Elevated levels of the acute-phase reactant CRP may reflect merely ongoing inflammation rather than a direct etiologic role for CRP in coronary artery disease.

Elevations in acute-phase reactants such as fibrinogen or CRP could reflect overall atherosclerotic burden and/or extravascular inflammation that potentiate atherosclerosis or its complications. In all likelihood, both

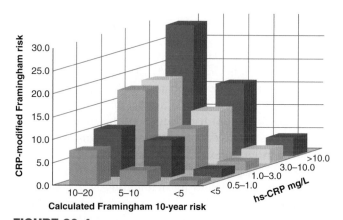

FIGURE 30-4

C-reactive protein (CRP) level adds to the predictive value of the Framingham score. hs-CRP, high-sensitivity measurement of CRP. (*Adapted from PM Ridker et al: Circulation 109:2818, 2004.*)

lesional and extravascular factors contribute to elevation of inflammatory markers in patients at risk for coronary events. Visceral adipose tissue releases pro-inflammatory cytokines that drive CRP production and may represent a major extravascular stimulus to elevation of inflammatory markers in obese and overweight individuals. Indeed, CRP levels rise with body mass index (BMI), and weight reduction lowers CRP levels. Infectious agents might also furnish inflammatory stimuli related to cardiovascular risk. However, the results of recent sufficiently powered randomized clinical trials do not support the use of antibiotics to reduce CHD risk.

Intriguing evidence suggests that lipid-lowering therapy reduces coronary events in part by muting the inflammatory aspects of the pathogenesis of atherosclerosis. A prespecified analysis of the Pravastatin or Atorvastatin Evaluation and Infection Therapy (PROVE-IT) trial, conducted in patients stabilized after acute coronary syndromes, showed that participants who achieved both below median LDL and CRP had fewer recurrent cardiovascular events than those who fell below only one of these cut points (**Fig. 30-5**). Those with both LDL and CRP above the median fared worst of all. The anti-inflammatory effect of statins appears independent of LDL lowering, as these two variables correlated very poorly in individual subjects in multiple clinical trials.

Lifestyle Modification

The prevention of atherosclerosis presents a long-term challenge to all health care professionals and for public health policy as well. Both individual practitioners and organizations providing health care should strive to help patients optimize their risk factor profile long before

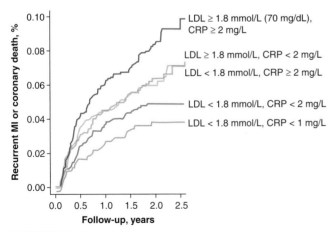

FIGURE 30-5
Evidence that both LDL-lowering and anti-inflammatory actions contribute to the benefit of statin therapy in survivors of acute coronary syndrome. See text for explanation. hs-CRP, high-sensitivity measurement of C-reactive protein (CRP); MI, myocardial infarction. (*Adapted from PM Ridker et al: N Engl J Med 352:20, 2005.*)

atherosclerotic disease becomes manifest. The current accumulation of cardiovascular risk in youth and in certain minority populations presents a particularly vexing concern from a public health perspective.

The care plan for all patients seen by internists should include measures to assess and minimize cardiovascular risk. Physicians must counsel patients regarding the health risks of tobacco use and provide guidance and resources regarding smoking cessation. Likewise, physicians should advise all patients about prudent dietary and physical activity habits for maintaining ideal body weight. Both National Institutes of Health and AHA statements recommend at least 30 min of moderate-intensity physical activity per day. Obesity, particularly the male pattern of centripetal or visceral fat accumulation, can contribute to the elements of the metabolic syndrome (Table 30-3). Physicians should encourage their patients to take personal responsibility for behavior related to modifiable risk factors for development of premature atherosclerotic disease. Conscientious counseling and patient education may forestall the need for pharmacologic measures intended to reduce coronary risk.

Issues in Risk Assessment

A growing panel of markers of coronary risk presents a perplexing array to the practitioner. Markers measured in peripheral blood include size fractions of LDL particles and concentrations of homocysteine, Lp(a), fibrinogen, CRP, PAI-1, myeloperoxidase, and lipoprotein-associated phospholipase A_2, among many others. In general, such specialized tests add little to the information available from a careful history and physical examination combined with measurement of a plasma lipoprotein profile and fasting blood glucose. The high-sensitivity CRP measurement may well prove an exception in view of its robustness in risk prediction, its ease of reproducible and standardized measurement, its relative stability in individuals over time, and, most importantly, its ability to add to the risk information disclosed by standard measurements such as the components of the Framingham risk score (Fig. 30-4). Given the utility of high-sensitivity CRP measurement in predicting a gamut of important cardiovascular outcomes, this simple blood test may prove useful in the future in guiding therapy, particularly in primary prevention. Current advisories, however, recommend the use of this test only in individuals with intermediate risk of a CHD event (10–20%, 10-year risk). Clinical trials now under way will test the hypothesis that CRP levels can guide therapy. Results such as those from PROVE-IT (Fig. 30-5) suggest that CRP may prove a valid target of therapy, a proposition that requires more investigation before general adoption in practice.

Similar concerns pertain to the use of specialized radiographic estimations of coronary artery calcification and of the rapidly emerging computed tomographic coronary angiograms (CTA). Accumulating information indicates that the amount of calcium determined by such techniques as electron beam CT correlates with coronary risk; however, the utility of using such estimates of coronary artery calcium content as a guide to therapy remains unproven, particularly in asymptomatic individuals. Multidetector CTA provides visually appealing images of the epicardial coronary arteries yet still requires rigorous validation as a cardiovascular risk marker or guide to therapy. Inappropriate use of such imaging modalities might promote excessive invasive diagnostic and therapeutic procedures. Widespread application of such modalities for screening should await proof that clinical benefit derives from their application.

Progress in human genetics holds considerable promise for risk prediction and for individualization of cardiovascular therapy. Many reports have identified single nucleotide polymorphisms in candidate genes as predictors of cardiovascular risk. To date, the validation of such genetic markers of risk and drug-responsiveness in multiple populations has often proved disappointing. The advent of technology that permits relatively rapid and inexpensive genome-wide screens, and of powerful bioinformatics tools, should spur haplotype analyses and unbiased identification of risk and therapy-response genotypes in the future.

THE CHALLENGE OF IMPLEMENTATION: CHANGING PHYSICIAN AND PATIENT BEHAVIOR

Despite declining age-adjusted rates of coronary death, cardiovascular mortality is on the rise due to the overall aging of the population. There is a powerful global trend toward increased atherosclerotic disease. Enormous challenges remain regarding translation of the current evidence base into practice. We must learn how to help individuals adopt a healthy lifestyle and how to deploy our increasingly powerful pharmacologic tools most economically and effectively. The obstacles to implementation of current evidence-based prevention and treatment of atherosclerosis include economics, education, physician awareness, and patient adherence to recommended regimens. Future goals in the field of treatment of atherosclerosis should include more widespread implementation of the current evidence-based guidelines regarding risk-factor management and, when appropriate, drug therapy.

FURTHER READINGS

ALBERTI KG et al: Harmonizing the metabolic syndrome: A joint interim statement of the International Diabetes Federation Task Force on Epidemiology and Prevention; National Heart, Lung, and Blood Institute; American Heart Association; World Heart Federation; International Atherosclerosis Society; and International Association for the Study of Obesity. Circulation 120:1640, 2009

BAIGENT C et al: Efficacy and safety of cholesterol-lowering treatment: Prospective meta-analysis of data from 90,056 participants in 14 randomised trials of statins. Lancet 366:1267, 2005

BERLINER JA, WATSON AD: A role for oxidized phospholipids in atherosclerosis. N Engl J Med 353:9, 2005

D'AGOSTINO RB et al: General cardiovascular risk profile for use in primary care: The Framingham Heart Study. Circulation 117:743, 2008

DELAHOY PJ et al: The relationship between reduction in low-density lipoprotein cholesterol by statins and reduction in risk of cardiovascular outcomes: An updated meta-analysis. Clin Ther 31:236, 2009

GRODSTEIN F et al: Hormone therapy and coronary artery disease: The role of time since menopause and age at hormone initiation. J Women's Health 15:35, 2006

GRUNDY SM et al: Implications of recent clinical trials for the National Cholesterol Education Program Adult Treatment Panel III guidelines. Circulation 110:227, 2004

——— et al: Diagnosis and management of the metabolic syndrome: An American Heart Association/National Heart, Lung, and Blood Institute scientific statement. Circulation 112:2735, 2005

HAMSTEN A, ERIKSSON P: Identifying the susceptibility genes for coronary artery disease: From hyperbole through doubt to cautious optimism. J Intern Med 263:538, 2008

LIBBY P: The vascular endothelium and atherosclerosis, in The Handbook of Experimental Pharmacology, S Moncada, EA Higgs (eds). Berlin-Heidelberg, Springer-Verlag, 2006

———, RIDKER PM: Inflammation and atherothrombosis: From population biology and bench research to clinical practice. J Am Coll Cardiol 48(9 Suppl):A33–46, 2006

———, THEROUX P: Pathophysiology of coronary artery disease. Circulation 111:3481, 2005

——— et al: Inflammation in atherosclerosis: From pathophysiology to practice. J Am Coll Cardiol 54:2129, 2009

MILLER DT et al: Atherosclerosis: The path from genomics to therapeutics. J Am Coll Cardiol 49:1589, 2007

MOSCA L et al: Evidence-based guidelines for cardiovascular disease prevention in women: 2007 update. Circulation 115:1481, 2007

RIDKER PM et al: C-reactive protein and parental history improve global cardiovascular risk prediction: The Reynolds Risk Score for men. Circulation 118:2243, 2008

SHAO B, HEINECKE JW: HDL, lipid peroxidation, and atherosclerosis. J Lipid Res 50:599, 2009

CHAPTER 31

DISORDERS OF LIPOPROTEIN METABOLISM

Daniel J. Rader ■ Helen H. Hobbs

Lipoproteins are complexes of lipids and proteins that are essential for the transport of cholesterol, triglycerides, and fat-soluble vitamins. Previously, lipoprotein disorders were the purview of specialized lipidologists, but the demonstration that lipid-lowering therapy significantly reduces the clinical complications of atherosclerotic cardiovascular disease (ASCVD) has brought the diagnosis and treatment of these disorders into the domain of the internist. The number of individuals who are candidates for lipid-lowering therapy has continued to increase. The development of safe, effective, and well-tolerated pharmacologic agents has greatly expanded the therapeutic armamentarium available to the physician to treat disorders of lipid metabolism. Therefore, the appropriate diagnosis and management of lipoprotein disorders is of critical importance in the practice of medicine. This chapter will review normal lipoprotein physiology, the pathophysiology of primary (inherited) disorders of lipoprotein metabolism, the diseases and environmental factors that cause secondary disorders of lipoprotein metabolism, and the practical approaches to their diagnosis and management.

LIPOPROTEIN METABOLISM

LIPOPROTEIN CLASSIFICATION AND COMPOSITION

Lipoproteins are large macromolecular complexes that transport hydrophobic lipids (primarily triglycerides,

cholesterol, and fat-soluble vitamins) through body fluids (plasma, interstitial fluid, and lymph) to and from tissues. Lipoproteins play an essential role in the absorption of dietary cholesterol, long-chain fatty acids, and fat-soluble vitamins; the transport of triglycerides, cholesterol, and fat-soluble vitamins from the liver to peripheral tissues; and the transport of cholesterol from peripheral tissues to the liver.

Lipoproteins contain a core of hydrophobic lipids (triglycerides and cholesteryl esters) surrounded by hydrophilic lipids (phospholipids, unesterified cholesterol) and proteins that interact with body fluids. The plasma lipoproteins are divided into five major classes based on their relative density (Fig. 31-1 and Table 31-1): chylomicrons, very low density lipoproteins (VLDLs), intermediate-density lipoproteins (IDLs), low-density lipoproteins (LDLs), and high-density lipoproteins (HDLs). Each lipoprotein class comprises a family of particles that vary slightly in density, size, migration during electrophoresis, and protein composition. The density of a lipoprotein is determined by the amount of lipid per particle. HDL is the smallest and most dense lipoprotein, whereas chylomicrons and VLDLs are the largest and least dense lipoprotein particles. Most plasma triglyceride is transported in chylomicrons or VLDLs, and most plasma cholesterol is carried as cholesteryl esters in LDLs and HDLs.

The proteins associated with lipoproteins, called *apolipoproteins* (Table 31-2), are required for the assembly,

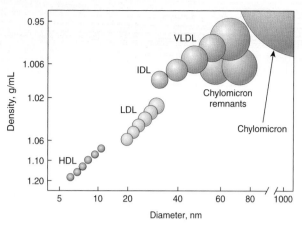

FIGURE 31-1

The density and size-distribution of the major classes of lipoprotein particles. Lipoproteins are classified by density and size, which are inversely related. VLDL, very low density lipoprotein; IDL, intermediate-density lipoprotein; LDL, low-density lipoprotein; HDL, high-density lipoprotein.

structure, and function of lipoproteins. Apolipoproteins activate enzymes important in lipoprotein metabolism and act as ligands for cell surface receptors. ApoA-I, which is synthesized in the liver and intestine, is found on virtually all HDL particles. ApoA-II is the second most abundant HDL apolipoprotein and is on approximately two-thirds of all HDL particles. ApoB is the major structural protein of chylomicrons, VLDLs, IDLs, and LDLs; one molecule of apoB, either apoB-48 (chylomicron) or apoB-100 (VLDL, IDL or LDL), is present on each lipoprotein particle. The human liver

synthesizes apoB-100, and the intestine makes apoB-48, which is derived from the same gene by mRNA editing. ApoE is present in multiple copies on chylomicrons, VLDL, and IDL, and it plays a critical role in the metabolism and clearance of triglyceride-rich particles. Three apolipoproteins of the C-series (apoC-I, apoC-II, and apoC-III) also participate in the metabolism of triglyceride-rich lipoproteins. The other apolipoproteins are listed in Table 31-2.

TRANSPORT OF DIETARY LIPIDS (EXOGENOUS PATHWAY)

The exogenous pathway of lipoprotein metabolism permits efficient transport of dietary lipids (**Fig. 31-2**). Dietary triglycerides are hydrolyzed by lipases within the intestinal lumen and emulsified with bile acids to form micelles. Dietary cholesterol, fatty acids, and fat-soluble vitamins are absorbed in the proximal small intestine. Cholesterol and retinol are esterified (by the addition of a fatty acid) in the enterocyte to form cholesteryl esters and retinyl esters, respectively. Longer-chain fatty acids (>12 carbons) are incorporated into triglycerides and packaged with apoB-48, cholesteryl esters, retinyl esters, phospholipids and cholesterol to form chylomicrons. Nascent chylomicrons are secreted into the intestinal lymph and delivered via the thoracic duct directly to the systemic circulation, where they are extensively processed by peripheral tissues before reaching the liver. The particles encounter lipoprotein lipase (LPL), which is anchored to proteoglycans that decorate the capillary endothelial surfaces of adipose tissue, heart and skeletal

TABLE 31-1

MAJOR LIPOPROTEIN CLASSES

LIPOPROTEIN	DENSITY, g/mL[a]	SIZE, nm[b]	ELECTROPHORETIC MOBILITY[c]	APOLIPOPROTEINS MAJOR	APOLIPOPROTEINS OTHER	OTHER CONSTITUENTS
Chylomicrons	0.930	75–1200	Origin	ApoB-48	A-I, A-IV, C-I, C-II, C-III	Retinyl esters
Chylomicron remnants	0.930–1.006	30–80	Slow pre-β	ApoB-48	E, A-I, A-IV, C-I, C-II, C-III	Retinyl esters
VLDL	0.930–1.006	30–80	Pre-β	ApoB-100	E, A-I, A-II, A-V, C-I, C-II, C-III	Vitamin E
IDL	1.006–1.019	25–35	Slow pre-β	ApoB-100	E, C-I, C-II, C-III	Vitamin E
LDL	1.019–1.063	18–25	β	ApoB-100		Vitamin E
HDL	1.063–1.210	5–12	α	ApoA-I	A-II, A-IV, E, C-III	LCAT, CETP paroxonase
Lp(a)	1.050–1.120	25	Pre-β	ApoB-100	Apo(a)	

All of the lipoprotein classes contain phospholipids, esterified and unesterified cholesterol, and triglycerides to varying degrees.
[a]The density of the particle is determined by ultracentrifugation.
[b]The size of the particle is measured using gel electrophoresis.
[c]The electrophoretic mobility of the particle on agarose gel electrophores reflects the size and surface charge of the particle, with β being the position of LDL and α being the position of HDL.
Note: VLDL, very low density lipoprotein; IDL, intermediate-density lipoprotein; LDL, low-density lipoprotein; HDL, high-density lipoprotein; Lp(a), lipoprotein A; LCAT, lecithin-cholesterol acyltransferase; CETP, cholesteryl ester transfer protein.

TABLE 31-2

MAJOR APOLIPOPROTEINS

APOLIPOPROTEIN	PRIMARY SOURCE	LIPOPROTEIN ASSOCIATION	FUNCTION
ApoA-I	Intestine, liver	HDL, chylomicrons	Structural protein for HDL Activates LCAT
ApoA-II	Liver	HDL, chylomicrons	Structural protein for HDL
ApoA-IV	Intestine	HDL, chylomicrons	Unknown
ApoA-V	Liver	VLDL, chylomicrons	Promotes LPL-mediated triglyceride lipolysis
ApoB-48	Intestine	Chylomicrons	Structural protein for chylomicrons
ApoB-100	Liver	VLDL, IDL, LDL, Lp(a)	Structural protein for VLDL, LDL, IDL, Lp(a) Ligand for binding to LDL receptor
ApoC-I	Liver	Chylomicrons, VLDL, HDL	Unknown
ApoC-II	Liver	Chylomicrons, VLDL, HDL	Cofactor for LPL
ApoC-III	Liver	Chylomicrons, VLDL, HDL	Inhibits lipoprotein binding to receptors
ApoD	Spleen, brain, testes, adrenals	HDL	Unknown
ApoE	Liver	Chylomicron remnants, IDL, HDL	Ligand for binding to LDL receptor
ApoH	Liver	Chylomicrons, VLDL, LDL, HDL	B_2 glycoprotein I
ApoJ	Liver	HDL	Unknown
ApoL	Unknown	HDL	Unknown
ApoM	Liver	HDL	Unknown
Apo(a)	Liver	Lp(a)	Unknown

Note: HDL, high-density lipoprotein; LCAT, lecithin-cholesterol acyltransferase; VLDL, very low density lipoprotein; IDL, intermediate-density lipoprotein; LDL, low-density lipoprotein; Lp(a), lipoprotein A; LPL, lipoprotein lipase.

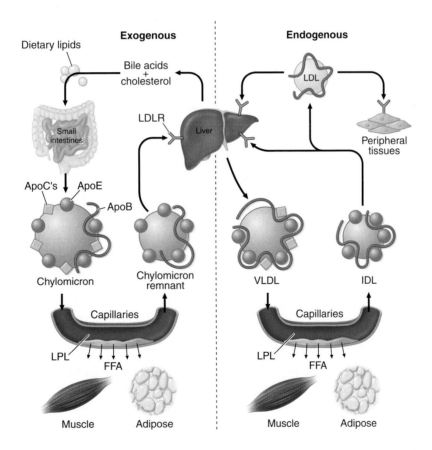

FIGURE 31-2

The exogenous and endogenous lipoprotein metabolic pathways. The exogenous pathway transports dietary lipids to the periphery and the liver. The endogenous pathway transports hepatic lipids to the periphery. LPL, lipoprotein lipase; FFA, free fatty acid; VLDL, very low density lipoprotein; IDL, intermediate-density lipoprotein; LDL, low-density lipoprotein; LDLR, low-density lipoprotein receptor.

muscle (Fig. 31-2). The triglycerides of chylomicrons are hydrolyzed by LPL, and free fatty acids are released. ApoC-II, which is transferred to circulating chylomicrons from HDL, acts as a cofactor for LPL in this reaction. The released free fatty acids are taken up by adjacent myocytes or adipocytes and either oxidized to generate energy or reesterified and stored as triglyceride. Some of the released free fatty acids bind albumin before entering cells and are transported to other tissues, especially the liver. The chylomicron particle progressively shrinks in size as the hydrophobic core is hydrolyzed and the hydrophilic lipids (cholesterol and phospholipids) and apolipoproteins on the particle surface are transferred to HDL, creating chylomicron remnants. Chylomicron remnants are rapidly removed from the circulation by the liver through a process that requires apoE as a ligand for receptors in the liver. Consequently, few, if any, chylomicrons or chylomicron remnants are present in the blood after a 12-h fast, except in patients with disorders of chylomicron metabolism.

TRANSPORT OF HEPATIC LIPIDS (ENDOGENOUS PATHWAY)

The endogenous pathway of lipoprotein metabolism refers to the hepatic secretion of apoB-containing lipoproteins and their metabolism (Fig. 31-2). VLDL particles resemble chylomicrons in protein composition but contain apoB-100 rather than apoB-48 and have a higher ratio of cholesterol to triglyceride (~1 mg of cholesterol for every 5 mg of triglyceride). The triglycerides of VLDL are derived predominantly from the esterification of long-chain fatty acids in the liver. The packaging of hepatic triglycerides with the other major components of the nascent VLDL particle (apoB-100, cholesteryl esters, phospholipids, and vitamin E) requires the action of the enzyme microsomal triglyceride transfer protein (MTP). After secretion into the plasma, VLDL acquires multiple copies of apoE and apolipoproteins of the C series by transfer from HDL. As with chylomicrons, the triglycerides of VLDL are hydrolyzed by LPL, especially in muscle and adipose tissue. After the VLDL remnants dissociate from LPL, they are referred to as IDLs, which contain roughly similar amounts of cholesterol and triglyceride. The liver removes approximately 40–60% of IDL by LDL receptor–mediated endocytosis via binding to apoE. The remainder of IDL is remodeled by hepatic lipase (HL) to form LDL. During this process, most of the triglyceride in the particle is hydrolyzed, and all apolipoproteins except apoB-100 are transferred to other lipoproteins. The cholesterol in LDL accounts for over half of the plasma cholesterol in most individuals. Approximately 70% of circulating LDL is cleared by LDL receptor–mediated endocytosis in the liver. *Lipoprotein(a)* [Lp(a)] is a lipoprotein similar to LDL in lipid and protein composition, but it contains an additional protein called *apolipoprotein(a)* [apo(a)]. Apo(a) is synthesized in the liver and attached to apoB-100 by a disulfide linkage. The major site of clearance of Lp(a) is the liver, but the uptake pathway is not known.

HDL METABOLISM AND REVERSE CHOLESTEROL TRANSPORT

All nucleated cells synthesize cholesterol, but only hepatocytes and enterocytes can effectively excrete cholesterol from the body, into either the bile or the gut lumen. In the liver, cholesterol is excreted into the bile, either directly or after conversion to bile acids. Cholesterol in peripheral cells is transported from the plasma membranes of peripheral cells to the liver and intestine by a process termed "reverse cholesterol transport" that is facilitated by HDL (Fig. 31-3).

Nascent HDL particles are synthesized by the intestine and the liver. Newly secreted apoA-I rapidly acquires phospholipids and unesterified cholesterol from its site of synthesis (intestine or liver) via efflux promoted by the membrane protein ATP-binding cassette protein A1 (ABCA1). This process results in the formation of discoidal HDL particles, which then recruit additional unesterified cholesterol from the periphery. Within the HDL particle, the cholesterol is esterified by lecithin-cholesterol acyltransferase (LCAT), a plasma enzyme associated with HDL, and the more hydrophobic cholesteryl ester moves to the core of the HDL particle. As HDL acquires more cholesteryl ester it becomes spherical, and additional apolipoproteins and lipids are transferred to the particles from the surfaces of chylomicrons and VLDLs during lipolysis.

HDL cholesterol is transported to hepatocytes by both an indirect and a direct pathway. HDL cholesteryl esters can be transferred to apoB-containing lipoproteins in exchange for triglyceride by the cholesteryl ester transfer protein (CETP). The cholesteryl esters are then removed from the circulation by LDL receptor–mediated endocytosis. HDL cholesterol can also be taken up directly by hepatocytes via the scavenger receptor class BI (SR-BI), a cell surface receptor that mediates the selective transfer of lipids to cells.

HDL particles undergo extensive remodeling within the plasma compartment by a variety of lipid transfer proteins and lipases. The phospholipid transfer protein has the net effect of transferring phospholipids from other lipoproteins to HDL. After CETP-mediated lipid exchange, the triglyceride-enriched HDL becomes a much better substrate for HL, which hydrolyzes the triglycerides and phospholipids to generate smaller HDL particles. A related enzyme called *endothelial lipase* hydrolyzes HDL phospholipids, generating smaller HDL particles that are catabolized faster. Remodeling of HDL influences the metabolism, function, and plasma concentrations of HDL.

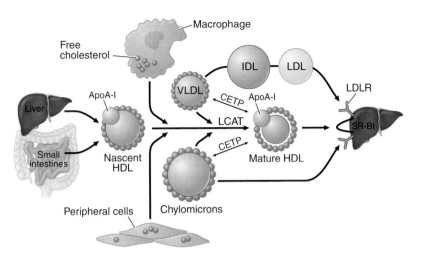

FIGURE 31-3

HDL metabolism and reverse cholesterol transport. This pathway transports excess cholesterol from the periphery back to the liver for excretion in the bile. The liver and the intestine produce nascent HDLs. Free cholesterol is acquired from macrophages and other peripheral cells and esterified by LCAT, forming mature HDLs. HDL cholesterol can be selectively taken up by the liver via SR-BI (scavenger receptor class BI). Alternatively, HDL cholesteryl ester can be transferred by CETP from HDLs to VLDLs and chylomicrons, which can then be taken up by the liver. LCAT, lecithin-cholesterol acyltransferase; CETP, cholesteryl ester transfer protein; VLDL, very low density lipoprotein; IDL, intermediate-density lipoprotein; LDL, low-density lipoprotein; HDL, high-density lipoprotein; LDLR, low-density lipoprotein receptor; TG, triglyceride.

DISORDERS OF LIPOPROTEIN METABOLISM

Frederickson and Levy classified hyperlipoproteinemias according to the type of lipoprotein particles that accumulate in the blood (type I–type V) (Table 31-3). A classification scheme based on the molecular etiology and pathophysiology of the lipoprotein disorders complements this system and forms the basis for this chapter. The identification and characterization of genes responsible for the genetic forms of hyperlipidemia have provided important molecular insights into the critical roles of structural apolipoproteins, enzymes, and receptors in lipid metabolism (Table 31-4).

PRIMARY DISORDERS OF ELEVATED ApoB-CONTAINING LIPOPROTEINS

A variety of genetic conditions are associated with the accumulation in plasma of specific classes of lipoprotein particles. In general, these can divide into those causing elevated LDL-cholesterol (LDL-C) with normal triglycerides and those causing elevated triglycerides (Table 31-4).

Lipid Disorders Associated with Elevated LDL-C with Normal Triglycerides

Familial Hypercholesterolemia (FH)

FH is an autosomal codominant disorder characterized by elevated plasma levels of LDL-C with normal triglycerides, tendon xanthomas, and premature coronary atherosclerosis. FH is caused by a large number (>900) of mutations in the LDL receptor gene. It has a higher incidence in certain founder populations, such as Afrikaners, Christian Lebanese, and French Canadians. The elevated levels of LDL-C in FH are due to an increase in the production of LDL from IDL and a delayed catabolism of LDL from the blood. There is a gene dose effect, in that individuals with two mutated LDL receptor alleles (FH homozygotes) are much more affected than those with one mutant allele (FH heterozygotes).

Homozygous FH occurs in approximately 1 in 1 million persons worldwide. Patients with homozygous FH can be classified into one of two groups based on the amount of LDL receptor activity measured in their skin fibroblasts: those patients with <2% of normal LDL receptor activity (receptor negative) and those patients with 2–25% of normal LDL receptor activity (receptor defective). Most patients with homozygous FH present in childhood with cutaneous xanthomas on the hands, wrists, elbows, knees, heels, or buttocks. Total cholesterol levels are usually >500 mg/dL and can be >1000 mg/dL. The devastating complication of homozygous FH is accelerated atherosclerosis, which can result in disability and death in childhood. Atherosclerosis often develops first in the aortic root, where it can cause aortic valvular or supravalvular stenosis, and typically extends into the coronary ostia, which become stenotic. Children with homozygous FH often develop symptomatic coronary atherosclerosis before puberty; symptoms can be atypical, and sudden death is common. Untreated, receptor-negative

TABLE 31-3

FREDERICKSON CLASSIFICATION OF HYPERLIPOPROTEINEMIAS

PHENOTYPE	I	IIA	IIB	III	IV	V
Lipoprotein, elevated	Chylomicrons	LDL	LDL and VLDL	Chylomicron and VLDL remnants	VLDL	Chylomicrons and VLDL
Triglycerides	++++	–	++	++ to +++	++	++++
Cholesterol	+ to ++	+++	++ to +++	++ to +++	– to +	++ to +++
LDL-cholesterol	↓	↑	↑	↓	↓	↓
HDL-cholesterol	+++	+	++	++	++	+++
Plasma appearance	Lactescent	Clear	Clear	Turbid	Turbid	Lactescent
Xanthomas	Eruptive	Tendon, tuberous	None	Palmar, tuberoeruptive	None	Eruptive
Pancreatitis	+++	0	0	0	0	+++
Coronary atherosclerosis	0	+++	+++	+++	+/–	+/–
Peripheral atherosclerosis	0	+	+	++	+/–	+/–
Molecular defects	LPL and apoC-II	LDL receptor, ApoB-100, PCSK9, ARH, ABCG5 and ABCG8	Unknown	ApoE	ApoA-V and Unknown	ApoA-V and Unknown
Genetic nomenclature	FCS	FH, FDB, ADH, ARH, sitosterolemia	FCHL	FDBL	FHTG	FHTG

Note: LPL, lipoprotein lipase; apo, apolipoprotein; FCS, familial chylomicronemia syndrome; FH, familial hypercholesterolemia; FDB, familial defective apoB; ARH, autosomal recessive hypercholesterolemia; ADH, autosomal dominant hypercholesterolemia; FCHL, familial combined hyperlipidemia; FDBL, familial dysbetalipoproteinemia; FHTG, familial hypertriglyceridemia.

patients with homozygous FH rarely survive beyond the second decade; patients with receptor-defective LDL receptor defects have a better prognosis but almost invariably develop clinically apparent atherosclerotic vascular disease by 30 years of age, and often much younger. Carotid and femoral disease develops later in life and is usually not clinically significant.

A careful family history should be taken, and plasma lipid levels should be measured in the parents and other first-degree relatives of patients with homozygous FH. The diagnosis of homozygous FH can be confirmed by obtaining a skin biopsy and measuring LDL receptor activity in cultured skin fibroblasts, or by quantifying the number of LDL receptors on the surfaces of lymphocytes using cell sorting technology. Molecular assays are also available to define the mutations in the LDL receptor by DNA sequencing.

Combination therapy with an HMG-CoA reductase inhibitor and a cholesterol absorption inhibitor sometimes results in relatively modest reductions in plasma LDL-C in the FH homozygote. Patients with homozygous FH invariably require additional lipid-lowering therapy. Since the liver is quantitatively the most important tissue for removing circulating LDLs via the LDL receptor, liver transplantation is effective in decreasing plasma LDL-C levels in this disorder. Liver transplantation, however, is associated with substantial risks, including the requirement for long-term immunosuppression. The current treatment of choice for homozygous FH is LDL apheresis (a process by which the LDL particles are selectively removed from the circulation), which can promote regression of xanthomas and may slow the progression of atherosclerosis. Initiation of LDL apheresis should generally be delayed until approximately 5 years of age, except when evidence of atherosclerotic vascular disease is present.

Heterozygous FH is caused by the inheritance of one mutant LDL receptor allele and occurs in ~1 in 500 persons worldwide, making it one of the most common single-gene disorders. It is characterized by elevated plasma levels of LDL-C (usually 200–400 mg/dL) and normal levels of triglyceride. Patients with heterozygous FH have hypercholesterolemia from birth, although the disease is often not detected until adulthood, usually due to the detection of hypercholesterolemia on routine screening, the appearance of tendon xanthomas, or the development of symptomatic coronary atherosclerotic disease (CAD). Since the disease is codominant in inheritance and has a high penetrance (>90%), one parent and ~50% of the patient's siblings usually also have hypercholesterolemia. The family history is frequently

TABLE 31-4

PRIMARY HYPERLIPOPROTEINEMIAS CAUSED BY KNOWN SINGLE GENE MUTATIONS

GENETIC DISORDER	GENE DEFECT	LIPOPROTEINS ELEVATED	CLINICAL FINDINGS	GENETIC TRANSMISSION	ESTIMATED INCIDENCE
Lipoprotein lipase deficiency	LPL (*LPL*)	Chylomicrons	Eruptive xanthomas, hepatosplenomegaly, pancreatitis	AR	1/1,000,000
Familial apolipoprotein C-II deficiency	ApoC-II (*APOC2*)	Chylomicrons	Eruptive xanthomas, hepatosplenomegaly, pancreatitis	AR	<1/1,000,000
ApoA-V deficiency	ApoA-V (*APOAV*)	Chylomicrons, VLDL	Eruptive xanthomas, hepatosplenomegaly, pancreatitis	AD	<1/1,000,000
Familial hepatic lipase deficiency	Hepatic lipase (*LIPC*)	VLDL remnants	Premature atherosclerosis, pancreatitis	AR	<1/1,000,000
Familial dysbetalipoproteinemia	apoE (*APOE*)	Chylomicron and VLDL remnants	Palmar and tuberoeruptive xanthomas, CHD, PVD	AR AD	1/10,000
Familial hypercholesterolemia	LDL receptor (*LDLR*)	LDL	Tendon xanthomas, CHD	AD	1/500
Familial defective apoB-100	apoB-100 (*APOB*) (Arg$_{3500}$ → Gln)	LDL	Tendon xanthomas, CHD	AD	<1/1000
Autosomal dominant hypercholesterolemia	PCSK9 (*PCSK9*)	LDL	Tendon xanthomas, CHD	AD	<1/1,000,000
Autosomal recessive hypercholesterolemia	ARH (*ARH*)	LDL	Tendon xanthomas, CHD	AR	<1/1,000,000
Sitosterolemia	*ABCG5* or *ABCG8*	LDL	Tendon xanthomas, CHD	AR	<1/1,000,000

Note: LPL, lipoprotein lipase; LDL, low-density lipoprotein; VLDL, very low density lipoprotein; ARH, autosomal recessive hypercholesterolemia; CHD, coronary heart disease; PVD, peripheral vascular disease; AR, autosomal recessive; AD, autosomal dominant.

positive for premature CAD on one side of the family. Corneal arcus is common, and tendon xanthomas involving the dorsum of the hands, elbows, knees, and especially the Achilles tendons are present in ~75% of patients. The age of onset of CAD is highly variable and depends in part on the molecular defect in the LDL receptor gene and also on coexisting cardiac risk factors. FH heterozygotes with elevated plasma levels of Lp(a) appear to be at greater risk for cardiovascular complications. Untreated men with heterozygous FH have a ~50% chance of having a myocardial infarction younger than 60 years. Although the age of onset of atherosclerotic heart disease is later in women with FH, coronary heart disease (CHD) is significantly more common in women with FH than in the general female population.

No definitive diagnostic test for heterozygous FH is available. Although FH heterozygotes tend to have reduced levels of LDL receptor function in skin fibroblasts, significant overlap with the LDL receptor activity levels in normal fibroblasts exists. Molecular assays have recently become available to identify the mutation in the DNA sequence, but the clinical utility of pinpointing the mutation has not been demonstrated. The clinical diagnosis is usually not problematic, but it is critical that hypothyroidism, nephrotic syndrome, and obstructive liver disease be excluded before initiating therapy.

FH patients should be aggressively treated to lower plasma levels of LDL-C. Initiation of a low-cholesterol, low-fat diet is recommended, but almost all heterozygous FH patients require lipid-lowering drug therapy. Statins are effective in heterozygous FH, but combination drug therapy with the addition of a cholesterol absorption inhibitor is frequently required, and even a third drug, such as bile acid sequestrant or nicotinic acid, is sometimes needed. Heterozygous FH patients who cannot be adequately controlled on combination drug therapy are candidates for LDL apheresis.

Familial Defective ApoB-100 (FDB)

This is a dominantly inherited disorder that clinically resembles heterozygous FH. FDB is a rare cause of hypercholesterolemia, except in populations with significant numbers of individuals of German descent where the frequency can be as high as 1 in 1000. The disease is characterized by elevated plasma LDL-C levels with normal triglycerides, tendon xanthomas, and an increased incidence of premature ASCVD. FDB is caused by mutations in the LDL receptor–binding domain of apoB-100. Most patients with FDB have a substitution of glutamine for arginine at position 3500 in apoB-100, although other rarer mutations have been reported to cause this disease. As a consequence of the mutation in apoB-100, LDL binds the LDL receptor with reduced affinity, and LDL is removed from the circulation at a reduced rate. Patients with FDB cannot be clinically distinguished from patients with heterozygous FH, although patients with FDB tend to have lower plasma levels of LDL-C than FH heterozygotes. The apoB-100 gene mutation can be detected directly, but genetic diagnosis is not currently encouraged since the recommended management of FDB and heterozygous FH is identical.

Autosomal Recessive Hypercholesterolemia (ARH)

ARH is a rare disorder (except on Sardinia, Italy) due to mutations in a protein (ARH, also called *LDLR adaptor protein*) involved in LDL receptor–mediated endocytosis in the liver. ARH clinically resembles homozygous FH and is characterized by hypercholesterolemia, tendon xanthomas, and premature coronary artery disease. The hypercholesterolemia tends to be intermediate between the levels seen in FH homozygotes and FH heterozygotes. LDL receptor function in cultured fibroblasts is normal or only modestly reduced in ARH, whereas LDL receptor function in lymphocytes and the liver is negligible. Unlike FH homozygotes, the hyperlipidemia responds partially to treatment with HMG-CoA reductase inhibitors, but these patients usually require LDL apheresis to lower plasma LDL-C to recommended levels.

Autosomal Dominant Hypercholesterolemia (ADH)

ADH is a rare disorder caused by gain-of-function mutations in proprotein convertase subtilisin/kexin type 9 (PCSK9). Increased activity of PCSK9 appears to cause dominant hypercholesterolemia by promoting the degradation of LDL receptors in the liver, thus reducing the clearance of circulating LDL. Interestingly, loss-of-function mutations in this gene cause low LDL-C levels (see later).

Sitosterolemia

This is a rare autosomal recessive disease caused by mutations in one of two members of the ATP-binding cassette (ABC) transporter family, ABCG5 and ABCG8. These genes are expressed in the intestine and liver, where they form a functional complex and pump plant sterols, such as sitosterol and campesterol, and animal sterols, predominantly cholesterol, from enterocytes into the gut lumen and from hepatocytes into the bile. In normal individuals, <5% of dietary plant sterols are absorbed by the proximal small intestine and delivered to the liver. Plant sterols that are carried to the liver on chylomicrons are preferentially secreted into the bile such that the plant sterol levels in plasma and tissues are normally very low. In sitosterolemia, the intestinal absorption of plant sterols is increased and biliary excretion of the sterols is reduced, resulting in increased plasma and tissue levels of sitosterol and other plant sterols.

The trafficking of cholesterol is also impaired in sitosterolemia. Patients with sitosterolemia usually have elevated plasma levels of LDL cholesterol. Patients develop tendon xanthomas as well as premature atherosclerosis and can be mistaken for FH patients. Episodes of hemolysis, presumably secondary to the incorporation of plant sterols into the red blood cell membrane, are a distinctive clinical feature of this disease. The hypercholesterolemia in subjects with sitosterolemia is unusually responsive to reductions in dietary cholesterol content. Sitosterolemia should be suspected in patients in whom the plasma cholesterol level falls more than 40% on a low-cholesterol diet.

Sitosterolemia is confirmed by demonstrating an increase in the plasma level of sitosterol using gas chromatography. The hypercholesterolemia does not respond to HMG-CoA reductase inhibitors; however, bile acid sequestrants and cholesterol-absorption inhibitors, such as ezetimibe, are effective in reducing plasma sterol levels in these patients.

Polygenic Hypercholesterolemia

This condition is characterized by hypercholesterolemia due to elevated LDL-C with a normal plasma level of triglyceride in the absence of secondary causes of hypercholesterolemia. Plasma LDL-C levels are generally not as elevated as they are in FH and FDB. Family studies are useful to differentiate polygenic hypercholesterolemia from the single-gene disorders described earlier; half of the first-degree relatives of patients with FH and FDB are hypercholesterolemic, whereas <10% of first-degree relatives of patients with polygenic hypercholesterolemia have hypercholesterolemia. Treatment of polygenic hypercholesterolemia is identical to that of other forms of hypercholesterolemia.

Lipid Disorders Associated with Elevated Triglycerides

Familial Chylomicronemia Syndrome (Type I Hyperlipoproteinemia; Lipoprotein Lipase and ApoC-II Deficiency)

As noted earlier, LPL is required for the hydrolysis of triglycerides in chylomicrons and VLDLs, and apoC-II is a cofactor for LPL (Fig. 31-2). Genetic deficiency or inactivity of either protein results in impaired lipolysis and profound elevations in plasma chylomicrons. These patients can also have elevated plasma levels of VLDL, but chylomicronemia predominates. The fasting plasma is turbid, and if left at 4°C for a few hours, the chylomicrons float to the top and form a creamy supernatant. In these disorders, called *familial chylomicronemia syndromes*, fasting triglyceride levels are almost invariably >1000 mg/dL. Fasting cholesterol levels are also usually elevated but to a much lesser degree.

LPL deficiency has autosomal recessive inheritance and has a frequency of ~1 in 1 million in the population.

ApoC-II deficiency is also recessive in inheritance pattern and is even less common than LPL deficiency. Multiple different mutations in the LPL and apoC-II genes cause these diseases. Obligate LPL heterozygotes have normal or mild-to-moderate elevations in plasma triglyceride levels, whereas individuals heterozygous for mutation in apoC-II do not have hypertriglyceridemia.

Both LPL and apoC-II deficiency usually present in childhood with recurrent episodes of severe abdominal pain due to acute pancreatitis. On fundoscopic examination the retinal blood vessels are opalescent (lipemia retinalis). Eruptive xanthomas, which are small, yellowish-white papules, often appear in clusters on the back, buttocks, and extensor surfaces of the arms and legs. The typically painless skin lesions may become puritic. Hepatosplenomegaly results from the uptake of circulating chylomicrons by reticuloendothelial cells in the liver and spleen. For unknown reasons, some patients with persistent and pronounced chylomicronemia never develop pancreatitis, eruptive xanthomas, or hepatosplenomegaly. Premature ASCVD is generally not a feature of familial chylomicronemia syndromes.

The diagnoses of LPL and apoC-II deficiency are established enzymatically in specialized laboratories by assaying triglyceride lipolytic activity in postheparin plasma. Blood is sampled after an intravenous heparin injection to release the endothelial-bound LPL. LPL activity is profoundly reduced in both LPL and apoC-II deficiency; in patients with apoC-II deficiency, it normalizes after the addition of normal plasma (providing a source of apoC-II).

The major therapeutic intervention in familial chylomicronemia syndromes is dietary fat restriction (to as little as 15 g/d) with fat-soluble vitamin supplementation. Consultation with a registered dietician familiar with this disorder is essential. Caloric supplementation with medium-chain triglycerides, which are absorbed directly into the portal circulation, can be useful but may be associated with hepatic fibrosis if used for prolonged periods. If dietary fat restriction alone is not successful in resolving the chylomicronemia, fish oils have been effective in some patients. In patients with apoC-II deficiency, apoC-II can be provided by infusing fresh frozen plasma to resolve the chylomicronemia. Management of patients with familial chylomicronemia syndrome is particularly challenging during pregnancy when VLDL production is increased and may require plasmapheresis to remove the circulating chylomicrons.

ApoA-V Deficiency

A newly discovered apolipoprotein called *ApoA-V* circulates at much lower concentrations than most other apolipoproteins. Individuals who are compound heterozygotes for a mutation that causes premature truncation of ApoA-V and a sequence variant associated with increased triglyceride levels have late-onset chylomicronemia.

The exact mechanism of action of ApoA-V is not known, but it appears to be required for the association of VLDL and chylomicrons with LPL.

Hepatic Lipase Deficiency

HL is a member of the same gene family as LPL and hydrolyzes triglycerides and phospholipids in remnant lipoproteins and HDLs. HL deficiency is a very rare autosomal recessive disorder characterized by elevated plasma levels of cholesterol and triglycerides (mixed hyperlipidemia) due to the accumulation of circulating lipoprotein remnants and either a normal or elevated plasma level of HDL-C. The diagnosis is confirmed by measuring HL activity in postheparin plasma. Because of the small number of patients with HL deficiency, the association of this genetic defect with ASCVD is not clearly known, but lipid-lowering therapy is recommended.

Familial Dysbetalipoproteinemia (type III Hyperlipoproteinemia)

Like HL deficiency, familial dysbetalipoproteinemia (FDBL) (also known as *type III hyperlipoproteinemia* or *familial broad β disease*) is characterized by a mixed hyperlipidemia due to the accumulation of remnant lipoprotein particles. ApoE is present in multiple copies on chylomicron and VLDL remnants and mediates their removal via hepatic lipoprotein receptors (Fig. 31-2). FDBL is due to genetic variations in apoE that interfere with its ability to bind lipoprotein receptors. The *APOE* gene is polymorphic in sequence, resulting in the expression of three common isoforms: apoE3, which is the most common; and apoE2 and apoE4, which both differ from apoE3 by a single amino acid. Although associated with slightly higher LDL-C levels and increased CHD risk, the apoE4 allele is not associated with FDBL. Patients with apoE4 have an increased incidence of late-onset Alzheimer's disease. ApoE2 has a lower affinity for the LDL receptor; therefore, chylomicron and VLDL remnants containing apoE2 are removed from plasma at a slower rate. Individuals who are homozygous for the E2 allele (the E2/E2 genotype) comprise the most common subset of patients with FDBL.

Approximately 0.5% of the general population are apoE2/E2 homozygotes, but only a small minority of these individuals develop FDBL. In most cases an additional, identifiable factor precipitates the development of hyperlipoproteinemia. The most common precipitating factors are a high-fat diet, diabetes mellitus, obesity, hypothyroidism, renal disease, estrogen deficiency, alcohol use, or certain drugs. Other mutations in apoE can cause a dominant form of FDBL where the hyperlipidemia is fully manifest in the heterozygous state, but these mutations are rare.

Patients with FDBL usually present in adulthood with xanthomas, premature coronary disease, and peripheral vascular disease. The disease seldom presents in women before menopause. Two distinctive types of xanthomas, tuberoeruptive and palmar, are seen in FDBL patients. Tuberoeruptive xanthomas begin as clusters of small papules on the elbows, knees, or buttocks and can grow to the size of small grapes. Palmar xanthomas (alternatively called *xanthomata striata palmaris*) are orange-yellow discolorations of the creases in the palms and wrists. In FDBL, the plasma levels of cholesterol and triglyceride are often elevated to a similar degree, the directly-measured LDL-C is low, and the HDL-C is usually normal (in contrast to the low HDL-C usually seen in patients with elevated triglyceride levels).

The traditional approaches to diagnosis of this disorder are lipoprotein electrophoresis (broad β band) or ultracentrifugation (ratio of VLDL-C to total plasma triglyceride >0.30). Protein methods (apoE phenotyping) or DNA-based methods (apoE genotyping) can be performed to confirm homozygosity for apoE2. However, absence of the apoE2/2 genotype does not rule out the diagnosis of FDBL, since other mutations in apoE can cause this condition.

Since FDBL is associated with increased risk of premature ASCVD, it should be treated aggressively. Subjects with FDBL have more peripheral vascular disease than is typically seen in FH. Other metabolic conditions that can worsen the hyperlipidemia (see above) should be actively treated. Patients with FDBL are typically very diet-responsive and can respond favorably to weight reduction and to low-cholesterol, low-fat diets. Alcohol intake should be curtailed. HMG-CoA reductase inhibitors, fibrates, and niacin are all generally effective in the treatment of FDBL, and sometimes combination drug therapy is required.

Familial Hypertriglyceridemia (FHTG)

FHTG is a relatively common (~1 in 500) autosomal dominant disorder of unknown etiology characterized by moderately elevated plasma triglycerides accompanied by more modest elevations in cholesterol. Since the major class of lipoproteins elevated in this disorder is VLDL, patients with this disorder are often referred to as having *type IV hyperlipoproteinemia* (Frederickson classification, Table 31-3). The elevated plasma levels of VLDL are due to increased production of VLDL, impaired catabolism of VLDL, or a combination of these mechanisms. Some patients with FHTG have a more severe form of hyperlipidemia in which both VLDLs and chylomicrons are elevated (type V hyperlipidemia), since these two classes of lipoproteins compete for the same lipolytic pathway. Increased intake of simple carbohydrates, obesity, insulin resistance, alcohol use, and estrogen treatment, all of which increase VLDL synthesis, can exacerbate this syndrome. FHTG appears not to be associated with increased risk of ASCVD in many families.

The diagnosis of FHTG is suggested by the triad of elevated levels of plasma triglycerides (250–1000 mg/dL),

normal or only mildly increased cholesterol levels (<250 mg/dL), and reduced plasma levels of HDL-C. Plasma LDL-C levels are generally not increased and are often reduced due to defective metabolism of the triglyceride-rich particles. The identification of other first-degree relatives with hypertriglyceridemia is useful in making the diagnosis. FDBL and familial combined hyperlipidemia (FCHL) should also be ruled out since these two conditions are associated with a significantly increased risk of ASCVD. The plasma apoB levels are lower and the ratio of plasma TG to cholesterol is higher in FHTG than in either FDBL or FCHL.

It is important to consider and rule out secondary causes of the hypertriglyceridemia (Table 31-5) before making the diagnosis of FHTG. Lipid-lowering drug therapy can frequently be avoided with appropriate dietary and lifestyle changes. Patients with plasma triglyceride levels >500 mg/dL after a trial of diet and exercise should be considered for drug therapy to avoid the development of chylomicronemia and pancreatitis. Fibrate drugs or fish oils (omega 3 fatty acids) are reasonable first-line approaches for FHTG, and niacin can also be considered in this condition.

Familial Combined Hyperlipidemia

FCHL is generally characterized by moderate elevations in plasma levels of triglycerides (VLDL) and cholesterol (LDL) and reduced plasma levels of HDL-C. It is the most common inherited lipid disorder, occurring in ~1 in 200 persons. Approximately 20% of patients who develop CHD younger than 60 years have FCHL. The disease is autosomal dominant in inheritance, and affected family members typically have one of three possible phenotypes: (1) elevated plasma levels of LDL-C, (2) elevated plasma levels of triglycerides due to elevation in VLDL-C, or (3) elevated plasma levels of both LDL-C and VLDL-C. A classic feature of FCHL is that the lipoprotein profile can switch among these three phenotypes over time and may depend on factors such as diet. FCHL can manifest in childhood but is usually not fully expressed until adulthood. A cluster of other metabolic risk factors are often found in association with this hyperlipidemia, including obesity, glucose intolerance, insulin resistance and hypertension (the so-called metabolic syndrome, Chap. 32). These patients do not develop xanthomas.

Patients with FCHL almost always have significantly elevated plasma levels of apoB. The levels of apoB are disproportionately high relative to the plasma LDL-C concentration, indicating the presence of small, dense LDL particles, which are characteristic of this syndrome. *Hyperapobetalipoproteinemia*, which has been used to describe the state of elevated plasma levels of apoB with normal plasma LDL-C levels, is probably a form of FCHL. Individuals with FCHL generally share the same metabolic defect, which is overproduction of VLDL by

TABLE 31-5

SECONDARY FORMS OF HYPERLIPIDEMIA

LDL		HDL		VLDL ELEVATED	IDL ELEVATED	CHYLOMICRONS ELEVATED	LP(a) ELEVATED
ELEVATED	**REDUCED**	**ELEVATED**	**REDUCED**				
Hypothyroidism	Severe liver disease	Alcohol	Smoking	Obesity	Multiple myeloma	Autoimmune disease	Renal insufficiency
Nephrotic syndrome	Malabsorption	Exercise	DM type 2	DM type 2	Monoclonal gammopathy	DM type 2	Inflammation
Cholestasis	Malnutrition	Exposure to chlorinated hydrocarbons	Obesity	Glycogen storage disease	Autoimmune disease		Menopause
Acute intermittent porphyria	Gaucher's disease	Drugs: estrogen	Malnutrition	Hepatitis	Hypothyroidism		Orchidectomy
Anorexia nervosa	Chronic infectious disease		Gaucher's disease	Alcohol			Hypothyroidism
Hepatoma	Hyperthyroidism		Drugs: anabolic steroids, beta blockers	Renal failure			Acromegaly
Drugs: thiazides, cyclosporin, tegretol	Drugs: niacin toxicity			Sepsis			Nephrosis
				Stress			Drugs: growth hormone, isotretinoin
				Cushing's syndrome			
				Pregnancy			
				Acromegaly			
				Lipodystrophy			
				Drugs: estrogen, beta blockers, glucocorticoids, bile acid binding resins, retinoic acid			

Note: LDL, low-density lipoprotein; HDL, high-density lipoprotein; VLDL, very low density lipoprotein; IDL, intermediate-density lipoprotein; Lp(a), lipoprotein A; DM, diabetes mellitus.

the liver. The molecular etiology of FCHL remains poorly understood, and it is likely that defects in several different genes can cause the phenotype of FCHL.

The presence of a mixed dyslipidemia (plasma triglyceride levels between 200–800 mg/dL and total cholesterol levels between 200–400 mg/dL, usually with HDL-C levels <40 mg/dL in men or <50 mg/dL in women) and a family history of hyperlipidemia and/or premature CHD strongly suggests the diagnosis of FCHL. The finding of an elevated plasma level of apoB level or the finding of an increased number of small, dense LDL particles in the plasma through advanced lipoprotein testing supports this diagnosis. FDBL should be considered and ruled out by beta quantification in suspected patients with a mixed hyperlipidemia.

Individuals with FCHL should be treated aggressively due to significantly increased risk of premature CHD. Decreased dietary intake of saturated fat and simple carbohydrates, aerobic exercise, and weight loss can all have beneficial effects on the lipid profile. Patients with diabetes should be aggressively treated to maintain good glucose control. Most patients with FCHL require lipid-lowering drug therapy to reduce lipoprotein levels to the recommended range and reduce the high risk of ASCVD. Statins are effective in this condition, but many patients will need a second drug (cholesterol absorption inhibitor, niacin, or fibrate) for optimal control of lipoprotein levels.

INHERITED CAUSES OF LOW LEVELS OF ApoB-CONTAINING LIPOPROTEINS

Abetalipoproteinemia

The synthesis and secretion of apoB-containing lipoproteins in the enterocytes of the proximal small bowel and in the hepatocytes of the liver involve a complex series of events that coordinate the coupling of various lipids with apoB-48 and apoB-100, respectively. Abetalipoproteinemia is a rare autosomal recessive disease caused by loss-of-function mutations in the gene encoding MTP, a protein that transfers lipids to nascent chylomicrons and VLDLs in the intestine and liver, respectively. Plasma levels of cholesterol and triglyceride are extremely low in this disorder, and chylomicrons, VLDLs, LDLs, and apoB are undetectable in plasma. The parents of patients with abetalipoproteinemia (obligate heterozygotes) have normal plasma lipid and apoB levels. Abetalipoproteinemia usually presents in early childhood with diarrhea and failure to thrive and is characterized clinically by fat malabsorption, spinocerebellar degeneration, pigmented retinopathy, and acanthocytosis. The initial neurologic manifestations are loss of deep-tendon reflexes, followed by decreased distal lower extremity vibratory and proprioceptive sense, dysmetria, ataxia, and the development of a spastic gait, often by the third or fourth decade. Patients with abetalipoproteinemia also develop a progressive pigmented retinopathy presenting with decreased night and color vision, followed by reductions in daytime visual acuity and ultimately progressing to near-blindness. The presence of spinocerebellar degeneration and pigmented retinopathy in this disease has resulted in some patients with abetalipoproteinemia being misdiagnosed as having Friedreich's ataxia. Rarely, patients with abetalipoproteinemia develop a cardiomyopathy with associated life-threatening arrhythmias.

Most clinical manifestations of abetalipoproteinemia result from defects in the absorption and transport of fat-soluble vitamins. Vitamin E and retinyl esters are normally transported from enterocytes to the liver by chylomicrons, and vitamin E is dependent on VLDL for transport out of the liver and into the circulation. As a consequence of the inability of these patients to secrete apoB-containing particles, patients with abetalipoproteinemia are markedly deficient in vitamin E and are also mildly to moderately deficient in vitamin A and vitamin K. Patients with abetalipoproteinemia should be referred to specialized centers for confirmation of the diagnosis and appropriate therapy. Treatment consists of a low-fat, high-caloric, vitamin-enriched diet accompanied by large supplemental doses of vitamin E. It is imperative that treatment be initiated as soon as possible to help forestall the development of the neurologic sequelae, which generally eventually progress even with appropriate therapy. New therapies for this serious disease are needed.

Familial Hypobetalipoproteinemia

Low plasma levels of LDL-C (the "beta lipoprotein") with a genetic or inherited basis are referred to generically as *familial hypobetalipoproteinemia*. Traditionally this term has been used to refer to the condition of low total cholesterol and LDL-C due to mutations in apoB. There is a range of mostly nonsense mutations in apoB that result in the translation of a truncated protein that has reduced secretion and/or accelerated catabolism. Individuals heterozygous for these mutations usually have LDL-C levels <80 mg/dL. They may be protected from the development of atherosclerotic vascular disease, though this has not been rigorously demonstrated. Some of these patients have evidence of increased hepatic fat. There are rare patients who have mutations in both apoB alleles and have plasma lipids similar to those in abetalipoproteinemia, but usually with a less severe neurologic phenotype. Patients with homozygous hypobetalipoproteinemia can be distinguished from individuals with abetalipoproteinemia by measuring the levels of LDL-C in the parents, which will also be low.

PCSK9 Deficiency

A phenocopy of familial hypobetalipoproteinemia has recently been shown to result from loss-of-function mutations in PCSK9, a protein that circulates in the blood and regulates LDL receptor levels. This condition is more common in people of African descent. Individuals bearing these mutations have lower plasma levels of LDL-C and have a substantial reduction in lifetime risk of CHD with no apparent adverse consequences. The mechanism of the low LDL-C appears to involve upregulation of the hepatic LDL receptor and thus increased catabolism of LDL.

GENETIC DISORDERS OF HDL METABOLISM

Mutations in certain genes encoding critical proteins in HDL synthesis and catabolism cause marked variations in plasma levels of HDL-C. Unlike the genetic forms of hypercholesterolemia, which are invariably associated with premature coronary atherosclerosis, genetic forms of hypoalphalipoproteinemia (low HDL-C) are not always associated with accelerated atherosclerosis.

INHERITED CAUSES OF LOW LEVELS OF HDL-C

ApoA-I Deficiency and Structural Mutations

Complete genetic deficiency of apoA-I due to deletion of the apoA-I gene results in the virtual absence of HDL from the plasma. The genes encoding apoA-I, apoC-III, apoA-IV, and apoA-V are clustered together on chromosome 11, and some of the patients with complete absence of apoA-I have deletions that include more than one of these genes in the complex. ApoA-I is required for LCAT function. Thus, plasma and tissue levels of free cholesterol are increased in this disease, resulting in the development of corneal opacities and planar xanthomas. Premature CHD is generally seen in the apoA-I deficient patients.

Missense and nonsense mutations in the apoA-I gene have been identified in selected patients with low plasma HDL levels (usually 15–30 mg/dL), but these are very rare causes of low HDL-C levels in the general population. Patients heterozygous for the apoA-I$_{Milano}$ Arg173Cys substitution have very low plasma levels of HDL due to the rapid catabolism of the mutant apolipoprotein, but they do not appear to have an increased risk of premature CHD. Most individuals with low plasma HDL-C levels due to missense mutations in apoA-I do not appear to have premature CHD or other clinical sequelae, though the disorder is too rare to study systematically. A few specific missense mutations in apoA-I cause systemic amyloidosis, and the mutant apoA-I has been found as the major component of the amyloid plaque.

Tangier Disease (ABCA1 Deficiency)

Tangier disease is a very rare autosomal codominant form of low plasma HDL-C caused by mutations in the gene encoding ABCA1, a cellular transporter that facilitates efflux of unesterified cholesterol and phospholipids from cells to apoA-I (Fig. 31-3). ABCA1 plays a critical role in the generation and stabilization of the mature HDL particle. In its absence, HDL is rapidly cleared from the circulation. Patients with Tangier disease have plasma HDL-C levels <5 mg/dL and extremely low circulating levels of apoA-I. The disease is associated with cholesterol accumulation in the reticuloendothelial system, resulting in hepatosplenomegaly and pathognomonic enlarged, grayish yellow or orange tonsils. An intermittent peripheral neuropathy (mononeuritis multiplex) or a sphingomyelia-like neurologic disorder can also be seen. Tangier disease is associated with increased risk of premature atherosclerotic disease, although not as great as might be anticipated, given the markedly decreased plasma levels of HDL-C and apoA-I. Patients with Tangier disease have low plasma levels of LDL-C, which may attenuate the atherosclerotic risk. Obligate heterozygotes for ABCA1 mutations have moderately reduced plasma HDL-C levels (15–30 mg/dL) and are also at increased risk of premature CHD. ABCA1 mutations may be a cause of low HDL-C in a nontrivial minority of low HDL-C patients.

LCAT Deficiency

This is a very rare autosomal recessive disorder caused by mutations in the gene encoding the plasma enzyme lecithin-cholesterol acyltransferase (Fig. 31-3). LCAT is synthesized in the liver and secreted into the plasma, where it circulates associated with lipoproteins. The enzyme mediates the esterification of cholesterol. Consequently, the proportion of free cholesterol in circulating lipoproteins is greatly increased (from ~25%–>70% of total plasma cholesterol) in this disorder. Lack of normal cholesterol esterification impairs the formation of mature HDL particles and therefore results in rapid catabolism of circulating apoA-I. Two genetic forms of LCAT deficiency have been described in humans: complete deficiency (also called *classic LCAT deficiency*) and partial deficiency (also called *fish-eye disease*). Progressive corneal opacification due to the deposition of free cholesterol in the lens, very low plasma levels of HDL-C (usually <10 mg/dL), and variable hypertriglyceridemia are characteristic of both types. In partial LCAT deficiency, there are no other known clinical sequelae. In contrast, complete LCAT deficiency is characterized by a hemolytic anemia and progressive renal insufficiency that eventually leads to end-stage renal disease (ESRD). Remarkably, despite the extremely low plasma levels of HDL-C and apoA-I, premature ASCVD is not a consistent feature of either complete or partial LCAT deficiency, once again exemplifying the complex relationship between low plasma levels of HDL-C and the development of ASCVD. The diagnosis can be confirmed in a specialized laboratory by assaying plasma LCAT activity.

Primary Hypoalphalipoproteinemia

Low plasma levels of HDL-C (the "alpha lipoprotein") is referred to as *hypoalphalipoproteinemia*. Primary hypoalphalipoproteinemia is defined as a plasma HDL-C level below the tenth percentile in the setting of relatively normal cholesterol and triglyceride levels, no apparent secondary causes of low plasma HDL-C, and no clinical signs of LCAT deficiency or Tangier disease. This syndrome is often referred to as *isolated low HDL*. A family history of low HDL-C facilitates the diagnosis of an inherited condition, which usually follows an autosomal dominant pattern. The metabolic etiology of this disease appears to be primarily accelerated catabolism of HDL and its apolipoproteins. Some of these patients may have ABCA1 mutations and therefore technically have heterozygous Tangier disease. Several kindreds with primary hypoalphalipoproteinemia have been described in association with an increased incidence of premature CHD, although this is not an invariant association. Association of hypoalphalipoproteinemia with premature CHD may depend on the specific nature of the gene defect or the underlying metabolic defect responsible for the low plasma HDL-C level.

INHERITED CAUSES OF HIGH LEVELS OF HDL-C

CETP Deficiency

Loss-of-function mutations in both alleles of the gene encoding cholesteryl ester transfer protein (CETP) cause substantially elevated HDL-C levels (usually >150 mg/dL). As noted earlier, CETP facilitates the transfer of cholesteryl esters from HDL to apoB-containing lipoproteins (Fig. 31-3). The absence of this transfer results in reduced catabolism of HDL and increased plasma concentrations of large, cholesterol-rich HDL particles. CETP deficiency occurs almost exclusively in persons of Japanese descent. The relationship of CETP deficiency to risk of ASCVD has not been definitively resolved and remains a matter of substantial debate. Heterozygotes for CETP deficiency have only modestly elevated HDL-C levels. Based on the phenotype of high HDL-C in CETP deficiency, pharmacologic inhibition of CETP is under development as a new therapeutic approach to the treatment of low HDL-C and ASCVD.

Familial Hyperalphalipoproteinemia

The condition of high plasma levels of HDL-C is referred to as *hyperalphalipoproteinemia* and is defined as a plasma HDL-C level above the 90th percentile. This trait runs in families, and outside of Japan it is unlikely to be due

to CETP deficiency. Most, but not all, persons with this condition appear to have a reduced risk of CHD and increased longevity. Other than CETP deficiency, the genetic basis of primary hyperalphalipoproteinemia is not known.

SECONDARY DISORDERS OF LIPOPROTEIN METABOLISM

Significant changes in plasma levels of lipoproteins are seen in a variety of diseases. It is critical that secondary causes of hyperlipidemias (Table 31-5) are considered prior to initiation of lipid-lowering therapy.

Obesity

Obesity is frequently accompanied by hyperlipidemia. The increase in adipocyte mass and accompanying decreased insulin sensitivity associated with obesity has multiple effects on lipid metabolism. More free fatty acids are delivered from the expanded adipose tissue to the liver, where they are reesterified in hepatocytes to form triglycerides, which are packaged into VLDLs for secretion into the circulation. The increased insulin levels promote fatty acid synthesis in the liver. Increased dietary intake of simple carbohydrates also drives hepatic production of VLDLs, resulting in elevations in VLDL and/or LDL in some obese subjects. Plasma levels of HDL-C tend to be low in obesity, due in part to reduced lipolysis. Weight loss is often associated with reductions in plasma levels of circulating apoB-containing lipoproteins and increases in the plasma levels of HDL-C.

Diabetes Mellitus

Patients with type 1 diabetes mellitus generally do not have hyperlipidemia if they remain under good glycemic control. Diabetic ketoacidosis is frequently accompanied by hypertriglyceridemia due to an increased hepatic influx of free fatty acids from adipose tissue. Patients with type 2 diabetes mellitus are usually dyslipidemic, even when under relatively good glycemic control. The high levels of insulin and insulin resistance associated with type 2 diabetes has multiple effects on fat metabolism: (1) a decrease in LPL activity resulting in reduced catabolism of chylomicrons and VLDLs, (2) an increase in the release of free fatty acid from the adipose tissue, (3) an increase in fatty acid synthesis in the liver, and (4) an increase in hepatic VLDL production. Patients with type 2 diabetes mellitus have several lipid abnormalities, including elevated plasma triglycerides (due to increased VLDL and lipoprotein remnants), elevated levels of dense LDL, and decreased plasma levels of HDL-C. In some diabetic patients, especially those with a genetic defect in lipid metabolism, the triglycerides can be extremely elevated, resulting in the development of pancreatitis. Elevated plasma LDL-C levels usually are not a feature of diabetes mellitus and suggest the presence of an underlying lipoprotein abnormality or may indicate the development of diabetic nephropathy. Patients with lipodystrophy, who have profound insulin resistance, have markedly elevated levels of VLDL and chylomicrons.

Thyroid Disease

Hypothyroidism is associated with elevated plasma LDL-C levels due primarily to a reduction in hepatic LDL receptor function and delayed clearance of LDL. Conversely, plasma levels of LDL-C are often reduced in the hyperthyroid patient. Hypothyroid patients also frequently have increased levels of circulating IDLs, and some patients with hypothyroidism also have mild hypertriglyceridemia. Because hypothyroidism is easily overlooked, all patients presenting with elevated plasma levels of LDL-C or IDL should be screened for hypothyroidism. Thyroid replacement therapy usually ameliorates the hypercholesterolemia; if not, the patient probably has a primary lipoprotein disorder and may require lipid-lowering drug therapy.

Renal Disorders

Nephrotic syndrome is often associated with pronounced hyperlipoproteinemia, which is usually mixed but can manifest as hypercholesterolemia or hypertriglyceridemia. The hyperlipidemia of nephrotic syndrome appears to be due to a combination of increased hepatic production and decreased clearance of VLDLs, with increased LDL production. Effective treatment of the underlying renal disease normalizes the lipid profile, but most patients with chronic nephrotic syndrome require lipid-lowering drug therapy.

ESRD is often associated with mild hypertriglyceridemia (<300 mg/dL) due to the accumulation of VLDLs and remnant lipoproteins in the circulation. Triglyceride lipolysis and remnant clearance are both reduced in patients with renal failure. Because the risk of ASCVD is increased in ESRD subjects with hyperlipidemia, they should be aggressively treated with lipid-lowering agents.

Patients with renal transplants usually have increased lipid levels due to the effect of the drugs required for immunosuppression (cyclosporine and glucocorticoids) and present a difficult management problem since HMG-CoA reductase inhibitors must be used cautiously in these patients.

Liver Disorders

Because the liver is the principal site of formation and clearance of lipoproteins, it is not surprising that liver diseases can profoundly affect plasma lipid levels in a variety of ways. Hepatitis due to infection, drugs, or alcohol is often associated with increased VLDL synthesis and mild to moderate hypertriglyceridemia. Severe hepatitis and liver failure are associated with dramatic reductions in plasma cholesterol and triglycerides due to reduced lipoprotein biosynthetic capacity. Cholestasis is associated with hypercholesterolemia, which can be very severe. A major pathway by which cholesterol is excreted from the body is via secretion into bile, either directly or after conversion to bile acids, and cholestasis blocks this critical excretory pathway. In cholestasis, free cholesterol, coupled with phospholipids, is secreted into the plasma as a constituent of a lamellar particle called *LP-X*. The particles can deposit in skin folds, producing lesions resembling those seen in patients with FDBL (xanthomata strata palmaris). Planar and eruptive xanthomas can also be seen in patients with cholestasis.

Alcohol

Regular alcohol consumption has a variable effect on plasma lipid levels. The most common effect of alcohol is to increase plasma triglyceride levels. Alcohol consumption stimulates hepatic secretion of VLDLs, possibly by inhibiting the hepatic oxidation of free fatty acids, which then promote hepatic triglyceride synthesis and VLDL secretion. The usual lipoprotein pattern seen with alcohol consumption is type IV (increased VLDLs), but persons with an underlying primary lipid disorder may develop severe hypertriglyceridemia (type V) if they drink alcohol. Regular alcohol use also raises plasma levels of HDL-C.

Estrogen

Estrogen administration is associated with increased VLDL and HDL synthesis, resulting in elevated plasma levels of both triglycerides and HDL-C. This lipoprotein pattern is distinctive since the levels of plasma triglyceride and HDL-C are typically inversely related. Plasma triglyceride levels should be monitored when birth control pills or postmenopausal estrogen therapy is initiated to ensure that the increase in VLDL production does not lead to severe hypertriglyceridemia. Use of low-dose preparations of estrogen or the estrogen patch can minimize the effect of exogenous estrogen on lipids.

Lysosomal Storage Diseases

Cholesteryl ester storage disease (due to deficiency in lysosomal acid lipase) and glycogen storage diseases such as von Gierke's disease (caused by mutations in glucose-6-phosphatase) are rare causes of secondary hyperlipidemias.

Cushing's Syndrome

Glucocorticoid excess is associated with increased VLDL synthesis and hypertriglyceridemia. Patients with Cushing's syndrome can also have mild elevations in plasma levels of LDL-C.

Many drugs have an impact on lipid metabolism and can result in significant alterations in the lipoprotein profile (Table 31-5).

SCREENING

(See also Chaps. 2 and 32) Guidelines for the screening and management of lipid disorders have been provided by an expert Adult Treatment Panel (ATP) convened by the National Cholesterol Education Program (NCEP) of the National Heart Lung and Blood Institute. The NCEP ATPIII guidelines published in 2001 recommend that all adults older than 20 years should have plasma levels of cholesterol, triglyceride, LDL-C, and HDL-C measured after a 12-hour overnight fast. In most clinical laboratories, the total cholesterol and triglycerides in the plasma are measured enzymatically, and then the cholesterol in the supernatant is measured after precipitation of apoB-containing lipoproteins to determine the HDL-C. The LDL-C is estimated using the following equation:

$$LDL\text{-}C = total\ cholesterol - (triglycerides/5) - HDL\text{-}C.$$

(The VLDL-C is estimated by dividing the plasma triglyceride by 5, reflecting the ratio of cholesterol to triglyceride in VLDL particles.) This formula is reasonably accurate if test results are obtained on fasting plasma and if the triglyceride level does not exceed ~300 mg/dL; by convention it cannot be used if the TGs are >400 mg/dL. The accurate determination of LDL-C levels in patients with triglyceride levels >300 mg/dL requires application of ultracentrifugation techniques or other direct assays for LDL-C. Further evaluation and treatment is based primarily on the plasma LDL-C level and the assessment of overall cardiovascular risk.

DIAGNOSIS

The critical first step in managing a lipid disorder is to determine the class or classes of lipoproteins that are increased or decreased in the patient. The Frederickson classification scheme for hyperlipoproteinemias (Table 31-3), though less commonly used now than in the past, can be helpful in this regard. Once the hyperlipidemia is accurately classified, efforts should be directed to rule out any possible secondary causes of the hyperlipidemia (Table 31-5). Although many patients with hyperlipidemia have a primary or genetic cause of their lipid disorder, secondary factors frequently contribute to the hyperlipidemia. A fasting glucose should be obtained in the initial work-up of all subjects with an elevated triglyceride level. Nephrotic syndrome and chronic renal insufficiency should be excluded by obtaining urine protein and serum creatinine. Liver function tests should be performed to rule out hepatitis and cholestasis.

Hypothyroidism should be ruled out by measuring serum TSH. Patients with hyperlipidemia, especially hypertriglyceridemia, who drink alcohol or are obese should be encouraged to decrease their intake. Sedentary lifestyle, obesity, and smoking are all associated with low HDL-C levels, and patients should be counseled about these issues.

Once secondary causes for the elevated lipoprotein levels have been ruled out, attempts should be made to diagnose the primary lipid disorder since the underlying etiology has a significant effect on the risk of developing CHD, on the response to drug therapy, and on the management of other family members. Often, determining the correct diagnosis requires a detailed family medical history and, in some cases, lipid analyses in family members.

If the fasting plasma triglyceride level is >1000 mg/dL, the patient almost always has chylomicronemia and either has type I or type V hyperlipoproteinemia (Table 31-3). The plasma triglyceride to cholesterol ratio helps distinguish between these two possibilities and is higher in type I than type V hyperlipoproteinemia. If the patient has type I hyperlipoproteinemia, a postheparin lipolytic assay should be performed to determine if the patient has LPL or apoC-II deficiency. type V is a much more frequent form of chylomicronemia in the adult patient. Often treatment of secondary factors contributing to the hyperlipidemia (diet, obesity, glucose intolerance, alcohol ingestion, estrogen therapy) will change a type V into a type IV pattern, reducing the risk of developing acute pancreatitis.

If the levels of LDL-C are very high (>95th percentile), it is likely the patient has a genetic form of hyperlipidemia. The presence of severe hypercholesterolemia, tendon xanthomas, and an autosomal dominant pattern of inheritance are consistent with the diagnosis of either FH, FDB, or ADH due to mutations in PCSK9. At the present time there is no compelling reason to perform molecular studies to further refine the molecular diagnosis, since the treatment of FH and FDB is identical. Patients with more moderate hypercholesterolemia that does not segregate in families as a monogenic trait likely have polygenic hypercholesterolemia. Recessive forms of severe hypercholesterolemia are rare; a clue to the diagnosis of sitosterolemia is the response of the hypercholesterolemia to reductions in dietary cholesterol content and to bile acid resins.

The most common error in the diagnosis and treatment of lipid disorders is in patients with a mixed hyperlipidemia without chylomicronemia. Elevations in the plasma levels of both cholesterol and triglycerides are seen in patients with increased plasma levels of IDL (type III) and of LDL and VLDL (type IIB) and in patients with increased levels of VLDL (type IV). The ratio of triglyceride to cholesterol is higher in type IV than the other two disorders. A beta quantification to determine the VLDL-C to triglyceride ratio in plasma (see discussion of FDBL) or a direct measurement of the plasma LDL-C should be performed at least once prior to initiation of lipid-lowering therapy to determine if the hyperlipidemia is due to the accumulation of remnants or to an increase in both LDL and VLDL.

℞ Treatment: LIPOPROTEIN DISORDERS

CLINICAL EVIDENCE THAT TREATMENT OF DYSLIPIDEMIA REDUCES RISK OF CHD

Multiple epidemiologic studies have demonstrated a strong relationship between serum cholesterol and CHD. A direct connection between plasma cholesterol levels and the atherosclerotic process was made in humans when aortic fatty streaks in young persons were shown to be strongly correlated with serum cholesterol levels. The elucidation of homozygous familial hypercholesterolemia was proof that high cholesterol itself caused atherosclerotic vascular disease. Moreover, PCSK9 deficiency proves that very low LDL-C levels are associated with substantial lifetime reduction in cardiovascular risk.

LDL-C Reduction Early clinical trials of cholesterol (mostly LDL-C) reduction utilized niacin, bile acid sequestrants, and even the surgical approach of partial ileal bypass to reduce serum cholesterol levels. Although most of these studies found a small but significant reduction in cardiac events, no decrease in total mortality was seen, which tempered enthusiasm for aggressive, population-based treatment of hypercholesterolemia. The discovery of more potent and well-tolerated cholesterol-lowering agents, namely HMG-CoA reductase inhibitors (statins), ushered in a series of large cholesterol reduction trials that unequivocally established the benefit of cholesterol reduction. Some of these trials were performed in patients with preexisting stable CHD. The Scandinavian Simvastatin Survival Study in hypercholesterolemic men with CHD showed reduced major coronary events by 44% and total mortality by 30% with simvastatin. The Cholesterol and Recurrent Events (CARE) study and the Long-Term Intervention with Pravastatin in Ischemic Heart Disease (LIPID) study demonstrated reduced cardiac events and cardiovascular deaths in women and men with established CHD and normal to only mildly elevated LDL-C levels. Some of the early statin trials were in individuals without preexisting CHD. In the West of Scotland Coronary Prevention Study (WOSCOPS) with pravastatin, subjects had significantly elevated baseline LDL-C levels, whereas in the Air Force/Texas Coronary Atherosclerosis Study (AFCAPS/TexCAPS) with lovastatin, baseline LDL-C levels were only modestly elevated. Both trials demonstrated significant reductions in cardiovascular events and clearly established that drug therapy for hypercholesterolemia is an effective method of decreasing risk of cardiovascular events even in persons who do not have preexisting symptomatic CHD.

More recent studies have enrolled subjects with average or subaverage LDL-C levels and have involved targeting the on-treatment LDL-C to ever lower levels. The Heart Protection Study (HPS) included 20,536 men and women, ages 40–80 years, who had either established ASCVD or were at high risk for the development of CHD (primarily diabetes); the only lipid entry criterion was a total plasma cholesterol level of >135 mg/dL. Treatment with simvastatin for an average of 5 years resulted in a 24% reduction in major coronary events and a highly significant 13% reduction in all-cause mortality. Importantly, the relative benefit of statin therapy was similar across tertiles of baseline LDL-C, and even the large subgroup of individuals with an LDL-C <100 mg/dL at baseline experienced significant benefit from therapy. This study demonstrated that statin therapy is beneficial in high-risk subjects, even if the baseline LDL-C level is below the currently recommended targeted goal; it also helped to shift the emphasis from simply treating elevated cholesterol to treating patients at high risk of CHD.

The Anglo-Scandinavian Cardiac Outcomes Trial Lipid-Lowering Arm (ASCOT-LLA) involved 19,342 hypertensive patients with at least three other cardiovascular risk factors and with total cholesterol levels <242 mg/dL. The lipid-lowering arm involved the intervention of atorvastatin 10 mg vs. placebo, and was terminated after 3.3 years because of a highly significant 36% relative risk reduction in major cardiovascular events. In the Collaborative Atorvastatin Diabetes Study (CARDS), 2838 patients with type 2 diabetes were randomized to atorvastatin 10 mg or placebo and was also terminated early due to a significant 37% reduction in major cardiovascular events. Both of these studies involved on-treatment LDL-C levels well below recommended targets for the patients, but still involved comparison to placebo.

The most compelling data supporting the concept that "lower is better" come from studies in which different statin regimens were directly compared. In the Treat to New Targets (TNT) trial, 10,001 patients with CHD and LDL-C <130 mg/dL were randomized to atorvastatin 80 mg vs 10 mg daily. Atorvastatin 80 mg was associated with a significant 22% reduction in major cardiovascular events and a mean on-treatment LDL-C level of 77 mg/dL (compared with 101 mg/dL for the 10 mg dose). In the Pravastatin or Atorvastatin Evaluation and Infection Therapy (PROVE-IT) study, patients presenting with acute coronary syndromes were randomized to atorvastatin 80 mg (more intensive) or pravastatin 40 mg (less intensive). Atorvastatin 80 mg was associated with a significant 16% relative risk reduction in major cardiovascular events compared with the less-intensive pravastatin 40 mg regimen. The mean on-treatment LDL-C levels were 62 mg/dL in the atorvastatin 80 mg group and 95 mg/dL in the pravastatin 40 mg group.

Based on several of these studies, a white paper was issued by the NCEP in 2004 establishing an "optional" LDL-C goal of <70 mg/dL in high-risk patients with CHD and of <100 mg/dL in very-high-risk patients without known CHD. These optional targets have been widely embraced, and clinical practice is clearly evolving to treating CHD and high-risk patients more aggressively for LDL reduction.

Treatment of the TG-HDL Axis Abnormalities of the TG-high-density lipoprotein (TG-HDL) axis are more common in patients with CHD or at risk for it than is elevated LDL-C. Yet the data supporting pharmacologic intervention in the TG-HDL axis is less abundant and compelling than the data supporting LDL-C reduction. Fibric acid derivatives (fibrates), nicotinic acid (niacin), and omega 3 fatty acids (fish oils) are the primary agents currently available for intervention regarding the TG-HDL axis. Fibrates have been used as lipid-lowering drugs for several decades and are more effective in reducing plasma TG levels and relatively less effective in increasing plasma HDL-C levels. The overall body of data with fibrates regarding cardiovascular outcomes trends is positive but mixed. The Helsinki Heart Study (HHS) compared gemfibrozil to placebo in hypercholesterolemic patients with no CHD and demonstrated a significant 36% reduction in coronary events. The Veteran Affairs High-Density Lipoprotein Cholesterol Intervention Trial (VA-HIT) examined the benefit of gemfibrozil in men with CHD, normal plasma levels of LDL-C levels, and low plasma levels of HDL-C levels and demonstrated a significant 22% reduction in nonfatal myocardial infarction and coronary death with gemfibrozil therapy. However, the Bezafibrate Infarction Prevention (BIP) trial of bezafibrate vs placebo in CHD patients with low HDL-C failed to demonstrate a statistically significant reduction in coronary events, though there was a positive trend. Similarly, the Fenofibrate Intervention and Event Lowering in Diabetes (FIELD) trial of fenofibrate in 9795 patients with type 2 diabetes also failed to show a significant reduction in its primary endpoint of nonfatal myocardial infarction and coronary death, though there was a positive trend (11% relative risk reduction) and significant reductions in total cardiovascular disease events. There was significantly greater "drop-in" of the placebo group into lipid-lowering therapy, mostly statins, making the interpretation complicated. Nevertheless, the overall body of data with fibrates and CVD risk reduction is mixed. Interestingly, despite the fact that fibrates are most effective in lowering triglycerides, no fibrate trial has ever been performed specifically in subjects with hypertriglyceridemia subjects; in addition, the benefit of the addition of a fibrate to baseline statin therapy has never been tested.

Although, niacin is the most effective HDL-raising drug currently available, it has never been tested for its ability to reduce cardiovascular risk in a trial in subjects with low HDL-C patients. The Coronary Drug Project showed that niacin modestly reduced cardiovascular events, but this was performed in hypercholesterolemic men with CHD. The AIM-HIGH trial is an ongoing study of the effect of niacin added to baseline statin therapy in patients with CHD and low HDL-C. Finally, while low-dose fish oils have been shown to reduce cardiovascular events, higher doses that reduce triglyceride levels have not been tested for their ability to reduce cardiovascular events. Definitive proof that treating the TG-HDL axis reduces cardiovascular events is likely to come from new therapies that are more effective in targeting these abnormalities.

LIPID-MODIFYING THERAPY The major goal of lipid-modifying therapy in most patients with disorders of lipid metabolism is to prevent ASCVD and its complications. Management of lipid disorders should be based on clinical trial data demonstrating that treatment reduces cardiovascular morbidity and mortality, although reasonable extrapolation of these data to specific subgroups is sometimes required. Clearly, elevated plasma levels of LDL-C are strongly associated with increased risk of ASCVD and treatment to lower the levels of plasma LDL-C decreases risk of clinical cardiovascular events in both secondary and primary prevention. Although the proportional benefit accrued from reducing plasma LDL-C appears to be similar over the entire range of LDL-C values, the absolute risk reduction depends on the baseline level of cardiovascular risk. The treatment guidelines developed by NCEP ATPIII incorporate these principles. As noted above, abnormalities in the TG-HDL axis (elevated TG, low HDL-C, or both) are commonly seen in patients with CHD or at high risk for developing it, but clinical trial data supporting the treatment of these abnormalities is much less compelling, and the pharmacologic tools for their management are more limited. Importantly, the NCEP ATPIII guidelines promote the use of the "non-HDL-C" as a secondary target of therapy in patients with TG levels >200 mg/dL. The goals for non-HDL-C are 30 mg/dL higher than the goals for LDL-C. Thus, many patients with abnormalities of the TG-HDL axis require additional therapy for reduction of non-HDL-C to recommended goals.

NONPHARMACOLOGIC TREATMENT

Diet Dietary modification is an important component in the management of dyslipidemia. The physician should assess the content of the patient's diet and provide suggestions for dietary modifications. In the patient with elevated LDL-C, dietary saturated fat and cholesterol should be restricted. For individuals with hypertriglyceridemia, the intake of simple carbohydrates should be curtailed. For severe hypertriglyceridemia (>1000 mg/dL), restriction of total fat intake is critical.

The most widely used diet to lower the LDL-C level is the "Step I diet" developed by the American Heart Association. Most patients have a relatively modest (<10%) decrease in plasma levels of LDL-C on a step I diet in the absence of any associated weight loss. Almost all persons experience a decrease in plasma HDL-C levels with a reduction in the amount of total and saturated fat in their diet.

Foods and Additives Certain foods and dietary additives are associated with modest reductions in plasma cholesterol levels. Plant stanol and sterol esters are available in a variety of foods such as spreads, salad dressings, and snack bars. Plant sterol and sterol esters interfere with cholesterol absorption and reduce plasma LDL-C levels by ~10% when taken three times per day. The addition to the diet of psyllium, soy protein, or Chinese red yeast rice (which contains lovastatin) can have modest cholesterol-lowering effects. Other herbal approaches such as guggulipid have not been shown to reduce LDL-C. No controlled studies have been performed in which several of these nonpharmacologic options have been combined to address their additive or synergistic effects.

Weight Loss and Exercise The treatment of obesity, if present, can have a favorable impact on plasma lipid levels and should be actively encouraged. Plasma triglyceride levels tend to fall and HDL-C levels tend to increase in obese subjects after weight reduction. Regular aerobic exercise can also have a positive effect on lipids, in large measure due to the associated weight reduction. Aerobic exercise has a very modest elevating effect on plasma levels of HDL-C in most individuals but also has cardiovascular benefits that extend beyond the effects on plasma lipid levels.

PHARMACOLOGIC TREATMENT The decision to use drug therapy depends on the level of cardiovascular risk. Drug therapy for hypercholesterolemia in patients with established CHD is well supported by clinical trial data, as reviewed earlier. Even patients with CHD or risk factors who have "average" LDL-C levels benefit from treatment. Drug treatment to lower LDL-C levels in patients with CHD is also highly cost-effective. Patients with diabetes mellitus without known CHD have similar cardiovascular risk to those without diabetes but with preexisting CHD. An effective way to estimate absolute risk of a cardiovascular event over 10 years is to use a scoring system based on the Framingham Heart Study database. Patients with a 10-year absolute CHD risk of >20% are considered "CHD risk equivalents." Current NCEP ATPIII guidelines call for drug therapy to reduce LDL-C to <100 mg/dL in patients with established CHD, other ASCVD (aortic aneurysm, peripheral vascular disease, or cerebrovascular disease), diabetes mellitus, or CHD risk equivalents; and "optionally" to reduce LDL-C to <70 mg/dL in high-risk CHD patients. Based on these guidelines, virtually all CHD and CHD risk-equivalent patients require cholesterol-lowering drug therapy. Moderate risk patients with two or more risk factors and a 10-year absolute risk of 10–20% should be treated to a goal LDL-C of <130 mg/dL or "optionally" to LDL-C <100 mg/dL.

Persons with markedly elevated plasma levels of LDL-C levels (>190 mg/dL) should be strongly considered for drug therapy even if their 10-year absolute CHD risk is not particularly elevated. The decision of whether to initiate drug treatment in individuals with plasma LDL-C levels between 130 and 190 mg/dL can be difficult. Although it is desirable to avoid drug treatment in patients who are unlikely to develop CHD, a very high proportion of patients who eventually develop CHD have plasma LDL-C levels that are in this range. Other clinical information can assist in the decision-making process. For example, a low plasma level of HDL-C (<40 mg/dL) supports a decision in favor of more aggressive therapy. Diagnosis of the metabolic syndrome also identifies a higher-risk individual who should be targeted for therapeutic lifestyle changes and might be a candidate for more aggressive drug therapy (Chap. 32). Other laboratory tests, such as an elevated plasma level of apoB, Lp(a) or high-sensitivity C-reactive protein, may help to identify additional high-risk individuals who should be considered for drug therapy when their LDL-C is in a "gray zone."

Drug treatment is also indicated in patients with triglycerides >1000 mg/dL who have been screened and treated for secondary causes of chylomicronemia. The goal is to reduce plasma triglycerides to <500 mg/dL to prevent the risk of acute pancreatitis. When triglycerides are 500–1000 mg/dL, the decision to use drug therapy depends on the assessment of cardiovascular risk. Most major clinical endpoint trials with statins have excluded persons with triglyceride levels >350–450 mg/dL, and there are therefore few data regarding the effectiveness of statins in reducing cardiovascular risk in persons with triglycerides higher than this threshold. More data are needed regarding the relative effectiveness of statins, fibrates, niacin, and fish oils for reducing cardiovascular risk in this setting. Combination therapy is often required for optimal control of mixed dyslipidemia.

HMG-CoA Reductase Inhibitors (Statins) HMG-CoA reductase is the rate-limiting step in cholesterol biosynthesis, and inhibition of this enzyme decreases cholesterol synthesis. By inhibiting cholesterol biosynthesis, statins lead to increased hepatic LDL receptor activity and accelerated clearance of circulating LDL, resulting in a dose-dependent reduction in plasma levels of LDL-C. There is wide interindividual variation in the initial response to a statin, but once a patient is on a statin, the doubling of the statin dose produces a 6% further reduction in the level of plasma LDL-C. The statins currently available differ in their LDL-C reducing effects (Table 31-6). Statins also reduce plasma triglycerides in a dose-dependent fashion, which is proportional to their LDL-C lowering effects (if the triglycerides are <400 mg/dL). Statins have a modest HDL-raising effect (5–10%), and this effect is not dose-dependent.

Statins are well tolerated and can be taken in tablet form once a day. Potential side effects include dyspepsia, headaches, fatigue, and muscle or joint pains. Severe myopathy and even rhabdomyolysis occur rarely with statin treatment. The risk of statin-associated myopathy is increased by the presence of older age, frailty, renal insufficiency, and coadministration of drugs that interfere with the metabolism of statins, such as erythromycin and related antibiotics, antifungal agents, immunosuppressive drugs, and fibric acid derivatives (particularly gemfibrozil). Severe myopathy can usually be avoided by careful patient selection, avoidance of interacting drugs, and instructing the patient to contact the physician immediately in the event of unexplained muscle pain. In the event of muscle symptoms, the plasma creatine kinase (CK) level should be obtained to document the myopathy. Serum CK levels need not be monitored on a routine basis in patients taking statins, as an elevated CK in the absence of symptoms does not predict the development of myopathy and does not necessarily suggest the need for discontinuing the drug.

Another consequence of statin therapy can be elevation in liver transaminases (ALT and AST). They should

TABLE 31-6

SUMMARY OF THE MAJOR DRUGS USED FOR THE TREATMENT OF HYPERLIPIDEMIA

DRUG	MAJOR INDICATIONS	STARTING DOSE	MAXIMAL DOSE	MECHANISM	COMMON SIDE EFFECTS
HMG-CoA reductase inhibitors (statins)	Elevated LDL-C			↓ Cholesterol synthesis, ↑ hepatic LDL receptors, ↓ VLDL production	Myalgias, arthralgias, elevated transaminases, dyspepsia
Lovastatin		20 mg daily	80 mg daily		
Pravastatin		40 mg qhs	80 mg qhs		
Simvastatin		20 mg qhs	80 mg qhs		
Fluvastatin		20 mg qhs	80 mg qhs		
Atorvastatin		10 mg qhs	80 mg qhs		
Rosuvastatin		10 mg qhs	40 mg qhs		
Cholesterol absorption inhibitors				↓ Intestinal cholesterol absorption	Elevated transaminases
Ezetimibe	Elevated LDL-C	10 mg daily	10 mg daily		
Bile acid sequestrants	Elevated LDL-C			↑ Bile acid excretion and ↑ LDL receptors	Bloating, constipation, elevated triglycerides
Cholestyramine		4 g daily	32 g daily		
Colestipol		5 g daily	40 g daily		
Colesevelam		3750 mg daily	4375 mg daily		
Nicotinic acid	Elevated LDL-C, low HDL-C, elevated TG			↓ VLDL hepatic synthesis	Cutaneous flushing, GI upset, elevated glucose, uric acid, and liver function tests
Immediate-release		100 mg tid	1 g tid		
Sustained-release		250 mg bid	1.5 g bid		
Extended-release		500 mg qhs	2 g qhs		
Fibric acid derivatives	Elevated TG, elevated remnants			↑ LPL, ↓ VLDL synthesis	Dyspepsia, myalgia, gallstones, elevated transaminases
Gemfibrozil		600 mg bid	600 mg bid		
Fenofibrate		145 mg qd	145 mg qd		
Omega 3 fatty acids	Elevated TG	3 g daily	6 g daily	↑ TG catabolism	Dyspepsia, diarrhea, fishy odor to breath

Note: LDL, low-density lipoprotein; VLDL, very low density lipoprotein; HDL, high-density lipoprotein; LDL-C, LDL-cholesterol; HDL-C, HDL-cholesterol; TG, triglyceride; LPL, lipoprotein lipase; GI, gastrointestinal.

be checked before starting therapy, at 2–3 months, and then annually. Substantial (greater than three times upper limit of normal) elevation in transaminases is relatively rare and mild to moderate (one–three times normal) elevation in transaminases in the absence of symptoms need not mandate discontinuing the medication. Severe clinical hepatitis associated with statins is exceedingly rare, and the trend is toward less frequent monitoring of transaminases in patients taking statins. The statin-associated elevation in liver enzymes resolves upon discontinuation of the medication.

Statins appear to be remarkably safe. Meta-analyses of large randomized controlled clinical trials with statins do not suggest an increase in any major noncardiac diseases. Statins are the drug class of choice for LDL-C reduction and are by far the most widely used class of lipid-lowering drugs.

Cholesterol Absorption Inhibitors Cholesterol within the lumen of the small intestine is derived from the diet (about one-third) and the bile (about two-thirds) and is actively absorbed by the enterocyte through a process that involves the protein NPC1L1. Ezetimibe (Table 31-6) is a cholesterol absorption inhibitor that binds directly to and inhibits NPC1L1 and blocks the intestinal absorption of cholesterol. In humans, ezetimibe at a dose of 10 mg was shown to inhibit cholesterol absorption by almost 60%. The result of inhibition of intestinal cholesterol absorption is likely to be reduction in hepatic cholesterol and an increase hepatic LDL receptor expression. The mean reduction in plasma LDL-C on ezetimibe (10 mg) is 18%, and the effect is additive when used in combination with a statin. Effects on TG and HDL-C levels are negligible, and no cardiovascular outcome data have been reported. When used in combination with a statin, monitoring of liver transaminases is recommended. Ezetimibe has become the preferred drug to add to a statin in patients who require further LDL-C reduction and is also widely used in patients who are statin-intolerant.

Bile Acid Sequestrants (Resins) Bile acid sequestrants bind bile acids in the intestine and promote their excretion in the stool. To maintain the bile acid pool size, the liver diverts cholesterol to bile acid synthesis. The decreased hepatic intracellular cholesterol content results in upregulation of the LDL receptor and enhanced LDL clearance from the plasma. Bile acid sequestrants, including cholestyramine, colestipol, and colesevelam (Table 31-6), primarily reduce plasma LDL-C levels and can cause an increase in plasma triglycerides. Therefore, patients with hypertriglyceridemia should not be treated with bile acid binding resins. Cholestyramine and colestipol are insoluble resins that must be suspended in liquids. Colesevelam is available as tablets but generally requires up to six to seven tablets per day

for effective LDL-C lowering. Most side effects of resins are limited to the gastrointestinal tract and include bloating and constipation. Since bile acid sequestrants are not systemically absorbed, they are very safe and the cholesterol-lowering drug of choice in children and in women of childbearing age who are lactating, pregnant, or could become pregnant. They are effective in combination with statins as well as in combination with ezetimibe and are particularly useful with one or both of these drugs for difficult-to-treat patients or those with statin intolerance.

Nicotinic Acid (Niacin) Nicotinic acid, or niacin, is a B-complex vitamin that has been used as a lipid-modifying agent for decades. It was previously shown to reduce the flux of nonesterified fatty acids (NEFAs) to the liver, resulting in reduced hepatic TG synthesis and VLDL secretion. Recently a receptor for nicotinic acid called GPR109A was discovered; it is expressed in adipocytes and, when activated, suppresses the release of NEFA by adipose. Niacin reduces plasma triglyceride and LDL-C levels and raises the plasma concentration of HDL-C (Table 31-6). Niacin is also the only currently available lipid-lowering drug that significantly reduces plasma levels of Lp(a). If properly prescribed and monitored, niacin is a safe and effective lipid-lowering agent.

The most frequent side effect of niacin is cutaneous flushing, which is mediated by activation of the same receptor GPR109A in the skin, leading to local generation of prostaglandin D2 production. Flushing can be reduced by formulations that slow the absorption and by taking aspirin prior to dosing. In addition, there is tachyphylaxis to the flushing. Niacin therapy is generally started at lower doses and titrated over time. Immediate-release crystalline niacin is generally administered three times per day, over-the-counter sustained-release niacin is taken twice a day, and a prescription form of extended release niacin is taken once a day. Mild elevations in transaminases occur in up to 15% of patients treated with any form of niacin, but these elevations may require stopping the medication. Niacin potentiates the effect of warfarin, and these two drugs should be prescribed together with caution. Acanthosis nigricans, a dark-colored coarse skin lesion, and maculopathy are infrequent side effects of niacin. Niacin is contraindicated in patients with peptic ulcer disease and can exacerbate the symptoms of esophageal reflux. It can also raise plasma levels of uric acid and precipitate gouty attacks in susceptible patients.

Niacin can raise fasting plasma glucose levels. However, in one study in type 2 diabetics, niacin treatment was associated with only a slight increase in fasting glucose and no significant change from baseline in the HbA1c. In another, low-dose niacin was found to effectively reduce triglycerides and raise HDL-C without adversely impacting on glycemic control. Thus, niacin can be used in diabetic patients, but every effort should be made to optimize the diabetes management before initiating niacin, and glucose should be carefully monitored in nondiabetic patients with impaired fasting glucose after initiation of niacin therapy.

Successful therapy with niacin requires careful education and motivation on the part of the patient. Its advantages are its low cost and long-term safety. It is the most effective drug currently available for raising HDL-C levels. It is particularly useful in patients with combined hyperlipidemia and low plasma levels of HDL-C and is effective in combination with statins.

Fibric Acid Derivatives (Fibrates) Fibric acid derivatives are agonists of PPARα, a nuclear receptor involved in the regulation of carbohydrate and lipid metabolism. Fibrates stimulate LPL activity (enhancing triglyceride hydrolysis), reduce apoC-III synthesis (enhancing lipoprotein remnant clearance), and may reduce VLDL production. Fibrates are the most effective drugs available for reducing triglyceride levels and also raise HDL-C levels modestly (Table 31-6). They have variable effects on LDL-C and in hypertriglyceridemic patients can sometimes be associated with increases in plasma LDL-C levels.

Fibrates are generally very well tolerated. The most common side effect is dyspepsia. Myopathy and hepatitis occur rarely in the absence of other lipid-lowering agents. Fibrates promote cholesterol secretion into bile and are associated with an increased risk of gallstones. Importantly, fibrates can potentiate the effect of warfarin and certain oral hypoglycemic agents, so the anticoagulation status and plasma glucose levels should be closely monitored in patients on these agents.

Fibrates are the drug class of choice in patients with severe hypertriglyceridemia (>1000 mg/dL) and are a reasonable consideration for first-line therapy in patients with moderate hypertriglyceridemia (500–1000 mg/dL) and FDBL. As noted earlier, the clinical trial data with fibrates overall suggests cardiovascular benefit, but the results are mixed. In patients with TG <500 mg/dL, the role of fibrates is primarily in combination with statins in selected patients with mixed dyslipidemia. In this setting, the risk of myopathy must be carefully weighed against the clinical benefit of the therapy.

Omega 3 Fatty Acids (Fish Oils) N-3 polyunsaturated fatty acids (n-3 PUFAs) are present in high concentration in fish and in flax seeds. The most widely used n-3 PUFAs for the treatment of hyperlipidemias are the two active molecules in fish oil: eicosapentaenoic acid (EPA) and decohexanoic acid (DHA). N-3 PUFAs have been concentrated into tablets and decrease fasting triglycerides in doses of 3–4 g/d. Fish oils can result in an increase in plasma LDL-C levels in some patients. Fish oil supplements can be used in combination with fibrates, niacin, or statins to treat hypertriglyceridemia. In general, fish oils are well tolerated and appear to be safe, at least at doses up to 3–4 g. Although fish oil administration is associated with a prolongation in the bleeding time, no increase in bleeding has been seen in clinical trials. A lower dose of omega 3 (about 1 g) has been associated with reduction in cardiovascular events in CHD patients and is used by some clinicians for this purpose.

Combination Drug Therapy This type of therapy is often required in patients who do not reach lipid targets on monotherapy. Combination drug therapy is frequently used for (1) patients unable to reach LDL-C and non-HDL-C goals on statin monotherapy, (2) patients with combined elevated LDL-C and abnormalities of the TG-HDL axis, and (3) patients with severe hypertriglyceridemia who do not achieve non-HDL-C goal on a fibrate or fish oils alone. Inability to achieve LDL-C (and non-HDL-C) goals is not uncommon on statin monotherapy. In this setting, a cholesterol absorption inhibitor or bile acid sequestrant can be added. Combination of niacin with a statin is an attractive option for high-risk patients who do not attain their target LDL-C level on statin monotherapy and who have a low HDL-C as their primary lipid abnormality. Conversely, in high-risk patients on statin therapy who have elevated TG levels as their primary remaining lipid abnormality, addition of a fibrate or fish oils is a reasonable consideration. Hypertriglyceridemic patients treated with a fibrate often fail to reach LDL-C and non-HDL-C goals and are therefore candidates for the addition of a statin. Coadministration of statins and fibrates has obvious appeal in patients with combined hyperlipidemia, but no clinical trials have assessed the effectiveness of a statin-fibrate combination compared with either a statin or a fibrate alone in reducing cardiovascular events, and the long-term safety of this combination is not known. Statin-fibrate combinations are known to be associated with an increased incidence of severe myopathy (up to 2.5%) and rhabdomyolysis, and therefore patients treated with these two drugs must be carefully counseled and monitored. This combination of drugs should be used cautiously in patients with underlying renal or hepatic insufficiency; in the elderly, frail, and chronically ill; and in those on multiple medications.

OTHER APPROACHES Occasionally, patients cannot tolerate any of the existing lipid-lowering drugs at doses required for adequate control of their lipid levels. A larger group of patients, most of whom have genetic lipid disorders, remain significantly hypercholesterolemic despite combination drug therapy. These patients are at high risk for development or progression of CHD and clinical CHD events. The preferred option for management of patients with severe refractory hypercholesterolemia is LDL apheresis. In this process, the patient's plasma is passed over a column that selectively removes the LDL, and the LDL-depleted plasma is returned to the patient. Patients on maximally tolerated combination drug therapy who have CHD and a plasma LDL-C level >200 mg/dL or no CHD and a plasma LDL-C level >300 mg/dL are candidates for every-other-week LDL apheresis and should be referred to a specialized lipid center.

MANAGEMENT OF LOW HDL-C Severely reduced plasma levels of HDL-C (<20 mg/dL) accompanied by triglycerides <400 mg/dL usually indicate the presence of a genetic disorder, such as a mutation in apoA-I, LCAT deficiency, or Tangier disease. HDL-C levels <20 mg/dL are common in the setting of severe hypertriglyceridemia, in which case the primary focus should be on the management of the triglycerides. HDL-C levels <20 mg/dL also occur in individuals using anabolic steroids. Secondary causes of more moderate reductions in plasma HDL (20–40 mg/dL) should be considered (Table 31-5). Smoking should be discontinued, obese persons should be encouraged to lose weight, sedentary persons should be encouraged to exercise, and diabetes should be optimally controlled. When possible, medications associated with reduced plasma levels of HDL-C should be discontinued. The presence of an isolated low plasma level of HDL-C in a patient with a borderline plasma level of LDL-C should prompt consideration of LDL-lowering drug therapy in high-risk individuals. Statins increase plasma levels of HDL-C only modestly (~5–10%). Fibrates also have only a modest effect on plasma HDL-C levels (increasing levels ~5–15%), except in patients with coexisting hypertriglyceridemia, where they can be more effective. Niacin is the most effective available HDL-C–raising therapeutic agent and can be associated with increases in plasma HDL-C by up to ~30%, although some patients do not respond to niacin therapy.

The issue of whether pharmacologic intervention should be used to specifically raise HDL-C levels has not been adequately addressed in clinical trials. In persons with established CHD and low HDL-C levels whose plasma LDL-C levels are at or below the goal, it may be reasonable to initiate therapy (with a fibrate or niacin) directed specifically at reducing plasma triglyceride levels and raising the level of plasma HDL-C. More data are required before broad recommendations are made to use drug therapy to specifically raise HDL-C levels to prevent cardiovascular events. New HDL-raising approaches are under development that may help to address this important issue.

FURTHER READINGS

BAIGENT C et al: Efficacy and safety of cholesterol-lowering treatment: Prospective meta-analysis of data from 90,056 participants in 14 randomised trials of statins. Lancet 366:1267, 2005

BRUNZELL JD: Clinical practice. Hypertriglyceridemia. N Engl J Med 357(10):1009, 2007

CANNON CP et al: Intensive versus moderate lipid lowering with statins after acute coronary syndromes. N Engl J Med 350:1495, 2004

CARLSON LA: Nicotinic acid: The broad-spectrum lipid drug. A 50th anniversary review. J Intern Med 258:94, 2005

DUFFY D, RADER DJ: Emerging therapies targeting high-density lipoprotein metabolism and reverse cholesterol transport. Circulation 113:1140, 2006

GRUNDY SM: The issue of statin safety: Where do we stand? Circulation 111:3016, 2005

——— et al: Implications of recent clinical trials for the National Cholesterol Education Program Adult Treatment Panel III guidelines. Circulation 110:227, 2004

LAROSA JC et al: Intensive lipid lowering with atorvastatin in patients with stable coronary disease. N Engl J Med 352:1425, 2005

NATIONAL CHOLESTEROL EDUCATION PROGRAM: Executive summary of the third report of the National Cholesterol Education Program (NCEP) Expert Panel on Detection, Evaluation, and Treatment of High Blood Cholesterol in Adults (Adult Treatment Panel III). JAMA 285:2486, 2001

RADER DJ et al: Monogenic hypercholesterolemia: New insights in pathogenesis and treatment. J Clin Invest 111:1795, 2003

SINGH IM et al: High-density lipoprotein as a therapeutic target: A systematic review. JAMA 298(7):786, 2007

CHAPTER 32

THE METABOLIC SYNDROME

Robert H. Eckel

The metabolic syndrome (syndrome X, insulin resistance syndrome) consists of a constellation of metabolic abnormalities that confer increased risk of cardiovascular disease (CVD) and diabetes mellitus (DM). The criteria for the metabolic syndrome have evolved since the original definition by the World Health Organization in 1998, reflecting growing clinical evidence and analysis by a variety of consensus conferences and professional organizations. The major features of the metabolic syndrome include central obesity, hypertriglyceridemia, low HDL cholesterol, hyperglycemia, and hypertension (Table 32-1).

EPIDEMIOLOGY

Prevalence of the metabolic syndrome varies across the globe, in part reflecting the age and ethnicity of the populations studied and the diagnostic criteria applied. In general, the prevalence of metabolic syndrome increases with age. The highest recorded prevalence worldwide is in Native Americans, with nearly 60% of women aged 45–49 years and 45% of men aged 45–49 years meeting National Cholesterol Education Program, Adult Treatment Panel III (NCEP:ATPIII) criteria. In the United States, metabolic syndrome is less common in African-American men but more common in Mexican-American women. Based on data from the National Health and Nutrition Examination Survey (NHANES) III, the age-adjusted prevalence of the metabolic syndrome in the United States is 34% for men and 35% for women.

In France, a 30–64-year-old cohort shows a <10% prevalence for each gender, although 17.5% are affected in the 60–64 age range. Greater industrialization worldwide is associated with rising rates of obesity, which is anticipated to dramatically increase prevalence of the metabolic syndrome, especially as the population ages. Moreover, the rising prevalence and severity of obesity in children is initiating features of the metabolic syndrome in a younger population.

The frequency distribution of the five components of the syndrome for the U.S. population (NHANES III) is summarized in (Fig. 32-1). Increases in waist circumference predominate in women whereas fasting triglycerides >150 mg/dL and hypertension are more likely in men.

RISK FACTORS

Overweight/Obesity

Although the first description of the metabolic syndrome occurred in the early twentieth century, the worldwide overweight/obesity epidemic has been the driving force for more recent recognition of the syndrome. Central adiposity is a key feature of the syndrome, reflecting the fact that the syndrome's prevalence is driven by the strong relationship between waist circumference and increasing adiposity. However, despite the importance of obesity, patients who are normal weight may also be insulin-resistant and have the syndrome.

TABLE 32-1

NCEP:ATPIII 2001 AND IDF CRITERIA FOR THE METABOLIC SYNDROME

NCEP:ATPIII 2001	IDF CRITERIA FOR CENTRAL ADIPOSITY[a]		
Three or more of the following:	**Waist Circumference**		
	Men	**Women**	**Ethnicity**
Central obesity: Waist circumference >102 cm (M), >88 cm (F)	≥ 94 cm	≥ 80 cm	Europid, Sub-Saharan African, Eastern & Middle Eastern
Hypertriglyceridemia: Triglycerides ≥150 mg/dL or specific medication	≥90 cm	≥80 cm	South Asian, Chinese, and ethnic South & Central American
Low HDL cholesterol: <40 mg/dL and <50 mg/dL, respectively, or specific medication	≥85 cm	≥90 cm	Japanese
Hypertension: Blood pressure ≥130 mm systolic or ≥85 mm diastolic or specific medication	**Two or more of the following:**		
Fasting plasma glucose ≥100 mg/dL or specific medication or previously diagnosed type 2 diabetes	Fasting triglycerides >150 mg/dL or specific medication		
	HDL cholesterol <40 mg/dL and <50 mg/dL for men and women, respectively, or specific medication		
	Blood pressure >130 systolic or >85 mm diastolic or previous diagnosis or specific medication		
	Fasting plasma glucose ≥100 mg/dL or previously diagnosed type 2 diabetes		

[a]In this analysis, the following thresholds for waist circumference were used: White men, ≥94 cm; African-American men, ≥94 cm; Mexican-American men, ≥90 cm; white women, ≥80 cm; African-American women, ≥80 cm; Mexican-American women, ≥80 cm. For participants whose designation was "other race—including multiracial," thresholds that were once based on Europid cut points (≥94 cm for men and ≥80 cm for women) and once based on South Asian cut points (≥90 cm for men and ≥80 cm for women) were used. For participants who were considered "other Hispanic," the IDF thresholds for ethnic South and Central Americans were used.

Note: NCEP:ATPIII, National Cholesterol Education Program, Adult Treatment Panel III; IDF, International Diabetes Foundation; HDL, high-density lipoprotein.

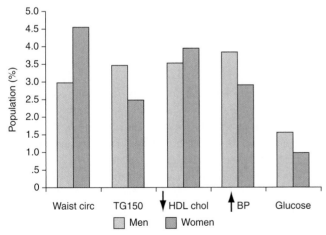

FIGURE 32-1

Prevalence of the metabolic syndrome components, from NHANES III. NHANES, National Health and Nutrition Examination Survey; TG, triglyceride; HDL, high-density lipoprotein; BP, blood pressure. *(From ES Ford et al: JAMA 287:356, 2002; with permission.)*

Sedentary Lifestyle

Physical inactivity is a predictor of CVD events and related mortality. Many components of the metabolic syndrome are associated with a sedentary lifestyle, including increased adipose tissue (predominantly central); reduced HDL cholesterol; and a trend toward increased triglycerides, blood pressure, and glucose in the genetically susceptible. In comparison with individuals who watched television or videos or used their computer <1 h daily, those who carried out these behaviors for >4 h daily have a twofold increased risk of the metabolic syndrome.

Aging

The metabolic syndrome affects 44% of the U.S. population older than 50 years. A greater percentage of women older than 50 years have the syndrome than men. The age dependency of the syndrome's prevalence is seen in most populations around the world.

Diabetes Mellitus

DM is included in both the NCEP and International Diabetes Foundation (IDF) definitions of the metabolic syndrome. It is estimated that the large majority (~75%) of patients with type 2 diabetes or impaired glucose tolerance (IGT) have the metabolic syndrome. The presence of the metabolic syndrome in these populations relates to a higher prevalence of CVD in comparison with patients with type 2 diabetes or IGT without the syndrome.

Coronary Heart Disease

The approximate prevalence of the metabolic syndrome in patients with coronary heart disease (CHD) is 50%, with a prevalence of 37% in patients with premature coronary artery disease (≤ 45 years), particularly in women. With appropriate cardiac rehabilitation and changes in lifestyle (e.g., nutrition, physical activity, weight reduction, and, in some cases, pharmacologic agents), the prevalence of the syndrome can be reduced.

Lipodystrophy

Lipodystrophic disorders in general are associated with the metabolic syndrome. Both genetic (e.g., Berardinelli-Seip congenital lipodystrophy, Dunnigan familial partial lipodystrophy) and acquired (e.g., HIV-related lipodystrophy in patients treated with highly active antiretroviral therapy) forms of lipodystrophy may give rise to severe insulin resistance and many of the metabolic syndrome's components.

ETIOLOGY

Insulin Resistance

The most accepted and unifying hypothesis to describe the pathophysiology of the metabolic syndrome is insulin resistance, caused by an incompletely understood defect in insulin action. The onset of insulin resistance is heralded by postprandial hyperinsulinemia, followed by fasting hyperinsulinemia and, ultimately, hyperglycemia.

An early major contributor to the development of insulin resistance is an overabundance of circulating fatty acids (**Fig. 32-2**). Plasma albumin-bound free fatty acids (FFAs) are derived predominantly from adipose tissue triglyceride stores released by hormone-sensitive lipase. Fatty acids are also derived through the lipolysis of triglyceride-rich lipoproteins in tissues by lipoprotein lipase (LPL). Insulin mediates both antilipolysis and the stimulation of LPL in adipose tissue. Of note, the inhibition of lipolysis in adipose tissue is the most sensitive pathway of insulin action. Thus, when insulin resistance develops, increased lipolysis produces more fatty acids, which further decrease the antilipolytic effect of insulin.

Excessive fatty acids enhance substrate availability and create insulin resistance by modifying downstream signaling. Fatty acids impair insulin-mediated glucose uptake and accumulate as triglycerides in both skeletal and cardiac muscle, whereas increased glucose production and triglyceride accumulation are seen in liver.

The oxidative stress hypothesis provides unifying theory for aging and the predisposition to the metabolic syndrome. In studies carried out in insulin-resistant subjects with obesity or type 2 diabetes, in the offspring of patients with type 2 diabetes, and in the elderly, a defect has been identified in mitochondrial oxidative phosphorylation, leading to the accumulation of triglycerides and related lipid molecules in muscle. The accumulation of lipids in muscle is associated with insulin resistance.

Increased Waist Circumference

Waist circumference is an important component of the most recent and frequently applied diagnostic criteria for the metabolic syndrome. However, measuring waist circumference does not reliably distinguish between a large waist caused by increases in subcutaneous adipose tissue vs. visceral fat; this distinction requires CT or MRI. With increases in visceral adipose tissue, adipose tissue-derived FFAs are directed to the liver. On the other hand, increases in abdominal subcutaneous fat release lipolysis products into the systemic circulation and avoid more direct effects on hepatic metabolism. Relative increases in visceral versus subcutaneous adipose tissue with increasing waist circumference in Asians and Asian Indians may explain the greater prevalence of the syndrome in these populations in contrast to African-American men in whom subcutaneous fat predominates. It is also possible that visceral fat is a marker for, but not the source of, excess postprandial FFAs in obesity.

Dyslipidemia

(See also Chap. 31) In general, FFA flux to the liver is associated with increased production of apoB–containing, triglyceride-rich very low density lipoproteins (VLDLs). The effect of insulin on this process is complex, but *hypertriglyceridemia* is an excellent marker of the insulin-resistant condition.

The other major lipoprotein disturbance in the metabolic syndrome is a *reduction in HDL cholesterol.* This reduction is a consequence of changes in HDL composition and metabolism. In the presence of hypertriglyceridemia, a decrease in the cholesterol content of HDL is a consequence of reduced cholesteryl ester content of the lipoprotein core in combination with cholesteryl ester transfer protein–mediated alterations in triglyceride making the particle small and dense. This change in lipoprotein composition also results in an increased clearance of HDL from the circulation. The relationships of these changes in

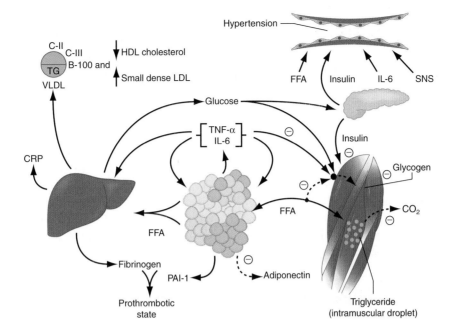

FIGURE 32-2

Pathophysiology of the metabolic syndrome. Free fatty acids (FFAs) are released in abundance from an expanded adipose tissue mass. In the liver, FFAs result in an increased production of glucose, triglycerides and secretion of very low density lipoproteins (VLDLs). Associated lipid/lipoprotein abnormalities include reductions in high-density lipoprotein (HDL) cholesterol and an increased density of low-density lipoproteins (LDLs). FFAs also reduce insulin sensitivity in muscle by inhibiting insulin-mediated glucose uptake. Associated defects include a reduction in glucose partitioning to glycogen and increased lipid accumulation in triglyceride (TG). Increases in circulating glucose, and to some extent FFA, increase pancreatic insulin secretion, resulting in hyperinsulinemia. Hyperinsulinemia may result in enhanced sodium reabsorption and increased sympathetic nervous system (SNS) activity and contribute to the hypertension, as might increased levels of circulating FFAs.

The proinflammatory state is superimposed and contributory to the insulin resistance produced by excessive FFAs. The enhanced secretion of interleukin 6 (IL-6) and tumor necrosis factor α (TNF-α) produced by adipocytes and monocyte-derived macrophages results in more insulin resistance and lipolysis of adipose tissue triglyceride stores to circulating FFAs. IL-6 and other cytokines also enhance hepatic glucose production, VLDL production by the liver, and insulin resistance in muscle. Cytokines and FFAs also increase the hepatic production of fibrinogen and adipocyte production of plasminogen activator inhibitor 1 (PAI-1), resulting in a prothrombotic state. Higher levels of circulating cytokines also stimulate the hepatic production of C-reactive protein (CRP). Reduced production of the anti-inflammatory and insulin sensitizing cytokine adiponectin are also associated with the metabolic syndrome. *(Reprinted from Eckel et al, with permission from Elsevier.)*

HDL to insulin resistance are likely indirect, occurring in concert with the changes in triglyceride-rich lipoprotein metabolism.

In addition to HDL, LDLs are also modified in composition. With fasting serum triglycerides >2.0 mM (~180 mg/dL), there is almost always a predominance of small dense LDLs. Small dense LDLs are thought to be more atherogenic. They may be toxic to the endothelium, and they are able to transit through the endothelial basement membrane and adhere to glycosaminoglycans. They also have increased susceptibility to oxidation and are selectively bound to scavenger receptors on monocyte-derived macrophages. Subjects with increased small dense LDL particles and hypertriglyceridemia also have increased cholesterol content of both VLDL1 and VLDL2 subfractions. This relatively cholesterol-rich VLDL particle may also contribute to the atherogenic risk in patients with metabolic syndrome.

Glucose Intolerance

The defects in insulin action lead to impaired suppression of glucose production by the liver and kidney and reduced glucose uptake and metabolism in insulin-sensitive tissues, i.e., muscle and adipose tissue. The relationship between impaired fasting glucose (IFG) or impaired glucose tolerance (IGT) and insulin resistance is well supported by human, nonhuman primate, and rodent studies. To compensate for defects in insulin action, insulin secretion and/or clearance must be modified to sustain euglycemia. Ultimately, this compensatory mechanism fails, usually because of defects in insulin secretion, resulting in progress from IFG and/or IGT to DM.

Hypertension

The relationship between insulin resistance and hypertension is well established. Paradoxically, under normal physiologic conditions, insulin is a vasodilator with secondary effects on sodium reabsorption in the kidney. However, in the setting of insulin resistance, the vasodilatory effect of insulin is lost, but the renal effect on sodium reabsorption is preserved. Sodium reabsorption is increased in whites with the metabolic syndrome but not in Africans or Asians. Insulin also increases the activity of the sympathetic nervous system, an effect that may also be preserved in the setting of the insulin resistance. Finally, insulin resistance is characterized by pathway-specific impairment in phosphatidylinositol 3-kinase signaling. In the endothelium, this may cause an imbalance between the production of nitric oxide and secretion of endothelin-1, leading to decreased blood flow. Although these mechanisms are provocative, when insulin action is assessed by levels of fasting insulin or by the Homeostasis Model Assessment (HOMA), insulin resistance contributes only modestly to the increased prevalence of hypertension in the metabolic syndrome.

Proinflammatory Cytokines

The increases in proinflammatory cytokines, including interleukin (IL) 1, IL-6, IL-18, resistin, tumor necrosis factor (TNF) α, and C-reactive protein (CRP), reflect overproduction by the expanded adipose tissue mass (Fig. 32-2). Adipose tissue-derived macrophages may be the primary source of proinflammatory cytokines locally and in the systemic circulation. It remains unclear, however, how much of the insulin resistance is caused by the paracrine vs. endocrine effects of these cytokines.

Adiponectin

Adiponectin is an anti-inflammatory cytokine produced exclusively by adipocytes. Adiponectin enhances insulin sensitivity and inhibits many steps in the inflammatory process. In the liver, adiponectin inhibits the expression of gluconeogenic enzymes and the rate of glucose production. In muscle, adiponectin increases glucose transport and enhances fatty acid oxidation, partially due to activation of AMP kinase. Adiponectin is reduced in the metabolic syndrome. The relative contribution of adiponectin deficiency versus overabundance of the proinflammatory cytokines remains unclear.

CLINICAL FEATURES

Symptoms and Signs

The metabolic syndrome is typically unassociated with symptoms. On physical examination, waist circumference may be expanded and blood pressure elevated. The presence of one or either of these signs should alert the clinician to search for other biochemical abnormalities that may be associated with the metabolic syndrome. Less frequently, lipoatrophy or acanthosis nigricans is found on examination. Because these physical findings are typically associated with severe insulin resistance, other components of the metabolic syndrome should be expected.

Associated Diseases

▬ Cardiovascular Disease

The relative risk for new-onset CVD in patients with the metabolic syndrome, in the absence of diabetes, averages between 1.5- and threefold. In an 8-year follow-up of middle-aged men and women in the Framingham Offspring Study (FOS), the population attributable risk for patients with the metabolic syndrome to develop CVD was 34% in men and 16% in women. In the same study, both the metabolic syndrome and diabetes predicted ischemic stroke with greater risk for patients with the metabolic syndrome than for diabetes alone (19% vs 7%), particularly in women (27% vs 5%). Patients with metabolic syndrome are also at increased risk for peripheral vascular disease.

▬ Type 2 Diabetes

Overall, the risk for type 2 diabetes in patients with the metabolic syndrome is increased three- to fivefold. In the FOS's 8-year follow-up of middle-aged men and women, the population-attributable risk for developing type 2 diabetes was 62% in men and 47% in women.

Other Associated Conditions

In addition to the features specifically associated with metabolic syndrome, insulin resistance is accompanied by other metabolic alterations. These included increases in apoB and C III, uric acid, prothrombotic factors (fibrinogen, plasminogen activator inhibitor 1), serum viscosity, asymmetric dimethylarginine, homocysteine, white blood cell count, proinflammatory cytokines, CRP, microalbuminuria, nonalcoholic fatty liver disease (NAFLD) and/or nonalcoholic steatohepatitis (NASH), polycystic ovarian disease (PCOS), and obstructive sleep apnea (OSA).

▬ Nonalcoholic Fatty Liver Disease

Fatty liver is relatively common. However, in NASH, both triglyceride accumulation and inflammation coexist. NASH is now present in 2–3% of the population in the United States and other Western countries. As the prevalence of overweight/obesity and the metabolic syndrome increases, NASH may become one of the more frequent causes of end-stage liver disease and hepatocellular carcinoma.

▬ Hyperuricemia

Hyperuricemia reflects defects in insulin action on the renal tubular reabsorption of uric acid, whereas the increase in asymmetric dimethylarginine, an endogenous inhibitor of nitric oxide synthase, relates to endothelial dysfunction. Microalbuminuria may also be caused by altered endothelial pathophysiology in the insulin-resistant state.

Polycystic Ovary Syndrome

PCOS is highly associated with the metabolic syndrome, with a prevalence between 40 and 50%. Women with PCOS are 2–4 times more likely to have the metabolic syndrome compared to women without PCOS.

Obstructive Sleep Apnea

OSA is commonly associated with obesity, hypertension, increased circulating cytokines, IGT, and insulin resistance. With these associations, it is not surprising that the metabolic syndrome is frequently present. Moreover, when biomarkers of insulin resistance are compared between patients with OSA and weight-matched controls, insulin resistance is more severe in patients with OSA. Continuous positive airway pressure (CPAP) treatment in OSA patients improves insulin sensitivity.

DIAGNOSIS

The diagnosis of the metabolic syndrome relies on satisfying the criteria listed in Table 32-1 using tools at the bedside and in the laboratory. Because the NCEP:ATPIII and IDF criteria are similar, either can be used. The medical history should include evaluation of symptoms for OSA in all patients and PCOS in premenopausal women. Family history will help determine risk for CVD and DM. Blood pressure and waist circumference measurements provide information necessary for the diagnosis.

Laboratory Tests

Fasting lipids and glucose are needed to determine if the metabolic syndrome is present. The measurement of additional biomarkers associated with insulin resistance must be individualized. Such tests might include apo B, high-sensitivity CRP, fibrinogen, uric acid, urinary microalbumin, and liver function tests. A sleep study should be performed if symptoms of OSA are present. If PCOS is suspected based on clinical features and anovulation, testosterone, luteinizing hormone, and follicle-stimulating hormone should be measured.

℞ Treatment:
THE METABOLIC SYNDROME

LIFESTYLE Obesity is the driving force behind the metabolic syndrome. Thus, weight reduction is the primary approach to the disorder. With weight reduction, the improvement in insulin sensitivity is often accompanied by favorable modifications in many components of the metabolic syndrome. In general, recommendations for weight loss include a combination of caloric restriction, increased physical activity, and behavior modification. For weight reduction, caloric restriction is the most important component, whereas increases in physical activity are important for maintenance of weight loss. Some, but not all, evidence suggests that the addition of exercise to caloric restriction may promote relatively greater weight loss from the visceral depot. The tendency for weight regain after successful weight reduction underscores the need for long-lasting behavioral changes.

Diet Before prescribing a weight-loss diet, it is important to emphasize that it takes a long time for a patient to achieve an expanded fat mass; thus, the correction need not occur quickly. On the basis of ~3500 kcal = 1 lb of fat, ~500 kcal restriction daily equates to a weight reduction of 1 lb per week. Diets restricted in carbohydrate typically provide a rapid initial weight loss. However, after one year, the amount of weight reduction is usually unchanged. Thus, adherence to the diet is more important than which diet is chosen. Moreover, there is concern about diets enriched in saturated fat, particularly for patients at risk for CVD. Therefore, a high quality of the diet—i.e., enriched in fruits, vegetables, whole grains, lean poultry, and fish—should be encouraged to provide the maximum overall health benefit.

Physical activity Before a physical activity recommendation is provided to patients with the metabolic syndrome, it is important to ensure that this increased activity does not incur risk. Some high-risk patients should undergo formal cardiovascular evaluation before initiating an exercise program. For the inactive participant, gradual increases in physical activity should be encouraged to enhance adherence and to avoid injury. Although increases in physical activity can lead to modest weight reduction, 60–90 min of daily activity is required to achieve this goal. Even if an overweight or obese adult is unable to achieve this level of activity, they still derive a significant health benefit from at least 30 min of moderate intensity daily activity. The caloric value of 30 min of a variety of activities can be found at *http://www.americanheart.org/presenter .runforward jhtml?identifier=3040364*. Of note, a variety of routine activities—such as gardening, walking, and housecleaning—require moderate caloric expenditure. Thus, physical activity need not be defined solely in terms of formal exercise such as jogging, swimming, or tennis.

Obesity In some patients with the metabolic syndrome, treatment options need to extend beyond lifestyle intervention. Weight-loss drugs come in two major classes: appetite suppressants and absorption inhibitors. Appetite suppressants approved by the Food and Drug Administration include phentermine (for short-term use only, 3 months) and sibutramine. Orlistat inhibits fat absorption by ~30% and is moderately effective compared to placebo (~5% weight loss). Orlistat has been shown to reduce the incidence of type 2 diabetes, an effect that was especially evident in patients with baseline IGT.

Bariatric surgery is an option for patients with the metabolic syndrome who have a body mass index (BMI) of >40 kg/m^2 or >35 kg/m^2 with comorbidities. Gastric bypass results in a dramatic weight reduction and improvement in the features of metabolic syndrome. At present, however, a survival benefit has yet to be realized.

LDL CHOLESTEROL (See also Chap. 31) The rationale for the NCEP:ATP III panel to develop criteria for the metabolic syndrome was to go beyond LDL cholesterol in identifying and reducing risk for CVD. The working assumption by the panel was that LDL cholesterol goals had already been achieved, and increasing evidence supports a linear reduction in CVD events with progressive lowering of LDL cholesterol. For patients with the metabolic syndrome and diabetes, LDL cholesterol should be reduced to <100 mg/dL and perhaps further in patients with a history of CVD events. For patients with the metabolic syndrome without diabetes, the Framingham risk score may predict a 10-year CVD risk that exceeds 20%. In these subjects, LDL cholesterol should also be reduced to <100 mg/dL. With a 10-year risk of <20%, however, the targeted LDL cholesterol goal is < 130 mg/dL.

Diets restricted in saturated fats (<7% of calories), trans fat (as few as possible), and cholesterol (<200 mg daily) should be applied aggressively. If LDL cholesterol remains above goal, then pharmacologic intervention is needed. Statins (HMG-CoA reductase inhibitors), which produce a 20–60% lowering of LDL cholesterol, are generally the first choice for medication intervention. Of note, for each doubling of the statin dose, there is only ~6% additional lowering of LDL cholesterol. Side effects are rare and include an increase in hepatic transaminases and/or myopathy. The cholesterol absorption inhibitor ezetimibe is well tolerated and should be the second choice. Ezetimibe typically reduces LDL cholesterol by 15–20%. The bile acid sequestrants cholestyramine and colestipol are more effective than ezetimibe but must be used with caution in patients with the metabolic syndrome because they often increase triglycerides. In general, bile sequestrants should not be administered when fasting triglycerides are >200 mg/dL. Side effects include gastrointestinal symptoms (palatability, bloating, belching, constipation, anal irritation). Nicotinic acid has modest LDL cholesterol–lowering capabilities (<20%). Fibrates are best employed to lower LDL cholesterol when both LDL cholesterol and nontriglycerides are elevated. Fenofibrate may be more effective than gemfibrozil in this group.

TRIGLYCERIDES The NCEP:ATPIII has focused on non-HDL cholesterol rather than triglycerides. However, a fasting triglyceride value of <150 mg/dL is recommended. In general, the response of fasting triglycerides relates to the amount of weight reduction achieved. A weight reduction of >10% is necessary to lower fasting triglycerides.

A fibrate (gemfibrozil or fenofibrate) is the drug of choice to lower fasting triglycerides and typically achieve a 35–50% reduction. Concomitant administration with drugs metabolized by the 3A4 cytochrome P450 system (including some statins) greatly increases the risk of myopathy. In these cases, fenofibrate may be preferable to gemfibrozil. In the Veterans Affairs HDL Intervention Trial (VA-HIT), gemfibrozil was administered to men with known CHD and levels of HDL cholesterol <40 mg/dL. A coronary disease event and mortality benefit was experienced predominantly in men with hyperinsulinemia and/or diabetes, many of whom retrospectively had the metabolic syndrome. Of note, the amount of triglyceride lowering in the VA-HIT did not predict benefit. Although levels of LDL cholesterol did not change, a decrease in LDL particle number related to benefit. Although several additional clinical trials have been performed, these have not shown clear evidence that fibrates reduce CVD risk as a consequence of triglyceride lowering.

Other drugs that lower triglycerides include statins, nicotinic acid, and high doses of omega-3 fatty acids. When choosing a statin for this purpose, the dose must be high for the "less potent" statins (lovastatin, pravastatin, fluvastatin) or intermediate for the "more potent" statins (simvastatin, atorvastatin, rosuvastatin). The effect of nicotinic acid on fasting triglycerides is dose-related and less than fibrates (~20–40%). In patients with the metabolic syndrome and diabetes, nicotinic acid may increase fasting glucose. Omega-3 fatty acid preparations that include high doses of docosahexaenoic acid and eicosapentaenoic acid (~3.0–4.5 g daily) lower fasting triglycerides by ~40%. No interactions with fibrates or statins occur, and the main side effect is eructation with a fishy taste. This can be partially blocked by ingesting the nutraceutical after freezing. Clinical trials of nicotinic acid or high-dose omega-3 fatty acids in patients with the metabolic syndrome have not been reported.

HDL CHOLESTEROL Beyond weight reduction, there are very few lipid-modifying compounds that increase HDL cholesterol. Statins, fibrates, and bile acid sequestrants have modest effects (5–10%), and there is no effect on HDL cholesterol with ezetimibe or omega-3 fatty acids. Nicotinic acid is the only currently available drug with predictable HDL cholesterol-raising properties. The response is dose-related and can increase HDL cholesterol ~30% above baseline. There is little evidence at present that raising HDL has a benefit on CVD events independent of lowering LDL cholesterol, particularly in patients with the metabolic syndrome.

BLOOD PRESSURE (See also Chap. 37) The direct relationship between blood pressure and all-cause mortality has been well established, including patients with hypertension (>140/90) versus prehypertension (>120/80 but <140/90) versus individuals with normal blood pressure (<120/80). In patients with the metabolic syndrome without diabetes, the best choice for the first antihypertensive should usually be an ACE inhibitor or an angiotensin II receptor blocker, as these two classes of drugs appear to reduce the incidence of new-onset type 2 diabetes. In all patients with hypertension, a sodium-restricted diet enriched in fruits and vegetables and low-fat dairy products should be advocated. Home monitoring of blood pressure may assist in maintaining good blood pressure control.

IMPAIRED FASTING GLUCOSE In patients with the metabolic syndrome and type 2 diabetes, aggressive glycemic control may favorably modify fasting triglycerides and/or HDL cholesterol. In those patients with IFG without a diagnosis of diabetes, a lifestyle intervention that includes weight reduction, dietary fat restriction, and increased physical activity has been shown to reduce the incidence of type 2 diabetes. Metformin has also been shown to reduce the incidence of diabetes, although the effect was less than that seen with lifestyle intervention.

INSULIN RESISTANCE Several drug classes [biguanides, thiazolidinediones (TZDs)] increase insulin sensitivity. If insulin resistance is the primary pathophysiologic mechanism for the metabolic syndrome, then representative drugs in these classes should reduce its prevalence. Both metformin and TZDs enhance insulin action in the liver and suppress endogenous glucose production. TZDs, but not metformin, also improve insulin-mediated glucose uptake in muscle and adipose tissue. Benefits of both drugs have also been seen in patients with NAFLD and PCOS, and they have been shown to reduce markers of inflammation and small dense LDL. In general, the beneficial effects of TZDs appear superior to those of metformin.

FURTHER READINGS

ALBERTI KG et al: The IDF Epidemiology Task Force Consensus Group. The metabolic syndrome—a new worldwide definition. Lancet 366:1059, 2005

ECKEL RH et al: The metabolic syndrome. Lancet 365:1415, 2005

EXPERT PANEL ON DETECTION EVALUATION, AND TREATMENT OF HIGH BLOOD CHOLESTEROL IN ADULTS: Executive summary of the third report of the National Cholesterol Education Program (NCEP) expert panel on detection, evaluation, and treatment of high blood cholesterol in adults (Adult Treatment Panel III). JAMA 285:2486, 2001

FORD ES: Prevalence of the metabolic syndrome defined by the International Diabetes Federation among adults in the U.S. Diabetes Care 28:2745, 2005

GRUNDY SM et al: Diagnosis and management of the metabolic syndrome. An American Heart Association/National Heart, Lung, and Blood Institute Scientific statement. Circulation 112:2735, 2005

————: Metabolic syndrome: Connecting and reconciling cardiovascular and diabetes worlds. J Am Coll Cardiol 47(6):1093, 2006

KAHN R et al: The metabolic syndrome: Time for a critical appraisal. Joint statement from the American Diabetes Association and the European Association for the Study of Diabetes. Diabetes Care 28:2289, 2005

CHAPTER 33

ISCHEMIC HEART DISEASE

Elliott M. Antman ■ Andrew P. Selwyn ■ Eugene Braunwald
■ Joseph Loscalzo

Ischemic heart disease (IHD) is a condition in which there is an inadequate supply of blood and oxygen to a portion of the myocardium; it typically occurs when there is an imbalance between myocardial oxygen supply and demand. The most common cause of myocardial ischemia is atherosclerotic disease of an epicardial coronary artery (or arteries) sufficient to cause a regional reduction in myocardial blood flow and inadequate perfusion of the myocardium supplied by the involved coronary artery.

EPIDEMIOLOGY

IHD causes more deaths and disability and incurs greater economic costs than any other illness in the developed world. IHD is the most common, serious, chronic, life-threatening illness in the United States, where 13 million persons have IHD, >6 million have angina pectoris, and >7 million have sustained a myocardial infarction (MI). A high-fat and energy-rich diet, smoking, and a sedentary lifestyle are associated with the emergence of IHD (Chap. 30). In the United States and western Europe, it is growing among low-income groups rather than high-income groups (who are adopting more healthful lifestyles), while primary prevention has delayed the disease to later in life in all socioeconomic groups.

Obesity, insulin resistance, and type 2 diabetes mellitus are increasing and are powerful risk factors for IHD. With urbanization in the developing world, the prevalence of risk factors for IHD is increasing rapidly in these regions such that a majority of the global burden of IHD is now occurring in low-income and middle-income countries. Population subgroups that appear to be particularly affected are men in South Asian countries, especially India. Given the projection of large increases in IHD throughout the world, IHD is likely to become the most common cause of death worldwide by 2020.

PATHOPHYSIOLOGY

Central to an understanding of the pathophysiology of myocardial ischemia is the concept of myocardial supply and demand. Under normal conditions, for any given level of a demand for oxygen, the myocardium will be supplied with oxygen-rich blood to prevent underperfusion of myocytes and the subsequent development of ischemia and infarction. The major determinants of myocardial oxygen demand (MVO$_2$) are heart rate, myocardial contractility, and myocardial wall tension (stress). An adequate supply of oxygen to the myocardium requires a satisfactory level of oxygen-carrying capacity of the blood (determined by the inspired level of oxygen, pulmonary function, and hemoglobin concentration and function) and an adequate level of coronary blood flow. Blood flows through the coronary arteries in a phasic fashion, with the majority occurring during diastole. About 75% of the total coronary resistance to flow occurs across three sets of arteries: (1) large epicardial arteries (Resistance 1 = R_1), (2) prearteriolar vessels (R_2), and (3) arteriolar and intramyocardial capillary vessels (R_3). In the absence of significant flow-limiting atherosclerotic obstructions, R_1 is trivial; the major determinant of coronary resistance is found in R_2 and R_3.

The normal coronary circulation is dominated and controlled by the heart's requirements for oxygen. This need is met by the ability of the coronary vascular bed to vary its resistance (and, therefore, blood flow) considerably while the myocardium extracts a high and relatively fixed percentage of oxygen. Normally, intramyocardial resistance vessels demonstrate an immense capacity for dilation (R_2 and R_3 decrease). For example, the changing oxygen needs of the heart with exercise and emotional stress affect coronary vascular resistance and in this manner regulate the supply of oxygen and substrate to the myocardium (*metabolic regulation*). The coronary resistance vessels also adapt to physiologic alterations in blood pressure in order to maintain coronary blood flow at levels appropriate to myocardial needs (*autoregulation*).

By reducing the lumen of the coronary arteries, atherosclerosis limits appropriate increases in perfusion when the demand for flow is augmented, as occurs during exertion or excitement. When the luminal reduction is severe, myocardial perfusion in the basal state is reduced. Coronary blood flow can also be limited by spasm (Chap. 34, Prinzmetal's Variant Angina), arterial thrombi, and, rarely, coronary emboli as well as by ostial narrowing due to aortitis. Congenital abnormalities, such as origin of the left anterior descending coronary artery from the pulmonary artery, may cause myocardial ischemia and infarction in infancy, but this cause is very rare in adults.

Myocardial ischemia can also occur if myocardial oxygen demands are markedly increased and when coronary blood flow may be limited, as occurs in severe left ventricular (LV) hypertrophy due to aortic stenosis. The latter can present with angina that is indistinguishable from that caused by coronary atherosclerosis largely owing to subendocardial ischemia (Chap. 20). A reduction in the oxygen-carrying capacity of the blood, as in extremely severe anemia or in the presence of carboxyhemoglobin, rarely causes myocardial ischemia by itself but may lower the threshold for ischemia in patients with moderate coronary obstruction.

Not infrequently, two or more causes of ischemia coexist, such as an increase in oxygen demand due to LV hypertrophy secondary to hypertension and a reduction in oxygen supply secondary to coronary atherosclerosis and anemia. Abnormal constriction or failure of normal dilation of the coronary resistance vessels can also cause

ischemia. When it causes angina, this condition is referred to as *microvascular angina*.

CORONARY ATHEROSCLEROSIS

Epicardial coronary arteries are the major site of atherosclerotic disease. The major risk factors for atherosclerosis [high plasma low-density lipoprotein (LDL), low plasma high-density lipoprotein (HDL), cigarette smoking, hypertension, and diabetes mellitus] (Chap. 30) disturb the normal functions of the vascular endothelium. These functions include local control of vascular tone, maintenance of an antithrombotic surface, and impairment of inflammatory cell adhesion and diapedesis. The loss of these defenses leads to inappropriate constriction, luminal thrombus formation, and abnormal interactions with blood leukocytes, especially monocytes, and platelets. Monocyte interaction ultimately results in the subintimal collections of fat, smooth-muscle cells, fibroblasts, and intercellular matrix (i.e., atherosclerotic plaques), which develop at irregular rates in different segments of the epicardial coronary tree and lead eventually to segmental reductions in cross-sectional area.

There is also a predilection for atherosclerotic plaques to develop at sites of increased turbulence in coronary flow, such as at branch points in the epicardial arteries. When a stenosis reduces the diameter of an epicardial artery by 50%, there is a limitation on the ability to increase flow to meet increased myocardial demand. When the diameter is reduced by ~80%, blood flow at rest may be reduced, and further minor decreases in the stenotic orifice area can reduce coronary flow dramatically and cause myocardial ischemia.

Segmental atherosclerotic narrowing of epicardial coronary arteries is caused most commonly by the formation of a plaque, which is subject to rupture or erosion of the cap separating the plaque from the bloodstream. Upon exposure of the plaque contents to blood, two important and interrelated processes are set in motion: (1) platelets are activated and aggregate; and (2) the coagulation cascade is activated, leading to deposition of fibrin strands. A thrombus composed of platelet aggregates and fibrin strands traps red blood cells and can reduce coronary blood flow, leading to the clinical manifestations of myocardial ischemia.

The location of the obstruction influences the quantity of myocardium rendered ischemic and determines the severity of the clinical manifestations. Thus, critical obstructions in vessels, such as the left main coronary artery or the proximal left anterior descending coronary artery, are particularly hazardous. Severe coronary narrowing and myocardial ischemia are frequently accompanied by the development of collateral vessels, especially when the narrowing develops gradually. When well developed, such vessels can, by themselves, provide sufficient blood flow to sustain the viability of the myocardium at rest but not during conditions of increased demand.

With progressive worsening of a proximal epicardial artery stenosis, the distal resistance vessels (when they function normally) dilate to reduce vascular resistance and maintain coronary blood flow. A pressure gradient develops across the proximal stenosis, and poststenotic pressure falls. When the resistance vessels are maximally dilated, myocardial blood flow becomes dependent on the pressure in the coronary artery distal to the obstruction. In these circumstances, ischemia, manifest clinically by angina or electrocardiographically by ST-segment deviation, can be precipitated by increases in myocardial oxygen demand caused by physical activity, emotional stress, and/or tachycardia. Changes in the caliber of the stenosed coronary artery due to physiologic vasomotion, loss of endothelial control of dilation (as occurs in diabetes mellitus), pathologic spasm (Prinzmetal's angina), or small platelet-rich plugs can also upset the critical balance between oxygen supply and demand and thereby precipitate myocardial ischemia.

EFFECTS OF ISCHEMIA

During episodes of inadequate perfusion caused by coronary atherosclerosis, myocardial tissue oxygen tension falls and may cause transient disturbances of the mechanical, biochemical, and electrical functions of the myocardium. Coronary atherosclerosis is a focal process that usually causes nonuniform ischemia. Regional disturbances of ventricular contractility cause segmental akinesia or, in severe cases, bulging (dyskinesia), which can greatly reduce myocardial pump function.

The abrupt development of severe ischemia, as occurs with total or subtotal coronary occlusion, is associated with almost instantaneous failure of normal muscle contraction and relaxation. The relatively poor perfusion of the subendocardium causes more intense ischemia of this portion of the wall (in comparison with the subepicardial region). Ischemia of large portions of the ventricle causes transient LV failure, and if the papillary muscle apparatus is involved, mitral regurgitation can occur. When ischemia is transient, it may be associated with angina pectoris; when it is prolonged, it can lead to myocardial necrosis and scarring with or without the clinical picture of acute MI (Chap. 35).

A wide range of abnormalities in cell metabolism, function, and structure underlie these mechanical disturbances during ischemia. The normal myocardium metabolizes fatty acids and glucose to carbon dioxide and water. With severe oxygen deprivation, fatty acids cannot be oxidized, and glucose is degraded to lactate; intracellular pH is reduced, as are the myocardial stores of high-energy phosphates, i.e., ATP and creatine phosphate. Impaired cell membrane function leads to the leakage of potassium and the uptake of sodium by myocytes, as well as an increase in cytosolic calcium. The severity and duration of the imbalance between myocardial oxygen supply and demand determine whether the damage is reversible (≤20 min for total occlusion in the absence of

collaterals) or whether it is permanent, with subsequent myocardial necrosis (>20 min).

Ischemia also causes characteristic changes in the electrocardiogram (ECG) such as repolarization abnormalities, as evidenced by inversion of T waves and, when more severe, by displacement of ST segments (Chap. 11). Transient T-wave inversion likely reflects nontransmural, intramyocardial ischemia; transient ST-segment depression often reflects subendocardial ischemia; and ST-segment elevation is thought to be caused by more severe transmural ischemia. Another important consequence of myocardial ischemia is electrical instability, which may lead to isolated ventricular premature beats or even ventricular tachycardia or ventricular fibrillation (Chap. 16). Most patients who die suddenly from IHD do so as a result of ischemia-induced ventricular tachyarrhythmias (Chap. 29).

ASYMPTOMATIC VERSUS SYMPTOMATIC IHD

Postmortem studies on accident victims and military casualties in western countries have shown that coronary atherosclerosis often begins to develop prior to 20 years of age and is widespread even among adults who were asymptomatic during life. Exercise stress tests in asymptomatic persons may show evidence of silent myocardial ischemia, i.e., exercise-induced ECG changes not accompanied by angina pectoris; coronary angiographic studies of such persons may reveal coronary artery plaques and previously unrecognized obstructions (Chap. 13). Postmortem examination of patients with such obstructions without a history of clinical manifestations of myocardial ischemia often shows macroscopic scars secondary to MI in regions supplied by diseased coronary arteries, with or without collateral circulation. According to population studies, ~25% of patients who survive acute MI may not come to medical attention, and these patients carry the same adverse prognosis as those who present with the classic clinical picture of acute MI (Chap. 35). Sudden death may be unheralded and is a common presenting manifestation of IHD (Chap. 29).

Patients with IHD can also present with cardiomegaly and heart failure secondary to ischemic damage of the LV myocardium that may have caused no symptoms prior to the development of heart failure; this condition is referred to as *ischemic cardiomyopathy*. In contrast to the asymptomatic phase of IHD, the symptomatic phase is characterized by chest discomfort due to either angina pectoris or acute MI (Chap. 35). Having entered the symptomatic phase, the patient may exhibit a stable or progressive course, revert to the asymptomatic stage, or die suddenly.

STABLE ANGINA PECTORIS

This episodic clinical syndrome is due to transient myocardial ischemia. Males constitute ~70% of all patients with angina pectoris and an even greater fraction of those younger than 50 years. Various diseases that cause myocardial ischemia as well as the numerous forms of discomforts with which it may be confused are discussed in Chap. 4.

HISTORY

The typical patient with angina is a man older than 50 years or a woman older than 60 years who complains of chest discomfort, usually described as heaviness, pressure, squeezing, smothering, or choking, and only rarely as frank pain. When the patient is asked to localize the sensation, he or she will typically place their hand over the sternum, sometimes with a clenched fist, to indicate a squeezing, central, substernal discomfort (Levine's sign). Angina is usually crescendo-decrescendo in nature, typically lasts 2–5 min, and can radiate to either shoulder and to both arms (especially the ulnar surfaces of the forearm and hand). It can also arise in or radiate to the back, interscapular region, root of the neck, jaw, teeth, and epigastrium. Angina is rarely localized below the umbilicus or above the mandible. A useful finding in assessing the patient with chest discomfort is the fact that myocardial ischemic discomfort does not radiate to the trapezius muscles; such a radiation pattern is more typical of pericarditis.

Although episodes of angina are typically caused by exertion (e.g., exercise, hurrying, or sexual activity) or emotion (e.g., stress, anger, fright, or frustration) and are relieved by rest, they may also occur at rest (Chap. 34) and while the patient is recumbent (angina decubitus). The patient may be awakened at night by typical chest discomfort and dyspnea. Nocturnal angina may be due to episodic tachycardia, diminished oxygenation as the respiratory pattern changes during sleep, or expansion of the intrathoracic blood volume that occurs with recumbency; the latter causes an increase in cardiac size (end-diastolic volume), in wall tension, and in myocardial oxygen demand that lead to ischemia and transient LV failure.

The threshold for the development of angina pectoris may vary by time of day and emotional state. Many patients report a fixed threshold for angina, which occurs predictably at a certain level of activity, such as climbing two flights of stairs at a normal pace. In these patients, coronary stenosis and myocardial oxygen supply are fixed, and ischemia is precipitated by an increase in myocardial oxygen demand; they are said to have *stable exertional angina*. In other patients, the threshold for angina may vary considerably within any given day and from day to day. In such patients, variations in myocardial oxygen supply, most likely due to changes in coronary vascular tone, may play an important role in defining the pattern of angina. A patient may report symptoms upon minor exertion in the morning (a short walk or shaving), yet, by midday, may be capable of much greater effort without symptoms. Angina may also be precipitated by unfamiliar tasks, a heavy meal, exposure to cold, or a combination.

Exertional angina is typically relieved by slowing or ceasing activities in 1–5 min and even more rapidly by rest and sublingual nitroglycerin (see later). Indeed, the diagnosis of angina should be suspect if it does not respond to the combination of these measures. The severity of angina can be conveniently summarized by the Canadian Cardiac Society functional classification (Table 33-1). Its impact on the patient's functional capacity can be described using the New York Heart Association functional classification (Table 33-1).

Sharp, fleeting chest pain or a prolonged, dull ache localized to the left submammary area is rarely due to myocardial ischemia. However, especially in women and diabetics, angina pectoris may be atypical in location and not strictly related to provoking factors. In addition, this symptom may exacerbate and remit over days, weeks, or months. Its occurrence can be seasonal, being more frequent in the winter in temperate climates. Anginal "equivalents" are symptoms of myocardial ischemia other than angina. These include dyspnea, nausea, fatigue, and faintness, and are more common in the elderly and in diabetic patients.

Systematic questioning of the patient with suspected IHD is important to uncover the features of an unstable syndrome associated with increased risk, such as angina occurring with less exertion than in the past or occurring at rest or awakening the patient from sleep. Since coronary atherosclerosis is often accompanied by similar lesions in other arteries, the patient with angina should be questioned and examined for peripheral arterial disease (intermittent claudication, Chap. 39), stroke, or transient ischemic attacks. It is also important to uncover a family history of premature IHD (<45 years in first-degree male relatives and <55 years in female relatives) and the presence of diabetes mellitus, hyperlipidemia, hypertension, cigarette smoking, and other risk factors for coronary atherosclerosis (Chap. 30). The history of typical angina pectoris establishes the diagnosis of IHD until proven otherwise. In patients with atypical angina (Chap. 4), the coexistence of advanced age, male gender, the postmenopausal state, and risk factors for atherosclerosis increase the likelihood of hemodynamically significant coronary disease.

PHYSICAL EXAMINATION

This is often normal in patients with stable angina when they are asymptomatic, but it may reveal evidence of atherosclerotic disease at other sites, such as an abdominal aortic aneurysm, carotid arterial bruits, and diminished arterial pulse in the lower extremities, or of risk factors for atherosclerosis, such as xanthelasmas and xanthomas (Chap. 30). Examination of the fundi may reveal an increased light reflex and arteriovenous nicking as evidence of hypertension. There may also be signs of anemia, thyroid disease, and nicotine stains on the fingertips from cigarette smoking. Palpation may reveal cardiac enlargement and abnormal contraction of the cardiac impulse (left ventricular akinesia or dyskinesia).

TABLE 33-1

CARDIOVASCULAR DISEASE CLASSIFICATION CHART

CLASS	NEW YORK HEART ASSOCIATION FUNCTIONAL CLASSIFICATION	CANADIAN CARDIOVASCULAR SOCIETY FUNCTIONAL CLASSIFICATION
I	Patients have cardiac disease but *without* the resulting *limitations* of physical activity. Ordinary physical activity does not cause undue fatigue, palpitation, dyspnea, or anginal pain.	Ordinary physical activity, such as walking and climbing stairs, *does not cause angina*. Angina present with strenuous or rapid or prolonged exertion at work or recreation.
II	Patients have cardiac disease resulting in *slight limitation* of physical activity. They are comfortable at rest. Ordinary physical activity results in fatigue, palpitation, dyspnea, or anginal pain.	*Slight limitation* of ordinary activity. Walking or climbing stairs rapidly, walking uphill, walking or stair climbing after meals, in cold, or when under emotional stress or only during the few hours after awakening. Walking more than two blocks on the level and climbing more than one flight of stairs at a normal pace and in normal conditions.
III	Patients have cardiac disease resulting in *marked limitation* of physical activity. They are comfortable at rest. Less than ordinary physical activity causes fatigue, palpitation, dyspnea, or anginal pain.	*Marked limitation* of ordinary physical activity. Walking one to two blocks on the level and climbing more than one flight of stairs in normal conditions.
IV	Patients have cardiac disease resulting in *inability* to carry on any physical activity without discomfort. Symptoms of cardiac insufficiency or of the anginal syndrome may be present even at rest. If any physical activity is undertaken, discomfort is increased.	*Inability* to carry on any physical activity without discomfort— anginal syndrome may be present at rest.

Source: Modified from L Goldman et al: Circulation 64:1227, 1981.

Auscultation can uncover arterial bruits, a third and/or fourth heart sound, and, if acute ischemia or previous infarction has impaired papillary muscle function, an apical systolic murmur due to mitral regurgitation. These auscultatory signs are best appreciated with the patient in the left lateral decubitus position. Aortic stenosis, aortic regurgitation (Chap. 20), pulmonary hypertension (Chap. 40), and hypertrophic cardiomyopathy (Chap. 21) must be excluded, since these disorders may cause angina in the absence of coronary atherosclerosis. Examination during an anginal attack is useful, since ischemia can cause transient LV failure with the appearance of a third and/or fourth heart sound, a dyskinetic cardiac apex, mitral regurgitation, and even pulmonary edema. Tenderness of the chest wall, localization of the discomfort with a single fingertip on the chest, or reproduction of the pain with palpation of the chest makes it unlikely that it is caused by myocardial ischemia.

LABORATORY EXAMINATION

Although the diagnosis of IHD can be made with a high degree of confidence from the clinical examination, a number of simple laboratory tests can be helpful. The urine should be examined for evidence of diabetes mellitus and renal disease (including microalbuminuria) since these conditions accelerate atherosclerosis. Similarly, examination of the blood should include measurements of lipids (cholesterol—total, LDL, HDL—and triglycerides), glucose, creatinine, hematocrit, and, if indicated based on the physical examination, thyroid function. A chest x-ray is important as it may show the consequences of IHD, i.e., cardiac enlargement, ventricular aneurysm, or signs of heart failure. These signs can support the diagnosis of IHD and are important in assessing the degree of cardiac damage.

ELECTROCARDIOGRAM

A 12-lead ECG recorded at rest may be normal in patients with typical angina pectoris, but there may also be signs of an old MI (Chap. 11). Although repolarization abnormalities—i.e., ST-segment and T-wave changes—as well as left ventricle (LV) hypertrophy and intraventricular conduction disturbances are suggestive of IHD, they are nonspecific since they can also occur in pericardial, myocardial, and valvular heart disease or, in the case of the former, transiently with anxiety, changes in posture, drugs, or esophageal disease. Dynamic ST-segment and T-wave changes that accompany episodes of angina pectoris and disappear thereafter are more specific.

STRESS TESTING

Electrocardiographic

The most widely used test for both the diagnosis of IHD and estimating the prognosis involves recording the 12-lead ECG before, during, and after exercise, usually on a treadmill (**Fig. 33-1**). The test consists of a standardized

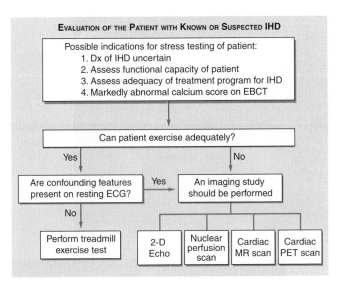

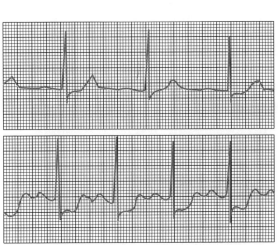

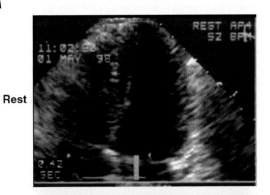

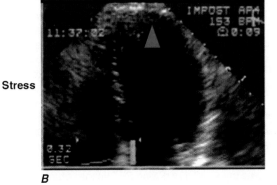

FIGURE 33-1

Evaluation of the patient with known or suspected ischemic heart disease. At the top of the figure is an algorithm for identifying patients who should be referred for stress testing and the decision pathway for determining if a standard treadmill exercise with ECG monitoring alone is adequate. A specialized imaging study is necessary if the patient cannot exercise adequately (pharmacologic challenge is given) or if there are confounding features on the resting ECG (symptom limited treadmill exercise may be used to stress the coronary circulation). At the bottom of the figure are examples of the data obtained with ECG monitoring and specialized imaging procedures. IHD, ischemic heart disease; EBCT, electron beam computed tomography; ECG, electrocardiogram; 2-D echo, two-dimensional echocardiography; MR, magnetic resonance; PET, positron emission tomography.

A. Lead V_4 at rest (*top*) and after 41/2 min of exercise (*bottom*). There is 3 mm (0.3 mV) of horizontal ST-segment depression, indicating a positive test for ischemia. [*Modified from BR Chaitman, in E Braunwald et al (eds): Heart Disease, 6th ed. Philadelphia, Saunders, 2001.*]

B. 45-year-old avid jogger who began experiencing classic substernal chest pressure underwent an exercise echo study. With exercise the patient's heart rate increased from 52 to 153 bpm. The left ventricular chamber dilated with exercise, and the septal and apical portions became akinetic to dyskinetic (*red arrow*). These findings are strongly suggestive of a significant flow limiting stenosis in the proximal left anterior descending coronary artery, which was confirmed at coronary angiography. [*Modified from SD Solomon, in E. Braunwald et al (eds): Primary Cardiology, 2d ed. Philadelphia, Saunders, 2003.*]

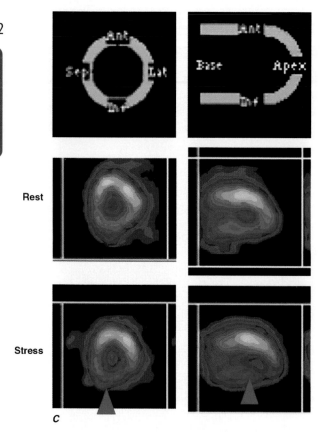

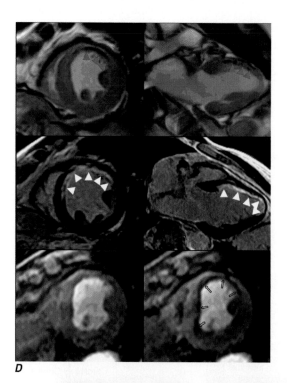

C

D

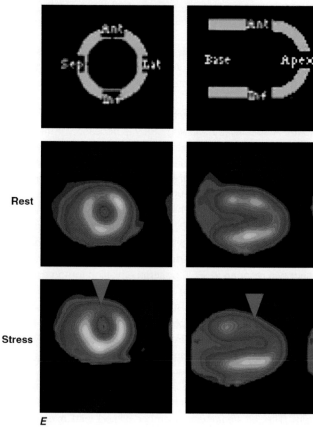

E

FIGURE 33-1 *(Continued)*

C. Stress and rest myocardial perfusion SPECT images obtained with Tc99m sestamibi in a patient with chest pain and dyspnea on exertion. The images demonstrate a medium size and severe stress perfusion defect involving the inferolateral and basal inferior walls, showing near complete reversibility, consistent with moderate ischemia in the right coronary artery territory (*red arrows*). *(Images provided by Dr. Marcello Di Carli, Nuclear Medicine Division, Brigham and Women's Hospital, Boston, MA.)*

D. A patient with a prior myocardial infarction (MI) presented with recurrent chest discomfort. On CMR cine imaging a large area of anterior akinesia was noted (marked by the arrows in the top left and right images, systolic frame only). This area of akinesia was matched by a larger extent of late gadolinium-DTPA enhancements consistent with a large transmural MI (marked by arrows in the middle left and right images). Resting (*bottom left*) and adenosine vasodilating stress (*bottom right*) first-pass perfusion images revealed reversible perfusion abnormality that extends to the inferior septum. This patient was found to have an occluded proximal left anterior descending coronary artery with extensive collateral formation. This case illustrates the utility of different modalities in a CMR examination in characterizing ischemic and infarcted myocardium. CMR, cardiac magnetic resonance; DTPA, diethylenetriamine pentaacetic acid. *(Images provided by Dr. Raymond Kwong, Cardiovascular Division, Brigham and Women's Hospital, Boston, MA.)*

E. Stress and rest myocardial perfusion PET images obtained with rubidium-82 in a patient with chest pain on exertion. The images demonstrate a large and severe stress perfusion defect involving the mid and apical anterior, anterolateral, and anteroseptal walls, and the LV apex, showing complete reversibility, consistent with extensive and severe ischemia in the mid left anterior descending coronary artery territory (*red arrows*). PET, positron emission tomography; LV, left ventricular. *(Images provided by Dr. Marcello Di Carli, Nuclear Medicine Division, Brigham and Women's Hospital, Boston, MA.)*

TABLE 33-2

RELATION OF METS TO STAGES IN VARIOUS TESTING PROTOCOLS

NYHA FUNCTIONAL CLASS	CLINICAL STATUS	O₂ COST mL/Kg PER MIN	METS	BRUCE MODIFIED 3 MIN STAGES		BRUCE 3 MIN STAGES	
				MPH	%GR	MPH	%GR
				6.0	22	6.0	22
				5.5	20	5.5	20
				5.0	18	5.0	18
Normal and I	Healthy, dependent on age, activity	56.0	16				
		52.5	15				
		49.0	14				
		45.5	13	4.2	16	4.2	16
		42.0	12				
	Sedentary healthy	38.5	11	3.4	14	3.4	14
		35.0	10				
		31.5	9				
		28.0	8				
		24.5	7	2.5	12	2.5	12
II		21.0	6				
	Limited	17.5	5	1.7	10	1.7	10
III		14.0	4				
	Symptomatic	10.5	3	1.7	5		
		7.0	2	1.7	0		
IV		3.5	1				

Source: Modified from GF Fletcher et al: Circulation 104:1694, 2001.

incremental increase in external workload (Table 33-2) while the symptoms, ECG, and arm blood pressure are monitored. Performance is usually symptom-limited, and the test is discontinued upon evidence of chest discomfort, severe shortness of breath, dizziness, severe fatigue, ST-segment depression >0.2 mV (2 mm), a fall in systolic blood pressure >10 mmHg, or the development of a ventricular tachyarrhythmia. This test seeks to discover any limitation in exercise performance, to detect typical ECG signs of myocardial ischemia, and to establish their relationship to chest discomfort. The ischemic ST-segment response is generally defined as flat or downsloping depression of the ST segment >0.1 mV below baseline (i.e., the PR segment) and lasting longer than 0.08 s (Fig. 33-1). Upsloping or junctional ST-segment changes are not considered characteristic of ischemia and do not constitute a positive test. Although T-wave abnormalities, conduction disturbances, and ventricular arrhythmias that develop during exercise should be noted, they are also not diagnostic. Negative exercise tests in which the target heart rate (85% of maximal predicted heart rate for age and sex) is not achieved are considered to be nondiagnostic.

When interpreting ECG stress tests, the probability that coronary artery disease (CAD) exists in the patient or population under study (i.e., pretest probability) should be considered. Overall, false-positive or false-negative results occur in one-third of cases. However, a positive result on exercise indicates that the likelihood of CAD is 98% in males >50 years with a history of typical angina pectoris and who develop chest discomfort during the test. The likelihood decreases if the patient has atypical or no chest pain by history and/or during the test.

The incidence of false-positive tests is significantly increased in patients with low probabilities of IHD, such as asymptomatic men younger than 40 years or in premenopausal women with no risk factors for premature atherosclerosis. It is also increased in patients taking cardioactive drugs, such as digitalis and antiarrhythmic agents, or in those with intraventricular conduction disturbances, resting ST-segment and T-wave abnormalities, ventricular hypertrophy, or abnormal serum potassium levels. Obstructive disease limited to the circumflex coronary artery may result in a false-negative stress test since the lateral portion of the heart which this vessel supplies is not well represented on the surface 12-lead ECG. Since the overall sensitivity of exercise stress electrocardiography is only ~75%, a negative result does not exclude CAD, although it makes the likelihood of three-vessel or left main CAD extremely unlikely.

The physician should be present throughout the exercise test, and it is important to measure total duration of exercise, the times to the onset of ischemic ST-segment change and chest discomfort, the external work performed (generally expressed as the stage of exercise), and the internal cardiac work performed, i.e., by the heart rate–blood pressure product. The depth of the ST-segment depression and the time needed for recovery of these ECG changes are also important. Because the risks of exercise testing are small but real—estimated at one fatality and two nonfatal complications per 10,000 tests—equipment for resuscitation should be available. Modified (heart rate–limited rather than symptom-limited) exercise tests can be performed safely in patients as early as 6 days after uncomplicated MI (Table 33-2). Contraindications to exercise stress testing include rest angina within 48 h, unstable rhythm, severe aortic stenosis, acute myocarditis, uncontrolled heart failure, severe pulmonary hypertension, and active infective endocarditis.

The normal response to graded exercise includes progressive increases in heart rate and blood pressure. Failure of the blood pressure to increase or an actual decrease with signs of ischemia during the test is an important adverse prognostic sign, since it may reflect ischemia-induced global LV dysfunction. The development of angina and/or severe (>0.2 mV) ST-segment depression at a low workload, i.e., before completion of stage II of the Bruce protocol, and/or ST-segment depression that persists for >5 min after the termination of exercise increases the specificity of the test and suggests severe IHD and a high risk of future adverse events.

Cardiac Imaging

(See also Chap. 12) When the resting ECG is abnormal (e.g., preexcitation syndrome, >1 mm of resting ST-segment depression, left bundle branch block, paced ventricular rhythm), information gained from an exercise test can be enhanced by stress myocardial radionuclide perfusion imaging after the intravenous administration of thallium 201 or technetium 99m (^{99m}Tc) sestamibi during exercise (or a pharmacologic) stress. Recent data also suggest positron emission tomography (PET) imaging (with exercise or pharmacologic stress) using N-13 ammonia or rubidium-82 nuclide as another technique for assessing perfusion. Images obtained immediately after cessation of exercise to detect regional ischemia are compared with those obtained at rest to confirm reversible ischemia and regions of persistent absent uptake that signify infarction.

A sizable fraction of patients who need noninvasive stress testing to identify myocardial ischemia and increased risk of coronary events cannot exercise because of peripheral vascular or musculoskeletal disease, exertional dyspnea, or deconditioning. In these circumstances an intravenous pharmacologic challenge is used in place of exercise. For example, dipyridamole or adenosine can be given to create a coronary "steal" by temporarily increasing flow in nondiseased segments of the coronary vasculature at the expense of diseased segments. Alternatively, a graded incremental infusion of dobutamine may be administered to increase MVO$_2$. A variety of imaging options are available to accompany these pharmacologic stressors (Fig. 33-1). The development of a transient perfusion defect with a tracer such as radioactive thallium or ^{99m}Tc sestamibi is used to detect myocardial ischemia.

Two-dimensional echocardiography can assess both global and regional wall motion abnormalities of the LV due to MI or persistent ischemia. Stress (exercise or dobutamine) echocardiography may cause the emergence of regions of akinesis or dyskinesis not present at rest. Stress echocardiography, like stress myocardial perfusion imaging, is more sensitive than exercise electrocardiography in the diagnosis of IHD. Cardiac magnetic resonance (CMR) stress testing is also evolving as an alternative to radionuclide, PET, or echocardiographic stress imaging. CMR stress testing performed with dobutamine infusion can be used to assess wall motion abnormalities accompanying ischemia, and myocardial perfusion CMR can be used to provide rather complete ventricular evaluation using multislice MR imaging studies. Ambulatory monitoring of the ECG can assess myocardial ischemia as episodes of ST-segment depression. Echocardiography or radionuclide angiography should be carried out to assess LV function in patients with chronic stable angina and in patients with a history of a prior MI, pathologic Q waves, or clinical evidence of heart failure.

Atherosclerotic plaques become progressively calcified over time, and coronary calcification in general increases with age. For this reason, methods for detecting coronary calcium have been developed as a measure of the presence of coronary atherosclerosis. These methods involve computed tomography (CT) applications that achieve rapid acquisition of images [ultrafast or electron beam (EBCT) and multidetector (MDCT)]. Coronary calcium detected by these imaging techniques is quantified using the Agatston score most commonly, which is based on the area and density of calcification. Although the diagnostic accuracy of this imaging method is high (sensitivity, 90–94%; specificity, 95–97%; negative predictive value, 93–99%), its prognostic utility and its role in the evaluative algorithm of patients with stable angina pectoris have not yet been defined.

CORONARY ARTERIOGRAPHY

(See also Chap. 13) This diagnostic method outlines the lumina of the coronary arteries and can be used to detect or exclude serious coronary obstruction. However, coronary arteriography provides no information regarding the arterial wall, and severe atherosclerosis that does not encroach on the lumen may go undetected. Of note, atherosclerotic plaques characteristically grow progressively in the intima and media of an epicardial coronary artery, at first without encroaching on the lumen, causing an outward bulging of the artery—a process referred to as negative remodeling (Chap. 30). Later in the course of the disease, further growth causes luminal narrowing.

Indications

Coronary arteriography is indicated in (1) patients with chronic stable angina pectoris who are severely symptomatic despite medical therapy and who are being considered for revascularization, i.e., a percutaneous coronary intervention (PCI) or coronary artery bypass grafting (CABG); (2) patients with troublesome symptoms that present diagnostic difficulties in whom there is a need to confirm or rule out the diagnosis of IHD; (3) patients with known or possible angina pectoris who have survived cardiac arrest; (4) patients with angina or evidence of ischemia on noninvasive testing with clinical or laboratory evidence of ventricular dysfunction; and (5) patients judged to be at high risk of sustaining coronary events based on signs of severe ischemia on noninvasive testing, regardless of the presence or severity of symptoms (see the following paragraphs).

Examples of other indications include:

1. Patients with chest discomfort suggestive of angina pectoris but a negative or nondiagnostic stress test who require a definitive diagnosis for guiding medical management, alleviating psychological stress, career or family planning, or insurance purposes.
2. Patients who have been admitted repeatedly to the hospital for a suspected acute coronary syndrome (Chaps. 34 and 35) but in whom this diagnosis has not been established and in whom the presence or absence of CAD should be determined.
3. Patients with careers that involve the safety of others (e.g., pilots, firefighters, police) who have questionable symptoms or suspicious or positive noninvasive tests, and in whom there are reasonable doubts about the state of the coronary arteries.
4. Patients with aortic stenosis or hypertrophic cardiomyopathy and angina in whom the chest pain could be due to IHD.
5. Male patients >45 years and females >55 years who are to undergo a cardiac operation, such as valve replacement or repair, and who may or may not have clinical evidence of myocardial ischemia.
6. Patients following MI, especially those who are at high risk after MI because of the recurrence of angina or the presence of heart failure, frequent ventricular premature contractions, or signs of ischemia on the stress test.
7. Patients with angina pectoris, regardless of severity, in whom noninvasive testing indicates a high risk of coronary events.
8. Patients in whom coronary spasm or another nonatherosclerotic cause of myocardial ischemia (e.g., coronary artery anomaly, Kawasaki's disease) is suspected.

Noninvasive alternatives to diagnostic coronary arteriography include CT angiography and cardiac MR angiography (Chap. 12). Although, these new imaging techniques can provide information about obstructive lesions in the epicardial coronary arteries, their exact role in clinical practice has not yet been rigorously defined. Important aspects of their use that should be noted include the substantially higher radiation exposure with CT angiography in comparison with conventional diagnostic arteriography and the limitations on cardiac MR imposed by cardiac movement during the cardiac cycle, especially at high heart rates.

PROGNOSIS

The principal prognostic indicators in patients known to have IHD are age, the functional state of the LV, the location(s) and severity of coronary artery narrowing, and the severity or activity of myocardial ischemia. Angina pectoris of recent onset, unstable angina (Chap. 34), early post-MI angina, and angina that is unresponsive or poorly responsive to medical therapy or is accompanied by symptoms of congestive heart failure all indicate an increased risk for adverse coronary events. The same is true for the physical signs of heart failure, episodes of pulmonary edema, transient third heart sounds, or mitral regurgitation, and for echocardiographic or radioisotopic (or roentgenographic) evidence of cardiac enlargement and reduced (<0.40) ejection fraction (EF).

Most importantly, any of the following signs during noninvasive testing indicate a high risk for coronary events: inability to exercise for 6 min, i.e., stage II (Bruce protocol) of the exercise test; a strongly positive exercise test showing onset of myocardial ischemia at low workloads (≥0.1 mV ST-segment depression before completion of stage II; ≥0.2 mV ST depression at any stage; ST depression for >5 min following the cessation of exercise; a decline in systolic pressure >10 mmHg during exercise; the development of ventricular tachyarrhythmias during exercise); the development of large or multiple perfusion defects or increased lung uptake during stress radioisotope perfusion imaging; and a decrease in LVEF during exercise on radionuclide ventriculography or during stress echocardiography. Conversely, patients who can complete stage III of the Bruce exercise protocol and have a normal stress perfusion scan or negative stress echocardiographic evaluation are at very low risk of future coronary events.

On cardiac catheterization, elevations of LV end-diastolic pressure and ventricular volume and reduced EF are the most important signs of LV dysfunction and are associated with a poor prognosis. Patients with chest discomfort but normal LV function and normal coronary arteries have an excellent prognosis. Obstructive lesions of the left main (>50% luminal diameter) or left anterior descending coronary artery proximal to the origin of the first septal artery are associated with a greater risk than are lesions of the right or left circumflex coronary artery because of the greater quantity of myocardium at risk. Atherosclerotic plaques in epicardial arteries with fissuring or filling defects indicate increased risk. These lesions go through phases of inflammatory cellular activity, degeneration, endothelial dysfunction, abnormal vasomotion, platelet aggregation, and fissuring or hemorrhage. These factors can temporarily worsen the stenosis and cause abnormal reactivity of the vessel wall, thus exacerbating the manifestations of ischemia. The recent onset of symptoms, the development of severe ischemia during stress testing (see earlier), and unstable angina pectoris (Chap. 34) all reflect episodes of rapid progression in coronary lesions.

With any degree of obstructive CAD, mortality is greatly increased when LV function is impaired; conversely, at any level of LV function, the prognosis is influenced importantly by the quantity of myocardium perfused by critically obstructed vessels. Therefore, it is useful to collect all the evidence substantiating past myocardial damage (evidence of MI on ECG, echocardiography, radioisotope imaging, or left ventriculography), residual LV function (EF and wall motion), and risk of future damage from coronary events (extent of coronary disease and severity of ischemia defined by noninvasive stress testing). The larger the quantity of established myocardial necrosis, the less the heart is able to withstand additional damage and the poorer the prognosis. All the above signs of past damage plus the risk of future damage should be considered indicators of risk.

The greater the number and severity of risk factors for coronary atherosclerosis [advanced age (>75 years), diabetes, morbid obesity, accompanying peripheral and/or cerebrovascular disease, previous MI], the worse the prognosis of the angina patient. Evidence exists that elevated levels of C-reactive protein in the plasma, extensive coronary calcification on EBCT (see earlier), and increased carotid intimal thickening on ultrasound examination also indicate an increased risk of coronary events.

℞ Treatment: STABLE ANGINA PECTORIS

Each patient must be evaluated individually with respect to his or her expectations and goals, control of symptoms, and prevention of adverse clinical outcomes, such as MI and premature death. The degree of disability as well as the physical and emotional stress that precipitates angina must be carefully recorded in order to set treatment goals. The management plan should include the following components: (1) explanation of the problem and reassurance about the ability to formulate a treatment plan, (2) identification and treatment of aggravating conditions, (3) recommendations for adaptation of activity as needed, (4) treatment of risk factors that will decrease the occurrence of adverse coronary outcomes, (5) drug therapy for angina, and (6) consideration of revascularization.

EXPLANATION AND REASSURANCE Patients with IHD need to understand their condition and to realize that a long and productive life is possible even though they suffer from angina pectoris or have experienced and recovered from an acute MI. Offering results of clinical trials showing improved outcomes can be of great value when encouraging patients to resume or maintain activity and return to their occupation. A planned program of rehabilitation can encourage patients to lose weight, improve exercise tolerance, and control risk factors with more confidence.

IDENTIFICATION AND TREATMENT OF AGGRAVATING CONDITIONS A number of conditions may either increase oxygen demand or decrease oxygen supply to the myocardium and may precipitate or exacerbate angina in patients with IHD. Aortic valve disease and hypertrophic cardiomyopathy may cause or contribute to angina and should be excluded or treated. Obesity, hypertension, and hyperthyroidism should be treated aggressively in order to reduce the frequency and severity of anginal episodes. Decreased myocardial oxygen supply may be due to reduced oxygenation of the arterial blood (e.g., in pulmonary disease or, when carboxyhemoglobin is present, due to cigarette or cigar smoking) or decreased oxygen-carrying capacity (e.g., in anemia). Correction of these abnormalities, if present, may reduce or even eliminate angina pectoris.

ADAPTATION OF ACTIVITY Myocardial ischemia is caused by a discrepancy between the demand of the heart muscle for oxygen and the ability of the coronary circulation to meet this demand. Most patients can be helped to understand this concept and utilize it in the rational programming of activity. Many tasks that ordinarily evoke angina may be accomplished without symptoms simply by reducing the speed at which they are performed. Patients must appreciate the diurnal variation in their tolerance of certain activities and should reduce their energy requirements in the morning, immediately after meals, and in cold or inclement weather.

On occasion, it may be necessary to recommend a change in employment or residence to avoid physical stress. However, with the exception of manual laborers, most patients with IHD can continue to function merely by allowing more time to complete each task. In some patients, anger and frustration may be the most important factors precipitating myocardial ischemia. If these cannot be avoided, training in stress management may be useful. A treadmill exercise test to determine the approximate heart rate at which ischemic ECG changes or symptoms develop may be helpful in the development of a specific exercise program.

Physical conditioning usually improves the exercise tolerance of patients with angina and exerts substantial

TABLE 33-3

377

CHAPTER 33

Ischemic Heart Disease

ENERGY REQUIREMENTS FOR SOME COMMON ACTIVITIES				
LESS THAN 3 METs	**3–5 METs**	**5–7 METs**	**7–9 METs**	**MORE THAN 9 METs**
Self-care				
Washing/shaving Dressing Light housekeeping Desk work Driving auto	Cleaning windows Raking Power lawn mowing Bed making/stripping Carrying objects (15–30 lb)	Easy digging in garden Level hand lawn mowing Carrying objects (30–60 lb)	Heavy shoveling Carrying objects (60–90 lb)	Carrying loads upstairs (objects more than 90 lb) Climbing stairs (quickly) Shoveling heavy snow
Occupational				
Sitting (clerical/ assembly) Desk work Standing (store clerk)	Stocking shelves (light objects) Light welding/ carpentry	Carpentry (exterior) Shoveling dirt Sawing wood	Digging ditches (pick and shovel)	Heavy labor
Recreational				
Golf (cart) Knitting	Dancing (social) Golf (walking) Sailing Tennis (doubles)	Tennis (singles) Snow skiing (downhill) Light backpacking Basketball Stream fishing	Canoeing Mountain climbing	Squash Ski touring Vigorous basketball
Physical Conditioning				
Walking (2 mph) Stationary bike Very light calisthenics	Level walking (3–4 mph) Level biking (6–8 mph) Light calisthenics	Level walking (4.5–5.0 mph) Bicycling (9–10 mph) Swimming, breast stroke	Level jogging (5 mph) Swimming (crawl stroke) Rowing machine Heavy calisthenics Bicycling (12 mph)	Running (>6 mph) Bicycling (>13 mph) Rope jumping Walking uphill (5 mph)

Source: Modified from WL Haskell: Rehabilitation of the coronary patient, in NK Wenger, HK Hellerstein (eds): *Design and Implementation of Cardiac Conditioning Program*. New York, Churchill Livingstone. 1978.

psychological benefits. A regular program of isotonic exercise that is within the limits of each patient's threshold for the development of angina pectoris and does not exceed 80% of the heart rate associated with ischemia on exercise testing should be strongly encouraged. Based on the results of an exercise test, the number of METS performed at the onset of ischemia can be estimated (Table 33-2) and a practical exercise prescription can be formulated to permit daily activities that will fall below the ischemic threshold (Table 33-3).

TREATMENT OF RISK FACTORS A *family history* of premature IHD is an important indicator of increased risk and should trigger a search for treatable risk factors such as hyperlipidemia, hypertension, and diabetes mellitus. *Obesity* impairs the treatment of other risk factors and increases the risk of adverse coronary events. In addition, obesity is often accompanied by three other risk factors—diabetes mellitus, hypertension, and hyperlipidemia. The treatment of obesity and these accompanying risk factors is an important component of any management plan. A diet low in saturated and *trans*-unsaturated fatty acids and a caloric intake to achieve optimal body weight is a cornerstone in the management of chronic IHD.

Cigarette smoking accelerates coronary atherosclerosis in both sexes and at all ages and increases the risk of thrombosis, plaque instability, MI, and death (Chap. 30). In addition, by increasing myocardial oxygen needs and reducing oxygen supply, it aggravates angina. Smoking cessation studies have demonstrated important benefits with a significant decline in the occurrence of these adverse outcomes. The physician's message must be clear and strong and supported by programs that achieve and monitor abstinence. *Hypertension* (Chap. 37) is associated with increased risk of adverse clinical events from coronary atherosclerosis as well as stroke. In addition, the LV hypertrophy that results from sustained hypertension aggravates ischemia. There is evidence that long-term, effective treatment of hypertension can decrease the occurrence of adverse coronary events. *Diabetes mellitus* accelerates coronary and peripheral atherosclerosis and is frequently associated with dyslipidemias and increases in the risk of angina, MI, and sudden coronary death. Aggressive control of the dyslipidemia (target LDL cholesterol <70 mg/dL) and hypertension (target BP ≤120/80) that are frequently found in diabetic patients is essential, as described below.

DYSLIPIDEMIA The treatment of dyslipidemia is central when aiming for long-term relief from angina, reduced need for revascularization, and reduction in MI and death. The control of lipids can be achieved by the combination of a diet low in saturated and *trans*-unsaturated fatty acids, exercise, and weight loss. Frequently, HMG-CoA reductase inhibitors (statins) are required and can lower LDL cholesterol (25–50%), raise HDL cholesterol (5–9%), and lower triglycerides (5–30%). Niacin or fibrates can be used to raise HDL cholesterol and lower triglycerides (Chaps. 30 and 31). Controlled trials with lipid-regulating regimens have shown equal proportional benefit for men, women, the elderly, diabetics, and even smokers.

Compliance with regard to the health-promoting behaviors listed earlier is generally very poor, and the conscientious physician must not underestimate the major effort required to meet this challenge. Fewer than one-half of patients in the United States discharged from the hospital with proven coronary disease receive treatment for dyslipidemia. Given the proof that treating dyslipidemia brings major benefits, physicians need to secure treatment pathways, monitor compliance, and follow up.

RISK REDUCTION IN WOMEN WITH IHD
The incidence of clinical IHD in premenopausal women is very low; however, following the menopause, the atherogenic risk factors increase (e.g., increased LDL, reduced HDL) and the rate of clinical coronary events accelerates to the levels observed in men. Women have not given up cigarette smoking as effectively as have men. Diabetes mellitus, which is more common in women, greatly increases the occurrence of clinical IHD

and amplifies the deleterious effects of hypertension, hyperlipidemia, and smoking. Cardiac catheterization and coronary revascularization are often applied more sparingly in women and at a later, and more severe, stage of the disease than in men. When cholesterol lowering, beta blockers after MI, and CABG are applied in the appropriate patient groups, women enjoy the same benefits of improved outcome as do men.

DRUG THERAPY The commonly used drugs for the treatment of angina pectoris are summarized in Tables 33-4–33-6. Pharmacotherapy for IHD is designed to reduce the frequency of anginal episodes and blunt the surge in the patient's heart rate and blood pressure with exertion so that they can perform daily activities without approaching the heart rate–blood pressure threshold that provokes ischemia. Antiplatelet therapy with aspirin is also used to reduce thrombotic events that may occur with destabilization of atherosclerotic plaques.

Nitrates The organic nitrates are a valuable class of drugs in the management of angina pectoris that have been in clinical use for over 125 years (**Table 33-4**). Their major mechanisms of action include systemic venodilation with concomitant reduction in LV end-diastolic volume and pressure, thereby reducing myocardial wall tension and oxygen requirements; dilation of epicardial coronary vessels; and increased blood flow in collateral vessels. The organic nitrates, when metabolized release nitric oxide (NO) which binds to guanylyl cyclase in vascular smooth-muscle cells, leading to an increase in cyclic guanosine monophosphate, which causes relaxation of vascular smooth muscle. Nitrates also exert antithrombotic activity by NO-dependent activation of platelet guanylyl cyclase and impairment of intraplatelet calcium flux, and platelet activation.

The absorption of these agents is most rapid and complete through the mucous membranes. For this reason, nitroglycerin is most commonly administered sublingually in tablets of 0.4 or 0.6 mg. Patients with angina should be instructed to take the medication both to relieve angina and also approximately 5 min before stress that is likely to induce an episode. The value of this prophylactic use of the drug cannot be overemphasized.

A pulsating feeling in the head or headache is the most common side effect of nitroglycerin and fortunately is only rarely disturbing at the doses usually required to relieve or prevent angina. Postural dizziness has also been reported. Nitroglycerin deteriorates with exposure to air, moisture, and sunlight, so that if the drug neither relieves discomfort nor produces a slight sensation of tingling at the sublingual site of absorption, the preparation may be inactive and a fresh supply should be obtained. If relief is not achieved by rest and within 2 or 3 min after up to three nitroglycerin tablets, the patient should consult a physician or report

TABLE 33-4

NITROGLYCERIN AND NITRATES FOR PATIENTS WITH ISCHEMIC HEART DISEASE

COMPOUND	ROUTE	DOSE	DURATION OF EFFECT
Nitroglycerin	Sublingual tablets	0.3–0.6 mg up to 1.5 mg	Approximately 10 min
	Spray	0.4 mg as needed	Similar to sublingual tablets
	Ointment	2% 6 × 6 in; 15 × 15 cm 7.5–40 mg	Effect up to 7 h
	Transdermal	0.2–0.8 mg/h every 12 h	8–12 h during intermittent therapy
	Oral sustained release	2.5–13 mg	4–8 h
	Intravenous	5–200 µg/min	Tolerance may be seen in 7–8 h
Isosorbide dinitrate	Sublingual	2.5–10 mg	Up to 60 min
	Oral	5–80 mg, 2–3 times daily	Up to 8 h
	Spray	1.25 mg daily	2–3 min
	Chewable	5 mg	2–2 1/2 h
	Oral slow release	40 mg 1–2 daily	Up to 8 h
	Intravenous	1.25–5.0 mg/h	Tolerance in 7–8 h
	Ointment	100 mg/24 h	Not effective
Isosorbide mononitrate	Oral	20 mg twice daily 60–240 mg once daily	12–24 h
Pentaerythritol tetranitrate	Sublingual	10 mg as needed	Not known

Source: Modified from RJ Gibbons et al.

promptly to a hospital emergency room for evaluation of possible unstable angina or acute MI (Chap. 35).

Nitrates improve exercise tolerance in patients with chronic angina and relieve ischemia in patients with unstable angina as well as in patients with Prinzmetal's variant angina (Chap. 34). A diary of angina and nitroglycerin use may be valuable for detecting changes in the frequency, severity, or threshold for discomfort that may signify the development of unstable angina pectoris and/or herald an impending MI.

Long-Acting Nitrates None of the long-acting nitrates is as effective as sublingual nitroglycerin for the acute relief of angina. These organic nitrate preparations can be swallowed, chewed, or administered as a patch or paste by the transdermal route (Table 33-4). They can provide effective plasma levels for up to 24 h, but the therapeutic response is highly variable. Different preparations and/or administration during the daytime should be tried only to prevent discomfort while avoiding side effects such as headache and dizziness. Individual dose titration is important in order to prevent side effects.

Useful preparations include isosorbide dinitrate (10–60 mg orally bid or tid) or mononitrate (30–120 mg orally qd), nitroglycerin ointment (0.5–2.0 in. qid), or sustained-release transdermal patches (5–25 mg/d). Tolerance with loss of efficacy develops within 12–24 h of continuous exposure to all of the long-acting nitrates.

The mechanism of development of nitrate tolerance is incompletely understood, but leading hypotheses include inadequate generation of reduced sulfhydryl groups required for biotransformation to NO, inhibition of mitochondrial aldehyde dehydrogenase (responsible for formation of NO), counterregulatory neurohormonal activation with vasoconstriction and fluid retention, and production of oxygen free radical species that inactivate NO and increase the sensitivity of vascular smooth muscle to circulating vasoconstrictors.

In order to minimize the effects of tolerance, the minimum effective dose should be used and a minimum of 8 h each day kept free of the drug so as to restore any useful response(s).

β-Adrenergic Blockers These drugs represent an important component of the pharmacologic treatment of angina pectoris (Table 33-5). They reduce myocardial oxygen demand by inhibiting the increases in heart rate, arterial pressure, and myocardial contractility caused by adrenergic activation. Beta blockade reduces these variables most strikingly during exercise while causing only small reductions at rest. Long-acting beta-blocking drugs or sustained release formulations offer the advantage of once daily dosage (Table 33-5). The therapeutic aims include relief of angina and ischemia. These drugs can also reduce mortality and reinfarction in patients after MI and are moderately effective antihypertensive agents.

TABLE 33-5

PROPERTIES OF BETA BLOCKERS IN CLINICAL USE FOR ISCHEMIC HEART DISEASE			
DRUGS	SELECTIVITY	PARTIAL AGONIST ACTIVITY	USUAL DOSE FOR ANGINA
Acebutolol	$\beta1$	Yes	200–600 mg twice daily
Atenolol	$\beta1$	No	50–200 mg/d
Betaxolol	$\beta1$	No	10–20 mg/d
Bisoprolol	$\beta1$	No	10 mg/d
Esmolol (intravenous)[a]	$\beta1$	No	50–300 μg/kg per min
Labetalol[b]	None	Yes	200–600 mg twice daily
Metoprolol	$\beta1$	No	50–200 mg twice daily
Nadolol	None	No	40–80 mg/d
Pindolol	None	Yes	2.5–7.5 mg 3 times daily
Propranolol	None	No	80–120 mg twice daily
Timolol	None	No	10 mg twice daily

Note: This list of β blockers that may be used to treat patients with angina pectoris is arranged alphabetically. The agents for which there is the greatest clinical experience include atenolol, metoprolol, and propranolol. It is preferable to use a sustained release formulation that may be taken once daily to improve the patient's compliance with the regimen.
[a]Esmolol is an ultrashort acting β blocker that is administered as a continuous intravenous infusion. Its rapid offset of action makes esmolol an attractive agent to use in patients with relative contraindications to β blockade.
[b]Labetolol is a combined alpha- and β blocker.
Source: Modified from RJ Gibbons et al.

Relative contraindications include asthma and reversible airway obstruction in patients with chronic lung disease, atrioventricular conduction disturbances, severe bradycardia, Raynaud's phenomenon, and a history of mental depression. Side effects include fatigue, reduced exercise tolerance, nightmares, impotence, cold extremities, intermittent claudication, bradycardia (sometimes severe), impaired atrioventricular conduction, LV failure, bronchial asthma, worsening claudication, and intensification of the hypoglycemia produced by oral hypoglycemic agents and insulin. Reducing the dose or even discontinuation may be necessary if these side effects develop and persist. Since sudden discontinuation can intensify ischemia, the doses should be tapered over 2 weeks.

Beta blockers with relative β_1-receptor specificity, such as metoprolol and atenolol, may be preferable in patients with mild bronchial obstruction and insulin-requiring diabetes mellitus.

Calcium Channel Blockers Calcium channel blockers (Table 33-6) are coronary vasodilators that produce variable and dose-dependent reductions in myocardial oxygen demand, contractility, and arterial pressure. These combined pharmacologic effects are advantageous and make these agents as effective as beta blockers in the treatment of angina pectoris. They are indicated when beta blockers are contraindicated, poorly tolerated, or ineffective. Verapamil and diltiazem may produce symptomatic disturbances in cardiac conduction and bradyarrhythmias. They also exert negative inotropic actions and are more likely to aggravate LV failure, particularly when used in patients with LV dysfunction, especially if they are also receiving beta blockers. Although useful effects are usually achieved when calcium channel blockers are combined with beta blockers and nitrates, careful individual titrations of the doses are essential with these combinations. Variant (Prinzmetal's) angina responds particularly well to calcium channel blockers (especially members of the dihydropyridine class), supplemented when necessary by nitrates (Chap. 34).

Verapamil should not ordinarily be combined with beta blockers because of the combined effects on heart rate and contractility. Diltiazem can be combined with beta blockers in patients with normal ventricular function and no conduction disturbances. Amlodipine and beta blockers have complementary actions on coronary blood supply and myocardial oxygen demands. While the former decreases blood pressure and dilates coronary arteries, the latter slows heart rate and decreases contractility. Amlodipine and the other second-generation dihydropyridine calcium antagonists (nicardipine, isradipine, long-acting nifedipine, and felodipine) are potent vasodilators and useful in the simultaneous treatment of angina and hypertension. Short-acting dihydropyridines should be avoided because of the risk of precipitating infarction, particularly in the absence of beta blockers.

TABLE 33-6   381

CALCIUM CHANNEL BLOCKERS IN CLINICAL USE FOR ISCHEMIC HEART DISEASE

DRUGS	USUAL DOSE	DURATION OF ACTION	SIDE EFFECTS
Dihydropyridines			
Amlodipine	5–10 mg qd	Long	Headache, edema
Felodipine	5–10 mg qd	Long	Headache, edema
Isradipine	2.5–10 mg bid	Medium	Headache, fatigue
Nicardipine	20–40 mg tid	Short	Headache, dizziness, flushing, edema
Nifedipine	Immediate release:[a] 30–90 mg/d orally Slow release: 30–180 mg orally	Short	Hypotension, dizziness, flushing, nausea, constipation, edema
Nisoldipine	20–40 mg qd	Short	Similar to nifedipine
Nondihydropyridines			
Diltiazem	Immediate release: 30–80 mg 4 times daily	Short	Hypotension, dizziness, flushing, bradycardia, edema
	Slow release: 120–320 mg qd	Long	
Verapamil	Immediate release: 80–160 mg tid	Short	Hypotension, myocardial depression, heart failure, edema, bradycardia
	Slow release: 120–480 mg qd	Long	

Note: This list of calcium channel blockers that may be used to treat patients with angina pectoris is divided into two broad classes, dihydropyridines and nondihydropyridines, and arranged alphabetically within each class. Among the dihydropyridines, the greatest clinical experience has been obtained with amlodipine and nifedipine. After the initial period of dose titration with a short-acting formulation, it is preferable to switch to a sustained release formulation that may be taken once daily to improve patient compliance with the regimen.
[a]May be associated with increased risk of mortality if administered during acute myocardial infarction.
Source: Modified from RJ Gibbons et al.

Choice between Beta Blockers and Calcium Channel Blockers for Initial Therapy

Because beta blockers have been shown to improve life expectancy following acute MI (Chaps. 34 and 35) whereas calcium channel blockers have not, the former may also be preferable in patients with chronic IHD. However, calcium channel blockers are indicated in patients with the following: (1) inadequate responsiveness to the combination of beta blockers and nitrates; many such patients do well with a combination of a beta blocker and a dihydropyridine calcium channel blocker; (2) adverse reactions to beta blockers such as depression, sexual disturbances, and fatigue; (3) angina and a history of asthma or chronic obstructive pulmonary disease; (4) sick-sinus syndrome or significant atrioventricular conduction disturbances; (5) Prinzmetal's angina; or (6) symptomatic peripheral arterial disease.

Antiplatelet Drugs Aspirin is an irreversible inhibitor of platelet cyclooxygenase activity and thereby interferes with platelet activation. Chronic administration of 75–325 mg orally per day has been shown to reduce coronary events in asymptomatic adult men, patients with chronic stable angina, and patients with or who have survived unstable angina and MI. There is a dose-dependent increase in bleeding when aspirin is used chronically. It is preferable to use an enteric-coated formulation in the range of 75–162 mg/d. Administration of this drug should be considered in all patients with IHD in the absence of gastrointestinal bleeding, allergy, or dyspepsia. Clopidogrel (300–600 mg loading and 75 mg/d maintenance) is an oral agent that blocks ADP receptor–mediated platelet aggregation. It provides similar benefits as aspirin in patients with stable chronic IHD and may be substituted for aspirin if aspirin causes the side effects listed earlier. Clopidogrel combined with aspirin reduces death and coronary ischemic events in patients with an acute coronary syndrome (Chap. 34) and also reduces the risk of thrombus formation in patients undergoing implantation of a stent in a coronary artery (Chap. 36).

(In order to reduce the risk of gastrointestinal bleeding, it is recommended that a proton pump inhibitor be prescribed to patients taking a combination of clopidogrel and aspirin.) While combined treatment with clopidogrel and aspirin for at least a year is recommended in patients with an acute coronary syndrome and following implantation of a drug-eluting stent, studies have not shown any benefit of the routine addition of clopidogrel to aspirin in patients with chronic stable IHD.

Other Therapies Angiotensin-converting enzyme (ACE) inhibitors are widely used in the treatment of survivors of MI; patients with hypertension or chronic IHD, including angina pectoris; and those at high risk of vascular disease, such as diabetes. The benefits of ACE inhibitors are most evident in IHD patients at increased risk, especially if diabetes mellitus or LV dysfunction is present, and in those who have not achieved adequate control of blood pressure and LDL cholesterol on beta blockers and statins. However, the routine administration of ACE inhibitors to IHD patients with normal LV function and who have achieved blood pressure and LDL goals on other therapies does not reduce events and therefore is not cost-effective.

Despite treatment with nitrates, beta blockers, or calcium channel blockers, some patients with IHD continue to experience angina, and additional medical therapy is now available to alleviate their symptoms. Ranolazine, a piperazine derivative, was approved for use in January 2006 for patients with chronic angina who continue to be symptomatic despite a standard medical regimen. The mechanism of the antianginal effect of ranolazine is not firmly established, but the leading theory is that the drug inhibits the late inward sodium current (I_{Na}). The benefits of I_{Na} inhibition include limitation of the Na overload of ischemic myocytes and prevention of Ca^{2+} overload via the Na^+-Ca^{2+} exchanger. Prevention of Ca^{2+} overload minimizes diastolic tension and blunts the reduction in coronary nutrient flow that results from compression of the intramyocardial arterioles. A dose of 500–1000 mg orally twice daily is usually well tolerated. Ranolazine is contraindicated in patients with hepatic impairment, with conditions or drugs associated with QT_c prolongation, and when drugs that inhibit the CYP3A metabolic system (e.g., ketoconazole, diltiazem, verapamil, macrolide antibiotics, HIV protease inhibitors, and large quantities of grapefruit juice) are being taken by the patient.

Use of nonsteroidal anti-inflammatory drugs (NSAIDs) in patients with IHD may be associated with a small but finite increased risk of MI and mortality. For this reason, they should generally be avoided in IHD patients. If they are required for symptom relief, it is advisable to coadminister aspirin and strive to use the lowest NSAID dose required for the shortest period of time.

Another class of agents that may be considered are potassium channel openers. These agents open ATP-sensitive potassium channels in myocytes, leading to hyperpolarization of the cell membrane and a reduction of free intracellular calcium ions. The major drug in this class is nicorandil, which is typically administered in a dose of 20 mg twice daily orally for prevention of angina. (Nicorandil is not available for use in the United States but is used in several other countries.) Tolerance to nicorandil's anti-anginal effect may develop with chronic dosing, but there is no cross-tolerance to the organic nitrates.

Angina and Heart Failure Transient LV failure with angina can be controlled by the use of nitrates. For patients with established congestive heart failure, the increased LV wall tension raises myocardial oxygen demand. Treatment of congestive heart failure with an angiotensin-converting enzyme inhibitor, diuretic, and digoxin (Chap. 17) reduces heart size, wall tension, and myocardial oxygen demand, which in turn helps to control angina and ischemia. If the symptoms and signs of heart failure are controlled, an effort should be made to use beta blockers not only for angina but because trials in heart failure have shown significant improvement in survival. A trial of the intravenous ultrashort acting beta blocker esmolol may be useful to establish the safety of beta blockade in individual patients. Nocturnal angina can often be relieved by the treatment of heart failure. Nitrates are useful and can simultaneously improve the disturbed hemodynamics of congestive heart failure by vasodilatation, thereby reducing preload, and relieve angina by preventing or reversing myocardial ischemia. The combination of congestive heart failure and angina in patients with IHD usually indicates a poor prognosis and warrants serious consideration of cardiac catheterization and coronary revascularization.

CORONARY REVASCULARIZATION

Although the basic management of patients with IHD is medical, as described above, many patients are improved by coronary revascularization procedures. *These interventions should be employed in conjunction with but do not replace the continuing need to modify risk factors and medical therapy.* An algorithm for integrating medical therapy and revascularization options in patients with IHD is shown in **Fig. 33-2**.

PERCUTANEOUS CORONARY INTERVENTION

(See also Chap. 36) PCI, involving balloon dilatation usually accompanied by coronary stenting, is widely used to achieve revascularization of the myocardium in patients with symptomatic IHD and suitable stenoses of epicardial coronary arteries. Whereas patients with stenosis of the left main coronary artery and those with three-vessel

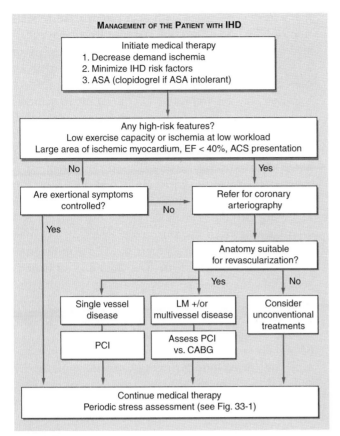

MANAGEMENT OF THE PATIENT WITH IHD

Initiate medical therapy
1. Decrease demand ischemia
2. Minimize IHD risk factors
3. ASA (clopidogrel if ASA intolerant)

Any high-risk features?
Low exercise capacity or ischemia at low workload
Large area of ischemic myocardium, EF < 40%, ACS presentation

No — Are exertional symptoms controlled?

Yes — Refer for coronary arteriography

No

Yes

Anatomy suitable for revascularization?

Yes — No

Single vessel disease — PCI

LM +/or multivessel disease — Assess PCI vs. CABG

Consider unconventional treatments

Continue medical therapy
Periodic stress assessment (see Fig. 33-1)

FIGURE 33-2

Algorithm for management of the patient with ischemic heart disease. All patients should receive the core elements of medical therapy as shown at the top of the algorithm. If high-risk features are present, as established by the clinical history, exercise test data, and imaging studies, the patient should be referred for coronary arteriography. Based on the number and location of the diseased vessels and their suitability for revascularization, the patient is treated with either a percutaneous coronary intervention (PCI), coronary artery bypass graft (CABG) surgery, or should be considered for unconventional treatments. See text for further discussion. IHD, ischemic heart disease; ASA, aspirin; EF, ejection fraction; ACS, acute coronary syndrome; LM, left main.

IHD (especially with diabetes and/or impaired LV function) who require revascularization are best treated with CABG, PCI is widely employed in patients with symptoms and evidence of ischemia due to stenoses of one or two vessels, and even in selected patients with three–vessel disease, and may offer many advantages over surgery.

Indications and Patient Selection

The most common clinical indication for PCI is angina pectoris, despite medical therapy, accompanied by evidence of ischemia during a stress test. PCI is more effective than medical therapy for the relief of angina. Whereas PCI improves outcomes in patients with unstable angina and MI, the value of this procedure in reducing

the occurrence of coronary death and MI in patients with chronic stable angina has not been established. PCI can be used to treat stenoses in native coronary arteries as well as in bypass grafts in patients who have recurrent angina following CABG.

Risks

When coronary stenoses are discrete and symmetric, two and even three vessels can be dilated in sequence. However, case selection is essential in order to avoid a prohibitive risk of complications, which are usually due to dissection or thrombosis with vessel occlusion, uncontrolled ischemia, and ventricular failure (Chap. 36). Oral aspirin, clopidogrel, and an antithrombin are given to reduce coronary thrombus formation. Left main coronary artery stenosis is generally regarded as a contraindication to PCI; such patients should be treated with CABG. In rare cases, such as patients with prohibitive surgical risks, PCI of an unprotected left main can be considered, but such a procedure should only be performed by a highly skilled operator; importantly, there are regional differences in the use of this approach internationally.

Efficacy

Primary success—i.e., adequate dilation (an increase in luminal diameter >20% to a residual diameter obstruction <50%) with relief of angina—is achieved in >95% of cases. Recurrent stenosis of the dilated vessels occurs in ~20% of cases within 6 months of PCI with bare metal stents, and angina will recur within 6 months in 10% of cases. Restenosis is more common in patients with diabetes mellitus, arteries with small caliber, incomplete dilation of the stenosis, occluded vessels, obstructed vein grafts, dilation of the left anterior descending coronary artery, and stenoses containing thrombi. In diseased vein grafts, procedural success has been improved by the use of capture devices or filters that prevent embolization, ischemia, and infarction.

It is usual clinical practice to administer aspirin indefinitely and clopidogrel for 1–3 months after the implantation of a bare metal stent. Although aspirin and the antiplatelet drug clopidogrel may help prevent coronary thrombosis during and shortly following PCI with stenting, there is no evidence that these medications reduce the incidence of restenosis. The use of drug-eluting stents that locally deliver antiproliferative drugs such as rapamycin or paclitaxel can reduce restenosis to near zero within the stent and 3–7% at its edges. Advances in PCI, especially the availability of drug–eluting stents, have vastly extended the use of this revascularization option in patients with IHD. Of note, however, the delayed endothelial healing in the region of a drug-eluting stent also extends the period during which the patient is at risk for subacute stent thrombosis. Current recommendations are to administer aspirin indefinitely and clopidogrel daily for at least 1 year after implantation of a drug-eluting stent. When a situation arises where temporary discontinuation of antiplatelet therapy is desirable, the clinical circumstances should be reviewed with the operator who performed the PCI and a coordinated plan should be established for minimizing the risk of late stent thrombus. Central to this plan is the discontinuation of antiplatelet therapy for the shortest acceptable period of time.

Successful PCI produces effective relief of angina in >95% of cases and has been shown to be more effective than medical therapy for up to 2 years. More than one-half of patients with symptomatic IHD who require revascularization can be treated initially by PCI. Successful PCI is less invasive and expensive than CABG, usually requires only 1–2 days in the hospital, and permits savings in the initial cost of care. Successful PCI also allows earlier return to work and the resumption of an active life. However, this economic benefit is reduced over time because of the greater need for follow-up and for repeat procedures.

CORONARY ARTERY BYPASS GRAFTING

Anastomosis of one or both of the internal mammary arteries or a radial artery to the coronary artery distal to the obstructive lesion is carried out. For additional obstructions that cannot be bypassed by an artery, a section of a vein (usually the saphenous) is used to form a connection between the aorta and the coronary artery distal to the obstructive lesion.

Although some indications for CABG are controversial, certain areas of agreement exist:

1. The operation is relatively safe, with mortality rates <1% in patients without serious comorbid disease and normal LV function, and when the procedure is performed by an experienced surgical team.
2. Intraoperative and postoperative mortality increase with the severity of ventricular dysfunction, comorbidities, age >80 years, and lack of surgical experience. The effectiveness and risk of CABG vary widely depending on case selection and the skill and experience of the surgical team.
3. Occlusion of *venous* grafts is observed in 10–20% of patients during the first postoperative year, in approximately 2% per year during 5- to 7-year follow-up, and in 4% per year thereafter. Long-term patency rates are considerably higher for internal mammary and radial artery implantations than saphenous vein grafts. In patients with left anterior descending coronary artery obstruction, survival is better when coronary bypass involves the internal mammary artery rather than a saphenous vein. Graft patency and outcomes are improved by meticulous treatment of risk factors, particularly dyslipidemia.
4. Angina is abolished or greatly reduced in ~90% of patients following complete revascularization. Although

this is usually associated with graft patency and restoration of blood flow, the pain may also have been alleviated as a result of infarction of the ischemic segment or a placebo effect. Within 3 years, angina recurs in about one-fourth of patients but is rarely severe.

5. Survival may be improved by operation in patients with stenosis of the left main coronary artery as well as in patients with three- or two-vessel disease with significant obstruction of the proximal left anterior descending coronary artery. The survival benefit is greater in patients with abnormal LV function (EF <50%). Survival may also be improved in the following patients: (1) those with obstructive CAD who have survived sudden cardiac death or sustained ventricular tachycardia; (2) those who have undergone previous CABG and who have multiple saphenous vein graft stenoses, especially of a graft supplying the left anterior descending coronary artery; and (3) those with recurrent stenosis following PCI and high-risk criteria on noninvasive testing.
6. Minimally invasive CABG through a small thoracotomy and/or off-pump surgery can reduce morbidity and shorten convalescence in suitable patients but does not appear to significantly reduce the risk of neurocognitive dysfunction postoperatively.

Indications for CABG are usually based on the severity of symptoms, coronary anatomy, and ventricular function. The ideal candidate is male, is <80 years of age, has no other complicating disease, has troublesome or disabling angina that is not adequately controlled by medical therapy or does not tolerate medical therapy and wishes to lead a more active life, and has severe stenoses of two or three epicardial coronary arteries with objective evidence of myocardial ischemia as a cause of the chest discomfort. Great symptomatic benefit can be anticipated in such patients. Congestive heart failure and/or LV dysfunction, advanced age (>80 years), reoperation, urgent need for surgery, and the presence of diabetes mellitus are all associated with a higher perioperative mortality.

LV dysfunction can be due to noncontractile or hypocontractile segments that are viable but are chronically ischemic (hibernating myocardium). As a consequence of chronic reduction in myocardial blood flow these segments downregulate their contractile function. These can be detected by using radionuclide scans of myocardial perfusion and metabolism, PET, CMR imaging, or delayed scanning with thallium-201; or by improvement of regional functional impairment, provoked by low-dose dobutamine. In such patients, revascularization improves myocardial blood flow, can return function, and can improve survival.

The Choice between PCI and CABG

A number of randomized clinical trials have compared PCI and CABG in patients with multivessel CAD who were suitable technically for both procedures. The redevelopment of angina requiring repeat coronary angiography and repeat revascularization is higher with PCI. This is a result of restenosis in the stented segment (a problem largely solved with drug-eluting stents) and the development of new stenoses in unstented portions of the coronary vasculature. It has been argued that PCI with stenting focuses on culprit lesions while a bypass graft to the target vessel also provides a conduit around future culprit lesions proximal to the anastomosis of the graft to the native vessel (**Fig. 33-3**).

Comparison of mortality rates in patients treated with CABG versus PCI is a complex issue. There is an early increased risk of mortality with CABG, but when considering a longer time horizon, such as 5 years, mortality is lower with CABG in comparison with PCI.

Based on available evidence, it is now recommended that patients with an unacceptable level of angina despite optimal medical management be considered for coronary revascularization. Patients with single- or two-vessel disease with normal LV function and anatomically suitable lesions are ordinarily advised to undergo PCI (Chap. 36). Patients with three-vessel disease (or two-vessel disease that includes the proximal left descending coronary artery) and impaired global LV function (LVEF <50%) or diabetes mellitus or those with left main coronary artery disease or other lesions unsuitable for catheter-based procedures should be considered for CABG as the initial method of revascularization.

UNCONVENTIONAL TREATMENTS FOR IHD

On occasion clinicians will encounter a patient with persistent disabling angina despite maximally tolerated medical therapy for whom revascularization is not an option (e.g., small diffusely diseased vessels not amenable to stent implantation or acceptable targets for bypass grafting). In such situations unconventional treatments should be considered.

Enhanced external counterpulsation utilizes pneumatic cuffs on the lower extremities to provide diastolic augmentation and systolic unloading of blood pressure in order to decrease cardiac work and oxygen consumption while enhancing coronary blood flow. Clinical trials have shown that regular application improves angina, exercise capacity, and regional myocardial perfusion.

Additional options include *transmyocardial laser revascularization* (to increase intramyocardial channels of blood flow), and the currently experimental approaches of gene and stem cell therapies are under study.

ASYMPTOMATIC (SILENT) ISCHEMIA

Obstructive CAD, acute MI, and transient myocardial ischemia are frequently asymptomatic. During continuous ambulatory ECG monitoring, the majority of ambulatory patients with typical chronic stable angina are found to have objective evidence of myocardial ischemia (ST-segment depression) during episodes of chest discomfort while they are active outside the hospital, but many of these patients have more frequent episodes of asymptomatic ischemia. In addition, there is a large (but as yet unknown) number of totally asymptomatic persons with severe coronary atherosclerosis who exhibit ST-segment changes during activity. Some of these patients exhibit higher thresholds to electrically induced pain, others show higher endorphin levels, and still others may be diabetics with autonomic dysfunction.

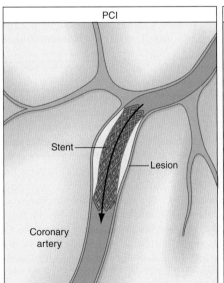

Stent addresses the existing lesion but not future lesions.

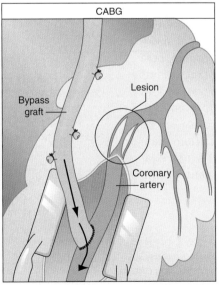

Bypass grafting addresses the existing lesion and also future culprit lesions.

FIGURE 33-3
Difference in the approach to the lesion with percutaneous coronary intervention (PCI) and coronary artery bypass grafting (CABG). PCI is targeted at the "culprit" lesion or lesions, whereas CABG is directed at the epicardial vessel, including the "culprit" lesion or lesions and future culprits, proximal to the insertion of the vein graft, a difference that may account for the superiority of CABG, at least in the intermediate term, in patients with multivessel disease. *(Reproduced from BJ Gersh et al: N Engl J Med 352:2235, 2005.)*

Frequent episodes of ischemia (symptomatic and asymptomatic) during daily life appear to be associated with an increased likelihood of adverse coronary events (death and MI). In addition, patients with asymptomatic ischemia after suffering a MI are at greater risk for a second coronary event. The widespread use of exercise ECG during routine examinations has also identified some of these heretofore unrecognized patients with asymptomatic CAD. Longitudinal studies have demonstrated an increased incidence of coronary events in asymptomatic patients with positive exercise tests.

Treatment: ASYMPTOMATIC ISCHEMIA

The management of patients with asymptomatic ischemia must be individualized. Thus, the physician should consider the following: (1) the degree of positivity of the stress test, particularly the stage of exercise at which ECG signs of ischemia appear, the magnitude and number of the ischemic zones of myocardium on imaging, and the change in LVEF which occurs on radionuclide ventriculography or echocardiography during ischemia and/or during exercise; (2) the ECG leads showing a positive response, with changes in the anterior precordial leads indicating a less favorable prognosis than changes in the inferior leads; and (3) the patient's age, occupation, and general medical condition.

Most would agree that an asymptomatic 45-year-old commercial airline pilot with 0.4-mV ST-segment depression in leads V$_1$ to V$_4$ during mild exercise should undergo coronary arteriography, whereas the asymptomatic, sedentary 75-year-old retiree with 0.1-mV ST-segment depression in leads II and III during maximal activity need not. However, there is no consensus about the appropriate procedure in the large majority of patients for whom the situation is less extreme. Asymptomatic patients with silent ischemia, three-vessel CAD, and impaired LV function may be considered appropriate candidates for CABG.

The treatment of risk factors, particularly lipid lowering as described above, and the use of aspirin, beta blockers, and statins have been shown to reduce events and improve outcomes in asymptomatic as well as symptomatic patients with ischemia and proven CAD. While the incidence of asymptomatic ischemia can be reduced by treatment with beta blockers, calcium channel blockers, and long-acting nitrates, it is not clear whether this is necessary or desirable in patients who have not suffered a MI.

FURTHER READINGS

Antman EM et al: Use of nonsteroidal anti-inflammatory drugs: An update for clinicians: A scientific statement from the American Heart Association. Circulation 115:1634, 2007; http://circ.ahajournals.org/cgi/content/full/115/12/1634

Bhatt DL et al: Clopidogrel and aspirin versus aspirin alone for the prevention of atherothrombotic events. N Engl J Med 354:1706, 2006

Boden WE et al: Optimal medical therapy with or without PCI for stable coronary disease. N Engl J Med 356:1503, 2007

Chaitman BR: Ranolazine for the treatment of chronic angina and potential use in other cardiovascular conditions. Circulation 113:2462, 2006

Cleeman JI et al: Executive summary of the Third Report of the National Cholesterol Education Program (NCEP) Expert Panel on Detection, Evaluation, and Treatment of High Blood Cholesterol in Adults (Adult Treatment Panel III). JAMA 285:2486, 2001

Defeyter PJ et al: Bypass surgery versus stenting for the treatment of multivessel disease in patients with unstable angina compared with stable angina. Circulation 105:2367, 2002

Frye RL et al: A randomized trial of therapies for type 2 diabetes and coronary artery disease. N Engl J Med 360:2503, 2009

Gibbons RJ et al: ACC/AHA 2002 guideline update for the management of patients with chronic stable angina: A report of the American College of Cardiology/American Heart Association Task Force on Practice Guidelines (Committee to Update the 1999 Guidelines for the Management of Patients with Chronic Stable Angina), 2002. http://acc.org/qualityandscience/clinical/guidelines/stable/update_index.htm

Goldschmidt-Clermont PJ et al: Atherosclerosis 2005: Recent discoveries and novel hypotheses. Circulation 112:3348, 2005

Kim MC et al: Refractory angina pectoris. Mechanism and therapeutic options. J Am Coll Cardiol 39:923, 2002

Lee TH et al: Noninvasive tests in patients with stable coronary artery disease. N Engl J Med 344:1840, 2001

Marasco SF et al: No improvement in neurocognitive outcomes after off-pump versus on-pump coronary revascularisation: a meta-analysis. Eur J Cardiothorac Surg 33:961, 2008

McQueen MJ et al: Lipids, lipoproteins, and apolipoproteins as risk markers of myocardial infarction in 52 countries (the INTERHEART study): a case-control study. Lancet 372:224, 2008

Mega JL et al: Cytochrome p-450 polymorphisms and response to clopidogrel. N Engl J Med 360:354, 2009

Morrow D et al: Chronic ischemic heart disease, in Braunwald's Heart Disease, 7th ed, D Zipes et al (eds). Philadelphia, Saunders, 2005

Morrow D et al: Chronic coronary artery disease, in Braunwald's Heart Disease, 8th ed, P Libby et al (eds). Philadelphia, Saunders, 2008

Opie LH et al: Controversies in stable coronary artery disease. Lancet 367:69, 2006

Pretre R et al: Choice of revascularization strategy for patients with coronary artery disease. JAMA 285:992, 2001

Serruys PW et al: Percutaneous coronary intervention versus coronary-artery bypass grafting for severe coronary artery disease. N Engl J Med 360:961, 2009

Smith SC Jr et al: ACC/AHA/SCAI 2005 guideline update for percutaneous coronary intervention: A report of the American College of Cardiology/American Heart Association Task Force on Practice Guidelines (ACC/AHA/SCAI Writing Committee to Update the 2001 Guidelines for Percutaneous Coronary Intervention). American College of Cardiology website. http://acc.org/qualityandscience/clinical/guidelines/percutaneous/update/index.pdf

Van den Brand MJBM et al: The effect of completeness of revascularization on event-free survival at one year in the ARTS trial. J Am Coll Cardiol 39:559, 2002

Weintraub WS et al: Predicting cardiovascular events with coronary calcium scoring. N Engl J Med 358:1394, 2008

CHAPTER 34

UNSTABLE ANGINA AND NON-ST-ELEVATION MYOCARDIAL INFARCTION

Christopher P. Cannon ■ Eugene Braunwald

Patients with ischemic heart disease fall into two large groups: patients with chronic coronary artery disease (CAD) who most commonly present with stable angina (Chap. 33) and patients with acute coronary syndromes (ACSs). The latter group, in turn, is composed of patients with acute myocardial infarction (MI) with ST-segment elevation on their presenting electrocardiogram (STEMI; Chap. 35) and those with unstable angina and non-ST-segment elevation MI (UA/NSTEMI; see Fig. 35-1). Every year in the United States, ~1.3 million patients are admitted to hospitals with UA/NSTEMI in comparison with ~300,000 patients with acute STEMI. The relative incidence of UA/NSTEMI in comparison with STEMI appears to be increasing. Almost one-half of patients with UA/NSTEMI are women, while more than three-fourths of patients with STEMI are men.

DEFINITION

The diagnosis of UA is based largely on the clinical presentation. *Stable* angina pectoris is characterized by chest or arm discomfort that may not be described as pain but is reproducibly associated with physical exertion or stress and is relieved within 5–10 min by rest and/or sublingual nitroglycerin (Chaps. 4 and 33). UA is defined as angina pectoris or equivalent ischemic discomfort with at least one of three features: (1) it occurs at rest (or with minimal exertion), usually lasting >10 min; (2) it is severe and of new onset (i.e., within the prior 4–6 weeks); and/or (3) it occurs with a crescendo pattern (i.e., distinctly more severe, prolonged, or frequent than previously). The diagnosis of NSTEMI is established if a patient with the clinical features of UA develops evidence of myocardial necrosis, as reflected in elevated cardiac biomarkers.

PATHOPHYSIOLOGY

UA/NSTEMI is most commonly caused by a reduction in oxygen supply and/or by an increase in myocardial oxygen demand superimposed on an atherosclerotic coronary plaque, with varying degrees of obstruction. Four pathophysiologic processes that may contribute to the development of UA/NSTEMI have been identified: (1) plaque rupture or erosion with superimposed nonocclusive thrombus, believed to be the most common cause—NSTEMI may occur with downstream embolization of platelet aggregates and/or atherosclerotic debris; (2) dynamic obstruction [e.g., coronary spasm, as in Prinzmetal's variant angina (p. 393)]; (3) progressive mechanical obstruction [e.g., rapidly advancing coronary atherosclerosis or restenosis following percutaneous coronary intervention (PCI)]; and (4) secondary UA related to increased myocardial oxygen demand and/or decreased supply (e.g., tachycardia, anemia). More than one of these processes may be involved.

Among patients with UA/NSTEMI studied at angiography, ~5% have left main stenosis, 15% have three-vessel CAD, 30% have two-vessel disease, 40% have single-vessel disease, and 10% have no critical coronary stenosis; some of the latter have Prinzmetal's variant angina (see later). The "culprit lesion" on angiography may show an eccentric stenosis with scalloped or overhanging edges and a narrow neck. Angioscopy may reveal "white" (platelet-rich) thrombi, as opposed to "red" thrombi, more often seen in patients with acute STEMI. Patients with UA/NSTEMI often have multiple plaques vulnerable to disruption.

CLINICAL PRESENTATION

History and Physical Examination

The clinical hallmark of UA/NSTEMI is chest pain, typically located in the substernal region or sometimes in the epigastrium that radiates to the neck, left shoulder, and left arm (Chap. 4). The discomfort is usually severe enough to be considered painful. Anginal "equivalents" such as dyspnea and epigastric discomfort may also occur, and these appear to occur more often in women. The examination resembles that in patients with stable angina (Chap. 33) and may be unremarkable. If the patient has a large area of myocardial ischemia or a large NSTEMI, the physical findings can include diaphoresis, pale cool skin, sinus tachycardia, a third and/or fourth heart sound, basilar rales, and sometimes hypotension, resembling the findings of large STEMI.

Electrocardiogram

In UA, ST-segment depression, transient ST-segment elevation, and/or T-wave inversion occur in 30–50% of patients, depending on the severity of the clinical presentation. In patients with the clinical features of UA, the presence of new ST-segment deviation, even of only 0.05 mV, is an important predictor of adverse outcome. T-wave changes are sensitive for ischemia but less specific, unless they are new, deep T-wave inversions (≥0.3 mV).

Cardiac Biomarkers

Patients with UA who have elevated biomarkers of necrosis, such as CK-MB and troponin (a much more specific and sensitive marker of myocardial necrosis), are at increased risk for death or recurrent MI. Elevated levels of these markers distinguish patients with NSTEMI from those with UA. There is a direct relationship between the degree of troponin elevation and mortality. However, in patients *without* a clear clinical history of myocardial ischemia, minor troponin elevations have been reported and can be caused by congestive heart failure, myocarditis,

or pulmonary embolism, or they may be false-positive readings. Thus, in patients with an *unclear* history, small troponin elevations may not be diagnostic of an ACS.

DIAGNOSTIC EVALUATION

(See also Chap. 4) Approximately 6–7 million persons per year in the United States present to hospital emergency departments (EDs) with a complaint of chest pain or other symptoms suggestive of ACS. A diagnosis of an ACS is established in 20–25% of such patients. The first step in evaluating patients with possible UA/NSTEMI is to determine the *likelihood* that CAD is the cause of the presenting symptoms. The American College of Cardiology/American Heart Association (ACC/AHA) Guidelines include, among the factors associated with a high likelihood of ACS, a clinical history typical of ischemic discomfort, a history of established CAD by angiography, prior MI, congestive heart failure, new electrocardiographic (ECG) changes, or elevated cardiac biomarkers. Factors associated with an intermediate likelihood of ACS in patients with the clinical features of this condition but without the above high-risk factors are: age >70 years, male gender, diabetes mellitus, known peripheral arterial or cerebrovascular disease, and old ECG abnormalities.

Diagnostic Pathways

Four major diagnostic tools are used in the diagnosis of UA/NSTEMI in the ED: the clinical history, the ECG, cardiac markers, and stress testing. The goals are to (1) recognize or exclude MI (using cardiac markers), (2) evaluate for rest ischemia (chest pain at rest, serial or continuous ECGs), and (3) evaluate for significant CAD (using provocative stress testing). Typical pathways begin with assessment of the likelihood that the presenting symptoms are due to ischemia. Patients with a low likelihood of ischemia are usually managed with an ED-based critical pathway (which in some institutions is carried out in a "chest pain unit" (Fig. 34-1). Evaluation of such patients includes clinical monitoring for recurrent ischemic discomfort, serial ECGs, and cardiac markers, typically performed at baseline and at 4–6 h and 12 h after presentation. If new elevations in cardiac markers (CK-MB and/or troponin) or ECG changes are noted, the patient is admitted to the hospital. If the patient remains pain-free and the markers are negative, the patient may go on to stress testing. This may be performed as early as 6 h after presentation in the ED or chest pain center, or on an outpatient basis within 72 h. For most patients, standard treadmill ECG stress testing is used, but for patients with fixed abnormalities on the ECG (e.g., left bundle branch block), perfusion or echocardiographic imaging is used. For patients who cannot walk, pharmacologic stress is used. By demonstrating normal myocardial perfusion, sestamibi or thallium imaging can reduce unnecessary hospitalizations by excluding acute ischemia. CT angiography is used with increasing frequency to exclude obstructive CAD (Chap. 12).

RISK STRATIFICATION AND PROGNOSIS

Patients with documented UA/NSTEMI exhibit a wide spectrum of early (30 days) risk of death, ranging from

1–10%, and of new or recurrent infarction of 3–10%. Assessment of "global risk" can be accomplished by clinical risk scoring systems such as that developed from in the Thrombolysis in Myocardial Infarction (TIMI) Trials, which includes seven independent risk factors: age ≥ 65 years, three or more risk factors for CAD, documented CAD at catheterization, development of UA/NSTEMI while on aspirin, more than two episodes of angina within the preceding 24 h, ST deviation ≥0.5 mm, and an elevated cardiac marker (**Fig. 34-2**). Other risk factors include diabetes mellitus, left ventricular dysfunction, and elevated levels of creatinine, atrial natriuretic peptides, and C-reactive protein. Early risk assessment (especially using troponin, ST-segment changes, and/or a global risk scoring system) is useful both in predicting the risk of recurrent cardiac events and in identifying those patients who would derive the greatest benefit from antithrombotic therapies more potent than unfractionated heparin, such as low-molecular-weight heparin (LMWH) and glycoprotein (GP)IIb/IIIa inhibitors, and from an early invasive strategy. For example, in the TACTICS-TIMI 18 Trial, an early invasive strategy conferred a 40% reduction in recurrent cardiac events in patients with a positive troponin level, whereas no benefit was observed in those with a negative troponin level.

C-reactive protein, a marker of vascular inflammation, and B-type natriuretic peptide, a marker of increased myocardial wall tension, correlate independently with increased mortality (and, in some studies, recurrent cardiac events) in patients presenting with UA/NSTEMI. Multimarker strategies are now gaining favor both to define the pathophysiologic mechanisms underlying a given patient's presentation more fully and to stratify the patient's risk further.

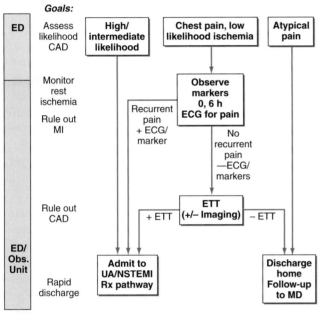

FIGURE 34-1

Diagnostic evaluation of patients presenting with suspected UA/NSTEMI. The first step is to assess the likelihood of coronary artery disease (CAD). Patients at *high* or *intermediate* likelihood are admitted to the hospital. Those with clearly atypical chest pain are sent home. Patients with a *low* likelihood of ischemia enter the pathway and are observed in a monitored bed in the emergency department (ED) or observation unit over a period of 6 h, and 12-lead electrocardiograms are performed if the patient has recurrent chest discomfort. A panel of cardiac markers (e.g., troponin and CK-MB) is drawn at baseline and 6 h later. If the patient develops recurrent pain, has ST-segment or T-wave changes, or has positive cardiac markers, he/she is admitted to the hospital and treated for UA/NSTEMI. If the patient has negative markers and no recurrence of pain, he/she is sent for exercise treadmill testing, with imaging reserved for patients with abnormal baseline electrocardiograms (e.g., left bundle branch block or left ventricular hypertrophy). If positive, the patient is admitted; if negative, the patient is discharged, with follow-up to his/her primary physician. ETT, exercise tolerance test; MI, myocardial infarction. [*Adapted from CP Cannon, E Braunwald, in Heart Disease: A Textbook of Cardiovascular Medicine, 6th ed, E Braunwald et al (eds). Philadelphia, Saunders, 2001.*]

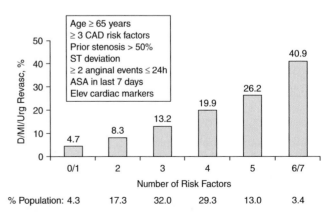

FIGURE 34-2

The TIMI Risk Score for UA/NSTEMI, a simple but comprehensive clinical risk stratification score to identify increasing risk of death, myocardial infarction, or urgent revascularization to day 14. CAD, coronary artery disease; ASA, aspirin. (*Adapted from Antman et al.*)

Treatment:
℞ UNSTABLE ANGINA AND NON-ST ELEVATION MYOCARDIAL INFARCTION

MEDICAL TREATMENT Patients with UA/NSTEMI should be placed at bed rest with continuous ECG monitoring for ST-segment deviation and cardiac rhythm. Ambulation is permitted if the patient shows no recurrence of ischemia (discomfort or ECG changes) and does not develop a biomarker of necrosis for 12–24 h. Medical therapy involves simultaneous anti-ischemic treatment and antithrombotic treatment.

ANTI-ISCHEMIC TREATMENT (Table 34-1) In order to provide relief and prevention of recurrence of chest pain, initial treatment should include bed rest, nitrates, and beta blockers.

Nitrates Nitrates should first be given sublingually or by buccal spray (0.3–0.6 mg) if the patient is experiencing ischemic pain. If pain persists after three doses given 5 min apart, intravenous nitroglycerin (5–10 μg/min using nonabsorbing tubing) is recommended. The rate of the infusion may be increased by 10 μg/min every 3–5 min until symptoms are relieved or systolic arterial pressure falls to <100 mmHg. Topical or oral nitrates (Chap. 33) can be used once the pain has resolved, or they may replace intravenous nitroglycerin when the patient has been pain-free for 12–24 h. The only absolute contraindications to the use of nitrates are hypotension or the use of sildenafil (Viagra) or other drugs in that class within the previous 24 h.

β-Adrenergic Blockade These agents are the other mainstay of anti-ischemic treatment. Intravenous beta blockade followed by oral beta blockade targeted to a heart rate of 50–60 beats/min is recommended. Heart rate–slowing calcium channel blockers, e.g., verapamil or diltiazem, are recommended in patients who have persistent or recurrent symptoms after treatment with full-dose nitrates and beta blockers and in patients with contraindications to beta blockade. Additional medical therapy includes angiotensin-converting enzyme (ACE) inhibition and HMG-CoA reductase inhibitors (statins) for long-term secondary prevention.

If pain persists despite intravenous nitroglycerin and beta blockade, morphine sulfate, 1–5 mg intravenously, can be administered every 5–30 min as needed.

ANTITHROMBOTIC THERAPY (Table 34-2) This is the other main component of treatment for UA/NSTEMI. Initial treatment should begin with the platelet cyclooxygenase inhibitor aspirin (Fig 34-3). The typical initial dose is 325 mg daily, with lower doses (75–162 mg daily) recommended for long-term therapy. "Aspirin resistance" has been noted in research studies in 5–10% of patients and more frequently in patients treated with lower doses of aspirin. No clear guidelines are available regarding evaluation or treatment, but the use of higher doses of aspirin and/or a thienopyridine (clopidogrel) appears to be logical in this situation.

The thienopyridine clopidogrel, which blocks the platelet $P2Y_{12}$ (adenosine) receptor (in combination with aspirin), was shown in the CURE trial to confer a 20% relative reduction in cardiovascular death, MI, or stroke, compared with aspirin alone in both low- and high-risk patients with UA/NSTEMI, but to be associated with a moderate (absolute 1%) increase in major bleeding, which is more common in patients who undergo coronary artery bypass grafting. Pretreatment with clopidogrel (a 300 or 600 mg loading dose, followed by 75 mg qd) has also been shown in three studies to reduce adverse outcomes associated with and following PCI and has a Class I, Grade A evidence recommendation in the PCI Guidelines (Chap. 36). Continued benefit of long-term (~1 year) treatment with the combination of clopidogrel and aspirin has been observed both in patients treated conservatively and in those who underwent a PCI. This combination is recommended for all patients with UA/NSTEMI who are not at excessive risk for bleeding.

Four options are available for anticoagulation therapy to be added to aspirin and clopidogrel. Unfractionated heparin (UFH) is the mainstay of therapy. The LMWH enoxaparin has been shown in several studies to be superior to UFH in reducing recurrent cardiac events, especially in conservatively managed patients. The Factor Xa inhibitor fondaparinux is equivalent for early efficacy compared with enoxaparin but appears to have a lower risk of major bleeding and thus may have the best benefit risk ratio. However, UFH, LMWH, or a direct thrombin inhibitor such as bivalirudin should be used during cardiac catheterization or PCI. Preliminary data indicate that bivalirudin is equivalent (for both efficacy and safety) to either UFH or enoxaparin among patients treated with a GP IIb/IIIa inhibitor, but use of bivalirudin alone had less bleeding than the combination of a heparin and GP IIb/IIIa inhibitor in patients with UA/NSTEMI undergoing PCI.

Intravenous GP IIb/IIIa inhibitors have also been shown to be beneficial in treating UA/NSTEMI. For "upstream" management of high-risk patients in whom an invasive management is intended (i.e., initiating therapy when the patient first presents to the hospital), the small molecule inhibitors eptifibatide and tirofiban show benefit, whereas the monoclonal antibody abciximab appears not to be effective in patients treated conservatively, (i.e., in those not undergoing coronary angiography or PCI). However, abciximab has been shown to be beneficial in patients with UA/NSTEMI undergoing PCI, even among troponin positive patients

TABLE 34-1

DRUGS COMMONLY USED IN INTENSIVE MEDICAL MANAGEMENT OF PATIENTS WITH UNSTABLE ANGINA AND NON-ST ELEVATION MI			
DRUG CATEGORY	**CLINICAL CONDITION**	**WHEN TO AVOID**[a]	**DOSAGE**
Nitrates	Administer intravenously when symptoms are not fully relieved with three sublingual nitroglycerin tablets and initiation of beta-blocker therapy	Hypotension patient receiving sildenafil or other PDE-5 inhibitor	5–10 µg/min by continuous infusion Titrated up to 75–100 µg/min until relief of symptoms or limiting side effects (headache or hypotension with a systolic blood pressure <90 mmHg or >30% below starting mean arterial pressure levels if significant hypertension is present) Topical, oral, or buccal nitrates are acceptable alternatives for patients without ongoing or refractory symptoms
Beta blockers[b]	Unstable angina	PR interval (ECG) >0.24 s 2° or 3° atrioventricular block Heart rate <60 beats/min Blood pressure <90 mmHg Shock Left ventricular failure with congestive heart failure Severe reactive airway disease	Metoprolol[c] 5-mg increments by slow (over 1–2 min IV administration) Repeated every 5 min for a total initial dose of 15 mg Followed in 1–2 h by 25–50 mg by mouth every 6 h If a very conservative regimen is desired, initial doses can be reduced to 1–2 mg Esmolol[c] Starting maintenance dose of 0.1 mg/kg per min IV Titration in increments of 0.05 mg/kg per min every 10–15 min as tolerated by blood pressure until the desired therapeutic response has been obtained, limiting symptoms develop, or a dose of 0.20 mg/kg per min is reached Optional loading dose of 0.5 mg/kg may be given by slow IV administration (2–5 min) for more rapid onset of action
Calcium channel blockers	Patients whose symptoms are not relieved by adequate doses of nitrates and beta blockers or in patients unable to tolerate adequate doses of one or both of these agents or in patients with variant angina	Pulmonary edema Evidence of left ventricular dysfunction (for diltiazem or verapamil)	Dependent on specific agent
Morphine sulfate	Patients whose symptoms are not relieved after three serial sublingual nitroglycerin tablets or whose symptoms recur with adequate anti-ischemic therapy	Hypotension Respiratory depression Confusion Obtundation	2–5 mg IV dose May be repeated every 5–30 min as needed to relieve symptoms and maintain patient comfort

[a]Allergy or prior intolerance is a contraindication for all categories of drugs listed in this chart.
[b]Choice of the specific agent is not as important as ensuring that appropriate candidates receive this therapy. If there are concerns about patient intolerance owing to existing pulmonary disease, especially asthma, left ventricular dysfunction, risk of hypotension or severe bradycardia, initial selection should favor a short-acting agent, such as propranolol or metoprolol or the ultra-short-acting agent esmolol. Mild wheezing or a history of chronic obstructive pulmonary disease should prompt a trial of a short-acting agent at a reduced dose (e.g., 2.5 mg IV metoprolol, 12.5 mg oral metoprolol, or 25 µg/kg per min esmolol as initial doses) rather than complete avoidance of beta-blocker therapy.
[c]Metoprolol and esmolol are two of several beta blockers that may be employed.
Note: Several recommendations in this guide suggest the use of agents for purposes or in doses other than those specified by the U.S. Food and Drug Administration. Such recommendations are made after consideration of concerns regarding nonapproved indications. Where made such recommendations are based on more recent clinical trials or expert consensus.
IV, intravenous; aPTT, activated partial thromboplastin time; ECG, electrocardiogram; 2Υ, second-degree; 3Υ, third-degree.
Source: Modified from E Braunwald et al: Circulation 1994;90:613–622.

TABLE 34-2

CLINICAL USE OF ANTITHROMBOTIC THERAPY

Oral Antiplatelet Therapy

Aspirin	Initial dose of 162–325 mg nonenteric formulation followed by 75–162 mg/d of an enteric or a nonenteric formulation
Clopidogrel (Plavix)	Loading dose of 300 mg followed by 75 mg/d

Intravenous Antiplatelet Therapy

Abciximab (ReoPro)	0.25 mg/kg bolus followed by infusion of 0.125 µg/kg per min (maximum 10 µg/min) for 12 to 24 h
Eptifibatide (Integrilin)	180 µg/kg bolus followed by infusion of 2.0 µg/kg per min for 72 to 96 h
Tirofiban (Aggrastat)	0.4 µg/kg per min for 30 min followed by infusion of 0.1 µg/kg per min for 48 to 96 h

Heparins[a]

Heparin (UFH)	Bolus 60–70 U/kg (maximum 5000 U) IV followed by infusion of 12–15 U/kg per h (initial maximum 1000 U/h) titrated to a PTT 50–70 s
Enoxaparin (Lovenox)	1 mg/kg SC every 12 h; the first dose may be preceded by a 30-mg IV bolus; renal adjustment to 1 mg/kg once daily if creatine Cl < 30 cc/min
Fondaparinux	2.5 mg SQ qd
Bivalirudin	Initial bolus intravenous bolus of 0.1 mg/kg and an infusion of 0.25 mg/kg per hour. Before PCI, an additional intravenous bolus of 0.5 mg/kg was administered, and the infusion was increased to 1.75 mg/kg per hour.

[a]Other LMWH exist beyond those listed.
Note: IV, intravenous; SC, subcutaneously; UFH, unfractionated heparin.
Source: Modified from E Braunwald et al: J Am Coll Cardiol 2000; 36:970–1056.

pretreated with clopidogrel. The ACC/AHA Guidelines note that these agents can be started either in the ED or during PCI. As with all antithrombotic agents, bleeding is the most important adverse effect of antiplatelet drugs, especially their combination. Thus, patients with a history of bleeding must be screened carefully and given fewer antithrombotic agents.

INVASIVE VERSUS CONSERVATIVE STRAT-EGY Multiple clinical trials have shown the benefit of an early invasive strategy in high-risk patients, i.e., patients with multiple clinical risk factors, ST-segment deviation, and/or positive biomarkers (Table 34-3). In

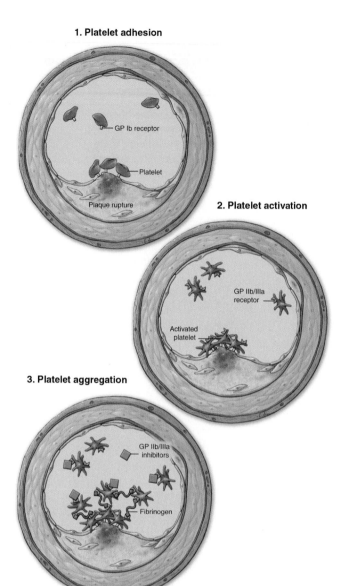

FIGURE 34-3

Platelets initiate thrombosis at the site of a ruptured plaque with denuded endothelium: *Platelet adhesion* occurs via (1) the GP 1b receptor in conjunction with von Willebrand factor. This is followed by *platelet activation* (2), which leads to a shape change in the platelet, degranulation of the alpha and dense granules, and expression of glycoprotein IIb/IIIa receptors on the platelet surface with activation of the receptor, such that it can bind fibrinogen. The final step is *platelet aggregation* (3), in which fibrinogen (or von Willebrand factor) binds to the activated GP IIb/IIIa receptors. Aspirin (ASA) and clopidogrel act to decrease platelet activation, whereas the GP IIb/IIIa inhibitors inhibit the final step of platelet aggregation. GP, glycoprotein. [*Modified from CP Cannon, E Braunwald, in Heart Disease: A Textbook of Cardiovascular Medicine, 8th ed, P Libby et al (eds). Philadelphia, Saunders, 2008.*]

TABLE 34-3

CLASS I RECOMMENDATIONS FOR USE OF AN EARLY INVASIVE STRATEGY[a]

Class I (level of evidence: a) indications

Recurrent angina at rest/low-level activity despite Rx
Elevated TnT or TnI
New ST-segment depression
Rec. angina/ischemia with CHF symptoms, rales, MR
Positive stress test
EF < 0.40
Decreased BP
Sustained VT
PCI < 6 months, prior CABG

[a]Any one of the high-risk indicators.
Note: TnT, troponin T; TnI, troponin I; Rec, recurrent; CHF, congestive heart failure; MR, mitral regurgitation; EF, ejection fraction; BP, blood pressure; VT, ventricular tachycardia; PCI, percutaneous coronary intervention; CABG, coronary artery bypass grafting.
Source: E Braunwald et al: Circulation 106:1893, 2002.

this strategy, following treatment with anti-ischemic and antithrombotic agents, coronary arteriography is carried out within ~48 h of admission, followed by coronary revascularization (PCI or coronary artery bypass grafting), depending on the coronary anatomy.

In low-risk patients, the outcomes from an invasive strategy are similar to those obtained from a conservative strategy, which consists of anti-ischemic and antithrombotic therapy followed by "watchful waiting," in which coronary arteriography is carried out only if rest pain or ST-segment changes recur or there is evidence of ischemia on a stress test.

LONG-TERM MANAGEMENT

The time of hospital discharge is a "teachable moment" for the patient with UA/NSTEMI, when the physician can review and optimize the medical regimen. Risk factor modification is key, and the physician should discuss with the patient the importance of smoking cessation, achieving optimal weight, daily exercise following an appropriate diet, blood pressure control, tight control of hyperglycemia (for diabetic patients), and lipid management, as recommended for patients with chronic stable angina (Chap. 33).

There is evidence of benefit with long-term therapy with five classes of drugs that are directed at different components of the atherothrombotic process. Beta blockers are appropriate anti-ischemic therapy and may help decrease triggers for MI. Statins (at a high dose, e.g., atorvastatin 80 mg/d) and ACE inhibitors are recommended for long-term plaque stabilization. Antiplatelet therapy, now recommended to be the combination of aspirin and

clopidogrel for at least 9–12 months, with aspirin continued thereafter, prevents or reduces the severity of any thrombosis that would occur if a plaque does rupture. Thus, a multifactorial approach to long-term medical therapy is directed at preventing the various components of atherothrombosis. This therapy should be begun early, i.e. within a week of the event, whenever possible.

Observational registries have shown that patients with UA/NSTEMI at high risk, including women and the elderly as well as racial minorities, are less likely to receive evidence-based pharmacologic and interventional therapies with resultant poorer clinical outcomes and quality of life.

PRINZMETAL'S VARIANT ANGINA

In 1959 Prinzmetal et al. described a syndrome of ischemic pain that occurs at rest but not usually with exertion and is associated with transient ST-segment elevation. The syndrome is due to focal spasm of an epicardial coronary artery, leading to severe myocardial ischemia. The exact cause of the spasm is not well defined, but it may be related to hypercontractility of vascular smooth muscle due to vasoconstrictor mitogens, leukotrienes, or serotonin. In some patients it is a manifestation of a vasospastic disorder and is associated with migraine, Raynaud's phenomenon, or aspirin-induced asthma.

Clinical and Angiographic Manifestations

Patients with variant angina are generally younger and have fewer coronary risk factors (with the exception of cigarette smoking) than patients with UA secondary to coronary atherosclerosis. The anginal discomfort is often extremely severe and has usually not progressed from a period of chronic stable angina. Cardiac examination is usually normal in the absence of ischemia.

The clinical diagnosis of variant angina is made with the detection of transient ST-segment *elevation* with rest pain. Many patients also exhibit multiple episodes of asymptomatic ST-segment elevation (*silent ischemia*). Small elevations of CK-MB and troponin may occur in patients with prolonged attacks of variant angina. Exercise testing in patients with variant angina is of limited value because the patients can demonstrate ST elevation, depression, or no ST changes.

Coronary angiography demonstrates transient coronary spasm as the diagnostic hallmark of Prinzmetal's angina. Atherosclerotic plaques, which do not usually cause critical obstruction, in at least one proximal coronary artery occur in the majority of patients, and in them spasm usually occurs within 1 cm of the plaque. Focal spasm is most common in the right coronary artery, and it may occur at one or more sites in one artery or in multiple arteries simultaneously. Ergonovine, acetylcholine, other vasoconstrictor medications, and hyperventilation have been used to provoke and demonstrate focal coronary stenosis to establish the diagnosis. Hyperventilation has also been used to provoke rest angina, ST-segment elevation, and spasm on coronary arteriography.

Rx Treatment: Prinzmetal's Variant Angina

Nitrates and calcium channel blockers are the main treatments for patients with variant angina. Sublingual or intravenous nitroglycerin often abolishes episodes of variant angina promptly, and long-acting nitrates are useful in preventing recurrences. Calcium antagonists are extremely effective in preventing the coronary artery spasm of variant angina, and they should be prescribed in maximally tolerated doses. Similar efficacy rates have been noted among the various types of calcium antagonists. Prazosin, a selective α-adrenoreceptor blocker, has also been found to be of value in some patients, while aspirin may actually increase the severity of ischemic episodes. The response to beta blockers is variable. Coronary revascularization may be helpful in patients with variant angina who also have discrete, proximal fixed obstructive lesions.

Prognosis

Many patients with Prinzmetal's angina pass through an acute, active phase, with frequent episodes of angina and cardiac events during the first 6 months after presentation. Long-term survival at 5 years is excellent (~90–95%). Patients with no or mild fixed coronary obstruction tend to experience a more benign course than do patients with associated severe obstructive lesions. Nonfatal MI occurs in up to 20% of patients by 5 years. Patients with variant angina who develop serious arrhythmias during spontaneous episodes of pain are at a higher risk for sudden death. In most patients who survive an infarction or the initial 3–6-month period of frequent episodes, the condition stabilizes, and there is a tendency for symptoms and cardiac events to diminish with time.

FURTHER READINGS

ALEXANDER KP et al: Excess dosing of antiplatelet and antithrombin agents in the treatment of non-ST-segment elevation acute coronary syndromes. JAMA 294:3108, 2005

ANDERSON JL et al: ACC/AHA 2007 guidelines for the management of patients with unstable angina/non-ST-Elevation myocardial infarction: a report of the American College of Cardiology/American Heart Association Task Force on Practice Guidelines. Circulation 116:e148, 2007

ANTMAN EM et al: The TIMI risk score for unstable angina/non-ST elevation MI: A method for prognostication and therapeutic decision making. JAMA 284:835, 2000

BRAUNWALD E et al: ACC/AHA 2002 guideline update for the management of patients with unstable angina and non-ST segment elevation myocardial infarction: A report of the American College of Cardiology/American Heart Association Task Force on Practice Guidelines (Committee on the Management of Unstable Angina). URL: *http://www.acc.org/qualityandscience/clinical/guidelines/unstable/update_index.htm*

CANNON CP, BRAUNWALD E: Unstable angina, in *Braunwald's Heart Disease*, 8th ed, P Libby et al (eds). Philadelphia, Saunders, 2008

———: Unstable angina, in *Braunwald's Heart Disease*, 9th ed, R Bonow et al (eds). Philadelphia, Saunders, 2010

——— et al: Intensive versus moderate lipid lowering with statins after acute coronary syndromes. N Engl J Med 350:1495, 2004

CLOPIDOGREL IN UNSTABLE ANGINA TO PREVENT RECURRENT EVENTS TRIAL INVESTIGATORS: Effects of clopidogrel in addition to aspirin in patients with acute coronary syndromes without ST-segment elevation. N Engl J Med 345:494, 2001

GIUGLIANO RP, BRAUNWALD E: The year in non-ST segment elevation acute coronary syndromes. J Am Coll Cardiol (in press)

——— et al: Early versus delayed, provisional eptifibatide in acute coronary syndromes. N Engl J Med 360:2176, 2009

KASTRATI A et al: Abciximab in patients with acute coronary syndromes undergoing percutaneous coronary intervention after clopidogrel pretreatment: The ISAR-REACT 2 randomized trial. JAMA 295:1531, 2006

MEHTA SR et al: Routine vs selective invasive strategies in patients with acute coronary syndromes: A collaborative meta-analysis of randomized trials. JAMA 293:2908, 2005

O'DONOGHUE M et al: Early invasive vs. conservative treatment strategies in women and men with unstable angina and non-ST-segment elevation myocardial infarction: a meta-analysis. JAMA 300:71, 2008

WALLENTIN LT et al: Ticagrelor versus clopidogrel in patients with acute coronary syndromes. N Engl J Med 361:1045, 2009

WIVIOTT SD et al: Prasugrel versus clopidogrel in patients with acute coronary syndromes. N Engl J Med 357:2001, 2007

YUSUF S et al: Comparison of fondaparinux and enoxaparin in acute coronary syndromes. N Engl J Med 354:1464, 2006

CHAPTER 35

ST-SEGMENT ELEVATION MYOCARDIAL INFARCTION

Elliott M. Antman ■ Eugene Braunwald

Acute myocardial infarction (AMI) is one of the most common diagnoses in hospitalized patients in industrialized countries. In the United States, approximately 650,000 patients experience a new AMI and 450,000 experience a recurrent AMI each year. The early (30-day) mortality rate from AMI is ~30%, with more than one-half of these deaths occurring before the stricken individual reaches the hospital. Although the mortality rate after admission for AMI has declined by ~30% over the past two decades, approximately 1 of every 25 patients who survives the initial hospitalization dies in the first year after AMI. Mortality is approximately fourfold higher in elderly patients (>75 years) in comparison with younger patients.

When patients with prolonged ischemic discomfort at rest are first seen, the working clinical diagnosis is that they are suffering from an acute coronary syndrome (Fig. 35-1). The 12-lead electrocardiogram (ECG) is a pivotal diagnostic and triage tool since it is at the center of the decision pathway for management. It permits discrimination of those patients presenting with ST-segment elevation from those presenting without ST-segment elevation. Serum cardiac biomarkers are obtained to distinguish unstable angina (UA) from non–ST-segment MI (NSTEMI) and to assess the magnitude of an ST-segment elevation MI (STEMI). This chapter focuses on the evaluation and management of patients with STEMI, while Chap. 34 discusses UA/NSTEMI.

PATHOPHYSIOLOGY: ROLE OF ACUTE PLAQUE RUPTURE

STEMI usually occurs when coronary blood flow decreases abruptly after a thrombotic occlusion of a coronary artery previously affected by atherosclerosis. Slowly developing, high-grade coronary artery stenoses do not typically precipitate STEMI because of the development of a rich collateral network over time. Instead, STEMI occurs when a coronary artery thrombus develops rapidly at a site of vascular injury. The injury is produced or facilitated by factors such as cigarette smoking,

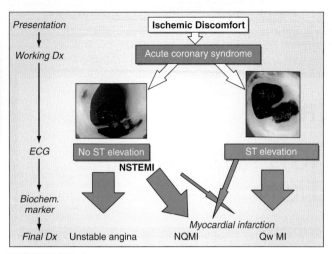

FIGURE 35-1

Acute coronary syndromes. Following disruption of a vulnerable plaque, patients experience ischemic discomfort resulting from a reduction of flow through the affected epicardial coronary artery. The flow reduction may be caused by a completely occlusive thrombus (*right*) or subtotally occlusive thrombus (*left*). Patients with ischemic discomfort may present with or without ST-segment elevation. Of patients with ST-segment elevation, the majority (*wide red arrow*) ultimately develop a Q-wave on the ECG (QwMI), while a minority (*thin red arrow*) do not develop Q-wave and in older literature where said to have sustained a non-Q-wave MI (NQMI). Patients who present without ST-segment elevation are suffering from either unstable angina or a non-ST-segment elevation MI (NSTEMI) (*wide green arrows*), a distinction that is ultimately made on the presence or absence of a serum cardiac marker such as CK-MB or a cardiac troponin detected in the blood. The majority of patients presenting with NSTEMI do not develop a Q-wave on the ECG; a minority develop a QwMI (*thin green arrow*). (*Adapted from CW Hamm et al: Lancet 358:1533, 2001, and MJ Davies: Heart 83:361, 2000; with permission from the BMJ Publishing Group.*)

hypertension, and lipid accumulation. In most cases, STEMI occurs when the surface of an atherosclerotic plaque becomes disrupted (exposing its contents to the blood) and conditions (local or systemic) favor thrombogenesis. A mural thrombus forms at the site of plaque disruption, and the involved coronary artery becomes occluded. Histologic studies indicate that the coronary plaques prone to disruption are those with a rich lipid core and a thin fibrous cap (Chap. 30). After an initial platelet monolayer forms at the site of the disrupted plaque, various agonists (collagen, ADP, epinephrine, serotonin) promote platelet activation. After agonist stimulation of platelets, thromboxane A_2 (a potent local vasoconstrictor) is released, further platelet activation occurs, and potential resistance to fibrinolysis develops.

In addition to the generation of thromboxane A_2, activation of platelets by agonists promotes a conformational change in the glycoprotein IIb/IIIa receptor. Once converted to its functional state, this receptor develops a high affinity for amino acid sequences on soluble adhesive proteins (i.e., integrins) such as fibrinogen. Since fibrinogen is a multivalent molecule, it can bind to two different platelets simultaneously, resulting in platelet cross-linking and aggregation.

The coagulation cascade is activated on exposure of tissue factor in damaged endothelial cells at the site of the disrupted plaque. Factors VII and X are activated, ultimately leading to the conversion of prothrombin to thrombin, which then converts fibrinogen to fibrin. Fluid-phase and clot-bound thrombin participate in an autoamplification reaction leading to further activation of the coagulation cascade. The culprit coronary artery eventually becomes occluded by a thrombus containing platelet aggregates and fibrin strands.

In rare cases STEMI may be due to coronary artery occlusion caused by coronary emboli, congenital abnormalities, coronary spasm, and a wide variety of systemic—particularly inflammatory—diseases. The amount of myocardial damage caused by coronary occlusion depends on (1) the territory supplied by the affected vessel; (2) whether or not the vessel becomes totally occluded; (3) the duration of coronary occlusion; (4) the quantity of blood supplied by collateral vessels to the affected tissue; (5) the demand for oxygen of the myocardium whose blood supply has been suddenly limited; (6) native factors that can produce early spontaneous lysis of the occlusive thrombus; and (7) the adequacy of myocardial perfusion in the infarct zone when flow is restored in the occluded epicardial coronary artery.

Patients at increased risk of developing STEMI include those with multiple coronary risk factors (Chap. 30) and those with unstable angina (Chap. 34). Less common underlying medical conditions predisposing patients to STEMI include hypercoagulability, collagen vascular disease, cocaine abuse, and intracardiac thrombi or masses that can produce coronary emboli.

CLINICAL PRESENTATION

In up to one-half of cases, a precipitating factor appears to be present before STEMI, such as vigorous physical exercise, emotional stress, or a medical or surgical illness. Although STEMI may commence at any time of the day or night, circadian variations have been reported such that clusters are seen in the morning within a few hours of awakening.

Pain is the most common presenting complaint in patients with STEMI. The pain is deep and visceral; adjectives commonly used to describe it are *heavy*, *squeezing*, and *crushing*, although occasionally it is described as stabbing or burning (Chap. 4). It is similar in character to the discomfort of angina pectoris (Chap. 33) but commonly occurs at rest, is usually more severe, and lasts longer. Typically the pain involves the central portion of the chest and/or the epigastrium, and on occasion it radiates to the arms. Less common sites of radiation include the abdomen, back, lower jaw, and neck. The frequent location of the pain beneath the xiphoid and epigastrium and the patients' denial that they may be suffering a heart attack are chiefly responsible for the common mistaken impression of indigestion. The pain of STEMI may radiate as high as the occipital area but not below the umbilicus. It is often accompanied by weakness, sweating, nausea, vomiting, anxiety, and a sense of impending doom. The pain may commence when the patient is at rest, but when it begins during a period of exertion, it does not usually subside with cessation of activity, in contrast to angina pectoris.

The pain of STEMI can simulate pain from acute pericarditis (Chap. 22), pulmonary embolism, acute aortic dissection (Chap. 38), costochondritis, and gastrointestinal disorders. These conditions should therefore be considered in the differential diagnosis. Radiation of discomfort to the trapezius is not seen in patients with STEMI and may be a useful distinguishing feature that suggests pericarditis is the correct diagnosis. However, *pain is not uniformly present in patients with STEMI*. The proportion of painless STEMIs is greater in patients with diabetes mellitus, and it increases with age. In the elderly, STEMI may present as sudden-onset breathlessness, which may progress to pulmonary edema. Other less common presentations, with or without pain, include sudden loss of consciousness, a confusional state, a sensation of profound weakness, the appearance of an arrhythmia, evidence of peripheral embolism, or merely an unexplained drop in arterial pressure.

PHYSICAL FINDINGS

Most patients are anxious and restless, attempting unsuccessfully to relieve the pain by moving about in bed, altering their position, and stretching. Pallor associated with perspiration and coolness of the extremities occurs commonly. The combination of substernal chest pain persisting for >30 min and diaphoresis strongly suggests STEMI. Although many patients have a normal pulse rate and blood pressure within the first hour of STEMI, about one-fourth of patients with anterior infarction have manifestations of sympathetic nervous system hyperactivity (tachycardia and/or hypertension), and up to one-half with inferior infarction show evidence of parasympathetic hyperactivity (bradycardia and/or hypotension).

The precordium is usually quiet, and the apical impulse may be difficult to palpate. In patients with anterior wall infarction, an abnormal systolic pulsation caused by dyskinetic bulging of infarcted myocardium may develop in the periapical area within the first days of the illness and then may resolve. Other physical signs of ventricular dysfunction include fourth and third heart sounds, decreased intensity of the first heart sound, and paradoxical splitting of the second heart sound (Chap. 9). A transient midsystolic or late systolic apical systolic murmur due to dysfunction of the mitral valve apparatus may be present. A pericardial friction rub is heard in many patients with transmural STEMI at some time in the course of the disease, if they are examined frequently. The carotid pulse is often decreased in volume, reflecting reduced stroke volume. Temperature elevations up to 38°C may be observed during the first week after STEMI. The arterial pressure is variable; in most patients with transmural infarction, systolic pressure declines by ~10–15 mmHg from the preinfarction state.

LABORATORY FINDINGS

Myocardial infarction (MI) progresses through the following temporal stages: (1) acute (first few hours–7 days); (2) healing (7–28 days); and (3) healed (≥29 days). When evaluating the results of diagnostic tests for STEMI, the temporal phase of the infarction must be considered. The laboratory tests of value in confirming the diagnosis may be divided into four groups: (1) ECG; (2) serum cardiac biomarkers; (3) cardiac imaging; and (4) nonspecific indices of tissue necrosis and inflammation.

ELECTROCARDIOGRAM

The electrocardiographic manifestations of STEMI are described in Chap. 11. During the initial stage, total occlusion of an epicardial coronary artery produces ST-segment elevation. Most patients initially presenting with ST-segment elevation ultimately evolve Q waves on the ECG (Figs. 35-1 and 11-13). However, Q waves in the leads overlying the infarct zone may vary in magnitude and even appear only transiently, depending on the reperfusion status of the ischemic myocardium and restoration of transmembrane potentials over time. A small proportion of patients initially presenting with ST-segment elevation will not develop Q waves when the obstructing thrombus is not totally occlusive, obstruction is transient, or if a rich collateral network is present. Among patients presenting with ischemic discomfort but *without* ST-segment elevation, if a serum cardiac biomarker of necrosis (see later) is detected, the diagnosis of NSTEMI is ultimately made (Fig. 35-1). A minority of patients who present initially without ST-segment elevation may develop a Q-wave MI. Previously it was believed that transmural MI is present if the ECG demonstrates Q waves or loss of R waves, and nontransmural MI may be present if the ECG shows only transient ST-segment and T-wave changes. However, electrocardiographic-pathologic correlations are far from perfect and terms such as *Q-wave MI, non-Q-wave MI,* transmural MI, and nontransmural MI, have been replaced by STEMI and NSTEMI (Fig. 35-1).

SERUM CARDIAC BIOMARKERS

Certain proteins, called serum cardiac biomarkers, are released from necrotic heart muscle after STEMI. The rate of liberation of specific proteins differs depending on their intracellular location, their molecular weight, and the local blood and lymphatic flow. Cardiac biomarkers become detectable in the peripheral blood once the capacity of the cardiac lymphatics to clear the interstitium of the infarct zone is exceeded and spillover into the venous circulation occurs. The temporal pattern of protein release is of diagnostic importance, but contemporary urgent reperfusion strategies necessitate making a decision (based largely on a combination of clinical and ECG findings) before the results of blood tests have returned from the laboratory. Rapid whole-blood bedside assays for serum cardiac markers are now available and may facilitate management decisions, particularly in patients with nondiagnostic ECGs.

Cardiac-specific troponin T (cTnT) and cardiac-specific troponin I (cTnI) have amino acid sequences different from those of the skeletal muscle forms of these proteins. These differences permitted the development of quantitative assays for cTnT and cTnI with highly specific monoclonal antibodies. Since cTnT and cTnI are not normally detectable in the blood of healthy individuals but may increase after STEMI to levels >20 times higher than the upper reference limit (the highest value seen in 99% of a reference population not suffering from MI), the measurement of cTnT or cTnI is of considerable diagnostic usefulness, and they are now the preferred biochemical markers for MI (Fig. 35-2). The cardiac troponins are particularly valuable when there is clinical suspicion of either skeletal muscle injury or a small MI that may be below the detection limit for creatine kinase (CK) also known as creatine phosphokinase and creatine kinase, myocardial bound (CK-MB) measurements, and they are therefore of particular value in distinguishing UA from NSTEMI. Levels of cTnI and cTnT may remain elevated for 7–10 days after STEMI.

Creatine phosphokinase (CK) rises within 4–8 h and generally returns to normal by 48–72 h (Fig. 35-2). An important drawback of total CK measurement is its lack of specificity for STEMI, as CK may be elevated with skeletal muscle disease or trauma, including intramuscular injection. The MB isoenzyme of CK has the advantage over total CK that it is not present in significant concentrations in extracardiac tissue and therefore is considerably more specific. However, cardiac surgery, myocarditis, and electrical cardioversion often result in elevated serum levels of the MB isoenzyme. A ratio (relative index) of CK-MB mass:CK activity ≥2.5 suggests but is not diagnostic of a myocardial rather than a skeletal muscle source for the CK-MB elevation.

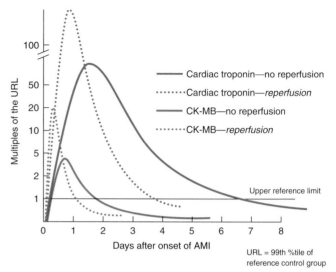

FIGURE 35-2

Typical cardiac biomarkers that are used to evaluate patients with STEMI include the MB isoenzyme of CK (CK-MB) and cardiac-specific troponins. The black horizontal line depicts the upper reference limit (URL) for the cardiac biomarker in the clinical chemistry laboratory. The kinetics of release of CK-MB and cardiac troponin in patients who do not undergo reperfusion are shown in the solid green and red curves as multiples of the URL. When patients with STEMI undergo reperfusion, as depicted in the dashed green and red curves, the cardiac biomarkers are detected sooner, rise to a higher peak value, but decline more rapidly, resulting in a smaller area under the curve and limitation of infarct size. *(Adapted from JS Alpert et al: J Am Coll Cardiol 36:959, 2000, and AH Wu et al: Clin Chem 45:1104, 1999.)*

Many hospitals are using cTnT or cTnI rather than CK-MB as the routine serum cardiac marker for diagnosis of STEMI, although any of these analytes remains clinically acceptable. It is *not* cost-effective to measure both a cardiac-specific troponin and CK-MB at all time points in every patient.

While it has long been recognized that the total quantity of protein released correlates with the size of the infarct, the peak protein concentration correlates only weakly with infarct size. Recanalization of a coronary artery occlusion (either spontaneously or by mechanical or pharmacologic means) in the early hours of STEMI causes earlier and higher peaking (at about 8–12 h after reperfusion) of serum cardiac biomarkers (Fig. 35-2) because of a rapid washout from the interstitium of the infarct zone, quickly overwhelming lymphatic clearance of the proteins.

The *nonspecific reaction* to myocardial injury is associated with polymorphonuclear leukocytosis, which appears within a few hours after the onset of pain and persists for 3–7 days; the white blood cell count often reaches levels of 12,000–15,000/μL. The erythrocyte sedimentation rate rises more slowly than the white blood cell count, peaking during the first week and sometimes remaining elevated for 1 or 2 weeks.

CARDIAC IMAGING

Abnormalities of wall motion on *two-dimensional echocardiography* (Chap. 12) are almost universally present. Although acute STEMI cannot be distinguished from an old myocardial scar or from acute severe ischemia by echocardiography, the ease and safety of the procedure make its use appealing as a screening tool in the emergency department setting. When the ECG is not diagnostic of STEMI, early detection of the presence or absence of wall motion abnormalities by echocardiography can aid in management decisions, such as whether the patient should receive reperfusion therapy [e.g., fibrinolysis or a percutaneous coronary intervention (PCI)]. Echocardiographic estimation of left ventricular (LV) function is useful prognostically; detection of reduced function serves as an indication for therapy with an inhibitor of the renin-angiotensin-aldosterone system. Echocardiography may also identify the presence of right ventricular (RV) infarction, ventricular aneurysm, pericardial effusion, and LV thrombus. In addition, Doppler echocardiography is useful in the detection and quantitation of a ventricular septal defect and mitral regurgitation, two serious complications of STEMI.

Several *radionuclide imaging techniques* (Chap. 12) are available for evaluating patients with suspected STEMI. However, these imaging modalities are used less often than echocardiography because they are more cumbersome and lack sensitivity and specificity in many clinical circumstances. Myocardial perfusion imaging with ^{201}Tl or ^{99m}Tc-sestamibi, which are distributed in proportion to myocardial blood flow and concentrated by viable myocardium (Chap. 33), reveal a defect ("cold spot") in most patients during the first few hours after development of a transmural infarct. Although perfusion scanning is extremely sensitive, it cannot distinguish acute infarcts from chronic scars and thus is not specific for the diagnosis of *acute* MI. Radionuclide ventriculography, carried out with ^{99m}Tc-labeled red blood cells, frequently demonstrates wall motion disorders and reduction in the ventricular ejection fraction in patients with STEMI. Although of value in assessing the hemodynamic consequences of infarction and in aiding in the diagnosis of RV infarction when the RV ejection fraction is depressed, this technique is nonspecific, as many cardiac abnormalities other than MI alter the radionuclide ventriculogram.

Myocardial infarction can be detected accurately with high-resolution cardiac magnetic resonance imaging (Chap. 12) using a technique referred to as late enhancement. A standard imaging agent (gadolinium) is administered and images are obtained after a 10-min delay. Since little gadolinium enters normal myocardium where there are tightly packed myocytes, but does percolate into the expanded intercellular region of the infarct zone, there is a bright signal in areas of infarction that appears in stark contrast to the dark areas of normal myocardium.

INITIAL MANAGEMENT

PREHOSPITAL CARE

The prognosis in STEMI is largely related to the occurrence of two general classes of complications: (1) electrical complications (arrhythmias) and (2) mechanical complications ("pump failure"). Most out-of-hospital deaths from STEMI are due to the sudden development of ventricular fibrillation. The vast majority of deaths due to ventricular fibrillation occur within the first 24 h of the onset of symptoms, and of these, over half occur in the first hour. Therefore, the major elements of prehospital care of patients with suspected STEMI include (1) recognition of symptoms by the patient and prompt seeking of medical attention; (2) rapid deployment of an emergency medical team capable of performing resuscitative maneuvers, including defibrillation; (3) expeditious transportation of the patient to a hospital facility that is continuously staffed by physicians and nurses skilled in managing arrhythmias and providing advanced cardiac life support; and (4) expeditious implementation of reperfusion therapy (Fig. 35-3). The biggest delay usually occurs not during transportation to the hospital but rather between the onset of pain and the patient's decision to call for help. This delay can best be reduced by health care professionals educating the public concerning the significance of chest discomfort and the importance of seeking early medical attention. Regular office visits with patients having a history of or who are at risk for ischemic heart disease are important "teachable moments" for clinicians to review the symptoms of STEMI and the appropriate action plan.

Increasingly, monitoring and treatment are carried out by trained personnel in the ambulance, further shortening the time between the onset of the infarction and appropriate treatment. General guidelines for initiation of fibrinolysis in the prehospital setting include the ability to transmit 12-lead ECGs to confirm the diagnosis, the presence of paramedics in the ambulance, training of paramedics in the interpretation of ECGs and management of STEMI, and online medical command and control that can authorize the initiation of treatment in the field.

MANAGEMENT IN THE EMERGENCY DEPARTMENT

In the emergency department, the goals for the management of patients with suspected STEMI include control of cardiac discomfort, rapid identification of patients who are candidates for urgent reperfusion therapy, triage

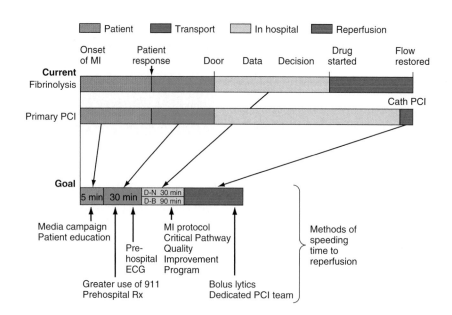

FIGURE 35-3

Major components of time delay between onset of symptoms from STEMI and restoration of flow in the infarct-related artery. Plotted sequentially from left to right are shown the times for patients to recognize symptoms and seek medical attention, transportation to the hospital, in-hospital decision-making, implementation of reperfusion strategy, and restoration of flow once the reperfusion strategy has been initiated. The time to initiate fibrinolytic therapy is the "door-to-needle" (D-N) time; this is followed by the period of time required for pharmacologic restoration of flow. More time is required to move the patient to the catheterization laboratory for a percutaneous coronary interventional (PCI) procedure, referred to as the "door-to-balloon" (D-B) time, but restoration of flow in the epicardial infarct-related artery occurs promptly after PCI. At the bottom are shown a variety of methods for speeding the time to reperfusion along with the goals for the time intervals for the various components of the time delay. (*Adapted from CP Cannon et al: J Thromb Thrombol 1:27, 1994.*)

of lower-risk patients to the appropriate location in the hospital, and avoidance of inappropriate discharge of patients with STEMI. Many aspects of the treatment of STEMI are initiated in the emergency department and then continued during the in-hospital phase of management.

Aspirin is essential in the management of patients with suspected STEMI and is effective across the entire spectrum of acute coronary syndromes (Fig. 35-1). Rapid inhibition of cyclooxygenase-1 in platelets followed by a reduction of thromboxane A_2 levels is achieved by buccal absorption of a chewed 160–325 mg tablet in the emergency department. This measure should be followed by daily oral administration of aspirin in a dose of 75–162 mg.

In patients whose arterial O_2 saturation is normal, supplemental O_2 is of limited if any clinical benefit and therefore is not cost-effective. However, when hypoxemia is present, O_2 should be administered by nasal prongs or face mask (2–4 L/min) for the first 6–12 h after infarction; the patient should then be reassessed to determine if there is a continued need for such treatment.

CONTROL OF DISCOMFORT

Sublingual *nitroglycerin* can be given safely to most patients with STEMI. Up to three doses of 0.4 mg should be administered at about 5-min intervals. In addition to diminishing or abolishing chest discomfort, nitroglycerin may be capable of both decreasing myocardial oxygen demand (by lowering preload) and increasing myocardial oxygen supply (by dilating infarct-related coronary vessels or collateral vessels). In patients whose initially favorable response to sublingual nitroglycerin is followed by the return of chest discomfort, particularly if accompanied by other evidence of ongoing ischemia such as further ST-segment or T-wave shifts, the use of intravenous nitroglycerin should be considered. Therapy with nitrates should be avoided in patients who present with low systolic arterial pressure (<90 mmHg) or in whom there is clinical suspicion of right ventricular infarction (inferior infarction on ECG, elevated jugular venous pressure, clear lungs, and hypotension). Nitrates should not be administered to patients who have taken the phosphodiesterase-5 inhibitor sildenafil for erectile dysfunction within the preceding 24 h since it may potentiate the hypotensive effects of nitrates. An idiosyncratic reaction to nitrates, consisting of sudden marked hypotension, sometimes occurs but can usually be reversed promptly by the rapid administration of intravenous atropine.

Morphine is a very effective analgesic for the pain associated with STEMI. However, it may reduce sympathetically mediated arteriolar and venous constriction, and the resulting venous pooling may reduce cardiac output and arterial pressure. These hemodynamic disturbances usually respond promptly to elevation of the legs, but in some patients volume expansion with intravenous saline is required. The patient may experience diaphoresis and nausea, but these events usually pass and are replaced by a feeling of well-being associated with the relief of pain. Morphine also has a vagotonic effect and may cause bradycardia or advanced degrees of heart block, particularly in patients with posteroinferior infarction. These side effects usually respond to atropine (0.5 mg intravenously). Morphine is routinely administered by repetitive (every 5 min) intravenous injection of small doses (2–4 mg) rather than by the subcutaneous administration of a larger quantity, because absorption may be unpredictable by the latter route.

Intravenous *beta blockers* are also useful in the control of the pain of STEMI. These drugs control pain effectively in some patients, presumably by diminishing myocardial O_2 demand and hence ischemia. More important, there is evidence that intravenous beta blockers reduce the risks of reinfarction and ventricular fibrillation (see Beta-Adrenoceptor Blockers, later in the chapter). A commonly employed regimen is metoprolol, 5 mg every 2–5 min for a total of 3 doses, provided the patient has a heart rate >60 beats/min, systolic pressure >100 mmHg, a PR interval <0.24 s, and rales that are no higher than 10 cm up from the diaphragm. Fifteen minutes after the last intravenous dose, an oral regimen is initiated of 50 mg every 6 h for 48 h, followed by 100 mg every 12 h.

Unlike beta blockers, calcium antagonists are of little value in the acute setting, and there is evidence that short-acting dihydropyridines may be associated with an increased mortality risk.

MANAGEMENT STRATEGIES

The primary tool for screening patients and making triage decisions is the initial 12-lead ECG. When ST-segment elevation of at least 2 mm in two contiguous precordial leads and 1 mm in two adjacent limb leads is present, a patient should be considered a candidate for *reperfusion therapy* (Fig. 35-4). The process of selecting patients for fibrinolysis versus primary PCI (angioplasty, or stenting; Chap. 36) is discussed later. In the absence of ST-segment elevation, fibrinolysis is not helpful, and evidence exists suggesting that it may be harmful.

LIMITATION OF INFARCT SIZE

The quantity of myocardium that becomes necrotic as a consequence of a coronary artery occlusion is determined by factors other than just the site of occlusion. While the central zone of the infarct contains necrotic tissue that is irretrievably lost, the fate of the surrounding ischemic myocardium may be improved by timely restoration of coronary perfusion, reduction of myocardial O_2 demands, prevention of the accumulation of noxious metabolites, and blunting of the impact of mediators of reperfusion injury (e.g., calcium overload and oxygen-derived free radicals). Up to one-third of patients with STEMI may achieve *spontaneous* reperfusion of the infarct-related coronary artery within 24 h and experience improved healing of infarcted tissue. Reperfusion, either pharmacologically (by fibrinolysis) or by PCI, accelerates the opening of infarct-related arteries in those patients in whom spontaneous fibrinolysis ultimately would have occurred and also greatly increases the number of patients in whom restoration of flow in the infarct-related artery is accomplished. Timely restoration of flow in the epicardial infarct–related artery combined with improved perfusion of the downstream zone of infarcted myocardium results in a limitation of infarct size. Protection of the ischemic myocardium by the maintenance of an optimal balance between myocardial O_2 supply and demand through pain control, treatment of congestive heart failure (CHF), and minimization of tachycardia and hypertension extends the "window" of time for the salvage of myocardium by reperfusion strategies.

Glucocorticoids and nonsteroidal anti-inflammatory agents, with the exception of aspirin, should be avoided in patients with STEMI. They can impair infarct healing and increase the risk of myocardial rupture, and their use may result in a larger infarct scar. In addition, they can increase coronary vascular resistance, thereby potentially reducing flow to ischemic myocardium.

Primary Percutaneous Coronary Intervention

(See also Chap. 36) PCI, usually angioplasty and/or stenting without preceding fibrinolysis, referred to as *primary PCI*, is effective in restoring perfusion in STEMI when carried out on an emergency basis in the first few hours of MI. It has the advantage of being applicable to patients who have contraindications to fibrinolytic therapy (see later) but otherwise are considered appropriate candidates for reperfusion. It appears to be more effective than fibrinolysis in opening occluded coronary arteries and, *when performed by experienced operators [≥75 PCI cases (not necessarily primary) per year] in dedicated medical centers (≥36 primary PCI cases per year)*, is associated with better short-term and long-term clinical outcomes. Compared with fibrinolysis, primary PCI is generally preferred when the diagnosis is in doubt, cardiogenic shock is present, bleeding risk is increased, or symptoms have been present for at least 2–3 h when the clot is more mature and less easily lysed by fibrinolytic drugs. However, PCI is expensive in terms of personnel and facilities, and its applicability is limited by its availability, around the clock, in only a minority of hospitals.

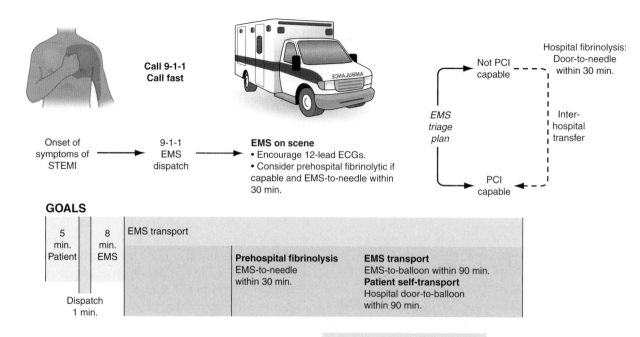

FIGURE 35-4

Options for transportation of patients with STEMI and initial reperfusion treatment. Patient transported by EMS after calling 911: Reperfusion in patients with STEMI can be accomplished by the pharmacologic (fibrinolysis) or catheter-based (primary PCI) approaches. Implementation of these strategies varies based on the mode of transportation of the patient and capabilities at the receiving hospital. Transport time to the hospital is variable from case to case, but the goal is to keep total ischemic time within 120 min. There are three possibilities: (1) If EMS has fibrinolytic capability and the patient qualifies for therapy, prehospital fibrinolysis should be started within 30 min of EMS arrival on scene; (2) If EMS is not capable of administering prehospital fibrinolysis and the patient is transported to a non–PCI-capable hospital, the hospital door-to-needle time should be within 30 min for patients in whom fibrinolysis is indicated; (3) If EMS is not capable of administering prehospital fibrinolysis and the patient is transported to a PCI-capable hospital, the hospital door-to-balloon time should be within 90 min. *Interhospital transfer*: It is also appropriate to consider emergency inter-hospital transfer of the patient to a PCI-capable hospital for mechanical revascularization if: (1) there is a contraindication to fibrinolysis; (2) PCI can be initiated promptly (within 90 minutes after the patient presented to the initial receiving hospital or within 60 min compared to when fibrinolysis with a fibrin-specific agent could be initiated at the initial receiving hospital); (3) fibrinolysis is administered and is unsuccessful (i.e., "rescue PCI"). Secondary nonemergency interhospital transfer can be considered for recurrent ischemia. *Patient self-transport*: Patient self-transportation is discouraged. If the patient arrives at a non-PCI–capable hospital, the door-to-needle time should be within 30 min. If the patient arrives at a PCI-capable hospital, the door-to-balloon time should be within 90 min. The treatment options and time recommended after first hospital arrival are the same. *[Reproduced with permission from Antman et al: ACC/AHA guidelines for the management of patients with ST-elevation myocardial infarction: A report of the American College of Cardiology/American Heart Association Task Force on Practice Guidelines (Committee to Revise the 1999 Guidelines for the Management of Patients with Acute Myocardial Infarction). Available at www.acc.org/clinical/guidelines/stemi/index.pdf.]*

Fibrinolysis

If no contraindications are present (see later), fibrinolytic therapy should ideally be initiated within 30 min of presentation (i.e., door-to-needle time ≤30 min). The principal goal of fibrinolysis is prompt restoration of full coronary arterial patency. The fibrinolytic agents tissue plasminogen activator (tPA), streptokinase, tenecteplase (TNK), and reteplase (rPA) have been approved by the U.S. Food and Drug Administration for intravenous use in patients with STEMI. These drugs all act by promoting the conversion of plasminogen to plasmin, which subsequently lyses fibrin thrombi. Although considerable emphasis was first placed on a distinction between more fibrin-specific agents, such as tPA, and non–fibrin-specific agents, such as streptokinase, it is now recognized that these differences are only relative, as some degree of systemic fibrinolysis occurs with the former agents. TNK and rPA are referred to as *bolus fibrinolytics* since their administration does not require a prolonged intravenous infusion.

When assessed angiographically, flow in the culprit coronary artery is described by a simple qualitative scale called the *thrombolysis in myocardial infarction (TIMI) grading system*: grade 0 indicates complete occlusion of the infarct-related artery; grade 1 indicates some penetration of the contrast material beyond the point of obstruction but without perfusion of the distal coronary bed; grade 2 indicates perfusion of the entire infarct vessel into the distal bed but with flow that is delayed compared with that of a normal artery; and grade 3 indicates full perfusion of the infarct vessel with normal flow. The latter is the goal of reperfusion therapy, because full perfusion of the infarct-related coronary artery yields far better results in terms of limiting infarct size, maintenance of LV function, and reduction of both short- and long-term mortality rates. Additional methods of angiographic assessment of the efficacy of fibrinolysis include counting the number of frames on the cine film required for dye to flow from the origin of the infarct-related artery to a landmark in the distal vascular bed (*TIMI frame count*) and determining the rate of entry and exit of contrast dye from the microvasculature in the myocardial infarct zone (*TIMI myocardial perfusion grade*). These methods have an even tighter correlation with outcomes after STEMI than the more commonly employed TIMI flow grade.

Fibrinolytic therapy can reduce the relative risk of in-hospital death by up to 50% when administered within the first hour of the onset of symptoms of STEMI, and much of this benefit is maintained for at least 10 years. When appropriately used, fibrinolytic therapy appears to reduce infarct size, limit LV dysfunction, and reduce the incidence of serious complications such as septal rupture, cardiogenic shock, and malignant ventricular arrhythmias. Since myocardium can be salvaged only before it has been irreversibly injured, the timing of reperfusion therapy, by fibrinolysis or a catheter-based approach, is of extreme importance in achieving maximum benefit. While the upper time limit depends on specific factors in individual patients, it is clear that "every minute counts" and that patients treated within 1–3 h of the onset of symptoms generally benefit most. Although reduction of the mortality rate is more modest, the therapy remains of benefit for many patients seen 3–6 h after the onset of infarction, and some benefit appears to be possible up to 12 h, especially if chest discomfort is still present and ST segments remain elevated. Compared with PCI for STEMI (primary PCI), fibrinolysis is generally the preferred reperfusion strategy for patients presenting in the first hour of symptoms, if there are logistical concerns about transportation of the patient to a suitable PCI center (experienced operator and team with a track record for a "door-to-balloon" time of <2 h), or there is an anticipated delay of at least 1 h between the time that fibrinolysis could be started versus implementation of PCI. Although patients <75 years achieve a greater relative reduction in the mortality rate with fibrinolytic therapy than do older patients, the higher *absolute* mortality rate

(15–25%) in the latter results in similar absolute reductions in the mortality rates for both age groups.

tPA and the other relatively fibrin-specific plasminogen activators, rPA and TNK, are more effective than streptokinase at restoring full perfusion—i.e., TIMI grade 3 coronary flow—and have a small edge in improving survival as well. The current recommended regimen of tPA consists of a 15 mg bolus followed by 50 mg intravenously over the first 30 min, followed by 35 mg over the next 60 min. Streptokinase is administered as 1.5 million units (MU) intravenously over 1 h. rPA is administered in a double-bolus regimen consisting of a 10-MU bolus given over 2–3 min, followed by a second 10-MU bolus 30 min later. TNK is given as a single weight-based intravenous bolus of 0.53 mg/kg over 10 s. In addition to the fibrinolytic agents discussed earlier, pharmacologic reperfusion typically involves adjunctive antiplatelet and antithrombotic drugs, as discussed subsequently.

Alternative pharmacologic regimens for reperfusion combine an intravenous glycoprotein IIb/IIIa inhibitor with a reduced dose of a fibrinolytic agent. Compared with fibrinolytic agents that involve a prolonged infusion (e.g., tPA), such combination reperfusion regimens facilitate the rate and extent of fibrinolysis by inhibiting platelet aggregation, weakening the clot structure, and allowing penetration of the fibrinolytic agent deeper into the clot. However, combination reperfusion regimens have similar efficacy as compared with bolus fibrinolytics and are associated with an increased risk of bleeding, especially in patients older than 75 years. Therefore, combination reperfusion regimens are not recommended for routine use. Glycoprotein IIb/IIIa inhibitors given alone (i.e., without any fibrinolytic agent) are being investigated as a preparatory pharmacologic regimen in STEMI patients who are referred promptly for PCI—an experimental strategy called *facilitated PCI*. Another experimental strategy that has been proposed but not yet rigorously evaluated is a *pharmacoinvasive* approach where STEMI patients are first treated with a pharmacologic reperfusion regimen followed by routine angiography and PCI after a delay of 12–24 h to minimize the risks of performing PCI while the effects of the lytic agent are still present.

Contraindications and Complications

Clear contraindications to the use of fibrinolytic agents include a history of cerebrovascular hemorrhage at any time, a nonhemorrhagic stroke or other cerebrovascular event within the past year, marked hypertension (a reliably determined systolic arterial pressure >180 mmHg and/or a diastolic pressure >110 mmHg) at any time during the acute presentation, suspicion of aortic dissection, and active internal bleeding (excluding menses). While advanced age is associated with an increase in hemorrhagic complications, the benefit of fibrinolytic therapy in the elderly appears to justify its use if no other contraindications are present and the amount of myocardium in jeopardy appears to be substantial.

Relative contraindications to fibrinolytic therapy, which require assessment of the risk: benefit ratio, include current use of anticoagulants (international normalized ratio ≥2), a recent (<2 weeks) invasive or surgical procedure or prolonged (>10 min) cardiopulmonary resuscitation, known bleeding diathesis, pregnancy, a hemorrhagic ophthalmic condition (e.g., hemorrhagic diabetic retinopathy), active peptic ulcer disease, and a history of severe hypertension that is currently adequately controlled. Because of the risk of an allergic reaction, patients should not receive streptokinase if that agent had been received within the preceding 5 days to 2 years.

Allergic reactions to streptokinase occur in ~2% of patients who receive it. Although a minor degree of hypotension occurs in 4–10% of patients given this agent, marked hypotension occurs, although rarely, in association with severe allergic reactions.

Hemorrhage is the most frequent and potentially the most serious complication. Because bleeding episodes that require transfusion are more common when patients require invasive procedures, unnecessary venous or arterial interventions should be avoided in patients receiving fibrinolytic agents. Hemorrhagic stroke is the most serious complication and occurs in ~0.5–0.9% of patients being treated with these agents. This rate increases with advancing age, with patients >70 years experiencing roughly twice the rate of intracranial hemorrhage as those <65 years. Large-scale trials have suggested that the rate of intracranial hemorrhage with tPA or rPA is slightly higher than with streptokinase.

Cardiac catheterization and coronary angiography should be carried out after fibrinolytic therapy if there is evidence of either (1) failure of reperfusion (persistent chest pain and ST-segment elevation >90 min), in which case a *rescue PCI* should be considered; or (2) coronary artery reocclusion (re-elevation of ST segments and/or recurrent chest pain) or the development of recurrent ischemia (such as recurrent angina in the early hospital course or a positive exercise stress test before discharge), in which case an *urgent PCI* should be considered. The potential benefits of routine angiography and *elective* PCI even in asymptomatic patients following administration of fibrinolytic therapy are controversial, but such an approach may have merit given the numerous technological advances that have occurred in the catheterization laboratory and the increasing number of skilled interventionalists. Coronary artery bypass surgery should be reserved for patients whose coronary anatomy is unsuited to PCI but in whom revascularization appears to be advisable because of extensive jeopardized myocardium or recurrent ischemia.

HOSPITAL PHASE MANAGEMENT

CORONARY CARE UNITS

These units are routinely equipped with a system that permits continuous monitoring of the cardiac rhythm of each patient and hemodynamic monitoring in selected patients. Defibrillators, respirators, noninvasive transthoracic pacemakers, and facilities for introducing pacing catheters and flow-directed balloon-tipped catheters are also usually available. Equally important is the organization of a highly trained team of nurses who can recognize arrhythmias; adjust the dosage of antiarrhythmic, vasoactive, and anticoagulant drugs; and perform cardiac resuscitation, including electroshock, when necessary.

Patients should be admitted to a coronary care unit early in their illness when it is expected that they will derive benefit from the sophisticated and expensive care provided. The availability of electrocardiographic monitoring and trained personnel outside the coronary care unit has made it possible to admit lower-risk patients (e.g., those not hemodynamically compromised and without active arrhythmias) to "intermediate care units."

The duration of stay in the coronary care unit is dictated by the ongoing need for intensive care. If symptoms are controlled with oral therapy, patients may be transferred out of the coronary care unit. Also, patients who have a confirmed STEMI but who are considered to be at low risk (no prior infarction and no persistent chest discomfort, CHF, hypotension, or cardiac arrhythmias) may be safely transferred out of the coronary care unit within 24 h.

Activity

Factors that increase the work of the heart during the initial hours of infarction may increase the size of the infarct. Therefore, patients with STEMI should be kept at bed rest for the first 12 h. However, in the absence of complications, patients should be encouraged, under supervision, to resume an upright posture by dangling their feet over the side of the bed and sitting in a chair within the first 24 h. This practice is psychologically beneficial and usually results in a reduction in the pulmonary capillary wedge pressure. In the absence of hypotension and other complications, by the second or third day patients typically are ambulating in their room with increasing duration and frequency, and they may shower or stand at the sink to bathe. By day 3 after infarction, patients should be increasing their ambulation progressively to a goal of 185 m (600 ft) at least three times a day.

Diet

Because of the risk of emesis and aspiration soon after STEMI, patients should receive either nothing or only clear liquids by mouth for the first 4–12 h. The typical coronary care unit diet should provide ≤30% of total calories as fat and have a cholesterol content of ≤300 mg/d. Complex carbohydrates should make up 50–55% of total calories. Portions should not be unusually large, and the menu should be enriched with foods that are high in potassium, magnesium, and fiber but low in sodium. Diabetes mellitus and hypertriglyceridemia are managed by restriction of concentrated sweets in the diet.

Bowels

Bed rest and the effect of the narcotics used for the relief of pain often lead to constipation. A bedside commode rather than a bedpan, a diet rich in bulk, and the routine use of a stool softener such as dioctyl sodium sulfosuccinate (200 mg/d) are recommended. If the patient remains constipated despite these measures, a laxative can be prescribed. Contrary to prior belief, it is safe to perform a gentle rectal examination on patients with STEMI.

Sedation

Many patients require sedation during hospitalization to withstand the period of enforced inactivity with tranquillity. Diazepam (5 mg), oxazepam (15–30 mg), or lorazepam (0.5–2 mg), given three or four times daily, is usually effective. An additional dose of any of the above medications may be given at night to ensure adequate sleep. Attention to this problem is especially important during the first few days in the coronary care unit, where the atmosphere of 24-h vigilance may interfere with the patient's sleep. However, sedation is no substitute for reassuring, quiet surroundings. Many drugs used in the coronary care unit, such as atropine, H_2 blockers, and narcotics, can produce delirium, particularly in the elderly. This effect should not be confused with agitation, and it is wise to conduct a thorough review of the patient's medications before arbitrarily prescribing additional doses of anxiolytics.

PHARMACOTHERAPY

ANTITHROMBOTIC AGENTS

The use of antiplatelet and antithrombin therapy during the initial phase of STEMI is based on extensive laboratory and clinical evidence that thrombosis plays an important role in the pathogenesis of this condition. The primary goal of treatment with antiplatelet and antithrombin agents is to establish and maintain patency of the infarct-related artery, in conjunction with reperfusion strategies. A secondary goal is to reduce the patient's tendency to thrombosis and thus the likelihood of mural thrombus formation or deep venous thrombosis, either of which could result in pulmonary embolization. The degree to which antiplatelet and antithrombin therapy

achieves these goals partly determines how effectively it reduces the risk of mortality from STEMI.

As noted previously (see Management in the Emergency Department, earlier), aspirin is the standard antiplatelet agent for patients with STEMI. The most compelling evidence for the benefits of antiplatelet therapy (mainly with aspirin) in STEMI is found in the comprehensive overview by the Antiplatelet Trialists' Collaboration. Data from nearly 20,000 patients with MI enrolled in 15 randomized trials were pooled and revealed a relative reduction of 27% in the mortality rate, from 14.2% in control patients to 10.4% in patients receiving antiplatelet agents.

Inhibitors of the $P2Y_{12}$ ADP receptor prevent activation and aggregation of platelets. The addition of the $P2Y_{12}$ inhibitor clopidogrel to background treatment with aspirin to STEMI patients reduces the risk of clinical events (death, reinfarction, stroke) and in patients receiving fibrinolytic therapy has been shown to prevent reocclusion of a successfully reperfused infarct artery (Fig. 35-5). Glycoprotein IIb/IIIa receptor inhibitors appear useful for preventing thrombotic complications in patients with STEMI undergoing PCI.

The standard antithrombin agent used in clinical practice is unfractionated heparin (UFH). The available data suggest that when UFH is added to a regimen of aspirin and a non-fibrin-specific thrombolytic agent such as streptokinase, additional mortality benefit occurs (about five lives saved per 1000 patients treated). It appears that the immediate administration of intravenous UFH, in addition to a regimen of aspirin and relatively fibrin-specific fibrinolytic agents (tPA, rPA, or TNK), helps to maintain patency of the infarct-related artery. This effect is achieved at the cost of a small increased risk of bleeding. The recommended dose of UFH is an initial bolus of 60 U/kg (maximum 4000 U) followed by an initial infusion of 12 U/kg per hour (maximum 1000 U/h). The activated partial thromboplastin time during maintenance therapy should be 1.5–2 times the control value.

An alternative to UFH for anticoagulation of patients with STEMI are the low-molecular-weight heparin (LMWH) preparations, which are formed by enzymatic or chemical depolymerization to produce saccharide chains of varying length but with a mean molecular weight of ~5000 Da. Advantages of LMWHs include high bioavailability permitting administration subcutaneously, reliable anticoagulation without monitoring, and greater antiXa:IIa activity. Enoxaparin has been shown to significantly reduce the composite endpoints of death/nonfatal reinfarction (Fig. 35-6) and death/nonfatal reinfarction/urgent revascularization compared with UFH in STEMI patients who receive fibrinolysis. Although treatment with enoxaparin is associated with higher rates of serious bleeding, net clinical benefit—a composite endpoint that combines efficacy and safety—strongly favors enoxaparin over UFH.

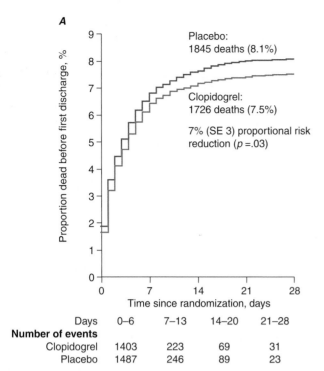

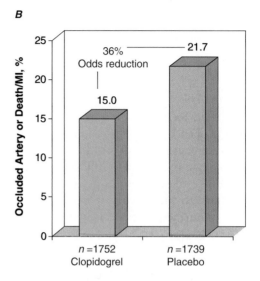

FIGURE 35-5

A. Effect of the addition of clopidogrel on in-hospital mortality after STEMI. These time-to-event curves show a 0.6% reduction in mortality in the group receiving clopidogrel plus aspirin (N = 22,961) compared to placebo plus aspirin (N = 22,891) in the COMMIT trial. SE, standard error. *(Reproduced with permission from ZM Chen et al: Lancet 366:1607, 2005.)* **B.** Effects of the addition of clopidogrel in patients receiving fibrinolysis for STEMI. Patients in the clopidogrel group (N = 1752) had a 36% reduction in the odds of dying, sustaining a recurrent infarction, or having an occluded infarct artery compared to the placebo group (N = 1739) in the CLARITY-TIMI 28 trial (p <001). *(Adapted from Sabatine MS et al: New Engl J Med 352:1179, 2005.)*

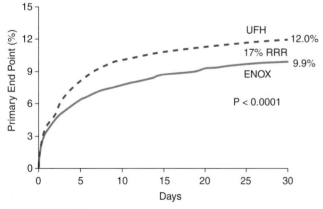

FIGURE 35-6

Enoxaparin is superior to unfractionated heparin in STEMI patients receiving fibrinolysis. In the ExTRACT-TIMI 25 trial, patients receiving the low-molecular-weight heparin enoxaparin in addition to a fibrinolytic agent plus aspirin (N = 10,256) had a significantly lower rate of the composite endpoint of death or nonfatal reinfarction compared to patients receiving unfractionated heparin in combination with a fibrinolytic plus aspirin (N = 10,223). RRR, relative risk reduction. *(Reproduced with permission from EM Antman et al: New Engl J Med 354:1477, 2006.)*

Patients with an anterior location of the infarction, severe LV dysfunction, heart failure, a history of embolism, two-dimensional echocardiographic evidence of mural thrombus, or atrial fibrillation are at increased risk of systemic or pulmonary thromboembolism. Such individuals should receive full therapeutic levels of antithrombin therapy (LMWH or UFH) while hospitalized, followed by at least 3 months of warfarin therapy.

BETA-ADRENOCEPTOR BLOCKERS

The benefits of beta blockers in patients with STEMI can be divided into benefits that occur immediately when the drug is given acutely and benefits that accrue over the long term when the drug is given for secondary prevention after an infarction. Acute intravenous beta blockade improves the myocardial O_2 supply-demand relationship, decreases pain, reduces infarct size, and decreases the incidence of serious ventricular arrhythmias. In patients who undergo fibrinolysis soon after the onset of chest pain, no incremental reduction in mortality rate is seen with beta blockers, but recurrent ischemia and reinfarction are reduced.

Thus, beta blocker therapy after STEMI is useful for most patients (including those treated with an ACE inhibitor) except those in whom it is specifically contraindicated (patients with heart failure or severely compromised LV function, heart block, orthostatic hypotension, or a history of asthma) and perhaps those whose excellent long-term prognosis (defined as an expected mortality rate of <1% per year, patients <55 years, no previous MI, with normal ventricular function, no complex ventricular ectopy, and no angina) markedly diminishes any potential benefit.

INHIBITION OF THE RENIN-ANGIOTENSIN-ALDOSTERONE SYSTEM

Angiotensin-converting enzyme (ACE) inhibitors reduce the mortality rate after STEMI, and the mortality benefits are additive to those achieved with aspirin and beta blockers. The maximum benefit is seen in high-risk patients (those who are elderly or who have an anterior infarction, a prior infarction, and/or globally depressed LV function), but evidence suggests that a short-term benefit occurs when ACE inhibitors are prescribed unselectively to all hemodynamically stable patients with STEMI (i.e., those with a systolic pressure >100 mmHg). The mechanism involves a reduction in ventricular remodeling after infarction (see Ventricular Dysfunction, later) with a subsequent reduction in the risk of congestive heart failure (CHF). The rate of recurrent infarction may also be lower in patients treated chronically with ACE inhibitors after infarction.

Before hospital discharge, LV function should be assessed with an imaging study. ACE inhibitors should be continued indefinitely in patients who have clinically evident CHF, in patients in whom an imaging study shows a reduction in global LV function or a large regional wall motion abnormality, or in those who are hypertensive.

Angiotensin receptor blockers (ARBs) should be administered to STEMI patients who are intolerant of ACE inhibitors and who have either clinical or radiological signs of heart failure. Long-term aldosterone blockade should be prescribed for STEMI patients without significant renal dysfunction (creatinine ≥2.5 mg/dL in men and ≥2.0 mg/dL in women) or hyperkalemia (potassium ≥5.0 mEq/L) who are already receiving therapeutic doses of an ACE inhibitor, an LV ejection fraction ≤40 percent, and either symptomatic heart failure or diabetes mellitus. A multidrug regimen for inhibiting the renin-angiotensin-aldosterone system has been shown to reduce both heart failure–related and sudden cardiac death–related cardiovascular mortality after STEMI, but has not been as thoroughly explored as ACE inhibitors in STEMI patients.

OTHER AGENTS

Favorable effects on the ischemic process and ventricular remodeling (see later) previously led many physicians to routinely use *intravenous nitroglycerin* (5–10 μg/min initial dose and up to 200 μg/min as long as hemodynamic stability is maintained) for the first 24–48 h after the onset of infarction. However, the benefits of routine use of intravenous nitroglycerin are less in the contemporary era where beta-adrenoceptor blockers and ACE inhibitors are routinely prescribed for patients with STEMI.

Results of multiple trials of different calcium antagonists have failed to establish a role for these agents in the treatment of most patients with STEMI. Therefore, the routine use of calcium antagonists cannot be recommended. Strict control of blood glucose in diabetic patients with STEMI has been shown to reduce the mortality rate. Serum magnesium should be measured in all patients on admission, and any demonstrated deficits should be corrected to minimize the risk of arrhythmias.

COMPLICATIONS AND THEIR MANAGEMENT

VENTRICULAR DYSFUNCTION

After STEMI, the left ventricle undergoes a series of changes in shape, size, and thickness in both the infarcted and noninfarcted segments. This process is referred to as *ventricular remodeling* and generally precedes the development of clinically evident CHF in the months to years after infarction. Soon after STEMI, the left ventricle begins to dilate. Acutely, this results from expansion of the infarct, i.e., slippage of muscle bundles, disruption of normal myocardial cells, and tissue loss within the necrotic zone, resulting in disproportionate thinning and elongation of the infarct zone. Later, lengthening of the noninfarcted segments occurs as well. The overall chamber enlargement that occurs is related to the size and location of the infarct, with greater dilation following infarction of the anterior wall and apex of the left ventricle and causing more marked hemodynamic impairment, more frequent heart failure, and a poorer prognosis. Progressive dilation and its clinical consequences may be ameliorated by therapy with ACE inhibitors and other vasodilators (e.g., nitrates). In patients with an ejection fraction <40%, regardless of whether or not heart failure is present, ACE inhibitors or ARBs should be prescribed (see Inhibition of the Renin-Angiotensin-Aldosterone System, earlier).

HEMODYNAMIC ASSESSMENT

Pump failure is now the primary cause of in-hospital death from STEMI. The extent of infarction correlates well with the degree of pump failure and with mortality, both early (within 10 days of infarction) and later. The most common clinical signs are pulmonary rales and S₃ and S₄ gallop sounds. Pulmonary congestion is also frequently seen on the chest roentgenogram. Elevated LV filling pressure and elevated pulmonary artery pressure are the characteristic hemodynamic findings, but these findings may result from a reduction of ventricular compliance (diastolic failure) and/or a reduction of stroke volume with secondary cardiac dilation (systolic failure) (Chap. 17).

A classification originally proposed by Killip divides patients into four groups: class I, no signs of pulmonary or venous congestion; class II, moderate heart failure as evidenced by rales at the lung bases, S_3 gallop, tachypnea, or signs of failure of the right side of the heart, including venous and hepatic congestion; class III, severe heart failure, pulmonary edema; and class IV, shock with systolic pressure <90 mmHg and evidence of peripheral vasoconstriction, peripheral cyanosis, mental confusion, and oliguria. When this classification was established in 1967, the expected hospital mortality rate of patients in these classes was as follows: class I, 0–5%; class II, 10–20%; class III, 35–45%; and class IV, 85–95%. With advances in management, the mortality rate in each class has fallen, perhaps by as much as one-third to one-half.

Hemodynamic evidence of abnormal global LV function appears when contraction is seriously impaired in 20–25% of the left ventricle. Infarction of ≥40% of the left ventricle usually results in cardiogenic shock (Chap. 28). Positioning of a balloon flotation (Swan-Ganz) catheter in the pulmonary artery permits monitoring of LV filling pressure; this technique is useful in patients who exhibit hypotension and/or clinical evidence of CHF. Cardiac output can also be determined with a pulmonary artery catheter. With the addition of intraarterial pressure monitoring, systemic vascular resistance can be calculated as a guide to adjusting vasopressor and vasodilator therapy. Some patients with STEMI have markedly elevated LV filling pressures (>22 mmHg) and normal cardiac indices [2.6–3.6 L/(min/m²)], while others have relatively low LV filling pressures (<15 mmHg) and reduced cardiac indices. The former patients usually benefit from diuresis, while the latter may respond to volume expansion.

Hypovolemia

This is an easily corrected condition that may contribute to the hypotension and vascular collapse associated with STEMI in some patients. It may be secondary to previous diuretic use, to reduced fluid intake during the early stages of the illness, and/or to vomiting associated with pain or medications. Consequently, hypovolemia should be identified and corrected in patients with STEMI and hypotension before more vigorous forms of therapy are begun. Central venous pressure reflects RV rather than LV filling pressure and is an inadequate guide for adjustment of blood volume, since LV function is almost always affected much more adversely than RV function in patients with STEMI. The optimal LV filling or pulmonary artery wedge pressure may vary considerably among patients. Each patient's ideal level (generally ~20 mmHg) is reached by cautious fluid administration during careful monitoring of oxygenation and cardiac output. Eventually the cardiac output level plateaus, and further increases in LV filling pressure only increase congestive symptoms and decrease systemic oxygenation without raising arterial pressure.

R̲X̲ Treatment:
CONGESTIVE HEART FAILURE

The management of CHF in association with STEMI is similar to that of acute heart failure secondary to other forms of heart disease (avoidance of hypoxemia, diuresis, afterload reduction, inotropic support) (Chap. 17), except that the benefits of digitalis administration to patients with STEMI are unimpressive. By contrast, diuretic agents are extremely effective, as they diminish pulmonary congestion in the presence of systolic and/or diastolic heart failure. LV filling pressure falls and orthopnea and dyspnea improve after the intravenous administration of furosemide or other loop diuretics. These drugs should be used with caution, however, as they can result in a massive diuresis with associated decreases in plasma volume, cardiac output, systemic blood pressure, and hence coronary perfusion. Nitrates in various forms may be used to decrease preload and congestive symptoms. Oral isosorbide dinitrate, topical nitroglycerin ointment, or intravenous nitroglycerin all have the advantage over a diuretic of lowering preload through venodilation without decreasing the total plasma volume. In addition, nitrates may improve ventricular compliance if ischemia is present, as ischemia causes an elevation of LV filling pressure. Vasodilators must be used with caution to prevent serious hypotension. As noted earlier, ACE inhibitors are an ideal class of drugs for management of ventricular dysfunction after STEMI, especially for the long term. (See Inhibition of the Renin-Angiotensin-Aldosterone System, earlier.)

CARDIOGENIC SHOCK

Prompt reperfusion, efforts to reduce infarct size, and treatment of ongoing ischemia and other complications of MI appear to have reduced the incidence of cardiogenic shock from 20% to about 7%. Only 10% of patients with this condition present with it on admission, while 90% develop it during hospitalization. Typically, patients who develop cardiogenic shock have severe multivessel coronary artery disease with evidence of "piecemeal" necrosis extending outward from the original infarct zone. The evaluation and management of cardiogenic shock and severe power failure after STEMI are discussed in detail in Chap. 28.

RIGHT VENTRICULAR INFARCTION

Approximately one-third of patients with inferior infarction demonstrate at least a minor degree of RV necrosis. An occasional patient with inferoposterior LV infarction also has extensive RV infarction, and rare patients present with infarction limited primarily to the RV. Clinically significant RV infarction causes signs of severe RV failure [jugular venous distention, Kussmaul's sign, hepatomegaly (Chap. 9)] with or without hypotension. ST-segment elevations of right-sided precordial ECG leads, particularly lead V_4R, are frequently present in the first 24 h in patients with RV infarction. Two-dimensional echocardiography is helpful in determining the degree of RV dysfunction. Catheterization of the right side of the heart often reveals a distinctive hemodynamic pattern resembling constrictive pericarditis (steep right atrial "y" descent and an early diastolic dip and plateau in RV waveforms) (Chap. 22). Therapy consists of volume expansion to maintain adequate RV preload and efforts to improve LV performance with attendant reduction in pulmonary capillary wedge and pulmonary arterial pressures.

ARRHYTHMIAS

(See also Chaps. 15 and 16) The incidence of arrhythmias after STEMI is higher in patients seen early after the onset of symptoms. The mechanisms responsible for infarction-related arrhythmias include autonomic nervous system imbalance, electrolyte disturbances, ischemia, and slowed conduction in zones of ischemic myocardium. An arrhythmia can usually be managed successfully if trained personnel and appropriate equipment are available when it develops. Since most deaths from arrhythmia occur during the first few hours after infarction, the effectiveness of treatment relates directly to the speed with which patients come under medical observation. The prompt management of arrhythmias constitutes a significant advance in the treatment of STEMI.

Ventricular Premature Beats

Infrequent, sporadic ventricular premature depolarizations occur in almost all patients with STEMI and do not require therapy. Whereas in the past, frequent, multifocal, or early diastolic ventricular extrasystoles (so-called warning arrhythmias) were routinely treated with antiarrhythmic drugs to reduce the risk of development of ventricular tachycardia and ventricular fibrillation, pharmacologic therapy is now reserved for patients with sustained ventricular arrhythmias. Prophylactic antiarrhythmic therapy (either intravenous lidocaine early or oral agents later) is contraindicated for ventricular premature beats in the absence of clinically important ventricular tachyarrhythmias, as such therapy may actually increase the mortality rate. Beta-adrenoceptor blocking agents are effective in abolishing ventricular ectopic activity in patients with STEMI and in the prevention of ventricular fibrillation. As described earlier (see Beta-Adrenoceptor Blockers, earlier), they should be used routinely in patients without contraindications. In addition, hypokalemia and hypomagnesemia are risk factors for ventricular fibrillation in patients with STEMI; the serum potassium concentration should be adjusted to ~4.5 mmol/L and magnesium to ~2.0 mmol/L.

Ventricular Tachycardia and Fibrillation

Within the first 24 h of STEMI, ventricular tachycardia and fibrillation can occur without prior warning arrhythmias. The occurrence of ventricular fibrillation can be reduced by prophylactic administration of intravenous lidocaine. However, prophylactic use of lidocaine has not been shown to reduce overall mortality from STEMI. In fact, in addition to causing possible noncardiac complications, lidocaine may predispose to an excess risk of bradycardia and asystole. For these reasons, and with earlier treatment of active ischemia, more frequent use of beta-blocking agents, and the nearly universal success of electrical cardioversion or defibrillation, routine prophylactic antiarrhythmic drug therapy *is no longer recommended.*

Sustained ventricular tachycardia that is well tolerated hemodynamically should be treated with an intravenous regimen of amiodarone (bolus of 150 mg over 10 min, followed by infusion of 1.0 mg/min for 6 h and then 0.5 mg/min); or procainamide (bolus of 15 mg/kg over 20–30 min; infusion of 1–4 mg/min); if it does not stop promptly, electroversion should be used (Chap. 16). An unsynchronized discharge of 200–300 J (monophasic wave form; ~50% of these energies with biphasic wave forms) is used immediately in patients with ventricular fibrillation or when ventricular tachycardia causes hemodynamic deterioration. Ventricular tachycardia or fibrillation that is refractory to electroshock may be more responsive after the patient is treated with epinephrine (1 mg intravenously or 10 mL of a 1:10,000 solution via the intracardiac route), or amiodarone (a 75–150 mg bolus).

Ventricular arrhythmias, including the unusual form of ventricular tachycardia known as torsades des pointes (Chap. 16), may occur in patients with STEMI as a consequence of other concurrent problems (such as hypoxia, hypokalemia, or other electrolyte disturbances) or of the toxic effects of an agent being administered to the patient (such as digoxin or quinidine). A search for such secondary causes should always be undertaken.

Although the in-hospital mortality rate is increased, the long-term survival is excellent in patients who survive to hospital discharge after *primary* ventricular fibrillation, i.e., ventricular fibrillation that is a primary response to acute ischemia that occurs during the first 48 h and is not associated with predisposing factors such as CHF, shock, bundle branch block, or ventricular aneurysm. This result is in sharp contrast to the poor prognosis for patients who develop ventricular fibrillation *secondary* to severe pump failure. For patients who develop ventricular tachycardia or ventricular fibrillation late in their hospital course (i.e., after the first 48 h), the mortality rate is increased both in-hospital and during long-term follow-up. Such patients should be considered for electrophysiologic study and implantation of a cardioverter/defibrillator (ICD) (Chap. 16). A more challenging issue is the prevention of sudden cardiac death from ventricular fibrillation late after STEMI in patients who have not exhibited sustained ventricular tachyarrhythmias during their index hospitalization. An algorithm for selection of patients who warrant prophylactic implantation of an ICD is shown in **Fig. 35-7**.

Accelerated Idioventricular Rhythm

Accelerated idioventricular rhythm (AIVR, "slow ventricular tachycardia"), a ventricular rhythm with a rate of

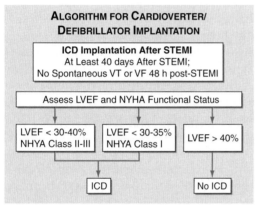

FIGURE 35-7

Algorithm for assessment of need for implantation of a cardioverter/defibrillator. The appropriate management is selected based upon measurement of left ventricular ejection fraction and assessment of the NYHA functional class. Patients with depressed left ventricular function at least 40 days post-STEMI are referred for insertion of an implantable cardioverter/defibrillator (ICD) if the LVEF is <30–40% and they are in NYHA class II–III or if the LVEF is <30–35% and they are in NYHA class I functional status. Patients with preserved left ventricular function (LVEF >40%) do not receive an ICD regardless of NYHA functional class. All patients are treated with medical therapy post-STEMI. [*Adapted from data contained in Zipes DP, Camm AJ, et al: ACC/AHA/ESC 2006 guidelines for management of patients with ventricular arrhythmias and the prevention of sudden cardiac death; a report of the American College of Cardiology/American Heart Association Task Force and the European Society of Cardiology Committee for Practice Guidelines (Writing Committee to Develop Guidelines for Management of Patients with Ventricular Arrhythmias and the Prevention of Sudden Cardiac Death). J Am Coll Cardiol 48:1064, 2006.*]

60–100 beats/min, occurs in 25% of patients with STEMI. It often occurs transiently during fibrinolytic therapy at the time of reperfusion. For the most part, AIVR is benign and does not presage the development of classic ventricular tachycardia. Most episodes of AIVR do not require treatment if the patient is monitored carefully, as degeneration into a more serious arrhythmia is rare.

Supraventricular Arrhythmias

Sinus tachycardia is the most common supraventricular arrhythmia. If it occurs secondary to another cause (such as anemia, fever, heart failure, or a metabolic derangement), the primary problem should be treated first. However, if it appears to be due to sympathetic overstimulation (e.g., as part of a hyperdynamic state), then treatment with a beta blocker is indicated. Other common arrhythmias in this group are atrial flutter and atrial fibrillation, which are often secondary to LV failure. Digoxin is usually the treatment of choice for supraventricular arrhythmias if heart failure is present. If heart failure is absent, beta blockers, verapamil, or diltiazem are suitable alternatives for controlling the ventricular rate, as they may also help to control ischemia. If the abnormal rhythm persists for >2 h with a ventricular rate >120 beats/min, or if tachycardia induces heart failure, shock, or ischemia (as manifested by recurrent pain or ECG changes), a synchronized electroshock (100–200 J monophasic wave form) should be used.

Accelerated junctional rhythms have diverse causes but may occur in patients with inferoposterior infarction. Digitalis excess must be ruled out. In some patients with severely compromised LV function, the loss of appropriately timed atrial systole results in a marked reduction of cardiac output. Right atrial or coronary sinus pacing is indicated in such instances.

Sinus Bradycardia

Treatment of sinus bradycardia is indicated if hemodynamic compromise results from the slow heart rate. Atropine is the most useful drug for increasing heart rate and should be given intravenously in doses of 0.5 mg initially. If the rate remains <50–60 beats/min, additional doses of 0.2 mg, up to a total of 2.0 mg, may be given. Persistent bradycardia (<40 beats/min) despite atropine may be treated with electrical pacing. Isoproterenol should be avoided.

Atrioventricular and Intraventricular Conduction Disturbances

(See also Chap. 15) Both the in-hospital mortality rate and the post-discharge mortality rate of patients who have complete atrioventricular (AV) block in association with anterior infarction are markedly higher than those of patients who develop AV block with inferior infarction. This difference is related to the fact that heart block in inferior infarction is commonly a result of increased vagal tone and/or the release of adenosine and therefore is transient. In anterior wall infarction, however, heart block is usually related to ischemic malfunction of the conduction system, which is commonly associated with extensive myocardial necrosis.

Temporary electrical pacing provides an effective means of increasing the heart rate of patients with bradycardia due to AV block. However, acceleration of the heart rate may have only a limited impact on prognosis in patients with anterior wall infarction and complete heart block in whom the large size of the infarct is the major factor determining outcome. It should be carried out if it improves hemodynamics. Pacing does appear to be beneficial in patients with inferoposterior infarction who have complete heart block associated with heart failure, hypotension, marked bradycardia, or significant ventricular ectopic activity. A subgroup of these patients, those with RV infarction, often respond poorly to ventricular pacing because of the loss of the atrial contribution to ventricular filling. In such patients, dual-chamber AV sequential pacing may be required.

External noninvasive pacing electrodes should be positioned in a "demand" mode for patients with sinus bradycardia (rate <50 beats/min) that is unresponsive to drug therapy, Mobitz II second-degree AV block, third-degree heart block, or bilateral bundle branch block (e.g., right bundle branch block plus left anterior fascicular block). Retrospective studies suggest that permanent pacing may reduce the long-term risk of sudden death due to bradyarrhythmias in the rare patient who develops combined persistent bifascicular and transient third-degree heart block during the acute phase of MI.

OTHER COMPLICATIONS
Recurrent Chest Discomfort

Recurrent angina develops in ~25% of patients hospitalized for STEMI. This percentage is even higher in patients who undergo successful fibrinolysis. Since recurrent or persistent ischemia often heralds extension of the original infarct or reinfarction in a new myocardial zone and is associated with a near tripling of mortality after STEMI, patients with these symptoms should be referred for prompt coronary arteriography and mechanical revascularization. Repeat administration of a fibrinolytic agent is an alternative to early mechanical revascularization.

Pericarditis

(See also Chap. 22) Pericardial friction rubs and/or pericardial pain are frequently encountered in patients with STEMI involving the epicardium. This complication can usually be managed with aspirin (650 mg four times daily). It is important to diagnose the chest pain of pericarditis accurately, since failure to recognize it may lead to the erroneous diagnosis of recurrent ischemic pain and/or infarct extension, with resulting inappropriate use of anticoagulants, nitrates, beta blockers, or coronary arteriography. When it occurs, complaints of pain radiating to either trapezius muscle is helpful since such a pattern of discomfort is typical of pericarditis but rarely occurs with ischemic discomfort. Anticoagulants potentially could cause tamponade in the presence of acute pericarditis (as manifested by either pain or persistent rub) and therefore should not be used unless there is a compelling indication.

Thromboembolism

Clinically apparent thromboembolism complicates STEMI in ~10% of cases, but embolic lesions are found in 20% of patients in necropsy series, suggesting that thromboembolism is often clinically silent. Thromboembolism is considered to be an important contributing cause of death in 25% of patients with STEMI who die after admission to the hospital. Arterial emboli originate from LV mural thrombi, while most pulmonary emboli arise in the leg veins.

Thromboembolism typically occurs in association with large infarcts (especially anterior), CHF, and a LV thrombus detected by echocardiography. The incidence of arterial embolism from a clot originating in the ventricle at the site of an infarction is small but real. Two-dimensional echocardiography reveals LV thrombi in about one-third of patients with anterior wall infarction but in few patients with inferior or posterior infarction. Arterial embolism often presents as a major complication, such as hemiparesis when the cerebral circulation is involved or hypertension if the renal circulation is compromised. When a thrombus has been clearly demonstrated by echocardiographic or other techniques or when a large area of regional wall motion abnormality is seen even in the absence of a detectable mural thrombus, systemic anticoagulation should be undertaken (in the absence of contraindications), as the incidence of embolic complications appears to be markedly lowered by such therapy. The appropriate duration of therapy is unknown, but 3–6 months is probably prudent.

Left Ventricular Aneurysm

The term *ventricular aneurysm* is usually used to describe *dyskinesis* or local expansile paradoxical wall motion. Normally functioning myocardial fibers must shorten more if stroke volume and cardiac output are to be maintained in patients with ventricular aneurysm; if they cannot, overall ventricular function is impaired. True aneurysms are composed of scar tissue and neither predispose to nor are associated with cardiac rupture.

The complications of LV aneurysm do not usually occur for weeks to months after STEMI; they include CHF, arterial embolism, and ventricular arrhythmias. Apical aneurysms are the most common and the most easily detected by clinical examination. The physical finding of greatest value is a double, diffuse, or displaced apical impulse. Ventricular aneurysms are readily detected by two-dimensional echocardiography, which may also reveal a mural thrombus in an aneurysm.

Rarely, myocardial rupture may be contained by a local area of pericardium, along with organizing thrombus and hematoma. Over time, this *pseudoaneurysm* enlarges, maintaining communication with the LV cavity through a narrow neck. Because a pseudoaneurysm often ruptures spontaneously, it should be surgically repaired if recognized.

POSTINFARCTION RISK STRATIFICATION AND MANAGEMENT

Many clinical and laboratory factors have been identified that are associated with an increase in cardiovascular risk after initial recovery from STEMI. Some of the most important factors include persistent ischemia (spontaneous or provoked), depressed LV ejection fraction (<40%), rales above the lung bases on physical examination or congestion on chest radiograph, and symptomatic ventricular arrhythmias. Other features associated with increased risk include a history of previous MI, older than 75 years, diabetes mellitus, prolonged sinus tachycardia, hypotension, ST-segment changes at rest without angina ("silent ischemia"), an abnormal signal-averaged ECG, nonpatency of the infarct-related coronary artery (if angiography is undertaken), and persistent advanced heart block or a new intraventricular conduction abnormality on the ECG. Therapy must be individualized on the basis of the relative importance of the risk(s) present.

The goal of preventing reinfarction and death after recovery from STEMI has led to strategies to evaluate risk after infarction. In stable patients, submaximal exercise stress testing may be carried out before hospital discharge to detect residual ischemia and ventricular ectopy and to provide the patient with a guideline for exercise in the early recovery period. Alternatively, or in addition, a maximal (symptom-limited) exercise stress test may be carried out 4–6 weeks after infarction. Evaluation of LV function is usually warranted as well. Recognition of a depressed LV ejection fraction by echocardiography or radionuclide ventriculography identifies patients who should receive medications to inhibit the renin-angiotensin-aldosterone system. Patients in whom angina is induced at relatively low workloads, those who have a large reversible defect on perfusion imaging or a depressed ejection fraction, those with demonstrable ischemia, and those in whom exercise provokes symptomatic ventricular arrhythmias should be considered at high risk for recurrent MI or death from arrhythmia (Fig. 35-7). Cardiac catheterization with coronary angiography and/or invasive electrophysiologic evaluation is advised.

Exercise tests also aid in formulating an individualized exercise prescription, which can be much more vigorous in patients who tolerate exercise without any of the above-mentioned adverse signs. Additionally, predischarge stress testing may provide an important psychological benefit, building the patient's confidence by demonstrating a reasonable exercise tolerance.

In many hospitals a cardiac rehabilitation program with progressive exercise is initiated in the hospital and continued after discharge. Ideally, such programs should include an educational component that informs patients about their disease and its risk factors.

The usual duration of hospitalization for an uncomplicated STEMI is about 5 days. The remainder of the convalescent phase may be accomplished at home. During the first 1–2 weeks, the patient should be encouraged to increase activity by walking about the house and outdoors in good weather. Normal sexual activity may be resumed during this period. After 2 weeks, the physician must regulate the patient's activity on the basis of exercise tolerance. Most patients will be able to return to work within 2–4 weeks.

SECONDARY PREVENTION

Various secondary preventive measures are at least partly responsible for the improvement in the long-term mortality and morbidity rates after STEMI. Long-term treatment with an antiplatelet agent (usually aspirin) after STEMI is associated with a 25% reduction in the risk of recurrent infarction, stroke, or cardiovascular mortality (36 fewer events for every 1000 patients treated). An alternative antiplatelet agent that may be used for secondary prevention in patients intolerant of aspirin is clopidogrel (75 mg orally daily). ACE inhibitors or ARBs and, in appropriate patients, aldosterone antagonists should be used indefinitely by patients with clinically evident heart failure, a moderate decrease in global ejection fraction, or a large regional wall motion abnormality to prevent late ventricular remodeling and recurrent ischemic events.

The chronic routine use of oral beta-adrenoceptor blockers for at least 2 years after STEMI is supported by well-conducted, placebo-controlled trials.

Evidence suggests that warfarin lowers the risk of late mortality and the incidence of reinfarction after STEMI. Most physicians prescribe aspirin routinely for all patients without contraindications and add warfarin for patients at increased risk of embolism (see "Thromboembolism," earlier). Several studies suggest that in patients older than 75 years a low dose of aspirin (75–81 mg/d) in combination with warfarin administered to achieve an INR >2.0 is more effective than aspirin alone for preventing recurrent MI and embolic cerebrovascular accident. However, there is an increased risk of bleeding and a high rate of discontinuation of warfarin that has limited clinical acceptance of combination antithrombotic therapy. There is increased risk of bleeding when warfarin is added to dual antiplatelet therapy (aspirin and clopidogrel). However, patients who have had a stent implanted and have an indication for anticoagulation should receive dual antiplatelet therapies in combination with warfarin. Such patients should also receive a proton pump inhibitor to minimize the risk of gastrointestinal bleeding and should have regular monitoring of their hemoglobin levels and stool hematest while on combination antithrombotic therapy.

Finally, risk factors for *atherosclerosis* (Chap. 1) should be discussed with the patient, and, when possible, favorably modified.

FURTHER READINGS

American Heart Association: *Heart and Stroke Facts: 2005 Statistical Supplement*. Dallas, American Heart Association, 2006

Antman EM: Time is muscle: Translation into practice. J Am Coll Cardiol 52:1216, 2008

———: *ST-Elevation Myocardial Infarction:* Management, in: P Libby, RO Bonow, DL Mann, DP Zipes (eds.) Braunwald's Heart Disease: A Textbook of Cardiovascular Medicine, 8th edition, Philadelphia, Saunders Elsevier, 1233-1299, 2008

———, Braunwald E: Acute myocardial infarction, in *Braunwald's Heart Disease*, 8th ed, P Libby et al (eds). Philadelphia, Saunders, 2008

Antman EM et al: 2007 Focused Update of the ACC/AHA 2004 Guidelines for the Management of Patients With ST-Elevation Myocardial Infarction: A report of the American College of Cardiology/American Heart Association Task Force on Practice Guidelines: developed in collaboration with the Canadian Cardiovascular Society endorsed by the American Academy of Family Physicians: 2007 Writing Group to Review New Evidence and Update the ACC/AHA 2004 Guidelines for the Management of Patients With ST-Elevation Myocardial Infarction, Writing on Behalf of the 2004 Writing Committee. Circulation 117:296, 2008

Braunwald E, Antman EM: *ST-Elevation Myocardial Infarction: Pathology, Pathophysiology, and Clinical Features* in P Libby, RO Bonow, DL Mann, DP Zipes (eds.) Braunwald's Heart Disease: A Textbook of Cardiovascular Medicine, 8th edition, Philadelphia, Saunders Elsevier, 1207-1232, 2008

Boersma E et al: Acute myocardial infarction. Lancet 361:847, 2003

Falk E et al: Coronary plaque disruption. Circulation 92:657, 1995

Jacobs AK et al: Development of systems of care for ST-elevation myocardial infarction patients: executive summary. *Circulation* 116:217, 2007

Lloyd-Jones D et al: Heart disease and stroke statistics—2009 update: a report from the American Heart Association Statistics Committee and Stroke Statistics Subcommittee. *Circulation* 119:e21, 2009

Mehran R et al: Bivalirudin in patients undergoing primary angioplasty for acute myocardial infarction (HORIZONS-AMI): 1-year results of a randomised controlled trial. Lancet 374:1149, 2009

Michaels AD, Goldschlager N: Risk stratification after acute myocardial infarction in the reperfusion era. Prog Cardiovasc Dis 42:273, 2000

Montalescot G et al: Platelet glycoprotein IIb/IIIa inhibition with coronary stenting for acute myocardial infarction. N Engl J Med 344:1895, 2001

White HD, Chew DP: Acute myocardial infarction. Lancet 372:570, 2008

Wiviott SD et al: Prasugrel versus clopidogrel in patients with acute coronary syndromes. N Engl J Med 357:2001, 2007

CHAPTER 36

PERCUTANEOUS CORONARY INTERVENTION

Donald S. Baim[†]

The introduction of *percutaneous transluminal coronary angioplasty* (PTCA) by Andreas Gruntzig in 1977 established this form of catheter-based therapy as an alternative to bypass surgery for providing coronary revascularization in selected patients. The limitations of early equipment, however, meant that PTCA was applicable to <10% of all coronary revascularization candidates. By 1990, progressive improvements in PTCA equipment led to improved results, expanded indications for use, and an explosive growth in the annual number of PTCA procedures (to ~300,000 in the United States), roughly matching the coronary revascularization provided by surgical bypass operations. Newer interventional devices including atherectomy (plaque removal), stents (plaque scaffolding), and drug–eluting stents were introduced subsequently, further improving the acute success, safety, and long-term durability of percutaneous coronary intervention (PCI). Today, >1 million procedures are performed annually, representing twice the annual number of coronary bypass operations. This dominant role of catheter-based intervention in the treatment of coronary artery disease (CAD) has led to creation of a separate area within the field of cardiovascular diseases known as *interventional cardiology*, with incremental fellowship requirements and Board certification of additional qualification based on training, ongoing experience, and a written examination.

All catheter-based interventions are derivatives of diagnostic cardiac catheterization (Chap. 13), in which catheters are introduced into the arterial circulation by needle puncture, advanced into the heart under fluoroscopic guidance, and used for pressure measurements and injections of radiopaque liquid contrast agents. Interventional procedures differ in that the catheter placed into the ostium of the narrowed coronary artery is then used to advance a flexible, steerable guidewire (diameter <0.4 mm) down the coronary artery lumen, through the narrowing, and into the vessel beyond. This guidewire then serves as a "rail" over which angioplasty balloons or other therapeutic devices can be advanced and used to enlarge the narrowed segment of coronary artery. Because PCI is performed under local anesthesia and requires only a short (1-day) hospitalization, its use in suitable patients can greatly decrease recovery time and expense compared to coronary bypass surgery.

While not all types of coronary narrowing are well suited to catheter-based intervention, PCI is the treatment of choice for the majority of patients with symptomatic coronary disease. To decide which patients should undergo revascularization (as opposed to continued medical management) and to select which patients should undergo catheter-based rather than surgical revascularization requires a detailed understanding of both clinical and coronary angiographic features, as well as the capabilities of

---

[†]Recently deceased.

various interventional techniques. The remaining anatomic restrictions relate to dealing with diffuse disease, chronic total occlusions, and bifurcation lesions, but even these challenges are yielding to improved interventional devices and techniques. Deciding between PCI and bypass surgery thus requires balancing the individual patient's coronary anatomy and technical challenges against any factors that limit potential completeness of surgical revascularization or increase its risk (advanced age, poor left ventricular function, and concomitant medical problems). Both patient and physician need to be aware that while catheter-based intervention is done under local anesthesia and has a lower elective mortality rate than bypass surgery (0.4–1.0%, compared to a rate of 1–3%), it is still an invasive procedure whose risks and benefits need to be weighed carefully for each individual patient.

INDICATIONS

The fundamental indication for PCI is the presence of one or more coronary stenoses thought to be responsible for a clinical syndrome, that warrant revascularization, are approachable by catheter-based techniques, with risks and benefits that compare favorably with those of bypass surgery. For most patients with stable angina, the main goal of either surgical or catheter-based revascularization is the relief of angina rather than improved survival. In patients with multivessel CAD, particularly those with reduced left ventricular function or diabetes, there may also be a survival advantage to surgical revascularization. Trials randomizing patients with multivessel disease in whom either balloon angioplasty or bypass surgery is possible have suggested that the two procedures have essentially equivalent in-hospital and 3- to 5-year mortality rates (except for patients with diabetes mellitus, in whom surgical treatment appears to offer improved 5- to 7-year survival compared to PCI). These trials, however, showed that up to 20% of patients who underwent balloon angioplasty needed a second revascularization procedure to treat renarrowing at the initial treatment site (restenosis). Recent advances in PCI technology (particularly drug-eluting stents) have dramatically reduced the incidence of repeat procedures to treat restenosis to <5%, and have made the durability of symptomatic relief by PCI nearly identical to that of surgery in anatomically suitable patients. Even patients with ostial or mid-shaft left main coronary artery lesions and near normal left ventricular function have 1 year event rates <3% with drug-eluting stenting, although bypass surgery is still the preferred revascularization modality in patients without factors that increase surgical risk.

The current clinical indications for PCI cover the spectrum of ischemic heart disease, from patients with silent ischemia to patients with unstable angina or acute myocardial infarction (MI). The detailed indications are summarized in the recent ACC/AHA guidelines, and the following discussion is thus more conceptual in nature. One clear indication for PCI is moderately *chronic stable angina*, which persists despite medical antianginal therapy and is caused by anatomically suitable lesions (Chap. 33). If multiple severe lesions are present, these can generally be treated during a single procedure. In patients with *acute coronary syndromes*, the benefits of PCI include reduced death and MI. In *unstable angina* and *non-ST-elevation MI* (STEMI) (Chap. 34), recent studies employing platelet IIb/IIIa receptor blockers and coronary stenting have shown >20% reduction in death or MI at 6 months, with a parallel reduction in hospital readmission, in comparison with a conservative strategy in which PCI was reserved for strongly positive exercise test results. In patients with *acute STEMI* (Chap. 35), trials comparing thrombolysis to primary angioplasty have consistently shown lower mortality (5.0 vs. 7.0%, $p = .0002$), less non-fatal reinfarction (3.0% vs. 7.0%, $p = .0003$, and less hemorrhagic stroke (0.05% vs. 1%, $p = .0001$), with primary angioplasty (both PTCA and stenting). The current PCI guidelines thus recommend that primary PCI should be performed in patients with STEMI who present within 12 h of symptom onset, if performed in a timely fashion (medical contact-to-balloon or door-to-balloon time within 90 min) by persons skilled in the procedure, working in an appropriate laboratory environment.

As the clinical indications for PCI have broadened, so have its anatomic capabilities. Largely through the introduction of newer interventional devices, PCI has advanced well beyond the treatment of proximal, discrete, subtotal, concentric, non-calcified lesions. Calcified, complex, or diffuse lesions respond well to coronary stent placement, sometimes after pretreatment with rotational atherectomy. Even chronically totally occluded coronary arteries can be crossed and dilated effectively and, when treated with drug-eluting stents, have a 90% long-term patency rate. In addition to lesions in the native coronary tree, obstructions in the saphenous vein bypass grafts can also be dilated successfully to treat recurrent post-bypass angina, making use of distal embolic protection devices to reduce the incidence of peri-procedural MI caused by the tendency of atheroembolic debris to be liberated during stenting of such lesions.

CURRENT TECHNIQUES

While conventional balloon angioplasty (PTCA) offered anatomic versatility and acceptable short- and long-term results, it had limited efficacy in certain anatomic lesion types (e.g., calcified eccentric, ostial, thrombus-containing, or bifurcation lesions). It was also plagued by the

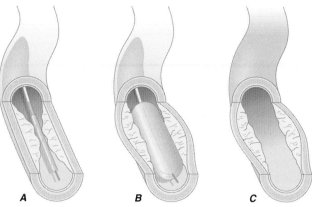

FIGURE 36-1

Proposed mechanism of angioplasty. *A.* Deflated balloon positioned across stenosis. ***B.*** Inflation of the balloon catheter within the stenotic segment causes cracking of the intimal plaque, stretching of the media and adventitia, and expansion of the outer diameter of the vessel. ***C.*** Following balloon deflation, there is partial elastic recoil of the vessel wall, leaving a residual stenosis of 30% and local plaque disruption that would be evident as haziness of the lumen contours on angiography. *[From JT Willerson (ed): Treatment of Heart Diseases, New York, Gower Medical, 1992.]*

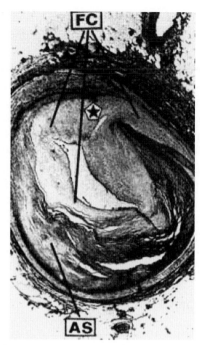

FIGURE 36-2

Mechanisms of restenosis. Cross section of a restenotic lesion in the left anterior descending artery 5 months after initial coronary angioplasty shows the original atherosclerotic plaque (AS), the crack in the medial layer induced by the original procedure (star), and the proliferation of fibrocellular tissues (FC) that constitutes the restenotic lesion. In stent restenosis, the mechanism is purely such proliferation, whereas in non-stent interventions such as balloon angioplasty there is frequently also a component due to shrinkage of the overall vessel diameter (unfavorable remodeling) at the treatment site. *(From PW Serruys, et al: Am J Cardiol 54:482, 1984.)*

problems of elastic recoil (**Fig. 36-1**), *intimal dissection* (which led to abrupt closure of the dilated segment in 3% of cases requiring emergency bypass surgery), and *restenosis* of 30–40% of the dilated segments within 6 months of initially successful treatment due to a combination of exaggerated neointimal hyperplasia and overall vessel contraction in response to the interventional injury (**Fig. 36-2**). These problems motivated the development of a number of newer, non-balloon techniques that entered routine clinical practice during the early 1990s. Stents (see later) increased acute procedural success to 98%, reduced the incidence of emergency surgery to 0.1%, and reduced the incidence of restenosis to 15–20%. The incidence of restenosis has been further reduced to 5% by the introduction of drug-eluting stents in 2003. In parallel, improvements in adjunctive pharmacotherapy (especially the acute use of platelet glycoprotein IIb/IIIa receptor blockers, and longer-term thienopyridine, i.e., clopidogrel) use have helped produce significant improvements in procedural safety. In large part, the progressive improvements in PCI results over the past 30 years, and thereby the growth of PCI to become the dominant coronary revascularization modality, lies in the progressive improvements in PCI devices and adjunctive pharmacology.

Stents

Stents are metallic scaffolds that are inserted into a diseased vessel segment in their collapsed form and are then deployed by balloon inflation. They overcome two

of the principal limitations of balloon dilatation—local dissection of the plaque and elastic recoil of the vessel wall—allowing stents to consistently provide an essentially normal-appearing vessel lumen in the treated segment. In 1994, the first two balloon-expandable stent designs were approved by the U.S. Food and Drug Administration (FDA), with a number of second- and third-generation stent designs introduced subsequently that offered easier delivery into tortuous or distal lesions (**Fig. 36-3**). In the early experience, metallic stents proved prone to thrombotic occlusion, either acute (<24 h) or subacute (1–14 days with a peak at 6 days), which was ameliorated by greater attention to full initial deployment and the use of dual antiplatelet therapy [aspirin indefinitely, plus the platelet P_2Y_{12}-receptor blockers (ticlopidine or clopidogrel) for 2–4 weeks]. In addition to controlling complications related to abrupt vessel closure, the fact that stenting provided a larger acute luminal area than balloon angioplasty alone reduced the incidence of subsequent restenosis. When in-stent restenosis did occur as the result of excessive neointimal

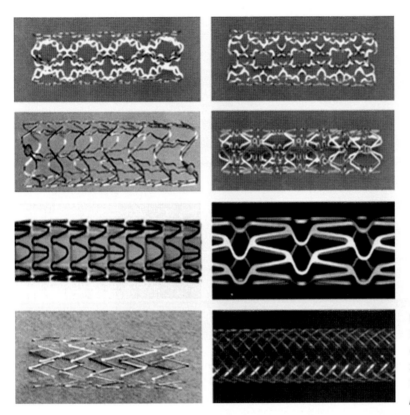

FIGURE 36-3

Examples of various coronary stent designs. Each design is shown in the expanded state. *[Modified from GW Stone. In D Baim (ed). Cardiac Catheterization, Angiography and Intervention, 7th ed, Philadelphia, Lippincott Williams & Wilkins, 2006.]*

hyperplasia within the stent, this could be treated by balloon dilatation followed by catheter-delivered local β or γ radiation (i.e., brachytherapy) to suppress subsequent neointimal regrowth. Despite the limitations of subacute stent thrombosis and in-stent restenosis, the major improvements in outcome led to the dominance of stent placement in catheter-based coronary revascularization, with placement of one or more stents in 85% of all procedures.

Since 2004, the concept of using stents as a local drug delivery platform to favorably modulate the neointimal healing process has entered clinical practice (Fig. 36-4). A wide variety of cytostatic, cytotoxic, and anti-inflammatory and anti-proliferative agents have been studied, but current drug-eluting stents utilize either sirolimus (or a derivative thereof) or paclitaxel released from a polymer coating applied to the stent surface. *Sirolimus* is a naturally occurring and immunosuppressive agent that arrests cell proliferation in the G_1 phase, and has been shown to reduce target-vessel failure (target vessel revascularization, death, or MI) to 8.6% vs. 21.0% for bare metal stents. *Paclitaxel* is an inhibitor of microtubules that can arrest cell division at the M phase in high concentrations, but can have cytostatic G_1, anti-migratory, and anti-inflammatory effects on smooth-muscle cells at lower concentrations. It has also been shown to reduce the incidence of ischemia-driven target-vessel revascularization at 12 months, to 7.1% vs. 17.1% for bare metal stents.

Subsequent trials and registries with both drug-eluting stents have supported their use in various vessel sizes and lesion lengths, total occlusions, vein grafts, as well as in patients with diabetes, with target lesion revascularization rates generally in the 4–6% range, and has brought the durability of PCI up to arguably match that of bypass surgery (Fig. 36-5). One consequence of the reduced neointimal hyperplasia with drug-eluting stents, however, is vulnerability to late stent thrombosis, extending to 3 years after implantation, and perhaps even longer. It is thus standard practice to prolong dual antiplatelet therapy (aspirin and clopidogrel) for at least 12 months after placement of a drug-eluting stent, to minimize the small (0.2–0.6% per year) risk of this potentially serious late complication. The risk of late stent thrombosis should always be kept in mind, however, should antiplatelet therapy need to be interrupted for bleeding or a noncardiac surgical procedure within the first year after drug-eluting stent implantation.

Other PCI Technologies

Whereas both balloon angioplasty and stent placement enlarge the coronary lumen by displacing plaque, *atherectomy catheters* enlarge the lumen by removing plaque mass from the treated lesion. Several mechanical atherectomy devices were developed in the 1990s, including directional, rotational, extraction, and laser atherectomy. Although each has certain applications, the greater technical difficulty and procedural complications associated with atherectomy in comparison with stenting has relegated these devices to niche roles (<5% adjunctive use

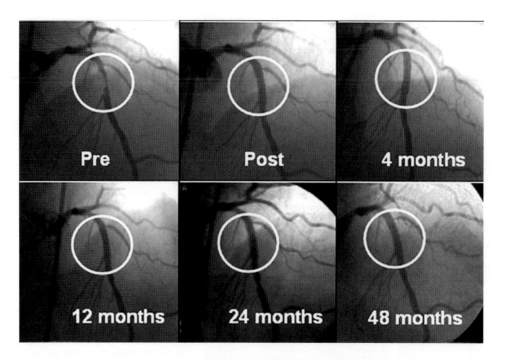

FIGURE 36-4

Long-term results from one of the first patients to receive a sirolimus-eluting stent in the early Sao Paulo experience. A high-grade stenosis in the proximal left anterior descending artery is stented with a single 3.0 mm sirolimus-eluting stent. Serial angiography shows sustained vessel patency with minimal late loss over a 4-year period. *[From GW Stone, in D Baim (ed): Cardiac Catheterization, Angiography and Intervention, 7th ed. Philadelphia, Lippincott Williams & Wilkins, 2006.]*

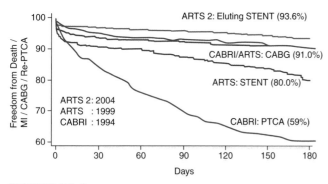

FIGURE 36-5

Improving results of percutaneous coronary intervention (PCI) compared to coronary artery bypass grafting (CABG). In a series of trials spanning a decade from 1994–2004, the 180-day event-free survival of bypass surgery has remained 91%. This was markedly superior to percutaneous transluminal coronary angioplasty (PTCA) in the CABRI trial (32% absolute difference) due to the effect of restenosis. In the ARTS trial, this deficit improved to 11% with the use of bare metal stenting. In the ARTS 2 trial, the event-free survival of drug-eluting stents was actually superior to that of bypass by 2.6%. Although the patient groups are not exactly comparable, the significant improvement in repeat revascularization with the drug-eluting stents may shift the balance further towards PCI. *(Courtesy of Prof. Patrick Serruys; with permission.)*

during current PCI). Various *thrombectomy* devices may be useful when large intracoronary thrombi are present (**Fig. 36-6**), although their routine use in acute MI PCI has failed to show any benefit in ST-segment resolution or final myocardial infarct size, and in one study their use has been associated with increased adverse events. *Embolic protection devices* (distal filters or occlusion/aspiration devices) may be useful adjuncts during the treatment of saphenous vein graft or other lesions prone to the liberation of debris that may compromise the distal myocardial microcirculation. Again, study of the routine use of distal embolic protection in STEMI has failed to show any improvement in myocardial salvage.

THE PCI PROCEDURE

The procedure begins with percutaneous insertion of an arterial sheath and coronary angiography (Chap. 13). The target lesions for PCI are identified, and the sequencing and strategy for each is planned. Anticoagulation is achieved using either unfractionated heparin [50–70 IU/kg, to an activated clotting time of 250–300 s (slightly less if a glycoprotein IIb/IIIa inhibitor is used concomitantly)] or a direct thrombin inhibitor such as bivalirudin. Aspirin pretreatment (325 mg/d) is begun before the procedure, and clopidogrel loading

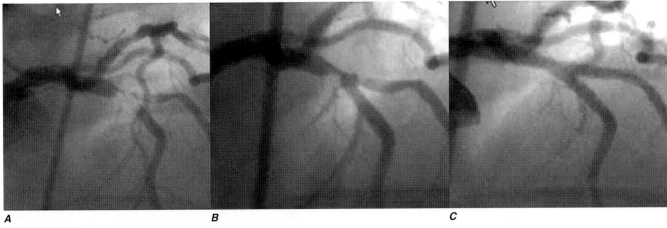

A   B   C

FIGURE 36-6

Diagnosis and treatment of an acute anterior wall myocardial infarction. In this patient, there is a subocclusive filling defect in the left anterior descending artery (**A**), which is removed by thrombectomy to show the underlying lesion (**B**), which is then treated by bifurcation stenting in the left anterior descending artery and the involved diagonal branch (**C**).

(300–600 mg) is administered either just before a planned PCI or otherwise at its conclusion. A guiding catheter, which may have the same 6 F (2 mm) outer diameter as a diagnostic coronary angiography catheter but a larger inner lumen to permit balloon and stent advancement, is placed in the involved coronary artery ostium. Under fluoroscopic guidance, a steerable 0.4-mm (0.014-in.) guidewire is advanced across the target stenosis and into the distal vessel beyond, to permit the advancement of a predilating balloon that is ~0.5 mm smaller than the estimated normal caliber of the target vessel, across the lesion. This balloon is inflated with dilute radiographic contrast to a pressure (usually 6–16 atm) to relieve any deformity in the balloon outline and thus partially relieve the stenosis.

If the lesion is heavily calcified, simple balloon predilation may be insufficient, and rotational atherectomy may be required to remove superficial luminal calcification and thereby improve lesion compliance. The guidewire is left in place as the predilating balloon is removed and a drug-eluting stent of appropriate size and length to cover the diseased segment plus a 5-mm margin on either side of the lesion is advanced into position. The angioplasty balloon on which the stent is mounted is then inflated to 14–16 atm to deploy the stent, which can then be further expanded at high pressure with a postdilating balloon as needed. The quality of the result is assessed with repeat angiography (and sometimes intravascular ultrasound) before moving on to treat other significant lesions. Lesions involving bifurcations may be treated either by placing a drug-eluting stent in the main vessel and "rescuing" a compromised branch by balloon dilation, or by any of several strategies to place drug-eluting stents in the main vessel and side branch.

A typical PCI may take 60–90 min, and utilize 150–250 mL of radiographic contrast, depending on the number and complexity of the lesions to be treated. At the end of the procedure, no further antithrombin therapy (heparin or bivalirudin) is given, although a IIb/IIIa receptor blocker may be continued for up to 18 h. The intraarterial sheath may be removed with manual pressure once the anticoagulated state has subsided (usually 2–4 h after the procedure) or may be removed immediately through the aid of a vascular entry sealing device (one of several collagen plugs, suture, or external clip devices). The patient is returned to an inpatient unit for overnight observation, before discharge the following day on dual antiplatelet therapy. A predischarge electrocardiogram (ECG) and biomarkers (CK-MB fraction) assessment are obtained to monitor for the occurrence of periprocedural non-Q wave myocardial necrosis. Elevation of CK-MB <5 times the laboratory upper limit of normal occur in 3–5% of procedures and should be noted, but it generally does not require changes in subsequent therapy. Larger elevations or the development of ECG changes, particularly if in the setting of ongoing or recurrent postprocedural chest pain, suggest a procedural complication such as vessel closure or loss of a side branch within the stented segment and may mandate repeat diagnostic coronary angiography to evaluate, exclude, or treat such problems.

Upon discharge, the need for ongoing dual antiplatelet therapy is reemphasized to the patient, who can generally return to work within 2–3 days. No specific follow-up of the interventional result is usually performed in the absence of a recurrence in chest pain suggestive of myocardial ischemia, but it is crucial to modify any existing coronary risk factors (generally including optimization of lipid

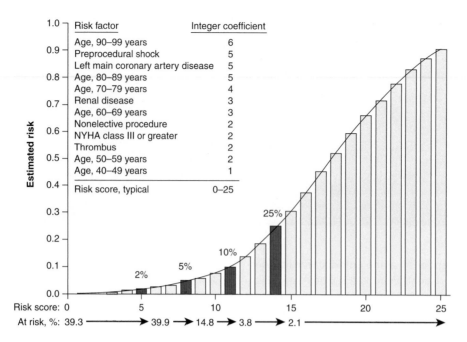

Risk factor	Integer coefficient
Age, 90–99 years	6
Preprocedural shock	5
Left main coronary artery disease	5
Age, 80–89 years	5
Age, 70–79 years	4
Renal disease	3
Age, 60–69 years	3
Nonelective procedure	2
NYHA class III or greater	2
Thrombus	2
Age, 50–59 years	2
Age, 40–49 years	1
Risk score, typical	0–25

At risk, %: 39.3 → 39.9 → 14.8 → 3.8 → 2.1 →

FIGURE 36-7

The Mayo Clinic risk score for mortality. This score assigns integer coefficients for each named clinical variable so that one can read the estimated mortality risk that corresponds to the total of the integer coefficients from the curve and the value on the *y* axis. The 2% of patients with a total score >14 thus have an expected procedural mortality of 25%. *(From M Singh et al, J Am Coll Cardiol 40:387, 2002, with permission.)*

status). The main cause of recurrent events in the 5 years after a successful stent-based PCI is, in fact, progression of disease at other (non-stented) coronary sites.

Serious complications of modern PCI are uncommon, with a mortality <0.3% for elective procedures (**Fig. 36-7**). As intervention has moved into more complex situations (multivessel disease, bifurcation lesions, vein graft, or unprotected left main lesions) in patients with acute coronary syndromes or poor baseline ventricular function, the average mortality of PCI has remained 1–1.5%. Abrupt vessel closure with emergency surgery has fallen to 0.1%, but current PCI guidelines still call for elective PCI to be performed in institutions that have on-site cardiac surgery support. Perforation of a coronary artery was an extremely rare complication of conventional balloon angioplasty but may occur in up to 1% of patients undergoing aggressive atherectomy procedures and may be seen with stenting. Even small perforations of the distal vessel by the angioplasty guidewire may lead to significant hemopericardium, requiring urgent pericardiocentesis in the setting of intense anticoagulant and antiplatelet therapy. PCI operators should thus be skilled in the management of such perforations using immediate balloon tamponade, placement of embolic vascular coils for small branch perforations, and placement of membrane-covered stents for perforations of major vessels. Finally, catheter-based interventions are subject to all of the complications of diagnostic catheterization, including local entry site complications, stroke, and

contrast nephropathy in sensitive patients. For most patients, however, catheter-based coronary revascularization offers a safe and effective alternative to surgical revascularization.

NONCORONARY INTERVENTIONS

Because atherosclerosis is a systemic disease (i.e., not limited to the coronary arteries), it is increasingly common for analogous percutaneous interventions to be performed in the carotid, renal, or lower extremity arteries. These procedures may be combined with PCI when clinically indicated. Catheter-based interventions may also be used to treat structural cardiac defects (e.g., atrial septal defect, patent foramen ovale) or valvular heart disease. Balloon valvuloplasty is now the dominant treatment for rheumatic mitral stenosis (Chap. 20), and various catheter-based modalities are being developed for percutaneous mitral valve repair for mitral regurgitation and for percutaneous aortic valve replacement for severe aortic stenosis in patients at prohibitive risk for surgical aortic valve replacement.

SUMMARY

The past 30 years have seen the development of new techniques (such as stent placement), new drug regimens, and refinements in practice driven by "evidence-based" medicine, allowing catheter-based revascularization (PCI) to develop from a procedural curiosity to what is now the dominant form of coronary revascularization. As short- and long-term results have improved and the number of procedures has continued to grow, the pace of development continues to accelerate. Similar catheter techniques are now being used elsewhere in the arterial circulation and for the correction of structural heart disease in selected patients.

FURTHER READINGS

ANTMAN EM et al: ACC/AHA guidelines for the management of patients with ST-elevation myocardial infarction—executive summary. A report of the American College of Cardiology/American Heart Association Task Force on Practice Guidelines (Writing Committee to revise the 1999 guidelines for the management of patients with acute myocardial infarction). J Am Coll Cardiol 44:671, 2004

BAIM DS: Percutaneous balloon angioplasty and general coronary intervention, in *Cardiac Catheterization, Angiography, and Intervention*, 7th ed, D Baim (ed). Philadelphia, Lippincott Williams & Wilkins, 2006

HIRSH AT et al: ACC/AHA 2005 practice guidelines for the management of patients with peripheral arterial disease (lower extremity, renal, mesenteric and abdominal aortic): Executive summary. Circulation 113, 1474, 2006

KEELEY EC et al: Should patients with acute myocardial infraction be transferred to a tertiary center for primary angioplasty or receive it at qualified hospitals in the community? The case for emergency transfer for primary percutaneous coronary intervention. Circulation 112:3520, 2005

MORENO R et al: Drug-eluting stent thrombosis: Results from a pooled analysis including 10 randomized studies. J Am Coll Cardiol 45:954, 2005

RESNIC F et al: Percutaneous coronary and valvular intervention, in *Braunwald's Heart Disease*, 8th ed, P Libby et al (eds). Philadelphia, Elsevier Saunders, 2008.

SERRUYS PW et al: Coronary-artery stents. N Engl J Med 354: 483, 2006

SMITH SC et al: ACC/AHA/SCAI 2005 guideline update for percutaneous coronary intervention—summary article. A report of the American College of Cardiology/American Heart Association Task Force on Practice Guidelines (ACC/AHA/SCAI Writing Committee to Update the 2001 Guidelines for Percutaneous Coronary Intervention). Circulation 113: 156, 2006

WHITE CJ: Catheter-based therapy for atherosclerotic renal artery stenosis. Circulation 113:1464, 2006

YADAV JS et al: Protected carotid-artery stenting versus endarterectomy in high-risk patients. N Eng J Med 351:1493, 2004

CHAPTER 37

HYPERTENSIVE VASCULAR DISEASE

Theodore A. Kotchen

Hypertension doubles the risk of cardiovascular diseases, including coronary heart disease (CHD), congestive heart failure (CHF), ischemic and hemorrhagic stroke, renal failure, and peripheral arterial disease. Hypertension is often associated with additional cardiovascular disease risk factors, and the risk of cardiovascular disease increases with the total burden of risk factors. Although antihypertensive therapy clearly reduces the risks of cardiovascular and renal disease, large segments of the hypertensive population are either untreated or inadequately treated.

EPIDEMIOLOGY

Blood pressure levels, the rate of age-related blood pressure increase, and the prevalence of hypertension vary among countries and among subpopulations within a country. Hypertension is present in all populations except for a small number of individuals living in primitive, culturally isolated societies. It has been estimated that hypertension accounts for 6% of deaths worldwide. In industrialized societies, blood pressure increases steadily during the first two decades. In children and adolescents, blood pressure is associated with growth and maturation. Blood pressure "tracks" over time in children and between adolescence and young adulthood. In the United States,

average systolic blood pressure is higher for men than for women during early adulthood, although among older individuals the age-related rate of rise is steeper for women. Consequently, among individuals 60 years and older, systolic blood pressures of women are higher than those of men. Among adults, diastolic blood pressure also increases progressively with age until approximately 55 years, after which it tends to decrease. The consequence is a widening of pulse pressure (the difference between systolic and diastolic blood pressure) beyond 60 years.

In the United States, based on results of the National Health and Nutrition Examination Survey (NHANES), 28.7% (age-adjusted prevalence) of U.S. adults, or ~58.4 million individuals, have hypertension (defined as any one of the following: systolic blood pressure ≥140 mmHg; diastolic blood pressure ≥90 mmHg; taking antihypertensive medications). Hypertension prevalence is 33.5% in non-Hispanic blacks, 28.9% in non-Hispanic whites, and 20.7% in Mexican Americans. The burden of hypertension increases with age, and among individuals aged ≥60, hypertension prevalence is 65.4%. Recent evidence suggests that the prevalence of hypertension in the United States may be increasing, possibly as a consequence of increasing obesity. The prevalence of hypertension and stroke mortality rates are higher in the southeastern United States than in other regions. In African Americans, hypertension appears earlier, is generally more severe, and results in higher rates of morbidity and mortality from stroke, left ventricular hypertrophy, CHF, and end-stage renal disease (ESRD) than in white Americans.

Both environmental and genetic factors may contribute to regional and racial variations of blood pressure and hypertension prevalence. Studies of societies undergoing "acculturation" and studies of migrants from a less to a more urbanized setting indicate a profound environmental contribution to blood pressure. Obesity and weight gain are strong, independent risk factors for hypertension. It has been estimated that 60% of hypertensive individuals are >20% overweight. Among populations, hypertension prevalence is related to dietary NaCl intake, and the age-related increase of blood pressure may be augmented by a high NaCl intake. Low dietary intakes of calcium and potassium may also contribute to the risk of hypertension. Additional environmental factors that may contribute to hypertension include alcohol consumption, psychosocial stress, and low levels of physical activity.

Adoption, twin, and family studies document a significant heritable component to blood pressure levels and hypertension. Family studies controlling for a common environment indicate that blood pressure heritabilities are in the range of 15–35%. In twin studies, heritability estimates of blood pressure are ~60% for males and 30–40% for females. High blood pressure before 55 years of age occurs 3.8 times more frequently among persons with a positive family history of hypertension. Although specific genetic etiologies have been identified for relatively rare causes of hypertension, this has not been the case for the large majority of hypertensive patients. For most individuals, it is likely that hypertension represents a polygenic disorder in which a single gene or combination of genes act in concert with environmental exposures to contribute only a modest effect on blood pressure.

GENETIC CONSIDERATIONS

Although specific genetic variants have been identified in rare Mendelian forms of hypertension (Table 37-5), these variants are not applicable to the vast majority (>98%) of patients with essential hypertension.

Blood pressure levels reflect the contributions of many susceptibility genes interacting with each other and with the environment. Essential hypertension is a polygenic disorder, and different patients may carry different subsets of genes that lead to elevated blood pressure and to different phenotypes associated with hypertension, e.g., obesity, dyslipidemia, insulin resistance.

Several strategies are being utilized in the search for specific hypertension-related genes. Animal models (including selectively bred rats and congenic rat strains) provide a powerful approach for evaluating genetic loci and genes associated with hypertension. Comparative mapping strategies allow for the identification of syntenic genomic regions between the rat and human genome that may be involved in blood pressure regulation. In linkage studies, polymorphic genetic markers are examined at regular distances along each chromosome. Linkage information is gathered family by family, and the minimum family unit comprises at least two relatives, often a pair of siblings. To date, genome scans for hypertension have yielded inconsistent results. In complementary association studies, different alleles (or combinations of alleles at different loci) of specific genes or chromosomal regions are compared in hypertensive patients and normotensive control subjects. Current evidence suggests that genes encoding components of the renin-angiotensin-aldosterone system, and angiotensinogen and angiotensin-converting enzyme (ACE) polymorphisms, may be related to hypertension and to blood pressure sensitivity to dietary NaCl. The alpha-adducin gene is also thought to be associated with increased renal tubular absorption of sodium, and variants of this gene may also be associated with hypertension and salt sensitivity of blood pressure. Other genes possibly related to hypertension include genes encoding the AT_1 receptor, aldosterone synthase, and the β_2-adrenoreceptor.

Preliminary evidence suggests that there may also be genetic determinants of target organ damage attributed to hypertension. Family studies indicate significant heritability of left ventricular mass, and there is considerable individual variation in the responses of the heart to hypertension. Family studies and variations in candidate genes associated with renal damage suggest that genetic factors may also contribute to hypertensive nephropathy. Specific genetic variants have been linked to CHD and stroke.

In the future, it is possible that DNA analysis will predict individual risk for hypertension and target organ damage and will identify responders to specific classes of antihypertensive agents. However, with the exception of the rare, monogenic hypertensive diseases, the genetic variants associated with hypertension remain to be confirmed, and the intermediate steps by which these variants affect blood pressure remain to be determined.

MECHANISMS OF HYPERTENSION

To provide a framework for understanding the pathogenesis and treatment options of hypertensive disorders, it is useful to understand factors involved in the regulation of both normal and elevated arterial pressure. Cardiac output and peripheral resistance are the two determinants of arterial pressure (Fig. 37-1). Cardiac output is determined by stroke volume and heart rate; stroke volume is related to myocardial contractility and to the size of the vascular compartment. Peripheral resistance is

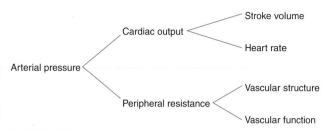

FIGURE 37-1
Determinants of arterial pressure.

determined by functional and anatomic changes in small arteries (lumen diameter 100–400 μm) and arterioles.

INTRAVASCULAR VOLUME

Vascular volume is a primary determinant of arterial pressure over the long term. Although the extracellular fluid space is composed of vascular and interstitial spaces, in general, alterations in total extracellular fluid volume are associated with proportional changes of blood volume. Sodium is predominantly an extracellular ion and is a primary determinant of the extracellular fluid volume. When NaCl intake exceeds the capacity of the kidney to excrete sodium, vascular volume initially expands and cardiac output increases. However, many vascular beds (including kidney and brain) have the capacity to autoregulate blood flow, and if constant blood flow is to be maintained in the face of increased arterial pressure, resistance within that bed must increase, since:

$$\text{Blood flow} = \frac{\text{pressure across the vascular bed}}{\text{vascular resistance}}$$

The initial elevation of blood pressure in response to vascular volume expansion is related to an increase of cardiac output; however, over time, peripheral resistance increases and cardiac output reverts toward normal. The effect of sodium on blood pressure is related to the provision of sodium with chloride; non-chloride salts of sodium have little or no effect on blood pressure. As arterial pressure increases in response to a high NaCl intake, urinary sodium excretion increases and sodium balance is maintained at the expense of an increase in arterial pressure. The mechanism for this "pressure-natriuresis" phenomenon may involve a subtle increase of glomerular filtration rate, decreased absorbing capacity of the renal tubules, and possibly hormonal factors such as atrial natriuretic factor. In individuals with an impaired capacity to excrete sodium, greater increases of arterial pressure are required to achieve natriuresis and sodium balance.

NaCl-dependent hypertension may be a consequence of a decreased capacity of the kidney to excrete sodium, due to either intrinsic renal disease or to increased production of a salt-retaining hormone (mineralocorticoid) resulting in increased renal tubular reabsorption of sodium.

Renal tubular sodium reabsorption may also be augmented by increased neural activity to the kidney. In each of these situations, a higher arterial pressure may be required to achieve sodium balance, i.e., the pressure-natriuresis phenomenon. Conversely, salt-wasting disorders are associated with low blood pressure levels. ESRD is an extreme example of volume-dependent hypertension. In ~80% of these patients, vascular volume and hypertension can be controlled with adequate dialysis; in the remainder 20%, the mechanism of hypertension is related to increased activity of the renin-angiotensin system and is likely to be responsive to pharmacologic blockade of renin-angiotensin.

AUTONOMIC NERVOUS SYSTEM

The autonomic nervous system maintains cardiovascular homeostasis via pressure, volume, and chemoreceptor signals. Adrenergic reflexes modulate blood pressure over the short term, and adrenergic function, in concert with hormonal and volume-related factors, contributes to the long-term regulation of arterial pressure. The three endogenous catecholamines are norepinephrine, epinephrine, and dopamine. All play important roles in tonic and phasic cardiovascular regulation. Adrenergic neurons synthesize norepinephrine and dopamine (a precursor of norepinephrine), which are stored in vesicles within the neuron. When the neuron is stimulated, these neurotransmitters are released into the synaptic cleft and to receptor sites on target tissues. Subsequently, the transmitter is either metabolized or taken up into the neuron by an active reuptake process. Epinephrine is synthesized in the adrenal medulla and released into the circulation upon adrenal stimulation.

The activities of the adrenergic receptors are mediated by guanosine nucleotide-binding regulatory proteins (G proteins) and by intracellular concentrations of downstream second messengers. In addition to receptor affinity and density, physiologic responsiveness to catecholamines may also be altered by the efficiency of receptor-effector coupling at a site "distal" to receptor binding. The receptor sites are relatively specific both for the transmitter substance and for the response that occupancy of the receptor site elicits. Norepinephrine and epinephrine are agonists for all adrenergic receptor subtypes, although with varying affinities. Based on their physiology and pharmacology, adrenergic receptors have been divided into two principal types: α and β. These types have been further differentiated into α_1, α_2, β_1, and β_2 receptors. Recent molecular cloning studies have identified several additional subtypes. α Receptors are more avidly occupied and activated by norepinephrine than by epinephrine, and the reverse is true for β receptors. α_1 Receptors are located on postsynaptic cells in smooth muscle and elicit vasoconstriction. α_2 Receptors are localized on presynaptic membranes of postganglionic nerve terminals that synthesize norepinephrine.

When activated by catecholamines, α_2 receptors act as negative feedback controllers, inhibiting further norepinephrine release. Different classes of antihypertensive agents either inhibit α_1 receptors or act as agonists of α_2 receptors and reduce systemic sympathetic outflow. Activation of myocardial β_1 receptors stimulates the rate and strength of cardiac contraction, and consequently increases cardiac output. β_1 receptor activation also stimulates renin release from the kidney. Another class of antihypertensive agents acts by inhibiting β_1 receptors. Activation of β_2 receptors by epinephrine relaxes vascular smooth muscle and results in vasodilation.

Circulating catecholamine concentrations may affect the number of adrenoreceptors in various tissues. Downregulation of receptors may be a consequence of sustained high levels of catecholamines and provides an explanation for decreasing responsiveness, or tachyphylaxis, to catecholamines. For example, orthostatic hypotension is frequently observed in patients with pheochromocytoma, possibly due to the lack of norepinephrine-induced vasoconstriction with assumption of the upright posture. Conversely, with chronic reduction of neurotransmitter substances, adrenoreceptors may increase in number, or be upregulated, resulting in increased responsiveness to the neurotransmitter. Chronic administration of agents that block adrenergic receptors may result in upregulation, and withdrawal of these agents may produce a condition of temporary hypersensitivity to sympathetic stimuli. For example, clonidine is an antihypertensive agent that is a centrally acting α_2 agonist that inhibits sympathetic outflow. Rebound hypertension may occur with the abrupt cessation of clonidine therapy, probably as a consequence of upregulation of α_1 receptors.

Several reflexes modulate blood pressure on a minute-to-minute basis. One arterial baroreflex is mediated by stretch-sensitive sensory nerve endings located in the carotid sinuses and the aortic arch. The rate of firing of these baroreceptors increases with arterial pressure, and the net effect is a decrease of sympathetic outflow, resulting in decreases of arterial pressure and heart rate. This is a primary mechanism for rapid buffering of acute fluctuations of arterial pressure that may occur during postural changes, behavioral or physiologic stress, and changes in blood volume. However, the activity of the baroreflex declines or adapts to sustained increases of arterial pressure such that the baroreceptors are reset to higher pressures. Patients with autonomic neuropathy and impaired baroreflex function may have extremely labile blood pressures with difficult-to-control episodic blood pressure spikes.

Pheochromocytoma is the most obvious example of hypertension related to increased catecholamine production, in this instance by a tumor. Blood pressure can be reduced by surgical excision of the tumor or by pharmacologic treatment with an α_1 receptor antagonist or with an inhibitor of tyrosine hydroxylase, the rate-limiting

step in catecholamine biosynthesis. Increased sympathetic activity may contribute to other forms of hypertension. Drugs that block the sympathetic nervous system are potent antihypertensive agents, indicating that the sympathetic nervous system plays a permissive, although perhaps not a causative, role in the maintenance of increased arterial pressure.

RENIN-ANGIOTENSIN-ALDOSTERONE

The renin-angiotensin-aldosterone system contributes to the regulation of arterial pressure primarily via the vasoconstrictor properties of angiotensin II and the sodium-retaining properties of aldosterone. Renin is an aspartyl protease that is synthesized as an enzymatically inactive precursor, prorenin. Most renin in the circulation is synthesized in the segment of the renal afferent renal arteriole (juxtaglomerular cells) that abuts the glomerulus and a group of sensory cells located at the distal end of the loop of Henle, the macula densa. Prorenin may be secreted directly into the circulation or may be activated within secretory cells and released as active renin. Although human plasma contains two- to fivefold times more prorenin than renin, there is no evidence that prorenin contributes to the physiologic activity of this system. There are three primary stimuli for renin secretion: (1) decreased NaCl transport in the thick ascending limb of the loop of Henle (macula densa mechanism), (2) decreased pressure or stretch within the renal afferent arteriole (baroreceptor mechanism), and (3) sympathetic nervous system stimulation of renin-secreting cells via β_1 adrenoreceptors. Conversely, renin secretion is inhibited by increased NaCl transport in the thick ascending limb of the loop of Henle, by increased stretch within the renal afferent arteriole, and by β_1 receptor blockade. In addition, renin secretion may be modulated by a number of humoral factors, including angiotensin II. Angiotensin II directly inhibits renin secretion due to angiotensin II type 1 receptors on juxtaglomerular cells, and renin secretion increases in response to pharmacologic blockade of either ACE or angiotensin II receptors.

Once released into the circulation, active renin cleaves a substrate, angiotensinogen, to form an inactive decapeptide, angiotensin I (**Fig. 37–2**). A converting enzyme, located primarily but not exclusively in the pulmonary circulation, converts angiotensin I to the active octapeptide, angiotensin II, by releasing the C-terminal histidyl-leucine dipeptide. The same converting enzyme cleaves a number of other peptides, including and thereby inactivating the vasodilator bradykinin. Acting primarily through angiotensin II type 1 (AT_1) receptors located on cell membranes, angiotensin II is a potent pressor substance, the primary trophic factor for the secretion of aldosterone by the adrenal zona glomerulosa, and a potent mitogen stimulating vascular smooth-muscle cell

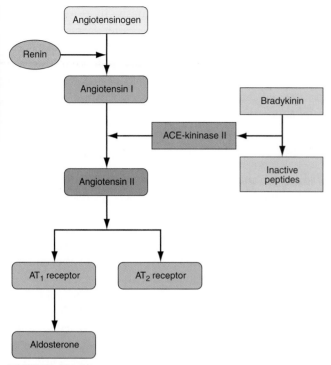

FIGURE 37-2

Renin-angiotensin-aldosterone axis.

and myocyte growth. Independent of its hemodynamic effects, angiotensin II may play a role in the pathogenesis of atherosclerosis through a direct cellular action on the vessel wall. An angiotensin II type 2 (AT$_2$) receptor has been characterized. It is widely distributed in the kidney and has the opposite functional effects of the AT$_1$ receptor. The AT$_2$ receptor induces vasodilation, sodium excretion, and inhibition of cell growth and matrix formation. Experimental evidence suggests that the AT$_2$ receptor improves vascular remodeling by stimulating smooth-muscle cell apoptosis and contributes to the regulation of glomerular filtration rate. AT$_1$ receptor blockade induces an increase in AT$_2$ receptor activity. Currently, the AT$_2$ receptor has a less well defined functional role than the AT$_1$ receptor.

Renin-secreting tumors are clear examples of renin-dependent hypertension. In the kidney, these include benign hemangiopericytomas of the juxtaglomerular apparatus, and infrequently renal carcinomas, including Wilms' tumors. Renin-producing carcinomas have also been described in lung, liver, pancreas, colon, and adrenals. In these instances, in addition to excision and/or ablation of the tumor, treatment of hypertension includes pharmacologic therapies targeted to inhibit angiotensin II production or action. Renovascular hypertension is another renin-mediated form of hypertension. Obstruction of the renal artery leads to decreased renal perfusion pressure, thereby stimulating renin secretion. Over time, as a consequence of secondary renal damage, this form of hypertension may become less renin dependent.

Angiotensinogen, renin, and angiotensin II are also synthesized locally in many tissues, including the brain, pituitary, aorta, arteries, heart, adrenal glands, kidneys, adipocytes, leukocytes, ovaries, testes, uterus, spleen, and skin. Angiotensin II in tissues may be formed by the enzymatic activity of renin or by other proteases, e.g., tonin, chymase, and cathepsins. In addition to regulating local blood flow, tissue angiotensin II is a mitogen that stimulates growth and contributes to modeling and repair. Excess tissue angiotensin II may contribute to atherosclerosis, cardiac hypertrophy, and renal failure and consequently may be a target for pharmacologic therapy to prevent target organ damage.

Angiotensin II is the primary trophic factor regulating the synthesis and secretion of aldosterone by the zona glomerulosa of the adrenal cortex. Aldosterone synthesis is also dependent on potassium, and aldosterone secretion may be decreased in potassium-depleted individuals. Although acute elevations of adrenocorticotropic hormone (ACTH) levels also increase aldosterone secretion, ACTH is not an important trophic factor for the chronic regulation of aldosterone.

Aldosterone is a potent mineralocorticoid that increases sodium reabsorption by amiloride-sensitive epithelial sodium channels (ENaC) on the apical surface of the principal cells of the renal cortical collecting duct. Electric neutrality is maintained by exchanging sodium for potassium and hydrogen ions. Consequently, increased aldosterone secretion may result in hypokalemia and alkalosis. Because potassium depletion may inhibit aldosterone synthesis, clinically, hypokalemia should be corrected before evaluating a patient for hyperaldosteronism.

Mineralocorticoid receptors are also expressed in the colon, salivary glands, and sweat glands. Cortisol also binds to these receptors but normally functions as a less potent mineralocorticoid than aldosterone because cortisol is converted to cortisone by the enzyme 11 β-hydroxysteroid dehydrogenase type 2. Cortisone has no affinity for the mineralocorticoid receptor. Primary aldosteronism is a compelling example of mineralocorticoid-mediated hypertension. In this disorder, adrenal aldosterone synthesis and release are independent of renin-angiotensin, and renin release is suppressed by the resulting volume expansion.

Aldosterone also has effects on nonepithelial targets. Independent of a potential effect on blood pressure, aldosterone may also play a role in cardiac hypertrophy and CHF. Aldosterone acts via mineralocorticoid receptors within the myocardium to enhance extracellular matrix and collagen deposition. In animal models, high circulating aldosterone levels stimulate cardiac fibrosis and left ventricular hypertrophy, and spironolactone (an aldosterone antagonist) prevents aldosterone-induced myocardial fibrosis. Pathologic patterns of left ventricular geometry have also been associated with elevations of plasma aldosterone concentration in patients with essential hypertension, as well as in patients with primary aldosteronism. In patients with CHF, low-dose spironolactone reduces the risk of progressive heart failure and sudden death from cardiac causes by 30%. Owing to a renal hemodynamic effect, in patients with primary aldosteronism, high circulating levels of aldosterone may also cause glomerular hyperfiltration and albuminuria. These renal effects are reversible after removal of the effects of excess aldosterone by adrenalectomy or spironolactone.

Increased activity of the renin-angiotensin-aldosterone axis is not invariably associated with hypertension. In response to a low-NaCl diet or to volume contraction, arterial pressure and volume homeostasis may be maintained by increased activity of the renin-angiotensin-aldosterone axis. Secondary aldosteronism (i.e., increased aldosterone secondary to increased renin-angiotensin), but not hypertension, is also observed in edematous states such as CHF and liver disease.

VASCULAR MECHANISMS

Vascular radius and compliance of resistance arteries are also important determinants of arterial pressure. Resistance to flow varies inversely with the fourth power of the radius, and consequently small decreases in lumen size significantly increase resistance. In hypertensive patients, structural, mechanical, or functional changes may reduce lumen diameter of small arteries and arterioles. Remodeling refers to geometric alterations in the vessel wall without changing vessel volume. Hypertrophic (increased cell number, increased cell size, and increased deposition of intercellular matrix) or eutrophic (no change in the amount of material in the vessel wall) vascular remodeling results in decreased lumen size and hence contributes to increased peripheral resistance. Apoptosis, low-grade inflammation, and vascular fibrosis also contribute to remodeling. Lumen diameter is also related to elasticity of the vessel. Vessels with a high degree of elasticity can accommodate an increase of volume with relatively little change of pressure, whereas in a semi-rigid vascular system, a small increment in volume induces a relatively large increment of pressure.

Hypertensive patients have stiffer arteries, and arteriosclerotic patients may have particularly high systolic blood pressures and wide pulse pressures as a consequence of decreased vascular compliance due to structural changes in the vascular wall. Recent evidence suggests that arterial stiffness has independent predictive value for cardiovascular events. Clinically, a number of devices are available to evaluate arterial stiffness or compliance, including ultrasound and MRI.

Ion transport by vascular smooth-muscle cells may contribute to hypertension-associated abnormalities of vascular tone and vascular growth, both of which are modulated by intracellular pH (pH_i). Three ion transport mechanisms participate in the regulation of pH_i: (1) Na^+-H^+ exchange, (2) Na^+-dependent HCO_3^--Cl^- exchange, and (3) cation-independent HCO_3^--Cl^- exchange. Based on measurements in cell types that are more accessible than vascular smooth muscle (e.g., leukocytes, erythrocytes, platelets, skeletal muscle), activity of the Na^+-H^+ exchanger is increased in hypertension, and this may result in increased vascular tone by two mechanisms. First, increased sodium entry may lead to increased vascular tone by activating Na^+-Ca^{2+} exchange and thereby increasing intracellular calcium. Second, increased pH_i enhances calcium sensitivity of the contractile apparatus, leading to an increase in contractility for a given intracellular calcium concentration. Additionally, increased Na^+-H^+ exchange might stimulate vascular smooth-muscle cell growth by enhancing sensitivity to mitogens.

Vascular endothelial function also modulates vascular tone. The vascular endothelium synthesizes and releases a spectrum of vasoactive substances, including nitric oxide, a potent vasodilator. Endothelium-dependent vasodilation is impaired in hypertensive patients. This impairment is often assessed with high-resolution ultrasonography as flow-mediated vasodilation of the brachial artery. Alternatively, endothelium-dependent vasodilation may be assessed with venous occlusion plethysmography in response to an intraarterially infused endothelium-dependent vasodilator, e.g., acetylcholine.

Presently, it is not known if these hypertension-related vascular abnormalities of ion transport and endothelial function are primary alterations or secondary consequences of elevated arterial pressure. Limited evidence suggests that vascular compliance and endothelium-dependent vasodilation may be improved by aerobic exercise, weight loss, and antihypertensive agents. It remains to be determined whether these interventions affect arterial structure and stiffness via a blood pressure–independent mechanism and whether different classes of antihypertensive agents preferentially affect vascular structure and function.

PATHOLOGIC CONSEQUENCES OF HYPERTENSION

Hypertension is a risk factor for all clinical manifestations of atherosclerosis. It is an independent predisposing factor for heart failure, coronary artery disease, stroke, renal disease, and peripheral arterial disease (PAD).

HEART

Heart disease is the most common cause of death in hypertensive patients. Hypertensive heart disease is the result of structural and functional adaptations leading to left ventricular hypertrophy, diastolic dysfunction, CHF, abnormalities of blood flow due to atherosclerotic coronary artery disease and microvascular disease, and cardiac arrhythmias.

Both genetic and hemodynamic factors contribute to left ventricular hypertrophy. Clinically, left ventricular hypertrophy can be diagnosed by electrocardiogram, although echocardiography provides a more sensitive measure of left ventricular wall thickness. Individuals with left ventricular hypertrophy are at increased risk for CHD, stroke, CHF, and sudden death. Aggressive control of hypertension can regress or reverse left ventricular hypertrophy and reduce the risk of cardiovascular disease. It is not clear if different classes of antihypertensive agents have an added impact on reducing left ventricular mass, independent of their blood pressure–lowering effect.

Abnormalities of diastolic function, ranging from asymptomatic heart disease to overt heart failure, are common in hypertensive patients. Patients with diastolic heart failure have a preserved ejection fraction, which is a measure of systolic function. Approximately one-third of patients with CHF have normal systolic function but abnormal diastolic function. Diastolic dysfunction is an early consequence of hypertension-related heart disease and is exacerbated by left ventricular hypertrophy and ischemia. Clinically, cardiac catheterization provides the most accurate assessment of diastolic function; however, this is an invasive procedure and generally not indicated for the assessment of diastolic function. Alternatively, diastolic function can be evaluated by several noninvasive methods, including echocardiography and radionuclide angiography.

BRAIN

Hypertension is an important risk factor for brain infarction and hemorrhage. Approximately 85% of strokes are due to infarction and the remainder are due to hemorrhage, either intracerebral hemorrhage or subarachnoid hemorrhage. The incidence of stroke rises progressively with increasing blood pressure levels, particularly systolic blood pressure in individuals >65 years. Treatment of hypertension convincingly decreases the incidence of both ischemic and hemorrhagic strokes.

Hypertension is also associated with impaired cognition in an aging population, and longitudinal studies support an association between mid-life hypertension and late-life cognitive decline. Hypertension-related cognitive impairment and dementia may be a consequence of a single infarct due to occlusion of a "strategic" larger vessel or multiple lacunar infarcts due to occlusive small vessel disease resulting in subcortical white matter ischemia. Several clinical trials suggest that antihypertensive therapy has a beneficial effect on cognitive function, although this remains an active area of investigation.

Cerebral blood flow remains unchanged over a wide range of arterial pressures (mean arterial pressure of 50–150 mmHg) through a process termed *autoregulation* of blood flow. In patients with the clinical syndrome of malignant hypertension, encephalopathy is related to failure of autoregulation of cerebral blood flow at the upper pressure limit, resulting in vasodilation and hyperperfusion. Signs and symptoms of hypertensive encephalopathy may include severe headache, nausea and vomiting (often of a projectile nature), focal neurologic signs, and alterations in mental status. Untreated, hypertensive encephalopathy may progress to stupor, coma, seizures, and death within hours. It is important to distinguish hypertensive encephalopathy from other neurologic syndromes that may be associated with hypertension, e.g., cerebral ischemia, hemorrhagic or thrombotic stroke, seizure disorder, mass lesions, pseudotumor cerebri, delirium tremens, meningitis, acute intermittent porphyria, traumatic or chemical injury to the brain, and uremic encephalopathy.

KIDNEY

Primary renal disease is the most common etiology of secondary hypertension. Conversely, hypertension is a risk factor for renal injury and ESRD. The increased risk associated with high blood pressure is graded, continuous, and present throughout the entire distribution of blood pressure above optimal. Renal risk appears to be more closely related to systolic than to diastolic blood pressure, and black men are at greater risk than white men for developing ESRD at every level of blood pressure.

The atherosclerotic, hypertension-related vascular lesions in the kidney primarily affect the preglomerular arterioles, resulting in ischemic changes in the glomeruli and postglomerular structures. Glomerular injury may also be a consequence of direct damage to the glomerular capillaries due to glomerular hyperperfusion. Glomerular pathology progresses to glomerulosclerosis, and eventually the renal tubules may also become ischemic and gradually atrophic. The renal lesion associated with malignant hypertension consists of fibrinoid necrosis of the afferent arterioles, sometimes extending into the glomerulus, and may result in focal necrosis of the glomerular tuft.

Clinically, macroalbuminuria (a random urine albumin/creatinine ratio >300 mg/g) or microalbuminuria (a random urine albumin/creatinine ratio 30–300 mg/g) are early markers of renal injury. These are also risk factors for renal disease progression and for cardiovascular disease.

PERIPHERAL ARTERIES

In addition to contributing to the pathogenesis of hypertension, blood vessels may be a target organ for atherosclerotic disease secondary to long-standing elevated blood pressure. Hypertensive patients with arterial disease of the lower extremities are at increased risk for future cardiovascular disease. Although patients with stenotic lesions of the lower extremities may be asymptomatic, intermittent claudication is the classic symptom of PAD. This is characterized by aching pain in the calves or buttocks while walking that is relieved by rest. The ankle-brachial index is a useful approach for evaluating PAD and is defined as the ratio of noninvasively assessed ankle to brachial (arm) systolic blood pressure. An ankle-brachial index <0.90 is considered diagnostic of PAD and is associated with >50% stenosis in at least one major lower limb vessel. Several studies suggest that an ankle-brachial index <0.80 is associated with elevated blood pressure, particularly systolic blood pressure.

DEFINING HYPERTENSION

From an epidemiologic perspective, there is no obvious level of blood pressure that defines hypertension. In adults, there is a continuous, incremental risk of cardiovascular disease, stroke, and renal disease across levels of both systolic and diastolic blood pressure. The Multiple Risk Factor Intervention Trial (MRFIT), which included >350,000 male participants, demonstrated a continuous and graded influence of both systolic and diastolic blood pressure on CHD mortality, extending down to systolic blood pressures of 120 mmHg. Similarly, results of a meta-analysis involving almost 1 million participants indicate that ischemic heart disease mortality, stroke mortality, and mortality from other vascular causes are directly related to the height of the blood pressure, beginning at 115/75 mmHg, without evidence of a threshold. Cardiovascular disease risk doubles for every 20-mmHg increase in systolic and 10-mmHg increase in diastolic pressure. Among older individuals, systolic blood pressure and pulse pressure are more powerful predictors of cardiovascular disease than diastolic blood pressure.

Clinically, hypertension might be defined as that level of blood pressure at which the institution of therapy reduces blood pressure–related morbidity and mortality. Current clinical criteria for defining hypertension are generally based on the average of two or more seated blood pressure readings during each of two or more outpatient visits. A recent classification recommends blood pressure criteria for defining normal blood pressure, prehypertension, hypertension (stages I and II), and isolated systolic hypertension, which is a common occurrence among the elderly (Table 37-1). In children and adolescents, hypertension is generally defined as systolic and/or diastolic blood pressure consistently >95th percentile for age, gender, and height. Blood pressures between the 90th and 95th percentiles are considered prehypertensive and are an indication for lifestyle interventions.

Home blood pressure and average 24-h ambulatory blood pressure measurements are generally lower than clinic blood pressures. Because ambulatory blood pressure recordings yield multiple readings throughout the day and night, they provide a more comprehensive assessment of the vascular burden of hypertension than a limited number of office readings. Increasing evidence

TABLE 37-1

BLOOD PRESSURE CLASSIFICATION

BLOOD PRESSURE CLASSIFICATION	SYSTOLIC, mmHg	DIASTOLIC, mmHg
Normal	<120	and <80
Prehypertension	120–139	or 80–89
Stage 1 hypertension	140–159	or 90–99
Stage 2 hypertension	≥160	or ≥100
Isolated systolic hypertension	≥140	and <90

Source: Adapted from Chobanian et al.

suggests that home blood pressures, including 24-h blood pressure recordings, more reliably predict target organ damage than office blood pressures. Blood pressure tends to be higher in the early morning hours, soon after waking, than at other times of day. Myocardial infarction and stroke are more frequent in the early morning hours. Nighttime blood pressures are generally 10–20% lower than daytime blood pressures, and an attenuated nighttime blood pressure "dip" is associated with increased cardiovascular disease risk. Blunting of the day-night blood pressure pattern occurs in several clinical conditions, including sleep apnea and autonomic neuropathy, and in certain populations, including African Americans. Recommended criteria for a diagnosis of hypertension are average awake blood pressure ≥135/85 mmHg and asleep blood pressure ≥120/75 mmHg. These levels approximate a clinic blood pressure of 140/90 mmHg.

Approximately 15–20% of patients with stage 1 hypertension (as defined in Table 37-1) based on office blood pressures have average ambulatory readings <135/85 mmHg. This phenomenon, so-called white coat hypertension, may also be associated with an increased risk of target organ damage (e.g., left ventricular hypertrophy, carotid atherosclerosis, overall cardiovascular morbidity), although to a lesser extent than individuals with elevated office and ambulatory readings. Individuals with white coat hypertension are also at increased risk for developing sustained hypertension.

CLINICAL DISORDERS OF HYPERTENSION

Depending on methods of patient ascertainment, ~80–95% of hypertensive patients are diagnosed as having "essential" hypertension (also referred to as primary or idiopathic hypertension). In the remaining 5–20% of hypertensive patients, a specific underlying disorder causing the elevation of blood pressure can be identified (Tables 37–2 and 37–3). In individuals with "secondary" hypertension, a specific mechanism for the blood pressure elevation is often more apparent.

TABLE 37-2

SYSTOLIC HYPERTENSION WITH WIDE PULSE PRESSURE
1. Decreased vascular compliance (arteriosclerosis)
2. Increased cardiac output
a. Aortic regurgitation
b. Thyrotoxicosis
c. Hyperkinetic heart syndrome
d. Fever
e. Arteriovenous fistula
f. Patent ductus arteriosus

ESSENTIAL HYPERTENSION

Essential hypertension tends to be familial and is likely to be the consequence of an interaction between environmental and genetic factors. The prevalence of essential hypertension increases with age, and individuals with relatively high blood pressures at younger ages are at increased risk for the subsequent development of hypertension. It is likely that essential hypertension represents a spectrum of disorders with different underlying pathophysiologies. In the majority of patients with established hypertension, peripheral resistance is increased and cardiac output is normal or decreased; however, in younger patients with mild or labile hypertension, cardiac output may be increased and peripheral resistance may be normal.

When plasma renin activity (PRA) is plotted against 24-h sodium excretion, ~10–15% of hypertensive patients have high PRA and 25% have low PRA. High-renin patients may have a vasoconstrictor form of hypertension, whereas low-renin patients may have a volume-dependent hypertension. Inconsistent associations between plasma aldosterone and blood pressure have been described in patients with essential hypertension. The association between aldosterone and blood pressure is more striking in African Americans, and PRA tends to be low in hypertensive African Americans. This raises the possibility that subtle increases of aldosterone may contribute to hypertension in at least some groups of patients who do not have overt primary aldosteronism. Furthermore, spironolactone, an aldosterone antagonist, may be a particularly effective antihypertensive agent for some patients with essential hypertension, including some patients with "drug-resistant" hypertension.

METABOLIC SYNDROME

(See also Chap. 32) Hypertension and dyslipidemia frequently occur together and in association with resistance to insulin-stimulated glucose uptake. This clustering of risk factors is often, but not invariably, associated with obesity, particularly abdominal obesity. Insulin resistance is also associated with an unfavorable imbalance in the endothelial production of mediators that regulate platelet aggregation, coagulation, fibrinolysis, and vessel tone. When these risk factors cluster, the risks for CHD, stroke, diabetes, and cardiovascular disease mortality are further increased.

TABLE 37-3

SECONDARY CAUSES OF SYSTOLIC AND DIASTOLIC HYPERTENSION	
Renal	Parenchymal diseases, renal cysts (including polycystic kidney disease), renal tumors (including renin-secreting tumors), obstructive uropathy
Renovascular	Arteriosclerotic, fibromuscular dysplasia
Adrenal	Primary aldosteronism, Cushing's syndrome, 17α-hydroxylase deficiency, 11β-hydroxylase deficiency, 11-hydroxysteroid dehydrogenase deficiency (licorice), pheochromocytoma
Aortic coarctation	
Obstructive sleep apnea	
Preeclampsia/eclampsia	
Neurogenic	Psychogenic, diencephalic syndrome, familial dysautonomia, polyneuritis (acute porphyria, lead poisoning), acute increased intracranial pressure, acute spinal cord section
Miscellaneous endocrine	Hypothyroidism, hyperthyroidism, hypercalcemia, acromegaly
Medications	High-dose estrogens, adrenal steroids, decongestants, appetite suppressants, cyclosporine, tricyclic antidepressants, monamine oxidase inhibitors, erythropoietin, nonsteroidal anti-inflammatory agents, cocaine
Mendelian forms of hypertension	(See Table 37-4)

Depending on the populations studied and the methodologies for defining insulin resistance, ~25–50% of non-obese, non-diabetic hypertensive persons are insulin resistant. The constellation of insulin resistance, hypertension, and dyslipidemia has been designated as the *metabolic syndrome*. As a group, first-degree relatives of patients with essential hypertension are also insulin resistant, and hyper-insulinemia (a surrogate marker of insulin resistance) may predict the eventual development of hypertension and cardiovascular disease. Although the metabolic syndrome may in part be heritable as a polygenic condition, the expression of the syndrome is modified by environmental factors, such as degree of physical activity and diet. Insulin sensitivity increases and blood pressure decreases in response to weight loss. The recognition that cardiovascular disease risk factors tend to cluster within individuals has important implications for the evaluation and treatment of hypertension. Evaluation of both hypertensive patients and individuals at risk for developing hypertension should include assessment of overall cardiovascular disease risk. Similarly, introduction of lifestyle modification strategies and drug therapies should address overall risk, and not simply focus on hypertension.

RENAL PARENCHYMAL DISEASES

Virtually all disorders of the kidney may cause hypertension (Table 37-3), and renal disease is the most common cause of secondary hypertension. Hypertension is present in >80% of patients with chronic renal failure. In general, hypertension is more severe in glomerular diseases than in interstitial diseases, such as chronic pyelonephritis. Conversely, hypertension may cause nephrosclerosis, and in some instances it may be difficult to determine whether hypertension or renal disease was the initial disorder. Proteinuria >1000 mg/day and an active urine sediment are indicative of primary renal disease. In either instance, the goals are to control blood pressure and retard the rate of progression of renal dysfunction.

Renovascular Hypertension

Hypertension due to obstruction of a renal artery, renovascular hypertension, is a potentially curable form of hypertension. The mechanism of hypertension is generally related to activation of the renin-angiotensin system. Two groups of patients are at risk for this disorder: older arteriosclerotic patients who have a plaque obstructing the renal artery, frequently at its origin, and patients with fibromuscular dysplasia. Although fibromuscular dysplasia may occur at any age, it has a strong predilection for young white women. The prevalence in females is eightfold that in males. There are several histologic variants of fibromuscular dysplasia, including medial fibroplasia, perimedial fibroplasia, medial hyperplasia, and intimal fibroplasia. Medial fibroplasia is the most common variant and accounts for approximately two-thirds of patients. The lesions of fibromuscular dysplasia are frequently bilateral, and in contrast to atherosclerotic renovascular disease, tend to affect more distal portions of the renal artery.

In addition to the age and gender of the patient, several clues from the history and physical examination suggest a diagnosis of renovascular hypertension. Patients should first be evaluated for evidence of atherosclerotic vascular disease. Although response to antihypertensive therapy does not exclude the diagnosis, severe or refractory hypertension, recent loss of hypertension control or recent onset of moderately severe hypertension, and unexplained deterioration of renal function or deterioration of renal function associated with an ACE inhibitor should raise the possibility of renovascular hypertension. Approximately 50% of patients with renovascular hypertension have an abdominal or flank bruit, and the bruit is more likely to be hemodynamically significant if it lateralizes or extends throughout systole into diastole.

If blood pressure is adequately controlled with a simple antihypertensive regimen and renal function remains stable, there may be little impetus to pursue an evaluation for renal artery stenosis, particularly in an older patient with atherosclerotic disease and comorbid conditions. Patients with long-standing hypertension, advanced renal insufficiency, or diabetes mellitus are less likely to benefit from renal vascular repair. The most effective medical therapies include an ACE inhibitor or an angiotensin II receptor blocker; however, these agents decrease glomerular filtration rate in the stenotic kidney owing to efferent renal arteriolar dilation. In the presence of bilateral renal artery stenosis or renal artery stenosis to a solitary kidney, progressive renal insufficiency may result from the use of these agents. Importantly, the renal insufficiency is generally reversible following discontinuation of the offending drug.

If renal artery stenosis is suspected, and if the clinical condition warrants an intervention such as percutaneous transluminal renal angioplasty (PTRA), placement of a vascular endoprosthesis (stent), or surgical renal revascularization, imaging studies should be the next step in the evaluation. As a screening test, renal blood flow may be evaluated with a radionuclide [^{131}I]-orthoiodohippurate (OIH) scan or glomerular filtration rate may be evaluated with [^{99m}Tc]-diethylenetriamine pentaacetic acid (DTPA) scan, before and after a single dose of captopril (or other ACE inhibitor). The following are consistent with a positive study: (1) decreased relative uptake by the involved kidney, which contributes <40% of total renal function; (2) delayed uptake on the affected side; or (3) delayed washout on the affected side. In patients with normal, or near-normal, renal function, a normal captopril renogram essentially excludes functionally significant renal artery stenosis; however its usefulness is limited in patients with renal insufficiency (creatinine clearance <20 mL/min) or bilateral renal artery stenosis.

Additional imaging studies are indicated if the scan is positive. Doppler ultrasound of the renal arteries produces reliable estimates of renal blood flow velocity and offers the opportunity to track a lesion over time. Positive studies are usually confirmed at angiography, whereas false-negative results occur frequently, particularly in obese patients. Gadolinium-contrast magnetic resonance angiography offers clear images of the proximal renal artery but may miss distal lesions. An advantage is the opportunity to image the renal arteries with an agent that is not nephrotoxic. Contrast arteriography remains the "gold standard" for evaluation and identification of renal artery lesions. Potential risks include nephrotoxicity, particularly in patients with diabetes mellitus or preexisting renal insufficiency.

Some degree of renal artery obstruction may be observed in almost 50% of patients with atherosclerotic disease, and there are several approaches for evaluating the functional significance of such a lesion to predict the effect of vascular repair on blood pressure control and renal function. Each approach has varying degrees of sensitivity and specificity, and no single test is sufficiently reliable to determine a causal relationship between a renal artery lesion and hypertension. On angiography, the presence of collateral vessels to the ischemic kidney suggests a functionally significant lesion. A lateralizing renal vein renin ratio (ratio >1.5 of affected side/contralateral side) has a 90% predictive value for a lesion that would respond to vascular repair; however, the false-negative rate for blood pressure control is 50–60%. Measurement of the pressure gradient across a renal artery lesion does not reliably predict the response to vascular repair.

In the final analysis, a decision concerning vascular repair vs. medical therapy and the type of repair procedure should be individualized for each patient. Patients with fibromuscular disease have more favorable outcomes than patients with atherosclerotic lesions, presumably owing to their younger age, shorter duration of hypertension, and less systemic disease. Because of its low risk-versus-benefit ratio and high success rate (improvement or cure of hypertension in 90% of patients and restenosis rate of 10%), PTRA is the initial treatment of choice for these patients. Surgical revascularization may be undertaken if PTRA is unsuccessful or if a branch lesion is present. In atherosclerotic patients, vascular repair should be considered if blood pressure cannot be adequately controlled with medical therapy or if renal function deteriorates. Surgery may be the preferred initial approach for younger atherosclerotic patients without comorbid conditions; however, for most atherosclerotic patients, depending on the location of the lesion, the initial approach may be PTRA and/or stenting. Surgical revascularization may be indicated if these approaches are unsuccessful, if the vascular lesion is not amenable to PTRA or stenting, or if concomitant aortic surgery is required, e.g., to repair an aneurysm.

PRIMARY ALDOSTERONISM

Excess aldosterone production due to primary aldosteronism is a potentially curable form of hypertension. In patients with primary aldosteronism, increased aldosterone production is independent of the renin-angiotensin system, and the consequences are sodium retention, hypertension, hypokalemia, and low PRA. The reported prevalence of this disorder varies from <2% to ~15% of hypertensive individuals. In part, this variation is related to the intensity of screening and to the criteria for establishing the diagnosis.

History and physical examination provide little information about the diagnosis. The age at the time of diagnosis is generally in the third through fifth decades. Hypertension is usually mild to moderate but occasionally may be severe; primary aldosteronism should be considered in all patients with refractory hypertension. Hypertension in these patients may be associated with glucose intolerance. Most patients are asymptomatic, although, infrequently, polyuria, polydypsia, paresthesias, or muscle weakness may be present as a consequence of hypokalemic alkalosis. The simplest screening test is measurement of serum potassium concentration. In a hypertensive patient with unprovoked hypokalemia (i.e., unrelated to diuretics, vomiting, or diarrhea), the prevalence of primary aldosteronism approaches 40–50%. In patients on diuretics, serum potassium <3.1 mmol/L (<3.1 meq/L) also raises the possibility of primary aldosteronism; however, serum potassium is an insensitive and nonspecific screening test. On initial presentation, serum potassium is normal in ~25% of patients subsequently found to have an aldosterone-producing adenoma, and higher percentages of patients with other etiologies of primary aldosteronism are not hypokalemic. Additionally, hypokalemic hypertension may be a consequence of secondary aldosteronism, other mineralocorticoid- and glucocorticoid-induced hypertensive disorders, and pheochromocytoma.

The ratio of plasma aldosterone to plasma renin activity (PA/PRA) is a useful screening test. These measurements are preferably obtained in ambulatory patients in the morning. A ratio >30:1 in conjunction with a plasma aldosterone concentration >555 pmol/L (>20 ng/dL) reportedly has a sensitivity of 90% and a specificity of 91% for an aldosterone-producing adenoma. In a Mayo Clinic series, an aldosterone-producing adenoma was subsequently surgically confirmed in >90% of hypertensive patients with a PA/PRA ratio ≥20 and a plasma aldosterone concentration ≥415 pmol/L (≥15 ng/dL). There are, however, several caveats to interpreting the ratio. The cutoff for a "high" ratio is laboratory- and assay-dependent. Although some antihypertensive agents may affect the ratio (e.g., aldosterone antagonists, angiotensin receptor antagonists, and ACE inhibitors may increase renin; aldosterone antagonists may increase aldosterone), the ratio has been reported to be useful as a screening test in measurements obtained with patients taking their usual antihypertensive medications. A high ratio in the absence of an elevated plasma aldosterone level is considerably less specific for primary aldosteronism since many patients with essential hypertension have low renin levels in this setting, particularly African Americans and elderly patients. In patients with renal insufficiency, the ratio may also be elevated because of decreased aldosterone clearance. In patients with an elevated PA/PRA ratio, the diagnosis of primary aldosteronism can be confirmed by demonstrating failure to suppress plasma aldosterone to <277 pmol/L (<10 ng/dL) after IV infusion of 2 L of isotonic saline over 4 h.

Several adrenal abnormalities may culminate in the syndrome of primary aldosteronism, and appropriate therapy depends on the specific etiology. Some 60–70% of patients have an aldosterone-producing adrenal adenoma. The tumor is almost always unilateral, and most measure <3 cm in diameter. Most of the remainder have bilateral adrenocortical hyperplasia (idiopathic hyperaldosteronism). Rarely, primary aldosteronism may be caused by an adrenal carcinoma or an ectopic malignancy, e.g., ovarian arrhenoblastoma. Most aldosterone-producing carcinomas, in contrast to adrenal adenomas and hyperplasia, produce excessive amounts of other adrenal steroids in addition to aldosterone. Functional differences in hormone secretion may assist in the differential diagnosis. Aldosterone biosynthesis is more responsive to ACTH in patients with adenoma and more responsive to angiotensin in patients with hyperplasia. Consequently, patients with adenoma tend to have higher plasma aldosterone in the early morning that decreases during the day, reflecting the diurnal rhythm of ACTH, whereas plasma aldosterone tends to increase with upright posture in patients with hyperplasia, reflecting the normal postural response of the renin-angiotensin-aldosterone axis.

Adrenal CT or MRI should be carried out in all patients diagnosed with primary aldosteronism. High-resolution CT may identify tumors as small as 0.3 cm and is positive for an adrenal tumor 90% of the time. If the CT or MRI is not diagnostic, an adenoma may be detected by adrenal scintigraphy with 6 β-[I^{131}]iodomethyl-19-norcholesterol after dexamethasone suppression (0.5 mg every 6 h for 7 days); however, this technique has decreased sensitivity for adenomas <1 cm. When results of functional and anatomic studies are inconclusive, bilateral adrenal venous sampling for aldosterone and cortisol levels in response to ACTH stimulation should be carried out. An ipsilateral/contralateral aldosterone ratio >10, with symmetric ACTH-stimulated cortisol levels, is diagnostic of an aldosterone-producing adenoma.

Hypertension is generally responsive to surgery in patients with adenoma but not in patients with bilateral adrenal hyperplasia. Unilateral adrenalectomy, often done via a laparoscopic approach, is curative in 40–70% of patients with an adenoma. Surgery should be undertaken after blood pressure has been controlled and hypokalemia corrected. Transient hypoaldosteronism may occur for up to 3 months postoperatively, resulting in hyperkalemia. Potassium should be monitored during this time, and hyperkalemia should be treated with potassium-wasting diuretics and with fludrocortisone, if needed. Patients with bilateral hyperplasia should be treated medically. The drug regimen for these patients, as well as for patients with an adenoma who are poor surgical candidates, should include an aldosterone antagonist and, if necessary, other potassium-sparing diuretics.

Glucocorticoid-remediable hyperaldosteronism is a rare, monogenic autosomal dominant disorder characterized by moderate to severe hypertension, often at an early age. Hypokalemia is usually mild or absent. Normally, angiotensin II stimulates aldosterone production by the adrenal zona glomerulosa, whereas ACTH stimulates cortisol production in the zona fasciculata. Owing to a chimeric gene on chromosome 8, ACTH also regulates aldosterone secretion by the zona fasciculata in patients with glucocorticoid-remediable hyperaldosteronism. The consequence is overproduction in the zona fasciculata of both aldosterone and hybrid steroids (18-hydroxycortisol and 18-oxocortisol) due to oxidation of cortisol. The diagnosis may be established by urine excretion rates of these hybrid steroids that are twenty to thirty times normal or by direct genetic testing. Therapeutically, suppression of ACTH with low-dose glucocorticoids corrects the hyperaldosteronism, hypertension, and hypokalemia. Spironolactone is also a therapeutic option.

CUSHING'S SYNDROME

Hypertension occurs in 75–80% of patients with Cushing's syndrome. The mechanism of hypertension may be related to stimulation of mineralocorticoid receptors by cortisol and increased secretion of other adrenal steroids. If clinically suspected, in patients not taking exogenous glucocorticoids, laboratory screening may be carried out with measurement of 24-h excretion rates of urine free cortisol or an overnight dexamethasone-suppression test. Recent evidence suggests that late night salivary cortisol is a sensitive and convenient screening test. Further evaluation is required to confirm the diagnosis and to identify the specific etiology of Cushing's syndrome. Appropriate therapy depends on the etiology.

PHEOCHROMOCYTOMA

Catecholamine-secreting tumors are located in the adrenal medulla (pheochromocytoma) or in extra-adrenal paraganglion tissue (paraganglioma) and account for hypertension in ~0.05% of patients. Approximately 20% of pheochromocytomas are familial with an autosomal dominant inheritance. Inherited pheochromocytomas may be associated with multiple endocrine neoplasia

TABLE 37-4

RARE MENDELIAN FORMS OF HYPERTENSION

DISEASE	PHENOTYPE	GENETIC CAUSE
Glucocorticoid-remediable hyperaldosteronism	Autosomal dominant, absent or mild hypokalemia	Chimeric 11β-hydroxylase/aldosterone gene on chromosome 8
17α-hydroxylase deficiency	Autosomal recessive Males: pseudohermaphroditism Females: primary amenorrhea, absent secondary sexual characteristics	Random mutations of the *CYP17* gene on chromosome 10
11β-hydroxylase deficiency	Autosomal recessive masculinization	Mutations of the *CYP11B1* gene on chromosome 8q21-q22
11β-hydroxysteroid dehydrogenase deficiency (apparent mineralocorticoid excess syndrome)	Autosomal recessive Hypokalemia, low renin, low aldosterone	Mutations in the 11β-hydroxysteroid dehydrogenase gene
Liddle's syndrome	Autosomal dominant Hypokalemia, low renin, low aldosterone	Mutation subunits of the epithelial sodium channel *SCNN1B* and *SCNN1C* genes
Pseudohypoaldosteronism type II (Gordon's syndrome)	Autosomal dominant Hyperkalemia, normal glomerular filtration rate	Linkage to chromosomes 1q31-q42 and 17p11-q21
Hypertension exacerbated in pregnancy	Autosomal dominant Severe hypertension in early pregnancy	Missense mutation with substitution of leucine for serine at codon 810 (MR_{L810})
Polycystic kidney disease	Autosomal dominant Large cystic kidneys, renal failure, liver cysts, cerebral aneurysms, valvular heart disease	Mutations in the *PKD1* gene on chromosome 16 and *PKD2* gene on chromosome 4
Pheochromocytoma	Autosomal dominant (a) Multiple endocrine neoplasia, type 2A Medullary thyroid carcinoma, hyperparathyroidism	(a) Mutations in the RET protooncogene
	(b) Multiple endocrine neoplasia, type 2B Medullary thyroid carcinoma, mucosal neuromas, thickened corneal nerves, alimentary ganglioneuromatoses, marfanoid habitus	(b) Mutations in the RET protooncogene
	(c) von Hippel–Lindau disease Retinal angiomas, hemangioblastomas of the cerebellum and spinal cord, renal cell carcinoma	(c) Mutations in the VHL tumor-suppressor gene
	(d) Neurofibromatosis type 1 Multiple neurofibromas, café au lait spots	(d) Mutations in the NF1 tumor-suppressor gene

(MEN) type 2A and type 2B (Table 37–4). If unrecognized, pheochromocytoma may result in lethal cardiovascular consequences. Clinical manifestations, including hypertension, are primarily related to increased circulating catecholamines, although some of these tumors may secrete a number of other vasoactive substances. In a small percent of patients, epinephrine is the predominant catecholamine secreted by the tumor, and these patients may present with hypotension rather than hypertension. The initial suspicion of the diagnosis is based on symptoms and/or the association of pheochromocytoma with other disorders (Table 37-4). Laboratory testing consists of measuring catecholamines in either urine or plasma.

Genetic screening is also available for evaluating patients and relatives suspected of harboring a pheochromocytoma associated with a familial syndrome. Surgical excision is the definitive treatment of pheochromocytoma and results in cure in ~90% of patients.

MISCELLANEOUS CAUSES OF HYPERTENSION

Hypertension due to *obstructive sleep apnea* is being recognized with increasing frequency. Independent of obesity, hypertension occurs in >50% of individuals with obstructive sleep apnea, the severe end of the sleep-disordered breathing syndrome. The severity of hypertension correlates with the severity of sleep apnea. Approximately 70% of patients with obstructive sleep apnea are obese. Hypertension related to obstructive sleep apnea should also be considered in patients with drug-resistant hypertension and in patients with a history of snoring. The diagnosis can be confirmed by polysomnography. In obese patients, weight loss may alleviate or cure sleep apnea and related hypertension. Continuous positive airway pressure (CPAP) administered during sleep is an effective therapy for obstructive sleep apnea. With CPAP, patients with apparently drug-resistant hypertension may be more responsive to antihypertensive agents.

Coarctation of the aorta is the most common congenital cardiovascular cause of hypertension (Chap. 19). The incidence is 1–8 per 1000 live births. It is usually sporadic but occurs in 35% of children with Turner's syndrome. Even when the anatomic lesion is surgically corrected in infancy, up to 30% of patients develop subsequent hypertension and are at risk of accelerated coronary artery disease and cerebrovascular events. Patients with less severe lesions may not be diagnosed until young adulthood. The physical findings are diagnostic, and include diminished and delayed femoral pulses and a systolic pressure gradient between the right arm and the legs, and, depending on the location of the coarctation, between the right and left arms. A blowing systolic murmur may be heard in the posterior left interscapular areas. The diagnosis may be confirmed by chest x-ray and transesophageal echocardiogram. Therapeutic options include surgical repair or balloon angioplasty, with or without placement of an intravascular stent. Subsequently, many patients do not have a normal life expectancy but may have persistent hypertension with death due to ischemic heart disease, cerebral hemorrhage, or aortic aneurysm.

Several additional endocrine disorders, including *thyroid diseases* and *acromegaly*, cause hypertension. Mild diastolic hypertension may be a consequence of hypothyroidism, whereas hyperthyroidism may result in systolic hypertension. *Hypercalcemia* of any etiology, the most common being primary hyperparathyroidism, may result in hypertension. Hypertension may also be related to a number of prescribed or over-the-counter *medications*.

MONOGENIC HYPERTENSION

A number of rare forms of monogenic hypertension have been identified (Table 37-4). These disorders may be recognized by their characteristic phenotypes, and in many instances the diagnosis may be confirmed by genetic analysis. Several inherited defects in adrenal steroid biosynthesis and metabolism result in mineralocorticoid-induced hypertension and hypokalemia. In patients with a 17α-hydroxylase deficiency, synthesis of sex hormones and cortisol is decreased (Fig. 37-3). Consequently, these individuals do not mature sexually; males may present with pseudohermaphroditism and females with primary amenorrhea and absent secondary sexual characteristics. Because cortisol-induced negative feedback on pituitary ACTH production is diminished, ACTH-stimulated adrenal steroid synthesis proximal to the enzymatic block is increased. Hypertension and

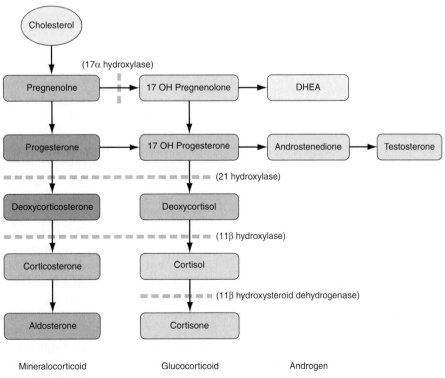

FIGURE 37-3
Adrenal enzymatic defects.

hypokalemia are consequences of increased synthesis of mineralocorticoids proximal to the enzymatic block, particularly desoxycorticosterone. Increased steroid production and, hence, hypertension may be treated with low-dose glucocorticoids. An 11β-hydroxylase deficiency results in a salt-retaining adrenogenital syndrome, occurring in 1 in 100,000 live births. This enzymatic defect results in decreased cortisol synthesis, increased synthesis of mineralocorticoids (e.g., desoxycorticosterone), and shunting of steroid biosynthesis into the androgen pathway. In the severe form, the syndrome may present early in life, including the newborn period, with virilization and ambiguous genitalia in females and penile enlargement in males, or in older children as precocious puberty and short stature. Acne, hirsutism, and menstrual irregularities may be the presenting features when the disorder is first recognized in adolescence or early adulthood. Hypertension is less common in the late-onset forms. Patients with an 11β-hydroxysteroid dehydrogenase deficiency have an impaired capacity to metabolize cortisol to its inactive metabolite, cortisone, and hypertension is related to activation of mineralocorticoid receptors by cortisol. This defect may be inherited or acquired, due to licorice-containing glyccherizic acid. This same substance is present in the paste of several brands of chewing tobacco. The defect in Liddle's syndrome results from constitutive activation of amiloride-sensitive epithelial sodium channels (ENaC) on the distal renal tubule, resulting in excess sodium reabsorption; the syndrome is ameliorated by amiloride. Hypertension exacerbated in pregnancy is due to activation of the mineralocorticoid receptor by progesterone. Approximately 20% of pheochromocytomas are familial and may be associated with distinctive phenotypes.

Approach to the Patient:
HYPERTENSION

HISTORY The initial assessment of the hypertensive patient should include a complete history and physical examination to confirm a diagnosis of hypertension, screen for other cardiovascular disease risk factors, screen for secondary causes of hypertension, identify cardiovascular consequences of hypertension and other comorbidities, assess blood pressure–related lifestyles, and determine the potential for intervention.

Most patients with hypertension have no specific symptoms referable to their blood pressure elevation. Although popularly considered a symptom of elevated arterial pressure, headache generally occurs only in patients with severe hypertension. Characteristically, a "hypertensive headache" occurs in the morning and is localized to the occipital region. Other nonspecific symptoms that may be related to elevated blood

TABLE 37-5

PATIENT'S RELEVANT HISTORY
Duration of hypertension
Previous therapies: responses and side effects
Family history of hypertension and cardiovascular disease
Dietary and psychosocial history
Other risk factors: weight change, dyslipidemia, smoking, diabetes, physical inactivity
Evidence of secondary hypertension: history of renal disease; change in appearance; muscle weakness; spells of sweating, palpitations, tremor; erratic sleep, snoring, daytime somnolence; symptoms of hypo- or hyperthyroidism; use of agents that may increase blood pressure
Evidence of target organ damage: history of TIA, stroke, transient blindness; angina, myocardial infarction, congestive heart failure; sexual function
Other comorbidities

Note: TIA, transient ischemic attack.

pressure include dizziness, palpitations, easy fatigability, and impotence. When symptoms are present, they are generally related to hypertensive cardiovascular disease or to manifestations of secondary hypertension. Table 37-5 lists salient features that should be addressed in obtaining a history from a hypertensive patient.

MEASUREMENT OF BLOOD PRESSURE Reliable measurements of blood pressure depend on attention to the details of the technique and conditions of the measurement. Owing to recent regulations preventing the use of mercury because of concerns about its potential toxicity, most office measurements are made with aneroid instruments. The accuracy of automated blood pressure instruments should be confirmed. Before taking the blood pressure measurement, the individual should be seated quietly for 5 min in a private, quiet setting with a comfortable room temperature. The center of the cuff should be at heart level, and the width of the bladder cuff should equal at least 40% of the arm circumference; the length of the cuff bladder should encircle at least 80% of the arm circumference. It is important to pay attention to cuff placement, stethoscope placement, and the rate of deflation of the cuff (2 mmHg/s). Systolic blood pressure is the first of at least two regular "tapping" Korotkoff sounds, and diastolic blood pressure is the point at which the last regular Korotkoff sound is heard. In current practice, a diagnosis of hypertension is generally based on seated, office measurements.

Currently available ambulatory monitors are fully automated, use the oscillometric technique, and typically are programmed to take readings every 15–30 min. Ambulatory blood pressure monitoring is not, however, routinely used in clinical practice and is generally reserved for patients in whom white coat hypertension is suspected. The Seventh Report of the Joint National Committee on Prevention, Detection, Evaluation, and Treatment of High Blood Pressure (JNC 7) has also recommended ambulatory monitoring for treatment resistance, symptomatic hypotension, autonomic failure, and episodic hypertension.

PHYSICAL EXAMINATION Body habitus, including weight and height, should be noted. At the initial examination, blood pressure should be measured in both arms, and preferably in the supine, sitting, and standing positions to evaluate for postural hypotension. Even if the femoral pulse is normal to palpation, arterial pressure should be measured at least once in the lower extremity in patients in whom hypertension is discovered before age 30. Heart rate should also be recorded. Hypertensive individuals have an increased prevalence of atrial fibrillation. The neck should be palpated for an enlarged thyroid gland, and patients should be assessed for signs of hypo- and hyperthyroidism. Examination of blood vessels may provide clues about underlying vascular disease and should include funduscopic examination, auscultation for bruits over the carotid and femoral arteries, and palpation of femoral and pedal pulses. The retina is the only tissue in which arteries and arterioles can be examined directly. With increasing severity of hypertension and atherosclerotic disease, progressive funduscopic changes include increased arteriolar light reflex, arteriovenous crossing defects, hemorrhages and exudates, and, in patients with malignant hypertension, papilledema. Examination of the heart may reveal a loud second heart sound due to closure of the aortic valve and an S_4 gallop, attributed to atrial contraction against a noncompliant left ventricle. Left ventricular hypertrophy may be detected by an enlarged, sustained, and laterally displaced apical impulse. An abdominal bruit, particularly a bruit that lateralizes and extends throughout systole into diastole, raises the possibility of renovascular hypertension. Kidneys of patients with polycystic kidney disease may be palpable in the abdomen. The physical examination should also include evaluation for signs of CHF and a neurologic examination.

LABORATORY TESTING Table 37-6 lists recommended laboratory tests in the initial evaluation of hypertensive patients. Repeat measurements of renal function, serum electrolytes, fasting glucose, and lipids may be obtained after introducing a new antihypertensive agent and then annually, or more frequently if clinically indicated. More extensive laboratory testing is appropriate for patients with apparent drug-resistant hypertension or when the clinical evaluation suggests a secondary form of hypertension.

TABLE 37-6

BASIC LABORATORY TESTS FOR INITIAL EVALUATION

SYSTEM	TEST
Renal	Microscopic urinalysis, albumin excretion, serum BUN and/or creatinine
Endocrine	Serum sodium, potassium, calcium, TSH
Metabolic	Fasting blood glucose, total cholesterol, HDL and LDL (often computed) cholesterol, triglycerides
Other	Hematocrit, electrocardiogram

Note: BUN, blood urea nitrogen; TSH, thyroid-stimulating hormone; HDL, high-density lipoprotein; LDL, low-density lipoprotein.

℞ **Treatment:**
HYPERTENSION

LIFESTYLE INTERVENTIONS Implementation of lifestyles that favorably affect blood pressure has implications for both the prevention and treatment of hypertension. Health-promoting lifestyle modifications are recommended for individuals with pre-hypertension and as an adjunct to drug therapy in hypertensive individuals. These interventions should address overall cardiovascular disease risk. Although the impact of lifestyle interventions on blood pressure is more pronounced in persons with hypertension, in short-term trials, weight loss and reduction of dietary NaCl have also been shown to prevent the development of hypertension. In hypertensive individuals, even if these interventions do not produce a sufficient reduction of blood pressure to avoid drug therapy, the number of medications or dosages required for blood pressure control may be reduced. Dietary modifications that effectively lower blood pressure are weight loss, reduced NaCl intake, increased potassium intake, moderation of alcohol consumption, and an overall healthy dietary pattern (Table 37-7).

Prevention and treatment of obesity are important for reducing blood pressure and cardiovascular disease risk. In short-term trials, even modest weight loss can lead to a reduction of blood pressure and an increase of insulin sensitivity. Average blood pressure reductions of 6.3/3.1 mmHg have been observed with a reduction in mean body weight of 9.2 kg. Regular physical activity facilitates weight loss, decreases blood pressure, and reduces the overall risk of cardiovascular disease. Blood pressure may be lowered by 30 min of moderately intense physical activity, such as brisk walking, 6–7 days a week, or by more intense, less frequent workouts.

There is individual variability in the sensitivity of blood pressure to NaCl, and this variability may have a genetic basis. Based on results of meta-analyses,

TABLE 37-7

LIFESTYLE MODIFICATIONS TO MANAGE HYPERTENSION	
Weight reduction	Attain and maintain BMI <25 kg/m²
Dietary salt reduction	<6 g NaCl/d
Adapt DASH-type dietary plan	Diet rich in fruits, vegetables, and low-fat dairy products with reduced content of saturated and total fat
Moderation of alcohol consumption	For those who drink alcohol, consume ≤2 drinks/day in men and ≤1 drink/day in women
Physical activity	Regular aerobic activity, e.g., brisk walking for 30 min/d

Note: BMI, body mass index; DASH, Dietary Approaches to Stop Hypertension (trial).

lowering of blood pressure by limiting daily NaCl intake to 4.4–7.4 g (75–125 meq) results in blood pressure reductions of 3.7–4.9/0.9–2.9 mmHg in hypertensive and lesser reductions in normotensive individuals. Diets deficient in potassium, calcium, and magnesium are associated with higher blood pressures and a higher prevalence of hypertension. The urine sodium-to-potassium ratio is a stronger correlate of blood pressure than either sodium or potassium alone. Potassium and calcium supplementation have inconsistent, modest antihypertensive effects, and, independent of blood pressure, potassium supplementation may be associated with reduced stroke mortality. Alcohol use in persons consuming three or more drinks per day (a standard drink contains ~14 g ethanol) is associated with higher blood pressures, and a reduction of alcohol consumption is associated with a reduction of blood pressure. Mechanisms by which dietary potassium, calcium, or alcohol may affect blood pressure have not been established.

The DASH (Dietary Approaches to Stop Hypertension) trial convincingly demonstrated that over an 8-week period a diet high in fruits, vegetables, and low-fat dairy products lowers blood pressure in individuals with high-normal blood pressures or mild hypertension. Reduction of daily NaCl intake to <6 g (100 meq) augmented the effect of this diet on blood pressure. Fruits and vegetables are enriched sources of potassium, magnesium, and fiber, and dairy products are an important source of calcium.

PHARMACOLOGIC THERAPY Drug therapy is recommended for individuals with blood pressures ≥140/90 mmHg. The degree of benefit derived from antihypertensive agents is related to the magnitude of the blood pressure reduction. Lowering systolic blood pressure by 10–12 mmHg and diastolic blood pressure by 5–6 mmHg confers relative risk reductions of 35–40% for stroke and 12–16% for CHD within 5 years of initiating treatment. Risk of heart failure is reduced by >50%. There is considerable variation in individual responses to different classes of antihypertensive agents, and the magnitude of response to any single agent may be limited by activation of counterregulatory mechanisms that oppose the hypotensive effect of the agent. Selection of antihypertensive agents, and combinations of agents, should be individualized, taking into account age, severity of hypertension, other cardiovascular disease risk factors, comorbid conditions, and practical considerations related to cost, side effects, and frequency of dosing (Table 37-8).

Diuretics Low-dose thiazide diuretics are often used as first-line agents, alone or in combination with other antihypertensive drugs. Thiazides inhibit the Na⁺/Cl⁻ pump in the distal convoluted tubule and, hence, increase sodium excretion. Long term, they may also act as vasodilators. Thiazides are safe, efficacious, and inexpensive and reduce clinical events. They provide additive blood pressure–lowering effects when combined with beta blockers, ACE inhibitors, or angiotensin receptor blockers. In contrast, addition of a diuretic to a calcium channel blocker is less effective. Usual doses of hydrochlorothiazide range from 6.25–50 mg/d. Owing to an increased incidence of metabolic side effects (hypokalemia, insulin resistance, increased cholesterol), higher doses are generally not recommended. Two potassium-sparing diuretics, amiloride and triamterene, act by inhibiting epithelial sodium channels in the distal nephron. These agents are weak antihypertensive agents but may be used in combination with a thiazide to protect against hypokalemia. The main pharmacologic target for loop diuretics is the Na⁺-K⁺-2Cl⁻ cotransporter in the thick ascending limb of the loop of Henle. Loop diuretics are generally reserved for hypertensive patients with reduced glomerular filtration rates [reflected in serum creatinine >220 μmol/L (>2.5 mg/dL)], CHF, or sodium retention and edema for some other reason such as treatment with a potent vasodilator, e.g., minoxidil.

Blockers of the Renin-Angiotensin System ACE inhibitors decrease the production of angiotensin II, increase bradykinin levels, and reduce sympathetic nervous system activity. Angiotensin II receptor blockers provide selective blockade of AT₁ receptors, and the effect of angiotensin II on unblocked AT₂ receptors may augment the hypotensive effect. Both classes of agents are effective antihypertensive agents that may be used as monotherapy or in combination with diuretics, calcium antagonists, and alpha-blocking agents. Side effects of ACE inhibitors and angiotensin receptor blockers include functional renal insufficiency

TABLE 37-8

EXAMPLES OF ORAL DRUGS USED IN TREATMENT OF HYPERTENSION

DRUG CLASS	EXAMPLES	USUAL TOTAL DAILY DOSE[a] (DOSING FREQUENCY/DAY)	OTHER INDICATIONS	CONTRAINDICATIONS/ CAUTIONS
Diuretics				
Thiazides	Hydrochlorothiazide	6.25–50 mg (1–2)		Diabetes, dyslipidemia, hyperuricemia, gout, hypokalemia
	Chlorthalidone	25–50 MG (1)		
Loop diuretics	Furosemide	40–80 mg (2–3)	CHF, renal failure	Diabetes, dyslipidemia, hyperuricemia, gout, hypokalemia
	Ethacrynic acid	50–100 mg (2–3)		
Aldosterone antagonists	Spironolactone	25–100 mg (1–2)	CHF, primary aldosteronism	Renal failure, hyperkalemia
	Eplerenone			
K⁺ retaining	Amiloride	50–100 mg (1–2)		Renal failure, hyperkalemia
	Triamterene	5–10 mg (1–2)		
		50–100 mg (1–2)		
Beta blockers				Asthma, COPD, 2nd or 3rd degree heart block, sick-sinus syndrome
Cardioselective	Atenolol	25–100 mg (1)	Angina, CHF, post-MI, sinus tachycardia, ventricular tachyarrhythmias	
	Metoprolol	25–100 MG (1–2)		
Nonselective	Propranolol	40–160 mg (2)		
	Propranolol LA	60–180 (1)		
Combined alpha/ beta	Labetalol	200–800 mg (2)	Post-MI, CHF	
	Carvedilol	12.5–50 mg (2)		
Alpha antagonists				
Selective	Prazosin	2–20 mg (2–3)	Prostatism	
	Doxazosin	1–16 mg (1)		
	Terazosin	1–10 mg (1–2)		
Nonselective	Phenoxybenzamine	20–120 mg (2–3)	Pheochromocytoma	
Sympatholytics				
Central	Clonidine	0.1–0.6 mg (2)		
	Clonidine patch	0.1–0.3 mg (1/week)		
	Methyldopa	250–1000 mg (2)		
	Reserpine	0.05–0.25 mg (1)		
	Guanfacine	0.5–2 mg (1)		
ACE inhibitors	Captopril	25–200 mg (2)	Post-MI, CHF, nephropathy	Renal failure, bilateral renal artery stenosis, pregnancy, hyperkalemia
	Lisinopril	10–40 mg (1)		
	Ramipril	2.5–20 mg (1–2)		
Angiotensin II antagonists	Losartan	25–100 mg (1–2)	CHF, diabetic nephropathy, ACE inhibitor cough	Renal failure, bilateral renal artery stenosis, pregnancy, hyperkalemia
	Valsartan	80–320 mg (1)		
	Candesartan	2–32 mg (1–2)		
Calcium antagonists				Heart failure, 2nd or 3rd degree heart block
Dihydropyridines	Nifedipine (long acting)	30–60 mg (1)	Angina	
Nondihydropyridines	Verapamil (long acting)	120–360 mg (1–2)	Post-MI, supraventricular tachycardias, angina	
	Diltiazem (long-acting)	180–420 mg (1)		
Direct vasodilators	Hydralazine	25–100 mg (2)		Severe coronary artery disease
	Minoxidil	2.5–80 mg (1–2)		

[a] At the initiation of therapy, lower doses may be preferable for elderly patients and for select combinations of antihypertensive agents.

Note: CHF, congestive heart failure; COPD, chronic obstructive pulmonary disease; MI, myocardial infarction; ACE, angiotensin-converting enzyme.

due to efferent renal arteriolar dilatation in a kidney with a stenotic lesion of the renal artery. Additional predisposing conditions to renal insufficiency induced by these agents include dehydration, CHF, and use of nonsteroidal anti-inflammatory drugs. Dry cough occurs in ~15% of patients, and angioedema occurs in <1% of patients taking ACE inhibitors. Angioedema occurs most commonly in individuals of Asian ancestry and more commonly in

African Americans than in whites. Hyperkalemia due to hypoaldosteronism is an occasional side effect of both ACE inhibitors and angiotensin receptor blockers.

Aldosterone Antagonists Spironolactone is a nonselective aldosterone antagonist that may be used alone or in combination with a thiazide diuretic. It may be a particularly effective agent in patients with low-renin essential hypertension, resistant hypertension, and primary aldosteronism. In patients with CHF, low-dose spironolactone reduces mortality and hospitalizations for heart failure when given in addition to conventional therapy with ACE inhibitors, digoxin, and loop diuretics. Because spironolactone binds to progesterone and androgen receptors, side effects may include gynecomastia, impotence, and menstrual abnormalities. These side effects are circumvented by a newer agent, eplerenone, which is a selective aldosterone antagonist. Eplerenone has recently been approved in the United States for the treatment of hypertension.

Beta Blockers β-Adrenergic receptor blockers lower blood pressure by decreasing cardiac output, due to a reduction of heart rate and contractility. Other proposed mechanisms by which beta blockers lower blood pressure include a central nervous system effect, and inhibition of renin release. Beta blockers are particularly effective in hypertensive patients with tachycardia, and their hypotensive potency is enhanced by coadministration with a diuretic. In lower doses, some beta blockers selectively inhibit cardiac β_1 receptors and have less influence on β_2 receptors on bronchial and vascular smooth muscle cells; however, there seems to be no difference in the antihypertensive potencies of cardioselective and non-selective beta blockers. Certain beta blockers have intrinsic sympathomimetic activity, and it is uncertain whether this constitutes an overall advantage or disadvantage in cardiac therapy. Beta blockers without intrinsic sympathomimetic activity decrease the rate of sudden death, overall mortality, and recurrent myocardial infarction. In patients with CHF, beta blockers have been shown to reduce the risks of hospitalization and mortality. Carvedilol and labetalol block both β receptors and peripheral α-adrenergic receptors. The potential advantages of combined β- and α-adrenergic blockade in treating hypertension remain to be determined.

α-Adrenergic Blockers Postsynaptic, selective α-adrenoreceptor antagonists lower blood pressure by decreasing peripheral vascular resistance. They are effective antihypertensive agents, used either as monotherapy or in combination with other agents. However, in clinical trials of hypertensive patients, alpha blockade has not been shown to reduce cardiovascular morbidity and mortality or to provide as much protection against CHF as other classes of antihypertensive

agents. These agents are also effective in treating lower urinary tract symptoms in men with prostatic hypertrophy. Nonselective α-adrenoreceptor antagonists bind to postsynaptic and presynaptic receptors and are primarily used for the management of patients with pheochromocytoma.

Sympatholytic Agents Centrally acting α_2 sympathetic agonists decrease peripheral resistance by inhibiting sympathetic outflow. They may be particularly useful in patients with autonomic neuropathy who have wide variations in blood pressure due to baroceptor denervation. Drawbacks include somnolence, dry mouth, and rebound hypertension on withdrawal. Peripheral sympatholytics decrease peripheral resistance and venous constriction by depleting nerve terminal norepinephrine. Although potentially effective antihypertensive agents, their usefulness is limited by orthostatic hypotension, sexual dysfunction, and numerous drug-drug interactions.

Calcium Channel Blockers Calcium antagonists reduce vascular resistance through L-channel blockade, which reduces intracellular calcium and blunts vasoconstriction. This is a heterogeneous group of agents that includes drugs in the following three classes: phenylalkylamines (verapamil), benzothiazepines (diltiazem), and 1,4-dihydropyridines (nifedipine-like). Used alone and in combination with other agents (ACE inhibitors, beta blockers, α_1-adrenergic blockers), calcium antagonists effectively lower blood pressure; however, it is unclear if adding a diuretic to a calcium blocker results in a further lowering of blood pressure. Side effects of flushing, headache, and edema with dihydropyridine use are related to their potencies as arteriolar dilators; edema is due to an increase in transcapillary pressure gradients, not to net salt and water retention.

Direct Vasodilators These agents decrease peripheral resistance and concomitantly activate mechanisms that defend arterial pressure, notably the sympathetic nervous system, the renin-angiotensin-aldosterone system, and sodium retention. Usually, they are not considered first-line agents but are most effective when added to a combination that includes a diuretic and a beta blocker. Hydralazine is a potent direct vasodilator that has antioxidant and nitric-oxide enhancing actions, and minoxidil is a particularly potent agent and is most frequently used in patients with renal insufficiency who are refractory to all other drugs. Hydralazine may induce a lupus-like syndrome, and side effects of minoxidil include hypertrichosis and pericardial effusion.

COMPARISONS OF ANTIHYPERTENSIVES

Based on pooling results from clinical trials, meta-analyses of the efficacy of different classes of antihypertensive agents suggest essentially equivalent blood pressure–lowering effects of the following six major classes of antihypertensive agents when used as monotherapy: thiazide diuretics, beta blockers, ACE inhibitors, angiotensin II receptor blockers, calcium antagonists, and α_2 blockers. On average, standard doses of most antihypertensive agents reduce blood pressure by 8–10/4–7 mmHg; however, there may be subgroup differences in responsiveness. Younger patients may be more responsive to beta blockers and ACE inhibitors, whereas patients older than 50 years may be more responsive to diuretics and calcium antagonists. There is a limited relationship between plasma renin and blood pressure response. Patients with high-renin hypertension may be more responsive to ACE inhibitors and angiotensin II receptor blockers than to other classes of agents, whereas patients with low-renin hypertension are more responsive to diuretics and calcium antagonists. Hypertensive African Americans tend to have low renin and may require higher doses of ACE inhibitors and angiotensin II receptor blockers than whites for optimal blood pressure control, although this difference is abolished when these agents are combined with a diuretic. Beta blockers also appear to be less effective than thiazide diuretics in African Americans than in non-African Americans.

A number of clinical trials have evaluated the possibility that different classes of antihypertensive agents have cardiovascular and renal protective effects not totally accounted for by their capacity to lower blood pressure. ACE inhibitors may have particular advantages, beyond that of blood pressure control, in reducing cardiovascular and renal outcomes. ACE inhibitors and angiotensin II receptor blockers decrease proteinuria and retard the rate of progression of renal insufficiency in both diabetic and nondiabetic renal diseases. The renoprotective effect of these agents, compared with other antihypertensive drugs, is less obvious at lower blood pressures. In both hypertensive and normotensive individuals, ACE inhibitors improve symptomatology and risk of death from CHF and reduce morbidity and mortality in the post-myocardial infarction patient. Similar benefits in cardiovascular morbidity and mortality in patients with CHF have also been observed with the use of angiotensin II receptor blockers. ACE inhibitors provide better coronary protection than calcium channel blockers, whereas calcium channel blockers provide more stroke protection than either ACE inhibitors or beta blockers.

In most patients with hypertension and heart failure due to systolic and/or diastolic dysfunction, the use of diuretics, ACE inhibitors or angiotensin II receptor antagonists, and beta blockers is recommended to improve survival. Although the optimal target blood pressure in patients with heart failure has not been established, a reasonable goal is the lowest blood pressure that is not associated with evidence of hypoperfusion.

A recent summary compared the results of 15 large clinical trials on the effects of antihypertensive treatment with different classes of agents on cardiovascular morbidity and mortality. In 13 of these trials, the incidence of cardiovascular events was similar between treatment groups, and in the remaining 2 trials, the difference was only marginally significant. It is possible that drug-related differences in cardiovascular outcomes are minimized in these large trials because of patient dropout, unplanned crossover of patients between groups, and insufficient statistical power to detect subgroup differences. Nevertheless, it is clear that the greatest cardiovascular and renal protective effects of antihypertensive therapy are related to adequate control of hypertension.

BLOOD PRESSURE GOALS OF ANTIHYPERTENSIVE THERAPY

Based on clinical trial data, the maximum protection against combined cardiovascular endpoints is achieved with pressures <135–140 mmHg for systolic blood pressure and <80–85 mmHg for diastolic blood pressure; however, treatment has not reduced cardiovascular disease risk to the level in nonhypertensive individuals. More aggressive blood pressure targets for blood pressure control (e.g., office or clinic blood pressure <130/80 mmHg) may be appropriate for patients with diabetes, CHD, chronic kidney disease, or with additional cardiovascular disease risk factors. In diabetic patients, effective blood pressure control reduces the risk of cardiovascular events and death as well as the risk for microvascular disease (nephropathy, retinopathy). Risk reduction is greater in diabetic than in nondiabetic individuals.

To achieve recommended blood pressure goals, the majority of individuals with hypertension will require treatment with more than one drug. Three or more drugs are frequently needed in patients with diabetes and renal insufficiency. For most agents, reduction of blood pressure at half-standard doses is only ~20% less than at standard doses. Appropriate combinations of agents at these lower doses may have additive or almost additive effects on blood pressure with a lower incidence of side effects.

Despite theoretical concerns about decreasing cerebral, coronary, and renal blood flow by overly aggressive antihypertensive therapy, clinical trials have found no evidence for a "J-curve" phenomenon, i.e., at blood pressure reductions achieved in clinical practice, there does *not* appear to be a lower threshold for increasing cardiovascular risk. Even among patients with isolated systolic hypertension, further lowering of the diastolic blood pressure does not result in harm. However, relatively little information is available concerning the risk/benefit ratio of antihypertensive therapy in individuals older than 80 years, and, in this population, gradual blood pressure reduction to less aggressive target levels of control may be appropriate.

The term *resistant hypertension* refers to patients with blood pressures persistently >140/90 mmHg despite taking three or more antihypertensive agents, including a diuretic, in reasonable combination and at full doses. Resistant or difficult-to-control hypertension is more common in patients older than 60 years than in younger patients. Resistant hypertension may be related to "pseudoresistance" (high office blood pressures and lower home blood pressures), nonadherence to therapy, identifiable causes of hypertension (including obesity and excessive alcohol intake), and use of any of a number of nonprescription and prescription drugs (Table 37-3). Rarely, in older patients, pseudohypertension may be related to the inability to measure blood pressure accurately in severely sclerotic arteries. This condition is suggested if the radial pulse remains palpable despite occlusion of the brachial artery by the cuff (Osler maneuver). The actual blood pressure can be determined by direct intraarterial measurement. Evaluation of patients with resistant hypertension might include home blood pressure monitoring to determine if office blood pressures are representative of the usual blood pressure. A more extensive evaluation for a secondary form of hypertension should be undertaken if no other explanation for hypertension resistance becomes apparent.

HYPERTENSIVE EMERGENCIES Probably due to the widespread availability of antihypertensive therapy, in the United States there has been a decline in the numbers of patients presenting with "crisis levels" of blood pressure. Most patients who present with severe hypertension are chronically hypertensive, and in the absence of acute, end-organ damage, precipitous lowering of blood pressure may be associated with significant morbidity and should be avoided. The key to successful management of severe hypertension is to differentiate hypertensive crises from hypertensive urgencies. The degree of target organ damage, rather than the level of blood pressure alone, determines the rapidity with which blood pressure should be lowered. **Tables 37-9** and **37-10** list a number of

TABLE 37-9

PREFERRED PARENTERAL DRUGS FOR SELECTED HYPERTENSIVE EMERGENCIES	
Hypertensive encephalopathy	Nitroprusside, nicardipine, labetalol
Malignant hypertension (when IV therapy is indicated)	Labetalol, nicardipine, nitroprusside, enalaprilat
Stroke	Nicardipine, labetalol, nitroprusside
Myocardial infarction/unstable angina	Nitroglycerin, nicardipine, labetalol, esmolol
Acute left ventricular failure	Nitroglycerin, enalaprilat, loop diuretics
Aortic dissection	Nitroprusside, esmolol, labetalol
Adrenergic crisis	Phentolamine, nitroprusside
Postoperative hypertension	Nitroglycerin, nitroprusside, labetalol, nicardipine
Preeclampsia/eclampsia of pregnancy	Hydralazine, labetalol, nicardipine

Source: Adapted from DG Vidt, in S Oparil, MA Weber (eds): *Hypertension*, 2d ed. Philadelphia, Elsevier Saunders, 2005.

TABLE 37-10

USUAL INTRAVENOUS DOSES OF ANTIHYPERTENSIVE AGENTS USED IN HYPERTENSIVE EMERGENCIES[a]	
ANTIHYPERTENSIVE AGENT	**INTRAVENOUS DOSE**
Nitroprusside	Initial 0.3 (µg/kg)/min; usual 2–4 (µg/kg)/min; maximum 10 (µg/kg)/min for 10 min
Nicardipine	Initial 5 mg/h; titrate by 2.5 mg/h at 5–15 min intervals; max 15 mg/h
Labetalol	2 mg/min up to 300 mg *or* 20 mg over 2 min, then 40–80 mg at 10-min intervals up to 300 mg total
Enalaprilat	Usual 0.625–1.25 mg over 5 min every 6–8 h; maximum 5 mg/dose
Esmolol	Initial 80–500 µg/kg over 1 min, then 50–300 (µg/kg)/min
Phentolamine	5–15 mg bolus
Nitroglycerin	Initial 5 µg/min, then titrate by 5 µg/min at 3–5 min intervals; if no response is seen at 20 µg/min, incremental increases of 10–20 µg/min may be used
Hydralazine	10–50 mg at 30-min intervals

[a] Constant blood pressure monitoring is required. Start with the lowest dose. Subsequent doses and intervals of administration should be adjusted according to the blood pressure response and duration of action of the specific agent.

hypertension-related emergencies and recommended therapies.

Malignant hypertension is a syndrome associated with an abrupt increase of blood pressure in a patient with underlying hypertension or related to the sudden onset of hypertension in a previously normotensive individual. The absolute level of blood pressure is not as important as its rate of rise. Pathologically, the syndrome is associated with diffuse necrotizing vasculitis, arteriolar thrombi, and fibrin deposition in arteriolar walls. Fibrinoid necrosis has been observed in arterioles of kidney, brain, retina, and other organs. Clinically, the syndrome is recognized by progressive retinopathy (arteriolar spasm, hemorrhages, exudates, and papilledema), deteriorating renal function with proteinuria, microangiopathic hemolytic anemia, and encephalopathy. In these patients, historic inquiry should include questions about the use of monamine oxidase inhibitors and recreational drugs (e.g., cocaine, amphetamines).

Although blood pressure should be lowered rapidly in patients with hypertensive encephalopathy, there are inherent risks of overly aggressive therapy. In hypertensive individuals, the upper and lower limits of autoregulation of cerebral blood flow are shifted to higher levels of arterial pressure, and rapid lowering of blood pressure to below the lower limit of autoregulation may precipitate cerebral ischemia or infarction as a consequence of decreased cerebral blood flow. Renal and coronary blood flows may also decrease with overly aggressive acute therapy. The initial goal of therapy is to reduce mean arterial blood pressure by no more than 25% within minutes to 2 h or to a blood pressure in the range of 160/100–110 mmHg. This may be accomplished with IV nitroprusside, a short-acting vasodilator with a rapid onset of action that allows for minute-to-minute control of blood pressure. Parenteral labetalol and nicardipine are also effective agents for the treatment of hypertensive encephalopathy.

In patients with malignant hypertension without encephalopathy or some other catastrophic event, it is preferable to reduce blood pressure over hours or longer rather than minutes. This goal may effectively be achieved initially with frequent dosing of short-acting oral agents, such as captopril, clonidine, or labetalol.

Acute, transient blood pressure elevations, lasting days to weeks, frequently occur following thrombotic and hemorrhagic strokes. Autoregulation of cerebral blood flow is impaired in ischemic cerebral tissue, and higher arterial pressures may be required to maintain cerebral blood flow. Although specific blood pressure targets have not been defined for patients with acute cerebrovascular events, aggressive reductions of blood pressure are to be avoided. With the increasing availability of improved methods for measuring cerebral blood flow (using CT technology), studies are in progress to evaluate the effects of different classes of antihypertensive agents on both blood pressure and cerebral blood flow following an acute stroke. Currently, in the absence of other indications for acute therapy, for patients with cerebral infarction who are not candidates for thrombolytic therapy, one recommended guideline is to institute antihypertensive therapy only for those patients with a systolic blood pressure >220 mmHg or a diastolic blood pressure >130 mmHg. If thrombolytic therapy is to be used, the recommended goal blood pressure is <185 mmHg systolic pressure and <110 mmHg diastolic pressure. In patients with hemorrhagic stroke, suggested guidelines for initiating antihypertensive therapy are systolic >180 mmHg or diastolic pressure >130 mmHg. The management of hypertension after subarachnoid hemorrhage is controversial. Cautious reduction of blood pressure is indicated if mean arterial pressure is >130 mmHg.

In addition to pheochromocytoma, an adrenergic crisis due to catecholamine excess may be related to cocaine or amphetamine overdose, clonidine withdrawal, acute spinal cord injuries, and an interaction of tyramine-containing compounds with monamine oxidase inhibitors. These patients may be treated with phentolamine or nitroprusside.

Treatment of hypertension in patients with acute aortic dissection is discussed in Chap. 38.

FURTHER READINGS

ADROGUE JH, MADIAS NE: Sodium and potassium in the pathogenesis of hypertension. N Engl J Med 356:1966, 2007

ALLHAT COLLABORATIVE RESEARCH GROUP: Major outcomes in high-risk hypertensive patients randomized to angiotensin converting enzyme inhibitor or calcium channel blocker vs. diuretic: The Antihypertensive and Lipid-Lowering Treatment to Prevent Heart Attack Trial (ALLHAT). JAMA 288:2981, 2002

APPEL LJ et al: Dietary approaches to prevent and treat hypertension: A scientific statement from the American Heart Association. Hypertension 47:296, 2006

BATH PMW, SPRIGGS N: Control of blood pressure after stroke. Hypertension 48:203, 2006

BLOOD PRESSURE LOWERING TREATMENT TRIALISTS' COLLABORATION: Effects of ACE inhibitors, calcium antagonists, and other blood pressure-lowering drugs: Results of prospectively designed overviews of randomised trials. Lancet 355:1955, 2000

BLOOD PRESSURE LOWERING TREATMENT TRIALISTS' COLLABORATION: Effects of different blood pressure-lowering regimens on major cardiovascular events in individuals with and without diabetes mellitus. Arch Int Med 165:1410, 2005

CASAS JP et al: Effect of inhibitors of the renin-angiotensin system and other antihypertensive drugs on renal outcomes: Systematic review and meta-analysis. Lancet 366:2026, 2005

CHOBANIAN AV et al: The Seventh Report of the Joint National Committee on Prevention, Detection, Evaluation, and Treatment of High Blood Pressure: The JNC 7 Report. JAMA 289:2560, 2003

ENDOCRINE SOCIETY'S CLINICAL PRACTICE GUIDELINES: Case detection, diagnosis, and treatment of patients with primary aldosteronism: an Endocrine Society Clinical Practice Guideline. J Clin Endocrinol Metab 93:3266, 2008

444 HAAJAR IM, KOTCHEN TA: Trends in prevalence, awareness, treatment, and control of hypertension in the United States, 1988–2000. JAMA 290:199, 2003

LAW MR et al: Value of low dose combination treatment with blood pressure lowering drugs: Analysis of 354 randomised trials. BMJ 326:1427, 2003

LAWES CMM et al: Global burden of blood pressure-related disease, 2001. Lancet 371:1513, 2008

LIU W et al: Genome scan meta-analysis for hypertension. Am J Hypertens 17:1100, 2004

MANCIA G: Role of outcome trials in providing information on antihypertensive treatment: Importance and limitations. Am J Hypertens 19:1, 2006

MOSER M, Setano JF: Resistant or difficult-to-control hypertension. N Engl J Med 355:385, 2006

ONG KL et al: Prevalence, awareness, treatment, and control of hypertension among United States adults 1999-2004. Hypertension 49:69, 2007

PICKERING TG et al: Recommendations for blood pressure measurement in humans and experimental animals. Part 1: Blood pressure measurement in humans. A statement for professionals from the Subcommittee of Professional and Public Education of the American Heart Association Council on High Blood Pressure Research. Hypertension 45:142, 2005

——— et al: Ambulatory blood-pressure monitoring. N Engl J Med 3554:2368, 2006

STAESSEN JA et al: Cardiovascular prevention and blood pressure reduction: A quantitative overview updated until 1 March 2003. J Hypertens 21:1055, 2003

TEXTOR SC: Current approaches to renovascular hypertension. Med Clin N Am 93:717, 2009

WU J et al: A summary of the effects of antihypertensive medications on measured blood pressure. Am J Hypertens 18:935, 2005

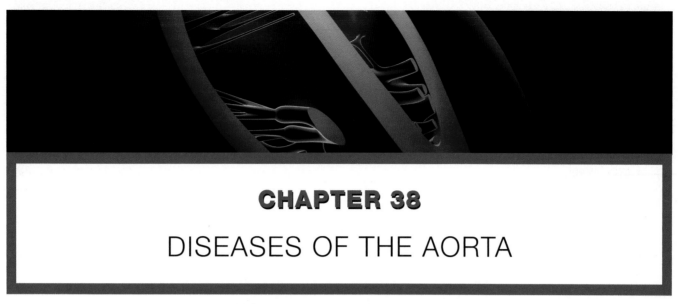

CHAPTER 38

DISEASES OF THE AORTA

Mark A. Creager ■ Joseph Loscalzo

The aorta is the conduit through which the blood ejected from the left ventricle is delivered to the systemic arterial bed. In adults, its diameter is approximately 3 cm at the origin and in the ascending portion, 2.5 cm in the descending portion in the thorax, and 1.8–2 cm in the abdomen. The aortic wall consists of a thin intima composed of endothelium, subendothelial connective tissue, and an internal elastic lamina; a thick tunica media composed of smooth-muscle cells and extracellular matrix; and an adventitia composed primarily of connective tissue enclosing the vasa vasorum and nervi vascularis. In addition to its conduit function, the viscoelastic and compliant properties of the aorta also subserve a buffering function. The aorta is distended during systole to enable a portion of the stroke volume and elastic energy to be stored, and it recoils during diastole so that blood continues to flow to the periphery. Because of its continuous exposure to high pulsatile pressure and shear stress, the aorta is particularly prone to injury and disease resulting from mechanical trauma (Table 38–1). The aorta is also more prone to rupture than any other vessel, especially with the development of aneurysmal dilatation, since its wall tension, as governed by Laplace's law (i.e., proportional to the product of pressure and radius), will be increased.

AORTIC ANEURYSM

An *aneurysm* is defined as a pathologic dilatation of a segment of a blood vessel. A *true aneurysm* involves all three layers of the vessel wall and is distinguished from a *pseudoaneurysm*, in which the intimal and medial layers are disrupted and the dilatation is lined by adventitia only and, at times, by perivascular clot. Aneurysms may also be classified according to their gross appearance. A *fusiform aneurysm* affects the entire circumference of a segment of the vessel, resulting in a diffusely dilated artery. In contrast, a *saccular aneurysm* involves only a portion of the circumference, resulting in an outpouching of the vessel wall. Aortic aneurysms are also classified according to location, i.e., abdominal versus thoracic. Aneurysms of the descending thoracic aorta are usually contiguous with infradiaphragmatic aneurysms and are referred to as *thoracoabdominal aortic aneurysms*.

ETIOLOGY

Aortic aneurysms result from conditions that cause degradation or abnormal production of the aortic wall's structural components, elastin and collagen. The causes

TABLE 38-1

DISEASES OF THE AORTA: ETIOLOGY AND ASSOCIATED FACTORS

Aortic aneurysm
  Degenerative/atherosclerosis
    Aging
    Cigarette smoking
    Male gender
    Family history
  Cystic medial necrosis
    Marfan syndrome
    Ehlers-Danlos syndrome type IV
    Familial etiology
    Bicuspid aortic valve
  Chronic aortic dissection
  Infective (see below)
  Trauma
Acute aortic syndromes (aortic dissection, acute intramural
  hematoma, penetrating atherosclerotic ulcer)
  Atherosclerosis
  Cystic medial necrosis (see above)
  Hypertension
  Vasculitis (see below)
  Pregnancy
  Trauma
Aortic occlusion
  Atherosclerosis
  Thromboembolism
Aortitis
  Vasculitis
    Takayasu's arteritis
    Giant cell arteritis
  Rheumatic
    HLA-B27–associated spondyloarthropathies
    Behçet's syndrome
    Cogan's syndrome
  Idiopathic retroperitoneal fibrosis
  Infective
    Syphilis
    Tuberculosis
  Mycotic (*Salmonella*, staphylococcal, streptococcal,
    fungal)

of aortic aneurysms may be broadly categorized as degenerative diseases, inherited or developmental diseases, infections, vasculitis, and trauma (Table 38-1). Inflammation, proteolysis, and biomechanical wall stress contribute to the degenerative processes that characterize most aneurysms of the abdominal and descending thoracic aorta. These are mediated by B and T cell lymphocytes, macrophages, inflammatory cytokines, and matrix metalloproteinases that degrade elastin and collagen and alter the tensile strength and ability of the aorta to accommodate pulsatile stretch. The associated histopathology demonstrates destruction of elastin and collagen, decreased vascular smooth muscle, in-growth of new blood vessels, and inflammation. Factors associated with degenerative aortic aneurysms include aging, cigarette smoking, hypercholesterolemia, male gender, and a family history of aortic aneurysms.

The most common pathologic condition associated with degenerative aortic aneurysms is *atherosclerosis*. Many patients with aortic aneurysms have coexisting risk factors for atherosclerosis (Chap. 30), as well as atherosclerosis in other blood vessels.

Cystic medial necrosis is the histopathologic term used to describe the degeneration of collagen and elastic fibers in the tunica media of the aorta, as well as the loss of medial cells that are replaced by multiple clefts of mucoid material. Cystic medial necrosis characteristically affects the proximal aorta, results in circumferential weakness and dilatation, and leads to the development of fusiform aneurysms involving the ascending aorta and the sinuses of Valsalva. This condition is particularly prevalent in patients with Marfan syndrome, Ehlers-Danlos syndrome type IV, hypertension, congenital bicuspid aortic valves, and familial thoracic aortic aneurysm syndromes. Sometimes it appears as an isolated condition in patients without any other apparent disease.

Familial clusterings of aortic aneurysms occur in 20% of patients, suggesting a hereditary basis for the disease. Mutations of the genes encoding fibrillin-1 and type III procollagen have been implicated in some cases of Marfan and Ehlers-Danlos type IV syndromes, respectively. Linkage analysis has identified loci on chromosomes 5q13–14, 11q23.3–q24, and 3p24–25 in several families, although the specific alleles have not been described.

The infectious causes of aortic aneurysms include syphilis, tuberculosis, and other bacterial infections. *Syphilis* is a relatively uncommon cause of aortic aneurysm. Syphilitic periaortitis and mesoaortitis damage elastic fibers, resulting in thickening and weakening of the aortic wall. Approximately 90% of syphilitic aneurysms are located in the ascending aorta or aortic arch. *Tuberculous aneurysms* typically affect the thoracic aorta and result from direct extension of infection from hilar lymph nodes or contiguous abscesses, or from bacterial seeding. Loss of aortic wall elasticity results from granulomatous destruction of the medial layer. A *mycotic aneurysm* is a rare condition that develops as a result of staphylococcal, streptococcal, *Salmonella* or other bacterial or fungal infections of the aorta, usually at an atherosclerotic plaque. These aneurysms are usually saccular. Blood cultures are often positive and reveal the nature of the infecting agent.

Vasculitides associated with aortic aneurysm include Takayasu's arteritis and giant cell arteritis, which may cause aneurysms of the aortic arch and descending thoracic aorta. Spondyloarthropathies, such as ankylosing spondylitis, rheumatoid arthritis, psoriatic arthritis, relapsing polychondritis, and Reiter's syndrome, are associated with dilatation of the ascending aorta. Behçet's syndrome causes thoracic and abdominal aortic aneurysms. *Traumatic aneurysms* may occur after penetrating or nonpenetrating chest trauma and most commonly affect the descending thoracic aorta just beyond the site of insertion of the ligamentum arteriosum. Chronic aortic dissections are associated with weakening of the aortic wall that may lead to the development of aneurysmal dilatation.

THORACIC AORTIC ANEURYSMS

The clinical manifestations and natural history of thoracic aortic aneurysms depend on their location. Cystic medial necrosis is the most common cause of ascending aortic aneurysms, whereas atherosclerosis is the condition most frequently associated with aneurysms of the aortic arch and descending thoracic aorta. The average growth rate of thoracic aneurysms is 0.1–0.2 cm per year. Thoracic aortic aneurysms associated with Marfan syndrome or aortic dissection may expand at a greater rate. The risk of rupture is related to the size of the aneurysm and the presence of symptoms, ranging approximately from 2–3% per year for thoracic aortic aneurysms <4.0 cm in diameter to 7% per year for those >6 cm in diameter. Most thoracic aortic aneurysms are asymptomatic; however, compression or erosion of adjacent tissue by aneurysms may cause symptoms such as chest pain, shortness of breath, cough, hoarseness, or dysphagia. Aneurysmal dilatation of the ascending aorta may cause congestive heart failure as a consequence of aortic regurgitation, and marked compression of the superior vena cava may produce congestion of the head, neck, and upper extremities.

A chest x-ray may be the first test to suggest the diagnosis of a thoracic aortic aneurysm (**Fig. 38-1**). Findings include widening of the mediastinal shadow

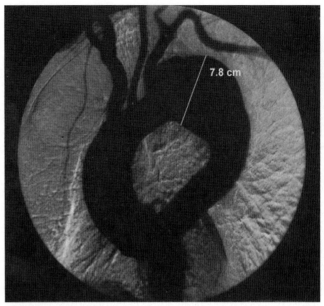

FIGURE 38-2
An aortogram demonstrating a large fusiform aneurysm of the descending thoracic aorta.

and displacement or compression of the trachea or left mainstem bronchus. Two-dimensional echocardiography, particularly transesophageal echocardiography, can be used to assess the proximal ascending aorta and descending thoracic aorta. Contrast-enhanced CT, MRI, and conventional invasive aortography are sensitive and specific tests for assessment of aneurysms of the thoracic aorta and involvement of branch vessels (**Fig. 38-2**). In asymptomatic patients whose aneurysms are too small to justify surgery, noninvasive testing with either contrast-enhanced CT or MRI should be performed at least every 6–12 months to monitor expansion.

℞ Treatment:
THORACIC AORTIC ANEURYSMS

Patients with thoracic aortic aneurysms, and particularly patients with Marfan syndrome who have evidence of aortic root dilatation, should receive long-term beta-blocker therapy. Additional medical therapy should be given, as necessary, to control hypertension. Operative repair with placement of a prosthetic graft is indicated in patients with symptomatic thoracic aortic aneurysms, and in those in whom the aortic diameter is >5.5–6 cm or has increased by >1 cm per year. In patients with Marfan syndrome or bicuspid aortic valve, thoracic aortic aneurysms >5 cm should be considered for surgery.

ABDOMINAL AORTIC ANEURYSMS

Abdominal aortic aneurysms occur more frequently in males than in females, and the incidence increases with age. Abdominal aortic aneurysms ≥4.0 cm may affect 1–2%

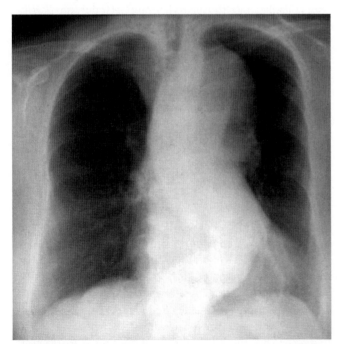

FIGURE 38-1
A chest x-ray of a patient with a thoracic aortic aneurysm.

of men older than 50 years. At least 90% of all abdominal aortic aneurysms >4.0 cm are related to atherosclerotic disease, and most of these aneurysms are below the level of the renal arteries. Prognosis is related to both the size of the aneurysm and the severity of coexisting coronary artery and cerebrovascular disease. The risk of rupture increases with the size of the aneurysm: the 5-year risk for aneurysms <5 cm is 1–2%, whereas it is 20–40% for aneurysms >5 cm in diameter. The formation of mural thrombi within aneurysms may predispose to peripheral embolization.

An abdominal aortic aneurysm commonly produces no symptoms. It is usually detected on routine examination as a palpable, pulsatile, expansile, and nontender mass, or it is an incidental finding during an abdominal x-ray or ultrasound study performed for other reasons. As abdominal aortic aneurysms expand, however, they may become painful. Some patients complain of strong pulsations in the abdomen; others experience pain in the chest, lower back, or scrotum. Aneurysmal pain is usually a harbinger of rupture and represents a medical emergency. More often, acute rupture occurs without any prior warning, and this complication is always life-threatening. Rarely, there is leakage of the aneurysm with severe pain and tenderness. Acute pain and hypotension occur with rupture of the aneurysm, which requires emergency operation.

Abdominal radiography may demonstrate the calcified outline of the aneurysm; however, about 25% of aneurysms are not calcified and cannot be visualized by plain x-ray. An abdominal ultrasound can delineate the transverse and longitudinal dimensions of an abdominal aortic aneurysm and may detect mural thrombus. Abdominal ultrasound is useful for serial documentation of aneurysm size and can be used to screen patients at risk for developing aortic aneurysm, such as those with affected siblings, peripheral atherosclerosis, or peripheral artery aneurysms. In one large study, ultrasound screening of men 65–74 years was associated with a risk reduction in aneurysm-related death by 42%. CT with contrast and MRI are accurate, noninvasive tests to determine the location and size of abdominal aortic aneurysms and to plan endovascular or open surgical repair (**Fig. 38-3**). Contrast aortography may be used for the evaluation of patients with aneurysms, but the procedure carries a small risk of complications, such as bleeding, allergic reactions, and atheroembolism. Since the presence of mural thrombi may reduce the luminal size, aortography may underestimate the diameter of an aneurysm.

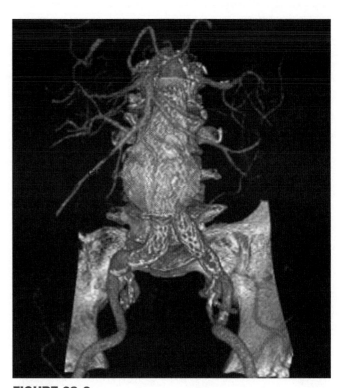

FIGURE 38-3

A computed tomographic angiogram (CTA) depicting a fusiform abdominal aortic aneurysm that has been treated with a bifurcated stent graft.

with symptoms. For asymptomatic aneurysms, operation is indicated if the diameter is >5.5 cm. In randomized trials of patients with abdominal aortic aneurysms <5.5 cm, there was no difference in the long-term (5- to 8-year) mortality rate between those followed with ultrasound surveillance and those undergoing elective aneurysm repair. Thus, serial noninvasive follow-up of smaller aneurysms (<5 cm) is an alternative to immediate surgery. Percutaneous placement of endovascular stent grafts (Fig. 38-3) for treatment of infrarenal abdominal aortic aneurysms is available for selected patients and is associated with lower short-term morbidity but comparable long-term mortality, compared with open surgical reconstruction.

In surgical candidates, careful preoperative cardiac and general medical evaluations (followed by appropriate therapy of complicating conditions) are essential. Preexisting coronary artery disease, congestive heart failure, pulmonary disease, diabetes, and advanced age add to the risk of surgery. β-adrenergic blockers decrease perioperative cardiovascular morbidity and mortality. With careful preoperative cardiac evaluation and postoperative care, the operative mortality rate approximates 1–2%. After acute rupture, the mortality rate of emergent operation is 45–50%. Endovascular repair with stent placement is an emerging approach but, at the current time, is associated with a mortality rate of approximately 40%.

℞ Treatment:
ABDOMINAL AORTIC ANEURYSMS

Operative repair of the aneurysm and insertion of a prosthetic graft are indicated for abdominal aortic aneurysms of any size that are expanding rapidly or are associated

ACUTE AORTIC SYNDROMES

The four major acute aortic syndromes include aortic rupture (discussed earlier), aortic dissection, intramural hematoma, and penetrating atherosclerotic ulcer. Aortic dissection is caused by a circumferential or, less frequently, transverse tear of the intima. It often occurs along the right lateral wall of the ascending aorta where the hydraulic shear stress is high. Another common site is the descending thoracic aorta just below the ligamentum arteriosum. The initiating event is either a primary intimal tear with secondary dissection into the media or a medial hemorrhage that dissects into and disrupts the intima. The pulsatile aortic flow then dissects along the elastic lamellar plates of the aorta and creates a false lumen. The dissection usually propagates distally down the descending aorta and into its major branches, but it may also propagate proximally. Distal propagation may be limited by atherosclerotic plaque. In some cases, a secondary distal intimal disruption occurs, resulting in the reentry of blood from the false to the true lumen.

There are at least two important pathologic and radiologic variants of aortic dissection: intramural hematoma without an intimal flap and penetrating atherosclerotic ulcer. Acute intramural hematoma is thought to result from rupture of the vasa vasorum with hemorrhage into the wall of the aorta. Most occur in the descending thoracic aorta. Acute intramural hematomas may progress to dissection and rupture. Penetrating atherosclerotic ulcers are caused by erosion of a plaque into the aortic media, are usually localized, and are not associated with extensive propagation. They are found primarily in the mid and distal portions of the descending thoracic aorta and are associated with extensive atherosclerotic disease. The ulcer can erode beyond the internal elastic lamina, leading to medial hematoma, and may progress to false aneurysm formation or rupture.

Several classification schemes have been developed for thoracic aortic dissections. DeBakey and colleagues initially classified aortic dissections as type I, in which an intimal tear occurs in the ascending aorta but involves the descending aorta as well; type II, in which the dissection is limited to the ascending aorta; and type III, in which the intimal tear is located in the descending aorta with distal propagation of the dissection (Fig. 38-4). Another classification (Stanford) is that of type A, in which the dissection involves the ascending aorta (proximal dissection), and type B, in which it is limited to the descending aorta (distal dissection). From a management standpoint, classification of aortic dissections and intramural hematomas into type A or B is more practical and useful, since DeBakey types I and II are managed in a similar manner.

The factors that predispose to aortic dissection include systemic hypertension, a coexisting condition in 70% of

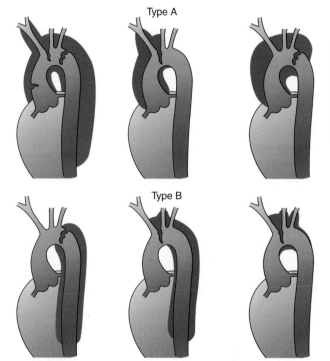

Type A

Type B

FIGURE 38-4

Classification of aortic dissections. Stanford classification: Type A dissections (*top panels*) involve the ascending aorta independent of site of tear and distal extension; type B dissections (*bottom panels*) involve transverse and/or descending aorta without involvement of the ascending aorta. DeBakey classification: Type I dissection involves ascending to descending aorta (*top left*); type II dissection is limited to ascending or transverse aorta, without descending aorta (*top center + top right*); type III dissection involves descending aorta only (*bottom left*). [From DC Miller, in RM Doroghazi, EE Slater (eds): Aortic Dissection. New York, McGraw-Hill, 1983, with permission.]

patients, and cystic medial necrosis. Aortic dissection is the major cause of morbidity and mortality in patients with Marfan syndrome and similarly may affect patients with Ehlers-Danlos syndrome. The incidence is also increased in patients with inflammatory aortitis (i.e., Takayasu's arteritis, giant cell arteritis), congenital aortic valve anomalies (e.g., bicuspid valve), coarctation of the aorta, and a history of aortic trauma. In addition, the risk of dissection is increased in otherwise normal women during the third trimester of pregnancy.

CLINICAL MANIFESTATIONS

The peak incidence of aortic dissection is in the sixth and seventh decades. Men are more affected than women by a ratio of 2:1. The presentations of aortic dissection and its variants are the consequences of intimal tear, dissecting hematoma, occlusion of involved arteries, and compression of adjacent tissues. Acute aortic dissection presents with the sudden onset of pain (Chap. 4), which is often described as very severe and tearing and is associated with diaphoresis. The pain may be localized to the front or back of the chest, often the interscapular region, and typically migrates with propagation of the dissection. Other symptoms include syncope, dyspnea, and weakness. Physical findings may include hypertension or hypotension, loss of pulses, aortic regurgitation, pulmonary edema, and neurologic findings due to carotid artery obstruction (hemiplegia, hemianesthesia) or spinal cord ischemia (paraplegia). Bowel ischemia, hematuria, and myocardial ischemia have all been observed. These clinical manifestations reflect complications resulting from the dissection occluding the major arteries. Furthermore, clinical manifestations may result from the compression of adjacent structures (e.g., superior cervical ganglia, superior vena cava, bronchus, esophagus) by the expanding dissection causing aneurysmal dilatation, and include Horner's syndrome, superior vena cava syndrome, hoarseness, dysphagia, and airway compromise. Hemopericardium and cardiac tamponade may complicate a type A lesion with retrograde dissection. Acute aortic regurgitation is an important and common (>50%) complication of proximal dissection. It is the outcome of either a circumferential tear that widens the aortic root or a disruption of the annulus by dissecting hematoma that tears a leaflet(s) or displaces it, inferior to the line of closure. Signs of aortic regurgitation include bounding pulses, a wide pulse pressure, a diastolic murmur often radiating along the right sternal border, and evidence of congestive heart failure. The clinical manifestations depend on the severity of the regurgitation.

In dissections involving the ascending aorta, the chest x-ray often reveals a widened superior mediastinum. A pleural effusion (usually left-sided) also may be present. This effusion is typically serosanguineous and not indicative of rupture unless accompanied by hypotension and falling hematocrit. In dissections of the descending thoracic aorta, a widened mediastinum may also be observed on chest x-ray. In addition, the descending aorta may appear to be wider than the ascending portion. An electrocardiogram that shows no evidence of myocardial ischemia is helpful in distinguishing aortic dissection from myocardial infarction. Rarely, the dissection involves the right or, less commonly, left coronary ostium and causes acute myocardial infarction.

The diagnosis of aortic dissection can be established by noninvasive techniques such as echocardiography, CT, or MRI. Aortography is used less commonly because of the accuracy of these noninvasive techniques. Transthoracic echocardiography can be performed simply and rapidly and has an overall sensitivity of 60–85% for aortic dissection. For diagnosing proximal ascending aortic dissections, its sensitivity exceeds 80%; it is less useful for detecting dissection of the arch and descending thoracic aorta. Transesophageal echocardiography requires greater skill and patient cooperation but is very accurate in identifying dissections of the ascending and descending thoracic aorta, but not the arch, achieving 98% sensitivity and approximately 90% specificity. Echocardiography also provides important information regarding the presence and severity of aortic regurgitation and pericardial effusion. CT and MRI are both highly accurate in identifying the intimal flap and the extent of the dissection and involvement of major arteries; each has a sensitivity and specificity >90%. They are useful in recognizing intramural hemorrhage and penetrating ulcers. MRI can also detect blood flow, which may be useful in characterizing antegrade versus retrograde dissection. The relative utility of transesophageal echocardiography, CT, and MRI depends on the availability and expertise in individual institutions as well as on the hemodynamic stability of the patient, with CT and MRI obviously less suitable for unstable patients.

℞ Treatment: AORTIC DISSECTION

Medical therapy should be initiated as soon as the diagnosis is considered. The patient should be admitted to an intensive care unit for hemodynamic monitoring. Unless hypotension is present, therapy should be aimed at reducing cardiac contractility and systemic arterial pressure, and thereby shear stress. For acute dissection, unless contraindicated, β-adrenergic blockers should be administered parenterally, using intravenous propranolol, metoprolol, or the short-acting esmolol to achieve a heart rate of ~ 60 beats/min. This should be accompanied by sodium nitroprusside infusion to lower systolic blood pressure to ≤120 mmHg. Labetalol (Chap. 38), a drug with both β- and α-adrenergic blocking properties, may also be used as a parenteral agent in the acute therapy of dissection.

The calcium channel antagonists verapamil and diltiazem may be used intravenously if nitroprusside or β-adrenergic blockers cannot be employed. The addition of a parenteral angiotensin-converting enzyme (ACE) inhibitor, such as enalaprilat, to a β-adrenergic blocker also may be considered. Isolated use of direct vasodilators, such as diazoxide and hydralazine, is contraindicated because these agents can increase hydraulic shear and may propagate dissection.

Emergent or urgent surgical correction is the preferred treatment for acute ascending aortic dissections and intramural hematomas (type A) and for complicated type B dissections, including those characterized by propagation, compromise of major aortic branches, impending rupture, or continued pain. Surgery involves excision of the intimal flap, obliteration of the false lumen, and placement of an interposition graft. A composite valve-graft conduit is used if the aortic valve is disrupted. The overall in-hospital mortality rate after surgical treatment of patients with aortic dissection is reported to be 15–25%. The major causes of perioperative mortality and morbidity include myocardial infarction, paraplegia, renal failure, tamponade, hemorrhage, and sepsis. Reports of the use of endoluminal stent grafts in selected patients with type B dissection are encouraging. Other transcatheter techniques, such as fenestration of the intimal flaps and stenting of narrowed branch vessels to increase flow to compromised organs, are investigational approaches used in selected patients. For uncomplicated and stable distal dissections and intramural hematomas (type B), medical therapy is the preferred treatment. The in-hospital mortality rate of medically treated patients with type B dissection is 10–20%. Long-term therapy for patients with aortic dissection and intramural hematomas (with or without surgery) consists of the control of hypertension and reduction of cardiac contractility with the use of beta blockers plus other antihypertensive agents, such as ACE inhibitors or calcium antagonists. Patients with chronic type B dissection and intramural hematomas should be followed on an outpatient basis every 6–12 months by contrast-enhanced CT or MRI to detect propagation or expansion. Patients with Marfan syndrome are at high risk for postdissection complications. The long-term prognosis for patients with treated dissections is generally good with careful follow-up; the 10-year survival rate is ~60%.

AORTIC OCCLUSION

CHRONIC ATHEROSCLEROTIC OCCLUSIVE DISEASE

Atherosclerosis may affect the thoracic and abdominal aorta. Occlusive aortic disease caused by atherosclerosis is usually confined to the distal abdominal aorta below the renal arteries. Frequently the disease extends to the iliac arteries (Chap. 39). Claudication characteristically involves the buttocks, thighs, and calves and may be associated with impotence in males (Leriche syndrome). The severity of the symptoms depends on the adequacy of collaterals. With sufficient collateral blood flow, a complete occlusion of the abdominal aorta may occur without the development of ischemic symptoms. The physical findings include absence of femoral and other distal pulses bilaterally, and the detection of an audible bruit over the abdomen (usually at or below the umbilicus) and the common femoral arteries. Atrophic skin, loss of hair, and coolness of the lower extremities are usually observed. In advanced ischemia, rubor on dependency and pallor on elevation can be seen.

The diagnosis is usually established by physical examination and noninvasive testing, including leg pressure measurements, Doppler velocity analysis, pulse volume recordings, and duplex ultrasonography. The anatomy may be defined by MRI, CT, or conventional aortography, typically performed when considering revascularization. Catheter-based endovascular or operative treatment is indicated in patients with lifestyle-limiting or debilitating symptoms of claudication and in patients with critical limb ischemia.

ACUTE OCCLUSION

Acute occlusion in the distal abdominal aorta constitutes a medical emergency because it threatens the viability of the lower extremities; it usually results from an occlusive embolus that almost always originates from the heart. Rarely, acute occlusion may occur as the result of in situ thrombosis in a preexisting severely narrowed segment of the aorta.

The clinical picture is one of acute ischemia of the lower extremities. Severe rest pain, coolness, and pallor of the lower extremities and the absence of distal pulses bilaterally are the usual manifestations. Diagnosis should be established rapidly by MRI, CT, or aortography. Emergency thrombectomy or revascularization is indicated.

AORTITIS

Aortitis, a term referring to inflammatory disease of the aorta, may be caused by large vessel vasculitides such as Takayasu's arteritis and giant cell arteritis, rheumatic and HLA-B27–associated spondyloarthropathies, Behçet's syndrome, ANCA-associated vasculitides, Cogan's syndrome, and infections, such as syphilis, tuberculosis, and *Salmonella*, or may be associated with retroperitoneal fibrosis. Aortitis may result in aneurysmal dilatation and aortic regurgitation, occlusion of the aorta and its branch vessels, or acute aortic syndromes.

TAKAYASU'S ARTERITIS

This inflammatory disease often affects the ascending aorta and aortic arch, causing obstruction of the aorta and its major arteries. Takayasu's arteritis is also termed *pulseless disease* because of the frequent occlusion of the large arteries originating from the aorta. It may also involve the descending thoracic and abdominal aorta and occlude large branches such as the renal arteries. Aortic aneurysms may also occur. The pathology is a panarteritis, characterized by mononuclear cells and occasionally giant cells, with marked intimal hyperplasia, medial and adventitial thickening, and, in the chronic form, fibrotic occlusion. The disease is most prevalent in young females of Asian descent but does occur in women of other geographic and ethnic origins and also in young men. During the acute stage, fever, malaise, weight loss, and other systemic symptoms may be evident. Elevations of the erythrocyte sedimentation rate and C-reactive protein are common. The chronic stages of the disease, which is intermittently active, present with symptoms related to large artery occlusion, such as upper extremity claudication, cerebral ischemia, and syncope. Since the process is progressive and there is no definitive therapy, the prognosis is usually poor. Glucocorticoids and immunosuppressive agents have been reported to be effective in some patients during the acute phase. Surgical bypass or endovascular intervention of a critically stenotic artery may be necessary.

GIANT CELL ARTERITIS

This vasculitis occurs in older individuals and affects women more often than men. Primarily large and medium-sized arteries are affected. The pathology is that of focal granulomatous lesions involving the entire arterial wall; it may be associated with polymyalgia rheumatica. Obstruction of medium-sized arteries (e.g., temporal and ophthalmic arteries) and of major branches of the aorta and the development of aortitis and aortic regurgitation are important complications of the disease. High-dose glucocorticoid therapy may be effective when given early.

RHEUMATIC AORTITIS

Rheumatoid arthritis, ankylosing spondylitis, psoriatic arthritis, Reiter's syndrome, relapsing polychondritis, and inflammatory bowel disorders may all be associated with aortitis involving the ascending aorta. The inflammatory lesions usually involve the ascending aorta and may extend to the sinuses of Valsalva, the mitral valve leaflets, and adjacent myocardium. The clinical manifestations are aneurysm, aortic regurgitation, and involvement of the cardiac conduction system.

SYPHILITIC INFECTIVE AORTITIS

Infective aortitis may result from direct invasion of the aortic wall by bacterial pathogens, such as *Staphylococcus*, *Streptococcus*, and *Salmonella*, or by fungi. These bacteria cause aortitis by infecting the aorta at sites of atherosclerotic plaque. Bacterial proteases lead to degradation of collagen, and the ensuing destruction of the aortic wall leads to formation of a saccular aneurysm, referred to as a mycotic aneurysm. Mycotic aneurysms have a predilection for the suprarenal abdominal aorta. The pathologic characteristics of the aortic wall include acute and chronic inflammation, abscesses, hemorrhage, and necrosis. Mycotic aneurysms typically affect the elderly and occur in men three times more frequently than in women. Patients may present with fever, sepsis, and chest, back, or abdominal pain; there may have been a preceding diarrheal illness. Blood cultures are positive in the majority of patients. Both CT and MRI are useful to diagnose mycotic aneurysms. Treatment includes antibiotic therapy and surgical removal of the affected part of the aorta, and revascularization of the lower extremities with grafts placed in uninfected tissue.

Syphilitic aortitis is a late manifestation of luetic infection that usually affects the proximal ascending aorta, particularly the aortic root, resulting in aortic dilatation and aneurysm formation. Syphilitic aortitis may occasionally involve the aortic arch or the descending aorta. The aneurysms may be saccular or fusiform and are usually asymptomatic, but compression of and erosion into adjacent structures may result in symptoms; rupture may also occur.

The initial lesion is an obliterative endarteritis of the vasa vasorum, especially in the adventitia. This is an inflammatory response to the invasion of the adventitia by the spirochetes. Destruction of the aortic media occurs as the spirochetes spread into this layer, usually via the lymphatics accompanying the vasa vasorum. Destruction of collagen and elastic tissues leads to dilation of the aorta, scar formation, and calcification. These changes account for the characteristic radiographic appearance of linear calcification of the ascending aorta.

The disease typically presents as an incidental chest radiographic finding 15–30 years after initial infection. Symptoms may result from aortic regurgitation, narrowing of coronary ostia due to syphilitic aortitis, compression of adjacent structures (e.g., esophagus), or rupture. Diagnosis is established by a positive serologic test, i.e., rapid plasmin reagin (RPR) or fluorescent treponemal antibody. Treatment includes penicillin and surgical excision and repair.

FURTHER READINGS

ASHTON HA et al: The Multicentre Aneurysm Screening Study (MASS) into the effect of abdominal aortic aneurysm screening on mortality in men: A randomized controlled trial. The Multicentre Aneurysm Screening Study Group. Lancet 360:1531, 2002

BARIL DT et al: Surgery insight: Advances in endovascular repair of abdominal aortic aneurysm. Nat Clin Pract Cardiovasc Med 4:206, 2007

BLANKENSTEIJN JD et al: Two-year outcomes after conventional or endovascular repair of abdominal aortic aneurysms. N Engl J Med 352:2398, 2005

BROOK BS et al: Angiotensin II blockade and aortic-root dilation in Marfan's syndrome. N Engl J Med 358: 2787, 2008

CREAGER MA et al (eds): *Vascular Medicine: A Companion to Braunwald's Heart Disease*. 1st ed. Philadelphia, Saunders, 2006

FLEMING C et al: Screening for abdominal aortic aneurysm: A best-evidence systematic review for the U.S. Preventive Services Task Force. Ann Intern Med 142:203, 2005

GOLLEDGE J, EAGLE KA: Acute aortic dissection. Lancet 372:55, 2008

GORNIK HL, CREAGER MA: Diseases of the Aorta, in E. Topol (ed) Textbook of Cardiovascular Medicine, 3d ed., Philadelphia, Lippincott, Williams & Wilkins, 2007

GORNIK HL, CREAGER MA: Aortitis. Circulation 117:3039, 2008

GRECO C et al: Outcomes of endovascular treatment of ruptured abdominal aortic aneurysms. J Vasc Surg 43:453, 2006

HAGAN PG et al: The International Registry of Acute Aortic Dissection (IRAD): New insights into an old disease. JAMA 283:897, 2000

HIRSCH AT et al: ACC/AHA 2005 Practice Guidelines for the management of patients with peripheral arterial disease (lower extremity, renal, mesenteric, and abdominal aortic). Circulation 113:e463, 2006

ISSELBACHER EM: Thoracic and abdominal aortic aneurysms. Circulation 111:816, 2005

LEDERLE FA et al: Immediate repair compared with surveillance of small abdominal aortic aneurysms. The Aneurysm Detection and Management Veterans Affairs Cooperative Study Group. N Engl J Med 346:1437, 2002

LEDERLE FA et al: Systematic review: repair of unruptured abdominal aortic aneurysm. Ann Intern Med 146:735, 2007

PATEL HJ, DEEB GM: Ascending and arch aorta: pathology, natural history, and treatment. Circulation 118:188, 2008

SCHERMERHORN ML et al: Endovascular vs. open repair of abdominal aortic aneurysms in the Medicare population. N Engl J Med 358:464, 2008

UNITED KINGDOM SMALL ANEURYSM TRIAL PARTICIPANTS: Long-term outcomes of immediate repair compared with surveillance of small abdominal aortic aneurysms. N Engl J Med 346:1445, 2002

TSAI TT et al: Acute aortic syndromes. Circulation 112:3802, 2005

CHAPTER 39

VASCULAR DISEASES OF THE EXTREMITIES

Mark A. Creager ■ Joseph Loscalzo

ARTERIAL DISORDERS

PERIPHERAL ARTERIAL DISEASE

Peripheral arterial disease (PAD) is defined as a clinical disorder in which there is a stenosis or occlusion in the aorta or arteries of the limbs. Atherosclerosis is the leading cause of PAD in patients >40 years. Other causes include thrombosis, embolism, vasculitis, fibromuscular dysplasia, entrapment, cystic adventitial disease, and trauma. The highest prevalence of atherosclerotic PAD occurs in the sixth and seventh decades of life. As in patients with atherosclerosis of the coronary and cerebral vasculature, there is an increased risk of developing PAD in cigarette smokers and in persons with diabetes mellitus, hypercholesterolemia, hypertension, or hyperhomocysteinemia.

Pathology

(See also Chap. 30) Segmental lesions causing stenosis or occlusion are usually localized to large- and medium-sized vessels. The pathology of the lesions includes atherosclerotic plaques with calcium deposition, thinning of the media, patchy destruction of muscle and elastic fibers, fragmentation of the internal elastic lamina, and thrombi composed of platelets and fibrin. The primary sites of involvement are the abdominal aorta and iliac arteries (30% of symptomatic patients), the femoral and popliteal arteries (80–90% of patients), and the more distal vessels, including the tibial and peroneal arteries (40–50% of patients). Atherosclerotic lesions occur preferentially at arterial branch points, sites of increased turbulence, altered shear stress, and intimal injury. Involvement of the distal vasculature is most common in elderly individuals and patients with diabetes mellitus.

Clinical Evaluation

Less than 50% of patients with PAD are symptomatic, although many have a slow or impaired gait. The most common *symptom* is intermittent claudication, which is defined as a pain, ache, cramp, numbness, or a sense of fatigue in the muscles; it occurs during exercise and is relieved by rest. The site of claudication is distal to the location of the occlusive lesion. For example, buttock, hip, and thigh discomfort occur in patients with aortoiliac disease, whereas calf claudication develops in patients with femoral-popliteal disease. Symptoms are far more common in the lower than in the upper extremities because of the higher incidence of obstructive lesions in the former region. In patients with severe arterial occlusive disease in whom resting blood flow cannot accommodate basal nutritional needs of the tissues, critical limb ischemia may develop. Patients will complain of rest pain or a feeling of cold or numbness in the foot and toes. Frequently, these symptoms occur at night when the legs are horizontal and improve when the legs are in a dependent position. With severe ischemia, rest pain may be persistent.

Important *physical findings* of PAD include decreased or absent pulses distal to the obstruction, the presence of bruits over the narrowed artery, and muscle atrophy. With more severe disease, hair loss, thickened nails, smooth and shiny skin, reduced skin temperature, and pallor or cyanosis are frequent physical signs. In patients with critical limb ischemia, ulcers or gangrene may occur. Elevation of the legs and repeated flexing of the calf muscles produce pallor of the soles of the feet, whereas rubor, secondary to reactive hyperemia, may develop when the legs are dependent. The time required for rubor to develop or for the veins in the foot to fill when the patient's legs are transferred from an elevated to a dependent position is related to the severity of the ischemia and the presence of collateral vessels. Patients with severe ischemia may develop peripheral edema because they keep their legs in a dependent position much of the time. Ischemic neuropathy can result in numbness and hyporeflexia.

Noninvasive Testing

The history and physical examination are often sufficient to establish the diagnosis of PAD. An objective assessment of the presence and severity of disease is obtained by noninvasive techniques. Arterial pressure can be recorded noninvasively in the legs by placement of sphygmomanometric cuffs at the ankles and use of a Doppler device to auscultate or record blood flow from the dorsalis pedis and posterior tibial arteries. Normally, systolic blood pressure in the legs and arms is similar. Indeed, ankle pressure may be slightly higher than arm pressure due to pulse-wave amplification. In the presence of hemodynamically significant stenoses, the systolic blood pressure in the leg is decreased. Thus, the ratio of the ankle and brachial artery pressures [termed the *ankle/brachial index* (ABI)] is ≥1.0 in normal individuals and <1.0 in patients with peripheral arterial disease; a ratio of <0.5 is consistent with severe ischemia.

Other noninvasive tests include segmental pressure measurements, pulse volume recordings, Doppler flow velocity waveform analysis, duplex ultrasonography (which combines B-mode imaging and pulse-wave Doppler examination), transcutaneous oximetry, and stress testing (usually using a treadmill). Placement of pneumatic cuffs enables assessment of systolic pressure along the legs. The presence of pressure gradients between sequential cuffs provides evidence of the presence and location of hemodynamically significant stenoses. Also, the volume displacement in the leg is decreased with each pulse, and the Doppler velocity contour becomes progressively blunted in the presence of significant PAD. Duplex ultrasonography is used to image and detect stenotic lesions in native arteries and bypass grafts.

Treadmill testing allows the physician to assess functional limitations objectively. Decline of the ABI immediately after exercise provides further support for the diagnosis of PAD in patients with equivocal symptoms and findings on examination.

Magnetic resonance angiography (MRA), computed tomographic angiography (CTA), and conventional contrast angiography should not be used for routine diagnostic testing but are performed prior to potential revascularization. Each test is useful in defining the anatomy to assist planning for catheter-based and surgical revascularization procedures.

Prognosis

The natural history of patients with PAD is influenced primarily by the extent of coexisting coronary artery and cerebrovascular disease. Approximately one-third to one-half of patients with symptomatic PAD have evidence of coronary artery disease based on clinical presentation and electrocardiogram, and over one-half have significant coronary artery disease by coronary angiography. Patients with PAD have a 15–30% 5-year mortality rate and a two- to sixfold increased risk of death from coronary heart disease. Mortality is highest in those with the most severe PAD. The likelihood of symptomatic progression of PAD appears less than the chance of succumbing to coronary artery disease. Approximately 75–80% of nondiabetic patients who present with mild to moderate claudication remain symptomatically stable. Deterioration is likely to occur in the remainder, with ~1–2% of the group ultimately developing critical limb ischemia. Approximately 25–30% of patients with critical limb ischemia survive and undergo amputation within 1 year. The prognosis is worse in patients who continue to smoke cigarettes or who have diabetes mellitus.

℞ **Treatment:**
PERIPHERAL ARTERIAL DISEASE

Patients with PAD should receive therapies to reduce the risk of associated cardiovascular events, such as myocardial infarction (MI) and death, and to improve limb symptoms, prevent progression to critical limb ischemia, and preserve limb viability. Risk factor modification and antiplatelet therapy should be initiated to improve cardiovascular outcomes. The importance of discontinuing cigarette smoking cannot be overemphasized. The physician must assume a major role in this lifestyle modification. Counseling and adjunctive drug therapy with the nicotine patch, bupropion, or varenicline increase smoking cessation rates and reduce recidivism. It is important to control blood pressure in hypertensive patients. Angiotensin-converting enzyme inhibitors may reduce the risk of cardiovascular events in patients with symptomatic PAD. β-Adrenergic blockers do not worsen claudication and may be used to treat hypertension, especially in patients with coexistent coronary artery disease. Treatment of hypercholesterolemia with statins is advocated to reduce the risk of MI, stroke and death. The National Cholesterol Education Program Adult Treatment Panel considers PAD to be a coronary heart disease equivalent and recommends treatment to reduce LDL cholesterol to <100 mg/dL. Platelet inhibitors, particularly aspirin, reduce the risk of adverse cardiovascular events in patients with peripheral atherosclerosis. Clopidogrel, a drug that inhibits platelet aggregation via its effect on adenosine diphosphate–dependent platelet-fibrinogen binding, appears to be more effective than aspirin in reducing cardiovascular morbidity and mortality in patients with PAD. There is insufficient evidence of efficacy to support the routine use of dual antiplatelet therapy with both aspirin and clopidogrel in patients with PAD. The anticoagulant warfarin is not indicated to improve outcome in patients with chronic PAD.

Therapies for intermittent claudication and critical limb ischemia include supportive measures, medications, nonoperative interventions, and surgery. Supportive measures include meticulous care of the feet, which should be kept clean and protected against excessive drying with moisturizing creams. Well-fitting and protective shoes are advised to reduce trauma. Elastic support hose should be avoided, as they reduce blood flow to the skin. In patients with critical limb ischemia, shock blocks under the head of the bed together with a canopy over the feet may improve perfusion pressure and ameliorate some of the rest pain.

Patients with claudication should be encouraged to exercise regularly and at progressively more strenuous levels. Supervised exercise training programs for 30–45 min sessions, three to five times per week for at least 12 weeks, prolong walking distance. Patients also should be advised to walk until near-maximum claudication discomfort occurs, then resting until the symptoms resolve before resuming ambulation. Pharmacologic treatment of PAD has not been as successful as the medical treatment of coronary artery disease (Chap. 33). In particular, vasodilators as a class have not proved to be beneficial. During exercise, peripheral vasodilation occurs distal to sites of significant arterial stenoses. As a result, perfusion pressure falls, often to levels less than that generated in the interstitial tissue by the exercising muscle. Drugs such as α-adrenergic blocking agents, calcium channel antagonists, papaverine, and other vasodilators have not been shown to be effective in patients with PAD.

Cilostazol, a phosphodiesterase inhibitor with vasodilator and antiplatelet properties, increases claudication distance by 40–60% and improves measures of quality of life. The mechanism of action accounting for its beneficial effects is not known. Pentoxifylline, a substituted xanthine derivative, has been reported to decrease blood viscosity and to increase red cell flexibility, thereby increasing blood flow to the microcirculation and enhancing tissue oxygenation. Although several placebo-controlled studies have found that pentoxifylline increases the duration of exercise in patients with claudication, its efficacy has not been confirmed in all clinical trials. Statins and propionyl-L-carnitine, a drug that affects skeletal muscle metabolic function, appear promising for treatment of intermittent claudication in initial clinical trials.

Several studies have suggested that long-term parenteral administration of vasodilator prostaglandins decreases pain and facilitates healing of ulcers in patients with critical limb ischemia. Clinical trials of angiogenic growth factors are proceeding. Intramuscular gene transfer of DNA encoding vascular endothelial growth factor, basic fibroblast growth factor, hepatocyte growth factor, or hypoxia-inducible factor-1α, and also administration of endothelial progenitor cells, may promote collateral blood vessel growth in patients with critical limb ischemia. Some trial results have been negative and others encouraging. The outcome of ongoing studies will further elucidate the potential role of therapeutic angiogenesis for PAD.

REVASCULARIZATION Revascularization procedures, including catheter-based and surgical interventions, are usually indicated for patients with disabling, progressive, or severe symptoms of intermittent claudication despite medical therapy, and for those with critical limb ischemia. MRA, CTA, or conventional contrast angiography should be performed to assess vascular anatomy in patients who are being considered for revascularization. Nonoperative interventions include percutaneous transluminal angiography (PTA), stent placement, and atherectomy (Chap. 36). PTA and stenting of the iliac artery are associated with higher success rates than PTA and stenting of the femoral and popliteal arteries. Approximately 90–95% of iliac PTAs are initially successful, and the 3-year patency rate is >75%. Patency rates may be higher if a stent is placed in the iliac artery. The initial success rates for femoral-popliteal PTA and stenting are ~80%, with 60% 3-year patency rates. Patency rates are influenced by the severity of pretreatment stenoses; the prognosis of occlusive lesions is worse than that of nonocclusive stenotic lesions. The role of drug-eluting stents in PAD is currently unclear.

Several operative procedures are available for treating patients with aortoiliac and femoral-popliteal artery disease. The preferred operative procedure depends on the location and extent of the obstruction(s) and general medical condition of the patient. Operative procedures for aortoiliac disease include aortobifemoral bypass, axillofemoral bypass, femoral-femoral bypass, and aortoiliac endarterectomy. The most frequently used procedure is the aortobifemoral bypass using knitted Dacron grafts. Immediate graft patency approaches 99%, and 5- and 10-year graft patency in survivors is >90% and 80%, respectively. Operative complications include MI and stroke, infection of the graft, peripheral embolization, and sexual dysfunction from interruption of autonomic nerves in the pelvis. Operative mortality ranges from 1–3%, mostly due to ischemic heart disease.

Operative therapy for femoral-popliteal artery disease includes in situ and reverse autogenous saphenous vein bypass grafts, placement of polytetrafluoroethylene (PTFE) or other synthetic grafts, and thromboendarterectomy. Operative mortality ranges from 1–3%. The long-term patency rate depends on the type of graft used, the location of the distal anastomosis, and the patency of runoff vessels beyond the anastomosis. Patency rates of femoral-popliteal saphenous vein bypass grafts approach 90% at 1 year and 70–80% at 5 years. Five-year patency rates of infrapopliteal saphenous vein bypass grafts are 60–70%. In contrast, 5-year patency rates of infrapopliteal PTFE grafts are <30%. Lumbar sympathectomy alone or as an adjunct to aortofemoral reconstruction has fallen into disfavor.

Preoperative cardiac risk assessment may identify individuals especially likely to experience an adverse cardiac event during the perioperative period. Patients with angina, prior MI, ventricular ectopy, heart failure, or diabetes are among those at increased risk. Noninvasive tests, such as treadmill testing (if feasible), dipyridamole or adenosine radionuclide myocardial perfusion imaging, dobutamine echocardiography, and ambulatory ischemia monitoring permit further stratification of patient risk (Chap. 36). Patients with abnormal test results require close supervision and adjunctive management with anti-ischemic medications. β-Adrenergic blockers reduce the risk of postoperative cardiovascular complications. Coronary angiography and coronary artery revascularization are not indicated in most patients undergoing peripheral vascular surgery, but cardiac catheterization should be considered in patients with unstable angina and angina refractory to medical therapy, as well as those suspected of having left main or three-vessel coronary artery disease.

FIBROMUSCULAR DYSPLASIA

This is a hyperplastic disorder affecting medium-sized and small arteries. It occurs predominantly in women and usually involves renal and carotid arteries but can affect extremity vessels, such as the iliac and subclavian arteries. The histologic classification includes intimal fibroplasia, medial dysplasia, and adventitial hyperplasia. Medial dysplasia is subdivided into medial fibroplasia, perimedial fibroplasia, and medial hyperplasia. Medial fibroplasia is the most common type and is characterized by alternating

areas of thinned media and fibromuscular ridges. The internal elastic lamina is usually preserved. The iliac arteries are the limb arteries most likely to be affected by fibromuscular dysplasia. It is identified angiographically by a "string of beads" appearance caused by thickened fibromuscular ridges contiguous with thin, less-involved portions of the arterial wall. When limb vessels are involved, clinical manifestations are similar to those for atherosclerosis, including claudication and rest pain. PTA and surgical reconstruction have been beneficial in patients with debilitating symptoms or threatened limbs.

THROMBOANGIITIS OBLITERANS

Thromboangiitis obliterans (Buerger's disease) is an inflammatory occlusive vascular disorder involving small and medium-sized arteries and veins in the distal upper and lower extremities. Cerebral, visceral, and coronary vessels may be affected rarely. This disorder develops most frequently in men <40 years. The prevalence is higher in Asians and individuals of eastern European descent. While the cause of thromboangiitis obliterans is not known, there is a definite relationship to cigarette smoking in patients with this disorder.

In the initial stages of thromboangiitis obliterans, polymorphonuclear leukocytes infiltrate the walls of the small and medium-sized arteries and veins. The internal elastic lamina is preserved, and a cellular, inflammatory, thrombus develops in the vascular lumen. As the disease progresses, mononuclear cells, fibroblasts, and giant cells replace the neutrophils. Later stages are characterized by perivascular fibrosis, organized thrombus, and recanalization.

The clinical features of thromboangiitis obliterans often include a triad of claudication of the affected extremity, Raynaud's phenomenon, and migratory superficial vein thrombophlebitis. Claudication is usually confined to the calves and feet or the forearms and hands because this disorder primarily affects distal vessels. In the presence of severe digital ischemia, trophic nail changes, painful ulcerations, and gangrene may develop at the tips of the fingers or toes. The physical examination shows normal brachial and popliteal pulses but reduced or absent radial, ulnar, and/or tibial pulses. Arteriography is helpful in making the diagnosis. Smooth, tapering segmental lesions in the distal vessels are characteristic, as are collateral vessels at sites of vascular occlusion. Proximal atherosclerotic disease is usually absent. The diagnosis can be confirmed by excisional biopsy and pathologic examination of an involved vessel.

There is no specific treatment except abstention from tobacco. The prognosis is worse in individuals who continue to smoke, but results are discouraging even in those who do stop smoking. Arterial bypass of the larger vessels may be used in selected instances, as well as local debridement, depending on the symptoms and severity of ischemia. Antibiotics may be useful; anticoagulants and glucocorticoids are not helpful. If these measures fail, amputation may be required.

VASCULITIS

Other vasculitides may affect the arteries supplying the upper and lower extremities.

ACUTE ARTERIAL OCCLUSION

This results in the sudden cessation of blood flow to an extremity. The severity of ischemia and the viability of the extremity depend on the location and extent of the occlusion and the presence and subsequent development of collateral blood vessels. There are two principal causes of acute arterial occlusion: embolism and thrombus in situ.

The most common sources of arterial emboli are the heart, aorta, and large arteries. Cardiac disorders that cause thromboembolism include atrial fibrillation, both chronic and paroxysmal; acute MI; ventricular aneurysm; cardiomyopathy; infectious and marantic endocarditis; thrombi associated with prosthetic heart valves; and atrial myxoma. Emboli to the distal vessels may also originate from proximal sites of atherosclerosis and aneurysms of the aorta and large vessels. Less frequently, an arterial occlusion results paradoxically from a venous thrombus that has entered the systemic circulation via a patent foramen ovale or other septal defect. Arterial emboli tend to lodge at vessel bifurcations because the vessel caliber decreases at these sites; in the lower extremities, emboli lodge most frequently in the femoral artery, followed by the iliac artery, aorta, and popliteal and tibioperoneal arteries.

Acute arterial thrombosis in situ occurs most frequently in atherosclerotic vessels at the site of an atherosclerotic plaque or aneurysm and in arterial bypass grafts. Trauma to an artery may also result in the formation of an acute arterial thrombus. Arterial occlusion may complicate arterial punctures and placement of catheters. Less-frequent causes include thoracic outlet compression syndrome, which causes subclavian artery occlusion, and entrapment of the popliteal artery by abnormal placement of the medial head of the gastrocnemius muscle. Polycythemia and hypercoagulable disorders are also associated with acute arterial thrombosis.

Clinical Features

The symptoms of an acute arterial occlusion depend on the location, duration, and severity of the obstruction. Often, severe pain, paresthesia, numbness, and coldness develop in the involved extremity within 1 h. Paralysis may occur with severe and persistent ischemia. Physical findings include loss of pulses distal to the occlusion, cyanosis or pallor, mottling, decreased skin temperature, muscle stiffening, loss of sensation, weakness, and/or absent deep tendon reflexes. If acute arterial occlusion occurs in

the presence of an adequate collateral circulation, as is often the case in acute graft occlusion, the symptoms and findings may be less impressive. In this situation, the patient complains about an abrupt decrease in the distance walked before claudication occurs or of modest pain and paresthesia. Pallor and coolness are evident, but sensory and motor functions are generally preserved. The diagnosis of acute arterial occlusion is usually apparent from the clinical presentation. Arteriography is useful for confirming the diagnosis and demonstrating the location and extent of occlusion.

℞ Treatment:
ACUTE ARTERIAL OCCLUSION

Once the diagnosis is made, the patient should be anticoagulated with intravenous heparin to prevent propagation of the clot. In cases of severe ischemia of recent onset, and particularly when limb viability is jeopardized, immediate intervention to ensure reperfusion is indicated. Endovascular or surgical thromboembolectomy or arterial bypass procedures are used to restore blood flow to the ischemic extremity promptly, particularly when a large proximal vessel is occluded.

Intraarterial thrombolytic therapy with recombinant tissue plasminogen activator or urokinase is often effective when acute arterial occlusion is caused by a thrombus in an atherosclerotic vessel or arterial bypass graft. Thrombolytic therapy may also be indicated when the patient's overall condition contraindicates surgical intervention or when smaller distal vessels are occluded, thus preventing surgical access. Meticulous observation for hemorrhagic complications is required during intraarterial thrombolytic therapy. Another endovascular approach for thrombus removal is percutaneous mechanical thrombectomy using devices that employ hydrodynamic forces or rotating baskets to fragment and remove the clot. These may be used alone but are usually used in conjunction with pharmacologic thrombolysis.

If the limb is not in jeopardy, a more conservative approach that includes observation and administration of anticoagulants may be taken. Anticoagulation prevents recurrent embolism and reduces the likelihood of thrombus propagation; it can be initiated with intravenous heparin and followed by oral warfarin. Recommended dosages are the same as those used for deep vein thrombosis (see later). Emboli resulting from infective endocarditis, the presence of prosthetic heart valves, or atrial myxoma often require surgical intervention to remove the cause.

ATHEROEMBOLISM

Atheroembolism constitutes a subset of acute arterial occlusion. In this condition, multiple small deposits of

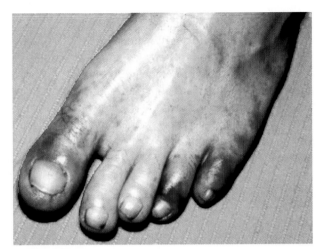

FIGURE 39-1
Atheroembolism causing cyanotic discoloration and impending necrosis of the toes (blue toe syndrome).

fibrin, platelets, and cholesterol debris embolize from proximal atherosclerotic lesions or aneurysmal sites. Large protruding aortic atheromas are a source of emboli that may lead to stroke and renal insufficiency as well as limb ischemia. Atheroembolism may occur after intraarterial procedures. Since the emboli tend to lodge in the small vessels of the muscle and skin and may not occlude the large vessels, distal pulses usually remain palpable. Patients complain of acute pain and tenderness at the site of embolization. Digital vascular occlusion may result in ischemia and the "blue toe" syndrome; digital necrosis and gangrene may develop (**Fig. 39-1**). Localized areas of tenderness, pallor, and livedo reticularis (see later) occur at sites of emboli. Skin or muscle biopsy may demonstrate cholesterol crystals.

Ischemia resulting from atheroemboli is notoriously difficult to treat. Usually neither surgical revascularization procedures nor thrombolytic therapy is helpful because of the multiplicity, composition, and distal location of the emboli. Some evidence suggests that platelet inhibitors prevent atheroembolism. Surgical intervention to remove or bypass the atherosclerotic vessel or aneurysm that causes the recurrent atheroemboli may be necessary.

THORACIC OUTLET COMPRESSION SYNDROME

This is a symptom complex resulting from compression of the neurovascular bundle (artery, vein, or nerves) at the thoracic outlet as it courses through the neck and shoulder. Cervical ribs, abnormalities of the scalenus anticus muscle, proximity of the clavicle to the first rib, or abnormal insertion of the pectoralis minor muscle may compress the subclavian artery, subclavian vein (see later), and brachial plexus as these structures pass from the thorax to the arm. Depending on the structures affected, thoracic outlet compression syndrome may be divided into arterial, venous, and neurogenic forms. Patients with neurogenic thoracic outlet compression may develop shoulder and arm pain, weakness, and paresthesias. Patients with arterial compression may experience claudication, Raynaud's phenomenon, and even ischemic tissue loss and gangrene. Venous compression may cause thrombosis of the subclavian and axillary veins; this is often associated with effort and referred to as *Paget-Schroetter syndrome*.

Approach to the Patient:
THORACIC OUTLET COMPRESSION SYNDROME

Examination of the patient with thoracic outlet compression syndrome is often normal unless provocative maneuvers are performed. Occasionally, distal pulses are decreased or absent and digital cyanosis and ischemia may be evident. Tenderness may be present in the supraclavicular fossa. In patients with axillo-subclavian venous thrombosis, the affected extremity typically is swollen. Dilated collateral veins may be apparent around the shoulder and upper arm.

Several maneuvers that support the diagnosis of thoracic outlet compression syndrome may be used to precipitate symptoms, cause a subclavian artery bruit, and diminish arm pulses. These include the abduction and external rotation test, in which the affected arm is abducted by 90° and the shoulder is externally rotated; the scalene maneuver (extension of the neck and rotation of the head to the side of the symptoms); the costoclavicular maneuver (posterior rotation of shoulders); and the hyperabduction maneuver (raising the arm 180°). A chest x-ray will indicate the presence of cervical ribs. Duplex ultrasonography, MRA, and contrast angiography can be performed during provocative maneuvers to demonstrate thoracic outlet compression of the subclavian artery. Duplex ultrasography, magnetic resonance venography, or contrast venography can be used to diagnose axillo-subclavian vein thrombosis. Neurophysiologic tests such as the electromyogram, nerve conduction studies, and somatosensory evoked potentials may be abnormal if the brachial plexus is involved, but the diagnosis of neurogenic thoracic outlet syndrome is not necessarily excluded if these tests are normal owing to their low sensitivity.

Treatment:
℞ **THORACIC OUTLET COMPRESSION SYNDROME**

Most patients can be managed conservatively. They should be advised to avoid the positions that cause symptoms. Many patients benefit from shoulder girdle exercises. Surgical procedures such as removal of the first rib or resection of the scalenus anticus muscle are necessary occasionally for relief of symptoms or treatment of ischemia.

ARTERIOVENOUS FISTULA

Abnormal communications between an artery and a vein, bypassing the capillary bed, may be congenital or acquired. Congenital arteriovenous fistulas are the result of persistent embryonic vessels that fail to differentiate into arteries and veins; they may be associated with birthmarks, can be located in almost any organ of the body, and frequently occur in the extremities. Acquired arteriovenous fistulas are either created to provide vascular access for hemodialysis or occur as a result of a penetrating injury such as a gunshot or knife wound or as complications of arterial catheterization or surgical dissection. An infrequent cause of arteriovenous fistula is rupture of an arterial aneurysm into a vein.

The clinical features depend on the location and size of the fistula. Frequently, a pulsatile mass is palpable, and a thrill and bruit lasting throughout systole and diastole are present over the fistula. With long-standing fistulas, clinical manifestations of chronic venous insufficiency, including peripheral edema; large, tortuous varicose veins; and stasis pigmentation become apparent because of the high venous pressure. Evidence of ischemia may occur in the distal portion of the extremity. Skin temperature is higher over the arteriovenous fistula. Large arteriovenous fistulas may result in an increased cardiac output with consequent cardiomegaly and high-output heart failure (Chap. 17).

Diagnosis

The diagnosis is often evident from the physical examination. Compression of a large arteriovenous fistula may cause reflex slowing of the heart rate (Nicoladoni-Branham sign). Duplex ultrasonography may detect an arteriovenous fistula, especially that which affects the femoral artery and vein at the site of catheter access. Computed tomographic and conventional angiography can confirm the diagnosis and are useful in demonstrating the site and size of the arteriovenous fistula.

R℞ Treatment:
ARTERIOVENOUS FISTULA

Management of arteriovenous fistulas may involve surgery, radiotherapy, or embolization. Congenital arteriovenous fistulas are often difficult to treat because the communications may be numerous and extensive, and new ones frequently develop after ligation of the most obvious ones. Many of these lesions are best treated conservatively using elastic support hose to reduce the consequences of venous hypertension. Occasionally, embolization with autologous material, such as fat or muscle, or with hemostatic agents, such as gelatin sponges or silicon spheres, is used to obliterate the fistula. Acquired arteriovenous fistulas are usually amenable to surgical treatment that involves division or excision of the fistula. Occasionally, autogenous or synthetic grafting is necessary to reestablish continuity of the artery and vein.

RAYNAUD'S PHENOMENON

Raynaud's phenomenon is characterized by episodic digital ischemia, manifested clinically by the sequential development of digital blanching, cyanosis, and rubor of the fingers or toes following cold exposure and subsequent rewarming. Emotional stress may also precipitate Raynaud's phenomenon. The color changes are usually well demarcated and are confined to the fingers or toes. Typically, one or more digits will appear white when the patient is exposed to a cold environment or touches a cold object. The blanching, or pallor, represents the ischemic phase of the phenomenon and results from vasospasm of digital arteries. During the ischemic phase, capillaries and venules dilate, and cyanosis results from the deoxygenated blood that is present in these vessels. A sensation of cold or numbness or paresthesia of the digits often accompanies the phases of pallor and cyanosis.

With rewarming, the digital vasospasm resolves, and blood flow into the dilated arterioles and capillaries increases dramatically. This "reactive hyperemia" imparts a bright red color to the digits. In addition to rubor and warmth, patients often experience a throbbing, painful sensation during the hyperemic phase. Although the triphasic color response is typical of Raynaud's phenomenon, some patients may develop only pallor and cyanosis; others may experience only cyanosis.

Pathophysiology

Raynaud originally proposed that cold-induced episodic digital ischemia was secondary to exaggerated reflex sympathetic vasoconstriction. This theory is supported by the fact that α-adrenergic blocking drugs as well as sympathectomy decrease the frequency and severity of Raynaud's phenomenon in some patients. An alternative hypothesis is that the digital vascular responsiveness to cold or to normal sympathetic stimuli is enhanced. It is also possible that normal reflex sympathetic vasoconstriction is superimposed on local digital vascular disease or that there is enhanced adrenergic neuroeffector activity.

Raynaud's phenomenon is broadly separated into two categories: the idiopathic variety, termed *Raynaud's disease*, and the secondary variety, which is associated with other disease states or known causes of vasospasm (Table 39-1).

TABLE 39-1

CLASSIFICATION OF RAYNAUD'S PHENOMENON

Primary or idiopathic Raynaud's phenomenon: Raynaud's disease Secondary Raynaud's phenomenon

    Collagen vascular diseases: scleroderma, systemic lupus erythematosus, rheumatoid arthritis, dermato-myositis, polymyositis

    Arterial occlusive diseases: atherosclerosis of the extremities, thromboangiitis obliterans, acute arterial occlusion, thoracic outlet syndrome

    Pulmonary hypertension

    Neurologic disorders: intervertebral disk disease, syringomyelia, spinal cord tumors, stroke, poliomyelitis, carpal tunnel syndrome

    Blood dyscrasias: cold agglutinins, cryoglobulinemia, cryofibrinogenemia, myeloproliferative disorders, Waldenström's macroglobulinemia

    Trauma: vibration injury, hammer hand syndrome, electric shock, cold injury, typing, piano playing

    Drugs: ergot derivatives, methysergide, β-adrenergic receptor blockers, bleomycin, vinblastine, cisplatin

Raynaud's Disease

This appellation is applied when the secondary causes of Raynaud's phenomenon have been excluded. More than 50% of patients with Raynaud's phenomenon have Raynaud's disease. Women are affected about five times more often than men, and the age of presentation is usually between 20 and 40 years. The fingers are involved more frequently than the toes. Initial episodes may involve only one or two fingertips, but subsequent attacks may involve the entire finger and may include all the fingers. The toes are affected in 40% of patients. Although vasospasm of the toes usually occurs in patients with symptoms in the fingers, it may happen alone. Rarely, the earlobes, the tip of the nose, and the penis are involved. Raynaud's phenomenon occurs frequently in patients who also have migraine headaches or variant angina. These associations suggest that there may be a common predisposing cause for the vasospasm.

Results of physical examination are often entirely normal; the radial, ulnar, and pedal pulses are normal. The fingers and toes may be cool between attacks and may perspire excessively. Thickening and tightening of the digital subcutaneous tissue (*sclerodactyly*) develop in 10% of patients. Angiography of the digits for diagnostic purposes is not indicated.

In general, patients with Raynaud's disease appear to have the milder forms of Raynaud's phenomenon. Less than 1% of these patients lose a part of a digit. After the diagnosis is made, the disease improves spontaneously in ~15% of patients and progresses in ~30%.

Secondary Causes of Raynaud's Phenomenon

Raynaud's phenomenon occurs in 80–90% of patients with systemic sclerosis (scleroderma) and is the presenting symptom in 30%. It may be the only symptom of scleroderma for many years. Abnormalities of the digital vessels may contribute to the development of Raynaud's phenomenon in this disorder. Ischemic fingertip ulcers may develop and progress to gangrene and autoamputation. Approximately 20% of patients with systemic lupus erythematosus (SLE) have Raynaud's phenomenon. Occasionally, persistent digital ischemia develops and may result in ulcers or gangrene. In most severe cases, the small vessels are occluded by a proliferative endarteritis. Raynaud's phenomenon occurs in about 30% of patients with dermatomyositis or polymyositis. It frequently develops in patients with rheumatoid arthritis and may be related to the intimal proliferation that occurs in the digital arteries.

Atherosclerosis of the extremities is a frequent cause of Raynaud's phenomenon in men >50 years. Thromboangiitis obliterans is an uncommon cause of Raynaud's phenomenon but should be considered in young men, particularly those who are cigarette smokers. The development of cold-induced pallor in these disorders may be confined to one or two digits of the involved extremity. Occasionally, Raynaud's phenomenon may follow acute occlusion of large- and medium-sized arteries by a thrombus or embolus. Embolization of atheroembolic debris may cause digital ischemia. The latter situation often involves one or two digits and should not be confused with Raynaud's phenomenon. In patients with thoracic outlet compression syndrome, Raynaud's phenomenon may result from diminished intravascular pressure, stimulation of sympathetic fibers in the brachial plexus, or a combination of both. Raynaud's phenomenon occurs in patients with primary pulmonary hypertension (Chap. 40); this is more than coincidental and may reflect a neurohumoral abnormality that affects both the pulmonary and digital circulations.

A variety of blood dyscrasias may be associated with Raynaud's phenomenon. Cold-induced precipitation of plasma proteins, hyperviscosity, and aggregation of red cells and platelets may occur in patients with cold agglutinins, cryoglobulinemia, or cryofibrinogenemia. Hyperviscosity syndromes that accompany myeloproliferative disorders and Waldenström's macroglobulinemia should also be considered in the initial evaluation of patients with Raynaud's phenomenon.

Raynaud's phenomenon occurs often in patients whose vocations require the use of vibrating hand tools, such as chain saws or jackhammers. The frequency of Raynaud's phenomenon also seems to be increased in pianists and keyboard operators. Electric shock injury to the hands or frostbite may lead to the later development of Raynaud's phenomenon.

Several drugs have been causally implicated in Raynaud's phenomenon. These include ergot preparations; methysergide; β-adrenergic receptor antagonists; and the chemotherapeutic agents bleomycin, vinblastine, and cisplatin.

℞ Treatment:
RAYNAUD'S PHENOMENON

Most patients with Raynaud's phenomenon experience only mild and infrequent episodes. These patients need reassurance and should be instructed to dress warmly and avoid unnecessary cold exposure. In addition to gloves and mittens, patients should protect the trunk, head, and feet with warm clothing to prevent cold-induced reflex vasoconstriction. Tobacco use is contraindicated.

Drug treatment should be reserved for the severe cases. Dihydropyridine calcium channel antagonists, such as nifedipine, isradipine, felodipine, and amlodipine, decrease the frequency and severity of Raynaud's phenomenon. Diltiazem may be considered but is less effective. The postsynaptic α_1-adrenergic antagonist prazosin has been used with favorable responses; doxazosin and terazosin may also be effective. Other sympatholytic agents, such as methyldopa, guanethidine, and phenoxybenzamine, may be useful in some patients, as may topical glyceryl trinitrate. Digital sympathectomy is helpful in some patients who are unresponsive to medical therapy.

ACROCYANOSIS

In this condition, there is arterial vasoconstriction and secondary dilation of the capillaries and venules with resulting persistent cyanosis of the hands and, less frequently, the feet. Cyanosis may be intensified by exposure to a cold environment. Acrocyanosis may be categorized as primary or secondary to an underlying condition. In primary acrocyanosis, women are affected much more frequently than men, and the age of onset is usually younger than 30 years. Generally, patients are asymptomatic but seek medical attention because of the discoloration. The prognosis is favorable, and pain, ulcers, and gangrene do not occur. Examination reveals normal pulses, peripheral cyanosis, and moist palms. Trophic skin changes and ulcerations do *not* occur. The disorder can be distinguished from Raynaud's phenomenon because it is persistent and not episodic, the discoloration extends proximally from the digits, and blanching does not occur. Ischemia secondary to arterial occlusive disease can usually be excluded by the presence of normal pulses. Central cyanosis and decreased arterial oxygen saturation are not present. Patients should be reassured and advised to dress warmly and avoid cold exposure. Pharmacologic intervention is not indicated.

Secondary acrocyanosis may result from hypoxemia, connective tissue diseases, atheroembolism, antiphospholipid antibodies, cold agglutinins, or cryoglobulins, and is associated with anorexia nervosa and orthostatic tachycardia syndrome. Treatment should be directed at the underlying disorder.

LIVEDO RETICULARIS

In this condition, localized areas of the extremities develop a mottled or rete (net-like) appearance of reddish to blue discoloration. The mottled appearance may be more prominent following cold exposure. There are primary and secondary forms of livedo reticularis. The primary, or idiopathic, form of this disorder may be benign or associated with ulcerations. The benign form occurs more frequently in women than in men, and the most common age of onset is in the third decade. Patients with the benign form are usually asymptomatic and seek attention for cosmetic reasons. These patients should be reassured and advised to avoid cold environments. No drug treatment is indicated. Primary livedo reticularis with ulceration is also called *atrophie blanche en plaque*. The ulcers are painful and may take months to heal. Secondary livedo reticularis can occur with atheroembolism (see earlier), SLE and other vasculitides, anticardiolipin antibodies, hyperviscosity, cryoglobulinemia, and Sneddon's syndrome (ischemic stroke and livedo reticularis). Rarely, skin ulcerations develop.

PERNIO (CHILBLAINS)

This is a vasculitic disorder associated with exposure to cold; acute forms have been described. Raised erythematous lesions develop on the lower part of the legs and feet in cold weather. These are associated with pruritus and a burning sensation, and they may blister and ulcerate. Pathologic examination demonstrates angiitis characterized by intimal proliferation and perivascular infiltration of mononuclear and polymorphonuclear leukocytes. Giant cells may be present in the subcutaneous tissue. Patients should avoid exposure to cold, and ulcers should be kept clean and protected with sterile dressings. Sympatholytic drugs may be effective in some patients.

ERYTHROMELALGIA

This disorder is characterized by burning pain and erythema of the extremities. The feet are involved more frequently than the hands, and men are affected more frequently than women. Erythromelalgia may occur at any age but is most common in middle age. It may be primary (also termed erythermalgia) or secondary. The most common causes of secondary erythromelalgia are myeloproliferative disorders such as polycythemia vera and essential thrombocytosis. Less-common causes include drugs, such as calcium channel blockers, bromocriptine, and pergolide; neuropathies; connective tissue diseases, such as systemic lupus erythematosus; and paraneoplastic syndromes. Patients complain of burning in the extremities that is precipitated by exposure to a warm environment and aggravated by a dependent position. The symptoms are relieved by exposing the affected area to cool air or water or by elevation. Erythromelalgia can be distinguished from ischemia secondary to peripheral arterial disorders and peripheral neuropathy because the peripheral pulses are present and the neurologic examination is normal. There is no specific treatment; aspirin may produce relief in patients with erythromelalgia secondary to myeloproliferative disease. Treatment of associated disorders in secondary erythromelalgia may be helpful.

FROSTBITE

In this condition, tissue damage results from severe environmental cold exposure or from direct contact with a very cold object. Tissue injury results from both freezing and vasoconstriction. Frostbite usually affects the distal aspects of the extremities or exposed parts of the face, such as the ears, nose, chin, and cheeks. Superficial frostbite involves the skin and subcutaneous tissue. Patients experience pain or paresthesia, and the skin appears white and waxy. After rewarming, there is cyanosis and erythema, wheal-and-flare formation, edema, and superficial blisters. Deep frostbite involves muscle, nerves, and deeper blood vessels. It may result in edema of the hand or foot, vesicles and bullae, tissue necrosis, and gangrene.

Initial treatment is rewarming, performed in an environment where reexposure to freezing conditions will not occur. Rewarming is accomplished by immersion of the affected part in a water bath at temperatures of 40°–44°C (104°–111°F). Massage, application of ice water, and extreme heat are contraindicated. The injured area should be cleansed with soap or antiseptic and sterile dressings applied. Analgesics are often required during rewarming. Antibiotics are used if there is evidence of infection. The efficacy of sympathetic blocking drugs is not established. Following recovery, the affected extremity may exhibit increased sensitivity to cold.

DISORDERS OF THE VEINS AND LYMPHATICS

VENOUS DISORDERS

Veins in the extremities can be broadly classified as either superficial or deep. In the lower extremity, the superficial venous system includes the greater and lesser saphenous veins and their tributaries. The deep veins of the leg accompany the major arteries. Perforating veins connect the superficial and deep systems at multiple locations.

Bicuspid valves are present throughout the venous system to direct the flow of venous blood centrally.

Venous Thrombosis

The presence of thrombus within a superficial or deep vein and the accompanying inflammatory response in the vessel wall is termed *venous thrombosis* or *thrombophlebitis*. Initially the thrombus is composed principally of platelets and fibrin. Red cells become interspersed with fibrin, and the thrombus tends to propagate in the direction of blood flow. The inflammatory response in the vessel wall may be minimal or characterized by granulocyte infiltration, loss of endothelium, and edema.

The factors that predispose to venous thrombosis were initially described by Virchow in 1856 and include stasis, vascular damage, and hypercoagulability. Accordingly, a variety of clinical situations are associated with increased risk of venous thrombosis (Table 39-2). Venous thrombosis may occur in >50% of patients having orthopedic surgical procedures, particularly those involving the hip or knee, and in 10–40% of patients who undergo abdominal or thoracic operations. The prevalence of venous thrombosis is particularly high in patients with cancer of the pancreas, lungs, genitourinary tract, stomach, and breast. Approximately 10–20% of patients with idiopathic deep vein thrombosis have or develop clinically overt cancer; there is no consensus on whether these individuals should be subjected to intensive diagnostic workup to search for occult malignancy.

The risk of thrombosis is increased following trauma, such as fractures of the spine, pelvis, femur, and tibia. Immobilization, regardless of the underlying disease, is a major predisposing cause of venous thrombosis. This fact may account for the relatively high incidence in patients with acute MI or congestive heart failure. The incidence of venous thrombosis is increased during pregnancy, particularly in the third trimester and in the first month postpartum, and in individuals who use oral contraceptives, postmenopausal hormone replacement therapy, or selective estrogen receptor modulators. A variety of clinical disorders that produce systemic hypercoagulability, including resistance to activated protein C (factor V Leiden); prothrombin G20210A gene mutation; antithrombin III, protein C, and protein S deficiencies; antiphospholipid syndrome; hyperhomocysteinemia; SLE; myeloproliferative diseases; dysfibrinogenemia; and disseminated intravascular coagulation, are associated with venous thrombosis. Venulitis occurring in thromboangiitis obliterans, Behçet's syndrome, and homocystinuria may also cause venous thrombosis.

Superficial Vein Thrombosis

Thrombosis of the greater or lesser saphenous veins or their tributaries—i.e., superficial vein thrombosis—does

TABLE 39-2

CONDITIONS ASSOCIATED WITH AN INCREASED RISK FOR DEVELOPMENT OF VENOUS THROMBOSIS

Surgery
  Orthopedic, thoracic, abdominal, and genitourinary
    procedures
Neoplasms
  Pancreas, lung, ovary, testes, urinary tract, breast,
    stomach
Trauma
  Fractures of spine, pelvis, femur, or tibia; spinal cord
    injuries
Immobilization
  Acute myocardial infarction, congestive heart failure,
    stroke, postoperative convalescence
Pregnancy
Estrogen
  For replacement or contraception;
    Selective estrogen replacement modulators
Hypercoagulable states
  Resistance to activated protein C; prothrombin or
    20210 A gene mutation deficiencies of antithrombin III,
    protein C, or protein S; antiphospholipid antibodies;
    myeloproliferative diseases; dysfibrinogenemia; dis-
    seminated intravascular coagulation
Venulitis
  Thromboangiitis obliterans, Behçet's disease,
    homocysteinuria
Previous deep vein thrombosis

not result in pulmonary embolism. It is associated with intravenous catheters and infusions, occurs in varicose veins, and may develop in association with deep venous thrombosis (DVT). Migrating superficial vein thrombosis is often a marker for a carcinoma and may also occur in patients with vasculitides, such as thromboangiitis obliterans. The clinical features of superficial vein thrombosis are easily distinguished from those of DVT. Patients complain of pain localized to the site of the thrombus. Examination reveals a reddened, warm, and tender cord extending along a superficial vein. The surrounding area may be red and edematous.

℞ **Treatment:**
SUPERFICIAL VEIN THROMBOSIS

Treatment is primarily supportive. Initially, patients can be placed at bed rest with leg elevation and application of warm compresses. Nonsteroidal anti-inflammatory drugs may provide analgesia but may also obscure clinical evidence of thrombus propagation. If a thrombosis of the greater saphenous vein develops in the thigh and extends toward the saphenofemoral vein junction, it is reasonable to consider anticoagulant therapy to prevent extension of the thrombus into the deep system and a possible pulmonary embolism.

Varicose Veins

Varicose veins are dilated, tortuous superficial veins that result from defective structure and function of the valves of the saphenous veins, from intrinsic weakness of the vein wall, from high intraluminal pressure, or, rarely, from arteriovenous fistulas. Varicose veins can be categorized as primary or secondary. Primary varicose veins originate in the superficial system and occur two to three times as frequently in women as in men. Approximately half of patients have a family history of varicose veins. Secondary varicose veins result from deep venous insufficiency and incompetent perforating veins or from deep venous occlusion causing enlargement of superficial veins that are serving as collaterals.

Patients with venous varicosities are often concerned about the cosmetic appearance of their legs. Symptoms consist of a dull ache or pressure sensation in the legs after prolonged standing; it is relieved with leg elevation. The legs feel heavy, and mild ankle edema develops occasionally. Extensive venous varicosities may cause skin ulcerations near the ankle. Superficial venous thrombosis may be a recurring problem, and, rarely, a varicosity ruptures and bleeds. Visual inspection of the legs in the dependent position usually confirms the presence of varicose veins.

Varicose veins can usually be treated with conservative measures. Symptoms often decrease when the legs are elevated periodically, when prolonged standing is avoided, and when elastic support hose are worn. External compression stockings provide a counterbalance to the hydrostatic pressure in the veins. Ablative procedures, including sclerotherapy, endovenous radiofrequency or laser ablation, and surgery may be considered to treat varicose veins in selected patients who have persistent symptoms, suffer recurrent superficial vein thrombosis, and/or develop skin ulceration. Ablative therapy may also be indicated for cosmetic reasons. Small, symptomatic varicose veins can be treated with sclerotherapy, in which a sclerosing solution is injected into the involved varicose vein and a compression bandage is applied. Percutaneous, endovenous delivery of radiofrequency or laser energy can be used to treat incompetent greater saphenous veins. Surgical therapy usually involves ligation and stripping of the greater and lesser saphenous veins.

Chronic Venous Insufficiency

Chronic venous insufficiency may result from DVT and/or valvular incompetence. Following DVT, the delicate valve leaflets become thickened and contracted so that they cannot prevent retrograde flow of blood; the vein becomes rigid and thick-walled. Although most veins recanalize after an episode of thrombosis, the large proximal veins may remain occluded. Secondary incompetence develops in distal valves because high pressures distend the vein and separate the leaflets. Primary deep venous valvular dysfunction may also occur without previous thrombosis. Patients with venous insufficiency often complain of a dull ache in the leg that worsens with prolonged standing and resolves with leg elevation. Examination demonstrates increased leg circumference, edema, and superficial varicose veins. Erythema, dermatitis, and hyperpigmentation develop along the distal aspect of the leg, and skin ulceration may occur near the medial and lateral malleoli. Cellulitis may be a recurring problem. Patients should be advised to avoid prolonged standing or sitting; frequent leg elevation is helpful. Graduated compression stockings should be worn during the day. These efforts should be intensified if skin ulcers develop. Ulcers should be treated with applications of wet to dry dressings or occlusive hydrocolloid dressings. Commercially available compressive dressings comprising paste with zinc oxide, calamine, glycerin, and gelatin may be applied and should be changed weekly until healing occurs. Recurrent ulceration and severe edema may be treated by surgical interruption of incompetent communicating veins. Subfascial endoscopic perforator surgery (SEPS) is a minimally invasive technique to interrupt incompetent communicating veins. Rarely, surgical valvuloplasty and bypass of venous occlusions are employed.

LYMPHATIC DISORDERS

Lymphatic capillaries are blind-ended tubes formed by a single layer of endothelial cells. The absent or widely fenestrated basement membrane of lymphatic capillaries allows access to interstitial proteins and particles. Lymphatic capillaries merge to form larger vessels that contain smooth muscle and are capable of vasomotion. Small and medium-sized lymphatic vessels empty into progressively larger channels, most of which drain into the thoracic duct. The lymphatic circulation is involved in the absorption of interstitial fluid and in the response to infection.

Lymphedema

Lymphedema may be categorized as primary or secondary (Table 39-3). The prevalence of primary lymphedema is 1 per 10,000 individuals. Primary lymphedema may be secondary to agenesis, hypoplasia, or obstruction of the lymphatic vessels. It may be associated with Turner's syndrome, Klinefelter's syndrome, Noonan's syndrome, yellow nail syndrome, intestinal lymphangiectasia syndrome, and lymphangiomyomatosis. Women are affected more frequently than men. There are three clinical subtypes: congenital lymphedema, which appears shortly after birth; lymphedema praecox, which has its onset at the time of puberty; and lymphedema tarda, which usually begins after age 35. Familial forms of congenital lymphedema (Milroy's

TABLE 39-3

CAUSES OF LYMPHEDEMA

Primary	Secondary
Congenital (includes Milroy's disease)	Recurrent lymphangitis
	Filariasis
Lymphedema praecox (includes Meige's disease)	Tuberculosis
	Neoplasm
	Surgery
Lymphedema tarda	Radiation therapy

disease) and lymphedema praecox (Meige's disease) may be inherited in an autosomal dominant manner with variable penetrance; autosomal or sex-linked recessive forms are less common.

Secondary lymphedema is an acquired condition resulting from damage to or obstruction of previously normal lymphatic channels (Table 39-3). Recurrent episodes of bacterial lymphangitis, usually caused by streptococci, are a very common cause of lymphedema. The most common cause of secondary lymphedema worldwide is filariasis. Tumors, such as prostate cancer and lymphoma, can also obstruct lymphatic vessels. Both surgery and radiation therapy for breast carcinoma may cause lymphedema of the upper extremity. Less-common causes include tuberculosis, contact dermatitis, lymphogranuloma venereum, rheumatoid arthritis, pregnancy, and self-induced or factitious lymphedema following application of tourniquets.

Lymphedema is generally a painless condition, but patients may experience a chronic dull, heavy sensation in the leg, and most often they are concerned about the appearance of the leg. Lymphedema of the lower extremity, initially involving the foot, gradually progresses up the leg so that the entire limb becomes edematous. In the early stages, the edema is soft and pits easily with pressure. In the chronic stages, the limb has a woody texture, and the tissues become indurated and fibrotic. At this point the edema may no longer be pitting. The limb loses its normal contour, and the toes appear square. Lymphedema should be distinguished from other disorders that cause unilateral leg swelling, such as DVT and chronic venous insufficiency. In the latter condition, the edema is softer, and there is often evidence of a stasis dermatitis, hyperpigmentation, and superficial venous varicosities.

The evaluation of patients with lymphedema should include diagnostic studies to clarify the cause. Abdominal and pelvic ultrasound and CTA can be used to detect obstructing lesions such as neoplasms. MRI may reveal edema in the epifascial compartment and identify lymph nodes and enlarged lymphatic channels. Lymphoscintigraphy and lymphangiography are rarely indicated, but either can be used to confirm the diagnosis or to differentiate primary from secondary lymphedema. Lymphoscintigraphy involves the injection of radioactively labeled technetium-containing colloid into the distal subcutaneous tissue of the affected extremity. In lymphangiography, contrast material is injected into a distal lymphatic vessel that has been isolated and cannulated. In primary lymphedema, lymphatic channels are absent, hypoplastic, or ectatic. In secondary lymphedema, lymphatic channels are usually dilated, and it may be possible to determine the level of obstruction.

℞ **Treatment:**
LYMPHEDEMA

Patients with lymphedema of the lower extremities must be instructed to take meticulous care of their feet to prevent recurrent lymphangitis. Skin hygiene is important, and emollients can be used to prevent drying. Prophylactic antibiotics are often helpful, and fungal infection should be treated aggressively. Patients should be encouraged to participate in physical activity; frequent leg elevation can reduce the amount of edema. Physical therapy, including massage to facilitate lymphatic drainage, may be helpful. Patients can be fitted with graduated compression hose to reduce the amount of lymphedema that develops with upright posture. Occasionally, intermittent pneumatic compression devices can be applied at home to facilitate reduction of the edema. Diuretics are contraindicated and may cause depletion of intravascular volume and metabolic abnormalities. Microsurgical lymphatico-venous anastomotic procedures have been performed to rechannel lymph flow from obstructed lymphatic vessels into the venous system.

FURTHER READINGS

BERGAN JJ et al: Chronic venous disease. N Engl J Med 355:488, 2006

CREAGER MA (ed): Atlas of Vascular Disease, 3d ed. Philadelphia, Current Medicine Group, 2007

——— et al (eds): *Vascular Medicine*. Philadelphia, Saunders Elsevier, 2006

——— et al: Atherosclerotic Peripheral Vascular Disease Symposium II: Executive summary. Circulation 118:2811, 2008

FAXON DP et al: Atherosclerotic Vascular Disease Conference: Executive summary: Atherosclerotic Vascular Disease Conference proceeding for healthcare professionals from a special writing group of the American Heart Association. Circulation 109:2595, 2004

FOWKES FG et al: Ankle brachial index combined with Framingham Risk Score to predict cardiovascular events and mortality: a meta-analysis. JAMA 300:197, 2008

GOLOMB BA et al: Peripheral arterial disease: Morbidity and mortality implications. Circulation 114:688, 2006

HANKEY GJ et al: Medical treatment of peripheral arterial disease. JAMA 295:547, 2006

HIRSCH AT et al: ACC/AHA 2005 guidelines for the management of patients with peripheral arterial disease (lower extremity, renal, mesenteric, and abdominal aortic). J Am Coll Cardiol 47:1239, 2006

MCDERMOTT MM et al: The ankle brachial index is associated with leg function and physical activity: The Walking and Leg Circulation Study. Ann Intern Med 136:873, 2002

NORGREN L et al: Inter-Society Consensus for the Management of Peripheral Arterial Disease (TASC II). J Vasc Surg 45:S5, 2007

OLIN JW: Thromboangiitis obliterans (Buerger's disease). N Engl J Med 343:864, 2000

RAJU S, Neglen P: Clinical practice. Chronic venous insufficiency and varicose veins. N Engl J Med 360:2319, 2009

ROCKSON SG: Lymphedema. Current Treat Options Cardiovasc Med 8:129, 2006

WHITE C: Clinical practice. Intermittent claudication. N Engl J Med 356:1241, 2007

WIGLEY FM: Clinical practice. Raynaud's phenomenon. N Engl J Med 347:1001, 2002

CHAPTER 40

PULMONARY HYPERTENSION

Stuart Rich

Pulmonary hypertension, an abnormal elevation in pulmonary artery pressure, may be the result of left heart failure, pulmonary parenchymal or vascular disease, thromboembolism, or a combination of these factors. Whether the pulmonary hypertension arises from cardiac, pulmonary, or intrinsic vascular disease, it generally is a feature of advanced disease. Because the causes of pulmonary hypertension are so diverse, it is essential that the etiology underlying the pulmonary hypertension be clearly determined before embarking on treatment.

Cor pulmonale (Chap. 17) is a term used to indicate right ventricular (RV) enlargement secondary to any underlying cardiac or pulmonary disease. Pulmonary hypertension is the most common cause of cor pulmonale. Advanced cor pulmonale is associated with the development of RV failure.

PATHOPHYSIOLOGY

The right ventricle responds to an increase in resistance within the pulmonary circulation by increasing RV systolic pressure as necessary to preserve cardiac output. Over time, chronic changes occur in the pulmonary circulation that result in progressive remodeling of the vasculature, which can sustain or promote pulmonary hypertension even if the initiating factor is removed.

The ability of the RV to adapt to increased vascular resistance is influenced by several factors, including age and the rapidity of the development of pulmonary hypertension. For example, a large acute pulmonary thromboembolism can result in RV failure and shock, whereas chronic thromboembolic disease of equal severity may result in only mild exercise intolerance. Coexisting hypoxemia can impair the ability of the ventricle to compensate. Several studies support the concept that RV failure occurs in pulmonary hypertension when the RV myocardium becomes ischemic due to excessive demands and inadequate right ventricular coronary blood flow to the RV. The onset of clinical RV failure, usually manifest by peripheral edema, is associated with a poor outcome.

DIAGNOSIS

The most common symptom attributable to pulmonary hypertension is exertional dyspnea. Other common symptoms are fatigue, angina pectoris that may represent RV ischemia, syncope, near syncope, and peripheral edema.

The physical examination typically reveals increased jugular venous pressure, a reduced carotid pulse, and a palpable RV impulse. Most patients have an increased pulmonic component of the second heart sound, a right-sided fourth heart sound, and tricuspid regurgitation (Chap. 9). Peripheral cyanosis and/or edema tend to occur in later stages of the disease.

Laboratory Findings

(Fig. 40-1) The chest x-ray generally shows enlarged central pulmonary arteries. The lung fields may or may not reveal other pathology. The electrocardiogram usually shows right axis deviation and RV hypertrophy. The echocardiogram commonly demonstrates RV and right atrial enlargement, a reduction in left ventricular (LV)

cavity size, and a tricuspid regurgitant jet that can be used to estimate RV systolic pressure. Pulmonary function tests are helpful in documenting underlying obstructive airways disease, whereas high-resolution chest CT is preferred to diagnose restrictive lung disease. Hypoxemia and an abnormal diffusing capacity for carbon monoxide are common features of pulmonary hypertension of many causes. A perfusion lung scan is almost always abnormal in patients with thromboembolic pulmonary hypertension. However, diffuse defects of a nonsegmental nature can often be seen in long-standing pulmonary hypertension in the absence of thromboemboli. Laboratory tests should include antinuclear antibody and HIV testing. Because of the high frequency of thyroid abnormalities in patients with idiopathic pulmonary hypertension, it is recommended that the thyroid-stimulating hormone level be determined periodically.

Cardiac Catheterization

This procedure is mandatory for accurate measurement of pulmonary artery pressure, cardiac output, and LV filling pressure, as well as for exclusion of an underlying cardiac shunt. Care should be taken to measure pressures only at end expiration. It is also recommended that patients with pulmonary arterial hypertension undergo drug testing with a short-acting pulmonary vasodilator at the time of cardiac catheterization to determine the extent of pulmonary vasodilator reactivity (Fig. 40-2). Inhaled nitric oxide, intravenous adenosine, and intravenous epoprostenol appear to have comparable effects in reducing pulmonary artery pressure acutely. Nitric oxide is administered via inhalation in 10–20 parts per million. Adenosine is given in doses of 50 μg/kg per min and increased every 2 min until side effects develop. Epoprostenol is given in doses of 2 ng/kg per min and increased every 30 min until side effects develop. Patients who respond can often be treated with calcium channel blockers and have a more favorable prognosis.

PULMONARY ARTERIAL HYPERTENSION

There are many causes of pulmonary arterial hypertension (PAH) (Table 40-1). Patients with PAH share a common histopathology characterized by medial hypertrophy, eccentric and concentric intimal fibrosis, recanalized thrombi appearing as fibrous webs, and plexiform lesions.

PATHOBIOLOGY

Abnormalities in molecular pathways regulating the pulmonary vascular endothelial and smooth-muscle cells have been described as underlying PAH. These include inhibition of the voltage-regulated potassium channel,

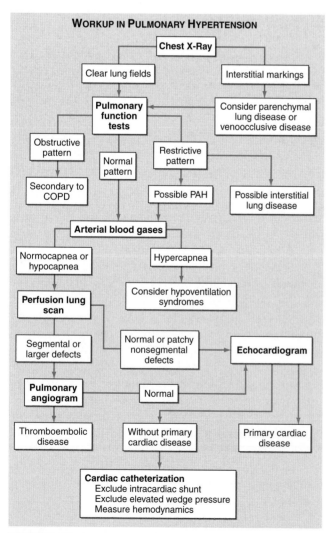

FIGURE 40-1

An algorithm for the workup of a patient with unexplained pulmonary hypertension. (*Adapted with permission from Rich.*)

ALGORITHM FOR DRUG TREATMENT SELECTION

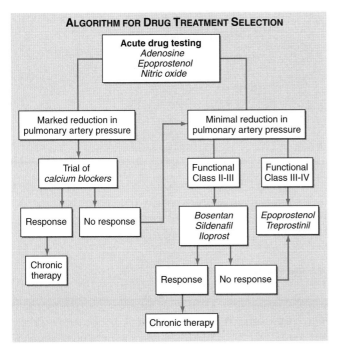

FIGURE 40-2

An algorithm for the selection of optimal drug treatment of a patient with pulmonary arterial hypertension. A marked reduction in pulmonary artery pressure from acute vasodilator testing is defined as a fall in mean pulmonary artery pressure (MPAP) ≥10 mmHg and a final MPAP that is <40 mmHg. (*Adapted with permission from S. Rich.*)

TABLE 40-1

CLINICAL CLASSIFICATION OF PULMONARY HYPERTENSION

1. **Pulmonary arterial hypertension (PAH)**
   1.1. Idiopathic (IPAH) (formerly PPH)
   1.2. Familial (FPAH)
   1.3. Associated with (APAH):
   1.3.1. Collagen vascular disease
   1.3.2. Congenital systemic-to-pulmonary shunts
   1.3.3. Portal hypertension
   1.3.4. HIV infection
   1.3.5. Drugs and toxins
   1.3.6. Other (thyroid disorders, glycogen storage disease, Gaucher disease, hereditary hemorrhagic telangiectasia, hemoglobinopathies, myeloproliferative disorders, splenectomy)
   1.4. Associated with significant venous or capillary involvement
   1.4.1. Pulmonary veno occlusive disease (PVOD)
   1.4.2. Pulmonary capillary hemangiomatosis (PCH)
   1.5. Persistent pulmonary hypertension of the newborn
2. **Pulmonary hypertension with left heart disease**
   2.1. Left-sided atrial or ventricular heart disease
   2.2. Left-sided valvular heart disease
3. **Pulmonary hypertension associated with lung diseases and/or hypoxemia**
   3.1. Chronic obstructive pulmonary disease
   3.2. Interstitial lung disease
   3.3. Sleep-disordered breathing
   3.4. Alveolar hypoventilation disorders
   3.5. Chronic exposure to high altitude
   3.6. Developmental abnormalities
4. **Pulmonary hypertension due to chronic thrombotic and/or embolic disease**
   4.1. Thromboembolic obstruction of proximal pulmonary arteries
   4.2. Thromboembolic obstruction of distal pulmonary arteries
   4.3. Nonthrombotic pulmonary embolism (tumor, parasites, foreign material)
5. **Miscellaneous**
   Sarcoidosis, histiocytosis X, lymphangiomatosis, compression of pulmonary vessels (adenopathy, tumor, fibrosing mediastinitis)

Source: From G Simonneau et al: Clinical classification of pulmonary hypertension. J Am Coll Cardiol 43:S5, 2004.

mutations in the bone morphogenetic protein-2 receptor, increased serotonin uptake in the smooth-muscle cells, increased angiopoietin expression in the smooth-muscle cells, and excessive thrombin deposition related to a procoagulant state. As a result there appears to be loss of apoptosis of the smooth-muscle cells allowing their proliferation, and the emergence of apoptosis-resistant endothelial cells which can obliterate the vascular lumen.

IDIOPATHIC PULMONARY ARTERIAL HYPERTENSION

Idiopathic pulmonary arterial hypertension (IPAH), formerly referred to as primary pulmonary hypertension is uncommon, with an estimated incidence of two cases per million. There is a strong female predominance, with most patients presenting in the fourth and fifth decades, although the age range is from infancy to >60 years.

Familial IPAH accounts for up to 20% of cases of IPAH and is characterized by autosomal dominant inheritance, variable age of onset, and incomplete penetrance. The clinical and pathologic features of familial and sporadic IPAH are identical. Heterozygous germline mutations that involve the gene coding the type II bone morphogenetic protein receptor (BMPR II), a member of the transforming growth factor (TGF)β superfamily,

appear to account for most cases of familial IPAH. The TGF-β superfamily comprise multifunctional proteins that initiate diverse cellular responses by binding to and activating serine/threonine kinase receptors. The low gene penetrance suggests that other risk factors or abnormalities are necessary to manifest clinical disease. Germline mutations in the activin-like kinase gene and endoglin gene, which have been linked to hereditary hemorrhagic telangiectasia (HHT) have been described to coexist in some patients with familial IPAH (**Fig. 40-3**).

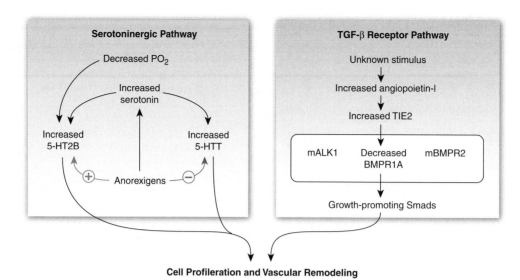

FIGURE 40-3

Mechanistic pathways promoting pulmonary arterial hypertension (PAH). External stimuli, such as hypoxia or anorexigens, can stimulate a serotoninergic pathway which, in concert with internal stimuli involving the TGF-β receptor pathway can produce PAH. 5-HT2B, serotonin receptor; 5-HTT, serotonin transporter; TGF-β, transforming growth factor β; TIE2, angiopoietin-1 receptor; BMPR1A, bone morphogenetic protein receptor 1A; mBMPR2, mutant form of bone morphogenetic protein receptor 2; mALK1, activin-receptor-like kinase. (*From Farber and Loscalzo, with permission.*)

NATURAL HISTORY

The natural history of IPAH is uncertain, and because the predominant symptom is dyspnea, which can have an insidious onset, the disease is typically diagnosed late in its course. Prior to current therapies, a mean survival of 2–3 years from the time of diagnosis was reported. Functional class remains a strong predictor of survival, with patients who are in New York Heart Association (NYHA) functional class IV having a mean survival of <6 months. The cause of death is usually RV failure, which is manifest by progressive hypoxemia, tachycardia, hypotension, and edema.

℞ **Treatment:**
PULMONARY ARTERIAL HYPERTENSION

Pulmonary arterial hypertension (PAH) refers to a variety of diseases, which includes IPAH, as noted in Table 40-1. The regulatory authorities have approved several treatments for PAH (reviewed later in this chapter) without making a distinction between the different types. However, physicians need to be mindful that the efficacy and side effects of these drugs might not be the same in all types of PAH (**Fig. 40-4**). Because the pulmonary artery pressure in PAH increases dramatically with exercise, patients should be cautioned against participating in activities that demand increased physical stress. Diuretic therapy relieves peripheral edema and may be useful in reducing RV volume overload in the presence of tricuspid regurgitation. Resting and exercise pulse oximetry should be obtained, as O$_2$ supplementation helps to alleviate dyspnea and RV ischemia in patients whose arterial O$_2$ saturation is reduced. Anticoagulant therapy is advocated for all patients with PAH based on retrospective and prospective studies demonstrating that warfarin increases survival of patients with PAH. The dose of warfarin is generally titrated to achieve an international normalized ration (INR) of 2–3 times control.

CALCIUM CHANNEL BLOCKERS Patients who have substantial reductions in pulmonary arterial pressure in response to short-acting vasodilators at the time of cardiac catheterization (a fall in mean pulmonary arterial pressure ≥10 mmHg and a final mean pressure <40 mmHg) should be treated initially with calcium channel blockers. Typically, patients require high doses (e.g., nifedipine, 240 mg/d, or amlodipine, 20 mg/d). Patients who respond favorably usually have dramatic reductions in pulmonary artery pressure and pulmonary vascular resistance associated with improved symptoms, regression of RV hypertrophy, and improved survival now documented to exceed 20 years. However, <20% of patients respond to calcium channel blockers in the long term. These drugs should not be given to patients who are unresponsive, as they can result in hypotension, hypoxemia, tachycardia, and worsening right heart failure. These agents have not been approved for the treatment of PAH by the U.S. Food and Drug Administration.

ENDOTHELIN RECEPTOR ANTAGONISTS
The nonselective endothelin receptor antagonist *bosentan* is an approved treatment of PAH for patients who

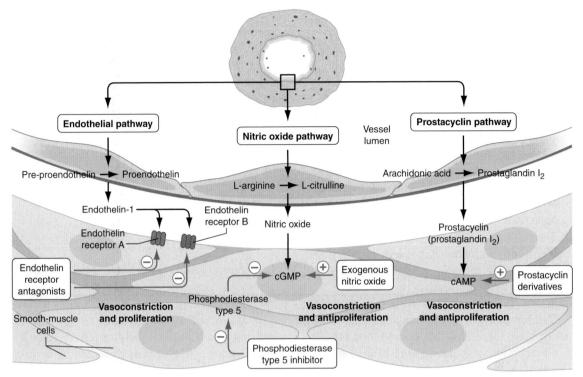

FIGURE 40-4

Current therapies target multiple growth factor pathways that appear to be involved in the pathogenesis of PAH. Whether treating multiple pathways simultaneously will yield better results is unknown. (*From Humbert et al., with permission.*)

are NYHA functional classes III and IV. In randomized clinical trials, bosentan improved symptoms and exercise tolerance as measured by an increase in 6-min walking distance. Therapy is initiated at 62.5 mg bid for the first month and then increased to 125 mg bid thereafter. Because of the high frequency of abnormal hepatic function tests associated with drug use, primarily an increase in transaminases, it is recommended that liver function be monitored monthly throughout the duration of use. Bosentan is also contraindicated in patients who are on cyclosporine or glyburide concurrently.

PHOSPHODIESTERASE-5 INHIBITORS *Sildenafil*, a phosphodiesterase-5 inhibitor, is approved for the treatment of PAH patients who are NYHA functional classes II and III. Phosphodiesterase-5 is responsible for the hydrolysis of cyclic GMP in pulmonary vascular smooth muscle, the mediator through which nitric oxide lowers pulmonary artery pressure and inhibits pulmonary vascular growth. Randomized clinical trials have shown that sildenafil improves symptoms and exercise tolerance in PAH. The recommended dose is 20 mg tid. The most common side effect is headache. Sildenafil should not be given to patients who are taking nitrate compounds.

PROSTACYCLINS *Iloprost*, a prostacyclin analogue, is approved via inhalation for PAH patients who are NYHA functional classes III and IV. It has been shown to improve symptoms and exercise tolerance. Therapy can be given at either 2.5 or 5 mcg per inhalation treatment. The inhaler must be given by a dedicated nebulizer. The most common side effects are flushing and cough. Because of the very short half-life (<30 min) it is recommended to administer treatments as often as every 2 h.

Epoprostenol is approved for the treatment of PAH patients who are NYHA functional class III or IV. Clinical trials have demonstrated an improvement in symptoms, exercise tolerance, and survival even if no acute hemodynamic response to drug challenge occurs. The drug is administered intravenously and requires placement of a permanent central venous catheter and infusion through an ambulatory infusion pump system. Side effects include flushing, jaw pain, and diarrhea, which are generally tolerated by most patients.

Treprostinil, an analogue of epoprostenol, is approved for patients with PAH who are NYHA functional classes II–IV. Treprostinil has a longer half-life than epoprostenol (4 h), is stable at room temperature, and may be given intravenously or subcutaneously through a small infusion pump that was originally developed for insulin. Clinical trials have demonstrated an improvement in symptoms and exercise capacity. The major problem with the subcutaneous administration has been local pain at the infusion site, which has caused many patients to discontinue therapy. Side effects are similar to those seen with epoprostenol.

The intravenous prostacyclins have the greatest efficacy as treatments for PAH, and are often effective in patients who have failed all other treatments. Favorable properties include vasodilation, platelet inhibition, inhibition of vascular smooth-muscle growth, and inotropic effects. It generally takes several months to titrate the dose of epoprostenol or treprostinil upwards to optimal clinical efficacy, which can be determined by symptoms, exercise testing, and catheterization. The optimal doses of these drugs have not been determined, but the typical doses of epoprostenol range from 25–40 ng/kg per min, and from 50–100 ng/kg per min for treprostinil. The major problem with intravenous therapy is infection related to the venous catheter, which requires close monitoring and diligence on behalf of the patient.

Although most clinical trials have focused on patients with advanced symptoms, it is recommended that every patient diagnosed with PAH be treated (Fig. 40-2). Although no treatment has been demonstrated to be superior as first-line therapy, patients often prefer to initiate their treatment with an oral or inhaled form of therapy. In the trials using bosentan, sildenafil, and iloprost, full clinical benefit was generally manifest within the first 2 months of therapy. Patients who fail to adequately improve should have the treatment discontinued and started on a different therapy. Equally important is that delaying a more effective treatment may allow the disease to progress and become less responsive. The use of these drugs in combination has become popular, but there are no randomized clinical trials demonstrating beneficial effects in combination.

LUNG TRANSPLANTATION Lung transplantation is considered for patients who, while on an intravenous prostacyclin, continue to manifest right heart failure. Acceptable results have been achieved with heart-lung, bilateral lung, and single-lung transplant. The availability of donor organs often influences the choice of procedure.

CONDITIONS ASSOCIATED WITH PULMONARY HYPERTENSION

COLLAGEN VASCULAR DISEASE

All of the collagen vascular diseases may be associated with PAH. This complication occurs commonly with the CREST syndrome (calcinosis, Raynaud's phenomenon, esophageal involvement, sclerodactyly, and telangiectasia) and in scleroderma, and less frequently in systemic lupus erythematosus, Sjögren's syndrome, dermatomyositis, polymyositis, and rheumatoid arthritis. It is usual for these patients to have some element of coexistent interstitial pulmonary fibrosis even though it may not be apparent on chest x-ray, CT, or pulmonary function tests. Consequently, these patients tend to have hypoxemia as an important clinical feature, along with the other classic findings of pulmonary hypertension.

Treatment of these patients is identical to that of patients with IPAH (see earlier) but is less effective. The treatment of the pulmonary hypertension, however, does not affect the natural history of the underlying collagen vascular disease.

CONGENITAL SYSTEMIC TO PULMONARY SHUNTS

It is common for large post-tricuspid cardiac shunts (e.g., ventricular septal defect, patent ductus arteriosus) to produce severe PAH (Chap. 19). Although less common, it may also occur in pre-tricuspid shunts (e.g., atrial septal defect, anomalous pulmonary venous drainage). In patients with uncorrected shunts, the clinical features include those associated with right-to-left shunting such as hypoxemia and peripheral cyanosis, which worsen dramatically with exertion (Chap. 6). PAH may occur years or even decades after surgical correction of these lesions, in which case there will be no associated right-to-left shunting. These patients present similarly to patients with IPAH but tend to have better long-term survival. The treatments are similar to those for IPAH.

PORTAL HYPERTENSION

Portal hypertension is associated with PAH, but the mechanism remains unknown. Patients with advanced cirrhosis can have the combined features of a high-output cardiac state in association with the features of pulmonary hypertension and RV failure. Thus, a normal cardiac output may actually reflect a marked impairment of RV function. The etiology of ascites and edema can be confusing in these patients since it can have both cardiac and hepatic causes. Patients with mild pulmonary hypertension who have a favorable response to epoprostenol have undergone successful liver transplantation with improvement of the pulmonary vascular disease.

ANOREXIGENS

A causal relationship has been established between exposure to several anorexigens, including aminorex and the fenfluramines, and the development of PAH. Often the pulmonary hypertension will not develop until years after the last exposure. Although the clinical features are identical to those of IPAH, the patients appear to be less responsive to medical treatments and have a poorer prognosis.

PULMONARY VENOOCCLUSIVE DISEASE

Pulmonary venoocclusive disease is a rare and distinct pathologic entity found in <10% of patients who present with unexplained pulmonary hypertension. Histologically it is manifest by intimal proliferation and fibrosis of the intrapulmonary veins and venules, occasionally extending to the arteriolar bed. The pulmonary venous obstruction explains the increase in pulmonary capillary wedge pressure observed in patients with advanced disease. These patients may develop orthopnea that can mimic LV failure. The therapy of this condition is not established.

PULMONARY CAPILLARY HEMANGIOMATOSIS

Pulmonary capillary hemangiomatosis is a very rare form of pulmonary hypertension. Histologically it is characterized by the presence of infiltrating thin-walled blood vessels throughout the pulmonary interstitium and walls of the pulmonary arteries and veins. The presenting symptoms are usually those of IPAH but often with hemoptysis as a clinical feature. The diagnosis can be made with pulmonary angiography. The clinical course is usually one of progressive deterioration leading to death. There is no established therapy.

PULMONARY VENOUS HYPERTENSION

Pulmonary hypertension occurs as a result of increased resistance to pulmonary venous drainage. It is often associated with diastolic dysfunction of the left ventricle; diseases affecting the pericardium or mitral or aortic valves; or rare entities such as cor triatriatum, left atrial myxoma, extrinsic compression of the central pulmonary veins from fibrosing mediastinitis, and pulmonary venoocclusive disease. Pulmonary venous hypertension affects the pulmonary veins and venules, producing arterialization of the external elastic lamina, medial hypertrophy, and focal eccentric intimal fibrosis. Microcirculatory lesions include capillary congestion, focal alveolar edema, and dilatation of the interstitial lymphatics. Although these lesions are potentially reversible, regression may take years after the underlying cause is removed. In some patients pulmonary venous hypertension triggers reactive vasoconstriction in the pulmonary arterial bed and results in proliferative changes of the intima and media that can produce severe elevations in pulmonary artery pressure. Clinically it may be confusing and appear as if two separate disease processes are occurring simultaneously. The discrimination is important, however, as treatments that are effective in PAH may make patients with pulmonary venous hypertension worse.

LEFT VENTRICULAR DIASTOLIC DYSFUNCTION

Pulmonary hypertension as a result of LV diastolic failure is common but often unrecognized (Chap. 17). It can occur with or without LV systolic failure. The most common causes are hypertensive heart disease; coronary artery disease; or impaired LV compliance related to age, diabetes, obesity, and hypoxemia. Symptoms of orthopnea and paroxysmal nocturnal dyspnea are prominent. Many patients improve considerably if LV end-diastolic pressure is lowered.

MITRAL VALVE DISEASE

Mitral stenosis and mitral regurgitation represent important causes of pulmonary hypertension (Chap. 20). These patients often have reactive pulmonary vasoconstriction resulting in marked elevations in pulmonary artery pressures. An echocardiogram usually shows abnormalities such as thickened mitral valve leaflets with reduced mobility or severe mitral regurgitation documented by Doppler echocardiography (Chap. 12). At cardiac catheterization, a pressure gradient between the pulmonary capillary wedge pressure and LV end-diastolic pressure is diagnostic of mitral stenosis.

In patients with mitral stenosis, corrective surgery of the mitral valve or mitral balloon valvuloplasty predictably results in a reduction in pulmonary artery pressure and pulmonary vascular resistance. Patients with mitral regurgitation, however, may not have as dramatic a response from surgery due to persistent elevations in LV end-diastolic pressure.

PULMONARY HYPERTENSION ASSOCIATED WITH LUNG DISEASE AND HYPOXEMIA

The mechanism of hypoxic pulmonary vasoconstriction involves the inhibition of potassium currents and membrane depolarization of pulmonary vascular smooth muscle as a result of the change in membrane sulfhydryl redox status. Increased calcium entry into the vascular smooth-muscle cells mediates hypoxic pulmonary vasoconstriction. Pulmonary vascular remodeling in response to chronic hypoxia is also mediated by a reduction in nitric oxide production; an increase in endothelin 1; and increased expression of platelet-derived growth factors, vascular endothelial growth factor, and angiotensin II. Chronic hypoxia results in muscularization of the arterioles with minimal effects on the intima. When it occurs as an isolated entity, the changes produced are potentially reversible.

Although chronic hypoxia is an established cause of pulmonary hypertension, it rarely leads to an increase in the systolic pulmonary artery pressure >50 mmHg. Polycythemia in response to the hypoxemia is a characteristic finding. Hypoxia may also occur in conjunction with other causes of pulmonary hypertension associated with more extensive vascular changes. Clinically, the hypoxia tends to have an added adverse effect. Patients with chronic hypoxia who have a marked elevation in pulmonary pressure should be evaluated for other causes of the pulmonary hypertension.

CHRONIC OBSTRUCTIVE LUNG DISEASE

Chronic obstructive lung disease (COLD) is associated with mild pulmonary hypertension in the advanced stages. Pulmonary hypertension has been attributed to multiple factors, including hypoxic pulmonary vasoconstriction, acidemia, hypercapnia, the mechanical effects of high lung volume on pulmonary vessels, the loss of small vessels in the vascular bed, and regions of emphysematous lung destruction.

The presence of pulmonary hypertension in patients with COLD confers a worse outcome. The only effective therapy is supplemental oxygen. Several large clinical trials have documented that continuous oxygen therapy relieves some of the pulmonary vasoconstriction, relieves chronic ischemia throughout the systemic and pulmonary vascular beds, and improves survival. Long-term oxygen therapy is indicated if the resting arterial P_{O_2} remains <55 mmHg.

INTERSTITIAL LUNG DISEASE

Pulmonary hypertension from interstitial lung disease is often associated with obliteration of the pulmonary vascular bed by lung destruction and fibrosis. In addition, hypoxemia and pulmonary vasculopathy can be contributory factors. Interstitial lung disease is often associated with the collagen vascular diseases. A large number of patients have pulmonary fibrosis of unknown etiology. Patients are commonly older than 50 years and report an insidious onset of progressive dyspnea and cough for months to years. It is uncommon for the mean pulmonary artery pressure to exceed 40 mmHg. While none of the medical treatments developed for PAH have been shown to be effective in these patients, their use may worsen the hypoxemia.

SLEEP-DISORDERED BREATHING

The incidence of pulmonary hypertension in the setting of *obstructive sleep apnea*, a common condition, appears to be <20% and is generally mild. Some patients, however, present with severe pulmonary hypertension in conjunction with sleep apnea, which may or may not be related. It is recommended that the sleep apnea and the PAH be treated as coexisting problems.

ALVEOLAR HYPOVENTILATION

Pulmonary hypertension can occur in patients with chronic hypoventilation and hypoxia secondary to thoracovertebral deformities. Symptoms are slowly progressive and related to hypoxemia. In patients with advanced disease, intermittent positive-pressure breathing and supplemental oxygen have been used successfully.

Pulmonary hypertension secondary to hypoxemia has been reported in patients with neuromuscular disease as a result of generalized weakness of the respiratory muscles and in patients with diaphragmatic paralysis, generally a result of trauma to the phrenic nerve. Patients with nontraumatic bilateral diaphragmatic paralysis may go unrecognized until they present with either respiratory failure or pulmonary hypertension.

PULMONARY HYPERTENSION DUE TO THROMBOEMBOLIC DISEASE

CHRONIC THROMBOEMBOLIC PULMONARY HYPERTENSION

Patients appropriately treated for acute pulmonary thromboembolism with intravenous heparin and chronic oral warfarin therapy usually do not develop chronic pulmonary hypertension. However, some patients have impaired fibrinolytic resolution of the thromboembolism, which leads to organization and incomplete recanalization and chronic obstruction of the pulmonary vascular bed. The entity of chronic thromboembolic pulmonary hypertension has been well characterized and often mimics PAH. In many patients, the initial pulmonary thromboembolism was undetected or untreated. Many of these patients have underlying thrombophilic disorders, such as the lupus anticoagulant/anticardiolipin antibody syndrome, prothrombin gene mutation, or factor V Leiden.

Diagnosis

The physical examination is typical of pulmonary hypertension but may include bruits heard over areas of the lung, representing blood flow through vessels with partial occlusion. A perfusion lung scan or contrast-enhanced spiral CT scan usually reveals multiple thromboemboli. However, pulmonary angiography is necessary to determine the precise location and proximal extent of the thromboemboli, and hence the potential for operability.

Treatment:
℞ **CHRONIC THROMBOEMBOLIC PULMONARY HYPERTENSION**

Pulmonary thromboendarterectomy is an established surgical treatment in patients whose thrombi are accessible to surgical removal. The operative mortality is fairly high, at ~12% in experienced centers. Postoperative survivors who have a good result can expect to realize an improvement in functional class and exercise tolerance. Lifelong anticoagulation using warfarin is mandatory. Thrombolytic therapy is rarely of help in patients with chronic thromboembolic pulmonary hypertension and may expose these patients to the increased risk of bleeding without potential benefit.

SICKLE CELL DISEASE

Cardiovascular system abnormalities are prominent in the clinical spectrum of sickle cell disease, including pulmonary hypertension. The etiology is multifactorial, including hemolysis, impaired nitric oxide bioavailability, hypoxemia, thromboembolism, chronic high cardiac output, and chronic liver disease. Regardless of the mechanism(s), the presence of pulmonary hypertension in patients with sickle cell disease is associated with a higher morbidity and mortality. Intensification of sickle cell disease–specific therapy appears to reduce the morbidity. The use of drugs to treat pulmonary hypertension is under clinical trials, but their efficacy remains unknown.

OTHER DISORDERS DIRECTLY AFFECTING PULMONARY VASCULATURE

SARCOIDOSIS

Sarcoidosis can produce severe pulmonary hypertension as a result of chronic severe fibrocystic lung involvement, or direct cardiovascular involvement. Consequently, patients with sarcoidosis who present with progressive dyspnea and clinical features of pulmonary hypertension need a thorough evaluation. There is a subset of patients with sarcoidosis who present with severe pulmonary hypertension believed to be due to direct pulmonary vascular involvement. Many of these patients exhibit a favorable response to intravenous epoprostenol therapy.

SCHISTOSOMIASIS

Although extremely rare in North America, schistosomiasis is the most common cause of pulmonary hypertension worldwide. The development of pulmonary hypertension often occurs in the setting of hepatosplenic disease and portal hypertension. Schistosome ova can embolize from the liver to the lungs, where they result in an inflammatory pulmonary vascular reaction and chronic changes. The diagnosis is confirmed by finding the parasite ova in the urine or stools of patients with symptoms, which can be difficult. The efficacy of therapies directed toward pulmonary hypertension in these patients is unknown.

HIV INFECTION

The mechanism by which HIV infection produces pulmonary hypertension remains unknown. Although it is uncommon for HIV infection to result in pulmonary hypertension, the marked rise in the prevalence of HIV infection worldwide could have a significant impact on the frequency that these entities are seen in combination. The evaluation and treatments are identical to those for IPAH. Treatment of the HIV infection does not appear to affect the severity or natural history of the underlying pulmonary hypertension.

FURTHER READINGS

CONDLIFFE R: Connective tissue disease-associated pulmonary arterial hypertension in the modern treatment era. Am J Respir Crit Care Med 179:151, 2009

DILLER GP, GATZOULIS MA: Pulmonary vascular disease in adults with congenital heart disease. Circulation 115:1039, 2007

FARBER HW, LOSCALZO J: Pulmonary arterial hypertension. N Engl J Med 351:1655, 2004

GALIE N, RUBIN LJ (eds): Pulmonary arterial hypertension. Epidemiology, pathobiology, assessment and therapy. J Amer Coll Cardiol 43:supplement S, 2004

HUMBERT M et al: Treatment of pulmonary arterial hypertension. N Engl J Med 351:1425, 2004

MACCHIA A: A meta-analysis of trials of pulmonary hypertension: A clinical condition looking for drugs and research methodology. Am Heart J 153:1037, 2007

MCLAUGHLIN VV: ACCF/AHA Expert consensus document on pulmonary hypertension. J Am Coll Cardiol 53:1573, 2009

PENALOZA D, ARIAS-STELLA J: The heart and pulmonary circulation at high altitudes: Healthy highlanders and chronic mountain sickness. Circulation 115:1132, 2007

RABINOVITCH M: Molecular pathogenesis of pulmonary arterial hypertension. J Clin Invest 118:2372, 2008

RAVIPATI G et al: Type 5 phosphodiesterase inhibitors in the treatment of erectile dysfunction and cardiovascular disease. Cardiol Rev 15:76, 2007

RICH S, MCLAUGHLIN VV: Pulmonary hypertension, in Braunwald's Heart Disease: A Textbook of Cardiovascular Medicine, 8th ed, P Libby et al (eds). Philadelphia, Elsevier Saunders, 2008

RICHTER A et al: Impaired transforming growth factor-beta signaling in idiopathic pulmonary arterial hypertension. Am J Respir Crit Care Med 170:1340, 2004

SITBON O et al: Long term response to calcium channel blockers in idiopathic pulmonary arterial hypertension. Circulation 111:3105, 2005

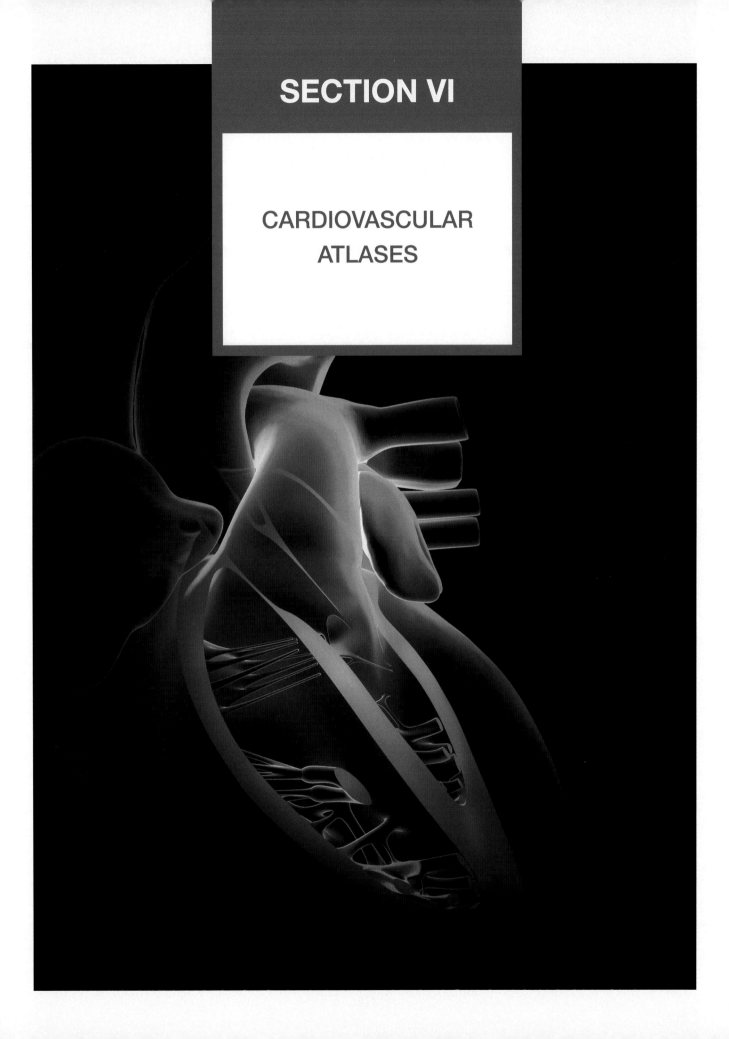

SECTION VI

CARDIOVASCULAR ATLASES

CHAPTER 41
ATLAS OF ELECTROCARDIOGRAPHY

Ary L. Goldberger

The electrocardiograms (ECGs) in this Atlas supplement those illustrated in Chap. 11. The interpretations emphasize findings of specific teaching value.

All of the figures are from ECG Wave-Maven, Copyright 2003, Beth Israel Deaconess Medical Center, Available at http://ecg.bidmc.harvard.edu. Case numbers are given in parentheses.

The abbreviations used in this chapter are as follows:

AF	atrial fibrillation
HCM	hypertrophic cardiomyopathy
LVH	left ventricular hypertrophy
MI	myocardial infarction
NSR	normal sinus rhythm
RBBB	right bundle branch block
RV	right ventricular
RVH	right ventricular hypertrophy

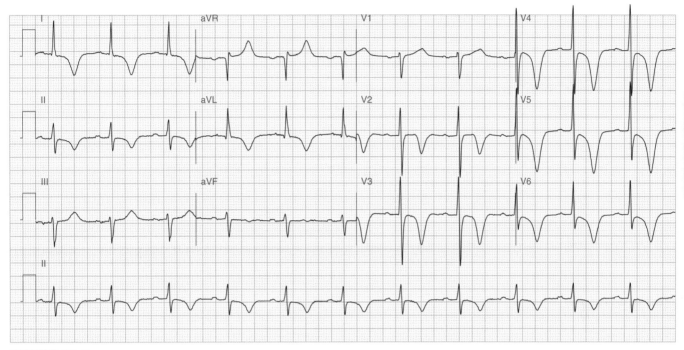

FIGURE 41-1
Anterior wall ischemia (deep T-wave inversions and ST-segment depressions in I, aVL, V_3–V_6) in a patient with **LVH** (increased voltage in V_2–V_5). (Case 11)

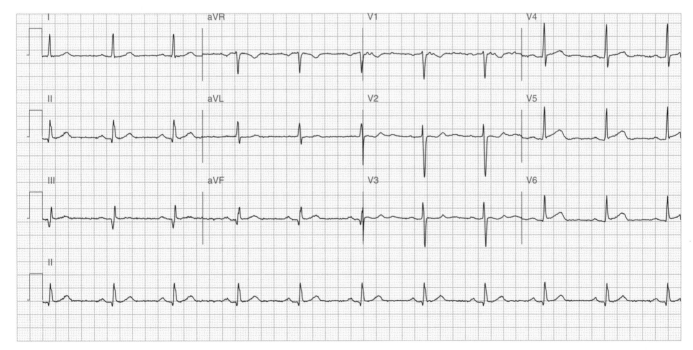

FIGURE 41-2
Acute anterolateral wall ischemia with ST elevations in V_4–V_6. Probable old inferior MI with Q waves in leads II, III and aVF. (Case 39)

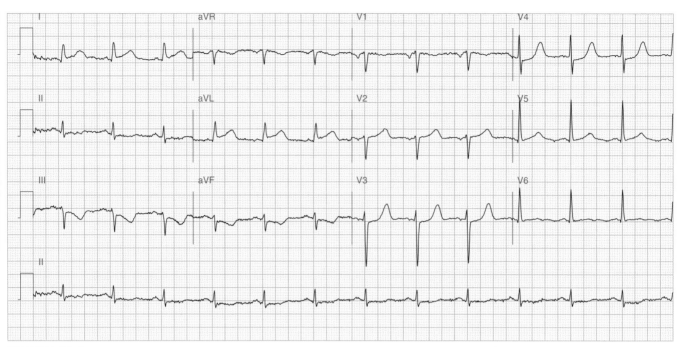

FIGURE 41-3

Acute lateral ischemia with ST elevations in I and aVL with probable reciprocal ST depressions inferiorly (II, III, and aVF). Ischemic ST depressions also in V₃ and V₄. **Left atrial abnormality.** (Case 72)

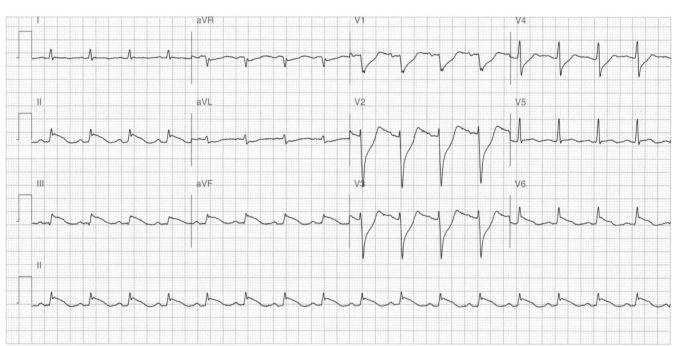

FIGURE 41-4

Sinus tachycardia. Marked ischemic ST-segment elevations in inferior limb leads (II, III, aVF) and laterally (V₆) suggestive of **acute inferolateral MI,** and prominent ST-segment depressions with upright T waves in V₁–V₄ consistent with **acute posterior MI.** (Case 208)

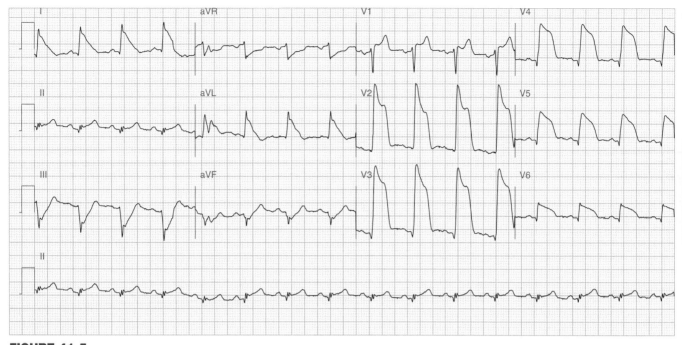

FIGURE 41-5

Acute MI with marked ST elevations in I, aVL, V$_1$–V$_6$ and small pathologic Q waves in V$_3$–V$_6$. Marked reciprocal ST-segment depressions in III and aVF. (Case 37)

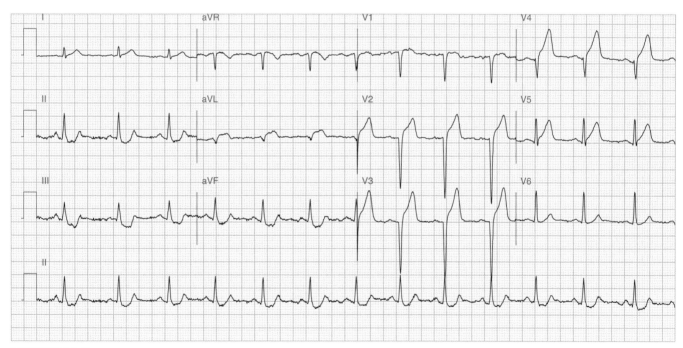

FIGURE 41-6

Acute anterior wall MI with ST elevations and Q waves in V$_1$–V$_4$ and aVL and reciprocal inferior ST depressions. (Case 86)

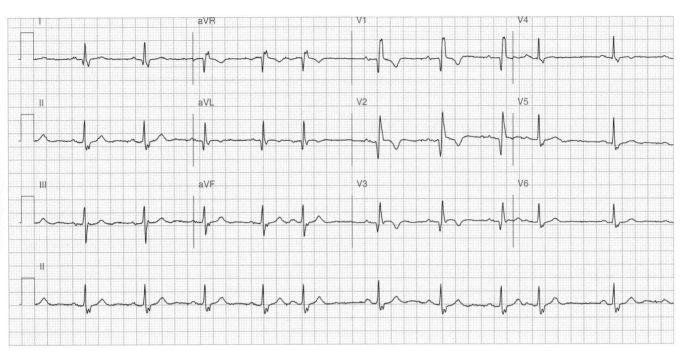

FIGURE 41-7

NSR with premature atrial complexes. **RBBB;** pathologic Q waves and ST elevation due to **acute anterior/septal MI** in V1–V3. (Case 63)

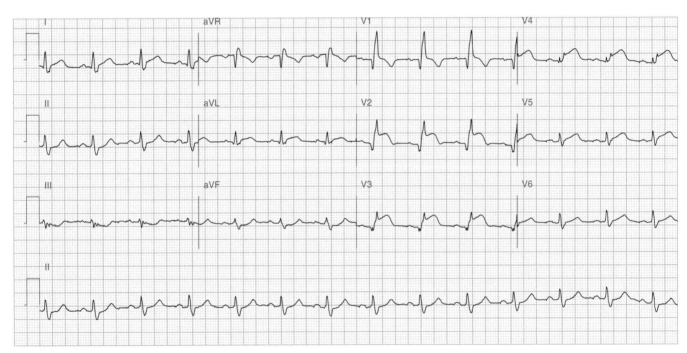

FIGURE 41-8

Acute anteroseptal MI (Q waves and ST elevations in V_1–V_4) with **RBBB** (see I, V_1). (Case 20)

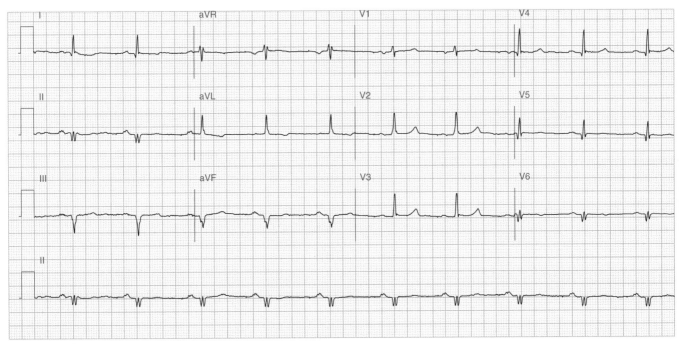

FIGURE 41-9

Extensive old MI involving inferior-posterior-lateral wall (Q waves in leads II, III, aVF, tall R waves in V₁, V₂, and Q waves in V₅, V₆). T-wave abnormalities in leads I and aVL, V₅, and V₆. (Case 33)

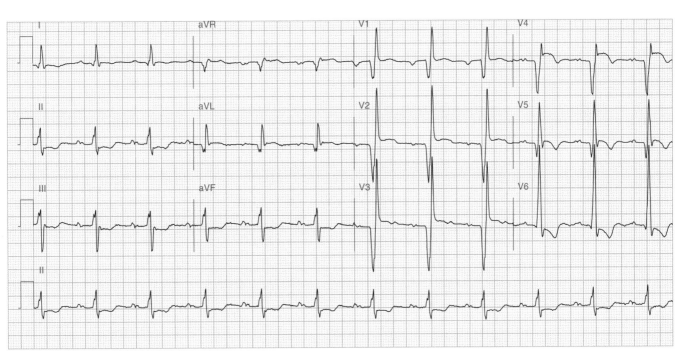

FIGURE 41-10

NSR with PR prolongation ("1st degree AV block"), left atrial abnormality, LVH, and RBBB. Pathologic Q waves in V₁–V₅ and aVL with ST elevations (a chronic finding in this patient). Findings compatible with **old anterolateral MI and LV aneurysm.** (Case 49)

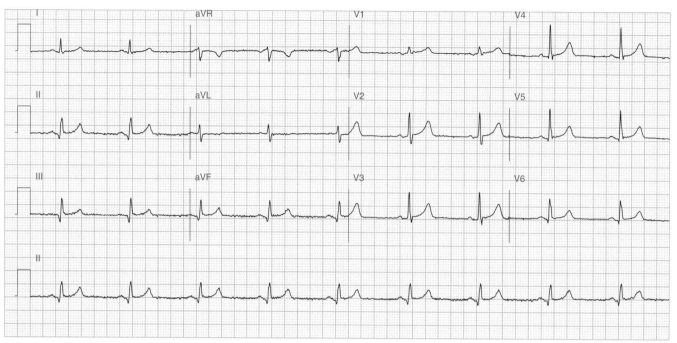

FIGURE 41-11

Old inferior-posterior MI. Wide (0.04 s) Q waves in the inferior leads (II, III, aVF); broad R wave in V_1 (a Q wave equivalent). Absence of right-axis deviation and the presence of upright T waves in V_1–V_2 are also against RVH. (Case 141)

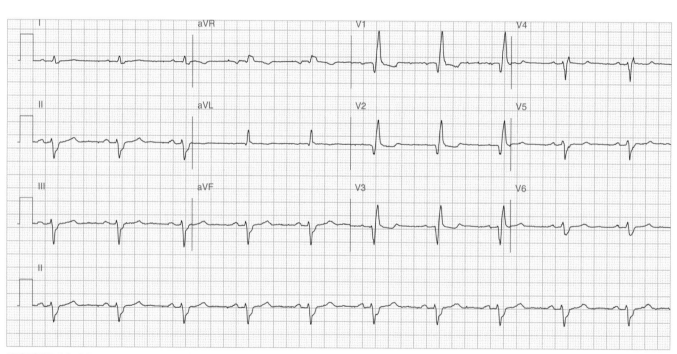

FIGURE 41-12

NSR with RBBB (broad terminal R wave in V_1) and left anterior hemiblock, pathologic anterior Q waves in V_1–V_3 with slow R wave progression. Patient had **severe multivessel coronary artery disease** with echocardiogram showing septal dyskinesis and apical akinesis. (Case 28)

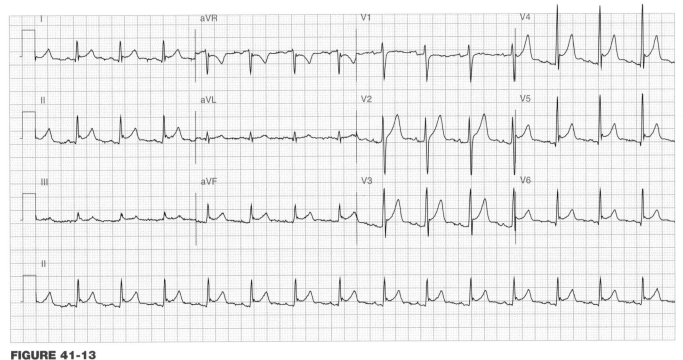

FIGURE 41-13
Acute pericarditis with diffuse ST elevations in I, II, III, aVF, V$_3$–V$_6$, without T-wave inversions. Also PR-segment elevation in aVR and PR depression in the inferolateral leads. (Case 3)

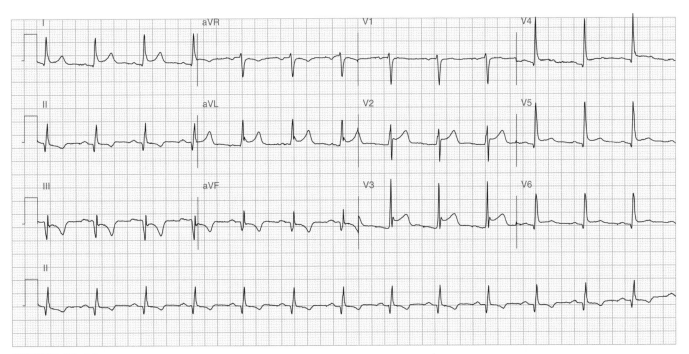

FIGURE 41-14
Sinus tachycardia; diffuse ST elevations (I, II, aVL, aVF, V$_2$–V$_6$) with associated PR deviations (elevated PR in aVR; depressed in V$_4$–V$_6$); borderline low voltage. Q-wave and T-wave inversions in II, III, and aVF. Diagnosis is **acute pericarditis with inferior Q wave MI.** (Case 34)

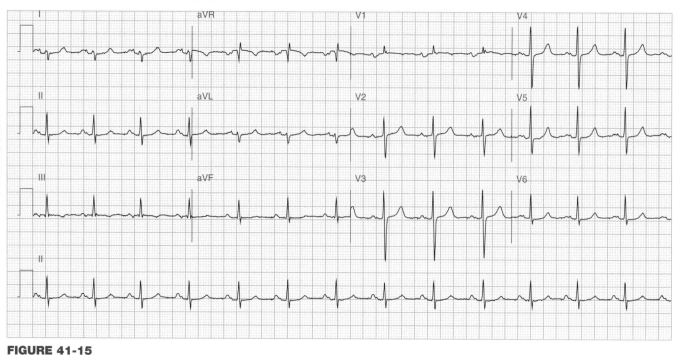

FIGURE 41-15

NSR, left atrial abnormality (see I, II, V₁), right-axis deviation and RVH (Rr' in V₁) in a patient with **mitral stenosis.** (Case 13)

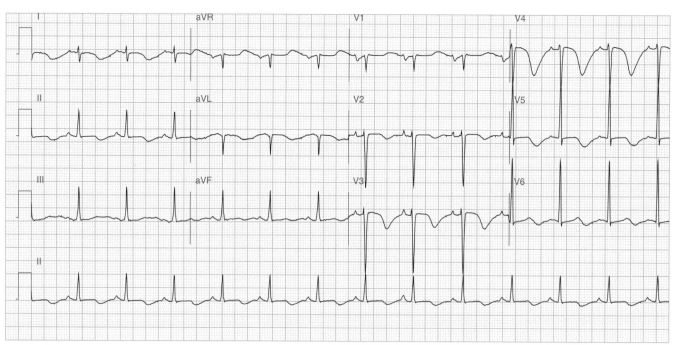

FIGURE 41-16

NSR, left atrial abnormality, and LVH by voltage criteria with borderline right-axis deviation in a patient with **mixed mitral stenosis** (left atrial abnormality and right-axis deviation) and **mitral regurgitation** (LVH). Prominent precordial T-wave inversions and QT prolongation also present. (Case 113)

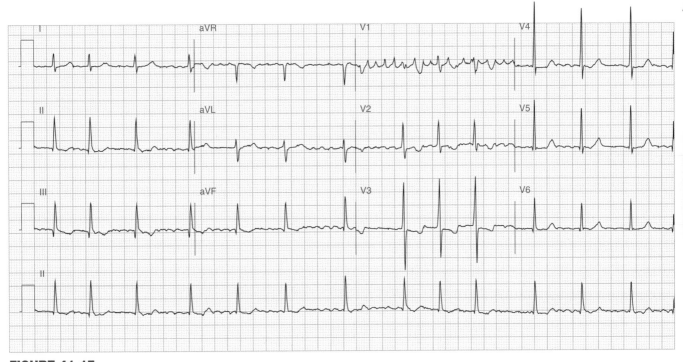

FIGURE 41-17

Coarse AF, tall R in V_2 with vertical QRS axis (positive R in aVF) indicating RVH. Tall R in V_4 may be due to concomitant LVH. Patient had **severe mitral stenosis with moderate mitral regurgitation.** (Case 85)

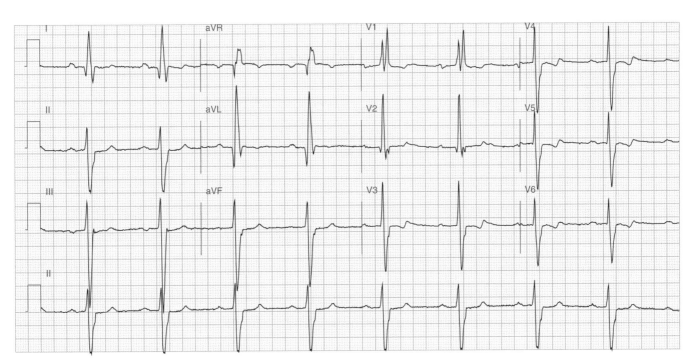

FIGURE 41-18

NSR; first-degree A-V block (P-R prolongation); LVH (tall R in aVL); RBBB (Rr') and left anterior fascicular block in a patient with **HCM.** Deep Q waves in I and aVL consistent with **septal hypertrophy.** (Case 17)

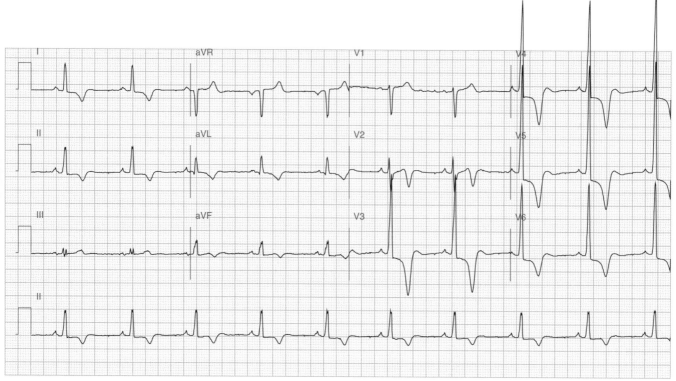

FIGURE 41-19

LVH with deep T-wave inversions in limb leads and precordial leads. Striking T-wave inversions in mid-precordial leads suggest **apical HCM.** (Case 14)

PULMONARY EMBOLISM AND CHRONIC PULMONARY HYPERTENSION

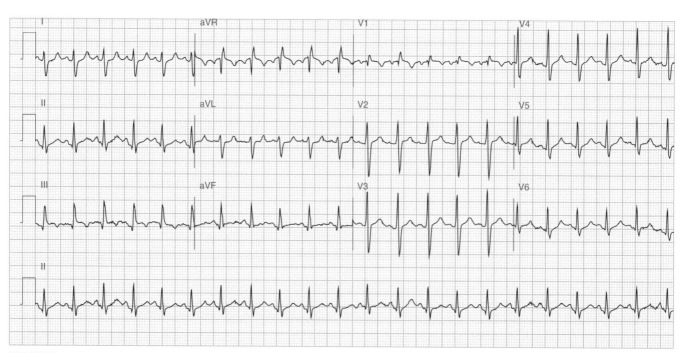

FIGURE 41-20

Sinus tachycardia with S1Q3T3 pattern (T-wave inversion in III), incomplete RBBB, and right precordial T-wave inversions consistent with acute RV overload in a patient with **pulmonary emboli.** (Case 77)

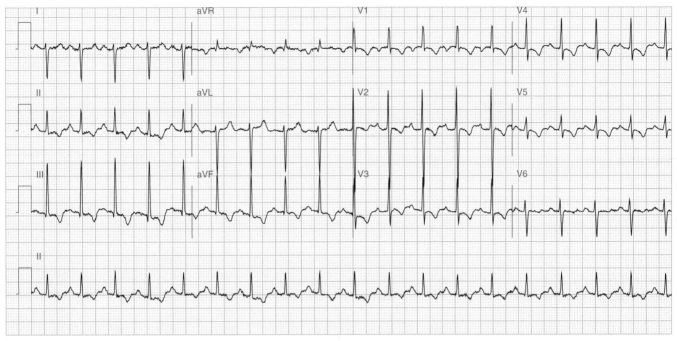

FIGURE 41-21

Sinus tachycardia, right-axis deviation, RVH with tall R in V₁ and deep S in V₆ and inverted T waves in II, III, aVF, and V₁–V₅ in a patient with **atrial septal defect and severe pulmonary hypertension.** (Case 168)

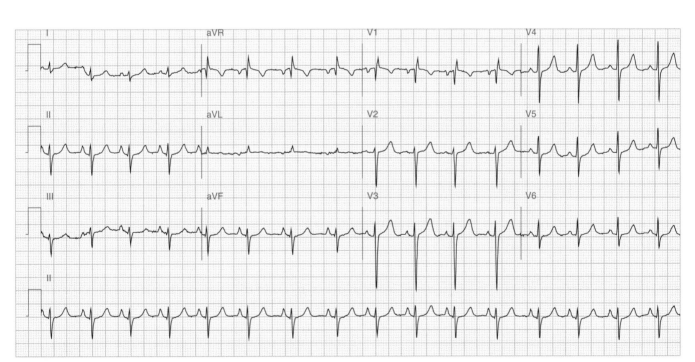

FIGURE 41-22

Signs of right atrial/RV overload in a patient with **chronic obstructive lung disease:** (1) peaked P waves in II; (2) QR in V₁ with narrow QRS; (3) delayed precordial transition, with terminal S waves in V₅/V₆; (4) superior axis deviation with an S₁-S₂-S₃ pattern. (Case 133)

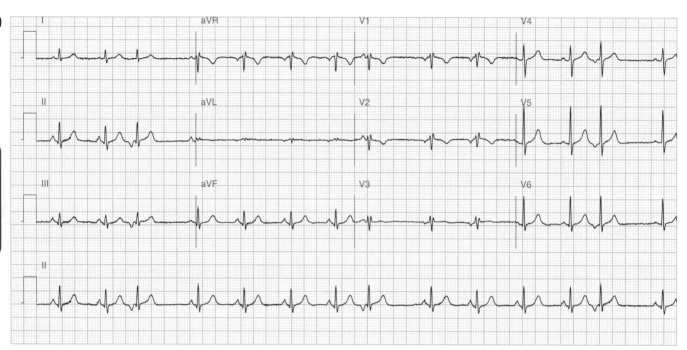

FIGURE 41-23

(1) Low voltage; (2) incomplete RBBB (rsr' in V_1–V_3); (3) borderline peaked P waves in lead II with vertical P-wave axis (probable right atrial overload); (4) slow R-wave progression in V_1–V_3; (5) prominent S waves in V_6; and (6) atrial premature beats. This combination is seen typically in **severe chronic obstructive lung disease.** (Case 125)

ELECTROLYTE DISORDERS

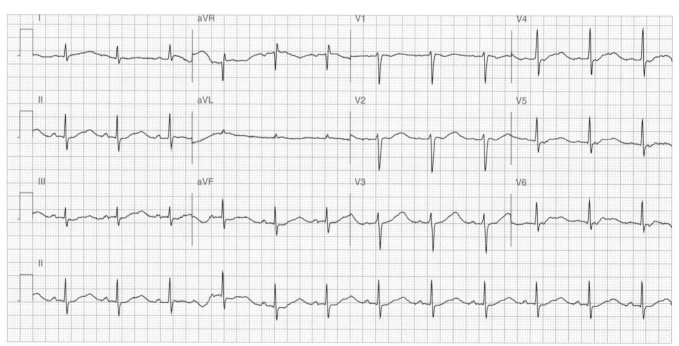

FIGURE 41-24

Prominent U waves (II, III, V_4–V_6) with Q-TU prolongation in a patient with **severe hypokalemia.** (Case 44)

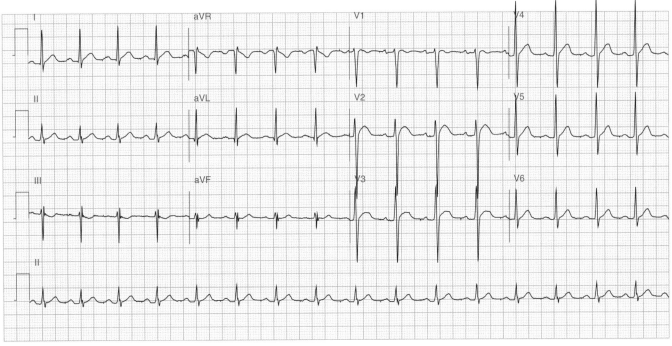

FIGURE 41-25

Abbreviated ST segment such that the T wave looks like it takes off directly from QRS in some leads (I, V₄, aVL, and V₅) in a patient with **hypercalcemia.** High take-off of ST segment in V₂/V₃. (Case 67)

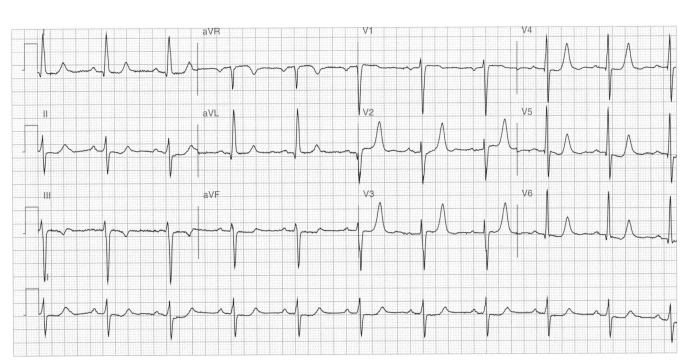

FIGURE 41-26

NSR with LVH, left atrial abnormality, and tall peaked T waves in the precordial leads with inferolateral ST depressions (II, III, aVF, and V₆); left anterior fascicular block and borderline prolonged QT interval in a patient with **renal failure, hypertension, and hyperkalemia;** prolonged QT is secondary to **associated hypocalcemia.** (Case 26)

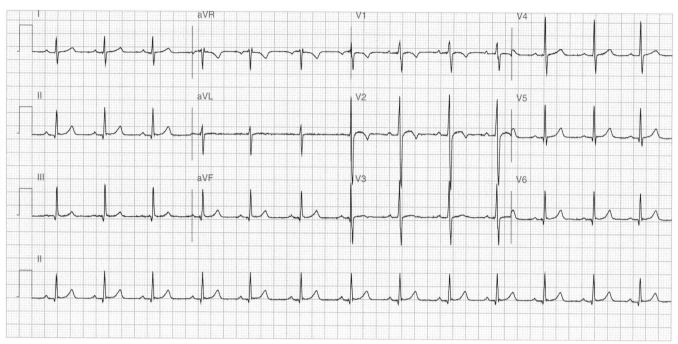

FIGURE 41-27

Normal ECG in an 11-year-old male. T-wave inversions in V_1–V_2. Vertical QRS axis (+90°) and early precordial transition between V_2 and V_3 are **normal findings in children.** (Case 107)

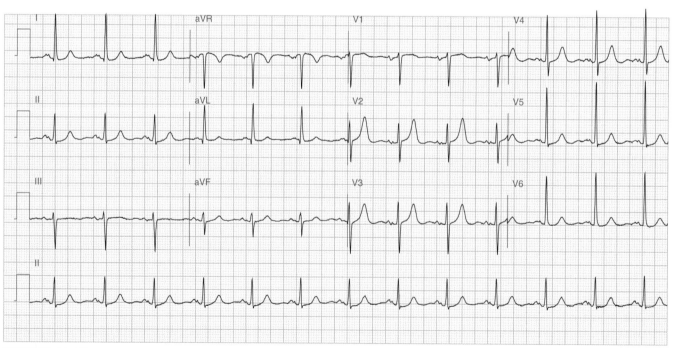

FIGURE 41-28

Left atrial abnormality and **LVH** in a patient with **long-standing hypertension.** (Case 225)

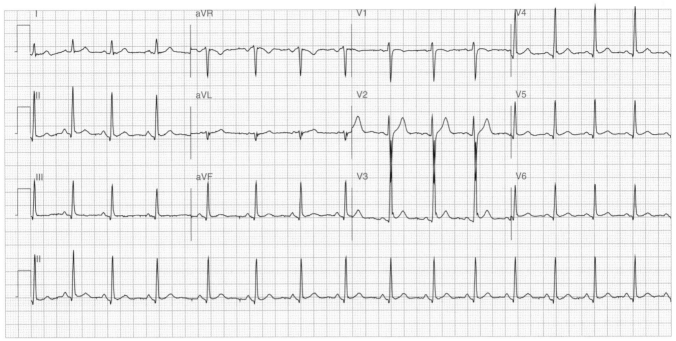

FIGURE 41-29

Normal variant ST-segment elevations in a healthy 21-year-old male (commonly referred to as *early repolarization pattern*). ST elevations exhibit upward concavity and are most apparent in V_3 and V_4. Precordial QRS voltages are prominent, but within normal limits for a young adult. No evidence of left atrial abnormality or ST depression/T wave inversions to go along with **LVH.** (Case 130)

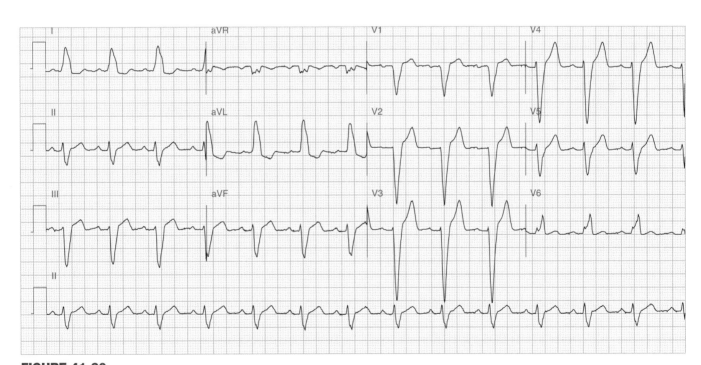

FIGURE 41-30

NSR with first-degree AV block (PR interval = 0.24 s), and complete **left bundle branch block.** (Case 151)

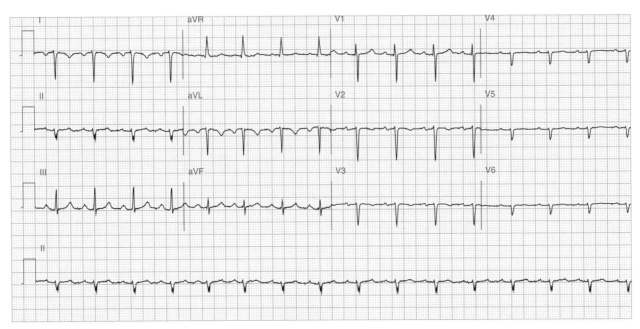

FIGURE 41-31

Dextrocardia with: (1) inverted P waves in I and aVL; (2) negative QRS complex and T wave in I; and (3) progressively decreasing voltage across the precordium. (Case 19)

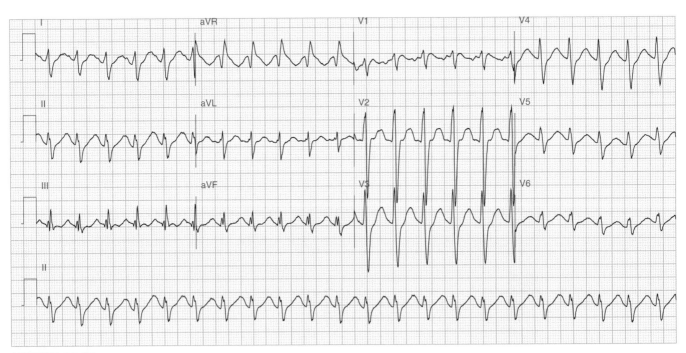

FIGURE 41-32

Sinus tachycardia; intraventricular conduction delay with a rightward QRS axis. QT interval is prolonged for the rate. The triad of sinus tachycardia, a wide QRS complex, and a long QT suggest **tricyclic antidepressant overdose.** Terminal S wave (rS) in I, and terminal R wave (qR) in aVR are also seen in this condition. (Case 100)

CHAPTER 42

ATLAS OF NONINVASIVE CARDIAC IMAGING

Rick A. Nishimura ■ Raymond J. Gibbons
■ James F. Glockner ■ A. Jamil Tajik

Noninvasive cardiac imaging is essential to the diagnosis and management of patients with known or suspected cardiovascular disease. Chapter 12 describes the principles and clinical applications of these important techniques. This atlas supplements Chap. 12. It provides additional static images.

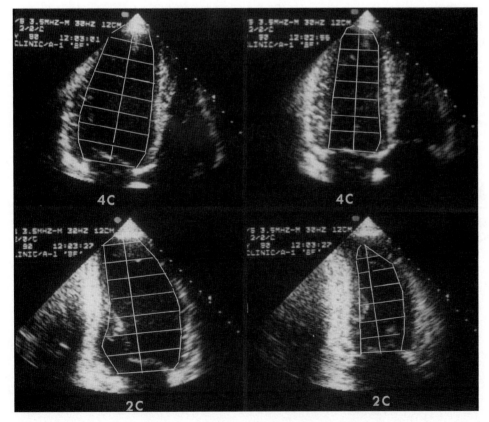

FIGURE 42-1

Still frame images of an echocardiogram in diastole *(left)* and systole *(right)*. Apical four-chamber view *(top)* and apical two-chamber view *(bottom)* comprise two orthogonal views. This illustrates the quantitative assessment of ejection fraction. The endocardial area is outlined and is used for calculation of ejection fraction.

With quantitative two-dimensional echocardiography, endocardial outlines of the left ventricle (LV) cavity are traced in systole and diastole and the LV cavity areas are then fitted to computer models of the LV to obtain systolic and diastolic volumes. The presence or absence of regional wall motion abnormalities can be assessed by examining endocardial motion as well as wall thickening.

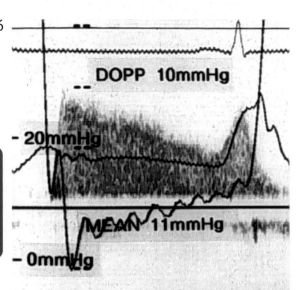

FIGURE 42-2

Continuous wave Doppler (DOPP) echocardiographic tracings across the mitral valve in a patient with mitral stenosis with simultaneous pressures in the left atrium (LA) and left ventricle (LV). The velocity of flow is high in early diastole, followed by a prolonged deceleration of transmitral mitral flow velocity, and a reacceleration during atrial systole (A). There is a mean gradient of 10 mmHg derived from the Doppler tracing, which corresponds to the simultaneous transmitral gradient of 11 mmHg derived from cardiac catheterization. These are consistent with the diagnosis of moderate mitral stenosis. LA, left atrial pressure; LV, left ventricular pressure; a, atrial contraction wave. *(From RA Nishimura et al: J Am Coll Cardiol 24:152, 1994.)*

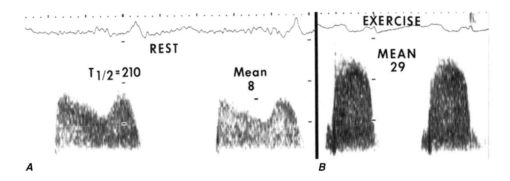

FIGURE 42-3

Continuous-wave Doppler echocardiogram across the mitral valve of a patient with mitral stenosis. In the resting state (**A**) there is a mean gradient of 8 mmHg. During exercise (**B**), the mean gradient rises to 29 mmHg, indicating hemodynamically significant mitral stenosis.

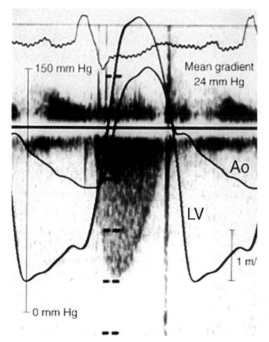

FIGURE 42-4

Continuous-wave Doppler tracings across the aortic valve in a patient with aortic stenosis. There is an increase in velocity to 3 m/s, with a mean transvalvular gradient calculated to be 24 mmHg. This corresponds to the simultaneous catheterization gradient of 24 mmHg between left ventricle (LV) and aorta (Ao).

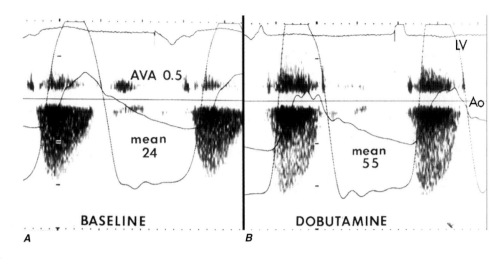

FIGURE 42-5

Continuous-wave Doppler echocardiogram across the aortic valve in a patient with low output–low gradient aortic stenosis and a reduced ejection fraction. **A.** At baseline, there is a mean left ventricular (LV)-aortic (Ao) gradient of 24 mmHg (by Doppler) with a calculated aortic valve area (AVA) of 0.5 cm². This presents a diagnostic dilemma as the reduced aortic valve area may be due to either critical aortic stenosis and secondary LV dysfunction or a low-output state, in which there is not enough force to open fully a mildly stenotic aortic valve. **B.** During dobutamine infusion, there is an increase in the transvalvular pressure gradient to 55 mmHg, with normalization of the stroke volume. This indicates the presence of severe aortic stenosis.

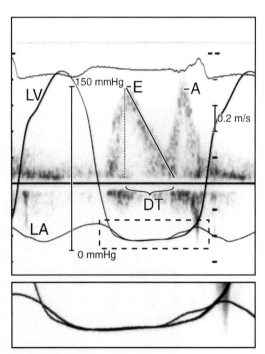

FIGURE 42-7

Pulsed-wave Doppler tracings of the mitral valve inflow velocities superimposed on left atrial (LA) and left ventricular (LV) pressures. The initial (early diastolic) velocity of mitral inflow (E) correlates with the driving pressure across the mitral valve. The deceleration time (DT) indicates the relative change in LA and LV pressures as blood begins to fill the LV. This increases LV pressure, which rises to meet the LA pressure. The A velocity on the mitral flow velocity curve is a reacceleration of flow due to atrial contraction. Normally, the E velocity exceeds the A velocity. In this patient, they are equal, suggestive of mild diastolic dysfunction (see Fig. 42-8).

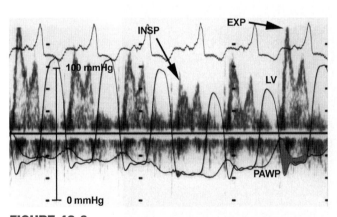

FIGURE 42-6

Pulsed-wave Doppler echocardiogram of transmitral flow recorded simultaneously with pulmonary artery wedge pressure (PAWP) and left ventricular (LV) pressure in a patient with constrictive pericarditis. There is a dissociation of intrathoracic and intracardiac pressures so that the PAWP has a larger inspiratory (INSP) fall than the LV pressure, causing a decrease in the driving force across the mitral valve. This results in a fall in the transmitral flow velocity. The opposite occurs during expiration (EXP).

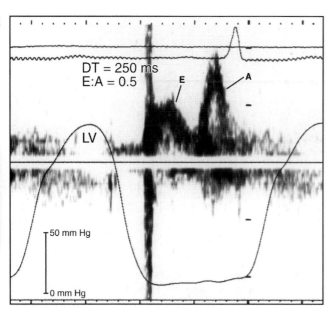

FIGURE 42-8

High-fidelity left ventricular (LV) pressure curve superimposed on a mitral inflow velocity curve obtained by Doppler echocardiography in a patient with stage I diastolic dysfunction. There is a decrease in the early diastolic filling and an increase with filling at atrial contraction, resulting in a low E:A ratio and prolonged deceleration time (DT). The LV diastolic pressure is normal at 12 mmHg.

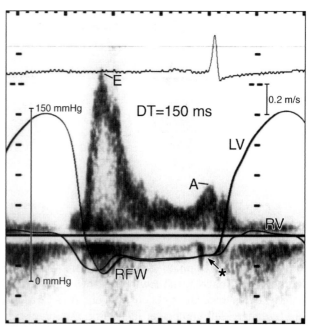

FIGURE 42-9

High-fidelity left ventricular (LV) and right ventricular (RV) pressure tracings superimposed on a Doppler mitral inflow velocity tracing in a patient with stage III diastolic dysfunction. There is a restriction to filling, in which there is a high early diastolic velocity [rapid filling wave (RFW)] and low velocity of atrial contraction resulting in a high E:A ratio with a short (150 ms) deceleration time (DT). Both ventricular diastolic pressures (*) are elevated.

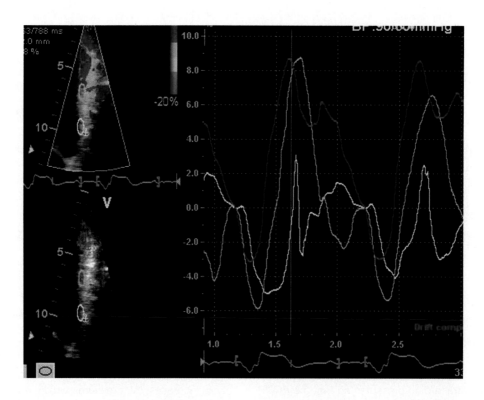

FIGURE 42-10

Strain rate images from a patient with severe left ventricular dysfunction illustrating dyssynchronous contraction.

Strain rate is a measure of regional deformation (or contraction). Strain rates can be used to examine the degree of dyssynchronous contraction of the ventricle, which may help in determining patients who would benefit from biventricular pacing. Shown are the different strain rates over time of the basal septum (yellow line), mid septum (blue line), and apical septum (red line).

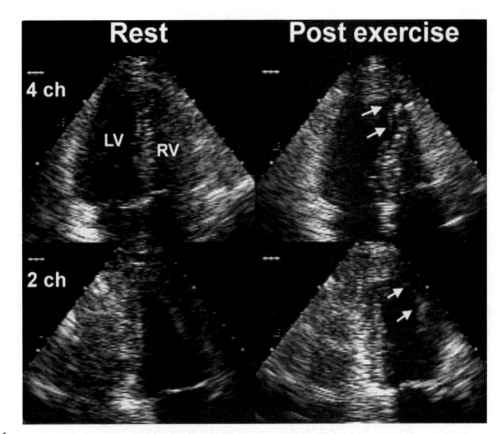

FIGURE 42-11

Still frame images demonstrating regional wall motion abnormalities during an exercise echocardiogram in a patient with known coronary artery disease. *Left.* The systolic frames in the resting state show symmetric contraction of all segments of the myocardium. The upper frame is from the apical four-chamber view and the lower frame is from the apical two-chamber view. *Right.* The systolic frames immediately after exercise show regional wall motion abnormalities in the anterior and apical segments (*arrows*). LV, left ventricle; RV, right ventricle *(From JK Oh et al: The Echo Manual, 2d ed. Philadelphia, Lippincott Williams & Wilkins, 1999, with permission.)*

Planar anterior stress

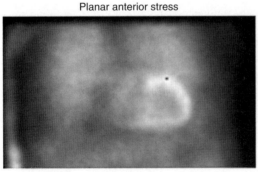

Increased

Planar anterior stress

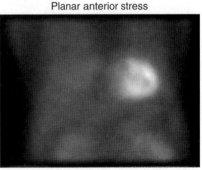

Normal

FIGURE 42-12

Anterior planar thallium images following stress, showing increased lung uptake on the left (count intensity in lung >50% of that in myocardium) and normal lung uptake on the right (count intensity in lung <50% of that in myocardium).

Increased lung uptake of thallium may be seen immediately after stress. It reflects increased pulmonary capillary wedge pressure and occurs in the presence of severe coronary artery disease and/or left ventricular dysfunction. It provides important adverse prognostic information that is incremental to other clinical, stress, and coronary angiographic variables.

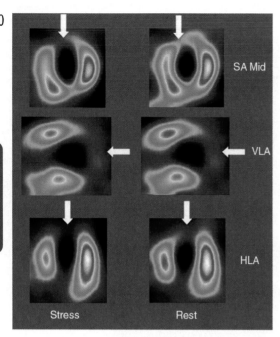

SA Mid

VLA

HLA

Stress   Rest

FIGURE 42-13

Adenosine ^{99m}Tc sestamibi scan in a 50-year-old male with a previous anterior infarct. The stress images (***left***) show a large defect involving the apex and anterior walls (*white arrows*) with little change from the rest images (*white arrows*), signifying a fixed defect without further ischemia during stress. SA, short axis in the middle of the left ventricle; VLA, vertical long axis; HLA, horizontal long axis.

The relative advantages of ^{201}Tl and 99^{m}Tc are detailed in Table 42-1. The better image quality and assessment of ventricular function permitted by ^{99m}Tc compounds have contributed to their more common use for stress imaging, although both ^{201}Tl- and ^{99m}Tc-labeled compounds provide clinically useful myocardial perfusion images in the majority of patients. A "dual-isotope" protocol is employed in some centers. This uses ^{201}Tl for the initial rest image and a ^{99m}Tc-labeled compound for the subsequent stress image, primarily for patient and scheduling convenience.

TABLE 42-1

RELATIVE ADVANTAGES OF THALLIUM 201 AND TECHNETIUM 99m
Thallium
Lower radiopharmaceutical cost Measurement of increased pulmonary uptake Less hepatobiliary and bowel uptake Detection of resting ischemia (hibernating myocardium)
Technetium
Better image quality (particularly in obese patients) Ventricular function assessment (gated SPECT) Shorter imaging time Shorter imaging protocols (patient/scheduling convenience) Acute imaging in myocardial infarction and unstable angina Superior quantification
SPECT, single photon emission computed tomography.

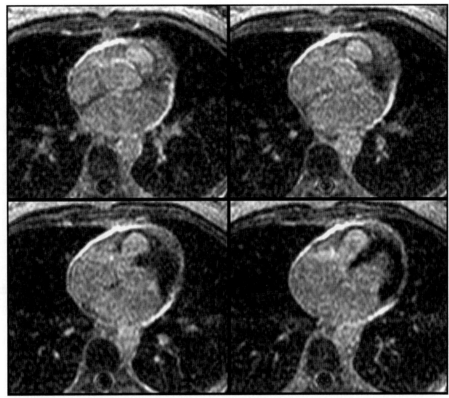

FIGURE 42-14
MR images with contrast enhancement of a patient with constrictive pericarditis, demonstrating abnormal pericardial thickening.

Top

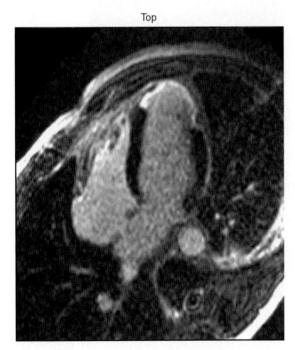

FIGURE 42-15
MR scan with delayed enhancement of a patient with an apical left ventricular infarction (*top*). Imaging the heart 10–20 min after gadolinium injection demonstrates enhancement of the infarcted tissue (visible as dense white image), as the tissue retains contrast by virtue of its large extracellular volume.

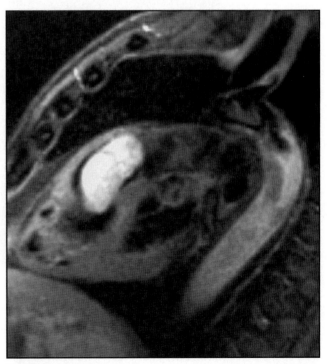

FIGURE 42-16
MR image of a patient with a right ventricular myxoma, which is shown as a bright oblong structure in the right ventricular outflow tract.

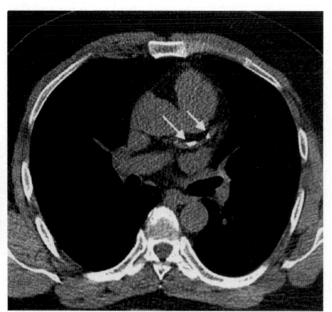

FIGURE 42-17

Noncontrast image from electron beam CT revealing two small foci of calcification in the left anterior descending artery (*arrows*).

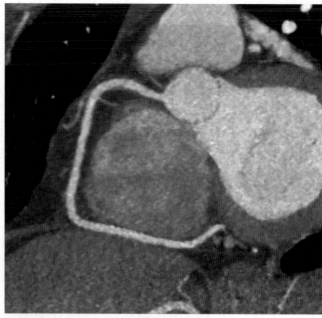

FIGURE 42-18

CT coronary angiogram showing a normal right coronary artery.

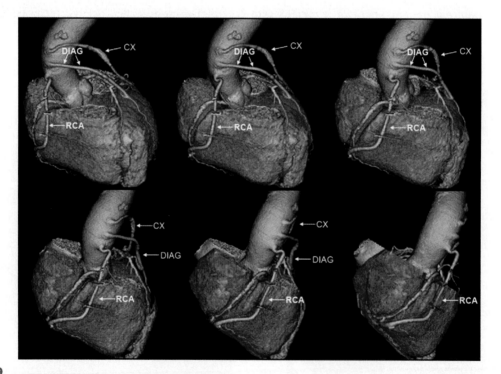

FIGURE 42-19

Three-dimensional reconstruction of a CT angiogram demonstrating three saphenous vein coronary artery bypass grafts in different views. In the upper left panel is an anterior-posterior view of the heart and grafts. The heart is sequentially rotated clockwise in the panels going from left to right to illustrate the ability of CT angiography to visualize the saphenous vein grafts. RCA, saphenous vein graft to the right coronary artery; CX, saphenous vein graft to the circumflex artery; DIAG, saphenous vein graft to the diagonal artery.

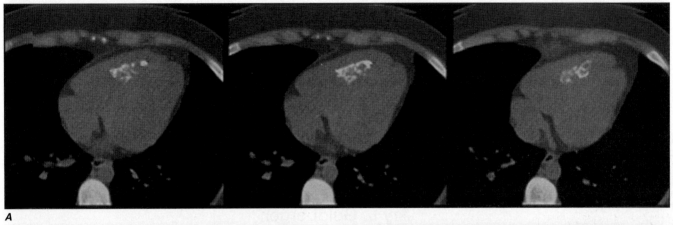

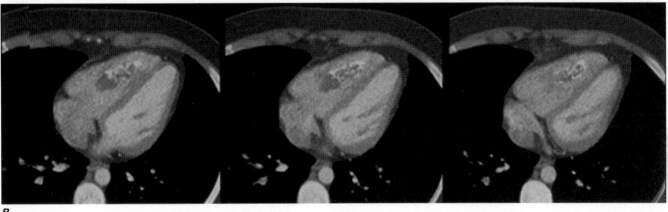

FIGURE 42-20
Cardiac CT images demonstrating a calcified mass in the right ventricle, which at pathologic examination was a chronic thrombus. Calcification is seen as a bright signal in both the noncontrast (**A**) and contrast-enhanced (**B**) images.

CHAPTER 43

ATLAS OF CARDIAC ARRHYTHMIAS

Ary L. Goldberger

The electrocardiograms in this atlas supplement those illustrated in Chaps. 15 and 16. The interpretations emphasize findings of specific teaching value.

All of the figures are from ECG Wave-Maven, Copyright 2003, Beth Israel Deaconess Medical Center, *http://ecg.bidmc.harvard.edu*. Case numbers are given in parentheses.

The abbreviations used in this chapter are as follows:

AF	atrial fibrillation
AV	atrioventricular
AVRT	atrioventricular reentrant tachycardia
LBBB	left bundle branch block
LV	left ventricular
LVH	left ventricular hypertrophy
MI	myocardial infarction
NSR	normal sinus rhythm
RBBB	right bundle branch block
VT	ventricular tachycardia
WPW	Wolff-Parkinson-White

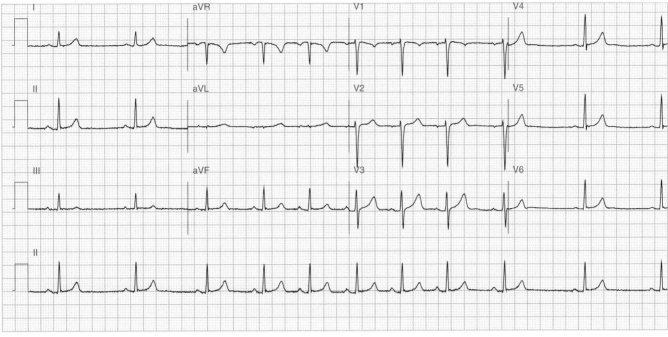

FIGURE 43-1

Respiratory sinus arrhythmias, a physiologic finding in a healthy young woman. The rate of the sinus pacemaker is slow at the beginning of the strip during expiration, then accelerates during inspiration and slows again with expiration. (Case 245)

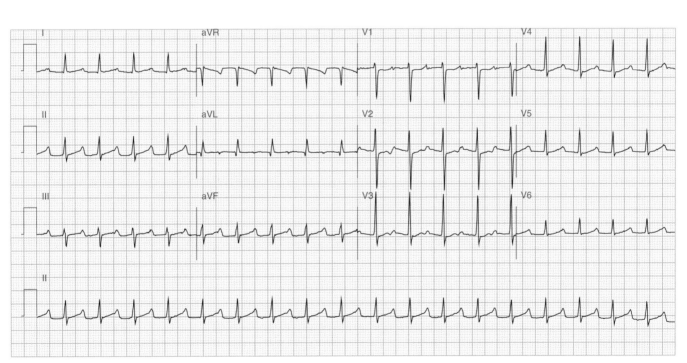

FIGURE 43-2

Sinus tachycardia (110/min) with first-degree AV block (PR interval = 0.28 s). The P wave is visible after the ST-T wave in V_1–V_3. Atrial tachycardia may produce a similar pattern. (Case 262)

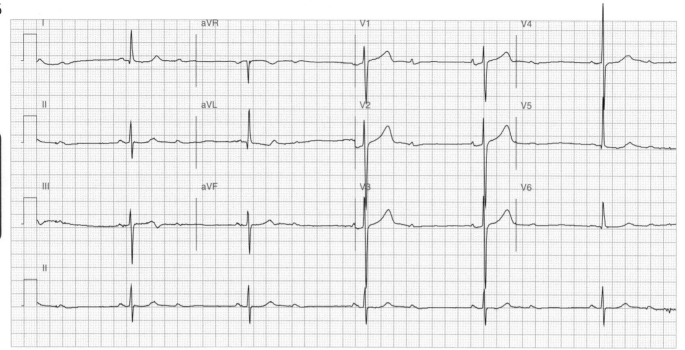

FIGURE 43-3
Sinus rhythm (pulse rate about 62/min) with 2:1 AV block causing marked bradycardia. (Case 5)

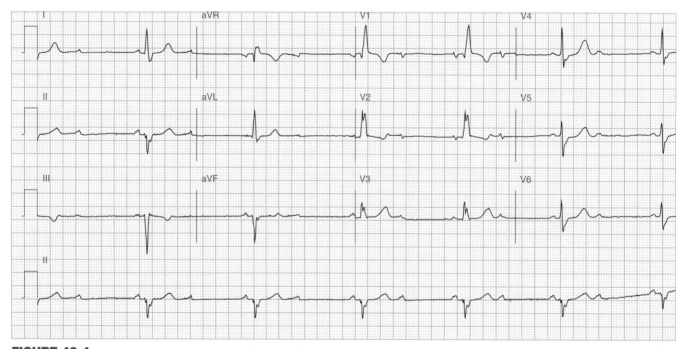

FIGURE 43-4
NSR with 2:1 AV block. Left atrial abnormality. **RBBB** with **left anterior fascicular block.** Possible **inferior myocardial infarction.** (Case 68)

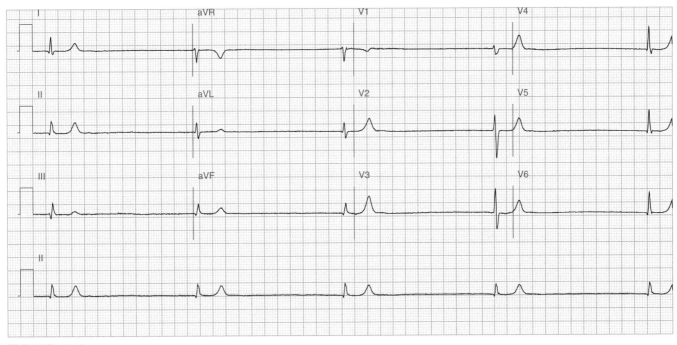

FIGURE 43-5

Marked junctional bradycardia (25 beats/min). Rate is regular, flat baseline between narrow QRS complexes without P waves. Patient was on atenolol, with **possible underlying sick sinus syndrome.** (Case 132)

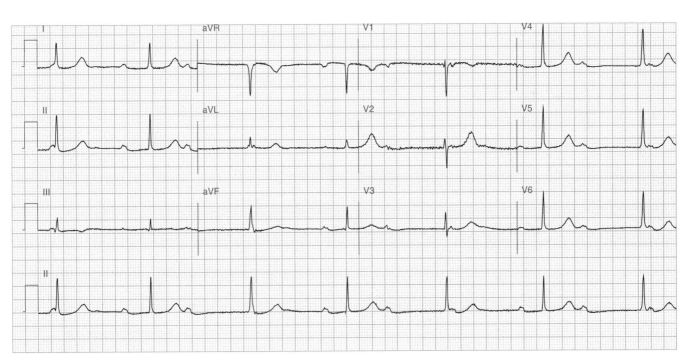

FIGURE 43-6

Sinus rhythm at a rate of 64/min with **third degree (complete) AV block** at a rate of 40/min. The narrow QRS complex indicates an A-V junctional pacemaker. **Left atrial abnormality.** (Case 219)

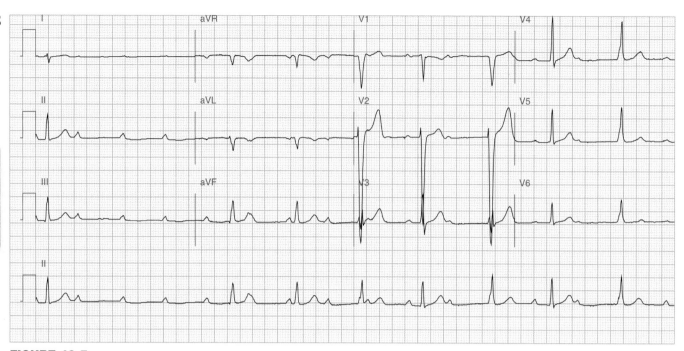

FIGURE 43-7

Sinus rhythm at a rate of 90/min with **third degree (complete) AV block** and an A-V junctional pacemaker at a rate of 60/min, with an occasional dropped beat, in a patients with **Lyme carditis.** (Case 161)

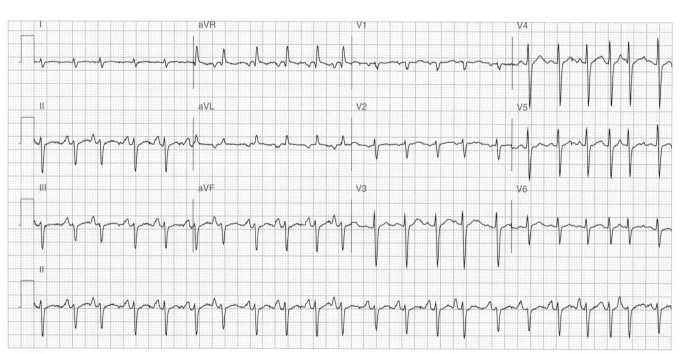

FIGURE 43-8

Multifocal atrial tachycardia with varying P-wave morphologies and P-P intervals; right atrial overload with peaked P waves in II, III, and aVF; superior axis; poor R-wave progression with delayed transition in precordial leads in patient with **severe obstructive lung disease.** (Case 42)

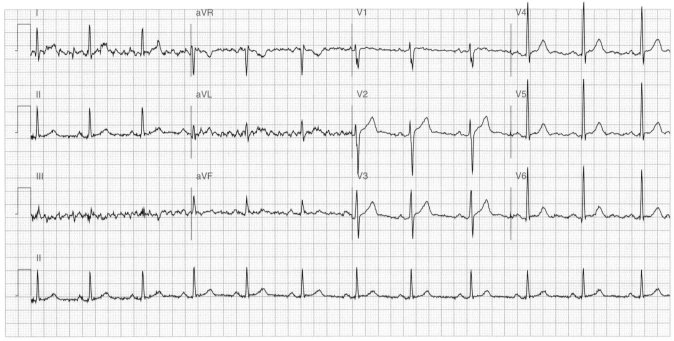

FIGURE 43-9

NSR in a patient with **Parkinson's disease.** Tremor artifact, best seen in limb leads. This **tremor artifact** may sometimes be confused with atrial flutter/fibrillation. (Case 76)

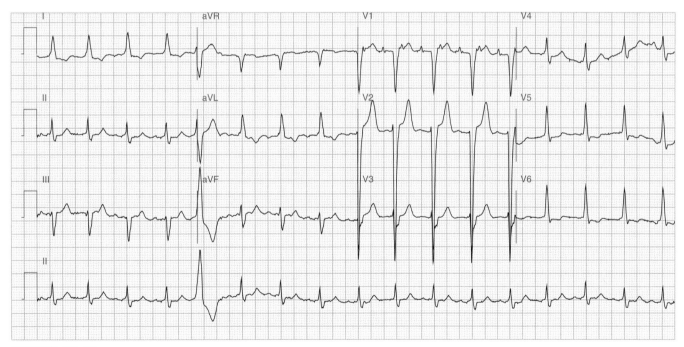

FIGURE 43-10

Atrial tachycardia with atrial rate 200/min (note lead V₁), **2:1 AV block,** and one premature ventricular complex. Also present: LVH with intraventricular conduction defect and slow precordial R-wave progression (cannot rule out old MI). (Case 83)

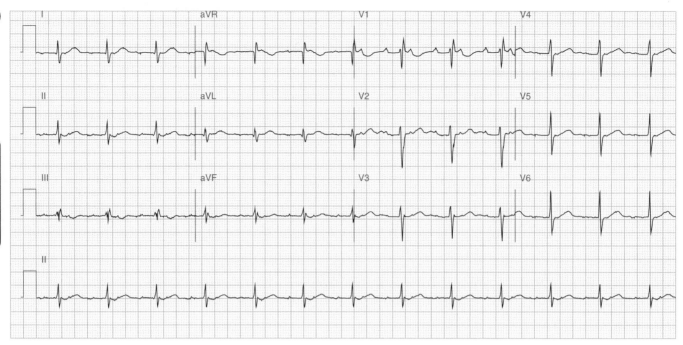

FIGURE 43-11

Atrial tachycardia with 2:1 block. The non-conducted ("extra") P waves just after the QRS complex are best seen in lead V1. Also, there is incomplete RBBB and borderline QT prolongation. (Case 61)

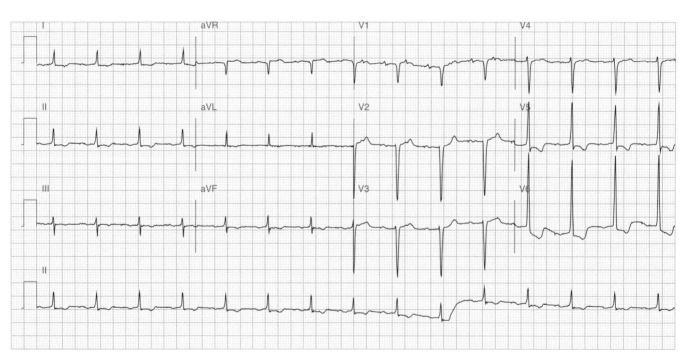

FIGURE 43-12

Atrial tachycardia [180/min with 2:1 AV block (see lead V₁)]. LVH by left precordial voltage. Slow R-wave progression (V₁–V₄) compatible with old anteroseptal MI. (Case 50)

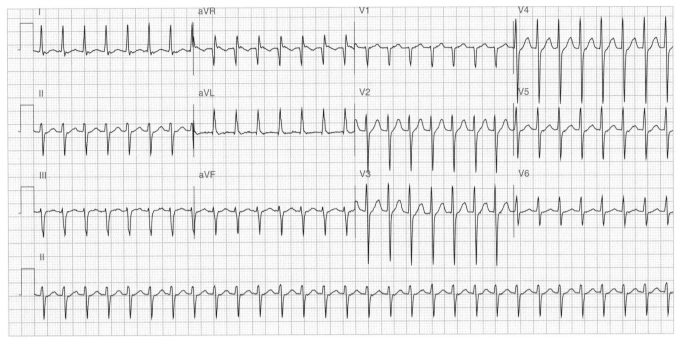

FIGURE 43-13
AV nodal reentrant tachycardia (AVNRT) at a rate of 150/min. (Case 7)

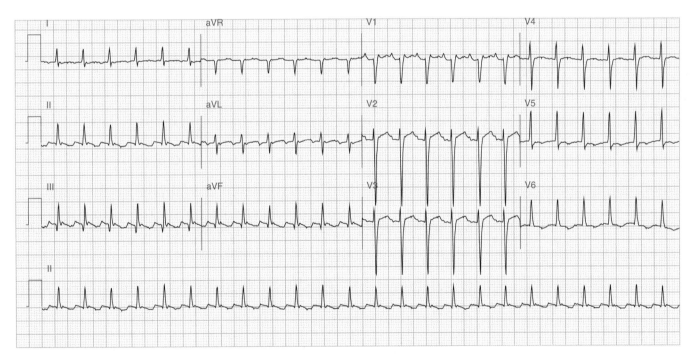

FIGURE 43-14
Atrial flutter with 2:1 conduction. Extra atrial waves in the early ST segment, seen, for example, in leads II and V_1. (Case 57)

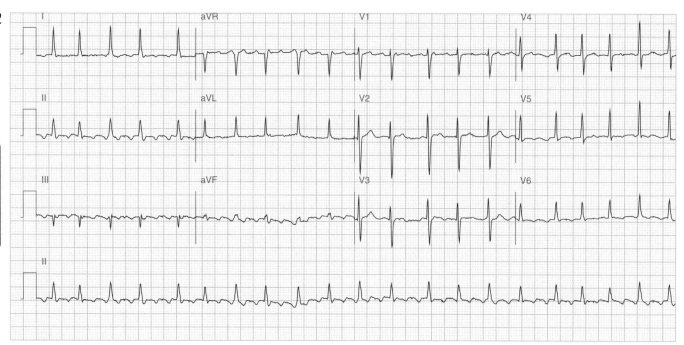

FIGURE 43-15

Atrial flutter with atrial rate 300/min and 2:1 or 3:1 conduction. Flutter waves best seen in lead II. (Case 35)

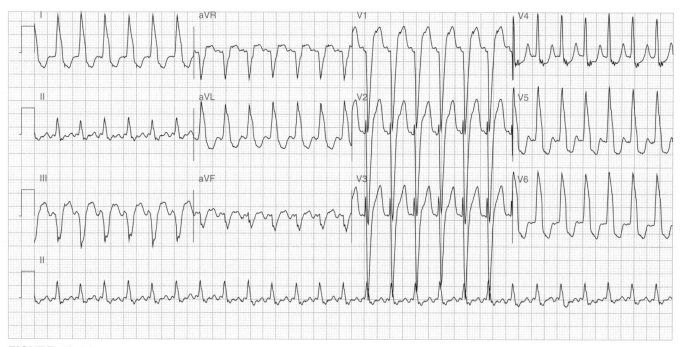

FIGURE 43-16

Wide complex tachycardia. Atrial flutter with 2:1 conduction and LBBB, not to be mistaken for VT. Atrial activity is present in lead II at rate of 320/min. (Case 64)

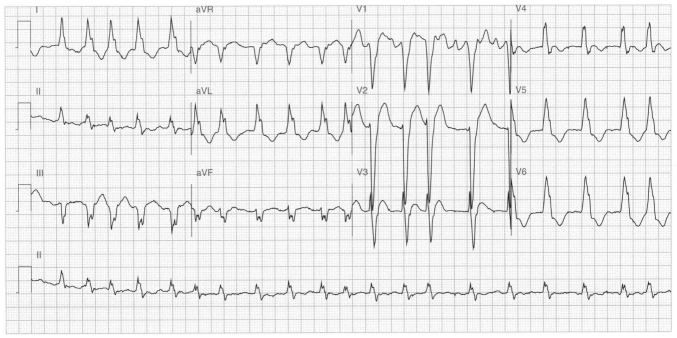

FIGURE 43-17

AF with LBBB. The ventricular rhythm is irregularly irregular. (Case 170)

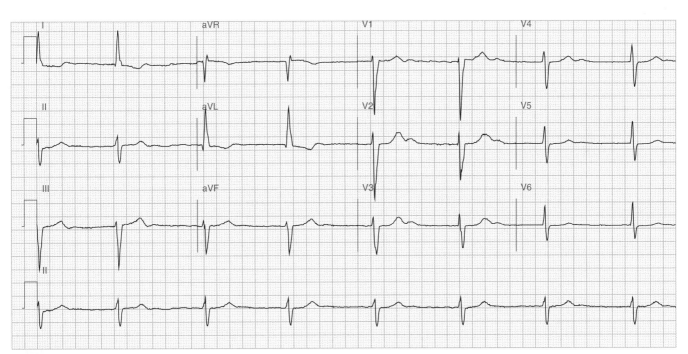

FIGURE 43-18

AF with complete heart block and a junctional escape mechanism causing a slow regular ventricular response (45/min). The QRS complexes show intraventricular conduction defect with left-axis deviation and LVH. Q-T (U) prolongation. (Case 73)

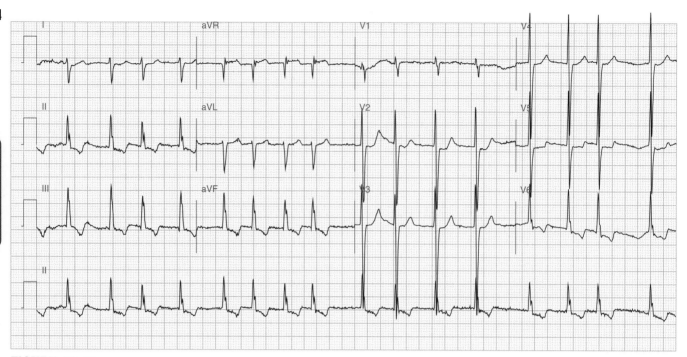

FIGURE 43-19

AF with right-axis deviation and LVH. Tracing suggests biventricular hypertrophy in a patient with **mitral stenosis and aortic valve disease.** (Case 74)

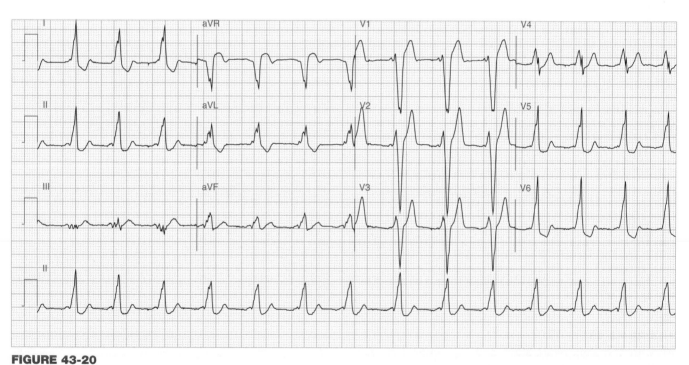

FIGURE 43-20

WPW pre-excitation pattern, with triad of short PR, wide QRS, and delta waves. Polarity of the delta waves (most positive in lead II and lateral chest leads) consistent with a right-sided bypass tract. (Case 97)

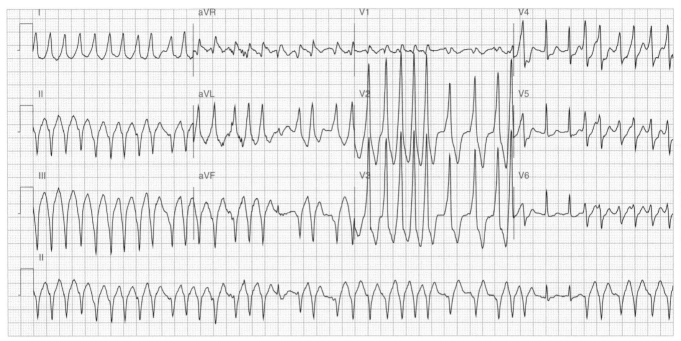

FIGURE 43-21

AF in patient with the WPW syndrome, and antegrade conduction down the bypass tract leading to a wide complex tachycardia. Rhythm is "irregularly irregular" and rate is extremely rapid (about 230/min). Not all beats are pre-excited. (Case 15)

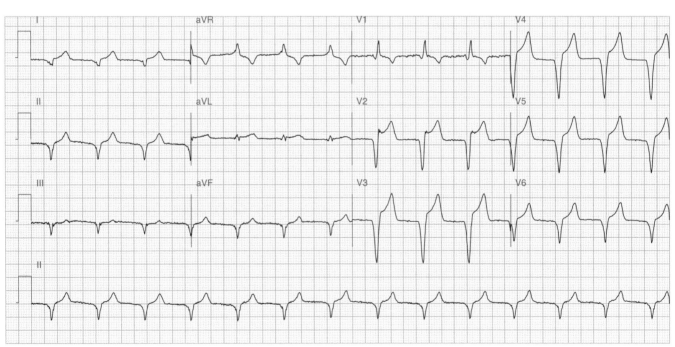

FIGURE 43-22

Accelerated idioventricular rhythm (AIVR) originating from the LV and accounting for RBBB morphology. ST elevations in the precordial leads from **underlying acute MI.** (Case 117)

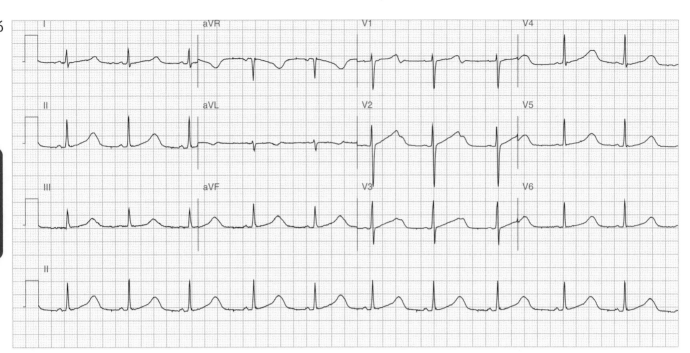

FIGURE 43-23

Prolonged (0.60 s) QT interval in a patient with **hereditary long-QT syndrome.** (Case 1)

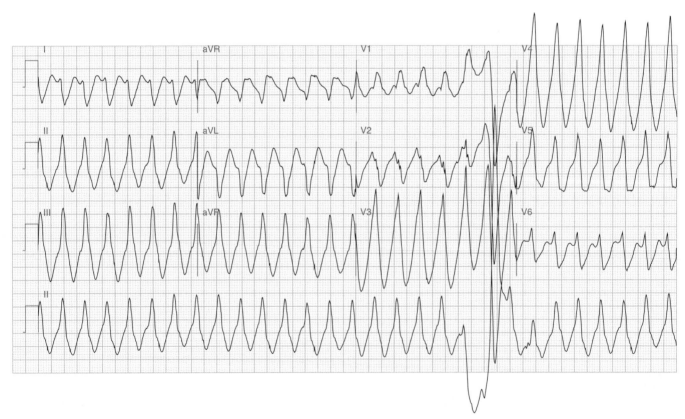

FIGURE 43-24

Monomorphic VT at rate of 170/min. The RBBB morphology in V₁ and the R:S ratio < 1 in V₆ are both suggestive of VT. The morphology of the VT is suggestive of origin from the left side of the heart, near the base (RBBB with inferior/rightward axis). Baseline artifact is present also in leads V₁–V₃. (Case 112)

CHAPTER 44

ATLAS OF PERCUTANEOUS REVASCULARIZATION

Donald S. Baim[†]

As indicated in Chap. 36, percutaneous coronary intervention (PCI) has assumed a major role in the management of coronary artery disease. It is used most commonly in patients with chronic stable angina, unstable angina, and primary therapy in acute ST segment elevation myocardial infarction.[1]

This chapter illustrates some complex uses of percutaneous techniques, including management of cardiogenic shock, stent thrombosis, management of distal coronary vascular disease, and stenting of a chronic totally occluded vessel. In addition, pressure tracings obtained at left heart catheterization in the diagnosis of obstructive hypertrophic cardiomyopathy are shown, as is the percutaneous insertion of an experimental aortic valve. The latter has not yet been approved for clinical use but demonstrates one of the future extensions of percutaneous techniques.

CASE 1: CARDIOGENIC SHOCK WITH LEFT MAIN CORONARY ARTERY OBSTRUCTION

- A 93-year-old man presented to the emergency room with 9 h of dyspnea and a sense of "dread"
- Prior subendocardial MI 2 months earlier managed medically (no catheterization done)
- Entry systolic pressure 70 mmHg, rales [2/3] way up, cool clammy extremities, arterial saturation 85% on 100% oxygen rebreathing mask
- Brought emergently to the catheterization laboratory—right heart catheterization performed

---

[†]Recently deceased.

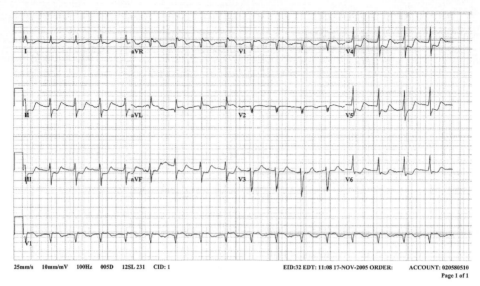

FIGURE 44-1

Presenting ECG—marked inferior and anterolateral ST depression.

LEFT MAIN CORONARY ARTERY STENOSIS WITH CARDIOGENIC SHOCK

- Cardiogenic shock requires emergent revascularization
- Right heart catheterization is useful to assess and monitor hemodynamics, in this case showing profound shock and probable ischemic mitral regurgitation
- Coronary angio showed the cause—a critical ulcerated stenosis of the distal left main and right coronary artery (RCA)

- With intraaortic balloon pump insertion via the contralateral groin, and double wire, "kissing" balloon and kissing stent implantation were performed via 8 Fr guide
- Because of ongoing shock, RCA stenting also performed
- This stabilized hemodynamics with PCW falling to 10 mmHg, and cardiac output normalizing over first 8 h in CCU
- Patient recovered despite a peak CPK of 2300, CKMB 274
- Discharged on day 7, despite a pre-procedure 85% estimated PCI mortality!

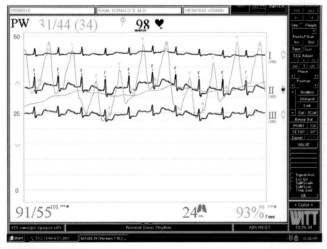

FIGURE 44-2

Cardiogenic shock is present. The mean pulmonary capillary wedge (PCW) pressure is elevated at 23 mmHg, with prominent *v* waves (peaking after the ECG T wave), suggestive of mitral regurgitation. Arterial pressure is reduced (91/55 mmHg) despite dopamine infusion, and the respiratory rate (24/min) plus arterial desaturation (93%) on 100% O_2 suggest incipient pulmonary edema.

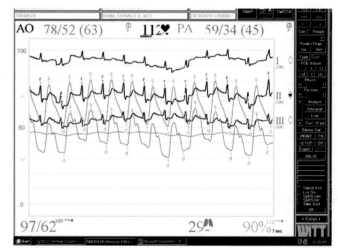

FIGURE 44-3

The aortic (Ao) pressure is reduced (78/52 mmHg), the pulmonary artery (PA) pressure is elevated (59/32 mmHg) and the PaO_2 saturation (32%) corresponds to a cardiac index of 1.4 (L/min)/m², confirming the cardiogenic shock state.

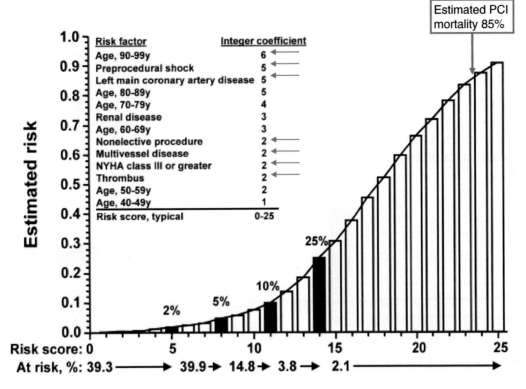

FIGURE 44-4
Estimation of risk of mortality of percutaneous coronary intervention (PCI). *(From M Singh et al: J Am Coll Cardiol 40:387, 2002.)*

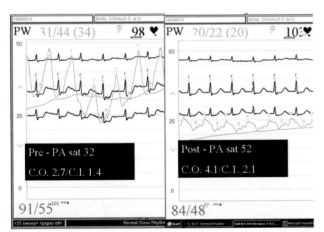

FIGURE 44-5
The PCW fell from 34 mmHg preintervention to 20 mmHg post-intervention with resolution of the tall v waves, and PA saturation increased from 32 to 52%, while cardiac index (CI) rose from 1.4 to 2.1 (L/min)/m².

CASE 2: INFERIOR MI WITH CARDIOGENIC SHOCK

- A 67-year-old man with no prior cardiac history has 20 min of chest pain
- He is hypotensive and hypoxic (oxygen saturation 85% on 100% O₂)

INFERIOR MI WITH CARDIOGENIC SHOCK

- Inferior MIs are usually more benign than anterior MIs
- When there *is* hypotension in an inferior MI, it may reflect right ventricular involvement as might have been the case here with the very proximal right coronary occlusion

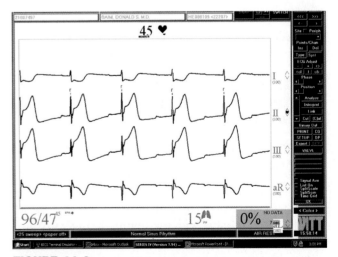

FIGURE 44-6
ECG shows sinus bradycardia, an accelerated idioventricular rhythm and isorhythmic dissociation, and profound inferior ST elevation.

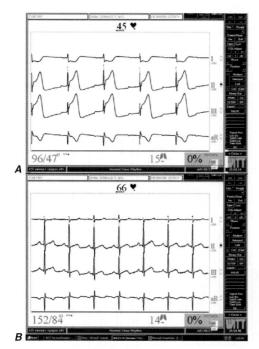

FIGURE 44-7

A. Preintervention. ***B.*** Postintervention. As soon as flow was restored, rhythm returned to normal sinus, ST elevation resolved, blood pressure rose to 152/84 mmHg despite discontinuation of dopamine, and oxygen saturation normalized (not shown). Right heart catheterization post-stent (not shown) revealed normal hemodynamics with wedge pressure of 12 mmHg and cardiac index of 2.4 (L/min)/m^2.

- The severity of the hypotension and coexistent hypoxia here, however, suggest associated global ischemia due to the left main disease
- The patient was clinically stable after the intervention on the right coronary artery, and an intraaortic balloon was placed preparatory to bypass surgery of the left system
- The very early presentation and rapid intervention virtually completely aborted this life-threatening MI

CASE 3: HYPERTROPHIC CARDIOMYOPATHY (HCM) WITH OBSTRUCTION

HYPERTROPHIC CARDIOMYOPATHY (HCM) WITH OBSTRUCTION

- Asymmetric hypertrophy of the upper septum can cause an intracavitary gradient within the LV due to contact of the anterior leaflet with the septum during systole
- While the LV-Ao pressure gradient may look superficially like that seen in aortic stenosis, the characteristic decrease in aortic or peripheral arterial pulse pressure and spike-and-dome pattern in a post-ventricular premature contraction are seen only in HCM with obstruction

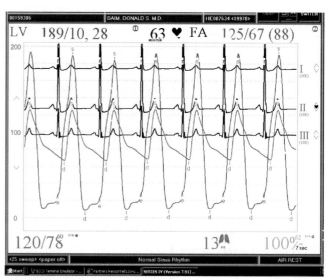

FIGURE 44-8

Simultaneous recording of the left ventricular (yellow) and femoral artery (orange) pressures shows a 60 mmHg pressure gradient. This could represent aortic stenosis, but this patient had a normal aortic valve on echo and asymmetric thickening of the upper left ventricular septum.

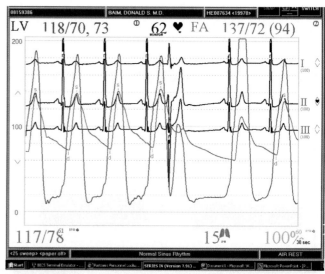

FIGURE 44-9

A spontaneous ventricular premature beat is followed by an augmented sinus beat marked by increased LV pressure and LV-Ao gradient, but a decrease in femoral artery pulse pressure, consistent with HCM with obstruction (Braunwald-Brockenbrough sign).

- An end-hole catheter positioned towards the LV apex allows recording this dynamic gradient, and intracavitary localization of the gradient during pull-back
- The diagnosis and evaluation of this disease, however, is more often made by echocardiography in current practice

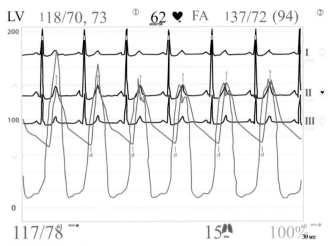

FIGURE 44-10

Slow pull-back of the end-hole catheter from the apex of the LV to the area just under the aortic valve shows disappearance of the pressure gradient.

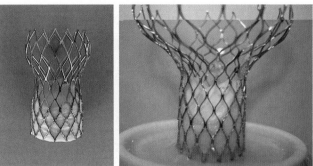

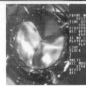

FIGURE 44-12

Self-expanding AV prosthesis: the CoreValve. A pericardium tissue valve fixed to the frame in a surgical manner.

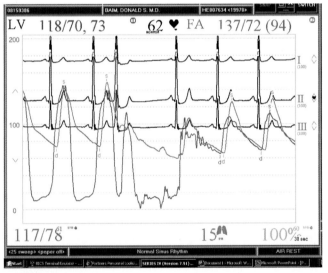

FIGURE 44-11

Continued pull-back into the aorta shows another VPB with reduced aortic pulse pressure and a "spike and dome" central aortic pressure tracing, again consistent with HCM with obstruction. Note that the femoral artery systolic pressure is slightly higher than the central aortic pressure due to peripheral augmentation.

CASE 4: PERCUTANEOUS AORTIC VALVE REPLACEMENT

- The preferred treatment for severe aortic stenosis is surgical replacement of the aortic valve
- Although the average surgical mortality for this procedure is ~4%, some patients are at significantly higher

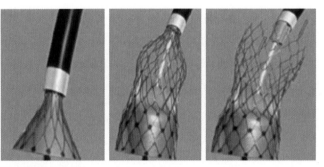

FIGURE 44-13

CoreValve delivery by sheath withdrawal.

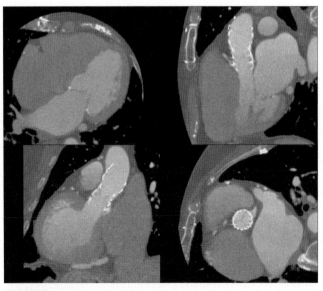

FIGURE 44-14

CoreValve follow-up: Post-implant morphologic assessment by CT scan.

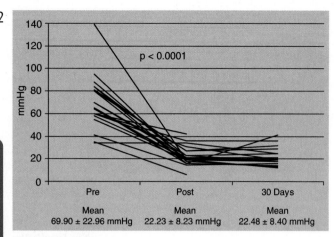

FIGURE 44-15

CoreValve study: Peak pressure gradients.

risk due to advanced age, poor LV function, or other comorbidities

- Percutaneous balloon valvuloplasty was evaluated in the late 1980s, and provided limited benefit
- A new class of investigational percutaneous aortic valve replacement techniques, using pericardial valves mounted in an outer stent, are now under investigation

The case and data shown here were provided by Dr. Eberhard Grube of Sieburg, Germany; with permission.

APPENDIX

LABORATORY VALUES OF CLINICAL IMPORTANCE

Alexander Kratz ■ Michael A. Pesce ■ Daniel J. Fink†

INTRODUCTORY COMMENTS

The following are tables of reference values for laboratory tests, special analytes, and special function tests. A variety of factors can influence reference values. Such variables include the population studied, the duration and means of specimen transport, laboratory methods and instrumentation, and even the type of container used for the collection of the specimen. The reference or "normal" ranges given in this appendix may therefore not be appropriate for all laboratories, and these values should only be used as general guidelines. Whenever possible, reference values provided by the laboratory performing the testing should be utilized in the interpretation of laboratory data. Values supplied in this Appendix reflect typical reference ranges in adults. Pediatric reference ranges may vary significantly from adult values.

In preparing the Appendix, the authors have taken into account the fact that the system of international units (SI, système international d'unités) is used in most countries and in some medical journals. However, clinical laboratories may continue to report values in "conventional" units. Therefore, both systems are provided in the Appendix. The dual system is also used in the text except for (1) those instances in which the numbers remain the same but only the terminology is changed (mmol/L for meq/L or IU/L for mIU/mL), when only the SI units are given; and (2) most pressure measurements (e.g., blood and cerebrospinal fluid pressures), when the conventional units (mmHg, mmH$_2$O) are used. In all other instances in the text the SI unit is followed by the traditional unit in parentheses.

---

†Deceased

REFERENCE VALUES FOR LABORATORY TESTS

TABLE A-1

HEMATOLOGY AND COAGULATION

ANALYTE	SPECIMEN[a]	SI UNITS	CONVENTIONAL UNITS
Activated clotting time	WB	70–180 s	70–180 seconds
Activated protein C resistance (Factor V Leiden)	P	Not applicable	Ratio >2.1
Alpha$_2$ antiplasmin	P	0.87–1.55	87–155%
Antiphospholipid antibody panel			
PTT-LA (Lupus anticoagulant screen)	P	Negative	Negative
Platelet neutralization procedure	P	Negative	Negative
Dilute viper venom screen	P	Negative	Negative
Anticardiolipin antibody	S		
IgG		0–15 arbitrary units	0–15 GPL
IgM		0–15 arbitrary units	0–15 MPL
Antithrombin III	P		
Antigenic		220–390 mg/L	22–39 mg/dL
Functional		0.7–1.30 U/L	70–130%
Anti-Xa assay (heparin assay)	P		
Unfractionated heparin		0.3–0.7 kIU/L	0.3–0.7 IU/mL
Low-molecular-weight heparin		0.5–1.0 kIU/L	0.5–1.0 IU/mL
Danaparoid (Orgaran)		0.5–0.8 kIU/L	0.5–0.8 IU/mL
Autohemolysis test	WB	0.004–0.045	0.4–4.50%
Autohemolysis test with glucose	WB	0.003–0.007	0.3–0.7%
Bleeding time (adult)		<7.1 min	<7.1 min
Bone marrow (see Table A-8)			
Clot retraction	WB	0.50–1.00/2 h	50–100%/2 h
Cryofibrinogen	P	Negative	Negative
D-Dimer	P	0.22–0.74 µg/mL	0.22–0.74 µg/mL
Differential blood count	WB		
Neutrophils		0.40–0.70	40–70%
Bands		0.0–0.05	0–5%
Lymphocytes		0.20–0.50	20–50%
Monocytes		0.04–0.08	4–8%
Eosinophils		0.0–0.6	0–6%
Basophils		0.0–0.02	0–2%
Eosinophil count	WB	150–300/µL	150–300/mm^3
Erythrocyte count	WB		
Adult males		4.30–5.60 × 10^{12}/L	4.30–5.60 × 10^6/mm^3
Adult females		4.00–5.20 × 10^{12}/L	4.00–5.20 × 10^6/mm^3
Erythrocyte life span	WB		
Normal survival		120 days	120 days
Chromium labeled, half life ($t_{1/2}$)		25–35 days	25–35 days
Erythrocyte sedimentation rate	WB		
Females		0–20 mm/h	0–20 mm/h
Males		0–15 mm/h	0–15 mm/h
Euglobulin lysis time	P	7200–14400 s	120–240 min
Factor II, prothrombin	P	0.50–1.50	50–150%
Factor V	P	0.50–1.50	50–150%
Factor VII	P	0.50–1.50	50–150%
Factor VIII	P	0.50–1.50	50–150%
Factor IX	P	0.50–1.50	50–150%
Factor X	P	0.50–1.50	50–150%
Factor XI	P	0.50–1.50	50–150%
Factor XII	P	0.50–1.50	50–150%
Factor XIII screen	P	Not applicable	Present
Factor inhibitor assay	P	< 0.5 Bethesda Units	<0.5 Bethesda Units
Fibrin(ogen) degradation products	P	0–1 mg/L	0–1 µg/mL
Fibrinogen	P	2.33–4.96 g/L	233–496 mg/dL
Glucose-6-phosphate dehydrogenase (erythrocyte)	WB	< 2400 s	<40 min

HEMATOLOGY AND COAGULATION

ANALYTE	SPECIMEN[a]	SI UNITS	CONVENTIONAL UNITS
Ham's test (acid serum)	WB	Negative	Negative
Hematocrit	WB		
Adult males		0.388–0.464	38.8–46.4
Adult females		0.354–0.444	35.4–44.4
Hemoglobin			
Plasma	P	6–50 mg/L	0.6–5.0 mg/dL
Whole blood	WB		
Adult males		133–162 g/L	13.3–16.2 g/dL
Adult females		120–158 g/L	12.0–15.8 g/dL
Hemoglobin electrophoresis	WB		
Hemoglobin A		0.95–0.98	95–98%
Hemoglobin A_2		0.015–0.031	1.5–3.1%
Hemoglobin F		0–0.02	0–2.0%
Hemoglobins other than A, A_2, or F		Absent	Absent
Heparin-induced thrombocytopenia antibody	P	Negative	Negative
Joint fluid crystal	JF	Not applicable	No crystals seen
Joint fluid mucin	JF	Not applicable	Only type I mucin present
Leukocytes			
Alkaline phosphatase (LAP)	WB	0.2–1.6 μkat/L	13–100 μ/L
Count (WBC)	WB	$3.54–9.06 \times 10^9$/L	$3.54–9.06 \times 10^3$/mm^3
Mean corpuscular hemoglobin (MCH)	WB	26.7–31.9 pg/cell	26.7–31.9 pg/cell
Mean corpuscular hemoglobin concentration (MCHC)	WB	323–359 g/L	32.3–35.9 g/dL
Mean corpuscular hemoglobin of reticulocytes (CH)	WB	24–36 pg	24–36 pg
Mean corpuscular volume (MCV)	WB	79–93.3 fL	79–93.3 μm^3
Mean platelet volume (MPV)	WB	9.00–12.95 fL	9.00–12.95 μm^3
Osmotic fragility of erythrocytes	WB		
Direct		0.0035–0.0045	0.35–0.45%
Index		0.0030–0.0065	0.30–0.65%
Partial thromboplastin time, activated	P	26.3–39.4 s	26.3–39.4 s
Plasminogen	P		
Antigen		84–140 mg/L	8.4–14.0 mg/dL
Functional		0.70–1.30	70–130%
Plasminogen activator inhibitor 1	P	4–43 μg/L	4–43 ng/mL
Platelet aggregation	PRP	Not applicable	>65% aggregation in response to adenosine diphosphate, epinephrine, collagen, ristocetin, and arachidonic acid
Platelet count	WB	$165–415 \times 10^9$/L	$165–415 \times 10^3$/mm^3
Platelet, mean volume	WB	6.4–11 fL	6.4–11.0 μm^3
Prekallikrein assay	P	0.50–1.5	50–150%
Prekallikrein screen	P		No deficiency detected
Protein C	P		
Total antigen		0.70–1.40	70–140%
Functional		0.70–1.30	70–130%
Protein S	P		
Total antigen		0.70–1.40	70–140%
Functional		0.65–1.40	65–140%
Free antigen		0.70–1.40	70–140%
Prothrombin gene mutation G20210A	WB	Not applicable	Not present
Prothrombin time	P	12.7–15.4 s	12.7–15.4 s
Protoporphyrin, free erythrocyte	WB	0.28–0.64 μmol/L of red blood cells	16–36 μg/dL of red blood cells
Red cell distribution width	WB	<0.145	<14.5%
Reptilase time	P	16–23.6 s	16–23.6 s
Reticulocyte count	WB		
Adult males		0.008–0.023 red cells	0.8–2.3% red cells
Adult females		0.008–0.020 red cells	0.8–2.0% red cells

(Continued)

TABLE A-1 (CONTINUED)

HEMATOLOGY AND COAGULATION

ANALYTE	SPECIMEN[a]	SI UNITS	CONVENTIONAL UNITS
Reticulocyte hemoglobin content	WB	>26 pg/cell	>26 pg/cell
Ristocetin cofactor (functional von Willebrand factor)	P		
Blood group O		0.75 mean of normal	75% mean of normal
Blood group A		1.05 mean of normal	105% mean of normal
Blood group B		1.15 mean of normal	115% mean of normal
Blood group AB		1.25 mean of normal	125% mean of normal
Sickle cell test	WB	Negative	Negative
Sucrose hemolysis	WB	<0.1	<10% hemolysis
Thrombin time	P	15.3–18.5 s	15.3–18.5 s
Total eosinophils	WB	150–300 × 10⁶/L	150–300/mm³
Transferrin receptor	S, P	9.6–29.6 nmol/L	9.6–29.6 nmol/L
Viscosity			
Plasma	P	1.7–2.1	1.7–2.1
Serum	S	1.4–1.8	1.4–1.8
Von Willebrand factor (vWF) antigen (factor VIII: R antigen)	P		
Blood group O		0.75 mean of normal	75% mean of normal
Blood group A		1.05 mean of normal	105% mean of normal
Blood group B		1.15 mean of normal	115% mean of normal
Blood group AB		1.25 mean of normal	125% mean of normal
Von Willebrand factor multimers	P	Normal distribution	Normal distribution
White blood cells: see "leukocytes"			

[a]P, plasma; JF, joint fluid; PRP, platelet-rich plasma; S, serum; WB, whole blood.

TABLE A-2

CLINICAL CHEMISTRY AND IMMUNOLOGY

ANALYTE	SPECIMEN[a]	SI UNITS	CONVENTIONAL UNITS
Acetoacetate	P	20–99 μmol/L	0.2–1.0 mg/dL
Adrenocorticotropin (ACTH)	P	1.3–16.7 pmol/L	6.0–76.0 pg/mL
Alanine aminotransferase (AST, SGPT)	S	0.12–0.70 μkat/L	7–41 U/L
Albumin	S		
Female		41–53 g/L	4.1–5.3 g/dL
Male		40–50 g/L	4.0–5.0 g/dL
Aldolase	S	26–138 nkat/L	1.5–8.1 U/L
Aldosterone (adult)			
Supine, normal sodium diet	S, P	55–250 pmol/L	2–9 ng/dL
Upright, normal sodium diet	S, P		2–5-fold increase over supine value
Supine, low-sodium diet	S, P		2–5-fold increase over normal sodium diet level
	U	6.38–58.25 nmol/d	2.3–21.0 μg/24 h
Alpha fetoprotein (adult)	S	0–8.5 μg/L	0–8.5 ng/mL
Alpha₁ antitrypsin	S	1.0–2.0 g/L	100–200 mg/dL
Ammonia, as NH₃	P	11–35 μmol/L	19–60 μg/dL
Amylase (method dependent)	S	0.34–1.6 μkat/L	20–96 U/L
Androstenedione (adult)	S	1.75–8.73 nmol/L	50–250 ng/dL
Angiotensin-converting enzyme (ACE)	S	0.15–1.1 μkat/L	9–67 U/L
Anion gap	S	7–16 mmol/L	7–16 mmol/L
Apo B/Apo A-1 ratio		0.35–0.98	0.35–0.98
Apolipoprotein A-1	S	1.19–2.40 g/L	119–240 mg/dL
Apolipoprotein B	S	0.52–1.63 g/L	52–163 mg/dL

CLINICAL CHEMISTRY AND IMMUNOLOGY

ANALYTE	SPECIMEN[a]	SI UNITS	CONVENTIONAL UNITS
Arterial blood gases			
[HCO_3]		22–30 mmol/L	22–30 meq/L
P_{CO_2}		4.3–6.0 kPa	32–45 mmHg
pH		7.35–7.45	7.35–7.45
P_{O_2}		9.6–13.8 kPa	72–104 mmHg
Aspartate aminotransferase (AST, SGOT)	S	0.20–0.65 μkat/L	12–38 U/L
Autoantibodies			
Anti-adrenal antibody	S	Not applicable	Negative at 1:10 dilution
Anti-double-strand (native) DNA	S	Not applicable	Negative at 1:10 dilution
Anti–glomerular basement membrane antibodies	S		
Qualitative		Negative	Negative
Quantitative		<5 kU/L	<5 U/mL
Anti-granulocyte antibody	S	Not applicable	Negative
Anti-Jo-1 antibody	S	Not applicable	Negative
Anti-La antibody	S	Not applicable	Negative
Anti-mitochondrial antibody	S	Not applicable	Negative
Antineutrophil cytoplasmic autoantibodies, cytoplasmic (C-ANCA)	S		
Qualitative		Negative	Negative
Quantitative (antibodies to proteinase 3)		<2.8 kU/L	<2.8 U/mL
Antineutrophil cytoplasmic autoantibodies, perinuclear (P-ANCA)	S		
Qualitative		Negative	Negative
Quantitative (antibodies to myeloperoxidase)		<1.4 kU/L	<1.4 U/mL
Antinuclear antibody	S	Not applicable	Negative at 1:40
Anti–parietal cell antibody	S	Not applicable	Negative at 1:20
Anti-Ro antibody	S	Not applicable	Negative
Anti-platelet antibody	S	Not applicable	Negative
Anti-RNP antibody	S	Not applicable	Negative
Anti-Scl 70 antibody	S	Not applicable	Negative
Anti-Smith antibody	S	Not applicable	Negative
Anti-smooth-muscle antibody	S	Not applicable	Negative at 1:20
Anti-thyroglobulin	S	Not applicable	Negative
Anti-thyroid antibody	S	<0.3 kIU/L	<0.3 IU/mL
B type natriuretic peptide (BNP)	P	Age and gender specific: <167 ng/L	Age and gender specific: <167 pg/mL
Bence Jones protein, serum	S	Not applicable	None detected
Bence Jones protein, urine, qualitative	U	Not applicable	None detected in 50× concentrated urine
Bence Jones Protein, urine, quantitative	U		
Kappa		<25 mg/L	<2.5 mg/dL
Lambda		<50 mg/L	<5.0 mg/dL
$β_2$-Microglobulin			
	S	<2.7 mg/L	<0.27 mg/dL
	U	<120 μg/d	<120 μg/day
Bilirubin	S		
Total		5.1–22 μmol/L	0.3–1.3 mg/dL
Direct		1.7–6.8 μmol/L	0.1–0.4 mg/dL
Indirect		3.4–15.2 μmol/L	0.2–0.9 mg/dL
C peptide (adult)	S, P	0.17–0.66 nmol/L	0.5–2.0 ng/mL
C1-esterase-inhibitor protein	S		
Antigenic		124–250 mg/L	12.4–24.5 mg/dL
Functional		Present	Present
CA 125	S	0–35 kU/L	0–35 U/mL
CA 19-9	S	0–37 kU/L	0–37 U/mL
CA-15-3	S	0–34 kU/L	0–34 U/mL
CA27-29	S	0–40 kU/L	0–40 U/mL

(*Continued*)

TABLE A-2 (*CONTINUED*)

CLINICAL CHEMISTRY AND IMMUNOLOGY

ANALYTE	SPECIMEN[a]	SI UNITS	CONVENTIONAL UNITS
Calcitonin	S		
Male		3–26 ng/L	3–26 pg/mL
Female		2–17 ng/L	2–17 pg/mL
Calcium	S	2.2–2.6 mmol/L	8.7–10.2 mg/dL
Calcium, ionized	WB	1.12–1.32 mmol/L	4.5–5.3 mg/dL
Carbon dioxide content (TCO$_2$)	P (sea level)	22–30 mmol/L	22–30 meq/L
Carboxyhemoglobin (carbon monoxide content)	WB		
Nonsmokers		0–0.04	0–4%
Smokers		0.04–0.09	4–9%
Onset of symptoms		0.15–0.20	15–20%
Loss of consciousness and death		>0.50	>50%
Carcinoembryonic antigen (CEA)	S		
Nonsmokers		0.0–3.0 μg/L	0.0–3.0 ng/mL
Smokers	S	0.0–5.0 μg/L	0.0–5.0 ng/mL
Ceruloplasmin	S	250–630 mg/L	25–63 mg/dL
Chloride	S	102–109 mmol/L	102–109 meq/L
Cholesterol (see Table A-5)			
Cholinesterase	S	5–12 kU/L	5–12 U/mL
Complement			
C3	S	0.83–1.77 g/L	83–177 mg/dL
C4	S	0.16–0.47 g/L	16–47 mg/dL
Total hemolytic complement (CH50)	S	50–150%	50–150%
Factor B	S	0.17–0.42 g/L	17–42 mg/dL
Coproporphyrins (types I and III)	U	150–470 μmol/d	100–300 μg/d
Cortisol			
Fasting, 8 A.M.–12 noon	S	138–690 nmol/L	5–25 μg/dL
12 noon–8 P.M.		138–414 nmol/L	5–15 μg/dL
8 P.M.–8 A.M.		0–276 nmol/L	0–10 μg/dL
Cortisol, free	U	55–193 nmol/24 h	20–70 μg/24 h
C-reactive protein	S	0.2–3.0 mg/L	0.2–3.0 mg/L
Creatine kinase (total)	S		
Females		0.66–4.0 μkat/L	39–238 U/L
Males		0.87–5.0 μkat/L	51–294 U/L
Creatine kinase-MB	S		
Mass		0.0–5.5 μg/L	0.0–5.5 ng/mL
Fraction of total activity (by electrophoresis)		0–0.04	0–4.0%
Creatinine	S		
Female		44–80 μmol/L	0.5–0.9 ng/mL
Male		53–106 μmol/L	0.6–1.2 ng/mL
Cryoproteins	S	Not applicable	None detected
Dehydroepiandrosterone (DHEA) (adult)			
Male	S	6.2–43.4 nmol/L	180–1250 ng/dL
Female		4.5–34.0 nmol/L	130–980 ng/dL
Dehydroepiandrosterone (DHEA) sulfate	S		
Male (adult)		100–6190 μg/L	10–619 μg/dL
Female (adult, premenopausal)		120–5350 μg/L	12–535 μg/dL
Female (adult, postmenopausal)		300–2600 μg/L	30–260 μg/dL
Deoxycorticosterone (DOC) (adult)	S	61–576 nmol/L	2–19 ng/dL
11-Deoxycortisol (adult) (compound S) (8:00 A.M.)	S	0.34–4.56 nmol/L	12–158 ng/dL
Dihydrotestosterone			
Male	S, P	1.03–2.92 nmol/L	30–85 ng/dL
Female		0.14–0.76 nmol/L	4–22 ng/dL
Dopamine	P	< 475 pmol/L	< 87 pg/mL
Dopamine	U	425–2610 nmol/d	65–400 μg/d
Epinephrine	P		
Supine (30 min)		<273 pmol/L	<50 pg/mL
Sitting		<328 pmol/L	<60 pg/mL
Standing (30 min)		<491pmol/L	<90 pg/mL

CLINICAL CHEMISTRY AND IMMUNOLOGY

ANALYTE	SPECIMEN[a]	SI UNITS	CONVENTIONAL UNITS
Epinephrine	U	0–109 nmol/d	0–20 µg/d
Erythropoietin	S	4–27 U/L	4–27 U/L
Estradiol	S, P		
Female			
Menstruating:			
Follicular phase		74–532 pmol/L	<20–145 pg/mL
Mid-cycle peak		411–1626 pmol/L	112–443 pg/mL
Luteal phase		74–885 pmol/L	<20–241 pg/mL
Postmenopausal		217 pmol/L	<59 pg/mL
Male		74 pmol/L	<20 pg/mL
Estrone	S, P		
Female			
Menstruating:			
Follicular phase		55–555 pmol/L	15–150 pg/mL
Luteal phase		55–740 pmol/L	15–200 pg/mL
Postmenopausal		55–204 pmol/L	15–55 pg/mL
Male		55–240 pmol/L	15–65 pg/mL
Fatty acids, free (nonesterified)	P	<0.28–0.89 mmol/L	<8–25 mg/dL
Ferritin	S		
Female		10–150 µg/L	10–150 ng/mL
Male		29–248 µg/L	29–248 ng/mL
Follicle stimulating hormone (FSH)	S, P		
Female			
Menstruating:			
Follicular phase		3.0–20.0 IU/L	3.0–20.0 mIU/mL
Ovulatory phase		9.0–26.0 IU/L	9.0–26.0 mIU/mL
Luteal phase		1.0–12.0 IU/L	1.0–12.0 mIU/mL
Postmenopausal		18.0–153.0 IU/L	18.0–153.0 mIU/mL
Male		1.0–12.0 IU/L	1.0–12.0 mIU/mL
Free testosterone, adult			
Female	S	2.1–23.6 pmol/L	0.6–6.8 pg/mL
Male		163–847 pmol/L	47–244 pg/mL
Fructosamine	S	<285 µmol/L	<285 µmol/L
Gamma glutamyltransferase	S	0.15–0.99 µkat/L	9–58 U/L
Gastrin	S	<100 ng/L	<100 pg/mL
Glucagon	P	20–100 ng/L	20–100 pg/mL
Glucose (fasting)	P		
Normal		4.2–6.1 mmol/L	75–110 mg/dL
Impaired glucose tolerance		6.2–6.9 mmol/L	111–125 mg/dL
Diabetes mellitus		>7.0 mmol/L	>125 mg/dL
Glucose, 2 h postprandial	P	3.9–6.7 mmol/L	70–120 mg/dL
Growth hormone (resting)	S	0.5–17.0 µg/L	0.5–17.0 ng/mL
Hemoglobin A$_{1c}$	WB	0.04–0.06 Hb fraction	4.0–6.0%
High-density lipoprotein (HDL) (see Table A-5)			
Homocysteine	P	4.4–10.8 µmol/L	4.4–10.8 µmol/L
Human chorionic gonadotropin (hCG)	S		
Non-pregnant female		<5 IU/L	<5 mIU/mL
1–2 weeks postconception		9–130 IU/L	9–130 mIU/mL
2–3 weeks postconception		75–2600 IU/L	75–2600 mIU/mL
3–4 weeks postconception		850–20,800 IU/L	850–20,800 mIU/mL
4–5 weeks postconception		4000–100,200 IU/L	4000–100,200 mIU/mL
5–10 weeks postconception		11,500–289,000 IU/L	11,500–289,000 mIU/mL
10–14 weeks postconception		18,300–137,000 IU/L	18,300–137,000 mIU/mL
Second trimester		1400–53,000 IU/L	1400–53,000 mIU/mL
Third trimester		940–60,000 IU/L	940–60,000 mIU/mL
β-Hydroxybutyrate	P	0–290 µmol/L	0–3 mg/dL
5-Hydroindoleacetic acid [5-HIAA]	U	10.5–36.6 µmol/d	2–7 mg/d

(*Continued*)

TABLE A-2 (*CONTINUED*)

CLINICAL CHEMISTRY AND IMMUNOLOGY

ANALYTE	SPECIMEN[a]	SI UNITS	CONVENTIONAL UNITS
17-Hydroxyprogesterone (adult)	S		
Male		0.15–7.5 nmol/L	5–250 ng/dL
Female			
Follicular phase		0.6–3.0 nmol/L	20–100 ng/dL
Midcycle peak		3–7.5 nmol/L	100–250 ng/dL
Luteal phase		3–15 nmol/L	100–500 ng/dL
Postmenopausal		≤2.1 nmol/L	≤70 ng/dL
Hydroxyproline	U, 24 h	38–500 µmol/d	38–500 µmol/d
Immunofixation	S	Not applicable	No bands detected
Immunoglobulin, quantitation (adult)			
IgA	S	0.70–3.50 g/L	70–350 mg/dL
IgD	S	0–140 mg/L	0–14 mg/dL
IgE	S	24–430 µg/L	10–179 IU/mL
IgG	S	7.0–17.0 g/L	700–1700 mg/dL
IgG_1	S	2.7–17.4 g/L	270–1740 mg/dL
IgG_2	S	0.3–6.3 g/L	30–630 mg/dL
IgG_3	S	0.13–3.2 g/L	13–320 mg/dL
IgG_4	S	0.11–6.2 g/L	11–620 mg/dL
IgM	S	0.50–3.0 g/L	50–300 mg/dL
Insulin	S, P	14.35–143.5 pmol/L	2–20 µU/mL
Iron	S	7–25 µmol/L	41–141 µg/dL
Iron-binding capacity	S	45–73 µmol/L	251–406 µg/dL
Iron-binding capacity saturation	S	0.16–0.35	16–35%
Joint fluid crystal	JF	Not applicable	No crystals seen
Joint fluid mucin	JF	Not applicable	Only type I mucin present
Ketone (acetone)	S, U	Negative	Negative
17 Ketosteroids	U	0.003–0.012 g/d	3–12 mg/d
Lactate	P, arterial	0.5–1.6 mmol/L	4.5–14.4 mg/dL
	P, venous	0.5–2.2 mmol/L	4.5–19.8 mg/dL
Lactate dehydrogenase	S	2.0–3.8 µkat/L	115–221 U/L
Lactate dehydrogenase isoenzymes	S		
Fraction 1 (of total)		0.14–0.26	14–26%
Fraction 2		0.29–0.39	29–39%
Fraction 3		0.20–0.25	20–25%
Fraction 4		0.08–0.16	8–16%
Fraction 5		0.06–0.16	6–16%
Lipase (method dependent)	S	0.51–0.73 µkat/L	3–43 U/L
Lipids: (see Table A-5)			
Lipoprotein (a)	S	0–300 mg/L	0–30 mg/dL
Low-density lipoprotein (LDL) (see Table A-5)			
Luteinizing hormone (LH)	S, P		
Female			
Menstruating			
Follicular phase		2.0–15.0 U/L	2.0–15.0 U/L
Ovulatory phase		22.0–105.0 U/L	22.0–105.0 U/L
Luteal phase		0.6–19.0 U/L	0.6–19.0 U/L
Postmenopausal		16.0–64.0 U/L	16.0–64.0 U/L
Male		2.0–12.0 U/L	2.0–12.0 U/L
Magnesium	S	0.62–0.95 mmol/L	1.5–2.3 mg/dL
Metanephrine	P	<0.5 nmol/L	<100 pg/mL
Metanephrine	U	30–211 mmol/mol creatinine	53–367 µg/g creatinine
Methemoglobin	WB	0.0–0.01	0–1%
Microalbumin urine	U		
24-h urine		0.0–0.03 g/d	0–30 mg/24 h
Spot urine		0.0–0.03 g/g creatinine	0–30 µg/mg creatinine

CLINICAL CHEMISTRY AND IMMUNOLOGY

ANALYTE	SPECIMEN[a]	SI UNITS	CONVENTIONAL UNITS
Myoglobin	S		
Male		19–92 µg/L	19–92 µg/L
Female		12–76 µg/L	12–76 µg/L
Norepinephrine	U	89–473 nmol/d	15–80 µg/d
Norepinephrine	P		
Supine (30 min)		650–2423 pmol/L	110–410 pg/mL
Sitting		709–4019 pmol/L	120–680 pg/mL
Standing (30 min)		739–4137 pmol/L	125–700 pg/mL
N-telopeptide (cross linked), NTx	S		
Female, premenopausal		6.2–19.0 nmol BCE	6.2–19.0 nmol BCE
Male		5.4–24.2 nmol BCE	5.4–24.2 nmol BCE
Bone collagen equivalent (BCE)			
N-telopeptide (cross linked), NTx	U		
Female, premenopausal		17–94 nmol BCE/mmol creatinine	17–94 nmol BCE/mmol creatinine
Female, postmenopausal		26–124 nmol BCE/mmol creatinine	26–124 nmol BCE/mmol creatinine
Male		21–83 nmol BCE/mmol creatinine	21–83 nmol BCE/mmol creatinine
Bone collagen equivalent (BCE)			
5′ Nucleotidase	S	0.02–0.19 µkat/L	0–11 U/L
Osmolality	P	275–295 mOsmol/kg serum water	275–295 mOsmol/kg serum water
	U	500–800 mOsmol/kg water	500–800 mOsmol/kg water
Osteocalcin	S	11–50 µg/L	11–50 ng/mL
Oxygen content	WB		
Arterial (sea level)		17–21	17–21 vol%
Venous (sea level)		10–16	10–16 vol%
Oxygen percent saturation (sea level)	WB		
Arterial		0.97	94–100%
Venous, arm		0.60–0.85	60–85%
Parathyroid hormone (intact)	S	8–51 ng/L	8–51 pg/mL
Phosphatase, alkaline	S	0.56–1.63 µkat/L	33–96 U/L
Phosphorus, inorganic	S	0.81–1.4 mmol/L	2.5–4.3 mg/dL
Porphobilinogen	U	None	None
Potassium	S	3.5–5.0 mmol/L	3.5–5.0 meq/L
Prealbumin	S	170–340 mg/L	17–34 mg/dL
Progesterone	S, P		
Female			
Follicular		<3.18 nmol/L	<1.0 ng/mL
Midluteal		9.54–63.6 nmol/L	3–20 ng/mL
Male		<3.18 nmol/L	<1.0 ng/mL
Prolactin	S	0–20 µg/L	0–20 ng/mL
Prostate-specific antigen (PSA)	S		
Male			
<40 years		0.0–2.0 µg/L	0.0–2.0 ng/mL
>40 years		0.0–4.0 µg/L	0.0–4.0 ng/mL
PSA, free; in males 45–75 years, with PSA values between 4 and 20 µg/mL	S	>0.25 associated with benign prostatic hyperplasia	>25% associated with benign prostatic hyperplasia
Protein fractions	S		
Albumin		35–55 g/L	3.5–5.5 g/dL (50–60%)
Globulin		20–35 g/L	2.0–3.5 g/dL (40–50%)
Alpha$_1$		2–4 g/L	0.2–0.4 g/dL (4.2–7.2%)
Alpha$_2$		5–9 g/L	0.5–0.9 g/dL (6.8–12%)
Beta		6–11 g/L	0.6–1.1 g/dL (9.3–15%)
Gamma		7–17 g/L	0.7–1.7 g/dL (13–23%)

(*Continued*)

CLINICAL CHEMISTRY AND IMMUNOLOGY

ANALYTE	SPECIMEN[a]	SI UNITS	CONVENTIONAL UNITS
Protein, total	S	67–86 g/L	6.7–8.6 g/dL
Pyruvate	P, arterial	40–130 μmol/L	0.35–1.14 mg/dL
	P, venous	40–130 μmol/L	0.35–1.14 mg/dL
Rheumatoid factor	S, JF	<30 kIU/L	<30 IU/mL
Serotonin	WB	0.28–1.14 μmol/L	50–200 ng/mL
Serum protein electrophoresis	S	Not applicable	Normal pattern
Sex hormone binding globulin (adult)	S		
Male		13–71 nmol/L	13–71 nmol/L
Female		18–114 nmol/L	18–114 nmol/L
Sodium	S	136–146 mmol/L	136–146 meq/L
Somatomedin-C (IGF-1) (adult)	S		
16–24 years		182–780 μg/L	182–780 ng/mL
25–39 years		114–492 μg/L	114–492 ng/mL
40–54 years		90–360 μg/L	90–360 ng/mL
>54 years		71–290 μg/L	71–290 ng/mL
Somatostatin	P	<25 ng/L	<25 pg/mL
Testosterone, total, morning sample	S		
Female		0.21–2.98 nmol/L	6–86 ng/dL
Male		9.36–37.10 nmol/L	270–1070 ng/dL
Thyroglobulin	S	0.5–53 μg/L	0.5–53 ng/mL
Thyroid-binding globulin	S	13–30 mg/L	1.3–3.0 mg/dL
Thyroid-stimulating hormone	S	0.34–4.25 mIU/L	0.34–4.25 μIU/mL
Thyroxine, free (fT_4)	S	10.3–21.9 pmol/L	0.8–1.7 ng/dL
Thyroxine, total (T_4)	S	70–151 nmol/L	5.4–11.7 μg/dL
(Free) thyroxine index	S	6.7–10.9	6.7–10.9
Transferrin	S	2.0–4.0 g/L	200–400 mg/dL
Triglycerides (see Table A-5)	S	0.34–2.26 mmol/L	30–200 mg/dL
Triiodothyronine, free (fT_3)	S	3.7–6.5 pmol/L	2.4–4.2 pg/mL
Triiodothyronine, total (T_3)	S	1.2–2.1 nmol/L	77–135 ng/dL
Troponin I	S		
Normal population, 99 %tile		0–0.08 μg/L	0–0.08 ng/mL
Cut-off for MI		>0.4 μg/L	>0.4 ng/mL
Troponin T	S		
Normal population, 99 %tile		0–0.1 μg/L	0–0.01 ng/mL
Cut-off for MI		0–0.1 μg/L	0–0.1 ng/mL
Urea nitrogen	S	2.5–7.1 mmol/L	7–20 mg/dL
Uric acid	S		
Females		0.15–0.33 μmol/L	2.5–5.6 mg/dL
Males		0.18–0.41 μmol/L	3.1–7.0 mg/dL
Urobilinogen	U	0.09–4.2 μmol/d	0.05–25 mg/24 h
Vanillylmandelic acid (VMA)	U, 24h	<30 μmol/d	<6 mg/d
Vasoactive intestinal polypeptide	P	0–60 ng/L	0–60 pg/mL

[a]P, plasma; S, serum; U, urine; WB, whole blood; JF, joint fluid.

TOXICOLOGY AND THERAPEUTIC DRUG MONITORING

DRUG	THERAPEUTIC RANGE		TOXIC LEVEL	
	SI UNITS	CONVENTIONAL UNITS	SI UNITS	CONVENTIONAL UNITS
Acetaminophen	66–199 µmol/L	10–30 µg/mL	>1320 µmol/L	>200 µg/mL
Amikacin				
Peak	34–51 µmol/L	20–30 µg/mL	>60 µmol/L	>35 µg/mL
Trough	0–17 µmol/L	0–10 µg/mL	>17 µmol/L	>10 µg/mL
Amitriptyline/Nortriptyline (Total Drug)	430–900 nmol/L	120–250 ng/mL	>1800 nmol/L	>500 ng/mL
Amphetamine	150–220 nmol/L	20–30 ng/mL	>1500 nmol/L	>200 ng/mL
Bromide	1.3–6.3 mmol/L	Sedation: 10–50 mg/dL	6.4–18.8 mmol/L	51–150 mg/dL: mild toxicity
	9.4–18.8 mmol/L	Epilepsy: 75–150 mg/dL	>18.8 mmol/L	
			>37.5 mmol/L	>150 mg/dL: Severe toxicity
				>300 mg/dL: Lethal
Carbamazepine	17–42 µmol/L	4–10 µg/mL	85 µmol/L	>20 µg/mL
Chloramphenicol				
Peak	31–62 µmol/L	10–20 µg/mL	>77 µmol/L	>25 µg/mL
Trough	15–31 µmol/L	5–10 µg/mL	>46 µmol/L	> 15 µg/mL
Chlordiazepoxide	1.7–10 µmol/L	0.5–3.0 µg/mL	>17 µmol/L	>5.0 µg/mL
Clonazepam	32–240 nmol/L	10–75 ng/mL	>320 nmol/L	>100 ng/mL
Clozapine	0.6–2.1 µmol/L	200–700 ng/mL	>3.7 µmol/L	>1200 ng/mL
Cocaine			>3.3 µmol/L	>1.0 µg/mL
Codeine	43–110 nmol/mL	13–33 ng/mL	>3700 nmol/mL	>1100 ng/mL (lethal)
Cyclosporine				
Renal Transplant				
0–6 months	208–312 nmol/L	250–375 ng/mL	>312 nmol/L	>375 ng/mL
6–12 months after transplant	166–250 nmol/L	200–300 ng/mL	>250 nmol/L	>300 ng/mL
>12 months	83–125 nmol/L	100–150 ng/mL	>125 nmol/L	>150 ng/mL
Cardiac Transplant				
0–6 months	208–291 nmol/L	250–350 ng/mL	>291 nmol/L	>350 ng/mL
6–12 months after transplant	125–208 nmol/L	150–250 ng/mL	>208 nmol/L	>250 ng/mL
>12 months	83–125 nmol/L	100–150 ng/mL	>125 nmol/L	150 ng/mL
Lung Transplant				
0–6 months	250–374 nmol/L	300–450 ng/mL	>374 nmol/L	>450 ng/mL
Liver Transplant				
0–7 days	249–333 nmol/L	300–400 ng/mL	>333 nmol/L	>400 ng/mL
2–4 weeks	208–291 nmol/L	250–350 ng/mL	>291 nmol/L	>350 ng/mL
5–8 weeks	166–249 nmol/L	200–300 ng/mL	>249 nmol/L	>300 ng/mL
9–52 weeks	125–208 nmol/L	150–250 ng/mL	>208 nmol/L	>250 ng/mL
>1 year	83–166 nmol/L	100–200 ng/mL	>166 nmol/L	>200 ng/mL
Desipramine	375–1130 nmol/L	100–300 ng/mL	>1880 nmol/L	>500 ng/mL
Diazepam (and Metabolite)				
Diazepam	0.7–3.5 µmol/L	0.2–1.0 µg/mL	>7.0 µmol/L	>2.0 µg/mL
Nordiazepam	0.4– 6.6 µmol/L	0.1–1.8 µg/mL	>9.2 µmol/L	>2.5 µg/mL
Digoxin	0.64–2.6 nmol/L	0.5–2.0 ng/mL	>3.1 nmol/L	>2.4 ng/mL
Disopyramide	>7.4 µmol/L	2.5 µg/mL	20.6 µmol/L	>7 µg/mL
Doxepin and Nordoxepin				
Doxepin	0.36–0.98 µmol/L	101–274 ng/mL	>1.8 µmol/L	>503 ng/mL
Nordoxepin	0.38–1.04 µmol/L	106–291 ng/mL	>1.9 µmol/L	>531 ng/mL
Ethanol				
Behavioral changes			>4.3 mmol/L	>20 mg/dL
Legal limit			≥17 mmol/L	≥80 mg/dL
Critical with acute exposure			>54 mmol/L	>250 mg/dL
Ethylene Glycol				
Toxic			>2 mmol/L	>12 mg/dL
Lethal			>20 mmol/L	>120 mg/dL
Ethosuximide	280–700 µmol/L	40–100 µg/mL	>700 µmol/L	>100 µg/mL
Flecainide	0.5–2.4 µmol/L	0.2–1.0 µg/mL	>3.6 µmol/L	>1.5 µg/mL

(Continued)

TABLE A-3 (*CONTINUED*)

TOXICOLOGY AND THERAPEUTIC DRUG MONITORING

DRUG	THERAPEUTIC RANGE		TOXIC LEVEL	
	SI UNITS	CONVENTIONAL UNITS	SI UNITS	CONVENTIONAL UNITS
Gentamicin				
Peak	10–21 µmol/mL	5–10 µg/mL	>25 µmol/mLµ	>12 µg/mL
Trough	0–4.2 µmol/mL	0–2 µg/mL	>4.2 µmol/mLµ	>2 µg/mL
Heroin (Diacetyl Morphine)			>700 µmol/L	>200 ng/mL (as morphine)
Ibuprofen	49–243 µmol/L	10–50 µg/mL	>97 µmol/L	>200 µg/mL
Imipramine (and metabolite)				
Desipramine	375–1130 nmol/L	100–300 ng/mL	>1880 nmol/L	>500 ng/mL
Total Imipramine+ Desipramine	563–1130 nmol/L	150–300 ng/mL	>1880 nmol/L	>500 ng/mL
Lidocaine	5.1–21.3 µmol/L	1.2–5.0 µg/mL	>38.4 µmol/L	>9.0 µg/mL
Lithium	0.5–1.3 meq/L	0.5–1.3 meq/L	>2 mmol/L	>2 meq/L
Methadone	1.3–3.2 µmol/L	0.4–1.0 µg/mL	>6.5 µmol/L	>2 µg/mL
Methamphetamine		20–30 ng/mL		0.1–1.0 µg/mL
Methanol			>6 mmol/L	>20 mg/dL
			>16 mmol/L	>50 mg/dL Severe
			>28 mmol/L	Toxicity
				>89 mg/dL Lethal
Methotrexate				
Low-dose	0.01–0.1 µmol/L	0.01–0.1 µmol/L	>0.1 mmol/L	>0.1 mmol/L
High-dose (24 h)	<5.0 µmol/L	<5.0 µmol/L	>5.0 µmol/L	>5.0 µmol/L
High-dose (48 h)	<0.50 µmol/L	<0.50 µmol/L	>0.5 µmol/L	>0.5 µmol/L
High-dose (72 h)	<0.10 µmol/L	<0.10 µmol/L	>0.1 µmol/L	>0.1 µmol/L
Morphine	35–250 µmol/L	10–70 ng/mL	180–14000 µmol/L	50–4000 ng/mL
Nitroprusside (as thiocyanate)	103–499 µmol/L	6–29 µg/mL	860 µmol/L	>50 µg/mL
Nortriptyline	190–569 nmol/L	50–150 ng/mL	>1900 nmol/L	>500 ng/mL
Phenobarbital	65–172 µmol/L	15–40 µg/mL	>215 µmol/L	>50 µg/mL
Phenytoin	40–79 µmol/L	10–20 µg/mL	>118 µmol/L	>30 µg/mL
Phenytoin, Free	4.0–7.9 µg/mL	1–2 µg/mL	>13.9 µg/mL	>3.5 µg/mL
% Free	.08–.14	8–14 %		
Primidone and Metabolite				
Primidone	23–55 µmol/L	5–12 µg/mL	>69 µmol/L	>15 µg/mL
Phenobarbital	65–172 µmol/L	15–40 µg/mL	>215 µmol/L	>50 µg/mL
Procainamide				
Procainamide	17 42 µmol/L	4–10 µg/mL	>51 µmol/L	>12 µg/mL
NAPA (N-acetylprocainamide)	22–72 µmol/L	6–120 µg/mL	>126 µmol/L	>35 µg/mL
Quinidine	>6.2–15.4 µmol/L	2.0 –5.0 µg/mL	>31 µmol/L	>10 µg/mL
Salicylates	145–2100 µmol/L	2–29 mg/dL	>2172 µmol/L	>30 mg/dL
Sirolimus (Trough Level)				
Kidney Transplant	4.4–13.1 nmol/L	4–12 ng/mL	>16 nmol/L	>15 ng/mL
Tacrolimus (FK506) (trough)				
Kidney and Liver				
0–2 months post transplant	12–19 nmol/L	10–15 ng/mL	>25 nmol/L	>20 ng/mL
>2 months post transplant	6–12 nmol/L	5–10 ng/mL		
Heart				
0–2 months post transplant	19–25 nmol/L	15–20 ng/mL	>25 nmol/L	>20 ng/mL
3–6 months post transplant	12–19 nmol/L	10–15 ng/mL		
>6 months post transplant	10–12 nmol/L	8–10 ng/mL		
Theophylline	56–111 µg/mL	10–20 µg/mL	>140 µg/mL	>25 µg/mL
Thiocyanate				
After nitroprusside infusion	103–499 µmol/L	6–29 µg/mL	860 µmol/L	>50 µg/mL
Nonsmoker	17–69 µmol/L	1–4 µg/mL		
Smoker	52–206 µmol/L	3–12 µg/mL		
Tobramycin				
Peak	11–22 µg/L	5–10 µg/mL	>26 µg/L	>12 µg/mL
Trough	0–4.3 µg/L	0–2 µg/mL	>4.3 µg/L	>2 µg/mL

TOXICOLOGY AND THERAPEUTIC DRUG MONITORING

DRUG	THERAPEUTIC RANGE		TOXIC LEVEL	
	SI UNITS	CONVENTIONAL UNITS	SI UNITS	CONVENTIONAL UNITS
Valproic acid	350–700 µmol/L	50–100 µg/mL	>1000 µmol/L	>150 µg/mL
Vancomycin				
Peak	14–28 µmol/L	20–40 µg/mL	>55µµmol/L	>80 µg/mL
Trough	3.5–10.4 µmol/L	5–15 µg/mL	>14 µmol/L	>20 µg/mL

TABLE A-4

VITAMINS AND SELECTED TRACE MINERALS

SPECIMEN	ANALYTE[a]	REFERENCE RANGE	
		SI UNITS	CONVENTIONAL UNITS
Aluminum	S	<0.2 µmol/L	<5.41 µg/L
	U, random	0.19–1.11 µmol/L	5–30 µg/L
Arsenic	WB	0.03–0.31 µmol/L	2–23 µg/L
	U, 24 h	0.07–0.67 µmol/L	5–50 µg/d
Cadmium	WB	<44.5 nmol/L	<5.0 µg/L
Coenzyme Q10 (ubiquinone)	P	433–1532 µg/L	433–1532 µg/L
B carotene	S	0.07–1.43 µmol/L	4–77 µg/dL
Copper			
	S	11–22 µmol/L	70–140 µg/dL
	U, 24 h	<0.95 µmol/d	<60 µg/d
Folic acid	RC	340–1020 nmol/L cells	150–450 ng/mL cells
Folic acid	S	12.2–40.8 nmol/L	5.4–18.0 ng/mL
Lead (adult)	S	<0.5 µmol/L	<10 µg/dL
Mercury			
	WB	3.0–294 nmol/L	0.6–59 µg/L
	U, 24 h	<99.8 nmol/L	<20 µg/L
Selenium	S	0.8–2.0 µmol/L	63–160 µg/L
Vitamin A	S	0.7–3.5 µmol/L	20–100 µg/dL
Vitamin B_1 (thiamine)	S	0–75 nmol/L	0–2 µg/dL
Vitamin B_2 (riboflavin)	S	106–638 nmol/L	4–24 µg/dL
Vitamin B_6	P	20–121 nmol/L	5–30 ng/mL
Vitamin B_{12}	S	206–735 pmol/L	279–996 pg/mL
Vitamin C (ascorbic acid)	S	23–57 µmol/L	0.4–1.0 mg/dL
Vitamin D_3, 1,25-dihydroxy	S	60–108 pmol/L	25–45 pg/mL
Vitamin D_3, 25-hydroxy	P		
Summer		37.4–200 nmol/L	15–80 ng/mL
Winter		34.9–105 nmol/L	14–42 ng/mL
Vitamin E	S	12–42 µmol/L	5–18 µg/mL
Vitamin K	S	0.29–2.64 nmol/L	0.13–1.19 ng/mL
Zinc	S	11.5–18.4 µmol/L	75–120 µg/dL

[a]P, plasma; RC, red cells; S, serum; WB, whole blood; U, urine.

TABLE A-5

CLASSIFICATION OF LDL, TOTAL, AND HDL CHOLESTEROL

LDL cholesterol, mg/dL (mmol/L)

<70 (<1.81)	Therapeutic option for very high risk patients
<100 (<2.59)	Optimal
100–129 (2.59–3.34)	Near optimal/above optimal
130–159 (3.36–4.11)	Borderline high
160–189 (4.14–4.89)	High
≥190 (≥4.91)	Very high

Total cholesterol, mg/dL (mmol/L)

<200 (<5.17)	Desirable
200–239 (5.17–6.18)	Borderline high
≥240 (≥6.21)	High

HDL cholesterol, mg/dL (mmol/L)

<40 (<1.03)	Low
≥60 (≥1.55)	High

Note: LDL, low-density lipoprotein; HDL, high-density lipoprotein.

Source: Executive summary of the third report of the National Cholesterol Education Program (NCEP) expert panel on detection, evaluation, and treatment of high blood cholesterol in adults (adult treatment panel III). JAMA 285:2486, 2001; and Implications of recent clinical trials for the National Cholesterol Education Program Adult Treatment Panel III Guidelines: SM Grundy et al for the Coordinating Committee of the National Cholesterol Education Program. Circulation 110:227, 2004.

REFERENCE VALUES FOR SPECIFIC ANALYTES

TABLE A-6

CEREBROSPINAL FLUID (CSF)[a]

	REFERENCE RANGE	
CONSTITUENT	**SI UNITS**	**CONVENTIONAL UNITS**
Osmolarity	292–297 mmol/kg water	292–297 mosmol/L
Electrolytes		
Sodium	137–145 mmol/L	137–145 meq/L
Potassium	2.7–3.9 mmol/L	2.7–3.9 meq/L
Calcium	1.0–1.5 mmol/L	2.1–3.0 meq/L
Magnesium	1.0–1.2 mmol/L	2.0–2.5 meq/L
Chloride	116–122 mmol/L	116–122 meq/L
CO_2 content	20–24 mmol/L	20–24 meq/L
P_{CO_2}	6–7 kPa	45–49 mmHg
pH	7.31–7.34	
Glucose	2.22–3.89 mmol/L	40–70 mg/dL
Lactate	1–2 mmol/L	10–20 mg/dL
Total protein		
Lumbar	0.15–0.5 g/L	15–50 mg/dL
Cisternal	0.15–0.25 g/L	15–25 mg/dL
Ventricular	0.06–0.15 g/L	6–15 mg/dL
Albumin	0.066–0.442 g/L	6.6–44.2 mg/dL
IgG	0.009–0.057 g/L	0.9–5.7 mg/dL
IgG index[b]	0.29–0.59	
Oligoclonal bands	<2 bands not present in matched serum sample	
Ammonia	15–47 µmol/L	25–80 µg/dL
Creatinine	44–168 µmol/L	0.5–1.9 mg/dL
Myelin basic protein	<4 µg/L	
CSF pressure		50–180 mmH₂O

TABLE A-6 (*CONTINUED*)

CEREBROSPINAL FLUID (CSF)[a]

	REFERENCE RANGE	
CONSTITUENT	SI UNITS	CONVENTIONAL UNITS
CSF volume (adult)	~150 mL	
Red blood cells	0	0
Leukocytes		
Total	0–5 mononuclear cells per μL	0–5 mononuclear cells per mm^3
Differential		
Lymphocytes	60–70%	
Monocytes	30–50%	
Neutrophils	None	

[a]Since cerebrospinal fluid concentrations are equilibrium values, measurements of the same parameters in blood plasma obtained at the same time are recommended. However, there is a time lag in attainment of equilibrium, and cerebrospinal levels of plasma constituents that can fluctuate rapidly (such as plasma glucose) may not achieve stable values until after a significant lag phase.
[b]IgG index = CSF IgG (mg/dL) × serum albumin (g/dL)/Serum IgG (g/dL) × CSF albumin (mg/dL).

TABLE A-7

URINE ANALYSIS

	REFERENCE RANGE	
	SI UNITS	CONVENTIONAL UNITS
Acidity, titratable	20–40 mmol/d	20–40 meq/d
Ammonia	30–50 mmol/d	30–50 meq/d
Amylase		4–400 U/L
Amylase/creatinine clearance ratio [(Cl$_{am}$/Cl$_{cr}$) × 100]	1–5	1–5
Calcium (10 meq/d or 200 mg/d dietary calcium)	<7.5 mmol/d	<300 mg/d
Creatine, as creatinine		
Female	<760 μmol/d	<100 mg/d
Male	<380 μmol/d	<50 mg/d
Creatinine	8.8–14 mmol/d	1.0–1.6 g/d
Eosinophils	<100,000 eosinophils/L	<100 eosinophils/mL
Glucose (glucose oxidase method)	0.3–1.7 mmol/d	50–300 mg/d
5-Hydroxyindoleacetic acid (5-HIAA)	10–47 μmol/d	2–9 mg/d
Iodine, spot urine		
WHO classification of iodine deficiency		
Not iodine deficient	>100 μg/L	>100 μg/L
Mild iodine deficiency	50–100 μg/L	50–100 μg/L
Moderate iodine deficiency	20–49 μg/L	20–49 μg/L
Severe iodine deficiency	<20 μg/L	<20 μg/L
Microalbumin		
Normal	0.0–0.03 g/d	0–30 mg/d
Microalbuminuria	0.03–0.30 g/d	30–300 mg/d
Clinical albuminuria	>0.3 g/d	>300 mg/d
Microalbumin/creatinine ratio		
Normal	0–3.4 g/mol creatinine	0–30 μg/mg creatinine
Microalbuminuria	3.4–34 g/mol creatinine	30–300 μg/mg creatinine
Clinical albuminuria	>34 g/mol creatinine	>300 μg/mg creatinine
Oxalate		
Male	80–500 μmol/d	7–44 mg/d
Female	45–350 μmol/d	4–31 mg/d
pH	5.0–9.0	5.0–9.0
Phosphate (phosphorus) (varies with intake)	12.9–42.0 mmol/d	400–1300 mg/d
Potassium (varies with intake)	25–100 mmol/d	25–100 meq/d

(Continued)

URINE ANALYSIS

	REFERENCE RANGE	
	SI UNITS	CONVENTIONAL UNITS
Protein	<0.15 g/d	<150 mg/d
Sediment		
Red blood cells	0–2/high power field	
White blood cells	0–2/high power field	
Bacteria	None	
Crystals	None	
Bladder cells	None	
Squamous cells	None	
Tubular cells	None	
Broad casts	None	
Epithelial cell casts	None	
Granular casts	None	
Hyaline casts	0–5/low power field	
Red blood cell casts	None	
Waxy casts	None	
White cell casts	None	
Sodium (varies with intake)	100–260 mmol/d	100–260 meq/d
Specific gravity	1.001–1.035	1.001–1.035
Urea nitrogen	214–607 mmol/d	6–17 g/d
Uric acid (normal diet)	1.49–4.76 mmol/d	250–800 mg/d

Note: WHO, World Health Organization.

TABLE A-8

DIFFERENTIAL NUCLEATED CELL COUNTS OF BONE MARROW ASPIRATES[a]

	OBSERVED RANGE, %	95% CONFIDENCE INTERVALS, %	MEAN, %
Blast cells	0–3.2	0–3.0	1.4
Promyelocytes	3.6–13.2	3.2–12.4	7.8
Neutrophil myelocytes	4–21.4	3.7–10.0	7.6
Eosinophil myelocytes	0–5.0	0–2.8	1.3
Metamyelocytes	1–7.0	2.3–5.9	4.1
Neutrophils			
Males	21.0–45.6	21.9–42.3	32.1
Females	29.6–46.6	28.8–45.9	37.4
Eosinophils	0.4–4.2	0.3–4.2	2.2
Eosinophils plus eosinophil myelocytes	0.9–7.4	0.7–6.3	3.5
Basophils	0–0.8	0–0.4	0.1
Erythroblasts			
Males	18.0–39.4	16.2–40.1	28.1
Females	14.0–31.8	13.0–32.0	22.5
Lymphocytes	4.6–22.6	6.0–20.0	13.1
Plasma cells	0–1.4	0–1.2	0.6
Monocytes	0–3.2	0–2.6	1.3
Macrophages	0–1.8	0–1.3	0.4
M:E ratio			
Males	1.1–4.0	1.1–4.1	2.1
Females	1.6–5.4	1.6–5.2	2.8

[a]Based on bone marrow aspirate from 50 healthy volunteers (30 men, 20 women).
Source: From BJ Bain: The bone marrow aspirate of healthy subjects. Br J Haematol 94(1):206, 1996.

TABLE A-9

STOOL ANALYSIS

	REFERENCE RANGE	
	SI UNITS	CONVENTIONAL UNITS
Amount	0.1–0.2 kg/d	100–200 g/24 h
Coproporphyrin	611–1832 nmol/d	400–1200 µg/24 h
Fat		
Adult		<7 g/d
Adult on fat-free diet		<4 g/d
Fatty acids	0–21 mmol/d	0–6 g/24 h
Leukocytes	None	None
Nitrogen	<178 mmol/d	<2.5 g/24 h
pH	7.0–7.5	
Occult blood	Negative	Negative
Trypsin		20–95 U/g
Urobilinogen	85–510 µmol/d	50–300 mg/24 h
Uroporphyrins	12–48 nmol/d	10–40 µg/24 h
Water	<0.75	<75%

Source: Modified from FT Fishbach, MB Dunning III: *A Manual of Laboratory and Diagnostic Tests*, 7th ed., Lippincott Williams & Wilkins, Philadelphia, 2004.

SPECIAL FUNCTION TESTS

TABLE A-10

RENAL FUNCTION TESTS

	REFERENCE RANGE	
	SI UNITS	CONVENTIONAL UNITS
Clearances (corrected to 1.72 m^2 body surface area)		
Measures of glomerular filtration rate		
Inulin clearance (Cl)		
Males (mean ± 1 SD)	2.1 ± 0.4 mL/s	124 ± 25.8 mL/min
Females (mean ± 1 SD)	2.0 ± 0.2 mL/s	119 ± 12.8 mL/min
Endogenous creatinine clearance	1.5–2.2 mL/s	91–130 mL/min
Measures of effective renal plasma flow and tubular function		
p-Aminohippuric acid clearance (Cl$_{PAH}$)		
Males (mean ± 1 SD)	10.9 ± 2.7 mL/s	654 ± 163 mL/min
Females (mean ± 1 SD)	9.9 ± 1.7 mL/s	594 ± 102 mL/min
Concentration and dilution test		
Specific gravity of urine		
After 12-h fluid restriction	>1.025	>1.025
After 12-h deliberate water intake	≤1.003	≤1.003
Protein excretion, urine	<0.15 g/d	<150 mg/d
Specific gravity, maximal range	1.002–1.028	1.002–1.028
Tubular reabsorption, phosphorus	0.79–0.94 of filtered load	79–94% of filtered load

TABLE A-11

CIRCULATORY FUNCTION TESTS

	RESULTS: REFERENCE RANGE	
TEST	**SI UNITS (RANGE)**	**CONVENTIONAL UNITS (RANGE)**
Arteriovenous oxygen difference	30–50 mL/L	30–50 mL/L
Cardiac output (Fick)	2.5–3.6 L/m^2 of body surface area per min	2.5–3.6 L/m^2 of body surface area per min
Contractility indexes		
Max. left ventricular dp/dt(dp/dt)/DP when DP = 5.3 kPa (40 mmHg) (DP, diastolic pressure)	220 kPa/s (176–250 kPa/s) (37.6 ± 12.2)/s	1650 mmHg/s (1320–1880 mmHg/s) (37.6 ± 12.2)/s
Mean normalized systolic ejection rate (angiography)	3.32 ± 0.84 end-diastolic volumes per second	3.32 ± 0.84 end-diastolic volumes per second
Mean velocity of circumferential fiber shortening (angiography)	1.83 ± 0.56 circumferences per second	1.83 ± 0.56 circumferences per second
Ejection fraction: stroke volume/end-diastolic volume (SV/EDV)	0.67 ± 0.08 (0.55–0.78)	0.67 ± 0.08 (0.55–0.78)
End-diastolic volume	70 ± 20.0 mL/m^2 (60–88 mL/m^2)	70 ± 20.0 mL/m^2 (60–88 mL/m^2)
End-systolic volume	25 ± 5.0 mL/m^2 (20–33 mL/m^2)	25 ± 5.0 mL/m^2 (20–33 mL/m^2)
Left ventricular work		
Stroke work index	50 ± 20.0 (g·m)/m^2 (30–110)	50 ± 20.0 (g·m)/m^2 (30–110)
Left ventricular minute work index	1.8–6.6 [(kg·m)/m^2]/min	1.8–6.6 [(kg·m)/m^2]/min
Oxygen consumption index	110–150 mL	110–150 mL
Maximum oxygen uptake	35 mL/min (20–60 mL/min)	35 mL/min (20–60 mL/min)
Pulmonary vascular resistance	2–12 (kPa·s)/L	20–130 (dyn·s)/cm^5
Systemic vascular resistance	77–150 (kPa·s)/L	770–1600 (dyn·s)/cm^5

Source: E Braunwald et al: *Heart Disease*, 6th ed, Philadelphia, Saunders, 2001.

TABLE A-12

GASTROINTESTINAL TESTS

	RESULTS	
TEST	**SI UNITS**	**CONVENTIONAL UNITS**
Absorption tests		
D-Xylose: after overnight fast, 25 g xylose given in oral aqueous solution		
Urine, collected for following 5 h	25% of ingested dose	25% of ingested dose
Serum, 2 h after dose	2.0–3.5 mmol/L	30–52 mg/dL
Vitamin A: a fasting blood specimen is obtained and 200,000 units of vitamin A in oil is given orally	Serum level should rise to twice fasting level in 3–5 h	Serum level should rise to twice fasting level in 3–5 h
Bentiromide test (pancreatic function): 500 mg bentiromide (chymex) orally; *p*-aminobenzoic acid (PABA) measured		
Plasma		>3.6 (±1.1) µg/mL at 90 min
Urine	>50% recovered in 6 h	>50% recovered in 6 h
Gastric juice		
Volume		
24 h	2–3 L	2–3 L
Nocturnal	600–700 mL	600–700 mL
Basal, fasting	30–70 mL/h	30–70 mL/h
Reaction		
pH	1.6–1.8	1.6–1.8
Titratable acidity of fasting juice	4–9 µmol/s	15–35 meq/h
Acid output		
Basal		
Females (mean ± 1 SD)	0.6 ± 0.5 µmol/s	2.0 ± 1.8 meq/h
Males (mean ± 1 SD)	0.8 ± 0.6 µmol/s	3.0 ± 2.0 meq/h

GASTROINTESTINAL TESTS

TEST	RESULTS	
	SI UNITS	CONVENTIONAL UNITS
Maximal (after SC histamine acid phosphate, 0.004 mg/kg body weight, and preceded by 50 mg promethazine, or after betazole, 1.7 mg/kg body weight, or pentagastrin, 6 µg/kg body weight)		
Females (mean ± 1 SD)	4.4 ± 1.4 µmol/s	16 ± 5 meq/h
Males (mean ± 1 SD)	6.4 ± 1.4 µmol/s	23 ± 5 meq/h
Basal acid output/maximal acid output ratio	≤0.6	≤0.6
Gastrin, serum	0–200 µg/L	0–200 pg/mL
Secretin test (pancreatic exocrine function): 1 unit/kg body weight, IV		
Volume (pancreatic juice) in 80 min	>2.0 mL/kg	>2.0 mL/kg
Bicarbonate concentration	>80 mmol/L	>80 meq/L
Bicarbonate output in 30 min	>10 mmol	>10 meq

TABLE A-13

NORMAL VALUES OF DOPPLER ECHOCARDIOGRAPHIC MEASUREMENTS IN ADULTS

	RANGE	MEAN
RVD (cm), measured at the base in apical 4-chamber view	2.6–4.3	3.5 ± 0.4
LVID (cm), measured in the parasternal long axis view	3.6–5.4	4.7 ± 0.4
Posterior LV wall thickness (cm)	0.6–1.1	0.9 ± 0.4
IVS wall thickness (cm)	0.6–1.1	0.9 ± 0.4
Left atrial dimension (cm), antero-posterior dimension	2.3–3.8	3.0 ± 0.3
Aortic root dimension (cm)	2.0–3.5	2.4 ± 0.4
Aortic cusps separation (cm)	1.5–2.6	1.9 ± 0.4
Percentage of fractional shortening	34–44%	36%
Mitral flow (m/s)	0.6–1.3	0.9
Tricuspid flow (m/s)	0.3–0.7	0.5
Pulmonary artery (m/s)	0.6–0.9	0.75
Aorta (m/s)	1.0–1.7	1.35

Note: RVD, right ventricular dimension; LVID, left ventricular internal dimension; LV, left ventricle; IVS, interventricular septum.

Source: From A Weyman: *Principles and Practice of Echocardiography*, 2d ed., Philadelphia, Lea & Febiger, 1994.

TABLE A-14

SUMMARY OF VALUES USEFUL IN PULMONARY PHYSIOLOGY

		TYPICAL VALUES	
	SYMBOL	MAN, AGE 40, 75 KG, 175 CM TALL	WOMAN, AGE 40, 60 KG, 160 CM TALL
Pulmonary Mechanics			
Spirometry—volume-time curves			
Forced vital capacity	FVC	5.1 L	3.6 L
Forced expiratory volume in 1 s	FEV_1	4.1 L	2.9 L
FEV_1/FVC	FEV_1%	80%	82%
Maximal midexpiratory flow	MMF (FEF 25–27)	4.8 L/s	3.6 L/s
Maximal expiratory flow rate	MEFR (FEF 200–1200)	9.4 L/s	6.1 L/s
Spirometry—flow-volume curves			
Maximal expiratory flow at 50% of expired vital capacity	V_{max} 50 (FEF 50%)	6.1 L/s	4.6 L/s
Maximal expiratory flow at 75% of expired vital capacity	V_{max} 75 (FEF 75%)	3.1 L/s	2.5 L/s
Resistance to airflow			
Pulmonary resistance	RL (R_L)	<3.0 (cmH₂O/s)/L	
Airway resistance	Raw	<2.5 (cmH₂O/s)/L	
Specific conductance	SGaw	>0.13 cmH₂O/s	
Pulmonary compliance			
Static recoil pressure at total lung capacity	Pst TLC	25 ± 5 cmH₂O	
Compliance of lungs (static)	CL	0.2 L cmH₂O	
Compliance of lungs and thorax	C(L + T)	0.1 L cmH₂O	
Dynamic compliance of 20 breaths per minute	C dyn 20	0.25 ± 0.05 L/cmH₂O	
Maximal static respiratory pressures			
Maximal inspiratory pressure	MIP	>90 cmH₂O	>50 cmH₂O
Maximal expiratory pressure	MEP	>150 cmH₂O	>120 cmH₂O
Lung Volumes			
Total lung capacity	TLC	6.7 L	4.9 L
Functional residual capacity	FRC	3.7 L	2.8 L
Residual volume	RV	2.0 L	1.6 L
Inspiratory capacity	IC	3.3 L	2.3 L
Expiratory reserve volume	ERV	1.7 L	1.1 L
Vital capacity	VC	5.0 L	3.4 L
Gas Exchange (Sea Level)			
Arterial O₂ tension	Pa_{O_2}	12.7 ± 0.7 kPa (95 ± 5 mmHg)	
Arterial CO₂ tension	Pa_{CO_2}	5.3 ± 0.3 kPa (40 ± 2 mmHg)	
Arterial O₂ saturation	Sa_{O_2}	0.97 ± 0.02 (97 ± 2%)	
Arterial blood pH	pH	7.40 ± 0.02	
Arterial bicarbonate	HCO_3^-	24 + 2 meq/L	
Base excess	BE	0 ± 2 meq/L	
Diffusing capacity for carbon monoxide (single breath)	DL_{CO}	0.42 mL CO/s/mmHg (25 mL CO/min/mmHg)	
Dead space volume	V_D	2 mL/kg body wt	
Physiologic dead space; dead space-tidal volume ratio	V_D/V_T		
Rest		≤ 35% V_T	
Exercise		≤ 20% V_T	
Alveolar-arterial difference for O₂	$P(A - a)_{O_2}$	≤ 2.7 kPa 20≤ kPa (≤ 20 mmHg)	

TABLE A-15

BODY FLUIDS AND OTHER MASS DATA

	REFERENCE RANGE	
	SI UNITS	CONVENTIONAL UNITS
Ascitic fluid		
Body fluid,		
Total volume (lean) of body weight	50% (in obese) to 70%	
Intracellular	0.3–0.4 of body weight	
Extracellular	0.2–0.3 of body weight	
Blood		
Total volume		
Males	69 mL per kg body weight	
Females	65 mL per kg body weight	
Plasma volume		
Males	39 mL per kg body weight	
Females	40 mL per kg body weight	
Red blood cell volume		
Males	30 mL per kg body weight	1.15–1.21 L/m^2 of body surface area
Females	25 mL per kg body weight	0.95–1.00 L/m^2 of body surface area
Body mass index	18.5–24.9 kg/m^2	18.5–24.9 kg/m^2

TABLE A-16

RADIATION-DERIVED UNITS

QUANTITY	OLD UNIT	SI UNIT	NAME FOR SI UNIT (AND ABBREVIATION)	CONVERSION
Activity	curie (Ci)	Disintegrations per second (dps)	becquerel (Bq)	1 Ci = 3.7 × 10^{10} Bq 1 mCi = 37 mBq 1 μCi = 0.037 MBq or 37 GBq 1 Bq = 2.703 × 10^{-11} Ci
Absorbed dose	rad	joule per kilogram (J/kg)	gray (Gy)	1 Gy = 100 rad 1 rad = 0.01 Gy 1 mrad = 10^{-3} cGy
Exposure	roentgen (R)	coulomb per kilogram (C/kg)	—	1 C/kg = 3876 R 1 R = 2.58 × 10^{-4} C/kg 1 mR = 258 pC/kg
Dose equivalent	rem	joule per kilogram (J/kg)	sievert (Sv)	1 Sv = 100 rem 1 rem = 0.01 Sv 1 mrem = 10 μSv

ACKNOWLEDGMENT

The authors acknowledge the contributions of Dr. Patrick M. Sluss, Dr. James L. Januzzi, and Dr. Kent B. Lewandrowski to this chapter in previous editions of Harrison's Principles of Internal Medicine.

FURTHER READINGS

KRATZ A et al: Case records of the Massachusetts General Hospital. Weekly clinicopathological exercises. Laboratory reference values. N Engl J Med 351(15):1548, 2004

LEHMAN HP, HENRY JB: SI units, in *Henry's Clinical Diagnosis and Management by Laboratory Methods*, 21st ed, RC McPherson, MR Pincus (eds). Philadelphia, Elsevier Saunders, 2007, pp 1404–1418

PESCE MA: Reference ranges for laboratory tests and procedures, in *Nelson's Textbook of Pediatrics*, 18th ed, RM Klegman et al (eds). Philadelphia, Elsevier Saunders, 2007, pp 2943–2949

SOLBERG HE: Establishment and use of reference values, in *Tietz Textbook of Clinical Chemistry and Molecular Diagnostics*, 4th ed, CA Burtis et al (eds). Philadelphia, Elsevier Saunders, 2006, pp 425–448

REVIEW AND SELF-ASSESSMENT*

Charles Wiener ■ Gerald Bloomfield ■ Cynthia D. Brown ■ Joshua Schiffer ■ Adam Spivak

QUESTIONS

DIRECTIONS: Choose the **one best** response to each question.

1. A 46-year-old white female presents to your office with concerns about her diagnosis of hypertension 1 month previously. She asks you about her likelihood of developing complications of hypertension, including renal failure and stroke. She denies any past medical history other than hypertension and has no symptoms that suggest secondary causes. She currently is taking hydrochlorothiazide 25 mg/d. She smokes one-half pack/day of cigarettes and drinks alcohol no more than once per week. Her family history is significant for hypertension in both parents. Her mother died of a cerebrovascular accident. Her father is alive but has coronary artery disease and is on hemodialysis. Her blood pressure is 138/90. Body mass index is 23. She has no retinal exudates or other signs of hypertensive retinopathy. Her point of maximal cardiac impulse is not displaced but is sustained. Her rate and rhythm are regular and without gallops. She has good peripheral pulses. An electrocardiogram (ECG) reveals an axis of −30 degrees with borderline voltage criteria for left ventricular hypertrophy. Creatinine is 1.0 mg/dL. Which of the following items in her history and physical examination is a risk factor for a poor prognosis in a patient with hypertension?

   A. Family history of renal failure and cerebrovascular disease
   B. Persistent elevation in blood pressure after the initiation of therapy
   C. Ongoing tobacco use
   D. Ongoing use of alcohol
   E. Presence of left ventricular hypertrophy on ECG

2. A 68-year-old male presents to your office for routine follow-up care. He reports that he is feeling well and has no complaints. His past medical history is significant for hypertension and hypercholesterolemia. He continues to smoke 1 pack/day of

2. (*Continued*)
   cigarettes. He is taking chlorthalidone 25 mg daily, atenolol 25 mg daily, and pravastatin 40 mg nightly. Blood pressure is 133/85 mmHg, and heart rate is 66 beats/min. Cardiac and pulmonary examinations are unremarkable. A pulsatile abdominal mass is felt just to the left of the umbilicus and measures ~4 cm. You confirm the diagnosis of abdominal aortic aneurysm by CT imaging. It is located infrarenally and measures 4.5 cm. All the following are true about the patient's diagnosis *except*

   A. The 5-year risk of rupture of an aneurysm of this size is 1–2%.
   B. Surgical or endovascular intervention is warranted because of the size of the aneurysm.
   C. Infrarenal endovascular stent placement is an option if the aneurysm experiences continued growth in light of the location of the aneurysm infrarenally.
   D. Surgical or endovascular intervention is warranted if the patient develops symptoms of recurrent abdominal or back pain.
   E. Surgical or endovascular intervention is warranted if the aneurysm expands beyond 5.5 cm.

3. A 45-year-old woman presents to the emergency department with complaints of progressive dyspnea on exertion and abrupt onset of painful ulcerations on her toes. She has noted the symptoms for the past 3 months. The dyspnea has progressed such that she is only able to walk about 1 block without stopping. Over this time, she has noticed a cough that occasionally produces thin, pink-tinged sputum. She also has reports that her breathing is worse at night. She sleeps on three pillows but awakens with dyspnea once or twice nightly. Over the past 2 days, she has developed painful ulcerations on toes 1 and 4 on her left foot. She reports that the areas started as reddish painful discoloration that ulcerated over the ensuing days. She denies fevers, chills, or weight loss. She has no history of chest pain, heart disease, or heart murmurs. She has been in good

*Questions and answers were taken from Wiener C, et al (eds). *Harrison's Principles of Internal Medicine Self-Assessment and Board Review, 17th ed.* New York: McGraw-Hill, 2008.

3. (*Continued*)
health until the past 3 months. She takes no medications. Her last dental visit was ~8 months ago. On physical examination, she appears in no distress. Vital signs: blood pressure is 145/92 mmHg, heart rate is 95 beats/min, respiratory rate is 24 breaths/min, temperature is 37.7°C, and SaO₂ is 95% on room air. The cardiovascular examination reveals a regular rate and rhythm. There is a III/VI mid-diastolic murmur with an occasional low-pitched mid-diastolic sound that occurs when the patient is in the upright position. The jugular venous pressure is measured at 10 cm above the sternal angle. A few bibasilar crackles are noted. There is 1+ pitting edema bilaterally to the knees. On her left great toe, there is an area of erythema with central ulceration covered by a black eschar. A similar area is present on her left fourth toe. The peripheral pulses are full and 2+. The patient undergoes an echocardiogram, shown in **Fig. 3**. What is the most appropriate plan of care for this patient?

A. Consult cardiac surgery for definitive therapy.
B. Initiate therapy with IV penicillin and gentamicin.
C. Obtain blood cultures and initiate therapy based upon results.
D. Obtain a positron emission tomographic scan to assess for primary malignancy.
E. Perform left heart catheterization and consider surgery based upon results.

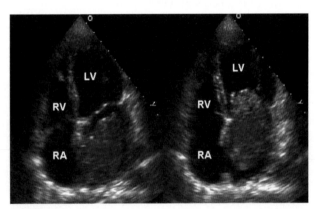

FIGURE 3

4. Your 57-year-old clinic patient is seeing you in follow-up for chronic stable angina. He is a former heavy tobacco smoker who maintained an unhealthy diet and exercise routine until recently. Since initiating a healthy diet and commencing an exercise regimen, he has lost weight and improved his blood pressure control. A cardiac catheterization 1 month ago showed two nonobstructive coronary lesions in the left circumflex artery. He still has angina, which is reproducible with moderate exercise

4. (*Continued*)
that is fully relieved by one sublingual nitroglycerin. Which of the following factors is least likely to be contributing to his angina?

A. Epicardial coronary artery resistance
B. Heart rate
C. Hemoglobin concentration
D. Diffusion capacity of the lung

5. In the tracing below (**Fig. 5**), what type of conduction abnormality is present and where in the conduction pathway is the block usually found?

A. First-degree AV block; intranodal
B. Second-degree AV block type 1; intranodal
C. Second-degree AV block type 2; infranodal
D. Second-degree AV block type 2; intranodal

6. A 62-year-old male loses consciousness in the street, and resuscitative efforts are undertaken. In the emergency room an electrocardiogram is obtained, part of which is shown below (**Fig. 6**). Which of the following disorders could account for this man's presentation?

A. Hypokalemia
B. Hyperkalemia
C. Intracerebral hemorrhage
D. Digitalis toxicity
E. Hypocalcemic tetany

7. You are seeing an 86-year-old male patient with severe aortic stenosis in follow-up. He has had severe aortic stenosis for 4 years without symptoms. Recently, he has scaled back his activities due to light-headedness with exertion. His wife reports one episode a week ago when he passed out briefly while gardening. On examination, his blood pressure is 150/85 mmHg, heart rate is 76 beats/min. He has a grade III/VI systolic ejection murmur that extends to S₂ with radiation to the carotids. S₂ is barely audible, consistent with his prior examinations. Carotid pulses are delayed as they have been in the past. He has femoral and abdominal aortic bruits. Peripheral pulses are 2+ bilaterally. Laboratory data show a creatinine of 0.9 mg/dL, low-density lipoprotein cholesterol of 75 mg/dL, high-density lipoprotein of 50 mg/dL. What is the next appropriate step in this patient's management?

A. Aortic valve surgery
B. Cardiac rehabilitation
C. End-of-life arrangements with hospice
D. Improved blood pressure control
E. Transthoracic echocardiogram

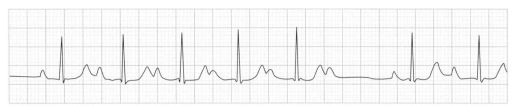

FIGURE 5

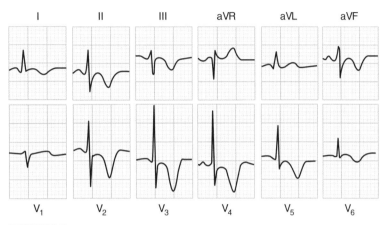

FIGURE 6

8. A 35-year-old man is evaluated for dyspnea. He first noticed shortness of breath with exertion ~12 months ago. It has become progressively worse such that he is only able to walk about 20 ft without stopping. In general, he rates his health as good, although he recalls being told when he was younger that he had a heart murmur. He has not seen a physician in 15 years. On examination, he is noted to be hypoxic with an SaO_2 of 85% on room air. His cardiac examination reveals a harsh machinery-like murmur that is continuous throughout systole and diastole with a palpable thrill. There is late systolic accentuation of the murmur at the upper left sternal angle. He is noted to have cyanosis and clubbing of his toes but not his fingers. What is the most likely cause of the patient's murmur?

A. Anomalous pulmonary venous return
B. Coarctation of the aorta
C. Patent ductus arteriosus
D. Tetralogy of Fallot
E. Ventricular septal defect

9. In the cardiac care unit, you are caring for a 69-year-old man with an inferior ST-segment elevation myocardial infarction (MI). He has undergone successful urgent percutaneous coronary intervention and is recovering. Later that day, he complains of shortness of breath and orthopnea. Vital signs: blood

9. (*Continued*)
pressure is 118/74 mmHg, heart rate is 63 beats/min, respiratory rate is 20 breaths/min, and SaO_2 is 91% on room air. Lung examination shows crackles bilaterally. On cardiac examination, the jugular venous pressure is elevated. There is a grade III/VI musical systolic murmur heard at the base of the heart with a crescendo-decrescendo pattern. The intensity of the murmur does not change with respiration. The murmur does not radiate to the axilla. A two-dimensional echocardiogram is requested. Which of the following echocardiographic findings is most likely?

A. Eccentric mitral regurgitant jet
B. High-frequency fluttering of the anterior mitral leaflet
C. Respiratory variation in velocity across the mitral valve
D. Systolic anterior motion of the aortic (anterior) mitral valve
E. Ventricular septal defect

10. A 44-year-old man with a history of hypertension that is poorly controlled presents to the emergency room with complaint of severe chest pain. The pain began abruptly this afternoon while at rest. He describes the pain as tearing and radiates to the back. He also complains of feeling lightheaded but

10. (*Continued*)

does not have nausea or vomiting. He has never had a similar episode of pain and is usually able to exercise at the gym without chest pain. In addition to hypertension, he also has a history of hypercholesterolemia. He has been prescribed felodipine, 10 mg once daily, and rosuvastatin, 10 mg once daily, but says that he only takes them intermittently. He smokes 1 pack/day of cigarettes and has done so since the age of 20. His family history is significant for coronary artery disease in his father, who had a heart attack at the age of 60. On physical examination, the patient appears uncomfortable and diaphoretic. Vital signs: blood pressure is 190/110 mmHg, heart rate is 112 beats/min, respiratory rate is 26 breaths/min, temperature is 36.3°C, and SaO$_2$ is 98% on room air. His carotid pulses are full and bounding. His cardiac examination reveals a hyperdynamic precordium. The rhythm is tachycardic but regular. An S$_4$ is present. There is a II/VI diastolic murmur heard at the lower left sternal border. An electrocardiogram (ECG) shows 1 mm of ST elevation in leads II, III, and aV$_F$. A contrast-enhanced chest CT shows a dissection of the ascending aorta with a small amount of pericardial fluid. What is the most appropriate management of the patient?

A. Emergent cardiac catheterization
B. Emergent cardiac surgery
C. Intravenous nitroprusside and esmolol alone
D. Intravenous nitroprusside and esmolol and cardiac surgery emergently
E. Thrombolysis with tenecteplase

11. A 29-year-old woman is in the intensive care unit with rhabdomyolysis due to compartment syndrome

11. (*Continued*)

of the lower extremities after a car accident. Her clinical course has been complicated by acute renal failure and severe pain. She has undergone fasciotomies and is admitted to the intensive care unit. An electrocardiogram (ECG) is obtained (shown in **Fig. 11**). What is the most appropriate course of action at this point?

A. 18-lead ECG
B. Coronary catheterization
C. Hemodialysis
D. Intravenous fluids and a loop diuretic
E. Ventilation/perfusion imaging

12. A 54-year-old male with type 2 diabetes mellitus reports 3 months of exertional chest pain. His physical examination is notable for obesity with a body mass index (BMI) of 32 kg/m^2, blood pressure of 150/90, an S$_4$, no cardiac murmurs, and no peripheral edema. Fasting glucose is 130 mg/dL, and serum triglycerides are 200 mg/dL. Which of the following is most likely in this patient?

A. Elevated high-density lipoprotein (HDL) cholesterol
B. Insulin resistance
C. Larger than normal LDL particles
D. Reduced serum endothelin level
E. Reduced serum homocysteine level

13. A 45-year-old man is admitted to the intensive care unit with symptoms of congestive heart failure. He is addicted to heroin and cocaine and uses both drugs daily via injection. His blood cultures have yielded methicillin-sensitive *Staphylococcus aureus* in four of four bottles within 12 h. His vital signs

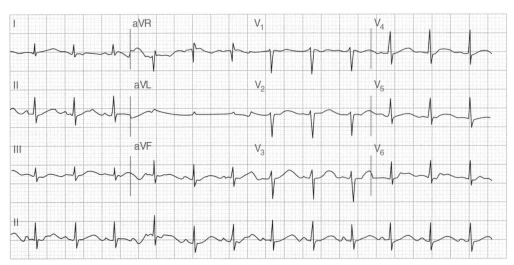

FIGURE 11

13. (*Continued*)

show a blood pressure of 110/40 mmHg and a heart rate of 132 beats/min. There is a IV/VI diastolic murmur heard along the left sternal border. A schematic representation of the carotid pulsation is shown in Fig. 13. What is the most likely cause of the patient's murmur?

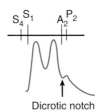

FIGURE 13

A. Aortic regurgitation
B. Aortic stenosis
C. Mitral stenosis
D. Mitral regurgitation
E. Tricuspid regurgitation

14. A 30-year-old male is transported to the emergency department after a motor vehicle accident. He has complaint of moderate chest pain. He becomes hypotensive, and his blood pressure pattern reveals a pulsus paradoxus. The heart sounds appear distant. An examination of the neck veins fails to reveal a Kussmaul's sign. An electrocardiogram is unremarkable, and a chest x-ray reveals an enlarged cardiac silhouette. A right heart catheter is placed. Which of the following values is consistent with the patient's diagnosis?

	PRESSURE, RA mmHg	PRESSURE, PA mmHg	PRESSURE, PCW mmHg
A	16	75/30	11
B	16	34/16	16
C	16	100/30	28
D	16	45/22	20
E	16	22/12	10
Normal values	0–5	12–28/3–13	3–11

Note: RA, atrial pressure; PA, pulmonary arterial; PCW, pulmonary capillary wedge.

15. You are treating a patient with stable angina pectoris. She is a postmenopausal woman with refractory angina despite therapy with metoprolol and isosorbide dinitrate, as well as her other anti-ischemic

15. (*Continued*)

medications. Past medical history is significant for coronary artery bypass grafting (CABG), chronic obstructive pulmonary disease, first-degree atrioventricular block, left bundle branch block, and dyslipidemia. A recent cardiac catheterization showed coronary artery disease not amenable to percutaneous intervention, and the patient is not interested in redo of the CABG. Renal function is normal. Her left ventricular ejection fraction is 15%, and she has New York Heart Association class II heart failure symptoms. Blood pressure and pulse allow for the addition of a calcium channel blocker to her regimen. Which calcium channel–blocking medication is appropriate for this patient?

A. Amlodipine
B. Diltiazem
C. Immediate-release nifedipine
D. Verapamil

16. A 30-year-old female is seen in the clinic before undergoing an esophageal dilation for a stricture. Her past medical history is notable for mitral valve prolapse with mild regurgitation. She takes no medications and is allergic to penicillin. Her physician should recommend which of the following?

A. Clarithromycin 500 mg PO 1 h before the procedure
B. Clindamycin 450 mg PO 1 h before the procedure
C. Vancomycin 1 g intravenously before the procedure
D. The procedure is low-risk, and therefore no prophylaxis is indicated.
E. Her valvular lesion is low-risk, and therefore no prophylaxis is indicated.

17. You are called to the bedside of a patient with Prinzmetal's angina who is having chest pain. The patient had a cardiac catheterization 2 days prior showing a 60% stenosis of the right coronary artery with associated spasm during coronary angiogram. At the patient's bedside, which finding is consistent with the diagnosis of Prinzmetal's angina?

A. Chest pain reproduced by palpation of the chest wall
B. Nonspecific ST-T-wave abnormalities
C. Relief of pain with drinking cold water
D. ST-segment elevation in II, III, and aV_F
E. ST-segment depression in I, aV_L, and V_6

18. A 38-year-old Bolivian male is admitted to the cardiac intensive care unit with decompensated heart failure. He has no known past medical history and takes no medications. He emigrated from Mexico 10 years ago and currently works in a retail store.

18. (*Continued*)

On physical examination, he has signs of congestion and poor perfusion. An ECG shows first-degree atrioventricular block and right bundle branch block. An echocardiogram shows dilated and thinned ventricles. He has an apical aneurysm in the left ventricle with thrombus formation. You treat his heart failure symptomatically and begin anticoagulation. A cardiac catheterization shows normal coronaries without atherosclerosis. Which statement is true regarding this patient's prognosis?

A. Aggressive lipid lowering (low-density lipoprotein <70 mg/dL) has been shown to be beneficial in this condition.

B. Calcium channel blockers will prevent progression of his disease.

C. Cardiac transplantation offers the only cure for this condition.

D. His cardiac function will improve over time.

E. Nifurtimox offers a reasonable chance for cure.

19. You are evaluating a 43-year-old female who has complaint of dyspnea on exertion. She was well until 2 months ago when she noticed decreasing exercise tolerance and fatigue. She denies chest pain but does have New York Heart Association class II symptoms. She has no orthopnea or paroxysmal nocturnal dyspnea. She has noticed bilateral ankle swelling that improves with recumbency. She has one child and has no other past medical history. On cardiac examination, the jugular venous pressure is slightly elevated. There is a prominent *a* wave. There is a right-ventricular tap felt along the left sternal border. S_1 is prominent and P_2 is accentuated. There is a sharp opening sound heard best during expiration just medial to the cardiac apex, which occurs shortly after S_2. A diastolic rumble is heard at the apex with the patient in the left lateral decubitus position. Hepatomegaly and ankle edema are present. The pulse is regular and blood pressure is 108/60 mmHg. The patient is at high risk for developing which of the following?

A. Atrial fibrillation
B. Left-ventricular dysfunction
C. Multifocal atrial tachycardia
D. Right bundle branch block
E. Right-ventricular outflow tract tachycardia

20. Which of the following conditions is not associated with sinus bradycardia?

A. Brucellosis
B. Leptospirosis

20. (*Continued*)

C. Hypothyroidism
D. Advanced liver disease
E. Typhoid fever

21. All of the following are common consequences of congenital heart disease in the adult *except*

A. Eisenmenger syndrome
B. erythrocytosis
C. infective endocarditis
D. pulmonary hypertension
E. stroke

22. Acute hyperkalemia is associated with which of the following electrocardiographic changes?

A. QRS widening
B. Prolongation of the ST segment
C. A decrease in the PR interval
D. Prominent U waves
E. T-wave flattening

23. All of the following clinical findings are consistent with severe mitral stenosis *except*

A. atrial fibrillation
B. opening snap late after S_2
C. pulmonary vascular congestion
D. pulsatile liver
E. right-ventricular heave

24. All the following patients should be evaluated for secondary causes of hypertension *except*

A. a 37-year-old male with strong family history of hypertension and renal failure who presents to your office with a blood pressure of 152/98 mmHg

B. a 26-year-old female with hematuria and a family history of early renal failure who has a blood pressure of 160/88 mmHg

C. a 63-year-old male with no past history with a blood pressure of 162/90 mmHg

D. a 58-year-old male with a history of hypertension since age 45 whose blood pressure has become increasingly difficult to control on four antihypertensive agents

E. a 31-year-old female with complaints of severe headaches, weight gain, and new-onset diabetes mellitus with a blood pressure of 142/89 mmHg

25. You are seeing a 71-year-old female patient with tachycardia-bradycardia syndrome in follow-up. She had a single-lead ventricular pacemaker implanted 2 years ago and has no new complaints. Past medical history also includes an old stroke with mild residual

25. (*Continued*)

left hand weakness and diabetes. Her last transthoracic echocardiogram (TTE) showed a left ventricular ejection fraction of 35–40% but no valvular abnormalities. The left atrium is mildly enlarged. Her medical regimen includes aspirin, metformin, metoprolol, lisinopril, lasix, and dipyridamole. What intervention, if any, should be considered for the patient at this time?

A. Anticoagulation
B. Cardiac catheterization
C. Discontinuation of dipyridamole
D. None, as she has no new complaints

26. A 64-year-old woman with known stage IV breast cancer presents to the emergency room with severe dyspnea and hypotension. Her blood pressure is 92/50 mmHg, and hear rate is 112 beats/min. She has distended neck veins that do not collapse with inspiration. Heart sounds are muffled. The systolic blood pressure drops to 70 with inspiration. An echocardiogram shows a large pericardial effusion with right ventricular diastolic collapse consistent with pericardial tamponade. Which of the following values most accurately demonstrate the expected values on right hear catheterization?

	RIGHT-ATRIAL PRESSURE, mmHg	RIGHT-VENTRICULAR PRESSURE, mmHg	PULMONARY ARTERY PRESSURE, mmHg	PULMONARY CAPILLARY WEDGE PRESSURE, mmHg
A.	5	20/5	25/10	12
B.	8	20/10	30/12	20
C.	17	40/17	45/17	17
D.	18	40/20	45/25	10

27. The electrocardiogram (ECG) (**Fig. 27**) most likely was obtained from which of the following patients?

27. (*Continued*)

A. A 33-year-old female with acute-onset severe headache, disorientation, and intraventricular blood on head CT scan
B. A 42-year-old male with sudden-onset chest pain while playing tennis
C. A 54-year-old female with a long history of smoking and 2 days of increasing shortness of breath and wheezing
D. A 64-year-old female with end-stage renal insufficiency who missed dialysis for the last 4 days
E. A 78-year-old male with syncope, delayed carotid upstrokes, and a harsh systolic murmur in the right second intercostal space

28. You are evaluating a new patient in your clinic who brings this electrocardiogram (ECG; **Fig. 28**) to the visit. The ECG was performed on the patient 2 weeks ago. What complaint do you expect to elicit from the patient?

A. Angina
B. Hemoptysis
C. Paroxysmal nocturnal dyspnea
D. Tachypalpitations

29. A patient is found to have a holosystolic murmur on physical examination. With deep inspiration, the intensity of the murmur increases. This is consistent with which of the following?

A. Atrial-septal defect
B. Austin Flint murmur
C. Carvallo's sign
D. Chronic mitral regurgitation
E. Gallavardin effect

30. A 37-year-old male with Wolff-Parkinson-White syndrome develops a broad-complex irregular tachycardia at a rate of 200 beats/min. He appears

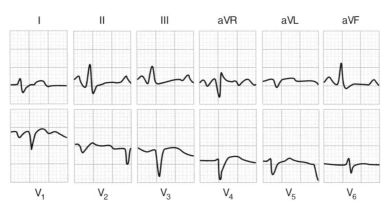

I   II   III   aVR   aVL   aVF

V₁   V₂   V₃   V₄   V₅   V₆

FIGURE 27

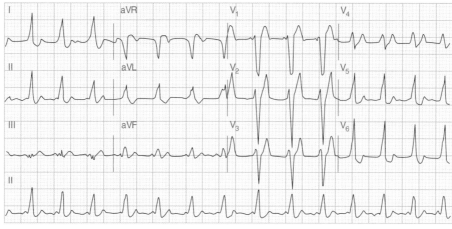

FIGURE 28

30. (*Continued*)
comfortable and has little hemodynamic impairment. Useful treatment at this point might include

A. digoxin
B. amiodarone
C. propranolol
D. verapamil
E. direct-current cardioversion

31. A 72-year-old male seeks evaluation for leg pain with ambulation. He describes the pain as an aching to crampy pain in the muscles of his thighs. The pain subsides within minutes of resting. On rare occasions, he has noted numbness of his right foot at rest and pain in his right leg has woken him at night. He has a history of hypertension and cerebrovascular disease. He previously had a transient ischemic attack and underwent right carotid endarterectomy 4 years previously. He currently takes aspirin, irbesartan, hydrochlorothiazide, and atenolol on a daily basis. On examination, he is noted to have diminished dorsalis pedis and posterior tibial pulses bilaterally. The right dorsal pedis pulse is faint. There is loss of hair in the distal extremities. Capillary refill is ~5 s in the right foot and 3 s in the left foot. Which of the following findings would be suggestive of critical ischemia of the right foot?

A. Ankle-brachial index <0.3
B. Ankle-brachial index <0.9
C. Ankle-brachial index >1.2
D. Lack of palpable dorsalis pedis pulse
E. Presence of pitting edema of the extremities

32. A 24-year-old male seeks medical attention for the recent onset of headaches. The headaches are described as "pounding" and occur during the day and night. He has had minimal relief with acetaminophen. Physical examination is notable for a

32. (*Continued*)
blood pressure of 185/115 mmHg in the right arm, a heart rate of 70 beats/min, arterioventricular (AV) nicking on funduscopic examination, normal jugular veins and carotid arteries, a pressure-loaded PMI with an apical S_4, no abdominal bruits, and reduced pulses in both lower extremities. Review of symptoms is positive only for leg fatigue with exertion. Additional measurement of blood pressure reveals the following:

Right arm	185/115
Left arm	188/113
Right thigh	100/60
Left thigh	102/58

Which of the following diagnostic studies is most likely to demonstrate the cause of the headaches?

A. MRI of the head
B. MRI of the kidney
C. MRI of the thorax
D. 24-h urinary 5-HIAA
E. 24-h urinary free cortisol

33. The patient described in Question 32 is most likely to have which of the following associated cardiac abnormalities?

A. Bicuspid aortic valve
B. Mitral stenosis
C. Preexcitation syndrome
D. Right bundle branch block
E. Tricuspid atresia

34. A 30-year-old female with a history of irritable bowel syndrome presents with complaint of palpitations. On further questioning, the symptoms

34. (*Continued*)

occur randomly throughout the day, perhaps more frequently after caffeine. The primary sensation is of her heart "flip-flopping" in her chest. The patient has never had syncope. Her vital signs and examination are normal. An electrocardiogram (ECG) is obtained, and it shows normal sinus rhythm with no other abnormality. A Holter monitor is obtained and shows premature ventricular contractions occurring approximately six times per minute. The next most appropriate step in her management is

A. referral to a cardiologist for electrophysiologic study
B. beta blocker administration
C. amiodarone administration
D. reassurance that this is not pathologic
E. verapamil administration

35. All the following electrocardiogram (ECG) findings are suggestive of left ventricular hypertrophy *except*

A. (S in V_1 + R in V_5 or V_6) >35 mm
B. R in aVL >11 mm
C. R in aVF >20 mm
D. (R in I + S in III) >25 mm
E. R in aVR >8 mm

36. A 27-year-old female is hospitalized in the intensive care unit (ICU) for Lyme disease. Complete heart block is noted and a single-lead pacemaker is implanted. She is discharged on a long-term course of antibiotics with a permanent pacemaker. She returns to see you in clinic complaining of inability to concentrate, fatigue, palpitations, and cough. On examination, her blood pressure is 121/72 mmHg; heart rate is 60 beats/min, respiratory rate is 18 breaths/min. She has an elevated jugular venous pressure with cannon *a* waves. She has rales on lung auscultation and an

36. (*Continued*)

S_3 on cardiac auscultation but no peripheral edema. Electrocardiogram (ECG) shows a ventricular paced rate at 60/min with repolarization abnormalities. These findings are most consistent with

A. acute myocardial infarction
B. ICU psychosis syndrome
C. Kearne-Sayer syndrome
D. pacemaker syndrome
E. pacemaker twiddler's syndrome

37. You are evaluating a new patient in clinic. He is a 72-year-old male who had a myocardial infarction (MI) and a stroke 3 years ago. He comes to your office to establish a primary care physician and because he ran out of medications (metoprolol, aspirin, lovastatin, lisinopril) 1 week ago. He brings with him an electrocardiogram (ECG) performed 1 year ago (Fig. 37). You obtain another tracing and it is not significantly changed. Other than occasional weakness in his right upper extremity, he has no complaint. He has not had any medications for 2 weeks. Which is the next most appropriate step?

A. Obtain chest radiograph in clinic today
B. Obtain a transthoracic echocardiogram
C. Refill medications and ask him to return to clinic in 6 months
D. Transfer him to the hospital for thrombolytic therapy
E. Transfer him to the hospital for cardiac catheterization

38. All the following disorders may be associated with thoracic aortic aneurysm *except*

A. osteogenesis imperfecta
B. Takayasu's arteritis
C. Ehlers-Danlos syndrome

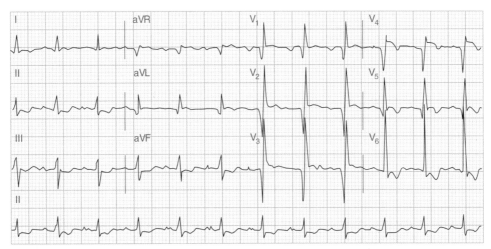

FIGURE 37

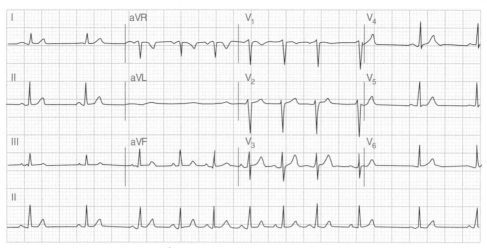

FIGURE 40

39. (*Continued*)
  D. ankylosing spondylitis
  E. Klinefelter's syndrome

39. All the following may cause elevation of serum troponin *except*

  A. congestive heart failure
  B. myocarditis
  C. myocardial infarction
  D. pneumonia
  E. pulmonary embolism

40. What is the correct interpretation of this electrocardiogram (ECG) tracing (**Fig. 40**)?

  A. Atrial fibrillation
  B. Complete heart block with junctional escape rhythm
  C. Idioventricular sinus arrhythmia
  D. Mobitz Type 2 AV Block
  E. Respiratory sinus arrhythmia

41. A 44-year-old male with history of HIV infection is brought to the emergency department by friends because of an altered mental status. They note that he has been coughing with worsening shortness of breath for the past 2–3 weeks. His antiretroviral therapy includes a protease inhibitor. In triage, his blood pressure is 110/74 mmHg; heart rate is 31 beats per minute, respiratory rate is 32 breaths/min, temperature is 38.7°C, and SaO$_2$ is 74% on room air. He appears well perfused. Chest radiograph shows bilateral fluffy infiltrates. An electrocardiogram (ECG) shows sinus bradycardia without ST changes. A chest CT scan shows no pulmonary embolus. After initiating oxygen and establishing an airway, you direct your attention to his bradycardia. Which is the most appropriate step at this time?

41. (*Continued*)
  A. Correct the oxygen deficit, check an arterial blood gas, and monitor closely
  B. Glucagon to reverse the effects of protease inhibitors
  C. Temporary transvenous pacemaker
  D. Urgent cardiac catheterization for percutaneous coronary intervention

42. A 55-year-old female is undergoing evaluation of dyspnea on exertion. She has a history of hypertension since age 32 and is also obese with a body mass index (BMI) of 44 kg/m^2. Her pulmonary function tests show mild restrictive lung disease. An echocardiogram shows a thickened left-ventricular wall, left-ventricular ejection fraction of 70%, and findings suggestive of pulmonary hypertension with an estimated right-ventricular systolic pressure of 55 mmHg, but the echocardiogram is technically difficult and of poor quality. She undergoes a right heart catheterization that shows the following results:

Mean arterial pressure	110 mmHg
Left-ventricular end-diastolic pressure	25 mmHg
Pulmonary artery (PA) systolic pressure	48 mmHg
PA diastolic pressure	20 mmHg
PA mean pressure	34 mmHg
Cardiac output	5.9 L/min

What is the most likely cause of the patient's dyspnea?

  A. Chronic thromboembolic disease
  B. Diastolic heart failure
  C. Obstructive sleep apnea

42. (*Continued*)

    D. Pulmonary arterial hypertension

    E. Systolic heart failure

43. Which of the following congenital cardiac disorders will lead to a left-to-right shunt, generally with cyanosis?

    A. Anomalous origin of the left coronary artery from the pulmonary trunk

    B. Patent ductus arteriosus without pulmonary hypertension

    C. Total anomalous pulmonary venous connection

    D. Ventricular septal defect

    E. Sinus venosus atrial septal defect

44. You are evaluating a new patient in clinic. On cardiac auscultation, there is a high-pitched, blowing, decrescendo diastolic murmur heard best in the third intercostal space along the left sternal border. A second murmur is heard at the apex, which is a low-pitched rumbling mid-diastolic murmur. Sustained hand-grip increases the intensity of the murmurs. The murmurs are heard best at end-expiration. There are also an S_3 and a systolic ejection murmur. The left ventricular impulse is displaced to the left and inferiorly. Radial pulses are brisk with a prominent systolic component. Blood pressure is 170/70 mmHg, heart rate is 98 beats/min, respiratory rate 18 breaths/min. An electrocardiogram (ECG) is obtained in clinic. Which of the following findings do you expect on the ECG tracing for this patient?

    A. Diffuse ST-segment elevation and PR-segment depression

    B. Inferior Q-waves

    C. Left-ventricular hypertrophy

    D. Low voltage

    E. Right-atrial enlargement

45. A 65-year-old male is seen in the emergency department with palpitations. His symptoms began 30 min before arrival. He has not had any dizziness, lightheadedness, or chest pain. His past medical history is notable for a myocardial infarct 2 years ago, chronic atrial fibrillation, and a three-vessel coronary artery bypass graft surgery 1 year ago. Medications include aspirin, metoprolol, warfarin, and lisinopril. An electrocardiogram (ECG) shows wide complex tachycardia at a rate of 170. Which of the following will prove definitively that his rhythm is ventricular tachycardia?

    A. Hypotension

    B. Cannon *a* waves

45. (*Continued*)

    C. An odd ECG with similar QRS morphology

    D. Irregular rhythm

    E. Syncope

46. You have referred your patient for an exercise-electrocardiography stress test. The report indicates that he walked for 7 min of the Bruce protocol and had no chest pain during or after the test. During the exercise, he had multiple premature ventricular complexes and reached 90% of maximum predicted heart rate. He had 2-mm upsloping ST-segment response during exercise. At the end of the protocol and during recovery, he had 1-mm ST-segment depressions, which lasted for 6 min. Blood pressure increased from 127/78 to 167/102 mmHg at maximal exertion. Which feature of this report is most suggestive of severe ischemic heart disease and a high risk of future events?

    A. Diastolic pressure >100 mmHg

    B. Not achieving 95% of maximum predicted heart rate

    C. Persistent ST-segment depressions into recovery

    D. Upsloping ST-segments during exercise

    E. Ventricular ectopy during exercise

47. A 45-year-old female who emigrated from Peru to the United States 10 years ago presents with dyspnea on exertion for the last 4 months. She denies chest pain but has noted significant accumulation of fluid in her abdomen and lower extremity edema. She has a history of tuberculosis, which was treated with a four-drug regimen when she was a child. Electrocardiography (ECG) shows normal sinus rhythm but no other abnormality. A CT of the chest is obtained and shows pericardial calcifications. In addition to an elevated jugular venous pressure and a third heart sound, which of the following is likely to be found on physical examination?

    A. Rapid *y* descent in jugular venous pulsations

    B. Double systolic apical impulse on palpation

    C. Loud, fixed split P_2 on auscultation

    D. Cannon *a* wave in jugular venous pulsations

    E. An opening snap on auscultation

48. During a yearly physical, a 55-year-old male is found to have a systolic murmur. The murmur is midsystolic and begins shortly after S_1 and peaks in midsystole. It is a low-pitched, rough murmur heard best at the base of the heart in the right second intercostal space. There is radiation to the carotids bilaterally. The rest of his physical examination is unremarkable, and you make a presumptive diagnosis of

48. (*Continued*)
aortic stenosis. Laboratory data show a hemoglobin A1C of 7.2%, high-density lipoprotein cholesterol 45 mg/dL, low-density lipoprotein cholesterol 144 mg/dL, and creatinine 1.2 mg/dL. Blood pressure is 159/85 mmHg, heart rate is 75 beats/min. Body mass index is 33 kg/m². What is the most likely etiology of this patient's aortic stenosis?

A. Age-related degeneration
B. Dyslipidemia
C. Glucose intolerance
D. Hypertension
E. Obesity

49. All the following are associated with a high risk of stroke in patients with atrial fibrillation *except*

A. diabetes mellitus
B. hypercholesterolemia
C. congestive heart failure
D. hypertension
E. age >65 years

50. A 54-year-old male with hypercholesterolemia and poorly controlled hypertension is admitted to the coronary care unit after coming to the emergency department with sudden chest pain. A coronary catheterization is performed, and complete occlusion of the posterior descending artery is identified. Percutaneous intervention fails and the patient is medically managed. Two days later he appears to be acutely ill. Physical examination reveals a new murmur. Which of the following would account for an early decrescendo systolic murmur in this patient?

A. Acute mitral regurgitation
B. Hypertrophic cardiomyopathy
C. Chronic mitral regurgitation
D. Severe aortic stenosis
E. Ventricular septal rupture

51. A 73-year-old female develops substernal chest pain, severe nausea, and vomiting while mowing the lawn. In the emergency department she has cool extremities, right arm and left arm blood pressure of 85/70 mmHg, heart rate of 65 beats/min, clear lungs, and no murmurs. She has no urine output. A Swan-Ganz catheter is placed and reveals cardiac index of 1.1 L/min per mm², PA pressure of 20/14 mmHg, PCW pressure of 6 mmHg, and RA pressure of 24 mmHg. The patient most likely has

A. Gram-negative sepsis
B. occlusion of the left main coronary artery

51. (*Continued*)
C. occlusion of the right coronary artery
D. perforated duodenal ulcer
E. ruptured aortic aneurysm

52. Which of the following patients with echocardiographic evidence of significant mitral regurgitation has the best indication for surgery with the most favorable likelihood of a positive outcome?

A. A 52-year-old male with an ejection fraction of 25%, New York Heart Association class III symptoms, and a left-ventricular end-systolic dimension of 60 mm
B. A 54-year-old male with an ejection fraction of 30%, New York Heart Association class II symptoms, and pulmonary hypertension
C. A 63-year-old male in sinus rhythm without symptoms, an ejection fraction of 65%, and a normal right heart catheterization
D. A 66-year-old male without symptoms, an ejection fraction of 50%, and left-ventricular end-systolic dimension of 45 mm
E. A 72-year-old asymptomatic female with newly discovered atrial fibrillation, ejection fraction of 60%, and end-systolic dimension of 35 mm

53. Which of the following patients meets criteria for the diagnosis of the metabolic syndrome?

A. A male with waist circumference of 110 cm, well-controlled diabetes mellitus with fasting plasma glucose of 98 mg/dL, and blood pressure of 140/75 mmHg
B. A female with triglycerides of 180 mg/dL, waist circumference of 75 cm, and polycystic ovary syndrome
C. A male with nonalcoholic liver disease, obstructive sleep apnea, and blood pressure of 135/90 mmHg
D. A female with high-density lipoprotein (HDL) of 54 mg/dL, blood pressure of 125/80 mmHg, and fasting plasma glucose of 85 mg/dL

54. In the maternity ward, 2 days following assisted vaginal delivery of a healthy boy, a 31-year-old African-American female has developed shortness of breath and wheezing. On examination, blood pressure is 113/78 mmHg, heart rate is 102 beats/min, and regular and jugular venous pressures are elevated. Chest auscultation shows rales 2/3 bilaterally without evidence of consolidation. Cardiac examination reveals an S_3. An echocardiogram shows a dilated left ventricle with an ejection fraction of 30%. A diagnosis of peripartum cardiomyopathy is made and she improves with treatment. Which of the following factors is predictive of her risk for developing peripartum cardiomyopathy or mortality with subsequent pregnancies?

54. *(Continued)*

    A. Age >30 years

    B. African ancestry

    C. Interpartum left ventricular function

    D. Male child

    E. Nadir ejection fraction

55. A 55-year-old male presents with complaint of 6 months of shortness of breath. He has new dyspnea on exertion and three-pillow orthopnea. Lung auscultation reveals rales 2/3 bilaterally. He has 2+ pitting lower extremity edema. Jugular venous pressure is estimated to be 14 cmH_2O measured at a 45°angle. Chest radiograph reveals pulmonary infiltrates and an enlarged cardiac silhouette. Electrocardiography (ECG) shows low-voltage in the precordial and limb leads. An echocardiogram shows a dilated left ventricle, ejection fraction of 20%, mild mitral regurgitation, and a small pericardial effusion. Which finding on cardiac examination would be consistent with this patient's diagnosis?

    A. Absent S_2

    B. Narrow pulse pressure

    C. Paradoxical splitting of S_2 with inspiration

    D. Pulsus bisferiens

56. A 49-year-old male is found to have persistently elevated total cholesterol and low-density lipoprotein (LDL) despite lifestyle modification. You prescribe an HMG-CoA reductase inhibitor to reduce the risk of coronary events. This medication will exert all the following beneficial effects *except*

    A. direct action on atheroma progression

    B. improvement in endothelial-dependent vasomotion

    C. long-term reduction of serum LDL

    D. regression of existing coronary stenosis

    E. stabilization of existing atherosclerotic lesions

57. Dipyridamole is often used during nuclear cardiac stress tests. Based on the pathophysiology of myocardial ischemia and the mechanism of action of dipyridamole, in which circumstance might the stress test underestimate the degree of ischemic tissue?

    A. Three-vessel high-grade obstruction

    B. Bradycardia

    C. Left bundle branch block

    D. Osteoarthritis

    E. Right coronary artery 99% occlusion

58. A 62-year-old female with a history of chronic left bundle branch block is admitted to the coronary care unit with 4 hours of substernal chest pain and shortness of breath. She has elevation of serum troponin-T. She receives urgent catheterization with angioplasty and stent placement of a left anterior descending (LAD) artery lesion. Three days after admission she develops recurrent chest pain. Which of the following studies is most useful for detecting new myocardial damage since the initial infarction?

    A. Echocardiogram

    B. Electrocardiogram

    C. Serum myoglobin

    D. Serum troponin-I

    E. Serum troponin-T

59. A 38-year-old female presents with complaints of fevers and chest pain. She is noted to have a widened mediastinum on chest radiograph, and a diastolic murmur is present at the lower left sternal border. She is hypertensive, with a blood pressure of 180/72 mmHg. All blood cultures are negative on three occasions from separate anatomic sites drawn 6 h apart. Further evaluation of the murmur demonstrates a dilation of the aortic root to 4 cm with subsequent aortic regurgitation. She is diagnosed with aortitis. Which of the following is the *least* likely cause of aortitis in this patient?

    A. Ankylosing spondylitis

    B. Giant cell arteritis

    C. Rheumatoid arthritis

    D. Syphilis

    E. Takayasu's arteritis

60. Echocardiogram of a patient with this electrocardiogram (ECG) tracing (**Fig. 60**) is likely to show which of the following?

    A. Catheter in the right ventricle

    B. Focal hypokinesis

    C. Global hypokinesis

    D. Small pericardial effusion

    E. Thickened left ventricle

61. A 54-year-old male is brought to the emergency department with 1 h of substernal crushing chest pain, nausea, and vomiting. He developed the pain while playing squash. The pain was improved with the administration of sublingual nitroglycerine in the field. His ECG is shown in **Fig. 61**. Emergent cardiac catheterization is most likely to show acute thrombus in which of the following vessels?

    A. Left anterior descending coronary artery

    B. Left circumflex coronary artery

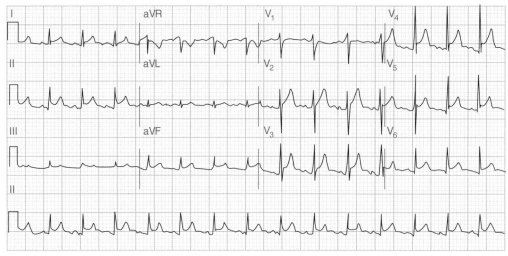

FIGURE 60

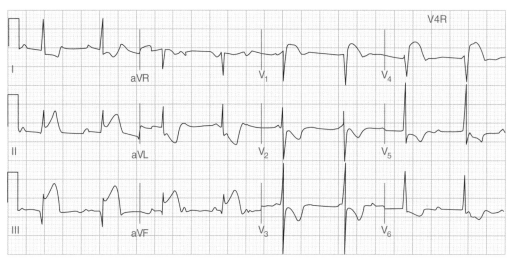

FIGURE 61

61. (*Continued*)
   C. Left main coronary artery
   D. Obtuse marginal coronary artery
   E. Right main coronary artery

62. A 54–year-old male presents to the emergency department with chest pain. He has had three episodes of chest pain in the past 24 h with exertion. Each episode has lasted 20–30 min and resolved with rest. His past medical history is significant for hypertension, hyperlipidemia, asthma, and chronic obstructive pulmonary disease. He currently smokes 1 pack/day of cigarettes. His family history is remarkable for early coronary artery disease in a sibling. Home medications include chlorthalidone, simvastatin, aspirin, albuterol, and home oxygen. In the emergency department, he becomes chest pain–free after

62. (*Continued*)
   receiving three sublingual nitroglycerin tablets and IV heparin. Electrocardiography (ECG) shows 0.8-mm ST-segment depression in V_5, V_6, lead I, and aV_L. Cardiac biomarkers are negative. An exercise stress test shows inducible ischemia. Which aspects of this patient's history add to the likelihood that he might have death, myocardial infarction (MI), or urgent revascularization in the next 14 days?

   A. Age
   B. Aspirin usage
   C. Beta-agonist usage
   D. Diuretic usage

63. A 62-year-old female presents to your office with dyspnea of 4-month duration. She has a history of

63. (*Continued*)
monoclonal gammopathy of unclear significance (MGUS) and has been lost to follow-up for the past 5 years. She is able to do only minimal activity before she has to rest but has no symptoms at rest. She has developed orthopnea but denies paroxysmal nocturnal dyspnea. She complains of fatigue, light headedness, and lower extremity swelling. On examination, blood pressure is 110/90 mmHg and heart rate is 94 beats/min. Jugular venous pressure is elevated, and the jugular venous wave does not fall with inspiration. An S_3 and S_4 are present, as well as a mitral regurgitation murmur. The point of maximal impulse is not displaced. Abdominal examination is significant for ascites and a large, tender, pulsatile liver. Chest radiograph shows bilateral pulmonary edema. An electrocardiogram (ECG) shows an old left bundle branch block. Which clinical features differentiate constrictive pericarditis from restrictive cardiomyopathy?

A. Elevated jugular venous pressure
B. Kussmaul's sign
C. Narrow pulse pressure
D. Pulsatile liver
E. None of the above

64. This electrocardiogram (ECG; **Fig. 64**) is obtained from a 47-year-old male after an exercise stress test. Which of the following additional tests would be important to obtain now?

A. 18-lead ECG
B. Chest CT scan with IV contrast
C. Chest radiograph
D. Erythrocyte sedimentation rate
E. Rhythm strip analysis

65. A 45-year-old male is evaluated following an episode of syncope. He has had occasional chest pain with exertion. Today, as he was climbing a flight of stairs in his home, he abruptly lost consciousness and fell two steps. His wife was home with him and heard the fall. He regained consciousness rapidly prior to arrival of emergency medical services but has no memory of the event. He is being treated for a broken radius that resulted from the fall. He has no history of childhood illnesses or previous history of heart murmur. His physical activity has not been limited until recently, because of anginal symptoms for which he has not sought evaluation. He has no history of hypertension or hypercholesterolemia and does not smoke. He last saw a physician ~8 years ago for a job-related physical examination and was told his health was good. You are asked to evaluate for a possible cardiac cause of syncope. On physical examination, his blood pressure is 160/90 mmHg and heart rate is 88 beats/min. He has a IV/VI harsh crescendo-decrescendo midsystolic murmur. His carotid upstroke is delayed. His electrocardiogram (ECG) shows left-ventricular hypertrophy with a strain pattern. You suspect aortic stenosis. What is the most likely cause of aortic stenosis in this individual?

A. Bicuspid aortic valve
B. Calcification of the aortic valve
C. Congenital aortic stenosis
D. Rheumatic fever

66. You are managing a patient with the metabolic syndrome. She is an obese female with poorly controlled diabetes and dyslipidemia. Her HbA_{1C} is 8.8% and

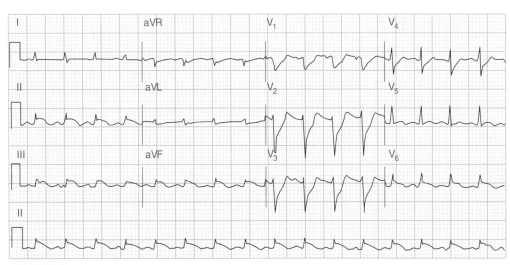

FIGURE 64

66. (*Continued*)

fasting plasma glucose is 195 mg/dL. Low-density lipoprotein (LDL) cholesterol is 98 mg/dL and triglycerides are 276 mg/dL. Her medications include insulin, atorvastatin, hydrochlorothiazide, and aspirin. What is the best option for a medication to treat this patient's hypertriglyceridemia?

A. Cholestyramine
B. Colestipol
C. Ezetimibe
D. Fenofibrate
E. Nicotinic acid

67. All of the following statements regarding percutaneous coronary interventions (PCI) accompanied by stenting for ischemic heart disease are true *except*

A. Coronary artery bypass grafting (CABG) is preferred over PCI in patients with isolated left main artery disease.
B. Compared to balloon angioplasty, PCI with stenting has higher target vessel patency rates at 6 months.
C. Drug-eluting stents delay endothelial healing and expose the patient to an increased risk of subacute stent thrombosis compared to bare metal stents.
D. PCI with stenting reduces the occurrence of coronary death and myocardial infarction (MI) in patients with symptomatic ischemic heart disease.

68. When treating a patient with a non-ST-segment elevation myocardial infarction (NSTEMI), risk stratification and timely administration of anti-ischemic and anti-thrombotic therapies are paramount. For a patient with unstable angina with negative biomarkers, which medication regimen is most appropriate as initial treatment?

A. Aspirin, beta blocker, spironolactone, HMG-CoA reductase inhibitor (statin)
B. Aspirin, clopidogrel, nitroglycerin, beta blocker, heparin
C. Aspirin, nitroglycerin, beta blocker, heparin, glycoprotein IIB/IIIa inhibitor
D. Aspirin, morphine, oxygen, nitrates

69. All the following are true about cardiac valve replacement *except*

A. Bioprosthetic valve replacement is preferred to mechanical valve replacement in younger patients because of the superior durability of the valve.
B. Bioprosthetic valves have a low incidence of thromboembolic complications.

69. (*Continued*)

C. The risk of thrombosis with mechanical valve replacement is higher in the mitral position than in the aortic position.
D. Mechanical valves are relatively contraindicated in patients who wish to become pregnant.
E. Double-disk tilting mechanical prosthetic valves offer superior hemodynamic characteristics over single-disk tilting valves.

70. A 35-year-old female undergoes a physical examination while obtaining new insurance coverage. She reports 1 year of slowly progressive dyspnea on exertion and a change in skin color. Her physical examination is notable for the presence of cyanosis, an elevated jugular venous pulse, a fixed split loud second heart sound, and peripheral edema. Arterial oxygen saturation is 84%. Chest radiography shows an enlarged heart and normal lung parenchyma. Ten years ago, at her last insurance physical examination, her physical examination, oxygen saturation, and chest radiogram were normal. Echocardiography most likely will reveal

A. atrial septal defect
B. Ebstein's anomaly
C. tetralogy of Fallot
D. truncus arteriosus
E. ventricular septal defect

71. A 28-year-old female has hypertension that is difficult to control. She was diagnosed at age 26. Since that time she has been on increasing amounts of medication. Her current regimen consists of labetalol 1000 mg bid, lisinopril 40 mg qd, clonidine 0.1 mg bid, and amlodipine 5 mg qd. On physical examination she appears to be without distress. Blood pressure is 168/100 mmHg and heart rate is 84 beats/min. Cardiac examination is unremarkable, without rubs, gallops, or murmurs. She has good peripheral pulses and has no edema. Her physical appearance does not reveal any hirsutism, fat maldistribution, or abnormalities of genitalia. Laboratory studies reveal a potassium of 2.8 mEq/dL and a serum bicarbonate of 32 mEq/dL. Fasting blood glucose is 114 mg/dL. What is the likely diagnosis?

A. Congenital adrenal hyperplasia
B. Fibromuscular dysplasia
C. Cushing's syndrome
D. Conn's syndrome
E. Pheochromocytoma

72. What is the best way to diagnose this disease?

A. Renal vein renin levels
B. 24-h urine collection for metanephrines
C. Magnetic resonance imaging of the renal arteries
D. 24-h urine collection for cortisol
E. Plasma aldosterone/renin ratio

73. You are evaluating a new patient in clinic. The 25-year-old male was diagnosed with "heart failure" in another state and has since relocated. He has New York Heart Association class II symptoms and denies angina. He presents for evaluation and management. On review of systems, the patient has been wheel-chair bound for many years and has severe scoliosis. He has no family history of hyperlipidemia. His physical examination is notable for bilateral lung crackles, an S_3, and no cyanosis. An electrocardiogram (ECG) is obtained in clinic and shows tall R waves in V_1 and V_2 with deep Qs in V_5 and V_6. An echocardiogram reports severe global left ventricular dysfunction with reduced ejection fraction. What is the most likely diagnosis?

A. Amyotrophic lateral sclerosis
B. Atrial septal defect
C. Chronic thromboembolic disease
D. Duchenne's muscular dystrophy
E. Ischemic cardiomyopathy

74. Which of the following congenital heart defects causes fixed splitting of the second heart sound?

A. Atrial septal defect
B. Epstein's anomaly
C. Patent foramen ovale
D. Tetralogy of Fallot
E. Ventricular septal defect

75. A 35-year-old female comes in for a routine visit. Her past medical history is significant for poorly controlled type 2 diabetes mellitus (HbA$_{1C}$ of 8.4%), obstructive sleep apnea, hypertension, and dyslipidemia. Her body mass index is 42 kg/m^2. Blood pressure in clinic is 154/87 mmHg and fasting plasma glucose is 130 mg/dL. Her medications include metformin, insulin, ramipril, hydrochlorothiazide, and atorvastatin. You have diagnosed her with the metabolic syndrome. Based on our current understanding of the metabolic syndrome, treating which of the following underlying conditions is the primary approach to treating this disorder?

A. Hyperglycemia
B. Hypercholesterolemia

75. (*Continued*)
C. Hypertension
D. Inflammatory cytokines
E. Obesity

76. A 24-year-old male is referred to cardiology after an episode of syncope while playing basketball. He has no recollection of the event, but he was told that he collapsed while running. He awakened lying on the ground and suffered multiple contusions resulting from the fall. He has always been an active individual but recently has developed some chest pain with exertion that has caused him to restrict his activity. His father died at age 44 while rock climbing. He believes his father's cause of death was sudden cardiac death and recalls being told his father had an enlarged heart. On examination, the patient has a III/VI midsystolic crescendo-decrescendo murmur. His electrocardiogram shows evidence of left ventricular hypertrophy. You suspect hypertrophic cardiomyopathy as the cause of the patient's heart disease. Which of the following maneuvers would be expected to cause an increase in the loudness of the murmur?

A. Handgrip exercise
B. Squatting
C. Standing
D. Valsalva maneuver
E. A and B
F. C and D

77. A patient is noted to have a crescendo-decrescendo midsystolic murmur on examination. The murmur is loudest at the left sternal border. The patient is asked to squat, and the murmur decreases in intensity. The patient stands and the murmur increases. Finally, the patient is asked to perform a Valsalva maneuver and the murmur increases in intensity. Which of the following is most likely to be the cause of this murmur?

A. Aortic stenosis
B. Chronic mitral regurgitation
C. Hypertrophic cardiomyopathy (HOCM)
D. Mitral valve prolapse
E. Pulmonic stenosis

78. A 40-year-old male with diabetes and schizophrenia is started on antibiotic therapy for chronic osteomyelitis in the hospital. His osteomyelitis has developed just underlying an ulcer where he has been injecting heroin. He is found unresponsive suddenly by the nursing staff. His electrocardiogram

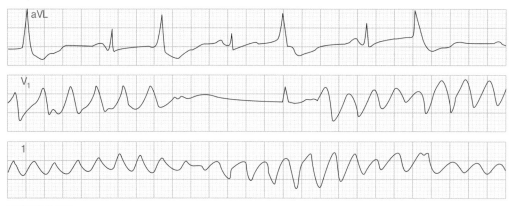

FIGURE 78

78. (*Continued*)

is shown in **Fig. 78**. The most likely cause of this rhythm is which of the following substances?

A. Furosemide
B. Metronidazole
C. Droperidol
D. Metformin
E. Heroin

79. Normal sinus rhythm is restored with electrical cardioversion. A 12-lead electrocardiogram (ECG) is notable for a prolonged QT interval. Besides stopping the offending drug, the most appropriate management for this rhythm disturbance should include intravenous administration of which of the following?

A. Amiodarone
B. Lidocaine
C. Magnesium
D. Metoprolol
E. Potassium

80. A 52-year-old male with a history of stable angina presents to the hospital with 30 min of chest pain. He reports that over the past 2 weeks, he has developed his typical anginal symptoms of chest pressure radiating to his jaw and left arm with progressively less exertion. He has been using sublingual nitroglycerin more frequently. His other medications include a beta blocker, aspirin, and lovastatin. On the day of admission, he developed pain at rest that was not relieved with three nitroglycerin tablets. On examination, he is anxious and short of breath. His vital signs are notable for a blood pressure of 140/88 mmHg; a heart rate of 110 beats/min, and a respiratory rate of 25 breaths/min. He has bilateral crackles halfway up both lung fields and has a

80. (*Continued*)

3/6 systolic murmur that radiates to his axilla. His electrocardiogram (ECG) shows 3-mm ST-segment depression in leads V_3–V_5. In addition to his outpatient medications, all of the following additional therapies are indicated *except*

A. cardiac catheterization
B. clopidogrel
C. enoxaparin
D. eptifibatide
E. tissue plasminogen activator

81. Which of the following patients with aortic dissection can be managed without surgical or endovascular intervention?

A. A 72-year-old male with a dissection of the descending aorta that begins just distal to the left subclavian artery and extends to below the left renal artery and with a baseline creatinine of 1.8 mg/dL that is not increasing
B. A 41-year-old male with an ascending aortic dissection that extends past the left common carotid artery after an automobile accident
C. A 42-year-old male with Marfan's syndrome with a distal aortic dissection beginning just below the left subclavian artery and an aortic root of 53 mm
D. A 72-year-old male with a chronic type B dissection with a CT that shows advancement of the dissection at 6 months
E. A 56-year-old male with a descending aortic dissection that encompasses the origin of the renal and iliac arteries with rest claudication

82. Based on the electrocardiogram (ECG) in **Fig. 82**, treating which condition might specifically improve this patient's tachycardia?

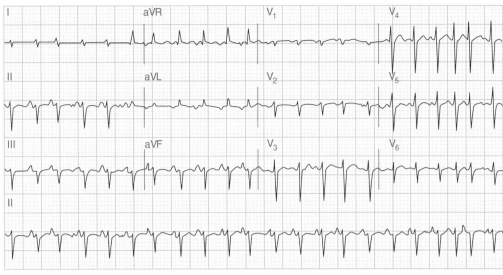

FIGURE 82

82. (*Continued*)

A. Anemia

B. Chronic obstructive pulmonary disease (COPD)

C. Myocardial ischemia

D. Pain

83. Each of these patients is alert and oriented and has a blood pressure of 110/60 mmHg. In which patient would adenosine constitute appropriate initial therapy?

A. A 65-year-old male with no ischemic heart disease and wide complex tachycardia

B. A 65-year-old female with known ischemic disease and narrow complex tachycardia

C. A 25-year-old female with known preexcitation syndrome and narrow complex tachycardia

D. A 28-year-old male with known preexcitation syndrome and wide complex tachycardia

E. A 44-year-old male with atrial fibrillation without a prior history of heart disease

84. A 68-year-old male with a history of coronary artery disease is seen in his primary care clinic for complaint of cough with sputum production. His care provider is concerned about pneumonia, so a chest radiograph is ordered. On the chest radiograph, the aorta appears tortuous with a widened mediastinum. A contrast-enhanced CT of the chest confirms the presence of a descending thoracic aortic aneurysm measuring 4 cm with no evidence of dissection. What is the most appropriate management of this patient?

84. (*Continued*)

A. Consult interventional radiology for placement of an endovascular stent.

B. Consult thoracic surgery for repair.

C. No further evaluation is needed.

D. Perform yearly contrast-enhanced chest CT and refer for surgical repair when the aneurysm size is >4.5 cm.

E. Treat with beta blockers, perform yearly contrast-enhanced chest CT, and refer for surgical repair if the aneurysm grows >1 cm/year.

85. A 55-year-old male presents with severe substernal chest pain for the last hour. It began at rest and is associated with dyspnea and nausea. The electrocardiogram (ECG) shows bradycardia with a Mobitz type II second-degree block. Chest plain film is normal. Which of the following is likely to be found in addition on the ECG?

A. ST elevation V_1–V_3

B. Wellen's T waves

C. ST elevation II, III, and aVF

D. ST depression in I and aVL

E. No other abnormality

86. A 44-year-old female presents to the emergency department with complaint of acute onset of chest pain. She describes the chest pain as 10/10 in intensity, with a sharp stabbing quality. The chest pain is worse when lying flat and better when sitting upright. The pain came on suddenly, awakening the patient from sleep. There is no

86. (*Continued*)

radiation of the pain and no nausea, vomiting, or lightheadedness. She has no other complaints. She has no history of hypertension, hypercholesterolemia, or diabetes mellitus. She does not smoke. On physical examination, she appears in distress moving in bed frequently. Her vital signs are: temperature 38.3°C, blood pressure 112/62 mmHg, heart rate 102 beats/min, respiratory rate 18 breaths/min, and SaO$_2$ 100% on room air. She has a regular tachycardia. There are no murmurs, rubs, or gallops. There is no pulsus paradoxus. The pulmonary, abdominal, extremity, and neurologic examinations are normal. An echocardiogram demonstrates a normal ejection fraction without an effusion. Initial troponin I level is 0.26 ng/mL (normal values <0.06–0.50 ng/mL). What is the most appropriate treatment for this patient? (See also Fig. 60.)

A. Anticoagulation with heparin and serial troponin measurements
B. Immediate cardiac catheterization with angioplasty and stent
C. Indomethacin, 50 mg three times daily
D. Reassurance only
E. Reteplase, 10 units IV now, followed by an additional dose in 30 min

87. A 22-year-old male collapses immediately after being hit in the chest with a ball while playing lacrosse. Emergency medical personnel were present during the game and noted the initial rhythm to be ventricular fibrillation. The patient underwent prompt defibrillation within 3 min, and normal sinus rhythm was restored. The patient has been transported to the emergency department and is stable with a blood pressure of 128/76 mmHg and heart rate of 112 beats/min. He has no prior history of syncope and no family history of sudden cardiac death. His electrocardiogram (ECG) is normal. There is no evidence of broken ribs or sternum by x-ray. What is the most likely diagnosis?

A. Brugada syndrome
B. Cardiac contusion
C. Commotio cordis
D. Hypertrophic cardiomyopathy
E. Right ventricular dysplasia

88. You are examining a new patient in clinic. On cardiac auscultation you palpate a double apical impulse. There is a III/VI harsh crescendo "diamond-shaped" murmur that begins well after the first heart sound. The murmur is best heard at

88. (*Continued*)

the lower left sternal border as well as at the apex. The murmur does not radiate to the neck. There is no respiratory variation. S$_1$ and S$_2$ are normal. With passive elevation of the legs, the murmur decreases in intensity. During the strain phase of the Valsalva maneuver, the murmur increases in intensity. With inhalation of amyl nitrate, the murmur increases in intensity. What is the etiology of this patient's murmur?

A. Aortic sclerosis
B. Aortic stenosis
C. Hypertrophic cardiomyopathy
D. Mitral regurgitation
E. Tricuspid regurgitation

89. Insulin resistance and fasting hyperglycemia are important when creating a treatment program for the metabolic syndrome. Often, lifestyle modifications will occur at the same time medications are prescribed. In addressing the treatment of insulin resistance and fasting hyperglycemia, which of the following statements is true?

A. Metformin is more effective than the combination of weight reduction, dietary fat restriction, and increased physical activity for the prevention of diabetes mellitus.
B. Metformin is superior to other drug classes for increasing insulin sensitivity.
C. Thiazolidinediones, but not metformin, improve insulin-mediated glucose uptake in muscle.
D. Lifestyle interventions alone are not effective in reducing the incidence of diabetes mellitus.

90. A 63-year-old male with end-stage ischemic cardiomyopathy is offered a heart transplant from a 20-year-old female with brain death after a skiing accident. Which of the following is not a risk that the patient should be advised about if he decides to accept the heart?

A. Increased risk of malignancy
B. Risk of rejection of transplanted organ
C. Coronary artery disease
D. Increased risk of infections
E. Increased risk of bradyarrhythmias

91. All the following interventions have demonstrated a decrease in macrovascular complications (coronary artery disease, stroke) in patients with diabetes and dyslipidemia *except*

A. ACE inhibitors
B. gemfibrozil therapy

91. (*Continued*)
    C. goal blood pressure <130/85
    D. HMG–CoA reductase therapy
    E. tight glycemic control

92. Pulsus paradoxus can be described by which of the following statements?

    A. Pulsus paradoxus can be seen in patients with acute asthma exacerbations in which the negative intrathoracic pressure decreases afterload of the heart with a resultant increase in systolic pressure during inspiration.
    B. Pulsus paradoxus has not been described in patients with superior vena cava syndrome.
    C. Pulsus paradoxus describes the finding of diminished pulses during inspiration, when the peripheral pulse is normally augmented during inspiration.
    D. A drop in systolic pressure during inspiration of more than 5 mmHg indicates the presence of pulsus paradoxus.
    E. Pulsus paradoxus occurs during cardiac tamponade when there is an exaggeration of the normal decrease in the systolic blood pressure during inspiration.

93. A 35-year-old female is admitted to the hospital with malaise, weight gain, increasing abdominal girth, and edema. The symptoms began about 3 months ago and gradually progressed. The patient reports an increase in waist size of ~15 cm. The swelling in her legs has gotten increasingly worse so that she now feels her thighs are swollen as well. She has dyspnea on exertion and two-pillow orthopnea. She has a past history of Hodgkin's disease diagnosed at age 18. She was treated at that time with chemotherapy and mediastinal irradiation. On physical examination, she has temporal wasting and appears chronically ill. Her current weight is 96 kg, an increase of 11 kg over the past 3 months. Her vital signs are normal. Her jugular venous pressure is ~16 cm, and the neck veins do not collapse on inspiration. Heart sounds are distant. There is a third heart sound heard shortly after aortic valve closure. The sound is short and abrupt and is heard best at the apex. The liver is enlarged and pulsatile. Ascites is present. There is pitting edema extending throughout the lower extremities and onto the abdominal wall. Echocardiogram shows pericardial thickening, dilatation of the inferior vena cava and hepatic veins, and abrupt cessation of ventricular filling in early diastole. Ejection fraction is 65%. What is the best approach for treatment of this patient?

    A. Aggressive diuresis only
    B. Cardiac transplantation

93. (*Continued*)
    C. Mitral valve replacement
    D. Pericardial resection
    E. Pericardiocentesis

94. A 52-year-old male is brought to the emergency department with complaint of shortness of breath, chest pain, and dizziness. The chest pain began acutely ~90 min ago. He had been working in the yard and thought he might have strained a muscle in his chest. He took an aspirin and lay down, but the symptoms worsened. He soon developed dizziness and shortness of breath. He called 911, and upon arrival to the emergency department, he was found to be hypotensive and tachycardic. His vital signs on presentation were: blood pressure 75/44 mmHg, heart rate 132 beats/min, respiratory rate 24 breaths/min, and SaO_2 88% on room air. On physical examination, he appears in distress and is diaphoretic. He is unable to speak in full sentences. His neck veins appear distended. There are crackles throughout both lung fields. The heart sounds are regular and tachycardic. There is no edema. The extremities are cool, and the pulses are thready. An electrocardiogram (ECG) shows ST elevations in leads V_2–V_6. Chest radiograph shows diffuse pulmonary edema. Emergency cardiac catheterization is scheduled, and it is estimated that the catheterization laboratory will be available in ~45 min. The patient remains hypotensive with a blood pressure that is now 68/38 mmHg, and the oxygen saturation has fallen to 82% on room air. What is the best management for the patient's hypotension?

    A. Aortic counterpulsation
    B. Dobutamine, 2.5 μg/kg per min IV
    C. Furosemide, 40 mg IV
    D. Metoprolol, 5 mg IV
    E. Norepinephrine, 4 μg/min IV

95. A 64-year-old female is admitted to the emergency department with hypotension and chest pain. The symptoms began 30 min ago, awakening the patient from sleep. She vomited twice and has felt dizzy and lightheaded. Upon arrival in the emergency department, her blood pressure was 80/40 mmHg, with a heart rate of 64 beats/min. She appears in distress and has another episode of emesis in the emergency department. The lungs are clear to auscultation. Pulses are thready. An electrocardiogram (ECG) demonstrates elevations in leads II, III, and aV_F. There are ST depressions in V_1 and V_2. The rhythm is sinus with occasional premature ventricular

95. (*Continued*)

contractions. A chest radiograph is clear. An echocardiogram shows normal left ventricular function and right ventricular dilatation. What is the best immediate treatment for this patient's hypotension?

A. Aortic counterpulsation
B. Dobutamine, 5 µg/kg per min
C. Dopamine, 5 µg/kg per min
D. Normal saline bolus, 500 mL
E. Transvenous pacemaker placement

96. All of the following statements regarding sudden cardiac death in the United States are true *except*

A. A strong parental history of sudden cardiac death as a presenting history of coronary artery disease increases the likelihood of a similar presentation in an offspring.
B. An estimated 50% of all cardiac deaths are sudden and unexpected.
C. As great as 70–75% of men who die of sudden cardiac death have evidence of acute myocardial infarction (MI), wheras only 20–30% have preexisting healed MIs.
D. By 5 min after sudden cardiac arrest, the estimated survival rates are no greater than 25–30% in the out-of-hospital setting.

97. A 64-year-old male collapses suddenly while playing the sousaphone with his alumni band during half-time of a football game. Emergency medical services with training in advanced cardiac life support are present within 2 min of collapse. Initial rhythm on cardiac monitor is ventricular fibrillation. What is the first step in the treatment of this patient?

A. Continue cardiopulmonary resuscitation (CPR) for a full 5 min prior to attempting defibrillation
B. Endotracheal intubation followed by rapid defibrillation
C. Immediate defibrillation at 300–360 J once, followed by CPR for 60–90 s before additional defibrillation
D. Obtain IV access and administer amiodarone, 150 mg
E. Obtain IV access and administer epinephrine, 1 mg

98. Which of the following therapies has been demonstrated to improve survival to hospital discharge with favorable neurologic outcome in out-of-hospital cardiac arrest?

A. Amiodarone
B. Epinephrine
C. Hypothermia

98. (*Continued*)

D. Time to initial defibrillation <10 min
E. Vasopressin

99. A 56-year-old male is admitted to the hospital for newly diagnosed heart failure. On cardiac examination his pulse is irregular, he has an S_3, and a laterally displaced point of maximal impulse. There is a high-pitched holosystolic murmur beginning with the first heart sound and extending to the second heart sound heard best in the axilla. Neurologic examination shows decreased sensation to pin prick in a stocking-glove distribution. Electrocardiogram (ECG) shows atrial fibrillation, low voltage in the limb leads, and first-degree atrioventricular block without evidence of prior myocardial infarction. Chest radiograph shows cardiomegaly. Blood chemistries show potassium 4.1 meq/L, magnesium 1.6 mg/dL, creatinine 0.8 mg/dL, calcium 11.4 mg/dL, albumin 3.7 mg/dL, total protein 8.4 mg/dL, AST 27 U/L, ALT 17 U/L, alkaline phosphatase 76 U/L. An echocardiogram is performed. Which finding on echocardiogram is most likely?

A. Akinesis of the inferior wall
B. Aortic stenosis
C. Protrusion of the left ventricular apex with hyper-contractility of the base
D. Systolic anterior motion of the mitral valve
E. Thickened interatrial septum

100. A cardiac biopsy is obtained from a 24-year-old male with new-onset heart failure during a right heart catheterization. Congo red staining shows positive birefringence characteristic of amyloid. Immunohistochemical staining of the biopsy reveals an abundance of the transthyretin protein. What is the next step in the management of this type of amyloidosis?

A. Bone marrow biopsy
B. Evaluation for underlying inflammatory disease
C. Family pedigree analysis
D. Neurocognitive testing
E. Urine for Bence-Jones protein

101. You are seeing a return patient in clinic. The patient is a 76-year-old male with a history of hypertension, remote cerebrovascular accident, diet-controlled diabetes, and congestive heart failure with left ventricular systolic dysfunction (ejection fraction = 30%). The patient reports no new complaints and feels well. On physical examination, you palpate an irregular pulse, and an electrocardiogram (ECG)

101. (*Continued*)

verifies atrial fibrillation. The patient does not have a history of atrial fibrillation. You and the patient are interested in a trial of direct current cardioversion (DCCV). What is the appropriate management of anticoagulation for this patient?

A. Initiate warfarin (with goal INR 2.0–3.0) following DCCV only if cardioversion is unsuccessful.
B. Give full-dose aspirin (325 mg daily) 3 weeks prior to DCCV, perform transesophageal echocardiogram (TEE) and DCCV (if not contraindicated), then discontinue aspirin if DCCV is successful.
C. Initiate IV heparin and warfarin, perform transesophageal echocardiogram (TEE) and DCCV (if not contraindicated), then discontinue warfarin if DCCV is successful.
D. Initiate IV heparin, perform TEE and DCCV (if not contraindicated), then continue warfarin for at least 1 month.

102. A 68-year-old male with a history of myocardial infarction and congestive heart failure is comfortable at rest. However, when walking to his car, he develops dyspnea, fatigue, and sometimes palpitations. He must rest for several minutes before the symptoms resolve. His New York Heart Association classification is which of the following?

A. Class I
B. Class II
C. Class III
D. Class IV

103. The husband of a 68-year-old female with congestive heart failure is concerned because his wife appears to stop breathing for periods of time when she sleeps. He has noticed that she stops breathing for ~10 s and then follows this with a similar period of hyperventilation. This does not wake her from sleep. She does not snore. She feels well rested in the morning but is very dyspneic with even mild activity. What is your next step in management?

A. Electroencephalography
B. Maximize heart failure management
C. Nasal continuous positive airway pressure (CPAP) during sleep
D. Obtain a sleep study
E. Prescribe bronchodilators

104. A 28-year-old male with long-standing cardiomyopathy presents with worsening dyspnea. Physical

104. (*Continued*)

examination reveals a blood pressure of 85/50 mmHg, heat rate of 112 beats/min, elevated jugular venous pressure, positive hepatojugular reflex, quiet S_1/S_2, apical S_3, no pulmonary rales, and 3+ lower extremity edema. Chest radiograph shows no pulmonary edema and a small left-sided pleural effusion. What information does the patient's pulmonary examination give you in regards to his likely pulmonary capillary wedge pressure?

A. It is likely to be elevated.
B. It is likely to be normal.
C. It is likely to be decreased.
D. No information.

105. All of the following findings on echocardiographic assessment of patients with congestive heart failure with preserved ejection fraction are relevant *except*

A. atrial fibrillation
B. left atrial dilatation
C. left ventricular wall thickness
D. left ventricular diastolic filling as measured by tissue Doppler
E. systolic anterior motion of the mitral valve

106. All of the following medications have been shown to worsen heart failure in patients with left ventricular systolic dysfunction *except*

A. angiotensin receptor blockers (ARBs)
B. calcium channel antagonists
C. nonsteroidal anti-inflammatory drugs (NSAIDs)
D. sotalol
E. thiazolidinediones

107. Which of the following is true regarding dose escalation of angiotensin-converting enzyme (ACE) inhibitors and beta blockers in patients newly diagnosed with congestive heart failure?

A. ACE inhibitors should be escalated on a daily basis to maximal tolerated doses, whereas beta blockers should be gently increased in dose over weeks, as tolerated.
B. Beta blockers should be escalated on a daily basis to maximal tolerated doses, whereas ACE inhibitors should be gently increased in dose over weeks, as tolerated.
C. Both should be escalated rapidly to maximally tolerated doses.
D. Both should be escalated slowly to maximally tolerated doses.
E. Both should be initiated at full doses.

108. In African Americans with New York Heart Association class II heart failure, which of the following drug combinations should be added to an angiotensin-converting enzyme (ACE) inhibitor and beta blocker?

A. Hydralazine/angiotensin receptor blockers
B. Hydrazaline/digoxin
C. Isosorbide dinitrate/angiotensin receptor blockers
D. Isosorbide dinitrate/digoxin
E. Isosorbide dinitrate/hydralazine

109. A 26-year-old male presents with severe bilateral pain in his hands, ankles, knees, and elbows. He is recovering from a sore throat and has had recent fevers to 38.9°C. Social history is notable for recent unprotected receptive oral intercourse with a man ~1 week ago. Physical examination reveals a well-developed male in moderate discomfort. He is afebrile. His pharynx is erythematous with pustular exudates on his tonsils. He has tender anterior cervical lymphadenopathy. His cardiac examination is notable for a normal S_1 and S_2 and a soft ejection murmur. His lungs are clear. Abdomen is benign with no organomegaly. He has no rash, and genital examination is normal. His bilateral proximal interphalangeal joints, metacarpophalangeal joints, wrists, ankles, and metatarsophalangeal joints are red, warm, and boggy with tenderness noted with both passive and active movement. A complete metabolic panel and complete blood count are all within normal limits. His erythrocyte sedimentation rate is 85 mm/h and C-reactive protein is 11 mg/dL. What is the most likely diagnosis?

A. Acute HIV infection
B. Acute rheumatic fever
C. Lyme disease
D. *Neisseria gonorrhoeae* infection
E. Poststreptococcal reactive arthritis

110. The parents of a 14-year-old boy want your opinion about treatment of their child's lipid disorder. The family emigrated from South Africa to the United States recently. The child has had cutaneous xanthomas on the hands, elbows, heels, and buttocks since childhood. In South Africa, he underwent thoracotomy for a problem with his aortic valve 3 years ago. He currently experiences exertional dyspnea, and his diet consists mostly of unhealthy, fatty foods. On examination, you appreciate bruits in the femoral arteries and abdominal aorta. His most recent lipid profile shows a total cholesterol of 734 mg/dL and a low-density

110. (*Continued*)
lipoprotein (LDL) of 376 mg/dL. What is the most appropriate step in this patient's evaluation?

A. Genetic test for familial defective apoB100
B. Rule out congenital syphilis
C. Rule out hypothyroidism
D. Screen the parents for Münchhausen-by-proxy syndrome

111. A 16-year-old male is brought to your clinic by his parents because of concern about his weight. He has not seen a physician for many years. He states that he has gained weight due to inactivity and that he is less active because of exertional chest pain. He takes no medications. He was adopted and his parents do not know the medical history of his biologic parents. Physical examination is notable for stage 1 hypertension and body mass index of 30 kg/m². He has xanthomas on his hands, heels, and buttocks. Laboratory testing shows a low-density lipoprotein (LDL) of 210 mg/dL, creatinine of 0.7 mg/dL, total bilirubin of 3.1 mg/dL, haptoglobin <6 mg/dL, and a glycosylated hemoglobin of 6.7%. You suspect a hereditary lipoproteinemia due to the clinical and laboratory findings. Which test would be diagnostic of the primary lipoprotein disorder in this patient?

A. Congo red staining of xanthoma biopsy
B. CT scan of the liver
C. Family pedigree analysis
D. Gas chromatography
E. LDL receptor function in skin biopsy

112. A 23-year-old female complains of dyspnea and substernal chest pain on exertion. Evaluation for this complaint 6 months ago included arterial blood gas testing, which revealed pH 7.48, P_{O_2} 79 mmHg, and P_{CO_2} 31 mmHg. Electrocardiography (ECG) then showed a right axis deviation. Chest x-ray now shows enlarged pulmonary arteries but no parenchymal infiltrates, and a lung perfusion scan reveals subsegmental defects that are thought to have a "low probability for pulmonary thromboembolism." Echocardiography demonstrates right heart strain but no evidence of primary cardiac disease. The most appropriate diagnostic test now would be

A. open lung biopsy
B. Holter monitoring
C. right-heart catheterization
D. transbronchial biopsy
E. serum α_1-antitrypsin level

ANSWERS

1. The answer is C.

(Chap. 37) Several factors have been shown to confer an increased risk of complications from hypertension. In the patient described here there is only one: ongoing tobacco use. Epidemiologic factors that have poorer prognosis include African-American ancestry, male sex, and onset of hypertension in youth. In addition, comorbid factors that independently increase the risk of atherosclerosis worsen the prognosis in patients with hypertension. These factors include hypercholesterolemia, obesity, diabetes mellitus, and tobacco use. Physical and laboratory examination showing evidence of end organ damage also may portend a poorer prognosis. This includes evidence of retinal damage or hypertensive heart disease with cardiac enlargement or congestive heart failure. Furthermore, electrocardiographic evidence of ischemia or left ventricular strain but not left ventricular hypertrophy alone may predict worse outcomes. A family history of hypertensive complications does not worsen the prognosis if diastolic blood pressure is maintained at <110 mmHg.

2. The answer is B.

(Chap. 38) Abdominal aortic aneurysms (AAAs) affect 1 to 2% of men >50 years. Most AAAs are asymptomatic and are found incidentally on physical examination. The predisposing factors for AAA are the same as those for other cardiovascular disease, with >90% being associated with atherosclerotic disease. Most AAAs are located infrarenally, and recent data suggest that an uncomplicated infrarenal AAA may be treated with endovascular stenting instead of the usual surgical grafting. Indications for proceeding to surgery include any patient with symptoms or an aneurysm that is growing rapidly. Serial ultrasonography or CT imaging is imperative, and all aneurysms larger than 5.5 cm warrant intervention because of the high mortality associated with repair of ruptured aortic aneurysms. The rupture rate of an AAA is directly related to size, with the 5-year risk of rupture being 1–2% with aneurysms less than 5 cm and 20–40% with aneurysms >5 cm. Mortality of patients undergoing elective repair is 1–2% and is >50% for emergent treatment of a ruptured AAA. Preoperative cardiac evaluation before elective repair is imperative as coexisting coronary artery disease is common.

3. The answer is A.

(Chap. 23) This patient is presenting with symptoms of congestive heart failure with evidence of systemic embolization. The physical examination suggests mitral valve stenosis with a positional low-pitched sound heard when the patient is in the upright position. This is characteristic of a "tumor plop," which should alert the physician to the possibility of a cardiac tumor. This is confirmed by the echocardiogram revealing a large left

atrium tumor, which is most likely an atrial myxoma. Myxomas are the most common type of benign primary cardiac tumors, accounting for more than three-quarters of surgically resected cardiac tumors. Myxomas generally present in between ages 20 and 50 and are seen more commonly in women. The clinical presentation of myxomas resembles that of valvular heart disease due either to obstruction of flow from the tumor obscuring valvular flow or to regurgitation due to abnormal valve closure. The tumor plop is heard in mid-diastole and results from the impact of the tumor against the valve or ventricular wall. Most tumors are solid masses located in the atria and measure 4–8 cm. They usually arise from the interatrial septum near the fossa ovalis. Histologically, they appear as gelatinous structures with scattered myxoma cells embedded in a glycosaminoglycan stromal matrix. They may embolize and can be mistaken for endocarditis, particularly as systemic symptoms, including fevers and weight loss, may be seen. Echocardiogram is useful to document tumor size and site of attachment. MRI or CT scanning may also be utilized for preoperative planning. However, cardiac catheterization is no longer considered mandatory prior to tumor resection, especially as catheterization of the chamber containing the tumor increases the likelihood of embolization. Primary surgical excision is the treatment of choice and should be performed regardless of tumor size as even small tumors can cause embolization or valvular obstruction. Surgical resection is generally curative with only a 1–2% recurrence rate in sporadic cases. Tumors metastatic to the heart are more common than primary cardiac tumors and occur with the highest incidence in metastatic melanoma. However, by absolute numbers of cases, breast and lung cancer account for the largest number of cases. Cardiac metastases usually occur in patients with known malignancies, are usually not the cause of presentation, and are found incidentally. Only 10% are clinically apparent at the time of presentation, and most are found at autopsy.

4. The answer is A.

(Chap. 33) Myocardial ischemia is determined by the balance between myocardial oxygen supply and demand. Myocardial oxygen demand ($M\dot{V}O_2$) is determined by heart rate, myocardial contractility, and myocardial wall tension. A normal oxygen supply to the myocardium requires adequate inspired oxygen, intact lung function (including diffusion capacity, which is abnormal in emphysema), normal hemoglobin concentration and function, and normal coronary blood flow. The resistance to coronary blood flow is determined by three vascular regions: large epicardial arteries, pre-arteriolar vessels, and arteriolar and intramyocardial capillaries. In the absence of significant flow-limiting atherosclerosis, the resistance in the epicardial arteries is negligible. The major determinant

of coronary-resistance is due to the pre-arteriolar, arteriolar, and intramyocardial capillary vessels.

5. The answer is B.

(Chap. 15) Second-degree AV block type 1 (Mobitz type 1) is characterized by a progressive lengthening of the PR interval preceding a pause. The pause in this tracing is between the third and fourth QRS complex. First-degree AV block is a slowing of conduction through the AV junction and is diagnosed when the PR interval >200 ms. Type 2 second-degree AV block is characterized by intermittent failure of conduction of the P wave without changes in the preceeding PR or RR intervals. Second-degree AV block type 2 usually occurs in the distal or infra-His conduction systems.

6. The answer is C.

(Chap. 11) The electrocardiographic T wave represents myocardial repolarization, and its configuration can be altered nonspecifically by metabolic abnormalities, drugs, neural activity, and ischemia through a dispersion effect on the activation or repolarization of action potentials. Although myocardial ischemia and subendocardial infarction can produce deep, symmetric T-wave inversions which would result in tachyarrhythmias and syncope, noncardiac phenomena such as intracerebral hemorrhage can similarly affect ventricular repolarization. Hyperkalemia is manifested by tall peaked T waves, not inverted ones. Hypocalcemia is manifested by prolonged QT intervals.

7. The answer is A.

(Chap. 20) Aortic stenosis (AS) may remain asymptomatic for many years. However, once symptoms develop, surgery is indicated owing to the increased mortality associated with symptomatic AS. The average time to death after onset of symptoms is as follows: angina pectoris, 3 years; syncope, 3 years; dyspnea, 2 years; congestive heart failure, 1.5–2 years. In addition, surgery is advocated when the ejection fraction falls below 50% or when severe calcification, rapid progression, or expected delays in surgery are present. There is no specific age cut-off or degree of left-ventricular function that precludes surgical correction. This is, in part, due to the fact that there are no good medical therapies to treat aortic stenosis. Percutaneous balloon valvuloplasty has been used as a bridge to surgery and in patients with severe left-ventricular dysfunction or who are otherwise too ill to tolerate surgery. Improving blood pressure will not improve this patient's symptomatic AS, and vasodilation to an excessive degree can precipitate syncope in these patients due to having a fixed cardiac output. Further characterization of the patient's AS will not alter management. An exercise regimen is likely to result in more episodes of syncope.

8. The answer is C.

(Chap. 19) The ductus arteriosus is an embryonic vessel connecting the pulmonary artery to the aorta just distal to the left subclavian artery, shunting blood from the fluid-filled lungs of the fetus. After birth, the ductus arteriosus closes as blood now circulates through the low-resistance pulmonary vascular bed. If the ductus arteriosus fails to close after birth, a left-to-right shunt develops between the aorta and the pulmonary vasculature. Because the pressure in the aorta is greater than that of the pulmonary artery through all portions of the cardiac cycle, the murmur of a patent ductus arteriosus is a continuous murmur. There is late systolic accentuation of the murmur at the upper left sternal angle. The murmur is described as "machinery"-like, and often a palpable thrill is present. If Eisenmenger syndrome occurs, as in this patient, the shunt changes directional flow and becomes a right-to-left shunt as a result of pulmonary hypertension. That is when patients will become cyanotic. Because of the anatomic location of the ductus arteriosus below the level of the left subclavian artery, a characteristic of Eisenmenger syndrome in those with patent ductus arteriosus is cyanosis and clubbing of the toes but not the fingers. Total anomalous pulmonary venous return occurs when all four pulmonary veins drain into the systemic venous circulation. This condition is fatal soon after birth if there is not also an atrial or ventricular septal defect or a patent foramen ovale. Most patients with this condition are identified shortly after birth because of cyanosis. Coarctation of the aorta is a relatively common congenital abnormality that is associated with a stricture of the aorta near the insertion site of the ligamentum arteriosus (the remnant of the ductus arteriosus). A patient with coarctation of the aorta frequently presents with headache. Upper extremity hypertension is present in association with low blood pressures in the lower extremities. Patients may also complain of claudication in the lower extremities. Tetralogy of Fallot is a congenital heart disease syndrome with ventricular septal defect, right-ventricular outflow obstruction, aortic override of the ventricular septal defect, and right-ventricular hypertrophy. This defect is almost always identified and corrected during childhood. Ventricular septal defect results in left-to-right shunt and a holosystolic murmur rather than a continuous murmur.

9. The answer is A.

(Chap. 20) In the post-MI setting, posterior (mural) mitral valve chordae rupture is more common than aortic (anterior) mitral valve rupture due to its singular blood supply. In contrast to functional mitral regurgitation, the regurgitant jet of valvular mitral regurgitation (MR) is eccentric and directed towards one wall of the atrium. The musical quality of the murmur has been described when the cause is a flail leaflet. Systolic anterior

motion (SAM) of the mitral valve is a finding on echocardiogram when MR is associated with hypertrophic cardiomyopathy. Acute ventricular septal defect can be seen within the first few days of an MI. These patients usually have hypotension and rapidly develop pulmonary hypertension and signs of cardiogenic shock. In the post-MI setting, ventricular free wall rupture into the pericardium is a catastrophic event that can cause tamponade and shock. Respiratory variation in mitral inflow velocity is an echocardiographic sign of tamponade physiology. High-frequency fluttering of the anterior mitral leaflet is the characteristic echocardiographic finding of acute aortic regurgitation, seen most commonly in primary aortic valvular disease, aortic dissection, infective endocarditis, or chest trauma.

10. The answer is D.

(Chap. 38) This patient presents with severe chest pain that is tearing in quality and associated with hypertension. These symptoms should raise the concern for aortic dissection as the cause of the chest pain, and prompt evaluation and treatment are essential to decrease mortality from this often fatal condition. In the presence of an aortic regurgitation murmur and ECG changes consistent with myocardial injury, an ascending aortic dissection should be considered with dissection of the right coronary artery. Aortic dissections are classified by either the DeBakey or Stanford classification. The DeBakey system classifies aortic dissections into three types. Type I is caused by an intimal tear in the ascending aorta and has propagated to include the descending aorta. A type II dissection involves only the ascending aorta, and a type III dissection involves only the descending aorta. The Stanford classification has only two categories: type A, which involves the ascending aorta, and type B, which involves only the descending aorta. Risk factors for developing an aortic dissection include systemic hypertension (70%), Marfan syndrome, inflammatory aortitis, congenital valve abnormalities, coarctation of the aorta, and trauma. Aortic dissections are a medical emergency with a high in-hospital mortality due to aortic rupture, pericardial tamponade, or visceral ischemia. Ascending aortic dissections have the highest mortality, and studies have demonstrated that medical management alone in an ascending aortic dissection has a mortality rate of >50% (PG Hagan et al, JAMA 283:897, 2000). The greatest mortality occurs early after presentation with the mortality reported at 1–2% per hour initially after symptoms onset (CA Nienaber, KA Eagle, Circulation 108:628, 2003). Because of the high associated mortality, it is imperative to evaluate and treat aggressively with early surgical intervention. Transesophageal echocardiography has 80% sensitivity for diagnosing ascending aortic dissections and will also provide information regarding valvular function and presence of pericardial tamponade. CT angiography and MRI both have sensitivities for diagnosing aortic dissection of >90%. The decision regarding which test to perform should be based on the rapid availability of testing and clinical stability of the patient. Management of an aortic dissection initially begins with medical therapy to stabilize the patient and decrease blood pressure. This should be occurring concurrently with surgical consultation to plan definitive operative repair on an emergent basis. Medical therapy should consist of antihypertensive therapy to rapidly reduce the systolic blood pressure to 100–120 mmHg. Most often this is accomplished with nitroprusside. In addition, use of a beta blocker to reduce cardiac contractility and heart rate is recommended. Surgery involves excision of the intimal flap, removal of the intramural hematoma, and placement of a graft. In some cases, replacement of the entire aortic root and aortic valve is necessary when the aortic valve is involved. With coronary artery involvement, coronary artery bypass may also be required. With prompt surgical intervention, mortality from ascending aortic dissection is ~15–25%.

11. The answer is D.

(Chap. 11) The ECG shows a short ST segment that is most prominent in V_2, V_3, V_4, and V_5. Hypercalcemia, by shortening the duration of repolarization, abbreviates the total time from depolarization through repolarization. This is manifested on the surface ECG by a short QT interval. In this scenario, the hypercalcemia is due to the rhabdomyolysis and renal failure. Fluids and a loop diuretic are an appropriate therapy for hypercalcemia. Hemodialysis is seldom indicated. Hemodialysis is indicated for significant hyperkalemia, which may also develop after rhabdomyolysis, manifest by "tenting" of the T waves or widening of the QRS. Classic ECG manifestations of a pulmonary embolus (S_1, Q_3, T_3 pattern) are infrequent in patients with pulmonary embolism (PE), though the changes may be seen with massive PE. There are no signs of myocardial ischemia on this ECG, which would make coronary catheterization and 18-lead ECG interpretation of low yield.

12. The answer is B.

(Chaps. 30 and 31) This patient meets the criteria for the metabolic syndrome. Patients with type 2 diabetes and an abnormal lipid profile have insulin resistance and a marked increase in cardiovascular risk. The LDL in these patients may not be markedly elevated, but the particles are smaller and denser. These small LDL particles are thought to be more atherogenic than are normal LDL particles. Patients with the metabolic syndrome have reduced HDL levels. Elevated serum endothelin levels may contribute to hypertension, and elevated homocysteine levels have been suggested as a cardiovascular risk factor. (See Table 30-3)

13. The answer is A.

(Chaps. 9 and 25) The presentation of this patient is consistent with the diagnosis of acute valvular dysfunction due to infective endocarditis. The presence of a widened pulse pressure and diastolic murmur heard best along the lower sternal border suggests aortic regurgitation. Figure 9-2 in panel *C* shows a typical bisferiens pulse that is characteristic of aortic regurgitation. With a bisferiens pulse, there are two distinct pulsations that can be palpated with systole. The initial pulse represents an exaggerated percussion wave reflecting the increased stroke volume that occurs in aortic regurgitation, with the second peak reflecting the tidal, or anacrotic, wave.

Infective endocarditis causes loss of valvular integrity and acutely causes valvular regurgitation. Of the other options, both mitral regurgitation and tricuspid regurgitation (choice E) would cause systolic and not diastolic murmurs. A hyperkinetic pulse may occur in these conditions, particularly if associated with fever or sepsis. With a hyperkinetic pulse the usual dichrotic notch is more pronounced as seen in panel *E* of the figure. Mitral stenosis causes a diastolic murmur but is not a common lesion associated with infective endocarditis, unless underlying valvular stenosis was present prior to acquiring the infection. It is not associated with a bisferiens pulse. Aortic stenosis is associated with pulsus parvus et tardus, with a delayed and prolonged carotid upstroke as shown here in panel *B* of the figure. Aortic stenosis has an associated harsh crescendo-decrescendo systolic murmur.

14. The answer is B.

(*Chap. 22*) This patient presents with pericardial tamponade. Patients often have distant heart sounds and on examination typically have pulsus paradoxus. Jugular veins are distended and typically show a prominent *x* descent and an absent *y* descent, as opposed to patients with constrictive pericarditis. In addition, Kussmaul's sign is absent in tamponade but present in constrictive pericarditis. The electrocardiogram is normal or shows low voltage. Rarely, electrical alternans may be present. Echocardiographic findings typically reveal right atrial collapse and right ventricular diastolic collapse. Cardiac catheterization will reveal equalization of diastolic pressures across the cardiac chambers. Therefore, the pulmonary capillary wedge pressure will be equal to the diastolic pulmonary arterial pressure, and this will be equal to the right atrial pressure. These catheterization findings are also present in a patient with constrictive pericarditis.

15. The answer is A.

(*Chap. 33*) Calcium channel blockers are potent coronary vasodilators, which also reduce myocardial oxygen demand, contractility, and arterial pressure. When beta blockers are ineffective or poorly tolerated, calcium channel blockers are indicated for the treatment of stable angina. Adverse effects of the calcium channel blockers include hypotension, conduction disturbances, and the propensity to exacerbate heart failure due to the negative

inotropic effects. In general, verapamil should not be used in conjunction with beta blockers because of the combined effect on heart rate and contractility. Diltiazem should not be used in patients taking beta blockers with conduction disturbances and a low ejection fraction. Immediate-release nifedipine and other short-acting dihydropyridines should be avoided due to the increased risk of precipitating myocardial infarction. Amlodipine and other second-generation dihydropyridines dilate coronary arteries and decrease blood pressure. In conjunction with beta blockers, which slow heart rate and decrease contractility, amlodipine has a favorable effect in the treatment of angina.

16. The answer is A.

(*Chap. 25*) Indications for endocarditis prophylaxis with procedures are assessed by taking into account the nature of the cardiac lesion and the risk posed by the procedure. High-risk cardiac lesions include prosthetic heart valves, a history of bacterial endocarditis, complex cyanotic congenital heart disease, patent ductus arteriosus, coarctation of the aorta, and surgically constructed systemic portal shunts. Moderate-risk patients include those with congenital cardiac malformations other than high-risk or low-risk lesions, acquired aortic or mitral valve dysfunction, hypertrophic cardiomyopathy with asymmetric septal hypertrophy, and mitral valve prolapse with valve thickening or regurgitation. Low-risk lesions include isolated secundum atrial septal defect (ASD), a surgically repaired ASD, ventricular septal defect (VSD), patent ductus arteriosis (PDA), prior coronary bypass graft, mitral valve prolapse without regurgitation or thickened valves, a history of rheumatic fever without valvular dysfunction, and cardiac pacemakers or implantable defibrillators. This patient falls into the moderate-risk category. Her procedure is an esophageal dilation, which, like dental procedures, calls for prophylaxis in the moderate- to high-risk groups. Amoxicillin 2 g PO 1 h before the procedure is the standard recommendation, but this patient may be penicillin-allergic. Acceptable alternatives include clarithromycin 500 mg PO 1 h before the procedure, clindamycin 600 mg PO 1 h before, or cephalexin 2 g PO 1 h before if the patient is able to tolerate cephalosporins.

17. The answer is D.

(*Chap. 34*) Prinzmetal and colleagues described a syndrome of angina that occurs at rest but not usually with exertion associated with transient ST-segment elevation. The pathophysiology is due to coronary artery vasospasm. Proximal nonobstructive coronary plaques are usually present. The vasospasm usually occurs within 1 cm of a coronary plaque and is associated with ST-segment elevations on the 12-lead surface electrocardiogram. Due to further vasospasm, cold water ingestion may exacerbate the patient's symptoms. Costochondritis or muscular strain can reproduce the patient's pain. By definition,

Prinzmetal's angina is associated with ST-segment elevation, not depression, during the anginal episode.

18. The answer is C.
(Chap. 27) This patient presents with the classic findings of chronic Chagas' disease with cardiomyopathy. Chagas' disease, or American trypanosomiasis, is due to infection with *Trypanosoma cruzi* and only occurs in the Americans. Acute Chagas' disease is usually a mild illness. A minority of chronically infected patients develop serious cardiac or gastrointestinal disease (megaesophagus or megacolon). This diagnosis should be considered in a person from Central or South America presenting with this degree of cardiomyopathy with conduction delays (most commonly right bundle branch block) and normal angiogram. Apical aneurysm and thrombus formation are common and may lead to systemic embolization, including stroke. Although, medical therapy for acute Chagas' improves mortality, the role in chronic Chagas' has not been proven. Treatment for coronary vasospasm and aggressive lipid lowering therapy do not have an established role in the treatment of Chagas' disease. Since the cardiomyopathy is considered irreversible, cardiac transplantation is the only viable option to improve function. The prognosis after cardiac transplantation tends to be favorable since this form of chronic Chagas' disease is usually limited to the heart. Many forms of acute viral myocarditis or stress cardiomyopathy are expected to improve with time.

19. The answer is A.
(Chap. 20) This patient has the opening snap, diastolic rumble, and signs of pulmonary hypertension indicative of mitral stenosis (MS). The most common cause is sequelae of rheumatic carditis, and symptoms of stenosis usually develop two decades after the onset of carditis. MS can remain asymptomatic for many years but be exaggerated when there is tachycardia, increased left-ventricular filling pressure, or reduced cardiac output (e.g., fever, excitement, anemia, atrial fibrillation, pregnancy, or thyrotoxicosis). Due to elevated left atrial pressure and concomitant left atrial dilation, these patients are at high risk for developing atrial fibrillation, pulmonary hypertension, and right-ventricular failure. Multifocal atrial tachycardia is commonly due to diseases of the lung parenchyma. Right-ventricular outflow tract tachycardia is unrelated to valvular pathology and is common in the young and women. Patients with MS do not develop primary left-ventricular dysfunction because the left ventricle is protected from the pressure and volume load by the diseased mitral valve. Patients with MS can develop right-ventricular hypertrophy and right-ventricular failure. Right bundle branch block is usually unrelated to MS.

20. The answer is B.
(Chap. 15) Although sinoatrial node dysfunction is seen most commonly in the elderly with no specific etiology

identified, certain disease states are associated with sinoatrial dysfunction, including infiltrative diseases such as amyloid and sarcoidosis. Additionally, multiple systemic disorders are associated with sinus bradycardia, for instance, hypothyroidism, advanced liver disease, hypoxemia, hypercapnia, acidemia, and acute hypertension. Finally, several infectious diseases are classically associated with sinus bradycardia, notably typhoid fever and brucellosis. Leptospirosis is not associated with sinus bradycardia.

21. The answer is E.
(Chap. 19) Congenital heart disease (CHD) affects ~1% of all live births, and >85% of affected individuals survive until adulthood. Currently, there are more adults than children living with CHD in the United States, and many of these individuals are unaware of the presence of CHD until other complications develop. Pulmonary hypertension may develop in individuals with a significant left-to-right shunt such as an undiagnosed atrial septal defect. Pulmonary hypertension is the result of increased blood flow across the pulmonary vascular bed, leading to obliteration of the vascular bed. With the development of significant pulmonary hypertension, Eisenmenger syndrome may develop. This occurs when a right-to-left shunt develops as a result of pulmonary hypertension. Patients will have cyanosis. Erythrocytosis due to chronic hypoxemia is a common feature of cyanotic congenital heart disease with a hematocrit of up to 65–70% commonly seen. However, symptoms of hyperviscosity rarely develop, and phlebotomy is not frequently required. The risk of infective endocarditis is increased in those with CHD, and prophylactic antibiotics are recommended for all individuals with CHD undergoing invasive procedures. Stroke is greatest in children <4 years but is not increased in adults unless there is inappropriate use of anticoagulants, concomitant atrial fibrillation, or infective endocarditis.

22. The answer is A.
(Chap. 11) Hyperkalemia leads to partial depolarization of cardiac cells. As a result, there is slowing of the upstroke of the action potential as well as reduced duration of repolarization. The T wave becomes peaked, the RS complex widens and may merge with the T wave (giving a sine-wave appearance), and the P wave becomes shallow or disappears. Prominent U waves are associated with hypokalemia; ST-segment prolongation is associated with hypocalcemia.

23. The answer is B.
(Chap. 20) The time interval between closure of the aortic valve (A_2) and the opening snap of mitral stenosis is inversely related to the severity of mitral stenosis. In severe mitral stenosis, the left atrial pressure is high. In a patient with elevated left atrial pressures, the mitral valve

opens quickly after closure of the aortic valve (A_2) due to the relatively low pressure gradient across the mitral valve in early diastole. If the left atrial pressure were lower, it would take longer for the pressure gradient across the mitral valve to cause mitral valve opening. A short interval between A_2 and the opening snap indicates very elevated left atrial pressures. Atrial fibrillation, pulmonary vascular congestion, pulmonary hypertension, and right-ventricular failure (elevated jugular pressure, pulsatile liver, peripheral edema) are all potential sequelae of severe mitral stenosis.

24. The answer is A.

(Chap. 37) Essential hypertension causes 92–94% of cases of hypertension in the general population, and screening for secondary causes of hypertension is not cost-effective in most instances. The abrupt onset of severe hypertension or the onset of any hypertension <35 years or >55 years should prompt evaluation for renovascular hypertension. In addition, patients should be evaluated for secondary causes if previously well-controlled blood pressure suddenly becomes increasingly difficult to control as this may indicate the development of renovascular disease. Any symptoms or physical findings of concern should be investigated further as well. In the scenarios presented in Question 27, (B) should signal concern for adult-onset polycystic kidney disease and (E) describes a woman with possible Cushing's disease. Other causes of secondary hypertension include pheochromocytoma, primary hyperaldosteronism, medication-induced, and vasculitis.

25. The answer is A.

(Chap. 15) One-third of patients with sinoatrial node dysfunction will develop supraventricular tachycardia, usually atrial fibrillation or atrial flutter. Patients with the tachycardia-bradycardia variant of sick sinus syndrome are at risk for thromboembolism. Those at greatest risk include age >65 years, prior history of stroke, valvular heart disease, left ventricular dysfunction, or atrial enlargement. These patients should be treated with anticoagulants. There is no reason to discontinue dypyridamole at this time as she is complaining of no side effects, and the absence of angina argues against the need for cardiac catheterization.

26. The answer is C.

(Chap. 22) Cardiac tamponade occurs with accumulation of fluid in the pericardial space such that the resulting pericardial pressure obstructs venous inflow and subsequently cardiac output. The most common causes of cardiac tamponade are neoplasm, renal failure, and idiopathic acute pericarditis. The amount of fluid required to cause cardiac tamponade varies widely, depending upon the acuity with which the effusion develops. Rapid accumulation of pericardial fluid will result in tamponade

with as little as 200 mL of fluid, whereas a slow accumulation of pericardial fluid may result in a pericardial effusion of ≥2000 mL. Cardiac tamponade can be rapidly fatal if not recognized and treated quickly with pericardiocentesis. Clinical features of pericardial tamponade are hypotension, muffled heart sounds, and jugular venous distention, with a rapid *x* descent but without a *y* descent. These symptoms collectively are known as Beck's triad. In more slowly accumulating effusions, symptoms may be those of heart failure, with dyspnea and orthopnea common. An elevated pulsus paradoxus is also present in cardiac tamponade. Normally, blood pressure falls during inspiration, due to an increase in blood flow into the right ventricle with displacement of the interventricular septum to the left, decreasing left-ventricular filling and cardiac output. This fall in blood pressure results in a fall in systolic blood pressure of ≤10 mmHg in normal individuals but is exaggerated in cardiac tamponade. On electrocardiogram, electrical alternans may be seen. Echocardiogram is frequently diagnostic, showing a large pericardial effusion with collapse of the right ventricle during diastole. A right heart catheterization demonstrates equalization of pressures in all chambers of the heart. This is exemplified in option C where the right-atrial pressure, right-ventricular diastolic pressure, pulmonary artery diastolic pressure, and pulmonary capillary wedge pressure are equal. Option A are normal values on right heart catheterization. Option B would be seen in congestive heart failure, and option D is seen in pulmonary arterial hypertension.

27. The answer is C.

(Chap. 11) The ECG shows slight right axis deviation and low voltage. These changes are typical of emphysema when the thorax is hyperinflated with air and the flattened diaphragm pulls the heart inferiorly and vertically. An acute central nervous system (CNS) event such as a subarachnoid hemorrhage may cause QT prolongation with deep, wide inverted T waves. Hyperkalemia will cause peaked narrowed T waves or a wide QRS complex. Patients with hypertrophic cardiomyopathy will have left ventricular hypertrophy and widespread deep, broad Q waves.

28. The answer is D.

(Chap. 11) This ECG tracing shows the triad of a short PR interval, wide QRS, and delta waves (seen best in leads I, II, and V_5), consistent with Wolff-Parkinson-White (WPW) syndrome. Patients with WPW syndrome are commonly diagnosed asymptomatically when an ECG is performed showing the classic findings. Symptoms are due to conduction via an accessory pathway and include tachypalpitations, light headedness, syncope, cardiopulmonary collapse, and sudden cardiac death. Life-threatening presentations are usually due the development of atrial fibrillation or atrial flutter with 1:1 conduction, which can both precipitate ventricular fibrillation.

29. The answer is C.

(Chap. 10) Causes of holosystolic murmurs include mitral regurgitation, tricuspid regurgitation, and ventricular septal defects. Carvallo's sign describes the increase in intensity of a tricuspid regurgitation murmur with inspiration. This occurs due to the increase in venous return during inspiration with falling pleural pressure. The Gallavardin effect occurs when the murmur of aortic stenosis is transmitted to the apex (and becomes higher pitched), approximating the murmur heard in mitral regurgitation. The Austin Flint murmur is a late diastolic murmur heard at the apex in aortic regurgitation. The murmur of chronic mitral regurgitation does not worsen with inspiration. Atrial septal defects cause a midsystolic murmur at the mid to upper left sternal border, with fixed splitting of S_2. There is no change with respiration.

30. The answer is E.

(Chap. 16) Persons who have Wolff-Parkinson-White syndrome are predisposed to develop two major types of atrial tachyarrhythmias. The first, which resembles paroxysmal supraventricular tachycardia (SVT) with reentry, involves the atrioventricular node in anterograde conduction and the bypass tract in retrograde conduction. This tachycardia typically has a narrow QRS complex and can be treated similarly to other forms of SVT. The other, more dangerous tachyarrhythmia (present in the patient described in this question) is atrial fibrillation, which usually is conducted anterograde down the bypass tract and has a wide QRS configuration. The ventricular rate in this situation is quite rapid, and cardiovascular collapse or ventricular fibrillation may result. The usual treatment is direct-current cardioversion, though quinidine may slow conduction through the bypass tract. Verapamil and propranolol have little effect on the bypass tract and may further depress ventricular function, which already is compromised by the rapid rate. Digoxin may accelerate conduction down the bypass tract and lead to ventricular fibrillation.

31. The answer is A.

(Chap. 39) Peripheral arterial disease (PAD) affects 5–8% of Americans with increasing incidence with age. Over the age of 65, the incidence of PAD rises to between 12 and 20%. The primary symptom of PAD is claudication. As this patient describes, claudication occurs with ambulation and is often described as a crampy to aching pain that is relieved with rest. On physical examination, those with PAD often have diminished peripheral pulses, delayed capillary refill, and hair loss in the distal extremities. The skin is often cool to touch with a thin, shiny appearance. In severe PAD, pain in the extremities occurs at rest. Diagnosis of PAD can be suggested by these findings and should be documented by determination of the ankle-brachial index (ABI), as physical examination

alone is insufficient to diagnose PAD. Although lack of a palpable pulse suggests critical ischemia, it is not diagnostic. To perform an ABI, blood pressures are determined in the arm and the lower extremities. Either the dorsalis pedis or posterior tibial pulses can be used. The ABI is calculated by dividing the ankle systolic pressure by the brachial systolic pressure. A resting ABI <0.9 is abnormal, but critical ischemia with rest pain does not occur until the ABI is <0.3. In individuals with heavily calcified blood vessels, the ABI can be abnormally elevated (ABI >1.2) when PAD is present. In this situation, toe pressures to determine ABI or employing imaging techniques such as MRI or arteriography should be considered. Lower extremity edema is suggestive of congestive heart failure, not PAD.

32 and 33. The answers are C and A.

(Chap. 19) This patient has a coarctation of the aorta presenting with marked hypertension proximal to the lesion. The narrowing most commonly occurs distal to the origin of the left subclavian artery, explaining the equal pressure in the arms and reduced pressure in the legs. Coarctations account for approximately 7% of congenital cardiac abnormalities, occur more frequently (2×) in men than in women, and are associated with gonadal dysgenesis and bicuspid aortic valves. Adults will present with hypertension, manifestations of hypertension in the upper body (headache, epistaxis), or leg claudication. Physical examination reveals diminished and/or delayed lower extremity pulses, enlarged collateral vessels in the upper body, or reduced development of the lower extremities. Cardiac examination may reveal findings consistent with left ventricular (LV) hypertrophy. There may be no murmur, a midsytolic murmur over the anterior chest and back, or an aortic murmur with a bicuspid valve. Transthoracic (suprasternal/parasternal) or transesophageal echocardiography, contrast CT or MRI of the thorax, or cardiac catheterization can be diagnostic. MRI of the head would not be useful diagnostically. The clinical picture is not consistent with renal artery stenosis, pheochromocytoma, carcinoid, or Cushing's syndrome.

34. The answer is D.

(Chap. 16) The patient is a young woman with no cardiac disease. In this population asymptomatic premature ventricular contractions (PVCs) require no specific therapy as they are not associated with increased mortality. In patients with symptoms such as palpitations, the primary therapy should be patient reassurance. If this is unsuccessful, beta blockers can be helpful, especially in patients whose symptoms are more prominent during stressful situations and patients with hyperthyroidism. Even in patients with myocardial infarction and PVCs there is no benefit to administering antiarrhythmic therapy with the goal of decreasing

the PVC rate. Trials such as CAST comparing ectopy suppression by encainide, flecainide, moricizine, or placebo showed that mortality was increased in all the drug groups compared with placebo at 2 years. Thus, it has become clear that PVC reduction cannot be used as a surrogate endpoint for reduction of risk from sudden cardiac death.

35. The answer is E.

(Chap. 11) The limb lead aVR generally has a negative deflection as the primary vector for ventricular depolarization is directed down and away from this lead. Therefore, in the case of left ventricular hypertrophy the negative deflection, or S wave, would be expected to be larger without an effect on the R wave. There are multiple criteria for diagnosing left ventricular hypertrophy on ECG. (See Fig. 11-9)

36. The answer is D.

(Chap. 15) Pacemaker syndrome occurs as a result of disrupted AV synchrony. The symptoms are similar to those in this scenario but can also include neck pulsation, confusion, exertional dyspnea, dizziness, and syncope. Signs on examination may suggest cardiac congestive failure. The management involves changing the pacing mode to restore AV synchrony. Lyme disease does not increase the risk of coronary artery diseases. The ECG shows only changes consistent with ventricular pacing, and there is no suggestion of ischemia. ICU psychosis is a cause of delirium among patients with prolonged stays in intensive care settings. Pacemaker twiddler's syndrome occurs when the pulse generator of the pacemaker rotates in its subcutaneous pocket, leading to lead dislodgement and failure to sense or pace. In this case, the stable paced rhythm at 60/min makes this unlikely. Kearne-Sayer syndrome is a rare syndrome caused by abnormal mitochondrial DNA in muscle, which can manifest as cardiac conduction delays.

37. The answer is B.

(Chap. 11) The ECG shows findings consistent with an old anterolateral MI. Given the patient's history and that the ST-segment elevations in aV_L and V_2–V_4 are unchanged from prior; this ECG is consistent with a left ventricular aneurysm. A transthoracic echocardiogram should be obtained to assess for severity as well as the presence of ventricular thrombus. Presence of left ventricular thrombus would warrant discussion of arrhythmogenic and embolic complications. Chest radiography may show an enlarged cardiac silhouette but will not be specific for the patient's pathology. As the patient's symptoms may be indicative of a more serious problem (i.e., left ventricular thrombus), it is not appropriate to schedule follow-up months from now. Without symptoms of chest pain and a stable electrocardiogram, neither cardiac catheterization nor thrombolysis is indicated.

38. The answer is E.

(Chap. 38) Aortic aneurysm results from numerous mechanisms. The vast majority are associated with atherosclerosis. The risk factors for atherosclerosis (hypertension, hypercholesterolemia, etc.) are also risk factors for aneurysm formation. It is unclear if atherosclerosis is the primary cause or a result of the same pathophysiologic mechanisms that lead to dilatation. Other etiologies include congenital causes. Marfan's syndrome and Ehlers-Danlos syndrome are the most frequently noted. However, there is also an association with osteogenesis imperfecta. Turner's syndrome is associated with coarctation of the aorta. Repair of coarctation may predispose to later dilation and aneurysm formation. Klinefelter's syndrome, however, is not associated with aneurysm formation. Chronic infectious causes include syphilis and mycotic aneurysm from bacterial endocarditis. Chronic inflammatory states such as Takayasu's arteritis, giant cell arteritis, and seronegative spondyloarthropathies such as Reiter's syndrome and ankylosing spondylitis are also associated with aneurysms.

39. The answer is D.

(Chap. 34) Although troponin is a commonly used biomarker for myocardial necrosis in the setting of acute myocardial infarction, it is also associated with and caused by a number of other clinical entities, including pulmonary embolism, myocarditis, and congestive heart failure. Troponin elevations are not known to be caused by pneumonia in the absence of myocardial necrosis.

40. The answer is E.

(Chap. 11) The ECG tracing shows a normal physiologic finding of respiratory sinus arrhythmia. The sinus pacemaker is slow at the beginning of the tracing, accelerates during inspiration in the middle of the tracing, and then slows again during expiration. In atrial fibrillation there are no discernable conducting P waves and the rate is irregularly irregular. In complete heart block, the QRS complexes are usually wider than normal and the R-R interval is regular; variability in the R-R interval rules out complete heart block. There are no nonconducted P waves in this tracing to suggest type 2 AV block. In a ventriculophasic sinus arrhythmia or idioventricular sinus arrhythmia, there is 2:1 AV block with two distinct P-P intervals, which appear to alternate with the QRS complexes.

41. The answer is A.

(Chap. 15) This patient's bradycardia may be symptomatic in that he has altered mental status, but he is also severely hypoxic with an active pulmonary infection. Correction of reversible etiologies is indicated since he is still able to generate enough pulse pressure to perfuse his vital organs. Although myocardial infarction due to right coronary artery disease can cause sinus bradycardia, there is no indication that this patient has any disease process other than his pulmonary infection. Glucagon can reverse the bradycardic effects of beta blockers. Temporary transvenous pacing is not indicated since the patient is well-perfused and reversible etiologies are yet to be corrected.

42. The answer is B.

(Chap. 40) In the diagnostic algorithm for pulmonary hypertension, the right heart catheterization is important to document the presence and degree of pulmonary hypertension. The right-ventricular systolic pressure (RVSP) on echocardiography provides an estimate of pulmonary arterial pressures, but accurate determination of the RVSP relies upon the presence of triscupid regurgitation and good quality echocardiography. In this patient, her body habitus is prohibitive in obtaining good windows for echocardiography. Thus, a right heart catheterization is imperative for documenting pulmonary hypertension as well as for determining the cause. The right heart catheterization demonstrates an elevated mean arterial pressure, elevated left-ventricular end-diastolic pressure (pulmonary capillary wedge pressure), and elevated mean pulmonary artery pressure. In the presence of a normal cardiac output and an elevated left-ventricular ejection fraction, this is consistent with the diagnosis of diastolic heart failure. Systolic heart failure is associated with similar indices on right heart catheterization, but left-ventricular function is depressed in systolic heart failure. The other causes listed as options are known causes of pulmonary hypertension but would not be expected to cause an increase in the left-ventricular end-diastolic pressure. Obstructive sleep apnea is usually associated only with mild elevations in pulmonary artery pressure. This patient's BMI puts her at risk for obstructive sleep apnea but would not be responsible for these right heart catheterization values. Both chronic thromboembolic disease and pulmonary arterial hypertension can cause severe elevations in the pulmonary arterial pressure but have a normal left atrial pressure.

43. The answer is C.

(Chap. 19; Brickner et al, 2000.) Left-to-right shunts occur in all types of atrial and ventricular septal defects but generally do not result in cyanosis, whereas large right-to-left shunts frequently do. The magnitude of the shunt depends on the size of the defect, the diastolic properties of both ventricles, and the relative impedance of the pulmonary and systemic circulations. Defects of the sinus venosus type occur high in the atrial septum near the entry of the superior vena cava or lower near the orifice of the inferior vena cava and may be associated with anomalous connection of the right inferior pulmonary vein to the right atrium. In the case of anomalous origin of the left coronary artery from the

pulmonary artery, as pulmonary vascular resistance declines immediately after birth, perfusion of the left coronary artery from the pulmonary trunk ceases and the direction of flow in the anomalous vessel reverses. Twenty percent of patients with this defect can survive to adulthood because of myocardial blood supply flowing totally through the right coronary artery. In the absence of pulmonary hypertension blood will flow from the aorta to the pulmonary artery throughout the cardiac cycle, resulting in a "continuous" murmur at the left sternal border. In total anomalous pulmonary venous connection all the venous blood returns to the right atrium; therefore, an interatrial communication is required and right-to-left shunts with cyanosis are common.

44. The answer is C.

(Chap. 20) This patient's murmur is consistent with chronic aortic regurgitation. The high-pitched blowing murmur in the left third intercostal space is commonly present, whereas the second diastolic murmur at the apex, resembling mitral stenosis (Austin Flint murmur), is not always present. Peripheral signs of chronic aortic regurgitation are manifestations of a widened pulse pressure and equalization of aortic and ventricular end-diastolic pressures. As pressure increases in the left ventricle, hypertrophy develops as a compensatory mechanism. Left atrial, but not right atrial, enlargement may be apparent on the ECG if there is concomitant mitral regurgitation. Inferior Q waves may be seen if there has been a myocardial infarction. ST-segment depressions may be seen in the lateral leads when there is significant left-ventricular hypertrophy. Low voltage on the ECG can be seen in obstructive lung diseases, pericardial effusions, and infiltrative diseases of the myocardium. Diffuse ST-segment elevation and PR-segment depression are seen in pericarditis.

45. The answer is B.

(Chap. 16) The differentiation of ventricular tachycardia from supraventricular tachycardia with an aberration of intraventricuar conduction can be challenging and has important implications for management. By definition, however, ventricular tachycardia is associated with atrioventricular (AV) dissociation. Cannon a waves are found in the jugular venous pulsations when the atria are contracting against a closed tricuspid valve. This can occur only with AV dissociation, thus proving ventricular tachycardia. Hypotension, irregular rhythm, and syncope can all be seen in both ventricular tachycardia and supraventricuar tachycardia with aberrancy.

46. The answer is C.

(Chap. 33) The ischemic ST-segment response during exercise is characterized by flat or downsloping ST-segment depression of at least 1 mm lasting for >0.08 s. Upsloping ST segments, ventricular arrhythmias, T-wave abnormalities, and conduction disturbances that develop during exercise should be noted, but are not diagnostic. A decrease in blood pressure or a failure to increase blood pressure with signs of ischemia on the stress test may be indicative of global dyskinesis and severe ischemic heart disease. The normal response to the graded exercise protocol is a gradual increase in blood pressure. Isolated hypertension during a stress test, despite its severity, is not indicative of myocardial ischemia. Developing angina at a low work-load (i.e., before completion of stage II of a Bruce protocol) or persistent ST-segment depressions lasting >5 min into recovery increase the specificity of the test and indicate a high risk of future events. The target heart rate for exercise stress tests is ≥85% of maximal predicted heart rate for age and sex.

47. The answer is A.

(Chap. 9) This patient presents with signs and symptoms consistent with congestive heart failure. Her history of tuberculosis puts her at risk for constrictive pericarditis, and indeed, chest CT shows the classic pericardial calcifications of this disorder. As she is relatively young and does not have enlarged chambers or ischemic changes on the electrocardiogram, dilated or ischemic cardiomyopathy is unlikely. Constrictive pericarditis has certain suggestive physical findings, notably the prominent and rapid *γ* descent in the jugular venous pulsations that represents early and rapid filling of the right ventricle during early diastole. Other findings that have been associated include rapid *x* descent, pericardial knock that is similar to a third heart sound, and impressive ascites, edema, and occasionally Kussmaul's sign (lack of inspiratory decline in jugular venous pressure). A double systolic apical impulse has been described in patients with hypertrophic cardiomyopathy. A loud and fixed split P_2 suggests pulmonary hypertension. Cannon *a* waves are most commonly seen in arrhythmias that cause atrioventricular dissociation. Finally, opening snaps are brief, high-pitched diastolic sounds that usually are due to mitral stenosis.

48. The answer is A.

(Chap. 20) Aortic stenosis in adults may be due to congenital degenerative calcification of the aortic cusps. Age-related degenerative calification is the most common cause of aortic stenosis (so-called senile aortic stenosis). Approximately 30% of persons >65 years have evidence of aortic valve sclerosis. Many have a murmur without obstruction, whereas 2% exhibit stenosis. The risk factors for developing aortic stenosis (dyslipidemia, chronic kidney disease, diabetes, etc.) are similar to those for developing atherosclerotic coronary artery disease. Pathology of the affected valves will show evidence of vascular inflammation, lipid deposition, and calcification. However, treating risk factors such as dyslipidemia has not been shown to improve severe aortic stenosis. There

is no effective medical therapy for aortic stenosis. In younger patients presenting with aortic stenosis, the aortic valve apparatus is commonly bicuspid.

49. The answer is B.

(Chap. 16) Atrial fibrillation is characterized by disorganized atrial activity with an irregular ventricular response to atrial activity. This lack of organization results in stasis of blood in the atria and puts the patient at risk for cardioembolic stroke. Several factors associated with increased stroke risk have been identified, including diabetes mellitus, hypertension, age >65 years, rheumatic heart disease, a prior stroke or transient ischemic attack, congestive heart failure, and a transesophageal echocardiogram showing spontaneous echo contrast in the left atrium, left atrial atheroma, or left atrial appendage velocity <20 cm/s. Hypercholesterolemia is not associated with an increased risk of stroke in patients with atrial fibrillation.

50. The answer is A.

(Chap. 10) This patient most likely experienced papillary muscle rupture, which led to acute mitral regurgitation. Other settings where acute mitral regurgitation may occur include rupture of chordae tendineae in the setting of myxomatous mitral valve disease, infective endocarditis, or chest wall trauma. The regurgitation into a normalsized noncompliant left atrium results in an early systolic descrescendo murmur heard best near the apical impulse. The decrescendo nature contrasts with chronic mitral regurgitation due to the rapid pressure rise in the left atrium during systole. Chronic mitral regurgitation causes a holosystolic murmur. Ventricular septal rupture also causes a holosystolic murmur and is associated with a systolic thrill at the left sternal border. Severe aortic stenosis and hypertrophic cardiomyopathy both present with a midsystolic murmur.

51. The answer is C.

(Chap. 35) This patient has a right ventricular infarction. The combination of findings consistent with bradycardia, cardiogenic shock, low normal left ventricular and PA pressures, and markedly elevated right atrial pressure is consistent with acute right ventricular (RV) failure. An acute pulmonary embolus may also cause acute RV failure, but the PA pressure is usually elevated. RV infarction is usually due to occlusion of the right coronary artery; the bradycardia is due to sinus or AV node ischemia. Right-sided precordial ECG will show ST-segment elevation. Occlusion of the left main artery will cause cardiogenic shock, but the PCW pressure will be elevated. Perforated duodenal ulcer and ruptured aortic aneurysm will cause hypovolemic shock with low RA and PCW pressures. Gram–negative sepsis will generally have a normal or increased cardiac index with normal filling pressures and low blood pressure.

52. The answer is D.

(Chap. 20) Indications for surgical repair of mitral regurgitation are dependent on left-ventricular function, ventricular size, and the presence of sequelae of chronic mitral regurgitation. The experience of the surgeon and the likelihood of successful mitral valve repair are also an important consideration. The management strategy for chronic severe mitral regurgitation depends on the presence of symptoms, left-ventricular function, left-ventricular dimensions, and the presence of complicating factors such as pulmonary hypertension and atrial fibrillation. With very depressed left-ventricular function (<30% or end-systolic dimension >55 mm), the risk of surgery increases, left-ventricular recovery is often incomplete, and long-term survival is reduced. However, since medical therapy offers little for these patients, surgical repair should be considered if there is a high likelihood of success (>90%). When ejection fraction is between 30 and 60% and end-systolic dimension rises above 40 mm, surgical repair is indicated even in the absence of symptoms, owing to the excellent long-term results achieved in this group. Waiting for worsening left-ventricular function leads to irreversible left-ventricular remodeling. Pulmonary hypertension and atrial fibrillation are important to consider as markers for worsening regurgitation. For asymptomatic patients with normal left-ventricular function and dimensions, the presence of new pulmonary hypertension or atrial fibrillation in patients with normal ejection fraction and end-systolic dimensions are class IIa indications for mitral valve repair.

53. The answer is A.

(Chap. 32) The metabolic syndrome (according to the NCET:ATP III guidelines) is defined by three or more of the following: central obesity (men >102 cm; women >88 cm), hypertriglyceridemia (≥150 mg/dL or on specific medication), low HDL cholesterol (men <40 mg/dL; women <50 mg/dL), hypertension (systolic ≥130 mmHg or diastolic ≥85 mmHg, or on specific medication), and hyperglycemia (fasting plasma glucose ≥100 mg/dL, or previous diagnosis of diabetes mellitus, or on specific medication). The International Diabetes Foundation also has criteria that further subdivide the cut-offs of waist circumference based on ethnicity. Patients with the metabolic syndrome are at greater risk than patients without the syndrome for developing conditions such as atherosclerotic cardiovascular disease, type 2 diabetes mellitus, peripheral vascular disease, sleep apnea, and polycystic ovary syndrome. The presence of one of the criteria should prompt the clinician to search for other criteria and treat the conditions as necessary.

54. The answer is C.

(Chap. 21) Peripartum cardiomyopathy can develop in the last trimester of pregnancy or within 6 months of delivery. The cause is unknown and mortality is high (25–50%). Risk factors for developing the disease are African ancestry, age >30 years, and multiparity. Counseling patients with peripartum cardiomyopathy who are considering becoming pregnant in the future is important as it directly impacts maternal and fetal mortality. Some of these patients may become pregnant again; however, women whose ventricular function has not returned to normal usually are advised against pregnancy since the mortality can be as high as 50% during subsequent pregnancies in this population. Among all-comers, there is a 25–67% chance of having another bout of peripartum cardiomyopathy during future pregnancies. Sex of the child during the incident episode of peripartum cardiomyopathy, maternal age, or nadir ejection fraction is not known to be associated with future events. African ancestry is a risk for developing peripartum cardiomyopathy but subsequent risk of mortality depends on the resolution of the first episode.

55. The answer is B.

(Chap. 21) Varying degrees of cardiac enlargement and findings of congestion can be found in patients with dilated cardiomyopathies, depending on the chronicity of the illness. In severe left ventricular dilatation, the jugular venous pressure is elevated, murmurs of mitral and tricuspid regurgitation are common, and third or fourth heart sounds may be heard. Owing to the depressed cardiac output, systemic vascular resistance increases, and with it, diastolic blood pressure. Systolic blood pressure may decrease as a result of decreased cardiac output leading to a narrow pulse pressure. Conditions in which S_2 becomes absent include severe aortic stenosis and severe aortic insufficiency when the insufficiency murmur is louder than S_2. Paradoxical splitting occurs when P_2 and A_2 become closer during inspiration and can be seen in patients with left bundle branch block. Pulsus bisferiens (double-impulse pulse) is classically detected when aortic insufficiency exists in association with aortic stenosis, but it may also be found in isolated but severe aortic insufficiency and hypertrophic obstructive cardiomyopathy.

56. The answer is D.

(Chap. 30) HMG-CoA reductase inhibitors ("statins") clearly reduce cardiovascular events in patients with atherosclerosis. The mechanism appears to be more complex than simply the reduction of serum LDL. Lipid-lowering drugs do not appear to cause significant regression of fixed coronary lesions. The benefit of statins appears to be related to stabilization of plaques, long-term egress of lipids, and/or improved vasodilatory tone. The improved vasodilatory tone appears to be mediated by modulation of endothelial-dependent vasodilators such as nitric oxide. Thus, the beneficial effect of the statins probably consists of an early effect on vasomotion (or other mechanisms) and a long-term effect on serum and plaque lipids.

57. The answer is A.

(Chap. 33) Dipyridamole inhibits the activity of adenosine deaminase and phosphodiesterase, which cause an accumulation of adenosine and coronary artery vasodilation. Where there is significant obstructive coronary disease, there is a pressure gradient between prestenotic and poststenotic segments, and the poststenotic vascular bed dilates to allow for preserved coronary blood flow. Higher degrees of obstruction cause maximal poststenotic vasodilation. In nonaffected regions of myocardium, there is no distal vasodilation. Dipyridamole, by disproportionately dilating nonobstructed areas of myocardium, is useful as a pharmacologic agent to differentiate ischemic from nonischemic tissue. Where there is high-grade, three-vessel disease, the usefulness of dipyridamole or adenosine infusion is limited by (1) baseline maximal vasodilation, and (2) lack of ability to differentiate affected from nonaffected regions of myocardium. Dipyridamole testing is helpful in identifying ischemic tissue in a single-vessel territory. Intraventricular conduction abnormalities limit the use of electrocardiography or echocardiography as a stress-imaging technique. Dipyridamole, as a pharmacologic stressor, is not affected by heart rate and may be particularly useful for patients who are unable to exercise.

58. The answer is C.

(Chap. 35) Myoglobin is released from ischemic myocardial cells and appears in serum within hours. It has a very short half-life in serum as it is excreted rapidly in the urine. Serum myoglobin returns to normal within 24 h after an infarction. Therefore, in this patient a new elevation of myoglobin would be helpful in distinguishing new myocardial necrosis. Troponin-I and troponin-T are more specific markers of myocardial necrosis but have a long half-life in the circulation. They may remain elevated for over a week after an acute MI. Therefore, they are not as useful for detecting new or recurrent injury. In the presence of a preexisting left bundle branch ECG is of limited utility in detecting new ischemia. Serial echocardiograms may detect new wall motion abnormalities that suggest new ischemia or infarction, but in the absence of a prior study a single echocardiogram would have limited utility in this patient.

59. The answer is B.

(Chap. 38) Aortitis is an uncommon cause of an ascending aortic aneurysm and commonly presents with fevers and chest pain. Malaise and weight loss may also occur in association with underlying rheumatic disease. Physical examination frequently reveals evidence of aortic regurgitation. All of the listed choices can cause aortitis.

However, giant cell arteritis almost never occurs in individuals <50 years *(SM Levine, DB Hellmann: Curr Opin Rheumatol 14:3, 2002).*

60. The answer is D.

(Chap. 11) The ECG shows ST-segment elevation in all leads except for aV_L, aV_R and V_1. There is PR depression in the inferior leads and PR elevation in aV_R, consistent with acute pericarditis. Acute pericarditis can be due to infectious, neoplastic, autoimmune, cardiac, metabolic, or pharmacologic events. Most often, a causal factor is not identified. The ECG in acute pericarditis evolves through four stages. In stage 1 (hours to days), there are diffuse ST-segment elevations and PR-segment depressions. Stage 2 is characterized by normalization of the ST and PR segments. In stage 3, there are diffuse T-wave inversions. In stage 4, the tracing may become normal or the T-wave inversions may persist. Proximal main coronary artery occlusion can manifest as diffuse ST-segment elevations; however, PR-segment depression is highly specific for acute pericarditis. The echocardiogram will show a small to moderate amount of pericardial effusion with normal left ventricular function. Focal ST-segment elevations consistent with acute myocardial infarction would correlate with focal hypokinesis on echocardiography. This ECG does not meet any criteria for left ventricular hypertrophy. There are no pacemaker lead depolarizations or right bundle branch block, which might suggest a catheter irritating the right ventricular myocardium.

61. The answer is E.

(Chap. 11) The ECG shows a junctional rhythm with an atrioventricular (AV) block and ST-segment elevation in leads II, III, and aVF. There are also reciprocal changes in I and aVL. These changes are consistent with an acute inferior wall myocardial infarction. The ECG is more useful in localizing regions of ischemia in ST elevation than in non-ST elevation MI. Anteroseptal ischemia causes changes in V_1–V_3 and apical/lateral ischemia in V_4–V_6. The right coronary artery (RCA) generally supplies blood flow to the right ventricle and the AV node. The inferior-posterior region of the left ventricle is supplied by the right coronary artery or the left circumflex coronary artery. In approximately 60–70% of people it is supplied by the RCA (right dominant). In this case the presence of AV nodal dysfunction and inferior ischemia makes disease of the RCA most likely.

62. The answer is B.

(Chap. 34) Patients with unstable angina/non-ST-segment elevation myocardial infarction (UA/NSTEMI) exhibit a wide spectrum of risk of death, MI, or urgent revascularization. Risk stratification tools such as the TIMI risk score are useful for identifying patients who benefit from an early invasive strategy and those who are

best suited for a more conservative approach. The TIMI risk score is composed of seven independent risk factors: Age ≥65 years, three or more cardiovascular risk factors, prior stenosis >50%, ST-segment deviation ≥0.5mm, two or more anginal events in <24 h, aspirin usage in the past 7 days, and elevated cardiac markers. Aspirin resistance can occur in 5–10% of patients and is more common among those taking lower doses of aspirin. Having unstable angina despite aspirin usage suggests aspirin resistance. Use of a beta-agonist and a diuretic do not confer an independent risk for death, MI, or need for urgent revascularization.

63. The answer is E.

(Chap. 21) A common diagnostic dilemma is differentiating constrictive pericarditis from a restrictive cardiomyopathy. Elevated jugular venous pressure is almost universally present in both. Kussmaul's sign (increase in or no change in jugular venous pressure with inspiration) can be seen in both conditions. Other signs of heart failure do not reliably distinguish the two conditions. In restrictive cardiomyopathy, the apical impulse is usually easier to palpate than in constrictive pericarditis and mitral regurgitation is more common. These clinical signs, however, are not reliable to differentiate the two entities. In conjunction with clinical information and additional imaging studies of the left ventricle and pericardium, certain pathognomic findings increase diagnostic certainty. A thickened or calcified pericardium increases the likelihood of constrictive pericarditis. Conduction abnormalities are more common in infiltrating diseases of the myocardium. In constrictive pericarditis, measurements of diastolic pressures will show equilibrium between the ventricles, whereas unequal pressures and/or isolated elevated left ventricular pressures are more consistent with restrictive cardiomyopathy. The classic "square root sign" during right heart catheterization (deep, sharp drop in right ventricular pressure in early diastole, followed by a plateau during which there is no further increase in right ventricular pressure) can be seen in both restrictive cardiomyopathy and constrictive pericarditis. The presence of a paraprotein abnormality (MGUS, myeloma, amyloid) makes restrictive cardiomyopathy more common.

64. The answer is A.

(Chap. 11) The ECG demonstrates marked ST-segment elevations in the inferior leads (II, III, aV$_F$) and laterally (V$_6$) as well as prominent ST-segment depressions with upright T waves in V$_1$–V$_4$ consistent with an acute posterior and anterolateral myocardial infarction (MI). The 12-lead ECG is most useful for detecting infarctions in the inferior, lateral, and anterior walls of the left ventricle. As 40% of patients with inferior wall infarctions have right ventricular or posterior wall involvement, additional testing is recommended in the acute care of patients

with inferior MIs. The addition of right ventricular leads (V$_4$R, V$_5$R, V$_6$R) and posterior leads (V$_7$, V$_8$, V$_9$) improves both sensitivity and specificity for detecting infarctions in these territories. Although posterior infarctions predispose a patient to high-grade AV block, a specific rhythm strip analysis is not indicated. These patients should be monitored on telemetry. Chest radiography and CT scanning are not routinely obtained when a patient has an acute MI. Unnecessary testing will delay the time to reperfusion therapy, which has a direct impact on mortality and morbidity. Pericarditis may cause diffuse ST-segment elevation but not focal changes as described above.

65. The answer is A.

(Chap. 19) Given the young age of this patient, bicuspid aortic valve is the most likely cause of aortic stenosis. Bicuspid aortic valve is one of the most common abnormalities of the circulatory system, affecting 1–2% of the population. For unknown reasons, males are twice as likely as females to have a bicuspid aortic valve. Bicuspid aortic valves often are undetected until symptomatic aortic stenosis develops. This most commonly occurs between the fourth and fifth decades of life. Congenital aortic stenosis would be expected to present earlier in life. A murmur is often present from birth and requires valvular replacement before adulthood. Calcific aortic stenosis is the most common cause of aortic stenosis and most commonly presents in the seventh or eighth decade. Rheumatic heart disease as a result of rheumatic fever is also commonly associated with aortic valve disease. The age of presentation of rheumatic heart disease falls between that of bicuspid aortic valve and calcific aortic stenosis, usually around the sixth or seventh decade.

66. The answer is D.

(Chap. 32) According to the NCEP:ATP III guidelines, treating the dyslipidemia of the metabolic syndrome should first be directed towards LDL cholesterol goals (usually <100 mg/dL, depending on the presence of risk factors). If triglyceride levels are ≥200 mg/dL after the LDL goal is reached, the clinician should set a secondary goal for non–high-density lipoprotein cholesterol 30 points higher than the LDL goal. When triglyceride levels are between 200 and 499 mg/dL, options include nicotinic acid, a fibrate, or intensifying therapy with an HMG-CoA reductase inhibitor (statin). Average efficacy of these drug classes are as follows: nicotinic acid, 20–40%; fibrate, 35–50%; statin, 7–30%). Cholestyramine and colestipol are bile acid sequestrants. They lower cholesterol but often increase triglyceride levels and should not be used in patients with triglycerides >200 mg/dL. The effects of ezetimibe on hypertriglyceridemia are not well established. Nicotinic acid is effective for treating hypertriglyceridemia but may worsen

glucose control and therefore should be used cautiously in patients with the metabolic syndrome. Gemfibrozil is more likely to worsen statin myopathy than fenofibrate.

67. The answer is D.

(Chap. 33) The use of PCI with stenting relieves angina better than best medical therapy, but the salutary effects on coronary death or MI are not well established. In a recent large clinical trial (COURAGE trial) of patients with stable coronary artery disease, death rates with medical therapy were equivalent to death rates with PCI at 4 years of follow-up. Balloon angioplasty reocclusion rates are up to two times higher compared to restenosis with stenting. This type of restenosis is mediated by hyperproliferation of smooth muscle cells into the intima as they react to the vascular injury induced by the balloon angioplasty. However, due to the delayed endothelial healing that is achieved with drug-eluting stents, the patient is exposed to a higher risk of subacute in-stent restenosis. This type of restenosis is mediated by thrombus formation as the denuded endothelium is exposed to the circulation. Patients with left-main coronary occlusion, three-vessel disease, two-vessel disease including the left main, impaired left ventricular function, or diabetes should be considered for CABG.

68. The answer is B.

(Chap. 34) Unstable angina is defined as angina or ischemic discomfort with at least one of three factors: pain at rest lasting >10 min, severe recent pain (within 4–6 weeks), or crescendo angina. NSTEMI is diagnosed when a patient with unstable angina has positive cardiac biomarkers. Anti-ischemic therapy (nitrates, beta blockers) is important for symptom relief and to prevent recurrence of chest pain. Anti-thrombotic therapy is directed against the platelet aggregation at the site of the ruptured plaque. Initially, this therapy should consist of aspirin. Addition of clopidogrel confers an additional 20% risk reduction in both low- and high-risk NSTEMI patients, as demonstrated in the CURE trial. Continuation of treatment for up to 12 months confers additional benefit in patients treated conservatively and among those who underwent percutaneous coronary intervention. The glycoprotein IIb/IIIa inhibitors are usually reserved for high-risk (i.e., troponin-positive) patients and may not be beneficial for patients treated conservatively. Statin therapy is important for secondary prevention; however, spironolactone is not a first-line therapy for NSTEMI.

69. The answer is A.

(Chap. 20) Bioprosthetic valves are made from human, porcine, or bovine tissue. The major advantage of a bioprosthetic valve is the low incidence of thromboembolic phenomena, particularly 3 months after implantation. Although in the immediate postoperative period some anticoagulation may occur, >3 months there is no further need for anticoagulation or monitoring. The downside is the natural history and longevity of the bioprosthetic valve. Bioprosthetic valves tend to degenerate mechanically. Approximately 50% will need replacement at 15 years. Therefore, these valves are useful in patients with contraindications to anticoagulation, such as elderly patients with comorbidities and younger patients who desire to become pregnant. Elderly people may also be spared the need for repeat surgery as their life span may be shorter than the natural history of the bioprosthesis. Mechanical valves offer superior durability. Hemodynamic parameters are improved with double-disk valves compared with single-disk or ball-and-chain valves. However, thrombogenicity is high and chronic anticoagulation is mandatory. Younger patients with no contraindications to anticoagulation may be better served by mechanical valve replacement.

70. The answer is A.

(Chap. 40) This patient is presenting with Eisenmenger's syndrome. This designation is applied to patients with communications between the right and left circulations, pulmonary hypertension, and a predominantly right-to-left shunt. Eisenmenger's syndrome can develop in patients with communication at the atrial, ventricular, or aortopulmonary level. These shunts are initially left to right and therefore do not present with cyanosis. Pulmonary hypertension develops over years as a result of increased pulmonary flow, increased vascular tone, and erythrocytosis. Cyanosis develops when the pulmonary hypertension becomes so severe that it reverses the shunt. Atrial septal defects are most common in adults presenting with Eisenmenger's syndrome. This patient had no evidence of pulmonary hypertension or cyanosis 10 years ago. Ebstein's anomaly, tetralogy of Fallot, and truncus arteriosis all cause cyanosis.

71 and 72. The answers are D and E.

(Chap. 37) This patient presents at a young age with hypertension that is difficult to control, raising the question of secondary causes of hypertension. The most likely diagnosis in this patient is primary hyperaldosteronism, also known as Conn's syndrome. The patient has no physical features that suggest congenital adrenal hyperplasia or Cushing's syndrome. In addition, there is no glucose intolerance as is commonly seen in Cushing's syndrome. The lack of episodic symptoms and the labile hypertension make pheochromocytoma unlikely. The findings of hypokalemia and metabolic alkalosis in the presence of difficult to control hypertension yield the likely diagnosis of Conn's syndrome. Diagnosis of the disease can be difficult, but the preferred test is the plasma aldosterone/renin ratio. This test should be performed at 8 A.M., and a ratio >30–50 is diagnostic of primary hyperaldosteronism. Caution should be made in interpreting this test while the patient is on ACE inhibitor therapy as ACE inhibitors can falsely elevate plasma renin activity. However, a plasma renin level that is undetectable or an elevated aldosterone/renin ratio in the presence of an ACE inhibitor therapy is highly suggestive of primary hyperaldosteronism. Selective adrenal vein renin sampling may be performed after the diagnosis to help determine if the process is unilateral or bilateral. Although fibromuscular dysplasia is a common secondary cause of hypertension in young females, the presence of hypokalemia and metabolic alkalosis should suggest Conn's syndrome. Thus, magnetic resonance imaging of the renal arteries is unnecessary in this case. Measurement of 24-h urine collection for potassium wasting and aldosterone secretion can be useful in the diagnosis of Conn's syndrome. The measurement of metanephrines or cortisol is not indicated.

73. The answer is D.

(Chap. 21) Cardiac involvement is common in many of the neuromuscular diseases. The ECG pattern of Duchenne's muscular dystrophy is unique and consists of tall R waves in the right precordial leads with an R/S ratio >1.0, often with deep Q waves in the limb and precordial leads. These patients often have a variety of supraventricular and ventricular arrhythmias and are at risk for sudden death due to the intrinsic cardiomyopathy as well as the low ejection fraction. Implantable cardioverter defibrillators should be considered in the appropriate patient. Global left ventricular dysfunction is a common finding in dilated cardiomyopathies, whereas focal wall motion abnormalities and angina are more common if there is ischemic myocardium. This patient is at risk for venous thromboembolism; however, chronic thromboembolism would not account for the severity of the left heart failure and would present with findings consistent with pulmonary hypertension. Amyotrophic lateral sclerosis is a disease of motor neurons and does not involve the heart. This patient would be young for that diagnosis. An advanced atrial septal defect would present with cyanosis and heart failure (Eisenmenger's physiology).

74. The answer is A.

(Chap. 9) Splitting of the second heart sound normally occurs during inspiration when there is increased venous return to the right ventricle that increases its stroke volume and delays closure of the pulmonic valve. During inspiration, it is normal to hear the closing of the aortic valve (A_2) before the closing of the pulmonic valve (P_2). A fixed split of the second heart sound occurs in the setting of an atrial septal defect. With this congenital heart defect, the volume of blood that is shunted from the left atrium to the right atrium results in a stable right-ventricular stroke volume. Thus, there is no difference between inspiration and expiration, resulting in a fixed split of the second heart sound.

75. The answer is E.

(Chap. 32) The most accepted hypothesis to describe the pathophysiology of the metabolic syndrome involves an overabundance of free fatty acids and ensuing insulin resistance. Insulin resistance is thought to be a mediator of many of the other aspects of the metabolic syndrome, including hypertension and hyperglycemia. Free fatty acids are derived mainly from adipose tissue. Increases in visceral obesity are thought to be more harmful than subcutaneous stores because of the direct effect of free fatty acids on the liver from the visceral stores. The inflammatory milieu of the metabolic syndrome is enhanced by the overproduction of the proinflammatory cytokines by the expanded adipose tissue. Treating hypertension, hyperglycemia, dyslipidemia, and the oxidative stress of the proinflammatory state is important when treating metabolic syndrome. However, adipose tissue loss is the primary approach to treating the underlying cause of the disorder.

76. The answer is F.

(Chap. 9) When a murmur of uncertain cause is identified on physical examination, a variety of physiologic maneuvers can be used to assist in the elucidation of the cause. Commonly used physiologic maneuvers include change with respiration, Valsalva maneuver, position, and exercise. In hypertrophic cardiomyopathy, there is asymmetric hypertrophy of the interventricular septum, which creates a dynamic outflow obstruction. Maneuvers that decrease left-ventricular filling will cause an increase in the intensity of the murmur, whereas those that increase left-ventricular filling will cause a decrease in the murmur. Of the interventions listed, both standing and a Valsalva maneuver will decrease venous return and subsequently decrease left ventricular filling, resulting in an increase in the loudness of the murmur of hypertrophic cardiomyopathy. Alternatively, squatting increases venous return and thus decreases the murmur. Maximum handgrip exercise also results in a decreased loudness of the murmur.

77. The answer is C.

(Chap. 10) Causes of midsystolic murmurs include aortic stenosis, aortic sclerosis, hypertrophic cardiomyopathy (HOCM), coarctation of the aorta, and pulmonary valve stenosis. In the obstructive form of HOCM, maneuvers that increase the amount of outflow obstruction will increase the intensity of the murmur. Outflow obstruction is increased by decreasing preload, which occurs in standing, performing a Valsalva maneuver, or with the administration of vasodilators. Increasing preload by squatting or passive leg raise will lead to reduction of outflow tract obstruction and a diminished murmur. The murmur of HOCM will also decrease with increasing afterload (vasopressors) or decreasing contractility (beta blockers). The murmur of aortic stenosis is typically in the right second intercostal space and radiates to the

carotids. Valsalva maneuver will classically lead to a decreased aortic stenosis murmur. The murmur of congenital pulmonic stenosis is in the right second intercostal space. There is often a parasternal lift. Mitral valve prolapse causes a late systolic murmur usually introduced by an ejection click. It does not cause a crescendo-decrescendo murmur. Chronic mitral regurgitation causes a holosystolic murmur that radiates to the apex.

78 and 79. The answers are C and C.

(Chap. 16) The patient's rhythm is torsade de pointes, with polymorphic ventricular tachycardia and QRS complexes with variations in amplitude and cycle length giving the appearance of oscillation about an axis. Torsade de pointes is associated with a prolonged QT interval; thus, anything that is associated with a prolonged QT can potentially cause torsade. Most commonly, electrolyte disturbances such as hypokalemia and hypomagnesemia, phenothiazines, fluoroquinolones, antiarrhythmic drugs, tricyclic antidepressants, intracranial events, and bradyarrhythmias are associated with this malignant arrhythmia. Management, besides stabilization, which may require electrical cardioversion, consists of removing the offending agent. In addition, success in rhythm termination or prevention has been reported with the administration of magnesium as well as overdrive atrial or ventricular pacing, which will shorten the QT interval. Beta blockers are indicated for patients with congenital long QT syndrome but are not indicated in this patient.

80. The answer is E.

(Chap. 34) Standard therapy for a patient with unstable angina or non-ST-segment elevation myocardial infarction (NSTEMI) includes aspirin and clopidogrel. If an anticoagulant is added, enoxaparin has been shown to be superior to unfractionated heparin in reducing recurrent cardiac events. Glycoprotein IIb/IIIa inhibitors have also been shown to be beneficial in treating unstable angina/NSTEMI. Eptifibatide, tirofiban, and abciximab are beneficial for patients likely to receive percutaneous intervention. Clinical trials have shown benefit of early invasive strategy in the presence of high-risk factors such as recurrent rest angina, elevated troponin, new ST-segment depression, congestive heart failure symptoms, rales, mitral regurgitation, positive stress test, ejection fraction <0.40, decreased blood pressure, sustained ventricular tachycardia, or recent coronary intervention. The presence of ST depressions, rales, and mitral regurgitation puts this patient at high risk. Tissue plasminogen factor is beneficial in ST-segment elevation myocardial infarction, not NSTEMI.

81. The answer is A.

(Chap. 38) Ascending aortic dissections require surgical intervention, whereas descending aortic dissections that

are uncomplicated may be managed medically. Indications for intervention for descending dissections acutely include occlusion of a major aortic branch with symptoms. For example, paralysis may occur with occlusion of the spinal artery or worsening renal failure may occur in the case of dissection that involves the renal arteries. Once a descending dissection has been found, intensive medical management of blood pressure is imperative and should include agents that decrease cardiac contractility and aortic shear force. Follow-up with CT or MRI imaging every 6–12 months is recommended, and surgical intervention should be considered if there is continued advancement despite medical therapy. Finally, patients with Marfan's syndrome have increased complications with descending dissections and should be considered for surgical repair, especially if there is concomitant disease in the ascending aorta as demonstrated by aortic root dilation to greater than 50 mm.

82. The answer is B.

(Chap. 11) The ECG tracing shows multifocal atrial tachycardia (MAT), right atrial overload, a superior axis, and poor R-wave progression in the precordial leads. There are varying P-wave morphologies (more than three morphologies) and P-P intervals. MAT is most commonly caused by COPD, but other conditions associated with this arrhythmia include coronary artery disease, congestive heart failure, valvular heart disease, diabetes mellitus, hypokalemia, hypomagnesemia, azotemia, postoperative state, and pulmonary embolism. Anemia, pain, and myocardial ischemia are also causes of tachycardia that should be considered when managing a new tachycardia. These states are usually associated with sinus tachycardia.

83. The answer is B.

(Chap. 16; Camm and Garratt, 1991.) Adenosine is currently approved for the termination of paroxysmal supraventricular tachycardias at a dose of 6 mg or, if 6 mg fails, 12 mg. The primary mechanism of adenosine is to decrease conduction velocity through the atrioventricular (AV) node. Thus, it is an ideal drug for acute termination of regular reentrant supraventricular tachycardia involving the AV node. Side effects may include chest discomfort and transient hypotension. The half-life is extremely short, and the side effects tend to be brief. Patients with wide complex tachycardia suggestive of ventricular tachycardia or known preexcitation syndrome should be treated with agents that decrease automaticity, such as quinidine and procainamide. However, in patients with apparent ventricular tachycardia who have neither a history of ischemic heart disease nor preexcitation syndrome, adenosine may be a useful diagnostic agent to determine whether a patient has a reentrant tachycardia, in which case the drug may terminate it; an atrial tachycardia, in which case the atrial activity may

be unmasked; or a true, preexcited tachycardia, in which case adenosine will have no effect. Although adenosine is not the recommended primary therapy for patients with wide complex tachyarrhythmia, patients with junctional tachycardia who have evidence of poor ventricular function or concomitant β-adrenergic blockade may be reasonable candidates for its use.

84. The answer is E.

(Chap. 38) Descending aortic aneurysms are most commonly associated with atherosclerosis. The average growth rate is ~0.1–0.2 cm year. The risk of rupture and subsequent management are related to the size of the aneurysm as well as symptoms related to the aneurysm. However, most thoracic aortic aneurysms are asymptomatic. When symptoms do occur, they are frequently related to mechanical complications of the aneurysm causing compression of adjacent structures. This includes the trachea and esophagus, and symptoms can include cough, chest pain, hoarseness, and dysphagia. The risk of rupture is ~2–3% year for aneurysms <4 cm and rises to 7% per year once the size is >6 cm. Management of descending aortic aneurysms includes blood pressure control. Beta blockers are recommended because they decrease contractility of the heart and thus decrease aortic wall stress, potentially slowing aneurysmal growth. Individuals with thoracic aortic aneurysms should be monitored with chest imaging at least yearly, or sooner if new symptoms develop. This can include CT angiography, MRI, or transesophageal echocardiography. Operative repair is indicated if the aneurysm expands by >1 cm in a year or reaches a diameter of >5.5–6.0 cm. Endovascular stenting for the treatment of thoracic aortic aneurysms is a relatively new procedure with limited long-term results available. The largest study to date included >400 patients with a variety of indications for thoracic endovascular stents. In 249 patients, the indication for stent was thoracic aortic aneurysm. This study showed an initial success rate of 87.1%, with a 30-day mortality rate of 10%. However, if the procedure was done emergently, the mortality rate at 30 days was 28%. At 1 year, data were available on only 96 of the original 249 patients with degenerative thoracic aneurysms. In these individuals, 80% continued to have satisfactory outcomes with stenting and 14% showed growth of the aneurysm *(LJ Leurs, J Vasc Surg 40:670, 2004)*. Ongoing studies with long-term follow-up are needed before endovascular stenting can be recommended for the treatment of thoracic aortic aneurysms, although in individuals who are not candidates for surgery, stenting should be considered.

85. The answer is C.

(Chap. 15) The atrioventricular node is supplied by the posterior descending coronary artery in 90% of the population. Furthermore, this artery in the majority of

the population arises from the right coronary artery. Thus, a patient who presents as this one does with symptoms consistent with an acute coronary syndrome and who has a Mobitz type II second-degree block probably has significant ischemia in the right coronary artery. Right coronary artery transmural infarct is manifest most commonly by ST elevation in II, III, and aVF. Wellen's T waves are deep symmetric T-wave inversions that are seen in either significant left main coronary artery stenosis or proximal left anterior descending artery stenosis.

86. The answer is C.

(Chap. 22) The presentation of this patient is one of acute pericarditis. Acute pericarditis is the most common disease of the pericardium and typically presents as a sharp, intense anterior chest pain. It may be referred to the neck, arms, or left shoulder and may be pleuritic in nature. The positional nature of the pain is characteristic in acute pericarditis. The pain is worse with lying supine and improved with sitting up and leaning forward. A pericardial friction rub is present in 85% of cases of acute pericarditis. A pericardial friction rub is described as high-pitched, grating, or scratching and is heard throughout the cardiac cycle. The ECG, shown here, classically shows elevation of the ST segment in the limb leads and V_2–V_6 with reciprocal depression of the ST segment in aV_R and sometimes V_1. In addition, the PR segment is depressed in all leads except aV_R and V_1, where it may be elevated. Mild elevations in cardiac enzymes may be seen. An echocardiogram should be performed if there is suspicion of a possible effusion. Treatment of acute pericarditis involves rest and anti-inflammatory treatment. Aspirin or nonsteroidal anti-inflammatory drugs in high doses are most commonly used. Alternative treatments include colchicine, glucocorticoids, and intravenous immunoglobulin (IVIg). IVIg is indicated for pericarditis due to cytomegalovirus, adenovirus, or parvovirus. As this patient is in severe pain, reassurance only is not the best option but would be a possible treatment if panic attack were suspected. The other choices are utilized in the case of unstable angina and acute myocardial infarction and should not be utilized in this patient. Both heparin and reteplase would increase the risk of developing a hemorrhagic pericardial effusion. Cardiac catheterization is an unnecessary procedure.

87. The answer is C.

(Chap. 23) Commotio cordis occurs due to a blunt force injury to the chest wall that results in an often fatal arrhythmia, most frequently ventricular fibrillation. Although all of the diagnoses listed are causes of sudden cardiac death in young individuals, commotio cordis is the likely diagnosis because of the occurrence of the injury in relation to blunt trauma to the chest wall.

In contrast to cardiac contusion (contusion cordis), the force of the injury is insufficient to cause cardiac contusion or injury to the ribs or chest wall. All of the other choices would result in abnormalities in the ECG, and a family history of sudden cardiac death is frequent.

In animal studies, commotio cordis has been found to occur when the blunt force is applied at 20–50 mph and only during specific timing within the cardiac cycle (*C Madias et al: J Cardiovasc Electrophysiol 18:115, 2007; MS Link et al: N Engl J Med 338:1805, 1998*). If the force were delivered during the upstroke of the T wave (10–30 ms before the peak), ventricular fibrillation would frequently result. If the force were applied during the QRS (depolarization), transient complete heart block might occur (*MS Link et al: N Engl J Med 338:1805, 1998*). In reported case series, the survival of commotio cordis is only 15%. Defibrillation is most successful if applied within 3 min.

88. The answer is C.

(Chap. 21) This patient's murmur is due to hypertrophic cardiomyopathy (HCM). A normal S_2, the location of the murmur, the absence of radiation to the neck, and being loudest at the lower left sternal border make aortic sclerosis or aortic stenosis less likely. These murmurs are usually heard best in the second right intercostal space. Maneuvers such as going from standing to squatting and passively raising the legs decrease the gradient across the outflow tract and intensity of the murmur due to increased preload. Amyl nitrate causes a decrease in systemic vascular resistance and arterial pressure. The murmur of HCM increases in intensity while there is less regurgitation across the mitral valve and the murmur of mitral regurgitation gets softer. Right-sided murmurs, except for the pulmonic ejection "click" of pulmonary stenosis, usually increase in intensity during inspiration.

89. The answer is C.

(Chap. 32) Reversing insulin resistance and hyperglycemia can be achieved by lifestyle modifications, metformin or other biguanide medications, and/or thiazolidinedione medications. Of the medications, only the thiazolidinediones improve insulin-mediated glucose uptake in the muscle and adipose tissue. The mechanism of action of metformin is uncertain, but it appears to work by reducing hepatic gluconeogenesis and intestinal absorption of glucose. In a large trial of lifestyle modifications and metformin in the prevention of diabetes (Diabetes Prevention Program), subjects in the lifestyle arm of the trial had a more significant reduction in the incidence of diabetes than those assigned to metformin. In resource-poor settings and the developing world, lifestyle modifications have also been shown to be more cost-effective than metformin for preventing diabetes.

90. The answer is E.

(Chap. 18) Approximately 3000 heart transplants are performed each year in the United States. Generally the recipients do well, with survival rates of 76% at 3 years and an average transplant "half-life" of 9.3 years. However, certain complications are common with the necessary immunosuppression, including an increased risk of malignancy and infections. Additionally, patients are at risk of rejection of the transplanted organ that can be acute or chronic. Chronic cardiac transplant rejection manifests as coronary artery disease, with characteristic long, diffuse, and concentric stenosis seen on angiography. It is thought that these changes represent chronic rejection of the transplanted organ. The only definitive therapy is retransplantation. Bradyarrhythmias are not known to occur more frequently in transplant recipients.

91. The answer is E.

(Chap. 30) Although tight glycemic control clearly decreases the risk of the microvascular complications of diabetes (renal function, retinopathy), demonstration of a benefit for myocardial infarction or stroke is less compelling. However, other factors in the management of these patients have been shown to decrease risk. These factors include the use of HMG-CoA reductase inhibitors over all ranges of LDL cholesterol; gemfibrazil, particularly in patients with the metabolic syndrome; strict control of hypertension; and the use of an antihypertensive agent that inhibits the actions of angiotensin II, such as an ACE inhibitor or an angiotensin receptor blocker.

92. The answer is E.

(Chap. 9) During normal inspiration there is a small, <10 mmHg decrease in systolic pressure. In several disease states, notably severe obstructive lung disease, pericardial tamponade, and superior vena cava obstruction, an accentuation of this normal finding can occur. Indeed, in the most pronounced cases the peripheral pulse may not be palpable during inspiration.

93. The answer is D.

(Chap. 22) This patient's presentation and physical examination are most consistent with the diagnosis of constrictive pericarditis. The most common cause of constrictive pericarditis worldwide is tuberculosis, but given the low incidence of tuberculosis in the United States, constrictive pericarditis is a rare condition in this country. With the increasing ability to cure Hodgkin's disease with mediastinal irradiation, many cases of constrictive pericarditis in the United States are in patients who received curative radiation therapy 10–20 years prior. These patients are also at risk for premature coronary artery disease. Risks for these complications include dose of radiation and radiation windows that include the heart. Other rare causes of constrictive pericarditis are recurrent acute pericarditis, hemorrhagic pericarditis, prior cardiac

surgery, mediastinal irradiation, chronic infection, and neoplastic disease. Physiologically, constrictive pericarditis is characterized by the inability of the ventricles to fill because of the noncompliant pericardium. In early diastole, the ventricles fill rapidly, but filling stops abruptly when the elastic limit of the pericardium is reached. Clinically, patients present with generalized malaise, cachexia, and anasarca. Exertional dyspnea is common, and orthopnea is generally mild. Ascites and hepatomegaly occur because of increased venous pressure. In rare cases, cirrhosis may develop from chronic congestive hepatopathy. The jugular venous pressure is elevated, and the neck veins fail to collapse on inspiration (Kussmaul's sign). Heart sounds may be muffled. A pericardial knock is frequently heard. This is a third heart-sound that occurs 0.09–0.12 s after aortic valve closure at the cardiac apex. Right heart catheterization would show the "square root sign" characterized by an abrupt γ descent followed by a gradual rise in ventricular pressure. This finding, however, is not pathognomonic of constrictive pericarditis and can be seen in restrictive cardiomyopathy of any cause. Echocardiogram shows a thickened pericardium, dilatation of the inferior vena cava and hepatic veins, and an abrupt cessation of ventricular filling in early diastole. Pericardial resection is the only definitive treatment of constrictive pericarditis. Diuresis and sodium restriction are useful in managing volume status preoperatively, and paracentesis may be necessary. Operative mortality ranges from 5–10%. Underlying cardiac function is normal; thus, cardiac transplantation is not indicated. Pericardiocentesis is indicated for diagnostic removal of pericardial fluid and cardiac tamponade, which is not present on the patient's echocardiogram. Mitral valve stenosis may present similarly with anasarca, congestive hepatic failure, and ascites. However, pulmonary edema and pleural effusions are also common. Examination would be expected to demonstrate a diastolic murmur, and echocardiogram should show a normal pericardium and a thickened immobile mitral valve. Mitral valve replacement would be indicated if mitral stenosis were the cause of the patient's symptoms.

94. The answer is A.

(Chap. 28) This patient is presenting in pulmonary edema and cardiogenic shock due to acute myocardial infarction (MI). Given the distribution of ST-segment elevation, the left anterior descending artery is the most likely artery occluded. Initial management should include high-dose aspirin, heparin, and stabilization of blood pressure. Initial management of acute MI also includes use of nitroglycerin and beta blockers such as metoprolol in most individuals, but are contraindicated in this individuals because of his profound hypotension. In addition, use of furosemide for the treatment of pulmonary edema is also contraindicated because of the degree of hypotension. Intravenous fluids should be used with caution as the patient also has evidence of

pulmonary edema. The best choice for treatment of this patient's hypotension is aortic counterpulsation. Aortic counterpulsation requires placement of an intraaortic balloon pump percutaneously into the femoral artery. The sausage-shaped balloon inflates during early diastole, augmenting coronary blood flow, and collapses during early systole, markedly decreasing afterload. In contrast to vasopressors and inotropic agents, aortic counterpulsation decreases myocardial oxygen consumption. Both dobutamine and norepinephrine can increase myocardial oxygen demand and worsen ischemia.

95. The answer is D.

(Chap. 28) This patient is presenting with right ventricular (RV) myocardial infarction. The usual clinical features of right ventricular infarction are hypotension, elevated right heart filling pressures, absence of pulmonary congestion, and evidence of RV dilatation and dysfunction. In most cases of RV infarction, the vessel involved is the right coronary artery, which manifests as ST elevation in leads II, III, and aV_F. When RV infarction occurs, ST depression is commonly seen in V_1 and V_2. An electrocardiogram with the precordial leads placed on the right side of the chest demonstrates ST elevation in RV_4. The initial treatment of hypotension of RV infarction is IV fluids to raise the central venous pressure to 10–15 mmHg. If fluid administration fails to alleviate the hypotension, sympathomimetic agents or aortic counterpulsation can be used. However, care must be taken to avoid excess fluid administration, which would shift the interventricle septum to the left and further impede cardiac output. A transvenous pacemaker would be useful if the hypotension were related to heart block or profound bradycardia, which can be associated with right coronary artery ischemia.

96. The answer is C.

(Chap. 29) Sudden cardiac death (SCD) is defined as death due to cardiac causes heralded by the abrupt loss of consciousness within 1 h of onset of acute symptoms. Sudden cardiac death accounts for ~50% of all cardiac deaths, and of these, two-thirds are initial cardiac events or occur in populations with previously known heart disease who are considered to be relatively low risk. The most common electrical mechanism of SCD is ventricular fibrillation, accounting for 50–80% of cardiac arrests. The risk of SCD rises with age and is greater in men and individuals with a history of coronary artery disease. In addition, several inherited conditions increase the risk of SCD, including hypertrophic cardiomyopathy, right ventricular dysplasia, and long-QT syndromes, among others. A strong parental history of sudden cardiac death as a presenting history of coronary artery disease increases the likelihood of a similar presentation in an offspring. Interestingly, 70–80% of men who die from SCD have preexisting healed MIs whereas only 20–30% have had recent acute MI. On autopsy, individuals who die of SCD most commonly show longstanding atherosclerotic disease as well as evidence of an unstable coronary lesion. When this is considered with the fact that most individuals do not have pathologic evidence of an acute MI by pathology, this suggests that transient ischemia is the mechanism of onset of the fatal arrhythmia. Rapid intervention and restoration of circulation is important for survival in SCD. Within 5 min, the likelihood of surviving SCD is only 25–30% for out-of-hospital arrests.

97. The answer is C.

(Chap. 29) Immediate defibrillation should be the initial choice of action in the treatment of sudden cardiac arrest due to ventricular fibrillation (VF) or ventricular tachycardia (VT). Defibrillation should occur prior to endotracheal intubation or placement of intravenous access. If the time to potential defibrillation is <5 min, the medical team should proceed immediately to defibrillation at 300–360 J if a monophasic defibrillator is used (150 J if a biphasic defibrillator is used). If there is >5-min delay to defibrillation, then brief CPR should be given prior to defibrillation. A single shock should be given with immediate resumption of CPR for 60–90 s before delivering additional shocks. After each shock, CPR should be given without delay. Even if there is return of a perfusable rhythm, there is often a delayed return of pulse because of myocardial stunning. If the patient remains in VF or pulseless VT after initial defibrillation, the patient should be intubated and have IV access attained while CPR is performed. Once IV access is obtained, the initial drug of choice is either epinephrine, 1 mg, or vasopressin, 40 units. Amiodarone is a second-line agent.

98. The answer is C.

(Chap. 29; J Nolan et al: Circulation 108:118, 2003.) In 2002, two studies conducted in Europe and Australia confirmed the benefit of therapeutic hypothermia following out-of-hospital cardiac arrest. In these trials, patients were rapidly cooled to 32–34°C and maintained at these temperatures for the initial 12–24 h. Individuals who received therapeutic hypothermia were 40–85% more likely to have good neurologic outcomes upon hospital discharge. In addition, therapeutic hypothermia also decreased inhospital morality. Time to initial defibrillation of >5 min is associated with no more than a 25–30% survival rate, and survival continues to decrease linearly from 1–10 min. Defibrillation within 5 minutes has the greatest likelihood for good neurologic outcomes. Of the medications used in treatment of cardiac arrest due to ventricular fibrillation or pulseless ventricular tachycardia, none have been demonstrated to have any effects on neurologic outcome.

99. The answer is E.

(Chap. 24) Amyloidosis is in the differential diagnosis of a patient with newly diagnosed heart failure. The cardiac examination is not specific for cardiac amyloid, but accessory findings such as neurologic involvement, low voltage on the ECG and an elevated globulin fraction (total protein − albumin ≥4 mg/dL) are suggestive of cardiac amyloid. Echocardiographic findings include left ventricular hypertrophy, dilated atria, thickened interatrial septum, and a "starry-sky" appearance of the myocardium. The starry-sky appearance is rarely seen using contemporary ultrasound technology. Focal myocardial wall motion abnormalities (akinesis) are more suggestive of coronary artery disease. Valvular heart disease can cause heart failure if left uncorrected. This patient's murmur is characteristic of mitral regurgitation and is not consistent with aortic stenosis. Protrusion of the left ventricular apex with hypercontractility of the base is characteristic of stress cardiomyopathy, which is usually accompanied by clinical findings suggesting acute heart failure and ECG findings suggesting acute anterior myocardial infarction.

100. The answer is C.

(Chap. 24) Amyloidosis is a term for diseases that are due to the extracellular deposition of insoluble protein fibrils. The specific diseases are defined by the biochemical nature of the protein in the fibril deposits. Primary systemic amyloidosis (AL) is amyloid composed of immunoglobulin light chains and is usually due to a plasma cell dyscrasia. Bence-Jones protein is often in the urine of patients with plasma cell dyscrasia. Bone marrow biopsy is indicated when AL is diagnosed. AA (secondary amyloidosis) is due to an accumulation of serum amyloid A protein and occurs in the setting of chronic inflammatory or infectious diseases. Alzheimer's disease is caused by accumulation of Aβ protein. Neurocognitive testing may be helpful in patients diagnosed with early cognitive decline. There is currently no clinically available test for early accumulation of Aβ protein. Mutant transthyretin (prealbumin) is the protein usually found in the fibril deposits of the familial amyloidoses (AF). The disease is transmitted in an autosomal dominant fashion, although sporadic cases occur. Typical symptoms include neuropathy, cardiomyopathy, and autonomic neuropathy. Without intervention, survival is typically 5–15 years. Orthotopic liver transplantation removes the source of variant protein production and provides a source of normal protein production. Although neuropathy usually improves, cardiomyopathy may not. Screening family members is important for counseling family members who may also be affected.

101. The answer is D.

(Chap. 16) Anticoagulation is of particular importance for patients with atrial fibrillation for whom chemical or electrical cardioversion is considered. If the duration of atrial fibrillation is unknown or >24 h, there is an increased risk of an atrial appendage thrombus and subsequent

embolization. When DCCV is being considered, one of two strategies is used most often. Intravenous heparin can be initiated and transesophageal echocardiogram obtained. Once the activated partial thromboplastin time is at a therapeutic level, DCCV can be performed if there is no thrombus visualized on TEE. Alternatively, anticoagulation with warfarin can be initiated immediately and continued for at least 3 weeks. If the INR >1.8 on at least two separate occasions, DCCV can be safely performed. Using either strategy, anticoagulation must be continued for at least 1 month after DCCV if the duration of atrial fibrillation has been prolonged or unknown, due to the increased risk of thrombus formation and embolization after DCCV.

102. The answer is C.

(Chap. 17) The New York Heart Association classification is a tool to define criteria that describe the functional ability and clinical manifestations of patients in heart failure. It is also used in patients with pulmonary hypertension. The criteria have been shown to have prognostic value with worsening survival as class increases. They are also useful to clinicians when reading studies to understand the entry and exclusion criteria of large clinical trials. Class I includes patients with no limiting symptoms; class II includes patients with slight or mild limitation; class III includes patients are moderately limited with no symptoms at rest, but dyspnea or angina or palpitations with little exertion; class IV includes severely limited patients, so that even minimal activity causes symptoms. Treatment guidelines also frequently base recommendations on these clinical stages. This patient has symptoms with little exertion but is comfortable at rest; therefore he is New York Heart Association class III.

103. The answer is B.

(Chap. 17) Patients with severe congestive heart failure often exhibit Cheyne-Stokes breathing, defined as intercurrent short periods of hypoventilation and hyperventilation. The mechanism is thought to relate to the prolonged circulation time between the lungs and the respiratory control centers in the brain, leading to poor respiratory control of P_{CO_2}. The degree of Cheyne-Stokes breathing is related to the severity of heart failure. This pattern of breathing is different from obstructive sleep apnea, which is notable for periods of loud snoring, apnea, and sudden waking. Patients are also often hypersomnolent during the day. Although sleep apnea is managed with weight loss and overnight CPAP, Cheyne-Stokes breathing is difficult to address as it is often a sign of advanced systolic dysfunction and implies a poor prognosis. All efforts to further maximize heart failure management are indicated. A sleep study would demonstrate this pattern of breathing, but this history and clinical presentation is typical. There is no role for bronchodilators or an electroencephalogram.

104. The answer is D.

(Chap. 17) Patients with chronic congestive heart failure develop substantial lymphatic reserve in their lungs. Consequently, they may not display signs of pulmonary edema on physical examination or chest radiograph, even in the presence of a very elevated left ventricular filling pressure. The lack of these findings carries a very limited predictive value and does not rule out heart failure. This phenomenon also occurs in patients with chronic mitral stenosis so is likely an effect of long-standing elevation of pulmonary venous pressure. Acute heart failure will present with bilateral rales on pulmonary examination. However, noncardiac causes of pulmonary edema will also cause rales, so this finding is nonspecific.

105. The answer is E.

(Chap. 17) Heart failure with a preserved ejection fraction is very common but can be challenging to evaluate serially. Each of the described parameters gives important adjunct information regarding heart function in this type of patient. Left atrial dilatation often implies a chronic elevation in left ventricular diastolic pressures as the atria is relatively compliant and will dilate in this setting. Atrial fibrillation is easily seen on echocardiography and is problematic in these patients as they are often dependent on their atrial kick to maintain preload and therefore cardiac output. Left ventricular wall thickness and diastolic filling may imply severity and duration of disease. Systolic anterior motion of the mitral valve with asymmetric septal hypertrophy is a characteristic echocardiographic finding in hypertrophic cardiomyopathy.

106. The answer is A.

(Chap. 17) Angiotensin receptor blockers (ARBs) are useful in heart failure patients who do not tolerate angiotensin-converting enzyme inhibitors due to cough or other side effects. Inhibition of the renin-angiotensin pathway reduces left ventricular afterload and remodeling. They have been shown to improve symptoms and exercise capacity and to reduce need for hospitalization and mortality in patients with systolic heart failure. Calcium channel blockers, particularly first-generation medications, may worsen function in patients with systolic dysfunction. Thiazolidinediones (rosiglitazone, pioglitazone) are associated with fluid retention and may worsen heart failure. NSAID use in patients with a reduced cardiac output may cause acute renal failure. Sotalol has been shown to increase mortality in patients with left ventricular dysfunction.

107. The answer is A.

(Chap. 17) Because beta blockers take longer to achieve a steady state, can decrease inotropic function, and cause bradycardia or heart block, the dose of these medicines should be escalated slowly. ACE inhibitors are typically increased to doses achieved in clinical trials at a more rapid rate with careful monitoring of renal function.

108. The answer is E.

(Chap. 17; AL Taylor et al: N Eng J Med 351:2049, 2004.) Isosorbide dinitrate/hydralazine in a fixed combination (BiDil) was shown to decrease mortality and hospitalizations in African Americans with impaired left ventricular function (<35–45%) when added to standard heart failure therapy. The drug was approved by the U.S. Food and Drug Administration in 2005 as the first race-specific drug therapy.

109. The answer is E.

(Chap. 26) This patient has a small-joint, symmetric polyarthritis in the setting of a very recent sore throat. Although acute HIV commonly presents with a sore throat, other common features, such as rash, are missing. Moreover, the incubation period between this patient's high-risk sexual encounter and clinical syndrome would be too short for acute HIV infection. Certainly, this patient should be screened for HIV infection. The patient meets clinical criteria for group A *Streptococcus* throat infection given his recent fever, pustular exudates on examination, tender cervical lymph nodes, and lack of cough. His syndrome is consistent with a reactive arthritis, given the symmetric small-joint involvement and very short incubation period. Acute rheumatic fever is also seen with streptococcal throat infections but is very uncommon in the developed world. One would expect to see a latency period ranging between 1 and 5 weeks between resolution of sore throat and arthritis; asymmetric large-joint involvement; and possibly evidence of carditis, chorea, erythema marginatum, or subcutaneous nodules to suspect a diagnosis of acute rheumatic fever. Gonococcal infection can cause pharyngitis but is more commonly associated with single large-joint infection or enthesopathy, but not small-joint polyarthritis. Lyme disease is a clinical diagnosis contingent upon tick exposure, a classic target lesion rash, and, if present, a migratory large-joint arthritis.

110. The answer is C.

(Chap. 31) The child exhibits clinical and laboratory manifestations of homozygous familial hypercholesterolemia (FH). The presence of childhood xanthomas including hands, wrists, elbows, knees, and buttocks with evidence of premature atherosclerosis is characteristic. The atherosclerosis often develops initially in the aortic root, causing valvular or supravalvular stenosis. Drug therapy is often ineffective, and LDL apheresis is usually the necessary therapy. Before initiating therapy to reduce his LDL, it is necessary to rule out hypothyroidism, nephrotic syndrome, and obstructive liver disease. Although parental control of the patient's diet is also partly to blame, deliberate or unintentional ingestion of a poor diet is less likely to be responsible than a genetic disorder. Familial defective apoB100 is a dominantly

inherited disorder that may be confused with heterozygous FH, but not homozygous. These patients usually present with cardiovascular disease in adulthood. Syphilis can cause aortitis; however, it does not cause premature coronary artery disease.

111. The answer is D.

(Chap. 31) This patient has signs and symptoms of familial hypercholesterolemia (FH) with elevated plasma LDL, normal triglycerides, tendon xanthomas, and premature coronary artery disease. FH is an autosomal codominant lipoprotein disorder that is the most common of these syndromes caused by a single gene disorder. It has a higher prevalence in Afrikaners, Christian Lebanese, and French Canadians. There is no definitive diagnostic test for FH. FH may be diagnosed with a skin biopsy that shows reduced LDL receptor activity in cultured fibroblasts (although there is considerable overlap with normals). FH is predominantly a clinical diagnosis, although molecular diagnostics are being developed. Hemolysis is not a feature of FH. Sitosterolemia is distinguished from FH by episodes of hemolysis. It is a rare autosomal recessive disorder that causes a marked increase in the dietary absorption of plant sterols. Hemolysis is due to incorporation of plant sterols into the red blood cell membrane. Sitosterolemia is confirmed by demonstrating an increase in the plasma levels of sitosterol using gas chromatography. CT scanning of the liver does not sufficiently differentiate between the hyperlipoproteinemias. Many of the primary lipoproteinemias, including sitosterolemia, are inherited in an autosomal recessive pattern, and thus, a pedigree analysis would not be likely to isolate the disorder.

112. The answer is C.

(Chap. 40) Primary pulmonary hypertension is an uncommon disease that usually affects young females. Early in the illness affected persons often are diagnosed as psychoneurotic because of the vague nature of the presenting complaints, for example, dyspnea, chest pain, and evidence of hyperventilation without hypoxemia on arterial blood gas testing. However, progression of the disease leads to syncope in approximately one-half of cases and signs of right heart failure on physical examination. Chest x-ray typically shows enlarged central pulmonary arteries with or without attenuation of peripheral markings. The diagnosis of primary pulmonary hypertension is made by documenting elevated pressures by right heart catheterization and excluding other pathologic processes. Lung disease of sufficient severity to cause pulmonary hypertension would be evident by history and on examination. Major differential diagnoses include thromboemboli and heart disease; outside the United States, schistosomiasis and filariasis are common causes of pulmonary hypertension, and a careful travel history should be taken.

NOMENCLATURE AND CLASSIFICATION OF PULMONARY HYPERTENSION

Diagnostic Classification
1. Pulmonary arterial hypertension
   Primary pulmonary hypertension: sporadic and familial
   Related to
   a. Collagen-vascular disease
   b. Congenital systemic to pulmonary shunts
   c. Portal hypertension
   d. HIV infection
   e. Drugs/toxins: anorexigens and other
   f. Persistent pulmonary hypertension of the newborn
   g. Other
2. Pulmonary venous hypertension
   Left-side atrial or ventricular heart disease
   Left-side valvular heart disease
   Extrinsic compression of central pulmonary veins: fibrosing mediastinitis and adenopathy/tumors
   Pulmonary venoocclusive disease
   Other
3. Pulmonary hypertension associated with disorders of the respiratory system and/or hypoxemia
   Chronic obstructive pulmonary disease   Chronic exposure to high altitude
   Interstitial lung disease   Neonatal lung disease
   Sleep-disordered breathing   Alveolar-capillary dysplasia
   Alveolar hypoventilatory disorders   Other
4. Pulmonary hypertension due to chronic thrombotic and/or embolic disease
   Thromboembolic obstruction of proximal pulmonary arteries
   Obstruction of distal pulmonary arteries
   a. Pulmonary embolism (thrombus, tumor, ova and/or parasites, foreign material)
   b. In-situ thrombosis
   c. Sickle cell disease
5. Pulmonary hypertension due to disorders directly affecting the pulmonary vasculature
   Inflammatory: Schistosomiasis; Sarcoidosis; other
   Pulmonary capillary hemangiomatosis

INDEX

Bold number indicates the start of the main discussion of the topic; numbers with "f" and "t" refer to figure and table pages.